NCLEX-R
Q&A Plus!

made
Incredibly
Easy!®

Second Edition

NCLEX-PN®
Q&A Plus!

made
Incredibly
Easy!

Second Edition

Clinical Editor
Leigh W. Moore, MSN, RN, CNOR, CNE
Associate Professor of Nursing
Southside Virginia Community College
Alberta, Virginia

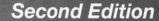 Wolters Kluwer

Philadelphia • Baltimore • New York • London
Buenos Aires • Hong Kong • Sydney • Tokyo

Senior Digital Product Manager, NCLEX: Renee A. Gagliardi
Associate Content Strategist: Dawn Lagrosa
Marketing Manager: Sarah Schuessler
Senior Production Project Manager: Cynthia Rudy
Design Coordinator: Elaine Kasmer
Manufacturing Coordinator: Kathleen Brown
Prepress Vendor: SPi Global

Second edition

9 8 7 6 5 4 3 2 1

Printed in China

Library of Congress Cataloging-in-Publication Data
Names: Moore, Leigh W., editor.
Title: NCLEX-PN Q&A plus! : made incredibly easy / clinical editor, Leigh W. Moore.
Other titles: NCLEX-PN questions and answers plus!
Description: Second edition. | Philadelphia : Wolters Kluwer, [2018] | Includes index.
Identifiers: LCCN 2016046553 | ISBN 9781496316721
Subjects: | MESH: Nursing, Practical | United States | Examination Questions
Classification: LCC RT55 | NLM WY 18.2 | DDC 610.73076--dc23 LC record available at https://lccn.loc.gov/2016046553

LWW.com

About the Editor

Leigh Moore, MSN, RN, CNOR, CNE, is a Registered Nurse and Associate Professor of Nursing in the Associate Degree program at Southside Virginia Community College in Alberta, Virginia. She graduated from a practical nursing program in 1978 and went on to further her education at Halifax Community College in Weldon, North Carolina, receiving an AAS degree in nursing. After many years of working in a variety of nursing settings—L&D, Newborn Nursery, Medical-Surgical, Intensive Care, Emergency, and Home Health—she found her home in the Perioperative Services department and achieved her CNOR. During this time, Leigh graduated with a BSN from Old Dominion University and went on to pursue her MSN, graduating in 2003.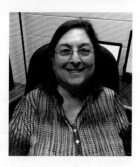
When she accepted a position teaching nursing at Southside Virginia Community College in 2002, it was the beginning of a new career. In 2008, she passed the certification examination to become a certified nurse educator (CNE).

Leigh has been married to her husband Robert for 36 years, and they reside in Emporia, Virginia. They have two children: son Justin Moore and his wife Alina, with granddaughter Mila Rose, and daughter Paula and her husband Timmy Moseley. Leigh enjoys spending time with her family and taking her granddaughter Mila on vacations. Traveling and reading are also hobbies that she enjoys.

Contributors

Kim Cooper, RN, MSN
Dean, School of Nursing
Ivy Tech Community College—Wabash Valley Region
Terre Haute, Indiana

Jackie Daniel, DNP, RNC, WHNP, FNP
Program Director, Associate Degree in Nursing and
    Assistant Dean of Nursing and Health Technologies
Southside Virginia Community College
Alberta, Virginia

Karen R. Ferguson, PhD, RNC, MSN, FNE
Associate Professor
Martin Methodist College
Pulaski, Tennessee

Maryann Foley, RN, BSN
Clinical Consultant
Flourtown, Pennsylvania

Felicia Hall-Grace, RN, MSN
Nursing Educator
Reid State Technical College
Evergreen, Alabama

Don Laurino, MSN, CCRN, CMSRN, PHN, RN-BC
Instructor, VN (RN)
American Career College at St. Francis
Lynwood, California

Lauren Winters, RN, BSN
PN Nursing Instructor
Nunez Community College
Chalmette, Louisiana

Felicia Omick, BSN, MSN, RN, CNE
Associate Professor of Nursing
Southside Virginia Community College
Alberta, Virginia

Mary B. Williams, MSN, RN
Associate Professor of Nursing
Nursing and Health Sciences
Gordon State College
Barnesville, Georgia

Mary Worrell, MSN, RN, CNE
Adjunct Nursing Faculty
Southside Virginia Community College
Alberta, Virginia

Patricia Zrelak, RN, PhD, NEA-BC, CNRN
Nurse Researcher
University of California Davis
Davis, California

Faculty

Krista L. Angell, RN, BSN, MEd
Willoughby-Eastlake School of
 Practical Nursing
Willoughby, Ohio

Janet Ballard, RN, BSN, MEd
EHOVE Career Center
Milan, Ohio

Mindy Barna, MSN, RN
College of Saint Mary
Omaha, Nebraska

Teresa Boyer, MSN, APN-BC
Motlow College
Lynchburg, Tennessee

Brittany L. Carson, MSN, RN
Chamberlain College of Nursing
Irving, Texas

Tomonica Clark, RN, MSN/Ed
Montana State University–
 Northern
Great Falls, Montana

Kim Clevenger, EdD, MSN, RN, BC
Morehead State University
Morehead, Kentucky

Sherri Comfort
Holmes Community College
Goodman, Missouri

Michele L. Comolli, RN, MA, CNE
Dutchess County BOCES
Poughkeepsie, New York

Jackie Daniel, DNP, RNC, WHNP, FNP
Southside Virginia Community
 College
Alberta, Virginia

Mattie Davis, DNP, UAB
JF Drake State Community and
 Technical College
Huntsville, Alabama

Nancy Delmont, BSN, RN
Bolivar Technical College
Bolivar, Missouri

Cheryl Dover, DNP, MS, RN, NE-BC
Prince George's Community
 College
Largo, Maryland

Penny Fauber, RN, BSN, MS, PhD
Dabney S. Lancaster Community
 College
Buena Vista, Virginia

Michele Faxel, EdD, MS, RN
Samuel Merritt University
Oakland, California

Nickole George, PhD, RN
University of Pittsburgh–
 Johnstown
Johnstown, Pennsylvania

Stacee Gillespie, RN, MS
Northeast Technology Center
Kansas, Oklahoma

Marion Goodman, RN, BSN, MS
Lone Star College
Cyprus, Texas

Shari Gould, MSN, RN
Victoria College
Victoria, Texas

Jennifer Holzer, BSN
Lincoln Technical Institute
Philadelphia, Pennsylvania

Carole L. Hoveland, MS, RN
Sheridan College
Sheridan, Wyoming

Nora James, MSN
Lee College
Baytown, Texas

Ruby Johnson, RN
Ozarka College
Melbourne, Arkansas

Laura Kanavy, MSN
Career Technology Center of
 Lackawanna County
Scranton, Pennsylvania

Cheryl Krieg, MSN, RNC-OB
Clearfield County Career and
 Technology Center
Clearfield, Pennsylvania

Jennifer Kuchta, MSN, MBA, RN
College of Saint Mary
Omaha, Nebraska

Annette Lane, RN, PhD
Athabasca University
Athabasca, Alberta

Freda Lawson, MSN
Pike County Career Technology
 Center
Piketon, Ohio

Alicia B. Lentz, MSNEd, RN
Mifflin Juniata Career and
 Technology Center
Lewistown, Pennsylvania

**Patricia Lewis, APRN, MSN, MSATE,
 FNPBC**
Academy of Careers and
 Technology
Beckley, West Virginia

Kimberly D. McCombs, MSN
Black Hawk College
Moline, Illinois

Janis McMillan, RN, MSN
Coconino Community College
Flagstaff, Arizona

Stephanie Miller, RN
Knoedler School of Practical
 Nurse Education
Jefferson, Ohio

Lauren Winters, RN, BSN
Nunez Community College
Chalmette, Louisiana

Melaine Moore, PhD, MSN, RN
Virginia Western Community
 College
Roanoke, Virginia

Sharon Nowak, BSN, MS
Jackson Community College
Jackson, Mississippi

Sherry Obert, MSN, RN NE-BC
Allegany College of Maryland at
 the Bedford County Campus
Everett, Pennsylvania

Felicia Omick, BSN, MSN
Southside Virginia Community
 College
Alberta, Virginia

Diana L. Rupert, RN, MSN, PhD
Indiana County Technical Center
Indiana, Pennsylvania

Eunice M. Scott, RN, BSN, MSNEd
Centura College Richmond
North Chesterfield, Virginia

Darla K. Shar, MSN, RN
Hannah E. Mullins School of
    Practical Nursing
Salem, Ohio

Wanda Spratt, MSN, RN
The College of Health Care
    Professions
Houston, Texas

Nancy Strassner, BS, MPA
Wayne-Finger Lakes BOCES
Newark, New York

Damien Unger, RN, BSN
James Rumsey Technical Institute
Atlanta, Georgia

Christina Warren, RN, MSNEd
Laramie County Community
    College
Laramie, Wyoming

Frances M. Warrick, MS, RN
El Centro College
Dallas, Texas

Kim Webb, RN, MN
Pioneer Technology Center
Ponca City, Oklahoma

**Augustene Weston, RN, MSN, PhD
    Counseling**
Tennessee Technology Center at
    Memphis
Memphis, Tennessee

Christina Wilson, BAN, RN, CMSRN
Anoka Technical College
Anoka, Minnesota

Stephanie Winsman, BSN, RN, CCE
Grand View Hospital
Souderton, Pennsylvania

Nicole B. Zeller, MSN, RN, CNE
Lake Land College
Mattoon, Illinois

Students

Michaella Barnes
Mildred Elley
Albany, New York

D'Andra Bell
Virginia College
Montgomery, Alabama

Chequitta Jackson
Johnson County Community
    College
Overland Park, Kansas

Tyler W. Johnson, LPN
Erie Business Center
Erie, Pennsylvania

Abbey Luckett
Christus St. Joseph's Home
Monroe, Louisiana

Jennifer Noe, LPN
St. Cloud Hospital
St. Cloud, Minnesota

Cydney Rosenthal, RN
Jersey College of Nursing
Tampa, Florida

Amber Stanley, RN
West Plains, Missouri

Adriana Torres, LVN
Kaiser Permanente
Los Angeles, California

Preface

I began as a Nurse Educator in 2002, teaching PN and RN labs and clinicals concurrently. In doing so, I had an appreciation for program outcomes and evaluation methods at both levels. Over time, my teaching methods have changed significantly, going from a lecture format, including PowerPoint presentations, to an active learning environment. I have found that when students are active and engaged in the classroom, they retain more information as well as develop a deeper understanding of the concepts. When these concepts are understood, they can be applied to any clinical situation or question.

It is important to practice NCLEX style questions not only at the end of your program, prior to taking NCLEX, but also throughout your program. Taking practice tests is only the beginning of practice. It is vitally important to remediate so that you have an understanding of why you got the question right or why you did not get it right. Read each question thoroughly and ask yourself, "What do I need to know to answer this question? What is the question asking me?" This resource is developed to help you take as many practice tests as possible to assist you in achieving your goal of NCLEX success. It is also designed to give you a brief overview of information that you may have covered in your program. The explanations will help you to understand not only why the answer is correct but also why the distractors are incorrect. Few questions are written at the comprehension level, with most at the application and analysis levels of Bloom's Taxonomy—just like the NCLEX. And the many alternate format questions will allow you practice for whatever questions your NCLEX contains.

I wish you success on your journey throughout the nursing program and your NCLEX. Strive for excellence and for being the best nurse that you can be. It is my sincere hope that you will find this profession a rewarding and satisfying career, as I have for 38 years.

—Leigh W. Moore, MSN, RN, CNOR, CNE

NCLEX-PN® Q&A Plus! Made Incredibly Easy!® will improve your knowledge while building your ability to apply that knowledge to real nursing scenarios. It also will strengthen your preparation for your licensure experience. Let's cut right to the chase! Here's how:

1. It will teach you all the important things you need to know about preparing for and passing the NCLEX. (And it will leave out all the fluff that wastes your time.)
2. It will direct your eye to the alternate-format questions.
3. It will help you remember what you've learned.
4. It will make you smile as it enhances your knowledge and skills.
   Don't believe it? Try these features on for size:

- Reliable NCLEX preparation guidelines and hundreds of test-taking hints and strategies
- 3,000 NCLEX-style questions within the book itself to test your knowledge in all areas tested on the real examination
- Two-column format with questions on the left and answers and rationales on the right
- Bookmark for you to hide the answers while reading the questions
- Red font for alternate-format questions and full-color photographs and illustrations for graphic and hot spot questions
- Accompanying Web site with 1,000 additional questions in an interactive format—including graphic and audio questions
  Plus, check out these updates:
- Alignment of all information with the 2017 NCLEX-PN test plan and NCSBN standards
- Full four-color design and art program integrated throughout
- Thorough content revision based on feedback from more than 70 nursing faculty and recent graduates across the United States to ensure the most up-to-date practices, highest quality questions, and appropriateness of content for review by students
- Question difficulty data derived from *Lippincott NCLEX-PN PassPoint*, an adaptive quizzing program that simulates the computerized adaptive testing experience
- Free 7-day trial of *Lippincott NCLEX-PN PassPoint*

Plus, look for Joy, Jake, and friends in the margins throughout this book. As always, they will be there to explain key concepts, provide important hints, and offer reassurance. And, if you don't mind, we'll be spicing up the pages with a bit of humor along the way, to teach and entertain in a way that no other resource can.

Contents

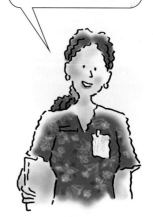

It may seem obvious, but one of the best ways to prepare for the NCLEX—or any important exam—is to understand exactly what you're facing.

Chapter 1

Preparing for the NCLEX®

Just the facts

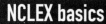

In this chapter, you'll learn:

◆ why you must take the NCLEX
◆ what you need to know about taking the NCLEX by computer
◆ strategies to use when answering NCLEX questions
◆ how to recognize and answer NCLEX alternate-format questions
◆ how to avoid common mistakes when taking the NCLEX.

NCLEX basics

Passing the National Council Licensure Examination (NCLEX®) is an important landmark in your career as a nurse. The first step on your way to passing the NCLEX is to understand what it is and how it's administered.

Exam structure

The NCLEX is a test written by registered nurses with a master's degree and clinical expertise in a particular area of nursing. Only one small difference distinguishes nurses who write NCLEX questions from those who are similarly qualified: They're trained to write questions in a style particular to this examination.

If you've completed an accredited nursing program, you've already taken numerous tests written by nurses with backgrounds and experiences similar to those of the nurses who write for the NCLEX. Therefore, the test-taking experience you've already gained will help you pass the NCLEX and your NCLEX review should be just that—a review of what you've already learned and should know.

What's the point?

The NCLEX is designed for one purpose: to determine whether it's appropriate for you to receive a license to practice as a nurse. By passing this exam, you demonstrate that you possess the minimum level of knowledge, understanding, and skills necessary to practice nursing safely.

Mix 'em up

In nursing school, you probably took courses organized according to the medical model. Courses were separated into such subjects as medical-surgical, pediatric, maternal-neonatal, and psychiatric nursing. In contrast, the NCLEX is integrated, which means that different subjects are mixed together.

As you answer NCLEX questions, you may encounter patients in any stage of life, from neonatal to geriatric. These patients—clients, in NCLEX lingo—may be of any background, may be completely well or extremely ill, and may have any of a variety of disorders.

Client needs, front and center

The NCLEX draws questions from four categories of client needs that were developed by the National Council of State Boards of Nursing (NCSBN), the organization that sponsors and manages the NCLEX. Client needs categories ensure that a wide variety of topics appears on every NCLEX.

1

Client needs categories

Each question on the NCLEX is assigned a category based on client needs. This chart lists client needs categories and subcategories and the percentages of each type of question that appear on the NCLEX.

Category	Subcategories	Percentage of questions
Safe and effective care environment	Coordinated care	18% to 24%
	Safety and infection control	10% to 16%
Health promotion and maintenance	—	6% to 12%
Psychosocial integrity	—	9% to 15%
Physiological integrity	Basic care and comfort	7% to 13%
	Pharmacological therapies	10% to 16%
	Reduction of risk potential	9% to 15%
	Physiological adaptation	7% to 13%

The NCSBN developed client needs categories after conducting a work-study analysis of new nurses. All aspects of nursing care observed in the study were broken down into four main categories, some of which were broken down further into subcategories. (See *Client needs categories.*)

The whole kit and caboodle

The categories and subcategories are used to develop the NCLEX test plan, the content guidelines for the distribution of test questions. Question writers and the people who put the NCLEX together use the test plan and client needs categories to make sure that a full spectrum of nursing activities is covered in the examination. Client needs categories appear in most NCLEX review and question-and-answer books, including this one. As a test-taker, you don't have to concern yourself with client needs categories. You'll see those categories for each question and answer in this book, but they'll be invisible on the actual NCLEX.

Testing by computer

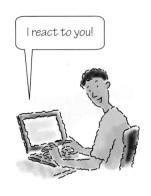

I react to you!

Like many standardized tests today, the NCLEX is administered by computer. That means you won't be filling in empty circles, sharpening pencils, or erasing frantically. It also means that you must become familiar with computer tests, if you aren't already. Fortunately, the skills required to take the NCLEX on a computer are simple enough to allow you to focus on the questions, not the keyboard.

Q&A formats—mixing them up

When you take the test, depending on the question format, you'll be presented with a question and four or more possible answers, a blank space in which to enter your answer, a figure on which you'll identify the correct area by clicking the mouse on it, a series of charts or exhibits you'll use to select the correct response, or items you must rearrange in priority order by dragging and dropping them in place.

Feeling smart? Think hard!

The NCLEX is a computer-adaptive test. When you respond to a question on the test, the computer supplies more difficult questions if you answer correctly and slightly easier questions if you answer incorrectly. This means each test is uniquely adapted to the individual test-taker.

A matter of time

You have a maximum of 5 hours to complete the test. That gives you the flexibility to spend extra time on more challenging questions. Just the same, it's important to keep an appropriate pace. Most students have plenty of time to finish the test. However, if you fail to correctly answer a set number of questions within 5 hours, the computer will determine that you lack minimum competency.

Most students have plenty of time to complete the test, so take as much time as you need to get the question right without wasting time. Keep moving at a decent pace to help maintain concentration.

Difficult items = good news

As you progress through the test, you may notice that the questions seem to be increasingly difficult. That's a good sign. The more questions you answer correctly, the more difficult the questions become.

Some students, knowing that questions get progressively harder, focus on the degree of difficulty of subsequent questions to figure out if they're answering questions correctly. Avoid this temptation and stay focused on selecting the best answer for each question.

Free at last!

The computer test ends when one of the following events occurs:
- You demonstrate minimum competency, according to the computer program.
- You demonstrate a lack of minimum competency, according to the computer program.
- You answer the maximum number of questions (205).
- You use the maximum time allowed (5 hours).

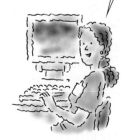

The harder it gets, the better I'm doing.

NCLEX® questions

Many questions on the NCLEX are standard four-option, multiple-choice questions with only one correct answer. However, some questions are presented in other formats. Being able to identify the different types of questions you might find on the NCLEX can help you understand them and answer them correctly.

Alternate formats

The types of alternate-format questions are multiple-response, fill-in-the-blank, hot spot, chart/exhibit, ordered response, graphic option, and audio.

Multiple, multiple: it's all or nothing

The first type of alternate-format question is the multiple-response question. Unlike a traditional multiple-choice question, each multiple-response question has, at a minimum, two correct answers. These questions do not have a maximum amount of correct answers, so all the choices may be correct. You'll recognize this type of question because it will ask you to select all of the correct answers that apply—not just the best answer.

Keep in mind that for each multiple-response question, you must select all of the correct answers for the item to be counted as correct. On the NCLEX, you don't receive partial credit in the scoring of these items.

Don't go blank!

The second type of alternate-format question is the fill-in-the-blank. In this type of question, you perform a calculation and type your answer (a number, without any words, commas, or spaces) in the blank space provided after the question. No answer options are presented.

Feeling hot, hot, hot

The third type of alternate-format question is one that asks you to identify an area on an illustration or graphic. For these so-called "hot-spot" questions, the computerized exam will ask you to place your cursor and click over the correct area on an illustration. Try to be as precise as possible when marking the location. As with the fill-in-the-blanks, these questions require extremely precise answers.

Take a look at that!

The fourth alternate-format type is the chart/exhibit format. For this question type, you'll be given a problem and then a series of small screens with additional information you'll need to answer the question. By clicking on the tabs on screen, you can access each chart or exhibit item. After viewing the chart or exhibit, you select your answer from four multiple-choice options.

Keep things in order!

Ordered response, the fifth type of alternate-format question, involves prioritizing actions or placing a series of statements in correct order using a drag-and-drop technique. To move an answer option from a list of unordered options into the correct sequence, click on it using the mouse. While still holding down the mouse button, drag the option to the ordered response part of the screen. Release the mouse button to "drop" the option into place. Repeat this process until you've moved all the available options into the correct order.

Now hear this

The sixth alternate-format item type is the audio item format. You'll be given a set of headphones and asked to listen to an audio clip and select the correct answer from four options. You'll need to select the correct answer on the computer screen as you would with the traditional multiple-choice questions.

Picture perfect

The final alternate-format item type is the graphic option question. This varies from the exhibit format type because in the graphic option, your answer choices will be graphics, such as ECG strips. You'll have to select the appropriate graphic to answer the question presented.

The standard is still the standard

The number of alternate-format questions will vary for each candidate. In fact, your exam may contain only one or may contain several. Keep in mind that standard four-option, multiple-choice questions constitute the bulk of the test. (See *Sample NCLEX questions*.)

Understanding the question

NCLEX® questions are commonly long. As a result, it's easy to become overloaded with information. To focus on the question and avoid becoming overwhelmed, apply these proven strategies for answering NCLEX questions:
- Determine what the question is asking.
- Determine relevant facts about the client.
- Rephrase the question in your mind.
- Choose the best option(s) before entering your answer.

Determine what the question is asking

Read the question twice. If the answer isn't apparent, rephrase the question in simpler, more personal terms. This strategy may help you to focus more effectively to determine the correct answer.

Give it a try

For example, a question might be, "An older adult client with a history of a myocardial infarction (MI) is admitted to the telemetry unit with heart failure and placed on 6 L of oxygen per minute and given furosemide. Which parameters should the nurse watch closely to monitor the client's response to furosemide?"

The answer options for this question might include:
1. Daily weight
2. 24-hour intake and output
3. Serum sodium levels
4. Hourly urine output

Hocus, focus on the question

Read the question again, ignoring all details except what's being asked. Focus on the last line of the question. It asks you to select the appropriate parameter for monitoring a client who received furosemide.

Determine what facts about the client are relevant

Next, sort out the relevant client information. Identify any irrelevant information provided about the client. For instance, do you need to know that the client has been

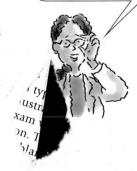

Focusing on what the question is really asking can help you choose the correct answer.

Sample NCLEX® questions

Sometimes, getting used to the format is as important as knowing the material. Try your hand at these sample questions, and you'll have a leg up when you take the real test!

Four-option, multiple-choice question

The nurse turns a client 4 days after abdominal surgery. When observing the incision, the nurse observes that part of the client's intestine is protruding. What is the **priority** action by the nurse?

1. Cover the incision and protruding intestine with a sterile dressing.
2. Irrigate the incision with normal saline solution.
3. Cover the incision and protruding intestine with gauze soaked in normal saline solution.
4. Attempt to reinsert the protruding intestine and cover it with an abdominal binder.

Correct answer: 3

Multiple-response question

A client is admitted with chronic obstructive pulmonary disease (COPD). Which findings are characteristic of COPD? Select all that apply.

1. Decreased respiratory rate
2. Dyspnea on exertion
3. Barrel chest
4. Shortened expiratory phase
5. Clubbed fingers
6. Fever

Correct answers: 2, 3, 5

Fill-in-the-blank, calculation question

The physician prescribes 600 mg of ceftriaxone oral suspension to be given once daily to a client with pneumonia. The nurse obtains the suspension from the pharmacy and reads the label, which indicates that the dosage strength is 125 mg/5 mL. How many milliliters of the medication should the nurse administer? Record your answer using a whole number.

_____ milliliters

Correct answer: 24

Hot-spot question

Orders for a client with cirrhosis request a daily measurement of abdominal girth. Identify the anatomical landmark where the tape measure should be placed to obtain this measurement.

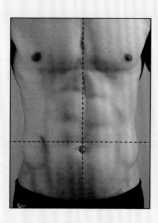

Correct answer:

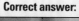
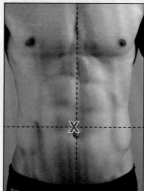

Chart/exhibit question

A preschooler is being admitted to the hospital and isolation precautions need to be implemented. Based on the progress note below, which isolation precautions would be used for this client?

(continued)

Sample NCLEX® questions *(continued)*

Progress notes	
4/15/2017	5-year-old with varicella admitted with high fever, dehydration, and pruritic rash on face and trunk with lesions in all stages. See graphic record for vital signs. IV started in L arm. Isolation precautions instituted.
	— J. Jefferson, RN.

1. Standard precautions
2. Airborne precautions
3. Droplet precautions
4. Contact precautions
Correct answer: 2

Ordered response question
The nurse thinks that a client may be in cardiac arrest. According to the 2015 American Heart Association guidelines, the nurse should perform the actions listed below in what order?
Unordered options:

Unordered options	Correct answer:
1. Activate the emergency response system.	**2.** Assess responsiveness
2. Assess responsiveness.	**1.** Activate the emergency response system.
3. Call for a defibrillator.	**3.** Call for a defibrillator.
4. Provide two breaths.	**5.** Assess pulse.
5. Assess pulse.	**6.** Begin cycles of 30 compressions.
6. Begin cycles of 30 chest compressions.	**4.** Provide two breaths.

Graphic option question
The nurse is assessing a client's respiratory pattern. Which graphic illustrates Kussmaul respirations?

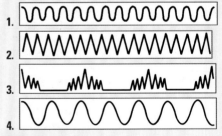

Correct answer: 2

Audio question (sample audio questions are available on thePoint)
Listen to the audio clip. What sound do you hear in the lung bases of this client with heart failure?

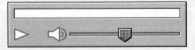

1. Crackles
2. Rhonchi
3. Wheezes
4. Pleural friction rub
Correct answer: 1

admitted to the telemetry unit? Probably not; the client's reaction to furosemide won't be affected by location in the hospital.

Determine what you do know about the client. In the example, you know that:
- the client just received a dose of the diuretic furosemide, a crucial fact
- the client has heart failure, the most fundamental aspect of the client's underlying condition
- the client is receiving oxygen at 6 L/minute, which suggests that heart failure is moderately severe
- the client is an older adult has had an MI, a fact that may or may not be relevant.

Rephrase the question

After you've determined relevant information about the client and the question being asked, consider rephrasing the question to make it clearer. Eliminate jargon and put the question in simpler, more personal terms. Here's how you might rephrase the question in the example: "My client has heart failure and requires 6 L/minute of oxygen. The client is an older adult and has had an MI. The client received a dose of furosemide. What parameter should I monitor?"

Choose the best option

Armed with all the information, it's time for you to select an option. You know that the client received a dose of furosemide. You know that monitoring fluid intake and output is a key nursing intervention for a client taking a diuretic, a fact that eliminates options 1 and 3 (daily weight and serum sodium levels) and narrows the answer down to options 2 and 4 (24-hour intake and output or hourly urine output).

Can I use a lifeline?

Monitoring the client's 24-hour intake and output would be appropriate for monitoring the effects of repeated doses of furosemide. Hourly urine output, however, is most appropriate in this situation because it monitors the more immediate effect of this drug.

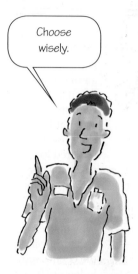

Choose wisely.

Key strategies

Regardless of the type of question, four key strategies will help you determine the correct answer for each question. (See *Strategies for success.*) These strategies include:
- considering the nursing process
- referring to Maslow hierarchy of needs
- reviewing client safety
- reflecting on principles of therapeutic communication.

Nursing process

One of the ways to answer a question is to apply the nursing process. Steps in the nursing process are implemented in this order:
- data collection
- planning
- implementation
- evaluation.

First things first

The nursing process may provide insights that help you analyze a question. According to the nursing process, data collection comes before planning, which comes before implementation, which comes before evaluation.

You're halfway to the correct answer when you encounter a four-option, multiple-choice question that asks you to collect data and then provides two data collection options and two implementation options. You can immediately eliminate the implementation options. This gives you, at worst, a 50-50 chance of selecting the correct answer. Use the following sample question to apply the nursing process:

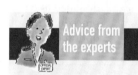

Advice from the experts

Strategies for success

Keeping a few main strategies in mind as you answer each NCLEX question can help ensure greater success. These four strategies are critical for answering NCLEX questions correctly:
- If the question asks what you should do in a situation, use the nursing process to determine which step in the process would be next.
- If the question asks what the client needs, use Maslow hierarchy to determine which need to address first.
- If the question indicates that the client doesn't have an urgent physiological need, focus on the client's safety.
- If the question involves communicating with a client, use the principles of therapeutic communication.

A client returns from an endoscopic procedure that required sedation. Before offering the client food, which action should the nurse take?
1. Monitor the client's respiratory status.
2. Check the client's gag reflex.
3. Place the client in a side-lying position.
4. Have the client drink a few sips of water.

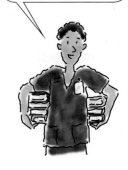

Say it 1,000 times: Studying for the NCLEX is fun... studying for the NCLEX is fun...

Collect data before intervening

According to the nursing process, the nurse must collect client data before performing an intervention. Does the question indicate that data have been properly collected? No, it doesn't. Therefore, you can eliminate options 3 and 4 because they're both interventions.

That leaves options 1 and 2, both of which demonstrate data collection. Your nursing knowledge should tell you the correct answer—in this case, option 2. The sedation required for an endoscopic procedure may impair the client's gag reflex, so you would check the gag reflex before giving food to the client to reduce the risk of aspiration and airway obstruction.

Final elimination

Why not select option 1, monitoring the client's respiratory status? The question is specifically asking about offering the client food, an action that wouldn't be taken if the client's respiratory status was at all compromised. In this case, you're making a judgment based on the phrase, "before offering the client food." If the question was designed to test your knowledge of respiratory depression following an endoscopic procedure, it probably wouldn't mention a function such as feeding a client. This option clearly occurs only after the client's respiratory status has been stabilized.

Maslow hierarchy

Knowledge of Maslow hierarchy of needs can be a vital tool for answering questions on the NCLEX that require you to establish priorities. Maslow theory states that physiological needs are the most basic human needs of all. Only after physiological needs have been met can safety concerns be addressed. Only after safety concerns are met can concerns involving love and belonging be addressed. Once concerns of love and belonging are met, an individual may explore the needs of self-esteem, then, ultimately, the needs of self-actualization. Apply the principles of Maslow hierarchy of needs to the following sample question:

A client reports severe pain 2 days after surgery. Which action should the nurse perform first?
1. Offer reassurance that the client will feel less pain tomorrow.
2. Allow time for the client to verbalize feelings.
3. Check the client's vital signs.
4. Administer an analgesic.

Phys before psych

In this example, options 3 and 4 address physiological needs. Options 1 and 2 address psychosocial concerns. According to Maslow, physiological needs must be met before psychosocial needs, so you can eliminate options 1 and 2.

Final elimination

Now, use your nursing knowledge to choose the best answer from the two remaining options. In this case, option 3 is correct because the client's vital signs should be checked before administering an analgesic (data collection before intervention). When prioritizing according to Maslow hierarchy, remember your ABCs—airway, breathing, circulation—to help you further prioritize. Check for a patent airway before addressing breathing. Check breathing before checking the health of the cardiovascular system.

One caveat...

Always examine your choice in light of your knowledge and experience. Ask yourself, "Does this choice make sense for this client?" Allow yourself to eliminate choices even ones that might normally take priority—if they don't make sense for a particular client's situation.

Client safety

As you might expect, client safety takes high priority on the NCLEX. You'll encounter many questions that can be answered by asking yourself, "Which answer will best ensure the safety of this client?" Use client safety criteria for situations involving laboratory values, drug administration, or nursing care procedures.

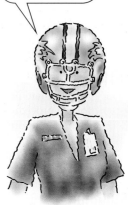

Client safety takes high priority on the NCLEX.

Client first, equipment second

You may encounter a question in which some options address the client and others address the equipment. When in doubt, select an option relating to the client; never place equipment before a client.

For instance, suppose a question asks what the nurse should do first when entering a client's room where an infusion pump alarm is sounding. If two options deal with the infusion pump, one with the infusion tubing, and another with the client's catheter insertion site, select the one relating to the client's catheter insertion site. Always check the client first; the equipment can wait.

Therapeutic communication

Some NCLEX questions focus on the nurse's ability to communicate effectively with the client. Therapeutic communication incorporates verbal or nonverbal responses and involves:
- listening to the client
- understanding the client's needs
- promoting clarification
- gaining insight into the client's condition.

Room for improvement

Like other NCLEX questions, those dealing with therapeutic communication commonly require choosing the best response. First, eliminate options that indicate the use of poor therapeutic communication techniques, such as those in which the nurse:
- tells the client what to do without regard to his or her feelings or desires (the "do this" response)
- asks a question that can be answered with a one-word response, such as "yes" or "no"
- seeks reasons for the client's behavior
- implies disapproval of the client's behavior
- offers false reassurances
- attempts to interpret the client's behavior rather than allow the client to verbalize feelings
- offers a response that focuses on the nurse, not the client.

Ah, that's better!

When answering NCLEX questions, look for responses that:
- allow the client time to think and reflect
- encourage the client to talk
- encourage the client to describe a particular experience
- reflect that the nurse has listened to the client through paraphrasing the client's response or another communication technique.

Avoiding pitfalls

Even the most knowledgeable students can be tripped up by certain NCLEX questions. Students commonly cite three areas that can be difficult for unwary test-takers:
1. knowing the difference between the NCLEX and the "real world"
2. delegating care
3. knowing laboratory values.

NCLEX® examination versus the real world

Some students who take the NCLEX have extensive practical experience in health care. For example, many test-takers have worked as nursing assistants. In that capacity, test-takers might have been exposed to less than optimal clinical practice and may carry those experiences over to the NCLEX.

However, the NCLEX is a textbook examination—not a test of clinical skills. Take the NCLEX with the understanding that what happens in the real world may differ from what the NCLEX and your nursing school recommend.

Don't take shortcuts

If you've had practical experience in health care, you may know a quicker way to perform a procedure or tricks to help you get by when you don't have the right equipment. Situations such as staff shortages may force you to improvise. On the NCLEX, such scenarios can lead to trouble. Always check your practical experiences against textbook nursing care and be sure to select the response that follows the textbook.

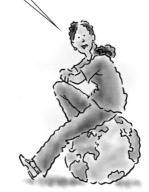

Remember, this is an exam, not the real world.

Delegating care

On the NCLEX, you may encounter questions that assess your ability to delegate care. Delegating care involves coordinating the efforts of other health care workers to provide effective care for your client. On the NCLEX, you may be asked to assign duties to nursing assistants and other support staff.

In addition, you'll be asked to decide when to notify a registered nurse, a physician or practitioner, a social worker, or another hospital staff member. In each case, you'll have to decide when, where, and how to delegate.

Shoulds and shouldn'ts

As a general rule, it's okay to delegate actions that involve stable clients or standard procedures. Bathing, feeding, dressing, and transferring clients are examples of procedures that can be delegated.

Be careful not to delegate complicated or complex activities. In addition, don't delegate activities that involve data collection, evaluation, or your own nursing judgment. On the NCLEX and in the real world, these duties fall squarely on your shoulders. Make sure that you take primary responsibility for collecting client data, evaluating the client, and making decisions about the client's care. Never hand off those responsibilities to someone with less training.

Calling in reinforcements

Notifying a registered nurse, a physician or practitioner, a social worker, or another hospital staff member is an important element of nursing care. On the NCLEX, however, choices that involve notifying the physician are usually incorrect. Remember that the NCLEX tests you, the nurse, at work.

When you're sure the correct answer is to notify the physician, first make sure the client's safety has been addressed. On the NCLEX, the client's safety has a higher priority than notifying other health care providers.

Knowing laboratory values

Some NCLEX questions supply laboratory results without indicating normal levels. As a result, answering questions involving laboratory values requires you to have the normal range of the most common laboratory values memorized to make an informed decision.

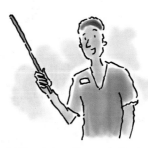

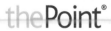® You can download charts and diagrams to help you prepare for the NCLEX®! View Commonly Used Abbreviations; Commonly Used English to Metric Conversion Equations; Normal Adult Laboratory Values; Normal Pediatric Laboratory Values; Erikson's Stages of Psychosocial Development; Sites for Cardiac Auscultation; Sites and Sequence for Posterior Auscultation; and Sites for Anterior Chest Palpation, Percussion, and Auscultation at **http://thePoint.lww.com**.

Chapter 2

Passing the NCLEX®

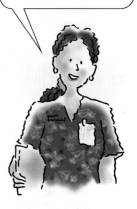

Just the facts

In this chapter, you'll review:

♦ how to properly prepare for the NCLEX
♦ how to concentrate during difficult study times
♦ how to make more effective use of your time
♦ how creative strategies can enhance study.

Study preparations

If you're like most people preparing to take the NCLEX®, you're probably feeling nervous, anxious, or concerned. Keep in mind that most test-takers pass the first time.

Passing the test won't happen by accident, though; you'll need to prepare carefully and efficiently. You should start studying sooner rather than later. To help jump-start your preparations:

• determine your strengths and weaknesses
• create a study schedule
• set realistic goals
• find an effective study space
• think positively.

Determine strengths and weaknesses

Most students recognize by the end of their nursing studies that they know more about some topics than others. Because the NCLEX covers a broad range of material, you should make some decisions about how intensively you'll review each subject.

Make a review list

Decide what to include in a comprehensive list of topics you need to study. Start with the contents page in the front of this book, which summarizes the information you covered in school. Divide a sheet of paper in half vertically. Label one side "know well" and label the other side "needs review." List each topic from the contents page in the appropriate column. Don't worry if one list is longer than the other. After you've studied, you'll feel strong in every area. Separating content areas this way helps you allocate your study time.

Schedule study time

Study when you're most alert. If you feel most alert and energized in the morning, for example, set aside sections of time early in the day for topics that need a lot of review. Then you can use the evening, a time of lesser alertness, to refresh your memory about more familiar topics. The opposite is true as well; if you're more alert in the evening, study difficult topics at that time.

What you'll do when

Set up a basic schedule for studying. Using a calendar or an organizer, determine how much time remains before you'll take the NCLEX. (See *2 to 3 months before the NCLEX.*) Fill in the remaining days with specific times and topics to study. For

2 to 3 months before the NCLEX®

Take these steps 2 to 3 months before you plan to take the examination:

• Establish a study schedule. Set aside ample time to study but leave time for social activities, exercise, family and personal responsibilities, and other matters.
• Become knowledgeable about the NCLEX: its content, the types of questions it asks, and the testing format.
• Begin studying your notes, websites, texts, and other appropriate materials.
• Take some NCLEX practice questions and online examinations to help you diagnose your strengths and weaknesses as well as to become familiar with NCLEX questions and computerized testing.

example, you might schedule the respiratory system on a Tuesday morning and the GI system that afternoon. Remember to schedule difficult topics during your most alert times.

Keep in mind that you shouldn't fill each day with studying. Be realistic and set aside time for normal activities. Try to create ample study time before the NCLEX and then stick to the schedule.

Set realistic goals

Part of creating a schedule means setting goals you can accomplish. You no doubt studied a great deal in nursing school, and by now you have a sense of your own capabilities. Ask yourself, "How much can I cover in a day?" Set aside that amount of time and then stay on task. You'll feel better about yourself—and your chances of passing the NCLEX—when you meet your goals regularly.

Find an effective study space

Find a space to study that is conducive to effective learning. Whatever you do, don't study with videos playing in the room or in an environment with multiple sources of distraction. Instead, find an inviting, quiet, convenient place, away from normal traffic patterns. Sit in a solid chair that encourages good posture. (Avoid studying in bed; you'll be more likely to fall asleep and not accomplish your goals.) The room should have comfortable, soft lighting with which you can see clearly without straining, a temperature between 65° and 70°F, flowers or green plants, familiar photos or paintings, and easy access to soft, instrumental background music.

Accentuate the positive

Consider taping positive messages around your study space. Make signs with words of encouragement, such as "You can do it!" and "Remember the goal!" These upbeat messages can help keep you going when your attention begins to waver.

Maintaining concentration

When you're faced with reviewing the amount of information covered by the NCLEX, it's easy to become distracted and lose your concentration. When you lose concentration, you make less effective use of valuable study time. To stay focused, keep these tips in mind:

- Alternate the order of the subjects you study to add variety to your day. Try alternating between topics you find more interesting and those you find less interesting.
- Approach your study with enthusiasm, sincerity, and determination.
- Begin studying on a schedule and don't let anything interfere with your thought processes after you've begun.
- Concentrate on accomplishing one task at a time, to the exclusion of everything else, such as going online and conversing with friends.
- Work continuously without interruption for a while but don't study for such a long period that the whole experience becomes grueling or boring.
- Take breaks to give yourself a change of pace. These breaks can ease your transition into studying a new topic.
- When studying in the evening, wind down from your studies slowly. Don't go directly from studying to sleeping.

Taking care of yourself

Never neglect your physical and mental well-being in favor of longer study hours. Maintaining physical and mental health is critical for success in taking the NCLEX. (See *4 to 6 weeks before the NCLEX*.)

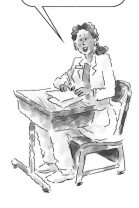

Approach your studying with enthusiasm, sincerity, and determination.

To-do list

4 to 6 weeks before the NCLEX®

Take these steps 4 to 6 weeks before you plan to take the examination:
- Focus on your areas of weakness, identified through online and book review and outcomes. Keep in mind that you'll have time to review these areas again before the test date.
- Find a study partner or form a study group.
- Take practice tests to gauge your skill level early. Use remediation tools offered through online resources and book rationales to address your learning gaps.
- Take time to eat, sleep, exercise, and socialize to avoid burnout.

A few simple rules

You can increase your likelihood of passing the test by following these simple health rules:

- Get plenty of rest. You can't think deeply or concentrate for long periods when you're tired.
- Eat nutritious meals and snacks. Maintaining your energy level is impossible when you're undernourished.
- Exercise regularly. Regular exercise helps you work harder and think more clearly. As a result, you'll study more efficiently and increase the likelihood of success on the all-important NCLEX.

Memory power!

If you're having trouble concentrating but would rather push through than take a break, try making your studying more active by reading out loud. Active studying can renew your powers of concentration. By reading review material out loud, you're engaging your ears as well as your eyes—and making your study a more active process. Hearing the material out loud fosters memory and subsequent recall.

You can also rewrite in your own words a few of the more difficult concepts you're reviewing. Explaining these concepts in writing forces you to think through the material and can jump-start your memory.

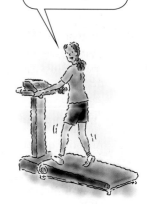

Regular exercise helps you work harder and think more clearly.

Study schedule

When you were creating your schedule, you might have asked yourself, "How long should I study? One hour at a stretch? Two hours? Three?" To make the best use of your study time, you'll need to answer those questions.

Optimal study time

Experts are divided about the optimal duration of study time. Some say you should study no more than 1 hour at a time several times per day. Their reasoning: You remember the material you study at the beginning and end of a session best and are less likely to remember material studied in the middle of the session.

Other experts say you should hold longer study sessions because you lose time in the beginning, when you're just warming up, and again at the end, when you're cooling down. That means a long, concentrated study period will allow you to cover more material.

To thine own self be true

So what's the best plan? It doesn't matter as long as you determine what's best for you. At the beginning of your NCLEX study schedule, try study periods of varying lengths. Pay close attention to those that seem more successful.

Remember that you're a trained nurse who competently collects data. Think of yourself as a client and collect data about your own progress. Then implement the strategy that works best for you.

Finding time to study

Regardless of the study plan you've chosen, remember that we all have periods in our day that might otherwise be dead time. These are perfect times to review for the NCLEX. However, you shouldn't cover new material because you may not have enough time to get deeply into it. Always keep your mobile device or tablet, flash cards, or a small notebook handy for situations when you have a few extra minutes. (See *1 week before the NCLEX*.)

You'll be amazed by how many short sessions you can find in a day and how much review you can do in 5 minutes. For example, the following occasions offer short stretches of time you can use for studying:

- eating breakfast
- waiting for a train or bus
- standing in line at the bank, post office, or bookstore

1 week before the NCLEX®

One week before the NCLEX, take these steps:
- Take a review test to measure your progress.
- Record key ideas and principles on your mobile device, tablet, note cards, or audiotapes.
- Rest, eat well, and avoid thinking about the examination during nonstudy times.
- Treat yourself to one special event. You've been working hard, and you deserve it!

Creative studying

Even when you study in a perfect place and concentrate better than ever, preparing for the NCLEX can get a little, well, dull. Even people with great study habits occasionally feel bored or sluggish. That's why it's important to have some creative tricks in your study bag to liven up those down times.

Creative studying doesn't have to be hard work. It involves making efforts to alter your study habits a bit. Some techniques that might help include alternating traditional book review with online adaptive quizzing programs, studying with a partner or group, and creating flash cards or other audiovisual study tools.

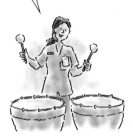

Studying getting dull? Get creative and liven it up.

Online adaptive quizzing

Adaptive quizzing programs such as *Lippincott NCLEX-PN PassPoint* can help keep you engaged with learning because the quizzes and exams are individualized to your level of understanding. The more correct knowledge you demonstrate, the more challenging the learning experience becomes. PassPoint gives you ongoing feedback about your strengths and weaknesses so you know how to prioritize your study plan. It gives you an opportunity to take NCLEX-style exams of varying lengths to help you build your endurance and become more familiar with a simulated computer adaptive testing environment. By alternating your book review and quizzing with online learning, you can stay energized and prepare for NCLEX using the different media available to you.

It isn't easy to find a partner who has the same study habits I do.

Study partners

Studying with a partner or group of students can be an excellent way to energize your studying. It allows you to test each other on the material you've reviewed and share ways of studying. You can also encourage and help each other to stay motivated. Perhaps most important, working with a partner can provide a welcome break from solitary studying.

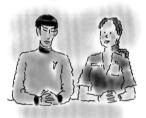

What to look for in a partner

Exercise care when choosing a study partner or assembling a study group. A partner who doesn't fit your needs won't help you make the most of your study time. Look for a partner who:
- possesses goals similar to yours—for example, someone taking the NCLEX at approximately the same date as you will likely feel the same sense of urgency as you and might make an excellent partner.
- possesses about the same level of knowledge as you—tutoring someone can help you learn, but each partner should add to the other's knowledge.
- studies without excess chatting or interruptions—socializing is an important part of creative study but you have to pass the NCLEX, so stay serious!

Audiovisual tools

Using flash cards and other audiovisual tools fosters retention and makes learning and reviewing fun.

Flash cards!

Flash cards can be an excellent study tool. The process of writing material on a flash card will help you remember it. In addition, flash cards are small and portable, perfect for those 5-minute slivers of time during the day.

Creating flash cards should be fun. Use magic markers, highlighters, and other colorful tools to make them visually stimulating. The more effort you put into creating your flash cards, the better you'll remember the material contained on them.

To-do list

The day before the NCLEX®

One day before the NCLEX, take these steps:
- Drive to the test site to check traffic patterns and find out where to park. If your drive occurs during heavy traffic or if you're expecting bad weather, set aside extra time to ensure your prompt arrival.
- Do something relaxing during the day.
- Avoid thinking too much about the test.
- Rest and eat well.
- Call a supportive friend or relative for some last-minute words of encouragement.

Other visual tools

Flowcharts, drawings, diagrams, and other image-oriented study aids can also help you learn material more effectively. Substituting images for text can be a great way to give your eyes a break and recharge your brain. Use vivid colors to make your creations visually engaging.

Hear's the thing

If you learn more effectively when you hear information rather than see it, consider recording key ideas using a voice memo–type app on your phone or tablet. Recording information helps promote memory because you say the information aloud and then listen to it as it plays back. Like flash cards, these portable recordings are perfect for those short study periods during the day. (See *The day before the NCLEX*.)

Practice questions

Practice questions should be an important part of your NCLEX study strategy. Practice questions can improve your studying by helping you review material and familiarize yourself with the exact style of questions you'll encounter on the test.

Practice at the beginning

Consider working through some practice questions as soon as you begin studying for the NCLEX. For example, you might try a few of the questions that appear at the end of each chapter in this book.

If you do well, you probably know that particular topic and can spend less time reviewing it. If you have trouble with the questions, spend extra study time on that topic.

I'm getting there

Practice questions can also provide an excellent means of marking your progress. Don't worry if you have trouble answering the first few practice questions; you'll need time to learn how the questions are asked. Eventually, you'll become accustomed to the question format and begin to focus more on the questions themselves.

If you make practice questions a regular part of your study regimen, you'll be able to recognize areas in which you're improving. You can then adjust your study time accordingly.

Practice makes perfect

As you near the examination date, you should increase the number of NCLEX practice questions you answer at one sitting. This will enable you to approximate the experience of taking the actual NCLEX. Using thePoint Web site that accompanies this resource (the code for which is found on this inside cover of this book), you can take practice tests with varying numbers of questions. Additionally, this code offers you a free 7-day trial of *Lippincott NCLEX-PN PassPoint*, which allows you to take adaptive quizzes across the curriculum as well as to take practice exams of varying lengths from 85 to 205 questions. These practice exams simulate the real NCLEX in every way. Note that 85 questions is the minimum number of questions you'll be asked on the actual NCLEX. By gradually tackling larger practice tests, you'll increase your confidence, build test-taking endurance, and strengthen the concentration skills that will enable you to succeed. (See *The day of the NCLEX*.)

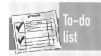

The day of the NCLEX®

On the day of the NCLEX:
• Get up early.
• Eat a nutritious breakfast.
• Wear comfortable clothes, preferably with layers you can add and remove to adjust to the room temperature.
• Leave your house early so you can arrive at the test site early.
• Avoid looking at your notes as you wait for your test computer.
• Listen carefully to the instructions given before entering the test room.

Taking lots of practice tests will help you succeed on the real exam!

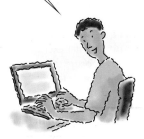

Chapter 3

Cardiovascular Disorders

Cardiovascular refresher

Abdominal aortic aneurysm

Stretched and bulging section of the wall of the aorta

Key signs and symptoms
- Commonly produces no symptoms

Key test results
- Abdominal x-ray shows an aneurysm
- Computed tomography (CT) scan reveals size

Key treatments
- Abdominal aortic aneurysm resection or repair
- Blood administration, as needed

Key interventions
- Monitor and record vital signs
- Monitor intake, output, and laboratory studies
- Observe for signs of hypovolemic shock from aneurysm rupture, such as:
  - anxiety and restlessness
  - severe back pain
  - decreased pulse pressure
  - increased thready pulse
  - pale, cool, moist, clammy skin

Angina

Chest pain caused by reduced blood flow to heart muscle

Key signs and symptoms
- Pain may be substernal, crushing, or compressing; may radiate to the arms, jaw, or back; usually lasts 3 to 5 minutes; usually occurs after exertion, emotional excitement, or exposure to cold but can also develop when at rest.

Key test results
- Electrocardiogram (ECG) shows ST-segment depression and T-wave inversion during anginal pain

Key treatments
- Percutaneous transluminal coronary angioplasty (PTCA) or coronary artery stent placement

Key interventions
- Administer medications as prescribed
- Withhold nitrates and notify health care provider if systolic blood pressure is less than 90 mm Hg
- Withhold beta-blockers and notify health care provider if heart rate is less than 60 beats/minute
- Monitor for chest pain; if present, evaluate its characteristics
- Obtain 12-lead ECG during an acute attack

Arrhythmias

Abnormal heart rhythm

Key signs and symptoms
Atrial fibrillation
- Commonly produces no symptoms
- Irregular pulse with no pattern to the irregularity

Asystole
- Apnea
- Cyanosis
- No palpable blood pressure
- Pulselessness

Ventricular fibrillation
- Apnea
- No palpable blood pressure
- Pulselessness

Ventricular tachycardia
- Diaphoresis
- Hypotension
- Weak pulse or pulselessness
- Dizziness

Key test results
Atrial fibrillation
- ECG shows:
  - irregular atrial rhythm
  - atrial rate greater than 400 beats/minute
  - irregular ventricular rhythm
  - QRS complexes of uniform configuration and duration
  - no discernible PR interval
  - no P waves, or P waves that appear as erratic, irregular baseline fibrillation waves

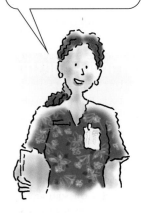
If you'd like to rummage through a Web site dedicated to cardiovascular disorders, check out the American Heart Association's *www.americanheart.org*. Go for it!

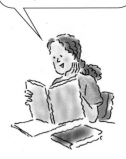
Do you remember the symptoms of angina?

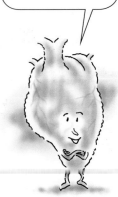
I've been feeling a little off my rhythm lately. What treatment would you recommend?

16

Asystole

- ECG shows no atrial or ventricular rate or rhythm, nor any discernible P waves, QRS complexes, or T waves

Ventricular fibrillation

- ECG shows ventricular activity that appears as fibrillatory waves with no recognizable pattern
- Atrial rate and rhythm and ventricular rhythm can't be determined because no pattern or regularity occurs
- The P wave, PR interval, QRS complex, T wave, and QT interval can't be determined

Ventricular tachycardia

- ECG shows ventricular rate of 100 to 250 beats/minute, wide and bizarre QRS complexes, and no discernible P waves
- May start or stop suddenly

Key treatments

Atrial fibrillation

- Antiarrhythmics: amiodarone, digoxin, diltiazem, procainamide
- Synchronized cardioversion (if client is unstable)

Asystole

- Cardiopulmonary resuscitation (CPR)
- Advanced cardiac life support (ACLS) protocol for endotracheal (ET) intubation and possible transcutaneous pacing
- Epinephrine per ACLS protocol

Ventricular fibrillation

- CPR
- Defibrillation
- ACLS protocol for ET intubation
- Amiodarone, epinephrine, lidocaine, magnesium sulfate, procainamide, vasopressin per ACLS protocol

Ventricular tachycardia

- CPR, if pulseless
- Defibrillation
- ACLS protocol for ET intubation
- Amiodarone, epinephrine, lidocaine, magnesium sulfate, procainamide

Key interventions

- Monitor ECG to detect arrhythmias and ischemia
- If pulse is abnormally rapid, slow, or irregular, watch for signs of hypoperfusion, such as hypotension and altered mental status
- When life-threatening arrhythmias develop, rapidly assess the level of consciousness (LOC), respirations, and pulse
- Initiate CPR, if indicated
- Administer medications as needed, and prepare for medical procedures (e.g., cardioversion) if indicated

- Monitor pulse oximetry. Provide adequate oxygen to reduce the heart's workload while carefully maintaining metabolic, neurologic, respiratory, and hemodynamic status

Arterial occlusive disease

Narrowing of the arteries that leads to decreased blood supply to muscles and tissues

Key signs and symptoms

Femoral, popliteal, or innominate arteries

- Mottling of the affected extremity
- Pallor
- Paralysis and paresthesia in the affected arm or leg
- Pulselessness distal to the occlusion
- Sudden and localized pain in the affected arm or leg (most common symptom)
- Temperature change distal to the occlusion

Internal and external carotid arteries

- Transient ischemic attacks (TIAs) that produce transient monocular blindness, dysarthria, hemiparesis, possible aphasia, confusion, decreased mentation, headache

Subclavian artery

- Subclavian steal syndrome (SSS) (characterized by the backflow of blood from the brain through the vertebral artery on the same side as the occlusion into the subclavian artery distal to the occlusion; clinical effects of vertebrobasilar occlusion and exercise-induced arm claudication)

Vertebral and basilar arteries

- TIAs that produce binocular vision disturbances, vertigo, dysarthria, and falling without loss of consciousness

Key test results

- Arteriography demonstrates the type (thrombus or embolus), location, degree of obstruction, and the status of collateral circulation.
- Doppler ultrasonography shows decreased blood flow distal to the occlusion.

Key treatments

- Surgery (for acute arterial occlusive disease): atherectomy, balloon angioplasty, bypass graft, embolectomy, laser angioplasty, patch grafting, stent placement, thromboendarterectomy, amputation
- Thrombolytic agents: alteplase

Key interventions

Preoperatively (during an acute episode)

- Check most distal pulses and inspect skin color and temperature
- Provide pain relief as needed

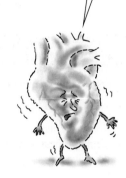

I'm sounding a little irregular. What could be wrong?

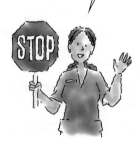

Your client is having a transient ischemic attack during an office visit. What signs should you look for?

- Maintain heparin infusion per protocol; monitor activated partial thromboplastin time (aPTT) and partial thromboplastin time (PTT)
- Watch for signs of fluid and electrolyte imbalance, and monitor intake and output for signs of renal failure (urine output less than 30 mL/hour)

Postoperatively

- Monitor vital signs. Continuously monitor circulatory function by inspecting skin color, taking temperature, and checking for distal pulses. While charting, compare earlier findings and observations. Watch closely for signs of hemorrhage (tachycardia, hypotension), and check dressings for excessive bleeding
- Check neurologic status frequently for changes in LOC, muscle strength, or pupil size
- With mesenteric artery occlusion, connect a nasogastric tube to low intermittent suction. Monitor intake and output. Check abdominal status
- With saddle block occlusion, check distal pulses for adequate circulation. Watch for signs of renal failure and mesenteric artery occlusion (severe abdominal pain)
- With iliac artery occlusion, monitor urine output for signs of renal failure from decreased perfusion to the kidneys as a result of surgery. Provide meticulous catheter care
- With femoral and popliteal artery occlusion, assist with early ambulation and discourage prolonged sitting

Cardiac tamponade

Accumulation of blood or fluids in space between the sac encasing the heart and the heart muscle

Key signs and symptoms

- Muffled heart sounds on auscultation
- Narrow pulse pressure
- Jugular vein distention
- Pulsus paradoxus (abnormal inspiratory drop in systemic blood pressure greater than 15 mm Hg)
- Restlessness
- Upright, leaning forward posture

Key test results

- Chest x-ray shows slightly widened mediastinum and cardiomegaly.
- Echocardiography identifies pericardial effusion with signs of right ventricular and atrial compression.
- ECG may reveal:
  - low-amplitude QRS complex and electrical alternans

  - alternating beat-to-beat change in the amplitude of the P wave, QRS complex, and T wave
  - generalized ST-segment elevation in all leads

Key treatments

- Supplemental oxygen
- Surgery: pericardiocentesis (needle aspiration of the pericardial cavity) or surgical creation of an opening to drain fluid (thoracotomy)
- Inotropic agent: dopamine

Key interventions

Pericardiocentesis

- Keep a pericardial aspiration needle attached to a 50-mL syringe by a three-way stopcock, an ECG machine, and an emergency cart with a defibrillator at the bedside. Keep the equipment turned on to be prepared for immediate use
- Position the client at a 45- to 60-degree angle
- Monitor blood pressure during and after pericardiocentesis to watch for complications such as hypotension, which may indicate cardiac chamber puncture
- Be alert for complications of pericardiocentesis, such as ventricular fibrillation, vasovagal response, or coronary artery or cardiac chamber puncture

Thoracotomy

- Explain the procedure and what to expect after the operation (chest tubes, drainage bottles, administration of oxygen). Teach how to turn, deep-breathe, and cough
- Maintain the chest drainage system, and observe for complications, such as hemorrhage and arrhythmias

Cardiogenic shock

Heart damaged so severely that it cannot supply enough blood to organs of the body

Key signs and symptoms

- Cold, clammy skin
- Hypotension (systolic pressure below 90 mm Hg)
- Narrow pulse pressure
- Tachycardia or other arrhythmias

Key test results

- ECG shows myocardial infarction (MI), as indicated by an enlarged Q wave and elevated ST segment

Key treatments

- Intra-aortic balloon pump
- Adrenergic agent: epinephrine

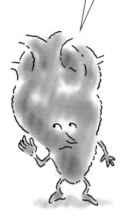

I'm sounding a little muffled. I wonder what that means?

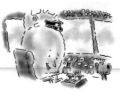

Monitor vital signs closely!

- Cardiac glycoside: digoxin
- Cardiac inotropic agents: dopamine, dobutamine, milrinone
- Diuretics: furosemide, bumetanide, metolazone
- Vasodilators: nitroprusside sodium, nitroglycerin
- Vasopressor: norepinephrine

Key interventions
- Monitor vital signs, heart sounds, capillary refill, skin temperature, and peripheral pulses
- Monitor ECG
- Monitor respiratory status, including breath sounds and arterial blood gas (ABG) levels
- Administer oxygen and medications as prescribed
- Maintain IV fluids

Cardiomyopathy
Progressive heart muscle disease

Key signs and symptoms
- Murmur
- S3 and S4 heart sounds

Key test results
- ECG shows left ventricular hypertrophy and nonspecific changes
- Echocardiogram shows dilated cardiomyopathy

Key treatments
- Dual chamber pacing (for hypertrophic cardiomyopathy)
- Beta-blockers: atenolol, propranolol, nadolol, metoprolol for hypertrophic cardiomyopathy
- Calcium channel blockers: amlodipine, diltiazem for hypertrophic cardiomyopathy
- Diuretics: furosemide, bumetanide, metolazone for dilated cardiomyopathy
- Inotropic agents: dobutamine, milrinone, digoxin for dilated cardiomyopathy
- Oral anticoagulant: warfarin for dilated or hypertrophic cardiomyopathy

Key interventions
- Monitor ECG
- Monitor vital signs
- Administer oxygen and medications, as prescribed

Coronary artery disease (CAD)
Plaque buildup in the arteries that supply blood to the heart

Key signs and symptoms
- Chest pain that may be substernal, crushing, or compressing; may radiate to the arms, jaw, or back; usually lasts 3 to 5 minutes; usually occurs after exertion, emotional excitement, or exposure to cold but can also develop when at rest.

Key test results
- Blood chemistry tests show increased cholesterol (decreased high-density lipoproteins [HDL] and increased low-density lipoproteins [LDL])
- ECG or Holter monitor shows ST-segment depression and T-wave inversion during an anginal episode

Key treatments
- Activity changes, including weight loss, if necessary
- Dietary changes, including establishing a low-sodium, low-cholesterol, low-fat diet with increased dietary fiber (low-calorie only if appropriate)
- Oxygen therapy
- Antilipemic agents: cholestyramine, lovastatin, simvastatin, nicotinic acid, gemfibrozil, colestipol

Key interventions
- Obtain ECG during anginal episodes
- Monitor vital signs
- Monitor ECG
- Monitor intake and output
- Administer nitroglycerin for anginal episodes

Endocarditis
Inflammation of the inside of the heart chambers and heart valves

Key signs and symptoms
- Chills
- Fatigue
- Loud, regurgitant murmur

Key test results
- Echocardiography may identify valvular damage
- ECG may show atrial fibrillation and other arrhythmias that accompany valvular disease
- Three or more blood cultures in a 24- to 48-hour period identify the causative organism in up to 90% of clients

Key treatments
- Maintaining sufficient fluid intake
- Antibiotics: based on causative organism
- Antiplatelet agent: aspirin

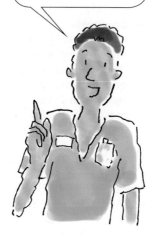

A client has been diagnosed with cardiomyopathy. What medications do you anticipate being ordered?

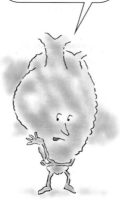

My arteries are feeling "gummed up" recently. What do you think the problem is?

Key interventions

- Monitor ECG
- Monitor cardiovascular status
- Watch for signs of embolization (hematuria, pleuritic chest pain, left-upper-quadrant pain, and paresis), a common occurrence during the first 3 months of treatment
- Monitor the client's renal status (blood urea nitrogen [BUN] level, creatinine clearance, and urine output)
- Observe for signs of heart failure, such as dyspnea, tachypnea, tachycardia, crackles, jugular vein distention, edema, and weight gain

Heart failure

Physiologic state when heart muscle is weakened and cannot pump enough blood to meet body's need of blood and oxygen

Key signs and symptoms

Left-sided failure

- Crackles
- Dyspnea
- Gallop rhythm: S3, S4 heart sounds

Right-sided failure

- Dependent edema
- Jugular vein distention
- Weight gain

Key test results

Left-sided failure

- B-type natriuretic peptide (BNP) levels elevated
- Chest x-ray shows increased pulmonary congestion and left ventricular hypertrophy.

Right-sided failure

- BNP levels elevated
- Chest x-ray reveals pulmonary congestion, cardiomegaly, and pleural effusion.

Key treatments

- Diuretics: furosemide, bumetanide, metolazone
- Human B-type natriuretic peptide: nesiritide
- Angiotensin-converting enzyme (ACE) inhibitors: captopril, enalapril, lisinopril
- Cardiac glycoside: digoxin
- Inotropic agents: dopamine, dobutamine
- Nitrates: isosorbide dinitrate, nitroglycerin
- Vasodilator: nitroprusside sodium

Key interventions

- Administer oxygen
- Monitor ECG
- Monitor vital signs
- Monitor respiratory status
- Keep the client in semi-Fowler position
- Weigh the client daily

Hypertension

Blood pressure in arteries is elevated; also known as high blood pressure

Key signs and symptoms

- Produces no symptoms

Key test results

- Blood pressure measurements result in sustained readings greater than 140/90 mm Hg

Key treatments

- Weight reduction
- Increased physical activity
- Dietary changes
- Reducing sodium intake
- Limiting alcohol intake
- ACE inhibitors: captopril, enalapril, Lisinopril

Key interventions

- Monitor vital signs. Take two or more blood pressure readings rather than relying on a single, possibly abnormal reading

Hypovolemic shock

Severe blood and fluid loss making the heart unable to pump enough blood to the body

Key signs and symptoms

- Cold, pale, clammy skin
- Decreased sensorium
- Hypotension with narrow pulse pressure
- Reduced urine output (less than 25 mL/hour)
- Tachycardia

Key test results

- Blood tests show:
  - elevated serum potassium, serum lactate, and BUN levels
  - increased urine specific gravity (greater than 1.020) and urine osmolality
  - decreased hemoglobin and hematocrit
  - decreased blood pH
- ABG analysis reveals metabolic acidosis

Key treatments

- Supplemental oxygen
- Blood and fluid replacement
- Control of bleeding

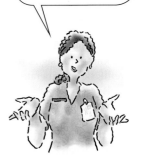

I'm hearing some crackles and galloping. What condition do you suspect?

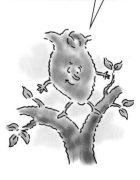

Exercise can help alleviate arterial blood pressure that is too high.

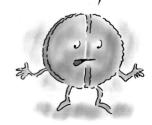

Relax! I'm an ACE inhibitor, and I'm here to help you decompress.

Key interventions

- Record blood pressure, pulse rate, peripheral pulses, respiratory rate, and pulse oximetry readings every 15 minutes, and monitor ECG continuously. A systolic blood pressure lower than 80 mm Hg usually results in inadequate coronary artery blood flow, cardiac ischemia, arrhythmias, and further complications of low cardiac output. When blood pressure drops below 80 mm Hg, increase the oxygen flow rate and notify the charge nurse or health care provider immediately
- Maintain IV lines with normal saline or lactated Ringer solution
- Indwelling urinary catheter may be inserted to measure urine output. If less than 30 mL/hour in adults, increase the fluid infusion rate but watch for signs of fluid overload. Notify the charge nurse or health care provider if urine output doesn't improve. An osmotic diuretic such as mannitol may be ordered
- During therapy, assess skin color and temperature; note any changes

Myocardial infarction

Irreversible necrosis of heart muscle secondary to prolonged ischemia; also known as heart attack

Key signs and symptoms

- Crushing substernal chest pain that may:
  - radiate to the jaw, back, and arms
  - last longer than anginal pain
  - not be relieved by rest or nitroglycerin
  - not be present (in silent MI—present atypically in women)

Key test results

- ECG shows an enlarged Q wave, an elevated or a depressed ST segment, and T-wave inversion
- Elevated cardiac biomarkers (myoglobin, troponin) confirm the diagnosis

Key treatments

- Antiplatelet aggregation: aspirin, abciximab, clopidogrel, eptifibatide
- Thrombolytic agents: reteplase (tissue plasminogen activator [t-PA]); given within 6 hours of onset of symptoms but most effective when started within 3 hours

Key interventions

- Monitor respiratory status
- Obtain an ECG reading during acute pain

Myocarditis

Inflammation of the heart muscle

Key signs and symptoms

- Arrhythmias (S3 and S4 gallops, faint S1)
- Dyspnea
- Fatigue
- Fever

Key test results

- ECG typically shows diffuse ST-segment and T-wave abnormalities (as in pericarditis), conduction defects (prolonged PR interval), and other supraventricular arrhythmias
- Endomyocardial biopsy confirms the diagnosis, but a negative biopsy *doesn't exclude* the diagnosis; repeat biopsy may be needed

Key treatments

- Bed rest
- Antiarrhythmics: amiodarone
- Antibiotics according to sensitivity of causative organism
- Cardiac glycoside: digoxin to increase myocardial contractility
- Diuretic: furosemide

Key interventions

- Observe breathing pattern and check lung status
- Stress the importance of bed rest. Assist the client with bathing as needed; provide a bedside commode. Reassure the client that activity limitations are temporary

Pericarditis

Inflammation of the sac covering the heart

Key signs and symptoms

Acute pericarditis
- Pericardial friction rub (grating sound heard as the heart moves)
- Sharp and (commonly) sudden pain that usually starts over the sternum and radiates to the neck, shoulders, back, and arms (unlike the pain of MI, pericardial pain is commonly pleuritic, increasing with deep inspiration and decreasing when the client sits up and leans forward, pulling the heart away from the diaphragmatic pleurae of the lungs).

Chronic pericarditis
- Pericardial friction rub
- Symptoms similar to those of chronic right-sided heart failure (fluid retention, ascites, hepatomegaly)

Key test results

- Echocardiography confirms the diagnosis when it shows an echo-free space between the ventricular wall and the pericardium (in cases of pleural effusion).
- ECG shows the following changes in acute pericarditis: elevation of ST segments in

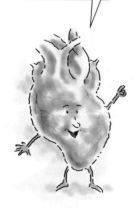

ECG and other tests can help to confirm a diagnosis.

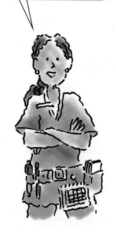

I keep key interventions in my tool belt when caring for a client who's had a heart attack.

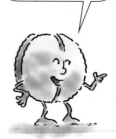

We antibiotics come in handy when your pericardium becomes infected.

the standard limb leads and most precordial leads without significant changes in QRS morphology that occur with MI; atrial ectopic rhythms such as atrial fibrillation; and diminished QRS voltage in pericardial effusion.

Key treatments
- Bed rest
- Surgery: pericardiocentesis (for cardiac tamponade), partial pericardiectomy (for recurrent pericarditis), and total pericardiectomy (for constrictive pericarditis)
- Antibiotics according to sensitivity of causative organism

Key interventions
- Provide complete bed rest
- Monitor pain related to respiration and body position
- Place client in an upright position
- Provide analgesics and oxygen, and reassure the client with acute pericarditis that condition is temporary and treatable

Pulmonary edema
Collection of excess fluid in the lungs

Key signs and symptoms
- Dyspnea, orthopnea, tachypnea

Key test results
- Chest x-ray shows pulmonary congestion

Key treatments
- Diuretics: furosemide, bumetanide, metolazone
- Cardiac glycoside: digoxin
- Inotropic agents: dobutamine, milrinone, nesiritide
- Nitrates: isosorbide dinitrate, nitroglycerin
- Vasodilator: nitroprusside sodium

Key interventions
- Administer oxygen
- Monitor vital signs and breathing pattern
- Place in high-Fowler position if blood pressure remains stable; if hypotensive, maintain in semi-Fowler position if tolerated
- Monitor ECG
- Monitor pulse oximetry readings

Raynaud disease
Reduced blood flow to fingers or toes in response to cold or emotional stress

Key signs and symptoms
- Numbness and tingling that are relieved by warmth

- Blanching of the skin on the fingers, which then become cyanotic before changing to red; typically occurs after exposure to cold or stress

Key test results
- Arteriography reveals vasospasm

Key treatments
- Activity changes: avoidance of cold
- Smoking cessation (if appropriate)
- Surgery (used in less than 25% of clients): sympathectomy
- Calcium channel blockers: diltiazem, nifedipine

Key interventions
- Advise client to avoid exposure to the cold, and to wear mittens/gloves in cold weather and when handling cold items

Rheumatic fever and rheumatic heart disease
Arises from complication of strep throat and can cause pain and swelling of joints and heart damage

Key signs and symptoms
- Temperature of 100.4° F (38° C) or higher
- Migratory joint pain or polyarthritis

Key test results
- Blood tests show elevated white blood cell count and erythrocyte sedimentation rate, as well as slight anemia during periods of inflammation
- Cardiac enzyme levels may increase in severe carditis
- C-reactive protein test is positive (especially during the acute phase)

Key treatments
- Bed rest (in severe cases)
- Surgery: corrective valvular surgery (in cases of persistent heart failure)
- Antibiotics: erythromycin, penicillin
- Nonsteroidal anti-inflammatory drugs (NSAIDs): aspirin, indomethacin

Key interventions
- Before giving penicillin, ask if client has ever had a hypersensitive reaction to it. Even if client has never had a reaction to penicillin, warn that such a reaction is possible
- Warn client to watch for, and immediately report signs of, recurrent streptococcal infection:
  - diffuse throat redness and oropharyngeal exudate
  - swollen and tender cervical lymph glands

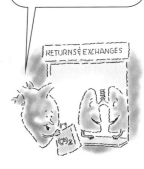

Could I get some oxygen out here please?

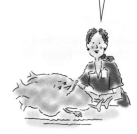

Wow—a temperature of 102°F, reports of pain and swelling in the joints, and recent history of strep throat. It might be rheumatic fever.

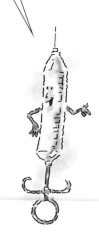

Make sure the client is not allergic to me before administering me!

- ○ pain on swallowing
- ○ temperature of 101° to 104° F (38.3° to 40° C)
- Urge client to avoid people with respiratory tract infections

Thoracic aortic aneurysm

Stretched and bulging area in the wall of the aorta

Key signs and symptoms

Ascending aneurysm
- Pain (described as severe, penetrating, and ripping; extending to the neck, shoulders, lower back, or abdomen)
- Unequal intensities of the right carotid pulse and left radial pulse

Descending aneurysm
- Pain (described as sharp and tearing, usually starting suddenly between the shoulder blades and possibly radiating to the chest)

Transverse aneurysm
- Dyspnea
- Pain (described as sharp and tearing and radiating to the shoulders)

Key test results
- Aortography, the definitive test, shows the lumen of the aneurysm, its size and location, and the false lumen in a dissecting aneurysm
- Chest x-ray shows widening of the aorta
- Computed tomography (CT) scan confirms and locates the aneurysm and may be used to monitor its progression

Key treatments
- Surgery: resection of aneurysm with a Dacron or Teflon graft replacement; possible replacement of aortic valve
- Blood product administration
- Oxygen therapy and possibly ET intubation and mechanical ventilation
- Analgesic: morphine
- Antihypertensives: nitroprusside sodium, labetalol
- Negative inotropic agent: propranolol

Key interventions
- Monitor blood pressure. Also evaluate pain; breathing; and carotid, radial, and femoral pulses
- Insert an indwelling urinary catheter. Maintain IV infusion of normal saline or lactated Ringer solution and antibiotics as needed
- When the health care provider suspects that an aneurysm is leaking, give any ordered whole-blood transfusion

- After repair of thoracic aneurysm:
  - ○ evaluate the client's LOC. Monitor vital signs, pulse rate, urine output, and pain
  - ○ check respiratory function. Carefully observe and record the type and amount of chest tube drainage, and frequently assess heart and breath sounds
  - ○ monitor IV therapy to prevent fluid excess, which may occur with rapid fluid replacement
  - ○ give medications as appropriate

Thrombophlebitis

Blood clot blocking one or more veins usually in legs

Key signs and symptoms
- Deep vein thrombosis
- Cramping calves
- Edema
- Tenderness to touch
- Superficial vein thrombosis
- Redness along vein
- Warmth and tenderness along vein

Key test results
- Photoplethysmography (PPG) shows venous-filling defects
- Ultrasound reveals decreased blood flow

Key treatments
- Activity changes: maintaining bed rest and elevating the affected extremity
- Anticoagulants: warfarin, heparin, dalteparin, enoxaparin sodium
- Antiplatelet aggregation agent: aspirin
- Fibrinolytic agent: reteplase (t-PA)

Key interventions
- Monitor breathing pattern and breath sounds
- Maintain bed rest and elevate the affected extremity
- Apply warm, moist compresses to improve circulation
- Perform neurovascular checks
- Monitor laboratory values

Valvular heart disease

Any disease involving one of four valves of the heart

Key signs and symptoms
Aortic insufficiency
- Angina
- Cough
- Dyspnea
- Fatigue
- Palpitations

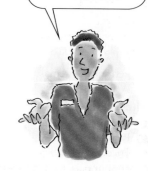

Thoracic aortic aneurysms can be extremely painful. What analgesic would be appropriate to administer?

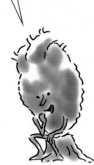

Coughing can be difficult post-surgery.

Mitral insufficiency
- Angina
- Dyspnea
- Fatigue
- Orthopnea
- Peripheral edema

Mitral stenosis
- Dyspnea on exertion
- Fatigue
- Orthopnea
- Palpitations
- Peripheral edema
- Weakness

Mitral valve prolapse
- May produce no symptoms
- Palpitations
- Tricuspid insufficiency
- Dyspnea
- Fatigue

Key test results

Aortic insufficiency
- Echocardiography shows left ventricular enlargement
- Chest x-ray shows left ventricular enlargement and pulmonary vein congestion

Mitral insufficiency
- Cardiac catheterization shows mitral regurgitation and elevated atrial and pulmonary artery wedge pressures

Mitral stenosis
- Cardiac catheterization shows diastolic pressure gradient across valve, and elevated left atrial and pulmonary artery wedge pressures

- Echocardiography shows thickened mitral valve leaflets
- ECG shows left atrial hypertrophy
- Chest x-ray shows left atrial and ventricular enlargement

Mitral valve prolapse
- ECG shows prolapse of the mitral valve into the left atrium
- Tricuspid insufficiency
- Echocardiography shows systolic prolapse of the tricuspid valve
- ECG shows right atrial or right ventricular hypertrophy
- Chest x-ray shows right atrial dilation and right ventricular enlargement

Key treatments
- Surgery: open-heart surgery using cardio-pulmonary bypass for valve replacement (in severe cases)
- Anticoagulant: warfarin to prevent thrombus formation around diseased or replaced valves

Key interventions
- Watch closely for signs of heart failure or pulmonary edema; watch for adverse effects of drug therapy
- Place in an upright position
- Maintain bed rest, and provide assistance with bathing, if necessary
- If client undergoes surgery, watch for hypotension, arrhythmias, and thrombus formation. Monitor vital signs, intake, output, daily weight, and blood chemistry values

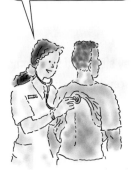

Listening to the client's heart and breathing can help you detect valvular heart disease.

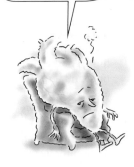

Bed rest is a key intervention for some cardiac disorders.

Cardiovascular questions, answers, and rationales

1. An older adult client is admitted to an acute care floor with the diagnosis of heart failure. Upon further workup the health care provider informs the nurse that the client has right-sided heart failure. Which symptom should the nurse expect to find in this client? Select all that apply.
- **1.** Dependent edema
- **2.** Jugular vein distention
- **3.** Weight loss
- **4.** Crackles
- **5.** Weight gain

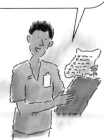

Right-sided heart failure has different symptoms from left-sided heart failure. Can you remember them?

1. **1, 2, 5.** Signs of right-sided heart failure include dependent edema, jugular vein distention, and weight gain. Crackles are a sign of left-sided heart failure. Weight loss is not an indication of heart failure.

CN: Physiological integrity; CNS: Physiological adaptation; CL: Analyze; DIFFICULTY: Challenge

2. A client is seen in the emergency department and the health care provider suspects an abdominal aortic aneurysm. Which nursing actions should be performed? Select all that apply.

1. Monitor and record vital signs.
2. Monitor intake, output and lab values.
3. Observe client for signs of hypovolemic shock.
4. Perform an abdominal x-ray.
5. Perform a CT scan to diagnose size.

2. 1, 2, 3. The nurse should monitor and record vital signs, monitor input and output (I&O) as well as lab values, and observe client for hypovolemic shock in case the aneurysm has ruptured. The nurse cannot perform an x-ray or CT scan.
CN: Physiological integrity; CNS: Physiological adaptation; CL: Apply; DIFFICULTY: Difficult

3. A nurse is screening clients for their risk of developing cardiovascular disease. The nurse identifies which clients to be at the **greatest** risk?

1. 40-year-old white female
2. 50-year-old white male
3. 40-year-old African American female
4. 50-year-old African American male

3. 4. African Americans are two to three times more likely to develop hypertension than whites. Males have more myocardial infarctions (MI) than women until women are postmenopause, when the risk of MI increases.
CN: Health promotion and maintenance; CNS: None; CL: Analyze; DIFFICULTY: Easy

4. The nursing student is caring for a client who is symptomatic for coronary artery disease (CAD). Which symptom does the student expect to find when obtaining data for this client? Select all that apply.

1. Chest pain
2. Arm pain
3. Jaw pain
4. Renal failure
5. Liver failure

4. 1, 2, 3. Chest pain, arm pain, jaw pain, and back pain are key signs and symptoms of CAD. These can occur after exertion, emotional stress, or exposure to cold—but can also develop when the client is at rest. Renal and liver failure are not normal symptoms.
CN: Physiological integrity; CNS: Physiological adaptation; CL: Analyze; DIFFICULTY: Moderate

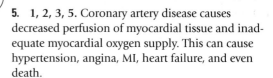

Warn your client that coronary artery disease can lead to many serious cardiovascular diseases.

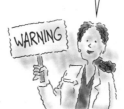

5. A client with a family history of heart disease is diagnosed with coronary artery disease. The client asks the nurse, "How it can affect my future health status?" What is the nurse's **best** response? Select all that apply.

1. It can lead to hypertension.
2. It can lead to angina.
3. It can lead to a myocardial infarction (MI).
4. It can lead to gastritis.
5. It can lead to heart failure.

5. 1, 2, 3, 5. Coronary artery disease causes decreased perfusion of myocardial tissue and inadequate myocardial oxygen supply. This can cause hypertension, angina, MI, heart failure, and even death.
CN: Physiological integrity; CNS: Physiological adaptation; CL: Apply; DIFFICULTY: Difficult

6. The nurse is obtaining data from a client who has just been diagnosed with coronary artery disease. Which findings does the nurse anticipate observing? Select all that apply.

1. Normal findings during asymptomatic progression
2. Chest pain
3. Palpitations
4. Confusion
5. Syncope
6. Excessive fatigue

6. 1, 2, 3, 5, 6. Symptoms for coronary artery disease occur when the artery is occluded to the point that inadequate blood supply to the muscle occurs. Assessment findings include possible normal findings during asymptomatic progression, chest pain, palpitations, syncope, and excessive fatigue.
CN: Physiological integrity; CNS: Physiological adaptation; CL: Apply; DIFFICULTY: Difficult

7. The client is informed that elevated serum total cholesterol levels significantly increases the risk of coronary artery disease (CAD)? Which intervention is **best** for the nurse to suggest to a client who has an elevated serum total cholesterol level?
- **1.** Change in diet
- **2.** Eating more protein
- **3.** Limiting amount of fruits
- **4.** Monitoring amount of vegetables

7. 1. A change in diet would be the best intervention and should include limited fats and carbohydrates. Total cholesterol levels above 200 mg/dL are considered borderline high; they require dietary restriction and, perhaps, medication. Eating more protein or limiting amount of fruits will not help decrease the level. Monitoring amount of vegetables consumed could be a good thing but does not guarantee a decrease in cholesterol.
CN: Physiological integrity; CNS: Reduction of risk potential; CL: Apply; DIFFICULTY: Easy

8. Which action by the nurse is the **priority** for a client exhibiting signs and symptoms of coronary artery disease?
- **1.** Decrease anxiety.
- **2.** Enhance myocardial oxygenation.
- **3.** Administer sublingual nitroglycerin.
- **4.** Educate the client about his symptoms.

8. 2. Enhancing myocardial oxygenation is always the priority when a client exhibits signs or symptoms of cardiac compromise. Without adequate oxygen, the myocardium suffers damage. Sublingual nitroglycerin dilates the coronary vessels to increase blood flow, but its administration isn't the priority. Although educating the client and decreasing anxiety are important in care delivery, neither are priorities when a client is compromised.
CN: Safe, effective care environment; CNS: Coordinated care; CL: Apply; DIFFICULTY: Moderate

9. The nurse explains to the client who has coronary artery disease (CAD) that there are different types of treatment for the disease. Which method of treatment is considered to be the initial treatment for coronary artery disease (CAD)?
- **1.** Cardiac catheterization
- **2.** Coronary artery bypass surgery
- **3.** Oral medication administration
- **4.** Percutaneous transluminal coronary angioplasty (PTCA)

9. 3. Oral medication administration is a noninvasive, medical treatment for CAD and is usually the initial treatment for coronary artery disease. Cardiac catheterization isn't a treatment but rather a diagnostic tool. Coronary artery bypass surgery and PTCA are invasive, surgical treatments.
CN: Physiological Integrity; CNS: Pharmacological Therapies; CL: Understand; DIFFICULTY: Difficult

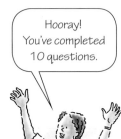

Hooray! You've completed 10 questions.

10. A client diagnosed with acute arterial occlusive disease is scheduled to undergo an atherectomy. What is the **priority** nursing intervention for this client immediately after the procedure?
- **1.** Monitor vital signs every 4 hours.
- **2.** Closely monitor catheter site for bleeding.
- **3.** Ambulate the client as soon as possible.
- **4.** Teach client about importance of exercise.

10. 2. Atherectomy is a surgical treatment used for acute arterial occlusive disease. After the procedure, the client should be monitored frequently for bleeding at the catheter site and vital signs should be taken every 15 minutes times four, and then every hour for the first few hours. Ambulation should be delayed for the first 12 hours and exercise is not a priority at this time.
CN: Physiological integrity; CNS: Physiological adaptation; CL: Analyze; DIFFICULTY: Easy

11. A client is suspected to be experiencing a myocardial infarction (MI). Which symptom reported by the client would lead the nurse to this conclusion?
- **1.** Chest pain
- **2.** Dyspnea
- **3.** Edema
- **4.** Palpitations

11. 1. The most common symptom of an MI is chest pain resulting from deprivation of oxygen to the heart. Dyspnea is the second most common symptom, related to an increase in the metabolic needs of the body during an MI. Edema is a later sign of heart failure, commonly seen after an MI. Palpitations may result from reduced cardiac output, producing arrhythmias.
CN: Safe, effective care environment; CNS: Coordinated care; CL: Apply; DIFFICULTY: Easy

12. The nursing student voices an understanding of correct anatomy when properly identifying the following areas on the precordium that are used for auscultation of heart sounds. Select all that apply.
1. Aortic area
2. Pulmonic area
3. Erb point
4. Mitral
5. Tricuspid area
6. Bronchial area

13. A client with coronary artery disease (CAD) comes to the clinic with an elevated total serum cholesterol level above 240. Which medication does the nurse expect the health care provider to prescribe? Select all that apply.
1. Cholestyramine
2. Lovastatin
3. Atenolol
4. Propranolol
5. Metoprolol

14. A client is hospitalized to rule out an acute myocardial infarction (MI). Laboratory studies indicate a normal lactate dehydrogenase level and an elevated troponin I level. The nurse enters the client's room and finds the client pacing the floor. Which statement by the nurse would be **most** appropriate in this situation?
1. "You've had a heart attack. Get back in bed."
2. "You seem upset. Why don't you get into bed and, if you wish, we can talk for a while."
3. "You sure have a lot of energy; do you want to play cards?"
4. "Your health care provider doesn't want you up. Would you please get back into your bed?"

15. The nurse is monitoring laboratory studies for a client that had a myocardial infarction. Which test will the nurse monitor that is **most** indicative of cardiac damage?
1. Arterial blood gas (ABG) levels
2. Complete blood count (CBC)
3. Complete chemistry
4. Creatine kinase isoenzymes (CK-MB)

16. A client has just had a myocardial infarction (MI) and the nurse is preparing to administer morphine. What is the **primary** reason for administering morphine to this client?
1. To sedate the client
2. To decrease the client's pain
3. To decrease the client's anxiety
4. To decrease oxygen demand on the client's heart

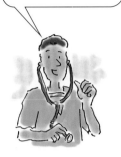

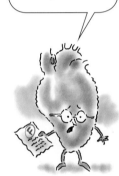

12. 1, 2, 3, 4, 5. The correct landmarks that can be used for auscultation of heart sounds are the aortic area, pulmonic area, Erb point, tricuspid area and mitral area. Bronchial area does not apply.
CN: Physiological integrity; CNS: Physiological adaptation; CL: Apply; DIFFICULTY: Difficult

13. 1, 2. Cholestyramine and lovastatin help to lower total cholesterol. Atenolol, propranolol, and metoprolol are not used to lower cholesterol, but rather are medications used for other cardiac problems when a beta-blocker is indicated.
CN: Physiological integrity; CNS: Pharmacological Therapies; CL: Analyze; DIFFICULTY: Moderate

14. 2. Given the laboratory data, especially the elevated troponin I level, the nurse should realize that the client probably had an MI and that he needs to lie down and rest his heart. However, the nurse should also realize the need to respond to the client's emotional distress by acknowledging his feelings and offering to discuss the situation. Telling the client that he had a heart attack would be giving a medical diagnosis that hasn't yet been made and would also be practicing outside the scope of nursing. A comment about his energy level acknowledges the client's pacing but not his underlying concerns. Stating the health care provider's preferences attempts to impose authority to control the client's behavior. It doesn't acknowledge the client's distress.
CN: Psychosocial integrity; CNS: None; CL: Apply; DIFFICULTY: Easy

15. 4. CK-MB isoenzymes are present in the blood after a myocardial infarction. These enzymes spill into the plasma when cardiac tissue is damaged. ABG levels are obtained to review respiratory function, a CBC is obtained to review blood counts, and a complete chemistry is obtained to review electrolytes.
CN: Health promotion and maintenance; CNS: None; CL: Apply; DIFFICULTY: Moderate

16. 2. Morphine is administered as analgesia because chest pain stimulates the sympathetic nervous system, leading to an increase in heart rate and vasoconstriction. In addition, morphine will reduce anxiety and the workload of the heart; however, the primary indication to administer morphine is to relieve chest pain.
CN: Physiological integrity; CNS: Pharmacological therapies; CL: Apply; DIFFICULTY: Moderate

17. When reinforcing education for the client about the importance of smoking cessation, which statements made by the client indicate understanding? Select all that apply.
1. "It causes the platelets in the blood to clump together and become sticky."
2. "It causes spasms in the coronary arteries."
3. "It lowers good cholesterol."
4. "It causes vasodilatation of the arteries."
5. "It reduces the amount of oxygen carried by the red blood cells."

18. An older adult client with heart failure and 2+ pitting edema is prescribed furosemide. Due to the effects of furosemide, which supplemental medication would the nurse expect to see ordered for this client?
1. Chloride
2. Digoxin
3. Potassium
4. Sodium

19. A client recently had a myocardial infarction (MI). Which finding does the nurse identify to be a normal metabolic change occurring after an MI?
1. Slowing of impulses through the atrioventricular (AV) node
2. Increased platelet aggregation
3. Decreased left ventricular ejection fraction
4. Increased serum glucose and free fatty acid protein levels

20. The nurse is auscultating the client's heart and identifies a third heart sound. Which complication does the nurse expect to be the cause of the third heart sound (S3)?
1. Ventricular dilation
2. Systemic hypertension
3. Aortic valve malfunction
4. Increased atrial contractions

21. A client who had an anterior wall myocardial infarction (MI) would have a greater risk for exhibiting crackles in the lungs related to which disorder?
1. Left-sided heart failure
2. Pulmonic valve malfunction
3. Right-sided heart failure
4. Tricuspid valve malfunction

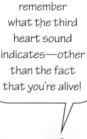

Can you remember what the third heart sound indicates—other than the fact that you're alive!

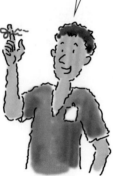

17. 1, 2, 3, 5. Smoking is the leading modifiable risk factor for developing coronary heart disease. Smoking causes the platelets of the blood to clump together, causes spasms in the coronary arteries, lowers good cholesterol, and reduces the amount of oxygen carried in the red blood cells.
CN: Physiological integrity; CNS: Physiological adaptation; CL: Apply; DIFFICULTY: Difficult

18. 3. Supplemental potassium is given with furosemide because of the potassium loss that occurs as a result of this diuretic. Chloride and sodium aren't lost during diuresis. Digoxin acts to increase contractility but isn't given routinely with furosemide.
CN: Physiological integrity; CNS: Pharmacological therapies; CL: Analyze; DIFFICULTY: Easy

19. 4. Glucose and fatty acids are metabolites whose levels increase after an MI. Slow conduction of impulses through the AV node is an electrophysiologic change. Hematologic changes affect the blood cells and platelets. Ejection fraction measures the mechanical pumping action of the heart.
CN: Physiological integrity; CNS: Physiological adaptation; CL: Analyze; DIFFICULTY: Difficult

20. 1. An S3 sound occurs when the ventricles are resistant to filling and is heard just after S2 when the atrioventricular valves open. Increased atrial contraction or systemic hypertension can result in a fourth heart sound. Aortic valve malfunction is heard as a murmur.
CN: Physiological integrity, CNS: Physiological adaptation; CL: Analyze; DIFFICULTY: Challenge

21. 1. The left ventricle is responsible for most of the cardiac output. An anterior wall MI may result in a decrease in left ventricular function. When the left ventricle doesn't function properly, resulting in left-sided heart failure, fluid accumulates in the interstitial and alveolar spaces in the lungs and causes crackles. Pulmonic and tricuspid valve malfunction causes right-sided heart failure.
CN: Physiological integrity; CNS: Physiological adaptation; CL: Analyze; DIFFICULTY: Easy

22. A client is admitted to the emergency department with chest discomfort, diaphoresis, and nausea. Suspecting possible myocardial infarction (MI), the nurse would anticipate the health care provider to prescribe which diagnostic test to quickly determine myocardial damage?
1. Cardiac catheterization
2. Cardiac enzymes
3. Echocardiogram
4. Electrocardiogram (ECG)

23. What should be the nurse's **first** intervention for a client experiencing a myocardial infarction (MI)?
1. Administering morphine
2. Administering oxygen
3. Administering sublingual nitroglycerin
4. Obtaining an electrocardiogram (ECG)

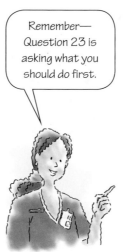

Remember—Question 23 is asking what you should do first.

24. A client has been diagnosed with left-sided heart failure. Which symptoms should the nurse expect to see? Select all that apply.
1. Syncope
2. Orthopnea
3. Jugular vein distention (JVD)
4. Peripheral edema
5. S3 heart gallop
6. Nocturia

25. A client is placed on several medications after having a myocardial infarction (MI). Which drug class is part of the medication regimen for this client that will protect the ischemic myocardium by decreasing catecholamines and sympathetic nerve stimulation?
1. Beta-blockers
2. Calcium channel blockers
3. Opioids
4. Nitrates

Ouch! I think I better go in and get an EKG.

26. A client who recently experienced a myocardial infarction (MI) is admitted to the hospital. Aware of the **most** common complication of an MI, the nurse would monitor this client closely for which condition?
1. Cardiogenic shock
2. Heart failure
3. Arrhythmias
4. Pericarditis

22. 4. ECG is the quickest, most accurate, and most widely used tool to diagnose MI. Cardiac enzymes also are used to diagnose MI, but the results can't be obtained as quickly. An echocardiogram is used most widely to view myocardial wall function after an MI has been diagnosed. Cardiac catheterization is an invasive study for determining coronary artery disease.
CN: Safe, effective care environment; CNS: Coordinated care; CL: Apply; DIFFICULTY: Moderate

23. 2. Administering supplemental oxygen to the client is the first priority of care. The myocardium is deprived of oxygen during an infarction, so additional oxygen is administered to assist in oxygenation and prevent further damage. Morphine and sublingual nitroglycerin are also used to treat MI, but they're more commonly administered after the oxygen. An ECG is the most common diagnostic tool used to evaluate MI.
CN: Physiological integrity; CNS: Pharmacological therapies; CL: Apply; DIFFICULTY: Moderate

24. 1, 2, 5. Left-sided heart failure causes decreased cardiac output and increases pulmonary congestion. Decreased cardiac output may cause a decrease in cerebral perfusion, resulting in syncope. Orthopnea is caused by pulmonary congestion. Development of an S3 gallop is caused by the left atria attempting to fill the distended left ventricle. JVD, peripheral edema, and nocturia are all observed with right-sided heart failure.
CN: Physiological integrity; CNS: Physiological adaptation; CL: Apply; DIFFICULTY: Difficult

25. 1. Beta-blockers work by decreasing catecholamines and sympathetic nerve stimulation. They protect the myocardium, helping to reduce the risk of another infarction by decreasing the heart's workload. Calcium channel blockers reduce workload by decreasing the heart rate and dilating arteries. Opioids reduce myocardial oxygen demand. Nitrates reduce myocardial oxygen consumption and decrease blood pressure.
CN: Physiological integrity; CNS: Pharmacological therapies; CL: Apply; DIFFICULTY: Moderate

26. 3. Arrhythmias, caused by oxygen deprivation to the myocardium, are the most common complication of an MI. Cardiogenic shock, another complication of MI, is defined as the end stage of left ventricular dysfunction. The condition occurs in approximately 15% of clients with MI. Because the pumping function of the heart is compromised by an MI, heart failure is the second most common complication. Pericarditis most commonly results from a bacterial or viral infection.
CN: Physiological integrity; CNS: Physiological adaptation; CL: Apply; DIFFICULTY: Difficult

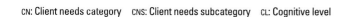

27. A nurse obtaining data from a client observes jugular vein distention (JVD). Which condition does the nurse suspect this client to have?
1. Abdominal aortic aneurysm
2. Heart failure
3. Myocardial infarction (MI)
4. Deep vein thrombosis

27. 2. Elevated venous pressure, exhibited as JVD, indicates the heart's failure to pump. This isn't a symptom of abdominal aortic aneurysm or deep vein thrombosis. An MI, if severe enough, can progress to heart failure; however, in and of itself, an MI doesn't cause JVD.
CN: Physiological integrity; CNS: Physiological adaptation;
CL: Analyze; DIFFICULTY: Easy

28. The client is prescribed a calcium channel blocker. Which primary actions should the nurse discuss with the client? Select all that apply.
1. Dilation of arteries
2. Decreases peripheral vascular resistance
3. Increases overload
4. Reduces afterload
5. Promotes calcium influx

28. 1, 2, 4. Calcium channel blockers inhibit calcium influx through the coronary arteries, causing arterial dilation and decreasing peripheral vascular resistance, which reduces afterload. Impulse conduction is slowed when calcium flow into cardiac cells is inhibited and contractility is decreased.
CN: Physiological integrity; CNS: Pharmacological therapies;
CL: Analyze; DIFFICULTY: Difficult

29. A nurse is about to administer digoxin to a client with heart failure. Which parameter should the nurse check before administering the medication?
1. Apical pulse
2. Blood pressure
3. Radial pulse
4. Respiratory rate

29. 1. An apical pulse is essential for accurately assessing the client's heart rate before administering digoxin. The apical pulse is the most accurate pulse point in the body. Blood pressure is usually only affected if the heart rate is too low, in which case the nurse would withhold digoxin. The radial pulse can be affected by cardiac and vascular disease and, therefore, won't always accurately depict the heart rate. Digoxin has no effect on respiratory function.
CN: Physiological integrity; CNS: Pharmacological therapies;
CL: Apply; DIFFICULTY: Easy

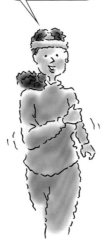

You're making great strides. Keep going!

30. A client is admitted to the hospital displaying sinus bradycardia, nausea, anorexia, and blurred vision. What should the nurse suspect this client to be experiencing?
1. Digoxin toxicity
2. Myocardial infarction
3. Hypertensive crisis
4. Cor pulmonale

30. 1. Digoxin toxicity typically causes bradycardia, nausea, anorexia, and vision disturbances. An MI, hypertensive crisis, and cor pulmonale usually do not cause vision disturbance.
CN: Physiological integrity; CNS: Pharmacological therapies;
CL: Apply; DIFFICULTY: Easy

31. An older adult client is newly diagnosed with left-sided heart failure. Which sign **most** commonly associated with this type of heart failure would the nurse expect to find when obtaining data for this client?
1. Crackles
2. Arrhythmias
3. Hepatic engorgement
4. Hypotension

31. 1. Crackles in the lungs are a classic sign of left-sided heart failure. These sounds are caused by fluid backing up into the pulmonary system. Arrhythmias can be associated with right- and left-sided heart failure. Hepatic engorgement is associated with right-sided heart failure. Left-sided heart failure causes hypertension secondary to an increased workload on the system.
CN: Physiological integrity; CNS: Physiological adaptation;
CL: Apply; DIFFICULTY: Easy

Want to see something shocking? Watch this.

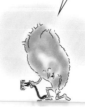

32. A client demonstrates signs of cardiogenic shock. Which medications should the nurse expect the health care provider to prescribe for this client? Select all that apply.
1. Digoxin
2. Dopamine
3. Furosemide
4. Clopidogrel
5. Nitroprusside sodium

32. 1, 2, 3, 5. Medications given for cardiogenic shock include a cardiac glycoside (digoxin), a cardiac inotropic agent (dopamine), a diuretic (furosemide), and a vasodilator (nitroprusside sodium). It does not indicate a need for an antiplatelet aggregate such as clopidogrel.
CN: Physiological integrity; CNS: Pharmacological Therapies;
CL: Analyze; DIFFICULTY: Difficult

33. Which symptom does the nurse expect a client with right-sided heart failure to exhibit? Select all that apply.
1. Jugular vein distention (JVD)
2. Peripheral edema
3. Hepatomegaly
4. Fatigue
5. Crackles

34. A nurse is monitoring a client with asthma taking atenolol. Which finding would indicate a potential complication associated with atenolol?
1. Baseline blood pressure of 166/88 mm Hg followed by a blood pressure of 138/74 mm Hg after two doses of medication
2. Baseline resting heart rate of 106 beats/minute followed by a resting heart rate of 88 beats/minute after two doses of medication
3. Development of audible expiratory wheezes
4. Serum potassium level of 4.2 mEq/L

35. A client is placed on a medication to stimulate the sympathetic nervous system. Which response should the nurse expect from this medication?
1. Heart rate decreased from 78 to 56 beats/minute
2. Heart rate increased from 60 to 88 beats/minute
3. Blood pressure decreased from 120/80 to 100/56
4. Decrease of myocardial contractility

36. A nurse receives a report on a client who has been diagnosed with an abdominal aortic aneurysm (AAA). The nurse would expect the client to have which underlying disease?
1. Atherosclerosis
2. Diabetes
3. Chronic obstructive pulmonary disease (COPD)
4. Renal failure

37. The nurse is caring for a client reporting weight gain, nausea, and decreased urine output. Which condition should the nurse suspect?
1. Angina pectoris
2. Cardiomyopathy
3. Left-sided heart failure
4. Right-sided heart failure

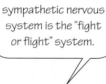

Remember—the sympathetic nervous system is the "fight or flight" system.

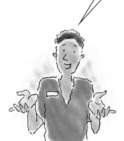

33. 1, 2, 3. During right-sided heart failure, the right ventricle fails to empty adequately, causing a back-up of blood into systemic blood vessels. This can lead to jugular vein distention, peripheral edema, and hepatomegaly. Crackles and fatigue are symptoms of left-sided heart failure.
CN: Physiological integrity; CNS: Physiological adaptation; CL: Analyze; DIFFICULTY: Challenge

34. 3. Audible wheezing may indicate serious bronchospasm, especially in clients with asthma or obstructive pulmonary disease. Decreases in blood pressure and heart rate are expected outcomes when beta-blockers are administered. A serum potassium level of 4.2 mEq/L is within normal limits.
CN: Physiological integrity; CNS: Pharmacological therapies; CL: Analyze; DIFFICULTY: Moderate

35. 2. Stimulation of the sympathetic nervous system causes tachycardia, or an increase in heart rate. This response causes an increase in contractility, which compensates for the response. The other symptoms listed are related to the parasympathetic nervous system, which is responsible for slowing the heart rate.
CN: Physiological integrity; CNS: Physiological adaptation; CL: Apply; DIFFICULTY: Moderate

36. 1. Atherosclerosis is linked to 75% of all AAAs. Plaque damages the wall of the artery and weakens it, causing an aneurysm. Although the other conditions are related to the development of aneurysm, none is a direct cause.
CN: Health promotion and maintenance; CNS: None; CL: Analyze; DIFFICULTY: Easy

37. 4. Weight gain, nausea, and a decrease in urine output are secondary effects of right-sided heart failure. Cardiomyopathy is usually identified as a symptom of left-sided heart failure. Left-sided heart failure causes primarily pulmonary symptoms rather than systemic ones. Angina pectoris doesn't cause weight gain, nausea, or a decrease in urine output.
CN: Physiological integrity; CNS: Physiological adaptation; CL: Apply; DIFFICULTY: Easy

38. A client is admitted to the emergency department with a diagnosis of an abdominal aortic aneurysm (AAA). Locate the area in which this would be found.

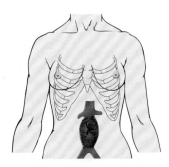

38. The portion of the aorta distal to the renal arteries is more prone to aneurysm formation, due to increased pressure as it divides into the iliac arteries. The aorta is proximal to the iliac arteries. There's no area adjacent to the aortic arch, which bends into the thoracic (descending) aorta. Aortic aneurysms proximal to the renal arteries are uncommon.

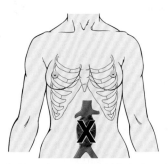

CN: Physiological integrity; CNS: Physiological adaptation;
CL: Apply; DIFFICULTY: Difficult

39. A client with pulmonary edema is given digoxin. What is the **most** direct effect on myocardial contraction due to digoxin in the failing heart?
1. Decreases cardiac output
2. Decreases ventricular emptying capacity
3. Increases circulating blood volume
4. Slows conduction of impulses through the atrioventricular (AV) node

39. 4. Digoxin's physiological effect on the heart slows impulse conduction through the AV node. Digoxin increases cardiac output and ventricular emptying capacity. Digoxin also promotes diuresis, thereby decreasing the circulating blood volume.
CN: Physiological integrity; CNS: Pharmacological therapies;
CL: Analyze; DIFFICULTY: Moderate

40. A client is admitted with acute pulmonary edema. Which signs and symptoms should the nurse expect to find when collecting data on this client?
1. Weight gain, abdominal distention, peripheral edema, jugular vein distention (JVD), tachycardia, and restlessness
2. Apprehension and restlessness, cough with frothy pink sputum, moist gurgling respirations with tachypnea, and orthopnea
3. Exertional dyspnea, cough with mucopurulent sputum, prolonged expiration with wheezing and crackles, and orthopnea
4. Sharp chest pain that worsens on inspiration, dyspnea, cyanosis, and tachycardia

Don't be apprehensive about question #40. I'm sure you can figure it out.

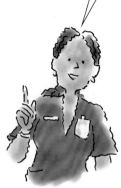

40. 2. Apprehension and restlessness with frothy pink sputum and moist breath sounds are typical findings in clients with acute pulmonary edema. Weight gain, edema, and JVD are signs and symptoms of right-sided heart failure. Exertional dyspnea and mucopurulent sputum are typical of emphysema. Chest pain that worsens with inspiration, dyspnea, cyanosis, and tachycardia are typical signs of acute pulmonary embolism.
CN: Physiological integrity; CNS: Physiological adaptation;
CL: Analyze; DIFFICULTY: Moderate

41. A client who's being treated for unilateral, lower-extremity deep vein thrombophlebitis is being discharged. Which statement indicates to the nurse that additional discharge education is needed?
1. "I should elevate my legs when sitting and should get up and walk around periodically."
2. "I need to take my warfarin exactly the way my health care provider ordered it."
3. "Tight compression hose rolled down behind the knee won't fall down, and improves the circulation in my legs."
4. "I should contact my health care provider immediately if I have frequent nosebleeds, bleeding from my gums, oozing from minor cuts, or if I see blood in my urine."

41. 3. Rolling the hose down behind the knee indicates improperly fitting hose that will impede venous return and cause venous stasis. Support hose should be smooth from the toes to the end of the hose. Elevating the legs while sitting promotes venous return. Warfarin must be taken exactly as prescribed, and the client must monitor himself for potential bleeding.
CN: Physiological integrity; CNS: Reduction of risk potential;
CL: Apply; DIFFICULTY: Easy

CN: Client needs category   CNS: Client needs subcategory   CL: Cognitive level

42. A client is admitted to the emergency department with a pulsating sensation in the abdomen and an audible bruit. Which diagnostic test would the nurse expect the health care provider to prescribe **first** to provide a definitive diagnosis?
1. Abdominal x-ray
2. Arteriogram
3. Computed tomography (CT) scan
4. Ultrasound

43. Which complication is of **greatest** concern when caring for a preoperative client with an abdominal aortic aneurysm?
1. Hypertension
2. Aneurysm rupture
3. Cardiac arrhythmias
4. Diminished pedal pulses

44. A client comes to the emergency department with symptoms of a myocardial infarction (MI). The health care provider prescribes reteplase. The nurse is aware that this medication will be **most** effective when given at which time?
1. Within 1 to 3 hours of onset of symptoms
2. Within 6 hours of onset of symptoms
3. Within 12 hours of onset of symptoms
4. Within 6 to 8 hours of onset of symptoms

45. Which precaution should a nurse take when caring for a client with a myocardial infarction (MI) who has received a thrombolytic agent?
1. Avoid puncture wounds.
2. Monitor potassium level.
3. Maintain a supine position.
4. Encourage fluids.

46. The student nurse correctly identifies which condition to cause the majority of abdominal aortic aneurysms?
1. Diabetes
2. Hypertension
3. Peripheral vascular disease
4. Syphilis

42. 4. Ultrasound is a noninvasive, cost-effective method of determining the presence of an AAA with 95% accuracy. Arteriograms and CT scans are more expensive, require the use of contrast agents and radiation, and are riskier to the client. An abdominal aneurysm would only be visible on an x-ray if it were calcified.
CN: Health promotion and maintenance; CNS: None; CL: Apply; DIFFICULTY: Difficult

43. 2. Rupture of the aneurysm is a life-threatening emergency and is of the greatest concern for the nurse caring for this type of client. Hypertension should be avoided and controlled because it can cause the weakened vessel to rupture. Diminished pedal pulses, a sign of poor circulation to the lower extremities, are associated with an aneurysm but aren't life-threatening. Cardiac arrhythmias aren't directly linked to an aneurysm.
CN: Physiological integrity; CNS: Reduction of risk potential; CL: Analyze; DIFFICULTY: Easy

44. 1. Thrombolytic agents such as reteplase can be given within 6 hours of onset of symptoms but will be most effective when started within 3 hours.
CN: Physiological integrity; CNS: Pharmacological therapies; CL: Apply; DIFFICULTY: Easy

45. 1. Thrombolytic agents are declotting agents that place the client at risk for hemorrhage from puncture wounds. All unnecessary needlesticks and invasive procedures should be avoided. The potassium level should be monitored in all cardiac clients, not just those receiving a thrombolytic agent. Although no specific position is required, most cardiac clients seem more comfortable in semi-Fowler position. The client's fluid balance must be carefully monitored, so it may be inappropriate to encourage fluids at this time.
CN: Physiological integrity; CNS: Reduction of risk potential; CL: Apply; DIFFICULTY: Moderate

46. 2. Continuous pressure on the vessel walls from hypertension causes the walls to weaken and an aneurysm to occur. Atherosclerotic changes can occur with peripheral vascular diseases and are linked to aneurysms, but the link isn't as strong as it is with hypertension. Only 1% of clients with syphilis experience an aneurysm. Diabetes isn't directly linked to aneurysm.
CN: Health promotion and maintenance; CNS: None; CL: Apply; DIFFICULTY: Challenge

47. A client has sudden cardiac death. Which arrhythmia commonly associated with sudden cardiac death does the nurse suspect this client may have experienced?
1. Atrial fibrillation
2. Ventricular fibrillation
3. Atrial tachycardia
4. Ventricular bigeminy

47. 2. Ventricular fibrillation is the arrhythmia most commonly associated with sudden cardiac death. Atrial fibrillation is associated with irregular heart rates; atrial tachycardia is associated with heart rates of over 100 beats/minute. Ventricular bigeminy is associated with ventricular irritability but not sudden cardiac death.
CN: Physiological integrity; CNS: Reduction of risk potential;
CL: Apply; DIFFICULTY: Easy

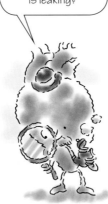

Hmm. What would be the clues that an aneurysm is leaking?

48. A nurse is caring for a client with a 7-cm infrarenal abdominal aortic aneurysm (AAA). The computed tomography (CT) scan indicates that the aneurysm may be leaking. When collecting data on the client, the nurse should be alert for which signs and symptoms? Select all that apply.
1. Constant, severe lower back pain
2. Constant, "tearing" abdominal pain
3. Hypotension
4. Increased red blood cell (RBC) count
5. Weak or absent bilateral leg pulses
6. Intermittent, severe lower back pain

48. 1, 2, 3, 5. Severe, constant lower back pain or constant, "tearing" abdominal pain indicates a leaking or ruptured aneurysm as blood enters the abdominal cavity and retroperitoneal space. The client's blood pressure and RBC count will fall as he becomes hypovolemic from hemorrhage. Diminished blood flow through the iliac and femoral arteries causes weak or absent bilateral leg pulses. Pain from a leaking or ruptured aneurysm is constant.
CN: Physiological integrity; CNS: Reduction of risk potential;
CL: Apply; DIFFICULTY: Difficult

49. A nurse is caring for a client who has a known 3-cm infrarenal abdominal aortic aneurysm (AAA). Which statements accurately characterize this disorder? Select all that apply.
1. AAA occurs more commonly above the level of the renal artery origins.
2. AAA occurs more commonly in men than women.
3. AAA is rarely linked to genetic factors.
4. A client with an AAA may also have "blue toe syndrome."
5. A 3-cm AAA rarely causes symptoms such as back pain.

49. 2, 4, 5. AAA is more than twice as common in men as women and up to 28% of these clients have a first-degree family member with an AAA. Small AAAs (less than 4 cm) are commonly identified coincidentally and are usually asymptomatic. Larger AAAs may be lined with an intraluminal thrombus, and "blue toe syndrome" occurs when the thrombus from the aneurysm microembolizes to the foot.
CN: Physiological integrity; CNS: Reduction of risk potential;
CL: Analyze; DIFFICULTY: Challenge

50. A nurse reviews the chart of a new client who recently underwent an abdominal aortic aneurysm resection. It's suspected that a hereditary disease is linked to this condition. Which hereditary disease linked to aneurysms would the nurse expect to find in the client's medical records?
1. Cystic fibrosis
2. Lupus erythematosus
3. Marfan syndrome
4. Myocardial infarction (MI)

50. 3. Marfan syndrome results in the degeneration of the elastic fibers of the aortic media. Therefore, clients with the syndrome are more likely to develop an aneurysm. Although cystic fibrosis is hereditary, it hasn't been linked to aneurysms. Lupus erythematosus isn't hereditary. MI is neither hereditary nor a disease.
CN: Health promotion and maintenance; CNS: None; CL: Analyze;
DIFFICULTY: Difficult

51. A client comes to the emergency department diagnosed with a ruptured aortic aneurysm. What is the **priority** action for this client?
1. Administer antihypertensive medication
2. Transport the client for an aortogram
3. Beta-blocker administration
4. Surgical intervention

51. 4. When the vessel ruptures, surgery is the only intervention that can repair it. Administration of antihypertensive medications and beta-blockers can help control hypertension, reducing the risk of rupture. An aortogram is a diagnostic tool used to detect an aneurysm.
CN: Physiological integrity; CNS: Reduction of risk potential;
CL: Apply; DIFFICULTY: Easy

52. A client is diagnosed with a 4.5-cm infrarenal abdominal aortic aneurysm (AAA). Which statements should the nurse include when reinforcing education to the client about the disease? Select all that apply.
1. Controlling blood pressure and lipid levels is beneficial in slowing aneurysm expansion.
2. An AAA will be monitored for expansion every 6 to 12 months.
3. Smoking has no effect on the rate of aneurysm expansion.
4. Genetic factors influence the development of AAA.
5. All AAAs need to be repaired as soon as they are identified.

53. A client is being discharged home with a diagnosis of hypertrophic cardiomyopathy (HCM). Which statement by the client **best** demonstrates an understanding of this disease process?
1. "I should start a vigorous aerobic exercise program to strengthen my heart function."
2. "Since this is a hereditary disorder, my family members should probably be evaluated for similar symptoms."
3. "Exercise or exertion of any kind could kill me. I should have a caretaker to perform my activities of daily living."
4. "I should keep a journal of my symptoms and take my prescribed medications only when I have symptoms."

54. A client is hospitalized with newly diagnosed hypertrophic cardiomyopathy (HCM). The nurse is reinforcing education about its causes and explains to the client about the abnormal thickening of the heart muscle. Which comment made by the client would indicate an understanding of the disease?
1. "This should not affect how well the pumping chamber works."
2. "I did not have this in childhood so I don't think I have this disease."
3. "I can see how this would make it harder for my heart to pump blood."
4. "Even though my father had the disease it is not hereditary so I might not have it."

55. The nurse is caring for a client with cardiomyopathy. What should the nurse monitor the client closely for?
1. Heart failure
2. Diabetes
3. Myocardial infarction (MI)
4. Pericardial effusion

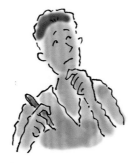

Hmm. What complication is most likely to occur with cardiomyopathy?

52. 1, 2, 4. Multiple factors lead to arterial wall damage and aneurysm formation. These include heredity, atherosclerosis, infection, smoking, and hypertension. Clients with AAAs of 4 to 5.4 cm should be monitored for expansion of the aneurysm using ultrasound or computed tomography (CT) scan every 6 to 12 months. The average aneurysm expansion rate is 10% per year but the rate of expansion is highly individual; many AAAs remain stable without expansion for many years.
CN: Safe, effective care environment; CNS: Coordinated care; CL: Apply; DIFFICULTY: Challenge

53. 2. Hypertrophic cardiomyopathy is a hereditary disease in which the heart muscle is abnormally thick and asymmetrical. In young clients, especially athletes, the first symptom may be sudden death during strenuous exercise. Strenuous physical exertion is restricted because it may precipitate arrhythmias or sudden cardiac death. The client is usually encouraged to perform normal activities of daily living after discussing restrictions with his health care provider. Medications, such as beta-blockers, calcium channel blockers, and antiarrhythmics, are usually prescribed and should be taken daily to help prevent complications.
CN: Physiological integrity; CNS: Reduction of risk potential; CL: Analyze; DIFFICULTY: Moderate

54. 3. Hypertrophic cardiomyopathy involves abnormal thickening of the heart muscle, particularly affecting the muscle of the heart's main pumping chamber (left ventricle). The thickened heart muscle can make it harder for the heart to pump blood.

Hypertrophic cardiomyopathy can develop at any age, but the condition tends to be more severe if it becomes apparent during childhood. Most affected people have a family history of the disease, and some genetic mutations have been linked to hypertrophic cardiomyopathy.
CN: Physiological integrity; CNS: Physiological adaptation; CL: Apply; DIFFICULTY: Easy

55. 1. Because the structure and function of the heart muscle is affected, heart failure most commonly occurs in clients with cardiomyopathy. MI results from atherosclerosis. Pericardial effusion is most predominant in clients with pericarditis. Diabetes is unrelated to cardiomyopathy.
CN: Physiological integrity; CNS: Physiological adaptation; CL: Apply; DIFFICULTY: Moderate

56. Which statement by the client **best** indicates an understanding on how to self-monitor while taking warfarin?
1. "I should use a soft toothbrush."
2. "I shouldn't worry if I see a lot of bruises as my blood thins."
3. "I should adjust my diet to eat less protein."
4. "I should use a safety razor to shave."

56. 1. A soft toothbrush will help prevent bleeding from friable gum tissue. Increased bruising should be reported to the health care provider. Dietary adjustments include consuming consistent amounts of dark green, leafy vegetables, which are high in vitamin K, but don't include protein restriction. Electric razors are recommended to reduce the risk of cutting the skin.
CN: Physiological integrity; CNS: Pharmacological therapies; CL: Apply; DIFFICULTY: Moderate

57. A nurse is caring for a client with cardiac tamponade. Which signs and symptoms should the nurse monitor for? Select all that apply.
1. Paradoxical chest movement
2. Tracheal deviation
3. Pulsus paradoxus
4. Widening pulse pressure
5. Narrowing pulse pressure
6. Muffled heart sounds

57. 3, 5, 6. Pulsus paradoxus is a symptom of cardiac tamponade caused by a marked decrease in cardiac output, which results in a diminished pulse and decreased blood pressure during inspiration. Narrowing pulse pressure and muffled heart sounds are additional signs of cardiac tamponade. Paradoxical chest movement occurs with flail chest. Tracheal deviation is seen with tension pneumothorax. Widening pulse pressure is found in increased intracranial pressure.
CN: Physiological integrity; CNS: Physiological adaptation; CL: Apply; DIFFICULTY: Difficult

58. A client has been diagnosed with pulmonary edema and is placed on a diuretic. Which medications will the nurse discuss with the client? Select all that apply.
1. Furosemide
2. Thiazide
3. Metolazone
4. Dobutamine
5. Nesiritide

58. 1, 2, 3. A key treatment for pulmonary edema is a diuretic which includes furosemide, thiazide, and metolazone. Dobutamine and nesiritide are both inotropic agents.
CN: Physiological integrity; CNS: Pharmacological therapies; CL: Apply; DIFFICULTY: Challenge

59. A nurse is caring for a client diagnosed with myocardial infarction (MI) who is prescribed a nitrate. What does the nurse identify as the purpose of giving a nitrate to this client?
1. Relieve pain.
2. Dilate coronary arteries.
3. Relieve headaches caused by other medications.
4. Calm and relax the client.

59. 2. Nitrates dilate the arteries, allowing oxygen to continue flowing to the myocardium. Nitrates can cause headaches but don't relieve pain, and they don't calm or relax the client.
CN: Physiological integrity; CNS: Pharmacological therapies; CL: Apply; DIFFICULTY: Easy

60. The nurse explains to the client that beta-blockers are most widely used in the treatment of cardiomyopathy. What are the main goals in the treatment of this condition that are accomplished by this class of medications? Select all that apply.
1. Improve cardiac output
2. Improve myocardial filling
3. Decrease myocardial filling
4. Increase blood pressure
5. Increase heart rate

60. 1, 2. The health care provider may prescribe medications to improve the heart's pumping ability and function, improve blood flow, lower blood pressure, slow the heart rate, remove excess fluid from the body, or keep blood clots from forming. By decreasing the heart rate and contractility, beta-blockers improve myocardial filling and cardiac output, which are primary goals in the treatment of cardiomyopathy.
CN: Physiological integrity; CNS: Pharmacological therapies; CL: Apply; DIFFICULTY: Difficult

61. A client who is very anxious often comes to the emergency department with reports of chest pain rated a 5 on a scale of 0 to 10. Which condition does the nurse anticipate this client may be experiencing?
1. Anxiety
2. Stable angina
3. Unstable angina
4. Variant angina

62. The telemetry monitor technician notifies the nurse that a client has sinus bradycardia with a heart rate of 42 beats/minute. What should the nurse do **first**?
1. Immediately review the client's current medical regimen to see if he is taking beta-blockers or calcium channel blockers.
2. Obtain a 12-lead electrocardiogram (ECG).
3. Notify the client's health care provider.
4. Check the client's level of consciousness (LOC), obtain vital signs, and ask the client about symptoms.

63. A client, 1 hour after undergoing a cardiac catheterization through a percutaneous femoral access site, calls the nurse to report that there's something wet under the buttocks. Upon entering the client's room, what step should the nurse take **first**?
1. Reinforce the groin dressing.
2. Obtain vital signs.
3. Help the client sit up so the wet area can be visualized.
4. Apply gloves and assess the femoral access site.

64. Which characteristic should a nurse expect to see on a normal cardiac rhythm strip obtained from an adult client?
1. PR interval of greater than 0.24 second
2. Heart rate of 88 beats/minute
3. Two P waves preceding each QRS complex
4. QRS complexes greater than 0.16 second that vary in configuration

65. A client comes to the emergency department reporting chest pain. Upon further evaluation the nurse suspects unstable angina. Which disease process should the nurse reinforce teaching this client about that is directly related to unstable angina?
1. Angina decubitus
2. Abdominal aortic aneurysm (AAA)
3. Nocturnal angina
4. Myocardial infarction (MI)

Congratulations! You're halfway done.

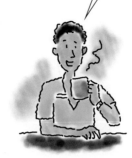

61. 2. The pain of stable angina is predictable in nature, builds gradually, and quickly reaches maximum intensity. Anxiety generally isn't described as painful. Unstable angina doesn't always need a trigger, is more intense, and lasts longer than stable angina. Variant angina usually occurs at rest—not as a result of exertion or stress.
CN: Physiological integrity; CNS: Physiological adaptation; CL: Analyze; DIFFICULTY: Moderate

62. 4. The priority is to gather data by assessing the client's LOC, obtaining vital signs, and determining the presence or absence of symptoms. Calling the health care provider and reviewing the medication record are necessary actions but not priorities. Obtaining a 12-lead ECG may be necessary but isn't the priority.
CN: Physiological integrity; CNS: Physiological adaptation; CL: Analyze; DIFFICULTY: Easy

63. 4. Observing standard precautions and assessing the femoral access site for potential bleeding is the priority. Reinforcing the groin dressing may be necessary after the site is assessed. Obtaining vital signs isn't the priority at this time. After a femoral puncture, the client is usually prescribed complete bed rest with his affected leg straight and immobilized for 2 to 4 hours to reduce the risk of bleeding.
CN: Physiological integrity; CNS: Reduction of risk potential; CL: Apply; DIFFICULTY: Easy

64. 2. The normal adult heart rate is between 60 and 100 beats/minute. The normal PR interval is 0.12 to 0.20 second. In a normal cardiac cycle, there should be one P wave preceding each QRS complex. A normal QRS complex should be less than 0.10 second.
CN: Physiological integrity; CNS: Reduction of risk potential; CL: Analyze; DIFFICULTY: Moderate

65. 4. Unstable angina progressively increases in frequency, intensity, and duration and is related to an increased risk of MI within 3 to 18 months. Angina decubitus, angina, nocturnal angina, and AAA aren't associated with an increased risk of MI.
CN: Physiological integrity; CNS: Physiological adaptation; CL: Apply; DIFFICULTY: Easy

66. When a client experiences chest pain during an acute anginal episode, the nurse should expect which form of nitroglycerin to be administered **first**?

1. Nitroglycerin IV drip at 10 mcg/minute
2. Application of 2 in (5 cm) of nitroglycerin paste to the chest wall
3. Metered buccal nitroglycerin spray, 0.4 mg/spray
4. Transdermal nitroglycerin patch, 0.2 mg/hour

67. Which statement by a client who has had a fasting lipoprotein profile indicates that further education is needed?

1. "Changing my diet has really helped! Now my LDL cholesterol level is 98 mg/dL."
2. "My total cholesterol level is optimal! It used to be 350 and now it is 250 mg/dL."
3. "My HDL cholesterol level is 60 mg/dL and that helps lower my risk of coronary heart disease."
4. "Even though my lipoprotein profile is normal this year, I know I'll need another one 5 years from now."

68. The nurse is reviewing the diagnostic test results for a client with reports of chest pain. Which diagnostic test result is **most** consistent with a diagnosis of angina?

1. Troponin level greater than 1.5 mg/mL
2. Creatine kinase isoenzymes (CK-MB) level of 45%
3. 12-lead electrocardiogram (ECG) with depressed, inverted, or downward slope to the T waves in leads II, III, and aVF
4. Transthoracic echocardiogram that shows a left ventricular ejection fraction of 30%

69. A client arrives in the emergency department and reports angina pain. What is the nurse's initial treatment for this client? Select all that apply.

1. Place on oxygen.
2. Administer ASA and nitroglycerin.
3. Give pain medicine.
4. Use guided imagery with client.
5. Obtain a chest x-ray.

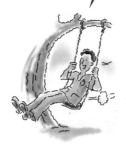

Looks like things are on the upswing. Great work!

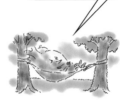

I hope the initial treatment for angina pain is napping.

66. 3. Sublingual or buccal nitroglycerin is the route of choice to quickly reduce myocardial oxygen demand and dilate coronary arteries. IV nitroglycerin is usually begun after a trial of sublingual or buccal spray nitroglycerin has proved unsuccessful in relieving the client's symptoms. Nitroglycerin paste and transdermal patches may be administered later because they have slower actions.
CN: Physiological integrity; CNS: Pharmacological therapies; CL: Analyze; DIFFICULTY: Moderate

67. 2. The National Cholesterol Education Program classifies a total cholesterol of 240 mg/dL or more as high, levels of 200 to 239 mg/dL as borderline high, and levels less than 200 mg/dL as desirable. LDL cholesterol levels of 100 mg/dL or less and HDL cholesterol levels 60 mg/dL or more are optimal. Adults should have a fasting lipoprotein profile every 5 years beginning at age 20.
CN: Physiological integrity; CNS: Reduction of risk potential; CL: Analyze; DIFFICULTY: Moderate

68. 3. The 12-lead ECG with abnormal T waves indicates ischemia. Elevated troponin and CK-MB levels indicate myocardial infarction, not ischemia. A decreased ejection fraction indicates heart failure.
CN: Physiological integrity; CNS: Reduction of risk potential; CL: Analyze; DIFFICULTY: Moderate

69. 1, 2, 3. The initial treatment consists of administration of oxygen, aspirin, nitroglycerin, morphine to relieve pain, and a beta-blocker. Given an altered, yet nondiagnostic ECG and no contraindications, further treatment with heparin (low-molecular weight or unfractionated), clopidogrel, or other antiplatelet agents may be initiated. Most often, an additional abnormal marker (e.g., an elevated serum troponin, myoglobin, or CPK level) will be verified prior to antiplatelet therapy. Guided imagery does not work on everyone and would not be an initial treatment. A chest x-ray is not indicated at this time.
CN: Physiological integrity; CNS: Physiological adaptation; CL: Apply; DIFFICULTY: Challenge

70. A client is experiencing chest pain at rest that's unresponsive to nitroglycerin. The health care provider diagnoses unstable angina and alerts the nurse that the client will require treatment with immediate surgical intervention. Which treatment does the nurse prepare the client for?
1. Cardiac catheterization
2. Echocardiogram
3. Heart transplantation
4. Percutaneous transluminal coronary angioplasty (PTCA)

71. The nurse identifies which intervention as the **priority** for a client experiencing chest pain while walking?
1. Sitting the client down
2. Getting the client back to bed
3. Obtaining an electrocardiogram (ECG)
4. Administering sublingual nitroglycerin

72. A client with heart failure is experiencing symptoms of cardiogenic shock. Which symptoms would the nurse expect this client to exhibit? Select all that apply.
1. Tachycardia
2. Decreased blood pressure
3. Bradycardia
4. Decreased peripheral pulses
5. Increased blood pressure

73. A nurse is caring for several clients on a medical floor. Which client does the nurse identify to have the **greatest** chance of developing cardiogenic shock?
1. A client with acute myocardial infarction (MI)
2. A client with coronary artery disease (CAD)
3. A client with a decreased hemoglobin level
4. A client with hypotension

74. A nurse is monitoring laboratory results for a client admitted with a possible myocardial infarction (MI). Which laboratory result would be used to rule out an MI?
1. Total white blood cell (WBC) count of 15,000/mm³
2. Troponin level of less than 0.2 ng/mL
3. Total red blood cell (RBC) count of 4.7 million/mm³
4. Mean corpuscular hemoglobin (MCH) of 27 pg/cell

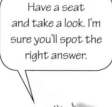
Have a seat and take a look. I'm sure you'll spot the right answer.

70. 4. PTCA can alleviate the blockage and restore blood flow and oxygenation. An echocardiogram is a noninvasive diagnostic test. Heart transplantation involves replacing the client's heart with a donor heart and is the treatment for end-stage cardiac disease. Cardiac catheterization is a diagnostic tool, not a treatment.
CN: Physiological integrity; CNS: Physiological adaptation; CL: Apply; DIFFICULTY: Challenge

71. 1. The priority is to decrease the oxygen consumption; this would be achieved by sitting the client down. An ECG can be obtained after the client is sitting down. After the ECG, sublingual nitroglycerin would be administered. When the client's condition is stabilized, he can return to bed.
CN: Physiological integrity; CNS: Basic care and comfort; CL: Apply; DIFFICULTY: Easy

72. 1, 2, 4. Cardiogenic shock is related to ineffective pumping of the heart and is an acute and serious complication of heart failure. Symptoms include tachycardia, decreased blood pressure, and decreased peripheral pulses. Bradycardia and high blood pressure is not associated with this disease process.
CN: Physiological integrity; CNS: Physiological adaptation; CL: Apply; DIFFICULTY: Difficult

73. 1. Of all clients with an acute MI, 15% suffer cardiogenic shock secondary to the myocardial damage and decreased function. CAD causes MI. Hypotension is the result of a reduced cardiac output produced by the shock state. A decreased hemoglobin level is a result of bleeding.
CN: Physiological integrity; CNS: Reduction of risk potential; CL: Apply; DIFFICULTY: Moderate

74. 2. Cardiac troponins are proteins that exist in cardiac muscle and are released with cardiac muscle injury. A troponin level of less than 0.2 ng/mL is considered normal. An elevated WBC count (15,000/mm³) is seen in many disease processes and with severe necrosis but doesn't specifically indicate MI. A total RBC count of 4.7 million/mm³ is within normal limits for males and females but isn't used to rule out an MI. MCH is an RBC index providing information about the hemoglobin concentration of RBCs and isn't used to rule out an MI.
CN: Physiological integrity; CNS: Reduction of risk potential; CL: Analyze; DIFFICULTY: Easy

75. The nurse is gathering data from a client, when the client mentions the heart races sometimes. The nurse should be especially vigilant to monitor this client for which life-threatening cardiac arrhythmia?
  * **1.** Ventricular fibrillation
  2. Sinus tachycardia
  3. Atrial fibrillation
  4. Atrial flutter

76. Which factor does the nurse determine is **most** useful in detecting a client's risk of developing cardiogenic shock?
  1. Decreased heart rate
  * **2.** Decreased cardiac index
  3. Decreased blood pressure
  4. Decreased cerebral blood flow

77. A client arrives in the emergency department with tachycardia, decreased urination, restlessness, and confusion. Auscultation reveals a fourth heart sound. What does the nurse suspect is occurring?
  1. Myocardial infarction
  2. Cardiogenic shock
  3. Peripheral vascular disease
  4. Abdominal aortic aneurysm (AAA)

78. A client with a history of chronic obstructive pulmonary disease (COPD) arrives in the Emergency Department with an oxygen saturation of 84%. Which diagnostic study does the nurse prepare the client for to evaluate cellular metabolism?
  * **1.** Arterial blood gas (ABG) analysis
  2. Complete blood count (CBC)
  3. Electrocardiogram (ECG)
  4. Lung scan

79. The nurse is reinforcing education for the client regarding the initial treatment goal of increasing myocardial oxygen supply for cardiogenic shock. The client demonstrates an understanding of this when making which statement?
  1. "Increasing my oxygen will cause me to become acidotic."
  2. "If I get less oxygen it will be easier on my body and I will get better quicker."
  3. "In a shock state I need less oxygen."
  4. "A balance must be maintained between oxygen supply and demand."

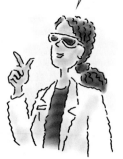

Looking good. Keep calm and carry on.

75. 1. Ventricular fibrillation is a life-threatening arrhythmia. It occurs when the ventricle fibrillates, failing to fully contract and pump blood through the heart. Sinus tachycardia, atrial fibrillation, and atrial flutter are arrhythmias that may require treatment but are not considered life-threatening.
CN: Physiological integrity; CNS: Physiological adaptation; CL: Apply; DIFFICULTY: Moderate

76. 2. The cardiac index, a figure derived by dividing the cardiac output by the client's body surface area, is used to identify whether the cardiac output is meeting a client's needs. Decreased cerebral blood flow, blood pressure, and heart rate are less useful in detecting the risk of cardiogenic shock.
CN: Physiological integrity; CNS: Physiological adaptation; CL: Analyze; DIFFICULTY: Difficult

77. 2. In cardiogenic shock initially the nurse would see a decrease in cardiac output resulting in a decrease in cerebral blood flow, which causes restlessness, agitation, or confusion. Tachycardia, decreased urine output, and an S4 heart sound are all later signs of shock. Peripheral vascular disease, AAA, and MI do not have these same signs.
CN: Physiological integrity; CNS: Basic care and comfort; CL: Analyze; DIFFICULTY: Difficult

78. 1. ABG levels reflect cellular metabolism and indicate hypoxia. A CBC is performed to determine various constituents of venous blood. An ECG shows the electrical activity of the heart. A lung scan is performed to view the lungs' function.
CN: Physiological integrity; CNS: Reduction of risk potential; CL: Apply; DIFFICULTY: Easy

79. 4. A balance must be maintained between oxygen supply and demand. In a shock state, the myocardium requires more oxygen. If it can't get more oxygen, the shock worsens. Increasing the oxygen will also help correct metabolic acidosis and hypoxia. Infarction typically causes the shock state, so prevention isn't an appropriate goal for this condition.
CN: Physiological integrity; CNS: Physiological adaptation; CL: Apply; DIFFICULTY: Easy

80. A client is suspected of having cardiogenic shock. Which medication does the nurse anticipate administering to improve myocardial contractility and blood flow?
- **1.** Dopamine
- **2.** Enalapril
- **3.** Furosemide
- **4.** Metoprolol

81. During a local wellness fair, a nurse takes some clients' blood pressures. Which client is at the highest risk for the diagnosis of essential (primary) hypertension?
- **1.** A 35-year-old pregnant female with a blood pressure of 126/80 mm Hg
- **2.** A 72-year-old female with a blood pressure of 142/88 mm Hg
- **3.** A 44-year-old male with end-stage renal failure and a blood pressure of 130/70 mm Hg
- **4.** A 76-year-old male with a systolic blood pressure of 136 mm Hg

> Taking a client's blood pressure can help determine the risk of primary hypertension.

82. Which is the **most** important instrument used as a diagnostic and monitoring tool for determining the severity of a client's shock state?
- **1.** Arterial line
- **2.** Indwelling urinary catheter
- **3.** Intra-aortic balloon pump (IABP)
- **4.** Pulmonary artery (PA) catheter

83. The nurse is obtaining the client's blood pressure and hears a faint, clear tapping sound. Which should be the nurse's next action?
- **1.** Continue listening, as this is normal.
- **2.** Immediately get the health care provider to come check this client.
- **3.** Call a rapid response.
- **4.** Ask the client if he has had an MI recently since this is not normal.

84. The nurse has reinforced education about angina to a client who has pain from angina. Which statement made by the client indicates a need for further teaching?
- **1.** "Angina pain can be relieved by nitroglycerin."
- **2.** "Angina pain can develop slowly or quickly."
- **3.** "Angina pain may radiate to shoulders, neck, arms or back."
- **4.** "Angina pain usually lasts less than 5 minutes."

80. 1. Dopamine, a sympathomimetic drug, improves myocardial contractility and blood flow through vital organs by increasing perfusion pressure. Enalapril is an angiotensin-converting enzyme (ACE) inhibitor that directly lowers blood pressure. Furosemide is a diuretic and doesn't have a direct effect on contractility or tissue perfusion. Metoprolol is a beta-blocker that slows the heart rate and lowers blood pressure, neither of which is a desired effect in the treatment of cardiogenic shock.
CN: Physiological integrity; CNS: Pharmacological therapies; CL: Apply; DIFFICULTY: Moderate

81. 2. Hypertension is defined by the Seventh Report of the Joint National Committee on Prevention, Detection, Evaluation and Treatment of High Blood Pressure as a sustained systolic blood pressure of 140 mm Hg or a diastolic blood pressure of 90 mm Hg. Secondary hypertension is attributed to an identifiable medical diagnosis, such as pregnancy-induced hypertension or renovascular disease. The 76-year-old male has prehypertension, which is defined as systolic blood pressure of 120 to 139 mm Hg or a diastolic pressure of 80 to 89 mm Hg.
CN: Physiological integrity; CNS: Reduction of risk potential; CL: Analyze; DIFFICULTY: Easy

82. 4. A PA catheter is used to give accurate pressure measurements within the heart, which aids in determining the course of treatment. An arterial line is used to directly assess blood pressure continuously. An indwelling urinary catheter is used to drain the bladder. An IABP is an assistive device used to rest the damaged heart.
CN: Physiological integrity; CNS: Reduction of risk potential; CL: Apply; DIFFICULTY: Difficult

83. 1. In phase I, auscultation produces a faint, clear tapping sound that gradually increases in intensity. Therefore, the nurse should continue to listen. It is not necessary to call the health care provider or call a rapid response.
CN: Physiological integrity; CNS: Basic care and comfort; CL: Apply; DIFFICULTY: Easy

84. 1. Angina pain if unstable may or may not be relieved by nitroglycerin. It can develop slowly or quickly, and it can radiate to arms, neck, shoulders and back. Angina pain usually lasts only 5 minutes but can last up to 15 to 20 minutes. It also can be described as mild or moderate.
CN: Physiological integrity; CNS: Physiological adaptation; CL: Apply; DIFFICULTY: Challenge

85. How do baroreceptors respond in a client with cardiogenic shock who experiences low blood pressure?
1. Stimulate the sympathetic nervous system
2. Stimulate the parasympathetic nervous system
3. Stimulate the chemoreceptors
4. Stimulate the renin–angiotensin–aldosterone system

86. A nurse is aware that the kidneys play an important role in regulating blood pressure. When hypertension occurs, which responses by the kidneys help normalize blood pressure?
1. The kidneys retain sodium and excrete water.
2. The kidneys excrete sodium and excrete water.
3. The kidneys retain sodium and retain water.
4. The kidneys excrete sodium and retain water.

87. A client is placed on an angiotensin-converting enzyme (ACE) inhibitor to reduce blood pressure. Which hormone in the renin–angiotensin–aldosterone system is associated with this medication and is responsible for preventing peripheral vasoconstriction? Select all that apply.
1. Angiotensin I
2. Angiotensin II
3. Epinephrine
4. Norepinephrine
5. Aldosterone

88. A client has recently been diagnosed with hypertension. The client has an elevated blood pressure with no symptoms and the cause is uncertain. Which term **best** describes this?
1. Accelerated hypertension
2. Malignant hypertension
3. Primary hypertension
4. Secondary hypertension

89. When gathering data from a client admitted with hypertension, the nurse should expect the client to report which symptom?
1. Blurred vision
2. Epistaxis
3. Headache
4. Peripheral edema

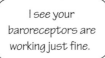

I see your baroreceptors are working just fine.

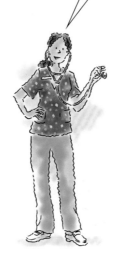

85. 1. Baroreceptors in the carotid arteries and the aorta sense pulsatile pressure and stimulate the sympathetic nervous system in response to low blood pressure. They do not stimulate the parasympathetic nervous system, chemoreceptors, or the renin–angiotensin–aldosterone system.
CN: Physiological integrity; CNS: Reduction of risk potential; CL: Analyze; DIFFICULTY: Moderate

86. 2. The kidneys respond to a rise in blood pressure by excreting sodium and excess water. This affects systolic blood pressure by regulating blood volume. Retaining sodium or water would only further increase blood pressure. Sodium and water must travel across the kidney membrane together; one can't travel without the other.
CN: Physiological integrity; CNS: Physiological adaptation; CL: Understand; DIFFICULTY: Moderate

87. 1, 2. An ACE inhibitor inhibits the renin–angiotensin–aldosterone system by blocking conversion of angiotensin I to angiotensin II and helps to prevent vasoconstriction.
CN: Physiological integrity; CNS: Pharmacological therapies; CL: Understand; DIFFICULTY: Difficult

88. 3. Characterized by a progressive, usually asymptomatic blood pressure increase over several years, primary hypertension is the most common type. Malignant hypertension, also known as accelerated hypertension, is rapidly progressive and uncontrollable and causes a rapid onset of complications. Secondary hypertension occurs secondary to a known, potentially correctable cause.
CN: Physiological integrity; CNS: Reduction of risk potential; CL: Analyze; DIFFICULTY: Easy

89. 3. An occipital headache is typical of hypertension owing to increased pressure in the cerebral vasculature. Blurred vision (due to arteriolar changes in the eye) and epistaxis (nosebleed) are far less common than headache but can also be diagnostic signs. Peripheral edema can occur from an increase in sodium and water retention, but it's usually a latent sign.
CN: Physiological integrity; CNS: Physiological adaptation; CL: Analyze; DIFFICULTY: Moderate

90. A nursing student is observed by the instructor obtaining a blood pressure. Which action by the student requires immediate intervention by the instructor?
1. Places the stethoscope over the brachial artery
2. Places the stethoscope over the brachioce-phalic artery
3. Uses the diaphragm of the stethoscope
4. Washes hands before taking a blood pressure

91. Which statement **best** explains why furosemide is administered to treat hypertension?
1. It dilates peripheral blood vessels.
2. It decreases sympathetic cardioacceleration.
3. It inhibits the angiotensin-converting enzyme.
4. It inhibits reabsorption of sodium and water in the loop of Henle.

92. A nurse is assisting with the teaching of a class for a group of teenagers at a local high school. What should the nurse include as risk factors for developing hypertension? Select all that apply.
1. Obesity
2. Smoking
3. Weight loss
4. Heredity
5. Daily exercise

93. A client is admitted for right leg vein ligation and stripping for varicose veins. Which nursing intervention postoperatively should the nurse include?
1. Ask the client to elevate the legs when sitting.
2. Ask the client to remain inactive until healing is complete.
3. Apply knee-high stockings over the dressing.
4. Apply ice to dressings to decrease swelling.

94. A healthy, pregnant woman is diagnosed with varicose veins. What should the nurse teach this client to help her avoid further development of the disease? Select all that apply.
1. Elevate legs
2. Change positions
3. Monitor weight
4. Avoid support stockings
5. Limit fluids to avoid constipation

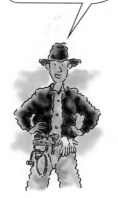

Ready for an adventure in assessment? First make sure you have all your tools and know how to use them.

90. 2. The brachial artery is typically used because of its easy accessibility and location. The brachio-cephalic artery isn't accessible for blood pressure measurement. The student uses standard precautions by washing hands whenever performing skills and the diaphragm is the correct part of stethoscope to use when taking a blood pressure. CN: Physiological integrity; CNS: Basic care and comfort; CL: Apply; DIFFICULTY: Easy

91. 4. Furosemide is a loop diuretic that inhib-its sodium and water reabsorption in the loop of Henle, thereby causing a decrease in blood pressure. Vasodilators cause dilation of peripheral blood vessels, directly relaxing vascular smooth muscle and decreasing blood pressure. Adrenergic blockers decrease sympathetic cardioaccelera-tion and decrease blood pressure. Angiotensin-converting enzyme inhibitors decrease blood pressure due to their action on angiotensin. CN: Physiological integrity; CNS: Pharmacological therapies; CL: Understand; DIFFICULTY: Easy

92. 1, 2, 4. Risk factors for hypertension include obesity, smoking, heredity and lack of exercise, among other factors. Weight loss and daily exercise are factors that help to *prevent* hypertension. CN: Health Promotion and Maintenance; CNS: None; CL: Apply; DIFFICULTY: Easy

93. 1. Postoperative nursing interventions must focus on maintaining peripheral circulation and venous return. Elevating the legs and early ambu-lation are encouraged to facilitate venous return. Applying knee-high stockings and ice would con-strict circulation. CN: Physiological integrity; CNS: Reduction of risk potential; CL: Apply; DIFFICULTY: Moderate

94. 1, 2, 3. Primary varicose veins have a gradual onset and progressively worsen. To help prevent or lessen the effects of varicose veins during pregnancy, the client should elevate legs to help promote circula-tion, change position frequently, and monitor weight, as high weight gain in a short period of time is hard on the veins. The client should use support panty hose or stockings to help, and should take steps to avoid constipation as this can lead to hemorrhoids. CN: Health promotion and maintenance; CNS: None; CL: Apply; DIFFICULTY: Moderate

95. Which client statement given when obtaining data is consistent with the diagnosis of varicose veins?
  1. "My legs feel tired and have a dull ache, especially when I walk or stand for long periods."
  2. "I have severe foot pain that awakens me, but it gets better if I dangle my foot off the edge of the bed."
  3. "My legs become numb and get weaker the farther I walk."
  4. "After I walk 1/2 mile (800 m) I get severe calf pain that goes away when I rest."

96. A client is admitted to the ICU after being seen in the emergency department with suspected cardiac tamponade. Which symptom should the nurse expect to see in the client? Select all that apply.
  1. Muffled heart sounds upon auscultation
  2. Wide pulse pressure
  3. Jugular vein distention
  4. Restlessness
  5. Pulsus paradoxus

97. Which client condition is caused by increased hydrostatic pressure and chronic venous stasis?
  1. Venous occlusion
  2. Cool extremities
  3. Nocturnal calf muscle cramps
  4. Diminished blood supply to the feet

98. The nurse is reinforcing discharge instructions for a client with varicose veins. Which statement by the client indicates a need for further instruction?
  1. "Exercise will make me feel better."
  2. "I have to elevate my legs."
  3. "Lying down can relieve my symptoms."
  4. "Wearing tight clothes will not affect me."

99. A client is diagnosed with valvular heart disease with a primary symptom of fatigue. Which disease process does the nurse suspect the client is experiencing? Select all that apply.
  1. Aortic insufficiency
  2. Mitral insufficiency
  3. Mitral valve prolapse
  4. Mitral stenosis
  5. Tricuspid insufficiency

100. A client is admitted with a diagnosis of post-thrombotic deep vein changes in both legs. Which signs and symptoms does the nurse expect to see in this client?
  1. Pallor and severe pain
  2. Severe pain and edema
  3. Edema and pigmentation
  4. Absent hair growth and pigmentation

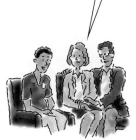

Remember to keep the client's family in the loop about the client's prognosis and treatment.

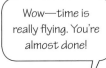

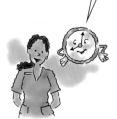

Wow—time is really flying. You're almost done!

95. 1. Fatigue, aching, and pressure are classic symptoms of varicose veins, secondary to increased blood volume and edema. Severe foot pain that awakens the client, as well as severe calf pain after walking that's relieved with rest, are symptoms of decreased peripheral arterial blood flow. Numbness and weakness that increase as the client walks are consistent with spinal stenosis.
CN: Physiological integrity; CNS: Physiological adaptation;
CL: Analyze; DIFFICULTY: Easy

96. 1, 3, 4, 5. Key signs and symptoms of cardiac tamponade are muffled heart sounds upon auscultation, narrow pulse pressure, jugular vein distention, pulsus paradoxus (an abnormal inspiratory drop in systemic blood pressure greater than 15 mm Hg), restlessness, and sitting upright or leaning forward.
CN: Physiological integrity; CNS: Reduction of risk potential;
CL: Apply; DIFFICULTY: Difficult

97. 3. Calf muscle cramps result from increased pressure and venous stasis secondary to varicose veins. An occlusion is a blockage of blood flow. Cool extremities and diminished blood supply to the feet are symptoms of decreased arterial blood flow.
CN: Health promotion and maintenance; CNS: None;
CL: Analyze; DIFFICULTY: Challenge

98. 4. Tight clothing, especially below the waist, increases vascular volume and impedes blood return to the heart. Exercise, leg elevations, and lying down usually relieve symptoms of varicose veins.
CN: Health promotion and maintenance; CNS: None;
CL: Apply, DIFFICULTY: Easy

99. 1, 2, 4, 5. A key sign and symptom of aortic insufficiency, mitral insufficiency, mitral stenosis, and tricuspid insufficiency is fatigue. Palpitations are usually the only symptom for mitral valve prolapse.
CN: Physiological Integrity; CNS: Physiological adaptation;
CL: Apply; DIFFICULTY: Difficult

100. 3. Blood clots in the deep veins of the leg typically cause permanent damage to the venous valves. Incompetent valves lead to impaired venous return, and edema and pigmentation result from venous stasis. Severe pain, pallor, and absent hair growth are symptoms of an altered arterial blood flow.
CN: Physiological integrity; CNS: Physiological adaptation;
CL: Apply; DIFFICULTY: Difficult

101. A client has undergone ligation of stripping of veins in the lower extremities. Which intervention will the nurse provide postoperatively?
1. Have the client sit for most of the day.
2. Maintain the client on strict bed rest.
3. Apply ice packs to the lower extremities.
4. Apply thigh-high elastic leg compression.

101. 4. Thigh-high elastic leg compression helps venous return to the heart, thereby decreasing venous stasis. Prolonged sitting and bed rest are contraindicated because both promote decreased blood return to the heart and venous stasis. Although ice packs would help reduce edema, they would also cause vasoconstriction and impede blood flow.
CN: Physiological integrity; CNS: Basic care and comfort;
CL: Apply; DIFFICULTY: Moderate

102. Which statement by a client **best** indicates that he understands the surgical procedure to remove varicose veins?
1. "The surgeon will tie off a large vein in my leg and then remove it."
2. "The surgeon will use a laser to prevent further varicose veins."
3. "A piece of vein will be removed and then used to replace my blocked artery."
4. "A cold solution will be infused to shrink the vein."

102. 1. Ligation and stripping surgically removes varicose veins. The use of laser ablation therapy won't prevent further varicose veins from developing. Veins can be used to create bypasses for blocked arteries, but this isn't a treatment for varicose veins. Infusion of a cold solution isn't used to treat varicose veins.
CN: Physiological integrity; CNS: Physiological adaptation;
CL: Analyze; DIFFICULTY: Difficult

103. A client who has been diagnosed with intermittent claudication is prescribed cilostazol. Which statement made by the client indicates a need for further education?
1. "Cilostazol works by increasing blood flow."
2. "Cilostazol works by decreasing stickiness of platelets."
3. "Cilostazol may be able to help my leg pain."
4. "Cilostazol works by decreasing blood flow."

103. 4. Cilostazol works by increasing blood flow into the legs and decreasing the stickiness of platelets. It also will help reduce some pain in the legs.
CN: Physiological integrity; CNS: Pharmacological therapies;
CL: Apply; DIFFICULTY: Difficult

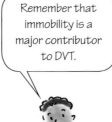

Remember that immobility is a major contributor to DVT.

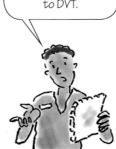

104. Which client is **most** at risk for developing deep vein thrombosis (DVT)?
1. A 62-year-old female recovering from a total hip replacement
2. A 35-year-old female 2 days postpartum
3. A 33-year-old male runner with Achilles tendonitis
4. An ambulatory 70-year-old male who's recovering from pneumonia

104. 1. DVT is more common in immobilized clients who have had surgical procedures such as total hip replacement. Pregnancy can cause varicose veins, which can lead to venous stasis, but it isn't a primary cause of DVT. Clients who are recovering from an injury or pneumonia may have decreased mobility, but these clients don't have the highest risk of developing DVT.
CN: Physiological integrity; CNS: Reduction of risk potential;
CL: Analyze; DIFFICULTY: Easy

105. A client who has a deep vein thrombosis (DVT) reports dyspnea, chest pain, and has diminished breath sounds. Which condition does the nurse prepare treatment for?
1. Hemothorax
2. Pneumothorax
3. Pulmonary embolism
4. Pulmonary hypertension

105. 3. The most common complication of a DVT is a pulmonary embolus. A pulmonary embolism is a thrombus that forms in a vein, travels to the lungs, and lodges in the pulmonary vasculature. Hemothorax refers to blood in the pleural space. Pneumothorax is caused by an opening in the pleura. Pulmonary hypertension is an increase in pulmonary artery pressure, which increases the workload of the right ventricle.
CN: Physiological integrity; CNS: Physiological adaptation;
CL: Analyze; DIFFICULTY: Easy

106. The nurse is reinforcing education to a client who has recently been diagnosed with a deep vein thrombosis (DVT). Which statement made by the client would indicate a need for further education?
1. "Hypercoagulability plays a role in the formation of DVT."
2. "Hypercoagulability, along with venous stasis and venous wall injury, accounts for the formation of deep vein thrombosis."
3. "An embolus is a blood clot or fatty globule that forms in one area and is carried through the bloodstream to another area."
4. "Hypercoagulability will cause the blood to coagulate slower than normal and therefore will cause the clotting factors to multiply."

106. 4. Hypercoagulability is the term that refers to the condition of blood coagulating faster than normal (not slower than normal), causing thrombin and other clotting factors to multiply. This condition, along with venous stasis and venous wall injury, accounts for the formation of deep vein thrombosis. An embolus is a blood clot or fatty globule that forms in one area and is carried through the bloodstream to another area.
CN: Physiological integrity; CNS: Physiological adaptation; CL: Apply; DIFFICULTY: Difficult

107. A client with a deep vein thrombosis (DVT) is admitted to the hospital for treatment. Which medication will the nurse administer orally to prevent further thrombus formation?
1. Warfarin
2. Heparin
3. Furosemide
4. Metoprolol

107. 1. Warfarin prevents vitamin K from synthesizing certain clotting factors. This oral anticoagulant can be given long term. Heparin is a parenteral anticoagulant that interferes with coagulation by readily combining with antithrombin; it can't be given by mouth. Neither furosemide nor metoprolol affect anticoagulation.
CN: Physiological integrity; CNS: Pharmacological therapies; CL: Apply; DIFFICULTY: Moderate

108. The nurse instructs the client with acute pulmonary edema that high Fowler's position is best to aid breathing. Which statement made by the client would indicate an understanding of this?
1. "This position will allow for better access if you need to do an assessment."
2. "It will cause constriction of all of my arteries that will help my breathing."
3. "This position reduces venous return and thus will help my breathing."
4. "It will increase my heart's workload and thus make breathing easier."

108. 3. High Fowler's position facilitates breathing by reducing venous return. It does not cause constriction of the arteries and it will not increase the workload of the heart. It may allow for better access but this is not the reason for the position.
CN: Physiological integrity; CNS: Basic care and comfort; CL: Apply; DIFFICULTY: Moderate

109. A postoperative client in the ICU begins exhibiting signs of hypovolemic shock. When gathering data on this client, which symptom does the nurse expect to see? Select all that apply.
1. Cold, pale, clammy skin
2. Decreased sensorium
3. Hypertension
4. Reduced urine output
5. Bradycardia

109. 1, 2, 4. Key signs and symptoms of hypovolemic shock are cold, pale, and clammy skin; decreased sensorium; hypotension; reduced urine output; and tachycardia.
CN: Physiological integrity; CNS: Physiological adaptation; CL: Analyze; DIFFICULTY: Challenge

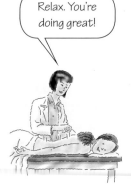

Relax. You're doing great!

110. A nurse is caring for an older adult client with sick sinus syndrome who's awaiting permanent pacemaker placement. Given this client's risk of decreased cardiac output, what findings would indicate that the client is experiencing an initial drop in cardiac output?
1. Decreased blood pressure
2. Altered level of consciousness (LOC)
3. Decreased blood pressure and diuresis
4. Increased blood pressure and fluid volume

110. 4. The body compensates for a decrease in cardiac output with a rise in blood pressure (due to the stimulation of the sympathetic nervous system) and an increase in fluid volume as the kidneys retain sodium and water. Blood pressure doesn't initially drop in response to the compensatory mechanism of the body. Alteration in LOC will occur only if decreased cardiac output persists.
CN: Physiological integrity; CNS: Physiological adaptation; CL: Analyze; DIFFICULTY: Difficult

111. Which nursing action is **priority** action for a client coughing up pink, frothy sputum?
1. Call for help.
2. Call the health care provider.
3. Start an IV line.
4. Suction the client.

112. A nurse recognizes that a client with severe hypertension will experience increased workload that can be attributed to which process?
1. Increased afterload
2. Increased cardiac output
3. Increased preload
4. Overload of the heart

113. What is the **best** action for the nurse to take when administering a new blood pressure medication to a client?
1. Administer the medication to the client without explanation.
2. Inform the client of the new drug only if he asks about it.
3. Inform the client of the new medication, its name, use, and the reason for the change.
4. Administer the medication and inform the client that the health care provider will explain the medication later.

114. Which statement by a nurse to an unlicensed assistive personnel (UAP) **best** explains the need to promptly report changes in respiratory rate for a client diagnosed with heart failure?
1. "Pulmonary edema, a life-threatening condition, can develop in minutes."
2. "Severe acute respiratory syndrome (SARS) is a common complication of heart failure."
3. "Pneumonia is a consequence of inadequate ventilation with heart failure."
4. "Pneumothorax, a life-threatening condition, can develop in minutes."

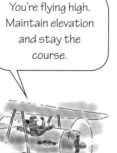

You're flying high. Maintain elevation and stay the course.

115. A client with a history of hypertension had a total hip replacement. The health care provider prescribes hydrochlorothiazide 35 mg oral solution by mouth once per day. The label on the solution reads hydrochlorothiazide 50 mg/5 mL. To administer the correct dose, how many milliliters should the nurse pour? Record your answer using one decimal place.

_____ mL

111. 1. Production of pink, frothy sputum is a classic sign of acute pulmonary edema. Because the client is at high risk for decompensation, the nurse should call for help but not leave the room. The other three interventions should immediately follow.
CN: Physiological integrity; CNS: Physiological adaptation; CL: Apply; DIFFICULTY: Challenge

112.1. Afterload refers to the resistance normally maintained by the aortic and pulmonic valves, the condition and tone of the aorta, and the resistance offered by the systemic and pulmonary arterioles. Hypertension increases afterload as the left ventricle has to work harder to eject blood against vasoconstriction. Cardiac output is the amount of blood expelled from the heart per minute. Preload is the volume of blood in the ventricle at the end of diastole. Overload refers to an abundance of circulating volume and can contribute to hypertension.
CN: Physiological integrity; CNS: Physiological adaptation; CL: Analyze; DIFFICULTY: Difficult

113. 3. Informing the client about the medication, its use, and the reason for the change is important to the care of the client. Educating the client about his treatment regimen promotes compliance. The other responses are inappropriate.
CN: Safe, effective care environment; CNS: Safety and infection control; CL: Apply; DIFFICULTY: Easy

114. 1. Pulmonary edema, a life-threatening complication of heart failure, can develop in minutes, secondary to a sudden fluid shift from the pulmonary vasculature to the lungs' interstitial alveoli. SARS and pneumonia are caused by infections. Pneumothorax is a collection of air or gas in the pleural space that causes the lung to collapse.
CN: Physiological integrity; CNS: Reduction of risk potential; CL: Apply; DIFFICULTY: Moderate

115. 3.5.
The correct formula to calculate a drug dosage is:
$$\text{Dose on hand} = \frac{\text{Dose desired}}{X}$$
In this example, the equation is:
$$50\ \text{mg}/5\ \text{mL} = \frac{35\ \text{mg}}{X}$$
$$X = 3.5\ \text{mL}$$

CN: Physiological integrity; CNS: Pharmacological therapies; CL: Analyze; DIFFICULTY: Easy

116. A client recovers from an episode of acute pulmonary edema and is prescribed enalapril. What does the nurse determine is the **most** important outcome of administration of this medication?
1. To decrease overload by promoting diuresis
2. To increase contractility of the heart
3. To decrease contractility of the heart
4. To decrease workload of the heart

117. An older adult client has a potassium level of 3.2 mEq/L. How should the nurse instruct the client in relation to diet?
1. Increase intake of bananas and oranges.
2. Avoid intake of bananas and oranges.
3. Increase intake of oatmeal and apples.
4. Avoid intake of oatmeal and apples.

118. A client has been hospitalized with a diagnosis of acute arterial occlusive disease. After surgery the health care provider orders heparin IV therapy for the client. What test does the nurse need to monitor for this client while on heparin?
1. PT
2. PTT
3. CBC
4. PSA
5. BUN

119. A nurse is obtaining data from a client who's at risk for cardiac tamponade due to chest trauma sustained in a motorcycle accident. What's the client's pulse pressure if the blood pressure is 108/82 mm Hg? Record your answer using a whole number.

_____ mm Hg

120. A client is admitted with a diagnosis of new-onset atrial fibrillation. To obtain an accurate pulse count, the nurse counts the apical heart rate. Identify the area where the nurse should place the stethoscope to **best** hear the apical rate.

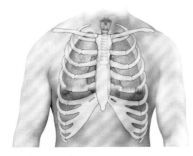

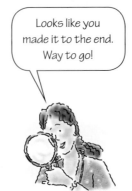

Looks like you made it to the end. Way to go!

116.4. Enalapril maleate is an angiotensin-converting enzyme (ACE) inhibitor that reduces blood pressure and decreases the workload of the heart. Diuretics are given to decrease circulating fluid volume. Inotropic agents increase cardiac contractility. Negative inotropic agents decrease cardiac contractility.
CN: Physiological integrity; CNS: Pharmacological therapies; CL: Apply; DIFFICULTY: Moderate

117. 1. A normal serum potassium blood level is 3.5 to 5 mEq/L in older adult clients. Bananas and oranges are high in potassium. Oatmeal and apples are high in fiber.
CN: Physiological integrity; CNS: Basic care and comfort; CL: Apply; DIFFICULTY: Easy

118.2. Partial Thromboplastin Time is used to monitor response to heparin therapy and is used to evaluate all the clotting factors of the intrinsic pathway. Both are monitored whenever a client is on heparin. Complete blood count is used to determine infection or inflammation. PSA is prostate-specific antigen used to screen for prostate cancer in men. Blood urea nitrogen is used to evaluate kidney function.
CN: Physiological integrity; CNS: Reduction of risk potential; CL: Apply; DIFFICULTY: Easy

119. 26.
Pulse pressure is the difference between systolic and diastolic pressures.

$$108 - 82 = 26.$$

Normally, systolic pressure exceeds diastolic pressure by about 40 mm Hg. Narrowed pulse pressure, a difference of less than 30 mm Hg, is a sign of cardiac tamponade.
CN: Physiological integrity; CNS: Physiological adaptation; CL: Analyze; DIFFICULTY: Easy

120. The apical heart rate is best heard at the point of maximal impulse, which is generally in the fifth intercostal space at the midclavicular line.

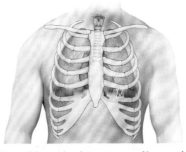

CN: Health promotion and maintenance; CNS: None; CL: Analyze; DIFFICULTY: Moderate

Chapter 4

Hematologic & Immune Disorders

Hematologic & immunologic refresher

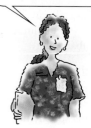

This challenging chapter covers HIV infection, AIDS, rheumatoid arthritis, DIC, and lots of other complex disorders. You can handle it, though; I know you can.

Acquired immunodeficiency syndrome (AIDS)

Immunologic disorder caused by human immunodeficiency virus (HIV) that lowers CD4 T-cell count, increases susceptibility to opportunistic infections, and is end stage of HIV infection

Key signs and symptoms

- Anorexia, weight loss, recurrent diarrhea, generalized lymphadenopathy
- Disorientation, confusion, dementia
- History of night sweats
- History of opportunistic infections

Key test results

- CD4+ T-cell level is less than 200 cells/μL
- Enzyme-linked immunosorbent assay shows positive human immunodeficiency virus antibody titer
- Western blot test is positive

Key treatments

- Transfusion therapy: fresh frozen plasma, platelets, and packed red blood cells (RBCs)
- Antibiotic: sulfamethoxazole and trimethoprim
- Antiprotozoal agent: pentamidine
- Combination therapy
- Non-nucleoside reverse transcriptase inhibitors: delavirdine, nevirapine, efavirenz
- Nucleoside reverse transcriptase inhibitors: lamivudine, zidovudine, abacavir, didanosine, emtricitabine, stavudine, tenofovir
- Protease inhibitors: indinavir, nelfinavir, ritonavir, saquinavir, atazanavir, fosamprenavir
- Fusion inhibitor: enfuvirtide

Key interventions

- Monitor for opportunistic infections
- Maintain the client's diet
- Provide mouth care
- Maintain standard precautions
- Make referrals to community agencies for support
- Monitor respiratory status

Anaphylaxis

Severe and life-threatening allergic reaction with massive release of histamine from the damaged cells

Key signs and symptoms

- Cardiovascular symptoms (hypotension, shock, cardiac arrhythmias) that may precipitate circulatory collapse if untreated
- Sudden physical distress within seconds or minutes after exposure to an allergen (may include feeling of impending doom or fright, weakness, sweating, sneezing, shortness of breath, nasal pruritus, urticaria, and angioedema, followed rapidly by symptoms in one or more target organs)
- Respiratory symptoms (nasal mucosal edema; profuse, watery rhinorrhea; itching; nasal congestion; sudden sneezing attacks; edema of the upper respiratory tract that causes hoarseness, stridor, and dyspnea [early sign of acute respiratory failure])

Key test results

- Rapid onset of severe respiratory or cardiovascular symptoms after an insect sting or after ingestion or injection of a drug, vaccine, diagnostic agent, food, or food additive

Key treatment

- Immediate subcutaneous (SQ) injection of epinephrine 1:1,000 aqueous solution, 0.1 to 0.5 mL, repeated every 10 to 15 minutes as necessary

Key interventions

- In early stages, give epinephrine IM or SQ and help it move into the circulation faster by massaging the injection site
- In severe reactions, epinephrine should be given IV
- Maintain airway patency
- Observe for early signs of laryngeal edema (stridor, hoarseness, and dyspnea)
- Prepare for endotracheal tube insertion or a tracheotomy and oxygen therapy
- Monitor blood pressure and urine output

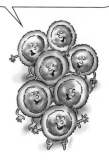

We're "packed red blood cells!"

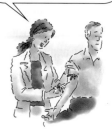

In anaphylaxis, epinephrine can be a life saver.

49

Ankylosing spondylitis

Inflammation of the spine causing abnormal fusion of vertebrae

Key signs and symptoms

- Intermittent lower back pain (the first indication), usually most severe in the morning or after a period of inactivity
- Mild fatigue, fever, anorexia, or weight loss; unilateral acute anterior uveitis
- Stiffness and limited motion of the lumbar spine

Key test results

- Typical symptoms, a family history, and the presence of HLA-B27 strongly suggest ankylosing spondylitis
- Confirmation requires characteristic x-ray findings:
  - blurring of the bony margins of joints in the early stage
  - bilateral sacroiliac involvement
  - patchy sclerosis with superficial bony erosions
  - eventual squaring of vertebral bodies
  - "bamboo spine" with complete ankylosis

Key treatments

- Good posture, stretching and deep-breathing exercises; in some clients, braces and lightweight supports to delay further deformity
- Anti-inflammatory agents: aspirin, ibuprofen, indomethacin, naproxen, sulfasalazine, sulindac to control pain and inflammation
- Tumor necrosis factor (TNF) blockers: adalimumab, etanercept, infliximab, golimumab

Key interventions

- Offer support and reassurance; keep in mind client's limited range of motion makes simple tasks difficult
- Administer medications as needed
- Apply local heat and provide massage; assess mobility and degree of discomfort frequently

Aplastic anemia

Decrease in production of red blood cells and other blood elements due to bone marrow suppression

Key signs and symptoms

- Dyspnea, tachypnea
- Epistaxis
- Melena
- Palpitations, tachycardia
- Purpura, petechiae, ecchymosis, pallor

Key test results

- Bone marrow biopsy shows decrease in activity or no cell production

Key treatments

- Transfusion of platelets and packed RBCs
- Antithymocyte globulin
- Hematopoietic growth factor: epoetin alfa

Key interventions

- Monitor for infection, bleeding, and bruising
- Administer oxygen
- Monitor transfusion therapy as prescribed
- Maintain protective precautions
- Avoid giving the client IM injections

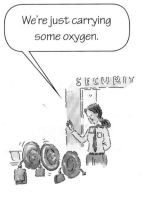

We're just carrying some oxygen.

Calcium imbalance

Hypocalcemia
- Decrease in blood calcium level

Hypercalcemia
- Increase in blood calcium level

Key signs and symptoms

Hypocalcemia

- Cardiac arrhythmias
- Chvostek sign
- Tetany
- Trousseau sign

Hypercalcemia
- Anorexia
- Decreased muscle tone
- Lethargy
- Muscle weakness
- Nausea
- Polydipsia
- Polyuria

Key test results

Because approximately one-half of serum calcium is bound to albumin, changes in serum protein must be considered when interpreting serum calcium levels

Hypocalcemia
- Serum calcium level less than 4.5 mEq/L
- Electrocardiogram reveals a lengthened QT interval, a prolonged ST segment, and arrhythmias

Hypercalcemia
- Serum calcium level greater than 5.5 mEq/L
- Electrocardiogram reveals a shortened QT interval and heart block

Key treatments

Hypocalcemia
- Diet: adequate intake of calcium, vitamin D, and protein

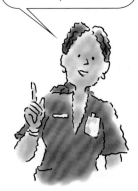

Encourage clients with hypocalcemia to increase their intake of calcium, vitamin D, and protein.

- Ergocalciferol (vitamin D_2), cholecalciferol (vitamin D_3), calcitriol, dihydrotachysterol (synthetic form of vitamin D_2) for severe deficiency
- Immediate correction by IV calcium gluconate or calcium chloride for acute hypocalcemia (an emergency)

Hypercalcemia
- Calcitonin
- Loop diuretics: ethacrynic acid and furosemide to promote calcium excretion (thiazide diuretics are contraindicated in hypercalcemia because they inhibit calcium excretion)

Key interventions
Hypocalcemia
- Monitor serum calcium levels every 12 to 24 hours. When giving calcium supplements, frequently check the pH level. Check for Trousseau and Chvostek signs

Hypercalcemia
- Monitor serum calcium levels frequently
- Increase fluid intake

Chloride imbalance
Hypochloremia
- Decrease in blood chloride level

Hyperchloremia
- Increase in blood chloride level

Key signs and symptoms
Hypochloremia
- Muscle hypertonicity (in conditions related to loss of gastric secretions)
- Muscle weakness
- Shallow, depressed breathing
- Twitching

Hyperchloremia
- Agitation
- Deep, rapid breathing
- Diminished cognitive ability
- Hypertension
- Pitting edema
- Tachycardia
- Weakness

Key test results
Hypochloremia
- Serum chloride level less than 98 mEq/L
- Supportive values with metabolic alkalosis include a serum pH greater than 7.45 and a serum carbon dioxide level greater than 32 mEq/L

Hyperchloremia
- Serum chloride level greater than 108 mEq/L

- With metabolic acidosis, serum pH is less than 7.35 and the serum carbon dioxide level is less than 22 mEq/L

Key treatments
Hypochloremia
- Acidifying agent: ammonium chloride
- Diet: salty broth
- Saline solution IV

Hyperchloremia
- Alkalinizing agent: sodium bicarbonate IV
- Lactated Ringer solution

Key interventions
Hypochloremia
- Monitor electrolyte levels
- Watch for excessive or continuous loss of gastric secretions

Hyperchloremia
- Monitor electrolyte levels
- Disseminated intravascular coagulation
- Overactivity of clotting cascade, resulting in widespread formation of clots in microcirculation with subsequent reduction of clotting factors

Disseminated intravascular coagulation (DIC)
Key signs and symptoms
- Abnormal bleeding without an accompanying history of serious hemorrhagic disorder
- Oliguria
- Shock

Key test results
- Blood tests show PT greater than 15 seconds; PTT greater than 60 seconds; fibrinogen levels less than 150 mg/dL; platelets less than 100,000/µL; and fibrin degradation products commonly greater than 100 mcg/mL
- A positive d-dimer test is specific for disseminated intravascular coagulation.

Key treatments
- Anticoagulant: heparin IV (heparin sodium injection)
- Bed rest
- Transfusion therapy: fresh frozen plasma, platelets, packed RBCs

Key interventions
- Enforce complete bed rest during bleeding episodes; pad the side rails if client becomes agitated
- Check all IV and venipuncture sites frequently for bleeding; apply pressure to injection sites for at least 10 minutes; alert other personnel to client's tendency to hemorrhage

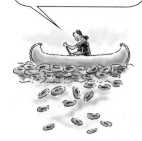

Excessive clotting and insufficient clotting are both problematic.

- Watch for transfusion reactions and signs of fluid overload
- Weigh the client daily, particularly in renal involvement
- Monitor the results of serial blood studies (particularly hematocrit [HCT], hemoglobin [Hb] level, and coagulation times)

Hemophilia

Group of hereditary bleeding disorders caused by lack of coagulation factor

Key signs and symptoms

- Hematuria
- Joint tenderness
- Pain and swelling in a weight-bearing joint
- Prolonged bleeding after major trauma or surgery (in mild hemophilia)
- Spontaneous or severe bleeding after minor trauma (in severe hemophilia)
- SQ and IM hematomas (in moderate hemophilia)
- Tarry stools

Key test results

- Factor VIII assay reveals 0% to 25% of normal factor VIII (hemophilia A)
- Factor IX assay shows deficiency (hemophilia B)

Key treatments

- Administration of factor VIII or cryoprecipitate antihemophilic factor (AHF) and lyophilized (dehydrated) AHF to encourage normal hemostasis (for hemophilia A)
- Administration of purified factor IX to promote hemostasis (for hemophilia B)
- Administration of analgesics to control joint pain (for both types)

Key interventions

- During bleeding episodes, monitor clotting factor or plasma administration; also administer analgesics
- Avoid IM injections
- Aspirin and aspirin-containing medications are contraindicated
- If the client has bled into a joint, immediately elevate the joint

Iron deficiency anemia

Anemia caused by inadequate intake of iron, malabsorption, and blood loss, which depletes iron stores

Key signs and symptoms

- Pallor
- Sensitivity to cold
- Weakness and fatigue

Key test results

- Hematology shows decreased Hb, HCT, iron, ferritin, reticulocytes, red cell indices, transferrin, and saturation; absent hemosiderin; increased iron-binding capacity

Key treatments

- Diet: high in iron, fiber, and protein with increased fluids; avoidance of teas and coffee, which reduce absorption of iron
- Vitamins: pyridoxine (vitamin B_6), ascorbic acid (vitamin C)
- Iron supplements: ferrous sulfate, iron dextran

Key interventions

- Monitor cardiovascular and respiratory status
- Monitor stool, urine, and vomitus for occult blood
- Administer medications as prescribed; administer iron injection deep into muscle using Z-track technique
- Provide mouth, skin, and foot care

Kaposi sarcoma

Red-brown to purplish skin lesion seen mainly in clients with acquired immunodeficiency syndrome (AIDS)

Key signs and symptoms

- One or more obvious lesions in various shapes, sizes, and colors (ranging from red-brown to dark purple) that appear most commonly on the skin, buccal mucosa, hard and soft palates, lips, gums, tongue, tonsils, conjunctivae, and sclerae
- Pain (if the sarcoma advances beyond the early stages or if lesion breaks down or impinges on nerves or organs)

Key test results

- Tissue biopsy identifies the lesion's type and stage

Key treatments

- High-calorie, high-protein diet
- Radiation therapy
- Antineoplastics: doxorubicin, etoposide, vinblastine, vincristine
- Antiemetics: dolasetron, trimethobenzamide

Key interventions

- Inspect client's skin every shift; look for new lesions and skin breakdown; help client into more comfortable position if lesions are painful
- Administer pain medications; suggest distractions and help client with relaxation techniques

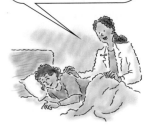

Use extra care when working with client's with hemophilia, as they bruise and bleed easily.

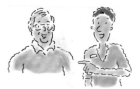

Encourage clients with iron deficiency anemia to consume plenty of protein.

- Urge client to share his feelings; provide encouragement
- Supply client with high-calorie, high-protein meals; provide client with frequent, smaller meals if regular meals not tolerated; consult with dietitian and plan meals around client's treatment
- Be alert for adverse reactions to radiation therapy or chemotherapy—such as anorexia, nausea, vomiting, and diarrhea; take steps to prevent or alleviate these reactions. Explain infection-prevention techniques; if necessary, demonstrate basic hygiene measures; advise client not to share toothbrush, razor, or other items that may be contaminated with blood (especially important if client also has HIV or AIDS)

Leukemia

Hematologic malignant disorder, resulting in an overproduction and overcrowding of immature leukocytes in the bone marrow

Key signs and symptoms
- Enlarged lymph nodes, spleen, and liver
- Frequent infections
- Bone pain
- Weakness and fatigue

Key test results
- Bone marrow biopsy shows large numbers of immature leukocytes

Key treatments
- Antimetabolites: fluorouracil, methotrexate
- Alkylating agents: busulfan, chlorambucil
- Vinca alkaloids: vinblastine, vincristine
- Antineoplastic antibiotics: doxorubicin, plicamycin
- Hematopoietic growth factor: epoetin alfa

Key interventions
- Monitor for bleeding
- Place client with epistaxis in upright position, leaning slightly forward
- Monitor for infection; promptly report temperature over 101° F (38.3° C) and decreased white blood cell (WBC) counts
- Monitor transfusion therapy for adverse reactions
- Provide gentle mouth and skin care

Lymphoma

Type of cancer of lymphoid tissue; two main types are Hodgkin lymphoma and non-Hodgkin lymphoma

Key signs and symptoms
- Predictable pattern of spread (Hodgkin lymphoma)
- Enlarged, nontender, firm, and movable lymph nodes in lower cervical regions (Hodgkin lymphoma)
- Less predictable pattern of spread (malignant lymphoma)
- Prominent, painless, generalized lymphadenopathy (malignant lymphoma)

Key test results
- Lymph node biopsy positive for Reed-Sternberg cells (Hodgkin lymphoma)
- Bone marrow aspiration and biopsy reveal small, diffuse, lymphocytic cells or large, follicular-type cells (malignant lymphoma)

Key treatments
- Radiation therapy
- Transfusion of packed RBCs
- Chemotherapy for Hodgkin lymphoma: mechlorethamine, vincristine, procarbazine, doxorubicin, bleomycin, vinblastine, dacarbazine
- Chemotherapy for malignant lymphoma: cyclophosphamide, vincristine, doxorubicin

Key interventions
- Monitor for bleeding, infection, jaundice, and electrolyte imbalance
- Provide mouth and skin care
- Encourage fluids
- Administer medications as prescribed and monitor for adverse effects
- Maintain transfusion therapy as prescribed and monitor for adverse reactions

Magnesium imbalance

Hypomagnesemia
- Decrease in blood magnesium level

Hypermagnesemia
- Increase in blood magnesium level

Key signs and symptoms
Hypomagnesemia
- Arrhythmias
- Neuromuscular irritability
- Chvostek sign
- Mood changes
- Confusion

Hypermagnesemia
- Diminished deep tendon reflexes
- Weakness
- Confusion
- Heart block
- Nausea
- Vomiting

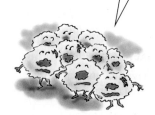

Overcrowding of the "good guys" can be an indicator of trouble brewing.

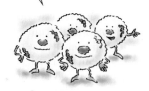

We're ready to spring into action!

Key test results

Hypomagnesemia
- Serum magnesium levels less than 1.5 mEq/L

Hypermagnesemia
- Serum magnesium levels greater than 2.5 mEq/L

Key treatments

Hypomagnesemia
- Daily magnesium supplements IM or by mouth
- High-magnesium diet
- Magnesium sulfate IV (10 to 40 mEq/L diluted in IV fluid) for severe cases

Hypermagnesemia
- Diet: low magnesium with increased fluid intake
- Loop diuretic: furosemide
- Magnesium antagonist: calcium gluconate (10%)
- Peritoneal dialysis or hemodialysis if renal function fails, or if excess magnesium can't be eliminated

Key interventions

Hypomagnesemia
- Monitor serum electrolyte levels (including magnesium, calcium, and potassium) daily for mild deficits (every 6 to 12 hours during replacement therapy)
- Measure intake and output frequently (urine output shouldn't fall below 25 mL/ hour or 600 mL/day)
- Monitor vital signs during IV therapy; infuse magnesium replacement slowly; watch for bradycardia, heart block, and decreased respiratory rate
- Have calcium gluconate IV available to reverse hypermagnesemia from overcorrection

Hypermagnesemia
- Frequently check level of consciousness (LOC), muscle activity, and vital signs
- Keep accurate intake and output records; provide sufficient fluids
- Correct abnormal serum electrolyte levels immediately
- Monitor the client receiving cardiac glycosides and calcium gluconate simultaneously

Metabolic acidosis
Accumulation of excess hydrogen ions in the body or excessive loss of bicarbonate from the body

Key signs and symptoms
- Central nervous system depression
- Kussmaul respirations
- Lethargy

Key test results
- Arterial blood gas (ABG) analysis: pH below 7.35; bicarbonate level less than 24 mEq/L

Key treatments
- Correction of underlying cause
- Sodium bicarbonate IV or orally

Key interventions
- Keep sodium bicarbonate ampules handy
- Frequently monitor vital signs, laboratory results, and LOC
- Record intake and output

Metabolic alkalosis
- Accumulation of excess bicarbonate in the body or excessive removal of acid from the body

Key signs and symptoms
- Atrial tachycardia
- Confusion
- Diarrhea
- Hypoventilation
- Twitching
- Vomiting

Key test results
- ABG analysis: pH greater than 7.45; bicarbonate level above 29 mEq/L

Key treatments
- Treatment of underlying cause
- Acidifying agent: ammonium chloride IV

Key interventions
- Monitor ammonium chloride 0.9% infusion
- Monitor vital signs and record intake and output

Multiple myeloma
Proliferation of malignant plasma cells in the bone marrow

Key signs and symptoms
- Anemia, thrombocytopenia, hemorrhage
- Constant, severe bone pain
- Pathologic fractures, skeletal deformities of the sternum and ribs, loss of height

Key test results
- Bence Jones protein assay is positive
- X-ray shows diffuse, round, punched-out bone lesions, osteoporosis, osteolytic

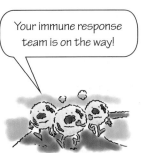

Your immune response team is on the way!

lesions of the skull; and widespread demineralization
- Bone marrow biopsy confirms diagnosis with the presence of sheets of plasma cells

Key treatments
- Orthopedic devices: braces, splints, casts
- Alkylating agents: melphalan, cyclophosphamide
- Androgen: fluoxymesterone
- Antibiotics: doxorubicin, plicamycin
- Antigout agent: allopurinol
- Antineoplastics: vinblastine, vincristine
- Glucocorticoid: prednisone
- Proteasome inhibiting agent: bortezomib

Key interventions
- Monitor renal status
- Evaluate bone pain
- Maintain IV fluids

Pernicious anemia
Vitamin B_{12} deficiency caused by lack of the intrinsic factor produced by gastric mucosa

Key signs and symptoms
- Paresthesia of hands and feet
- Weight loss, anorexia, dyspepsia
- Smooth, sore, bright red tongue
- Cheilosis

Key test results
- Bone marrow aspiration shows increased megaloblasts, few maturing erythrocytes, defective leukocyte maturation
- Schilling test
- Peripheral blood smear reveals oval, macrocytic, hyperchromic erythrocytes

Key treatment
- Vitamins: pyridoxine (vitamin B_6), ascorbic acid (vitamin C), cyanocobalamin (vitamin B_{12}), folic acid (vitamin B_9)

Key interventions
- Monitor cardiovascular status
- Administer medications as prescribed
- Provide mouth care before and after meals
- Prevent the client from falling

Phosphorus imbalance
Hypophosphatemia
- Decrease in blood phosphorus level

Hyperphosphatemia
- Increase in blood phosphorus level

Key signs and symptoms
Hypophosphatemia
- Muscle weakness

- Paresthesia
- Tremor

Hyperphosphatemia
- Usually produces no symptoms

Key test results
Hypophosphatemia
- Serum phosphorus level less than 1.7 mEq/L (or 2.5 mg/dL)
- Urine phosphorus level greater than 1.3 g/24 hours supports this diagnosis

Hyperphosphatemia
- Serum phosphorus level greater than 2.6 mEq/L (or 4.5 mg/dL)
- Supportive values include decreased levels of serum calcium (less than 9 mg/dL) and urine phosphorus (less than 0.9 g/24 hours)

Key treatments
Hypophosphatemia
- High-phosphorus diet
- Phosphate supplements

Hyperphosphatemia
- Low-phosphorus diet
- Calcium supplement: calcium acetate

Key interventions
Hypophosphatemia
- Record intake and output accurately; assess renal function; be alert for hypocalcemia when giving phosphate supplements
- Advise client to follow high-phosphorus diet containing milk and milk products, kidney, liver, turkey, and dried fruits

Hyperphosphatemia
- Monitor intake and output; notify health care provider immediately if urine output falls below 25 mL/hour or 600 mL/day
- Watch for signs of hypocalcemia (e.g., muscle twitching, tetany) which commonly accompany hyperphosphatemia
- Advise client to eat foods low in phosphorus (e.g., vegetables); obtain dietary consultation if condition results from chronic renal insufficiency

---

Polycythemia vera
Overproduction of erythrocytes in the bone marrow

Key signs and symptoms
- Clubbing of the digits
- Dizziness
- Headache
- Hypertension
- Ruddy cyanosis of the nose
- Thrombosis of smaller vessels
- Visual disturbances (blurring, diplopia, engorged veins of fundus and retina)

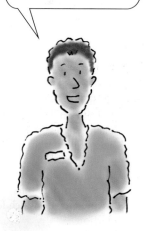

A deficiency of B_{12} is only pernicious without medical intervention.

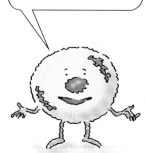

We immune cells sometimes get a little confused and attack your body ... sorry about that.

Key test results

- Elevated hemoglobin, RBC count, WBC count, platelet count, and leukocyte alkaline phosphatase, serum B_{12}, and uric acid levels; low levels of erythropoietin

Key treatments

- Phlebotomy: 350 to 500 mL of blood (typically) removed every other day until client's HCT is reduced to the low-normal range
- Antimetabolites: hydroxyurea
- Antiplatelet aggregation: anagrelide
- Plasmapheresis
- Antineoplastics: busulfan, chlorambucil, melphalan
- Antigout agent: allopurinol

Key interventions

- Check blood pressure, pulse rate, and respirations before and during phlebotomy
- During phlebotomy, make sure the client is lying down comfortably
- Stay alert for tachycardia, clamminess, or reports of vertigo; procedure should be stopped if these occur
- Check blood pressure and pulse rate after phlebotomy; Have client sit up for about 5 minutes before allowing him to walk; administer 24 oz (710 mL) of juice or water
- Tell client to watch for and report symptoms of iron deficiency (pallor, weight loss, weakness, glossitis)
- Give additional fluids, administer allopurinol, alkalinize the urine
- Warn client who develops leukopenia that resistance to infection is low; advise to avoid crowds, watch for symptoms of infection
- Tell client about possible adverse effects of alkylating agents (nausea, vomiting, risk of infection)
- Have client lie down during IV administration and for 15 to 20 minutes afterward

Rheumatoid arthritis

Chronic, systemic, autoimmune disease causing inflammation of the joints and related structures

Key signs and symptoms

- Painful, swollen joints; crepitus; morning stiffness
- Symmetrical joint swelling (mirror image of affected joints)

Key test results

- Antinuclear antibody test: Positive
- Rheumatoid factor test: Positive

Key treatments

- Cold therapy during acute episodes
- Heat therapy to relax muscles and relieve pain in chronic disease
- Disease-modifying antirheumatic drugs (DMARDs): etanercept, adalimumab, abatacept, cyclophosphamide, methotrexate, tofacitinib, hydroxychloroquine
- Cyclo-oxygenase-2 inhibitor: celecoxib
- Glucocorticoids: prednisone, hydrocortisone
- Nonsteroidal anti-inflammatory drugs (NSAIDs): indomethacin, ibuprofen, sulindac, piroxicam, flurbiprofen, diclofenac sodium, naproxen, diflunisal

Key interventions

- Check joints for swelling, pain, redness
- Splint inflamed joints
- Provide warm or cold therapy as prescribed

Scleroderma

Progressive, systemic, autoimmune disease involving fibrosis of the skin and connective tissue

Key signs and symptoms

- Pain
- Signs and symptoms of Raynaud phenomenon (e.g., blanching, cyanosis, erythema of the fingers and toes) in response to stress or exposure to cold
- Stiffness
- Swelling of fingers and joints
- Taut, shiny skin over the entire hand and forearm
- Tight and inelastic facial skin, causing masklike appearance and "pinching" of the mouth
- Signs and symptoms of renal involvement, usually accompanied by malignant hypertension, the main cause of death

Key test results

- Slightly elevated erythrocyte sedimentation rate (ESR), positive rheumatoid factor in 25% to 35% of clients, positive antinuclear antibody test
- Skin biopsy may show changes consistent with progress of the disease (e.g., marked thickening of the dermis, occlusive vessel changes)

Key treatments

- Physical therapy to maintain function and promote muscle strength
- Immunosuppressants: cyclosporine, cyclophosphamide, azathioprine, mycophenolate

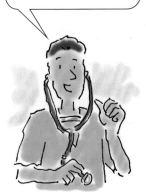

Blanching, cyanosis, and reddening of fingers and toes in the cold— what condition does this sound like?

Key interventions

- Evaluate: motion restrictions, pain, vital signs, intake and output, respiratory function, daily weight
- Teach client to monitor blood pressure at home, report any increases above baseline
- Whenever possible, let client participate in treatment

Septic shock

Type of shock that occurs in severe infection and sepsis

Key signs and symptoms

Early stage
- Chills
- Oliguria
- Sudden fever (over 101° F [38.3° C])

Late stage
- Altered LOC
- Anuria
- Hyperventilation
- Hypotension
- Hypothermia
- Restlessness
- Tachycardia
- Tachypnea

Key test results

- Blood cultures isolate the organism
- Decreased platelet count and leukocytosis (15,000 to 30,000/μL), increased blood urea nitrogen (BUN) and creatinine levels, decreased creatinine clearance, abnormal PT and PTT

Key treatments

- Removing and replacing any IV or urinary drainage catheters that may be the source of infection
- Oxygen therapy (may require endotracheal intubation and mechanical ventilation)
- Colloid or crystalloid infusion to increase intravascular volume
- Diuretic: furosemide after sufficient fluid volume has been replaced to maintain urine output above 20 mL/hour
- Antibiotics: according to sensitivity of causative organism
- Human-activated protein C: drotrecogin alfa
- Vasopressors: dopamine, norepinephrine, or phenylephrine, if fluid resuscitation fails to increase blood pressure

Key interventions

- Remove any IV or urinary drainage catheters and send to laboratory; new catheters can be reinserted

- Maintain IV infusion with normal saline solution or lactated Ringer solution, usually using large-bore (14G to 18G) catheter
- If systolic blood pressure drops below 80 mm Hg, increase oxygen flow rate and call health care provider immediately
- Keep accurate intake and output records
- Administer antibiotics IV and monitor drug levels

Sickle cell anemia

Chronic, severe, genetic type of anemia characterized by crescent-shaped red blood cells, causing decrease in tissue perfusion

Key signs and symptoms

- Aching bones
- Jaundice (worsens during painful crisis), pallor
- Unexplained dyspnea or dyspnea on exertion
- Tachycardia
- Severe pain (during sickle cell crisis)

Key test results

- Low RBC counts, elevated WBC and platelet counts, decreased ESR, increased serum iron levels, decreased RBC survival, reticulocytosis
- Hb electrophoresis shows hemoglobin S

Key treatments

- Iron and folic acid supplements to prevent anemia
- IV fluid therapy to prevent dehydration and vessel occlusion
- Analgesics: meperidine or morphine (to relieve pain from vaso-occlusive crises)

Key interventions

- Apply warm compresses to painful areas; cover client with blanket
- Maintain bed rest
- Encourage fluid intake and maintain prescribed IV fluids

Sodium imbalance

Hyponatremia
- Decrease in blood sodium level

Hypernatremia
- Increase in blood sodium level

Key signs and symptoms

Hyponatremia
- Abdominal cramps
- Cold, clammy skin
- Cyanosis
- Hypotension
- Oliguria or anuria
- Seizures
- Tachycardia

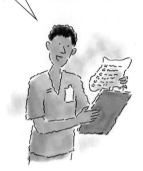

Sickle cell anemia—it's all in the genes.

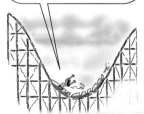

Hyper, hypo—with all these ups and downs, I must be experiencing an imbalance.

Hypernatremia
- Dry, sticky mucous membranes
- Excessive weight gain
- Flushed skin
- Hypertension
- Intense thirst
- Oliguria
- Pitting edema
- Rough, dry tongue
- Tachycardia

Key test results

Hyponatremia
- Serum sodium level less than 135 mEq/L

Hypernatremia
- Serum sodium level greater than 145 mEq/L

Key treatments

Hyponatremia
- IV infusion of saline solution
- Potassium supplement: potassium chloride (K-Lor)

Hypernatremia
- Diet: sodium restrictions
- Salt-free solution (such as dextrose in water), followed by infusion of 0.45% sodium chloride to prevent hyponatremia

Key interventions

Hyponatremia
- Watch for extremely low serum sodium and accompanying serum chloride levels; monitor urine specific gravity and other laboratory results; record fluid intake and output accurately; weigh client daily
- During administration of isosmolar or hyperosmolar saline solution, watch closely for signs of hypervolemia (dyspnea, crackles, engorged neck or hand veins)

Hypernatremia
- Measure serum sodium levels every 6 hours or at least daily; monitor vital signs for changes, especially for rising pulse rate; watch for signs of hypervolemia, especially in client receiving IV fluids
- Record fluid intake and output accurately, checking for body fluid loss; weigh client daily

Systemic lupus erythematosus

Chronic, systemic, inflammatory, autoimmune disease that can cause multiorgan failure

Key signs and symptoms
- Butterfly rash on face (rash may vary in severity from malar erythema to discoid lesions)
- Fatigue
- Migratory pain, joint stiffness and swelling

Key test result
- Lupus erythematosus cell preparation is positive

Key treatments
- Cytotoxic drug: methotrexate to delay or prevent deteriorating renal status
- Immunosuppressants: azathioprine, cyclophosphamide
- NSAIDs: indomethacin, ibuprofen, sulindac, piroxicam, flurbiprofen, diclofenac sodium, naproxen, diflunisal

Key interventions
- Evaluate musculoskeletal status
- Monitor renal status
- Provide prophylactic skin, mouth, and perineal care
- Maintain seizure precautions
- Minimize environmental stress, and provide rest periods

Vasculitis

Group of disorders that can cause inflammation of the blood vessels

Key signs and symptoms
- Wegener granulomatosis
- Cough
- Fever
- Malaise
- Signs and symptoms of pulmonary congestion
- Weight loss
- Temporal arteritis
- Fever
- Headache (associated with polymyalgia rheumatica syndrome)
- Jaw claudication
- Myalgia
- Visual changes
- Takayasu arteritis
- Arthralgias
- Bruits
- Loss of distal pulses
- Malaise
- Pain or paresthesia distal to affected area
- Syncope
- Weight loss

Key test results
- Wegener granulomatosis
- Tissue biopsy shows necrotizing vasculitis with granulomatous inflammation
- Temporal arteritis
- Tissue biopsy shows panarteritis with infiltration of mononuclear cells, giant cells within vessel wall, fragmentation of internal elastic lamina, proliferation of intima
- Takayasu arteritis

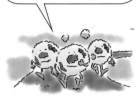

Immune cells of the body, charge! What do you mean we're going the wrong way?

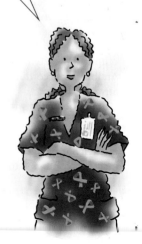

The word "-itis" refers to inflammation; so, what does "vasculitis" mean?

- Arteriography shows calcification and obstruction of affected vessels
- Tissue biopsy shows inflammation of adventitia and intima of vessels and thickening of vessel walls

Key treatments
- Removal of identified environmental antigen
- Diet: elimination of antigenic food, if identifiable

- Corticosteroid: prednisone
- Antineoplastic: cyclophosphamide

Key interventions
- Regulate environmental temperature
- Monitor vital signs. Use Doppler ultrasonic flowmeter, if available
- Monitor intake and output; check daily for edema; keep client well hydrated (3 L daily)

thePoint® You can download tables of drug information to help you prepare for the NCLEX®! View Generic Drug Names, Drug Classifications, Drug Actions, and Nursing Implications for the drugs discussed in this refresher at **http://thePoint.lww.com.**

Hematologic & immunologic questions, answers, and rationales

1. Which nutritional education should the nurse reinforce while teaching a client with acquired immunodeficiency syndrome (AIDS)? Select all that apply.
1. Thoroughly cook meats.
2. Choose foods low in fat.
3. Choose low calorie foods.
4. Weigh yourself weekly.
5. Eat small, frequent meals.

1. 1, 2, 5. To prevent food-borne illness, all meat and poultry should be cooked thoroughly. It's necessary to avoid foods high in fats because drugs used to treat AIDS may cause hyperlipidemia. Consuming small, frequent meals consisting of high-calorie, nutrient-dense food will help improve overall nutrition. Daily weights are important in determining patterns of weight loss.
CN: Physiological integrity; CNS: Basic care and comfort; CL: Apply; DIFFICULTY: Challenge

2. The nurse is caring for a client with Kaposi sarcoma with slight serous drainage. What should the nurse wear during the care of this client? Select all that apply.
1. Gloves
2. Gown
3. Surgical mask
4. Particulate mask
5. Shoe cover

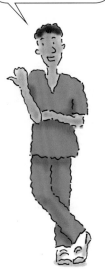

Before tackling serous drainage, you need gear up with all the right equipment.

2. 1, 2. Kaposi sarcoma is a type of skin cancer seen in clients with acquired immunodeficiency syndrome (AIDS). It is a red-brown to purplish skin lesion. The nurse should wear gloves and a gown when in contact with this client because of the serous drainage. Surgical mask is used for droplet precaution. Particulate mask is used for airborne precaution. Shoe cover is not necessary.
CN: Safe, effective care environment; CNS: Safety and infection control; CL: Apply; DIFFICULTY: Difficult

3. Immediately after giving an injection, a nurse is inadvertently stuck with the needle. When is the **best** time to test the nurse for human immunodeficiency virus (HIV) antibodies?
1. Immediately, and then again in 6 weeks
2. Immediately, and then again in 3 months
3. In 2 weeks, and then again in 6 months
4. In 2 weeks, and then again in 1 year

3. 2. The nurse should be tested immediately to determine whether a preexisting infection is present, and then again in 3 months to detect seroconversion as a result of the needlestick. Waiting 2 weeks to perform the first test is too late to detect preexisting infection. Retesting sooner than 3 months may yield false-negative results.
CN: Safe, effective care environment; CNS: Safety and infection control; CL: Apply; DIFFICULTY: Moderate

4. A nurse is assigned to a medical-surgical floor. Which client should the nurse see **first**?
1. A client with systemic lupus erythematosus (SLE) with a malar rash on face
2. A client with rheumatoid arthritis who is receiving adalimumab for inflammation
3. A client with Hodgkin lymphoma reporting fatigue and night sweats
4. A client with hemophilia who is receiving acetylsalicylic acid (ASA) for joint pain

4. 4. A client with hemophilia should be seen first because acetylsalicylic acid (ASA) or aspirin will further cause bleeding. It should not be given to a client with hemophilia. Malar rash or "butterfly" rash is usually seen in clients with SLE. Adalimumab is a tumor necrosis factor (TNF) inhibiting anti-inflammatory drug given to clients with rheumatoid arthritis. A client with Hodgkin lymphoma is expected to have fatigue and night sweats.
CN: Safe, effective care environment; CNS: Coordinated care; CL: Apply; DIFFICULTY: Moderate

CN: Client needs category   CNS: Client needs subcategory   CL: Cognitive level

5. A client with human immunodeficiency virus (HIV) experiences frequent bouts of diarrhea. The nurse determines dietary teaching is effective when the client states which food to avoid?
1. Milk
2. Red licorice
3. Chicken soup
4. Broiled meat

5. 1. Clients with chronic diarrhea may develop intolerance to lactose, which may worsen the diarrhea. Although red licorice (the candy) may be eaten, black licorice (the herb) should be avoided, as it may interfere with medications, especially corticosteroids. Other foods that the client should avoid include fatty foods, other lactose-containing foods, caffeine, and sugar. Chicken soup and broiled meat may be consumed.
CN: Physiological integrity; CNS: Reduction of risk potential; CL: Apply; DIFFICULTY: Easy

6. A disease-modifying antirheumatic drug (DMARD) is prescribed by the health care provider to a client with rheumatoid arthritis. Which medication does the nurse anticipate administering?
1. Aspirin
2. Methotrexate
3. Ferrous sulfate
4. Prednisone

6. 2. Methotrexate is considered as the first-line disease-modifying antirheumatic drug (DMARD) for most clients with RA. Ferrous sulfate isn't used to treat rheumatoid arthritis. Prednisone may be used to control inflammation when NSAIDs such as aspirin cannot be tolerated.
CN: Physiological integrity; CNS: Pharmacological therapies; CL: Apply; DIFFICULTY: Moderate

7. A client was admitted with rheumatoid arthritis. Which dietary recommendation may help reduce the inflammation associated with this disorder?
1. Consume more salmon.
2. Drink vitamin D–fortified milk.
3. Increase red meat consumption.
4. Consume more spinach.

7. 1. Salmon is high in omega-3 fatty acids. The therapeutic effect of fish oil suppresses inflammatory mediator production (such as prostaglandins); how it works is unknown. Iron-rich foods, such as spinach and red meats, are recommended to decrease the anemia associated with rheumatoid arthritis. Calcium and vitamin D found in milk may help reduce bone resorption.
CN: Physiological integrity; CNS: Physiological adaptation; CL: Apply; DIFFICULTY: Challenge

8. A client was admitted with human immunodeficiency virus (HIV). Which statement by a client would indicate the need for further education regarding safer sex practices?
1. "I should use plenty of oil-based lubricant to prevent latex condom tearing."
2. "I should inspect the condom for damage or defects before I use it."
3. "I must check the expiration date on the package before using the condom."
4. "Latex condoms are the best choice for preventing the spread of HIV."

I'll probably regret this later.

8. 1. Water-based lubricants should be used; oil- or petroleum-based products can damage latex condoms. Latex condoms or polyurethane (if the client has a latex allergy) condoms have been proven to decrease the spread of HIV. Checking for damaged, defective, or expired condoms ensures the integrity of the condoms and decreases the likelihood of HIV transmission.
CN: Health promotion and maintenance; CNS: None; CL: Analyze; DIFFICULTY: Moderate

9. The nurse is reviewing a client's complete blood count (CBC) and notes an erythrocyte count of $2.7 \times 10^6/\mu L$ ($2.70 \times 10^{12}/L$), leukocytes of $2,100/\mu L$ ($2.10 \times 10^9/L$), and thrombocytes of $90,000/\mu L$ ($90 \times 10^9/L$). The nurse interprets this as indicative of which condition?
1. Pernicious anemia
2. Aplastic anemia
3. Sickle cell anemia
4. Polycythemia

9. 2. Aplastic anemia is a pathology of bone marrow dysfunction. Bone marrow produces red blood cells, white blood cells, and platelets. Clients with aplastic anemia may have pancytopenia. Red blood cells, white blood cells, and platelets are all decreased. The normal erythrocyte (RBC) count for an adult male is $4.6 \times 10^6/\mu L$ ($4.60 \times 10^{12}/L$) to $6.2 \times 10^6/\mu L$ ($6.20 \times 10^{12}/L$) and female is $4.2 \times 10^6/\mu L$ ($4.20 \times 10^{12}/L$) to $5.4 \times 10^6/\mu L$ ($5.40 \times 10^{12}/L$). The normal leukocyte (WBC) is $4,500/\mu L$ ($4.50 \times 10^9/L$) to $11,000/\mu L$ ($11.00 \times 10^9/L$), and the normal thrombocytes (platelet) count is $150,000/\mu L$ ($150 \times 10^9/L$) to $400,000/\mu L$ ($400 \times 10^9/L$).
CN: Physiological integrity; CNS: Reduction of risk potential; CL: Analyze; DIFFICULTY: Moderate

10. Which instruction would be appropriate when reinforcing education to a client with human immunodeficiency virus (HIV) who is at high risk for altered oral mucous membranes?
  1. "Brush your teeth frequently with a firm toothbrush."
  2. "Use mouthwash that contains an astringent agent."
  3. "You always have to heat all your food."
  4. "It is important to lubricate your lips."

11. The nurse is caring for a client receiving chemotherapy. Which should the nurse consider the highest **priority**?
  1. Self-image
  2. Nutrition
  3. Family support
  4. Mobility

12. A client is admitted with hemophilia. Which sports should the nurse recommend for this client? Select all that apply.
  1. Basketball
  2. Swimming
  3. Baseball
  4. Golf
  5. Soccer

13. A client is receiving oral prednisolone. Which side effects should the nurse expect to see from prolonged use of this medication? Select all that apply.
  1. Weight loss
  2. Hyperglycemia
  3. Osteoporosis
  4. Hirsutism
  5. Cataract

14. A client with multiple myeloma was admitted with a calcium level of 14.6 mg/dL (3.65 mmol/L). Which signs and symptoms would the nurse anticipate during data collection? Select all that apply.
  1. Tetany
  2. Renal calculi
  3. Positive Chvostek sign
  4. Decreased bowel sounds
  5. Hyperactive deep tendon reflexes (DTR)

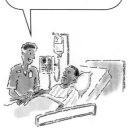

I have some ways to help you with your oral mucous membranes.

10. 4. Lubricating the lips will keep them moist and prevent cracking. A firm toothbrush would damage already sensitive gums. An astringent would be painful, as would foods that are too hot.
CN: Physiological integrity; CNS: Reduction of risk potential; CL: Apply; DIFFICULTY: Challenge

11. 2. The priority should be the client's nutritional needs because chemotherapy may cause nausea, vomiting, stomatitis, and diarrhea. All the other options are also important but not the priority. According to Maslow hierarchy of needs, physiologic needs should be met first before psychosocial needs.
CN: Physiological integrity; CNS: Basic care and comfort; CL: Analyze; DIFFICULTY: Easy

12. 2, 4. A client with hemophilia should avoid contact sports like soccer, baseball, and basketball because of the risk of bleeding with injury. The client can safely participate in noncontact sports such as swimming and golf.
CN: Safe, effective care environment; CNS: Safety and infection control; CL: Analyze; DIFFICULTY: Moderate

13. 2, 3, 4, 5. Prednisolone is a corticosteroid used for inflammation. Prolonged use of this drug will cause hyperglycemia, osteoporosis, hirsutism, and cataract formation. Client will have weight *gain* not weight loss due to fluid retention.
CN: Physiological integrity; CNS: Pharmacological therapies; CL: Apply; DIFFICULTY: Difficult

14. 2, 4. The client is having hypercalcemia. Normal calcium level is 8.5 to 10.5 mg/dL (2.1 to 2.6 mmol/L). Calcium acts like a sedative; therefore, too much calcium will cause sedative effects like lethargy, confusion, muscle weakness, decreased DTRs, and decreased bowel sounds. Renal calculi are formed because most kidney stones are calcium stones, usually in the form of calcium oxalate. Tetany and Chvostek sign are both signs of hypocalcemia where muscles are becoming tight due to a decrease in calcium. Chvostek sign is the twitching of the facial muscles in response to gentle tapping over the facial nerve in front of the ear.
CN: Physiological integrity; CNS: Physiological adaptation; CL: Apply; DIFFICULTY: Difficult

15. A nurse should be aware of the many complications that may occur as a result of human immunodeficiency virus (HIV) infection. Which scenario suggests that the client has acquired immunodeficiency syndrome (AIDS) wasting syndrome?

1. A 34-year-old male with oral pain, dysphagia, and yellow-white plaques in his mouth and throat
2. A 42-year-old female with recurrent vaginitis causing intense itching and white, thick vaginal discharge
3. A 52-year-old male with impaired memory, hallucinations, loss of balance, and personality changes
4. A 46-year-old female who has lost 12% of her body weight, with weakness, fever, and chronic diarrhea, for the past 35 days

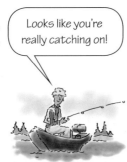

Looks like you're really catching on!

15. 4. AIDS wasting syndrome is diagnosed when there's a loss of 10% or more of body weight and the presence of one or more of the following for more than 30 days: fever, weakness, and at least two loose stools daily. Oral pain with visible yellow-white plaques and vaginitis with a white, cottage cheese-like discharge suggest infection with *Candida albicans*. Impaired intellect and motor functioning indicate HIV infection of the central nervous system with AIDS dementia complex.

CN: Physiological integrity; CNS: Physiological adaptation; CL: Analyze; DIFFICULTY: Easy

16. The nurse is making assignments for the unlicensed assistive personnel (UAP). Which tasks can be safely assigned to UAP? Select all that apply.

1. Assisting a client with a chest tube during ambulation
2. Feeding a client with swallowing difficulty
3. Teaching a client how to use the cane
4. Bathing a client with Alzheimer disease
5. Turning a client who is poorly nourished

16. 4, 5. Unlicensed assistive personnel (UAP) can safely perform bathing and turning a client. Unstable clients cannot be delegated to UAP. Assisting a client with chest tube and feeding a client with swallowing difficulty cannot be assigned to them. The registered nurse (RN) should only delegate routine tasks and tasks with lower priority. Teaching a client how to use the cane is not within their scope of UAP's practice.

CN: Safe, effective care environment; CNS: Coordinated care; CL: Apply; DIFFICULTY: Difficult

17. The nurse is collecting data on a client who has been experiencing black stools for the past month. The client suddenly reports chest and stomach pain. Which action should the nurse perform **first**?

1. Give nasal oxygen
2. Take vital signs
3. Begin cardiac monitoring
4. Draw blood for laboratory analysis

17. 2. The first step of nursing process is data collection. Taking vital signs would determine hemodynamic stability, and monitoring heart rhythm may be indicated based on data collected. Giving nasal oxygen and drawing blood require a health care provider's order and should not be part of a screening evaluation.

CN: Safe, effective care environment; CNS: Coordinated care; CL: Apply; DIFFICULTY: Moderate

18. A client arrives at the emergency department reporting chest and stomach pain and a history of black, tarry stools for the past 2 months. Which orders should the nurse anticipate?

1. Cardiac monitor, oxygen, creatine kinase, and lactate dehydrogenase (LD) levels
2. Prothrombin time (PT), partial thromboplastin time (PTT), fibrinogen, and fibrin split product values
3. ECG, complete blood count, testing for occult blood, and comprehensive serum metabolic panel
4. EEG, alkaline phosphatase and aspartate aminotransferase levels, and basic serum metabolic panel

18. 3. An ECG evaluates the report of chest pain, complete blood count (CBC) determines anemia, and the test for occult blood determines blood in the stool. Cardiac monitoring, oxygen, creatine kinase, and LD levels are appropriate for a cardiac primary problem. A basic metabolic panel (includes glucose, electrolytes, BUN, creatinine) and alkaline phosphatase and aspartate aminotransferase levels assess liver function. PT, PTT, fibrinogen, and fibrin split products are measured to verify bleeding dyscrasias. An EEG evaluates brain electrical activity.

CN: Physiological integrity; CNS: Reduction of risk potential; CL: Analyze; DIFFICULTY: Easy

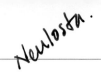

19. A nurse is reinforcing client teaching about the adverse effects of pegfilgrastim. The nurse should tell the client to immediately report which adverse effect of the drug?
1. Signs of thyroid crisis
2. Sickle cell crisis
3. Signs of addisonian crisis
4. Signs of hypertensive crisis

20. A nurse in a family health clinic is caring for a client with a hemoglobin level of 9 g/dL (90 g/L). What should the nurse inform the client?
1. Restrict activity as much as possible.
2. Eat foods high in calcium.
3. Have activities spaced to allow for rest periods.
4. Be supervised when ambulating.

21. A client is scheduled for a magnetic resonance imaging (MRI). Which situation would require further data collection?
1. The client has history of leukemia
2. The client is allergic to barium
3. The client is afraid of using elevators
4. The client is sensitive to light

22. Which client assigned to the nurse has the highest risk of developing anemia?
1. A client with a colostomy following colon resection
2. A client with gastroesophageal reflux disease (GERD)
3. A client who has had a gastrectomy
4. A client with dumping syndrome

23. A nurse is caring for a client who has had a bone marrow transplant. Which nursing intervention has the **priority**?
1. Assisting the client with daily hygiene needs
2. Listening to the breath sounds every 2 hours
3. Palpating the client's pulses every 2 hours
4. Administering pain medication as necessary

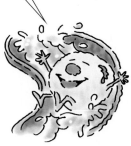

Leukocytes are delivered quickly to the site of an infection.

19. 2. Pegfilgrastim is a leukocyte growth factor used to stimulate the production of white blood cells (WBC). It is used to decrease the incidence of infection in clients with neutropenia. Adverse effects include severe allergic reactions, acute respiratory distress syndrome (ARDS), sickle cell crises, and spleen rupture. The other options are not related to pegfilgrastim use.
CN: Physiological integrity; CNS: Pharmacological therapies; CL: Apply; DIFFICULTY: Moderate

20. 3. The normal hemoglobin for male is 14-18 g/dL (140-180 g/L) and female is 12-16 g/dL (120-160 g/L). Clients with anemia become fatigued easily and need rest between activities to conserve energy. Activities don't need to be severely restricted for clients with anemia. The client needs to eat food that's high in iron (not calcium), such as lean red meat and fortified breakfast cereal. The client doesn't need close supervision when walking.
CN: Physiological integrity; CNS: Physiological adaptation; CL: Apply; DIFFICULTY: Easy

21. 3. During magnetic resonance imaging (MRI), the client will be confined in a small enclosed tube-shaped machine. The client who is afraid of using an elevator needs further data collection because that may indicate claustrophobia. The other options are not associated with MRI.
CN: Physiological integrity; CNS: Reduction of risk potential; CL: Apply; DIFFICULTY: Difficult

22. 3. Lack of intrinsic factor following gastrectomy would cause pernicious anemia due to the client's inability to absorb vitamin B_{12}. The presence of a colostomy, GERD, or dumping syndrome would not place a client at risk for developing anemia.
CN: Physiological integrity; CNS: Physiological adaptation; CL: Apply; DIFFICULTY: Moderate

23. 2. The two major complications of bone marrow transplantation are bleeding and infection. Listening to the client's breath sounds frequently, comparing them to his baseline, and reporting any congestion immediately will help prevent complications due to infection. Although hygiene and comfort needs should be addressed, they don't take priority over assessing for infection. Collecting data for potentially impaired peripheral circulation isn't a priority for clients after a bone marrow transplant.
CN: Physiological integrity; CNS: Reduction of risk potential; CL: Apply; DIFFICULTY: Challenge

24. In community health and epidemiologic studies, which definition of disease *prevalence* is correct?
1. The number of individuals affected by a particular disease at a specific time
2. The rate at which individuals without a specific disease develop that disease
3. The proportion of individuals affected by the disease who live for a particular period
4. The proportion of individuals without the disease who eventually develop the disease within a specific period

25. A nurse is reinforcing teaching instructions for a client with microcytic anemia about choosing combinations of foods to increase non-heme iron absorption. Which foods should the nurse include?
1. Enriched breakfast cereal and hot tea
2. Eggs and yogurt
3. Chicken and brown rice
4. Split pea soup with ham

26. A nurse has instructed a client about taking ferrous sulfate liquid preparation. Which statement by the client indicates the need for additional education?
1. "I should take the iron with an antacid to prevent gastric distress."
2. "I expect my stools to be dark green or black."
3. "I should rinse my mouth with water after taking the iron."
4. "I should add the iron to juice and drink it with a straw."

27. A nurse is caring for a client with rheumatoid arthritis. When should the nurse **best** schedule the client for ambulation?
1. When the client first awakens in the morning
2. After returning from physical therapy
3. After the client has a bath
4. Just before the noontime meal

28. The nurse is caring for a client who has just had a total hip replacement. Which condition is the client at greatest risk for developing?
1. Anemia
2. Polycythemia
3. Purpura
4. Thrombocytopenia

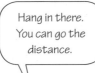

Hang in there. You can go the distance.

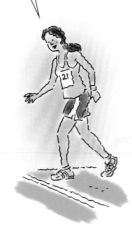

24. 1. *Prevalence* is the number of individuals affected by the disease at a specific time. *Risk* is the proportion of individuals without the disease who develop the disease within a particular period. *Incidence rate* is the rapidity with which individuals without the disease contract it. *Survival* is the proportion of individuals affected by the disease who live for a particular length of time.
CN: Health promotion and maintenance; CNS: None; CL: Understand; DIFFICULTY: Moderate

25. 4. Combining a non-heme iron source (split pea soup) with a heme iron source (ham) increases absorption of non-heme iron. Tea, calcium (in yogurt), and phytates (brown rice) block iron absorption.
CN: Physiological integrity; CNS: Basic care and comfort; CL: Analyze; DIFFICULTY: Difficult

26. 1. Antacids will interfere with absorption of iron and should be avoided. Dark green or black stools are a common adverse effect of iron supplements. Rinsing his mouth after swallowing liquid iron and drinking the liquid iron through a straw will help the client prevent discoloration of his teeth from contact with the iron preparation.
CN: Physiological integrity; CNS: Pharmacological therapies; CL: Apply; DIFFICULTY: Easy

27. 3. Warmth, and the movement of the extremities during a bath, eases the stiffness and pain of rheumatoid arthritis. Ambulation when the client first awakens is the worst time because pain and stiffness are greatest after long periods of immobility. The client may be too tired to walk soon after returning from therapy. There's no relationship between eating and ease of ambulation in rheumatoid arthritis.
CN: Physiological integrity; CNS: Basic care and comfort; CL: Understand; DIFFICULTY: Moderate

28. 1. Surgery is a risk factor for anemia. Polycythemia can occur from severe hypoxia due to congenital heart and pulmonary disease. Purpura and thrombocytopenia may result from decreased bone marrow production of platelets, but not from surgery.
CN: Physiological integrity; CNS: Reduction of risk potential; CL: Apply; DIFFICULTY: Challenge

29. The nurse is preparing medications for the client. Which prescriptions should the nurse question?
1. The clopidogrel to a client who is being prepared for a major surgery
2. The fondaparinux sodium to a client who had open reduction internal fixation (ORIF)
3. The pegfilgrastim to a client with a low white blood cell count
4. The emtricitabine to a client with acquired immunodeficiency syndrome

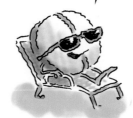

Sometimes you may need to give your medications a vacation for a while.

29. **1.** Clopidogrel is an anti-platelet drug that should be stopped 7 days prior to surgery because it can increase the risk of bleeding. Fondaparinux sodium can be given to a client who had ORIF to prevent blood clot formation. Pegfilgrastim is given to a client with low white blood cell (WBC) count. Emtricitabine is a non-nucleoside reverse transcriptase inhibitor (NNRTI) drug used for clients with HIV/AIDS.
CN: Physiological integrity; CNS: Pharmacological therapies; CL: Apply; DIFFICULTY: Difficult

30. A client was admitted with a platelet count of 95,000/µL (95×10^9/L). What would the nurse anticipate during data collection?
1. Weakness and fatigue
2. Dizziness and vomiting
3. Bruising and petechiae
4. Light-headedness and nausea

30. **3.** The normal thrombocytes (platelet) count is 150,000/µL (150×10^9/L) to 400,000/µL (400×10^9/L). The client has thrombocytopenia or low platelet count. Platelets are necessary for clot formation, so petechiae and bruising are signs of a decreased number of platelets. Weakness and fatigue are signs of anemia. Light-headedness, nausea, dizziness, and vomiting are *not* usual signs of thrombocytopenia.
CN: Physiological integrity; CNS: Reduction of risk potential; CL: Analyze; DIFFICULTY: Easy

31. The nurse has instructed the client on self-administration of heparin injections. The nurse determines that teaching is effective when the client makes which statement?
1. "Heparin slows the time it takes for the blood to clot."
2. "Heparin stops the blood from clotting."
3. "Heparin thins the blood."
4. "Heparin dissolves clots."

31. **1.** Heparin prolongs the time needed for blood to clot; however, it doesn't thin the blood. If given in large doses, heparin may stop the blood from clotting; however, this isn't why heparin is usually given. Heparin doesn't dissolve clots.
CN: Physiological integrity; CNS: Pharmacological therapies; CL: Apply; DIFFICULTY: Difficult

32. The health care provider prescribes a bone marrow biopsy and a platelet transfusion for a client with a bleeding disorder. When does the nurse anticipate the platelets will be administered?
1. Immediately following the bone marrow biopsy
2. 1 to 2 hours before the bone marrow biopsy
3. Immediately before the start of the bone marrow biopsy
4. Slowly during the bone marrow biopsy

32. **3.** Administering platelets immediately before beginning an invasive procedure increases the number of circulating platelets and therefore provides the greatest protection from potential hemorrhage. Administering platelets following the procedure may have some benefit but isn't as effective and may not prevent hemorrhage. Administering platelets too early may result in fewer circulating platelets during the procedure. Platelets are fragile and are administered as rapidly as the client can tolerate to minimize their destruction.
CN: Physiological integrity; CNS: Reduction of risk potential; CL: Analyze; DIFFICULTY: Difficult

33. A client with thrombocytopenia, secondary to leukemia, develops epistaxis. What should the nurse instruct the client to do?
1. Lie supine with his neck extended
2. Sit upright, leaning slightly forward
3. Tilt head backward while pinching the nose
4. Pinch nose while bending forward at the waist

33. **2.** The upright position, leaning slightly forward, avoids increasing the vascular pressure in the nose and helps the client avoid aspirating blood. Lying supine won't prevent aspiration of blood. Nose blowing can dislodge any clotting that has occurred. Bending at the waist increases vascular pressure and promotes bleeding rather than stopping it.
CN: Physiological integrity; CNS: Physiological adaptation; CL: Apply; DIFFICULTY: Moderate

34. A client is receiving oprelvekin. Which laboratory value shows the effectiveness of the drug?
1. Hemoglobin of 13 g/dL (130 g/L)
2. Hematocrit of 44% (0.44)
3. White blood cell count of 7,000/μL (7.00 × 10⁹/L)
 4. Platelet of 350,000/μL (350 × 10⁹/L)

35. A pregnant woman arrives at the emergency department with abruptio placentae at 34 weeks gestation. Which blood dyscrasia should the nurse closely monitor for?
1. Thrombocytopenia
2. Idiopathic thrombocytopenic purpura (ITP)
3. Disseminated intravascular coagulation (DIC)
4. Heparin-associated thrombocytopenia and thrombosis (HATT)

36. Which statement by a client with sickle cell disease indicates further education is needed to reinforce the therapeutic regimen?
1. "I should avoid vacationing or traveling in areas of high altitude."
2. "Cigarette smoking can cause a sickle cell crisis."
3. "I should drink 4 to 6 L of fluids each day."
4. "I should take one baby aspirin daily to help prevent sickle cell crisis."

37. Which laboratory test, besides a platelet count, is **best** for confirming the diagnosis of essential thrombocytopenia?
1. Bleeding time
2. Complete blood count (CBC)
3. Immunoglobulin (Ig) G level
4. Prothrombin time (PT) and International Normalized Ratio (INR)

38. Which statement is an example of passive acquired immunity?
1. A child receives the necessary immunizations before beginning school.
2. After having chickenpox, a teenager is unlikely to get the disease again.
3. A nurse who was inadvertently exposed to hepatitis B virus from a needlestick receives hepatitis B immune globulin.
4. An adult develops shingles.

Sir—you are just begging for a sickle cell crisis.

34. 4. Oprelvekin is given to a client with thrombocytopenia to stimulate the production of platelets. The other options are unrelated to the drug's effectiveness.
CN: Physiological integrity; CNS: Pharmacological therapies; CL: Apply; DIFFICULTY: Moderate

35. 3. Abruptio placentae is a cause of DIC because of activation of the clotting cascade after hemorrhage. Thrombocytopenia results from decreased bone marrow production. ITP can result in DIC but not because of abruptio placentae. A client with abruptio placentae wouldn't receive heparin and, as a result, wouldn't be at risk for HATT.
CN: Physiological integrity; CNS: Reduction of risk potential; CL: Apply; DIFFICULTY: Moderate

36. 4. Aspirin inhibits platelet aggregation and won't help prevent sickle cell crisis. Hydroxyurea is prescribed for some people to help prevent sickle cell crisis. High altitudes increase oxygen demand and therefore can also precipitate a crisis. Tobacco, alcohol, and dehydration can precipitate a sickle cell crisis and should be avoided.
CN: Physiological integrity; CNS: Reduction of risk potential; CL: Apply; DIFFICULTY: Moderate

37. 1. After a platelet count, the best test to determine thrombocytopenia is bleeding time. The platelet count is decreased and bleeding time is prolonged. IgG assays are nonspecific but may help determine the diagnosis. A CBC shows the hemoglobin levels, hematocrit, and white blood cell values. PT and INR evaluate the effect of warfarin therapy.
CN: Physiological integrity; CNS: Physiological adaptation; CL: Apply; DIFFICULTY: Challenge

38. 3. Immune globulin provides a temporary immunity that's passively acquired. Antibodies from one person are recovered and administered to another person to help prevent him from being infected. Since the recipient's immune system didn't make the antibodies, the immunity is considered to be passively acquired. Immunizations and actual disease processes, such as chickenpox, cause the body to manufacture antibodies against future exposure to these specific antigens; this is called *active immunity.* Active immunity produces antibodies that are either permanent or longer lasting than passively acquired immunity. Shingles develops when latent varicella zoster virus is activated. Varicella zoster is the virus that causes chickenpox.
CN: Physiological integrity; CNS: Reduction of risk potential; CL: Understand; DIFFICULTY: Difficult

39. The nurse is reviewing the client's laboratory report, noted below.

Laboratory results

Test	Result
Sodium	138 mEq/L (138 mmol/L)
Potassium	4.1 mEq/L (4.1 mmol/L)
Chloride	99 mEq/L (99 mmol/L)
Calcium	5.2 mg/dL (1.3 mmol/L)
Magnesium	1.5 mEq/L (0.75 mmol/L)
Phosphorus	3.1 mg/dL (1 mmol/L)

Based on the results, which interventions should the nurse anticipate to be included in the care plan? Select all that apply.
1. Administer sodium polystyrene per health care provider's order
2. Encourage client to eat sardines, tofu, rhubarb, and collard greens
3. Administer magnesium sulfate per health care provider's order
4. Observe for muscle cramps and hyperactive deep tendon reflexes
5. Limit fluid intake and monitor for jugular vein distension (JVD)

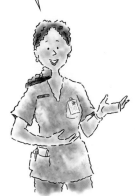

Can you spot which laboratory result is abnormal? That's the key to getting this one right.

39. 2, 4. The client has hypocalcemia. The normal calcium level is 8.5 to 10.5 mg/dL (2.1 to 2.6 mmol/L). The nurse should encourage the client to eat foods high in calcium like sardines, tofu, rhubarb, and collard greens. The nurse should also monitor the client for signs and symptoms of hypocalcemia, which includes muscle cramps, tetany, positive Chvostek sign, positive Trousseau sign, arrhythmias, and hyperactive deep tendon reflexes. All the other laboratory results are normal. Sodium polystyrene sulfonate is used to lower potassium in clients with hyperkalemia. It is not necessary to administer magnesium sulfate since the magnesium level is normal. The client has no fluid volume overload so there's no need to limit fluid and monitor for jugular vein distension (JVD).

CN: Physiological integrity; CNS: Reduction of risk potential; CL: Analyze; DIFFICULTY: Difficult

40. A nurse is reinforcing teaching instructions to a client about saquinavir. Which adverse effects would the nurse include in the teaching?
1. Hypoglycemia
2. Thrombocytopenia
3. Leukocytosis
4. Hypolipidemia

40. 2. Saquinavir is an antiretroviral-protease inhibitor drug used in combination with other antiretroviral medications to help manage human immunodeficiency virus (HIV) infection. Adverse effects include hyperglycemia, bone loss, hypersensitivity reaction, hyperlipidemia, thrombocytopenia, and leukopenia.

CN: Physiological integrity; CNS: Pharmacological therapies; CL: Apply; DIFFICULTY: Difficult

41. The nurse is making assignments for the next shift. Which clients can be assigned to a licensed practical nurse/licensed vocational nurse (LPN/LVN)? Select all that apply.
1. A client who just had coronary artery bypass graft (CABG)
2. A client who needs initial admission assessment
3. A client who needs assistance with colostomy irrigation
4. A client who is receiving insulin glargine subcutaneously
5. A client who has C3 to C5 spine injury

41. 3, 4. An LPN/LVN can perform colostomy irrigation and administer subcutaneous injections. A client who just had CABG is unstable and needs to be monitored by an RN. The initial admission assessment should also be performed by an RN. C3 to C5 injury may cause respiratory compromise. Possible paralysis of diaphragm due to phrenic nerve involvement may occur. This client is unstable and should be assigned to an RN.

CN: Safe, effective care environment; CNS: Coordinated care; CL: Apply; DIFFICULTY: Moderate

42. A client was admitted with *Pneumocystis jirovecii* pneumonia. Which vital piece of information would the nurse expect to see from the client's chart?
1. History of diabetes
2. History of heart failure
3. History of COPD
4. History of AIDS

42. 4. *Pneumocystis jirovecii* pneumonia (PJP), formerly known as *Pneumocystis carinii* pneumonia (PCP) is a type of pneumonia caused by a fungus called Pneumocystis jirovecii. It is one of the opportunistic infections seen in clients who are immunocompromised, particularly in clients with HIV/AIDS.

CN: Safe, effective care environment; CNS: Safety and infection control; CL: Analyze; DIFFICULTY: Challenge

43. Following a kidney transplantation, a client is prescribed a combination of medications that includes steroids and cyclosporine. Which client education should the nurse reinforce?
1. Avoid eating home-canned foods.
● 2. Avoid being in crowded places.
3. Stop the medication when bleeding occurs.
4. Take acetaminophen when having fever.

43. **2.** The client should avoid situations in which infections can be transmitted because his ability to resist pathogens is diminished. Steroids impair the immune system, and cyclosporine is given to suppress the immune response and decrease the chance of transplant organ rejection. Home-canned foods should be boiled for 20 minutes and inspected before being consumed but generally pose no greater risk of infection than commercially canned foods. Steroids and cyclosporine aren't associated with bleeding tendencies and should never be stopped abruptly. Even mild febrile episodes should be reported immediately because the client's immune system is impaired, and taking medications such as acetaminophen could mask the presence of serious infections.
CN: Physiological integrity; CNS: Pharmacological therapies; CL: Apply; DIFFICULTY: Challenge

44. A nurse is caring for an older adult client. While reviewing the client's chart, the nurse noticed the laboratory results, noted below.

Laboratory results	
Test	Result
Hematocrit	61% (0.61)
BUN	32 mg/dL (11.4 mmol/L)
Sodium	159 mEq/L (159 mmol/L)

Based on the client's laboratory results, which interventions should the nurse anticipate in the care plan? Select all that apply.
1. Check for distended neck vein
2. Test urine for specific gravity
3. Weigh the client daily
4. Record input and output
5. Limit fluid intake

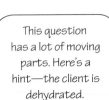

This question has a lot of moving parts. Here's a hint—the client is dehydrated.

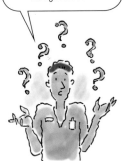

44. **2, 3, 4.** The client is experiencing dehydration. Signs and symptoms include thirst, poor skin turgor, flat neck veins, weight loss, confusion, decreased urine output, increased heart rate, thready pulse, and postural hypotension. Fluid volume deficit will cause hemoconcentration. Hematocrit, BUN, and sodium will increase whenever the blood is concentrated. The normal hematocrit for males is 40-54% (0.40-0.54) and for female is 37-47% (0.37-0.47). The normal blood urea nitrogen (BUN) is from 8-23 mg/dL (2.9-8.2 mmol/L). Sodium level normal range is from 135-145 mEq/L (135-145 mmol/L). The kidneys will compensate by conserving the remaining fluid in the body leading to a decrease in urine output. Urine specific gravity will increase because the urine is concentrated. The nurse should encourage the client to increase fluid intake.
CN: Physiological integrity; CNS: Physiological adaptation; CL: Analyze; DIFFICULTY: Difficult

45. A client diagnosed with uncomplicated rheumatoid arthritis is receiving naproxen. Which medication that the client is also taking with naproxen should the nurse discuss with the health care provider?
1. Cimetidine
2. Gabapentin
● 3. Dabigatran
4. Etanercept

45. **3.** Naproxen is a nonsteroidal anti-inflammatory drug (NSAID) used for clients with rheumatoid arthritis. NSAIDs are aspirin and aspirin-like medications that may increase the risk of bleeding when taken with an anticoagulant like dabigatran. Histamine H_2 receptor antagonist drugs used for peptic ulcer disease (such as cimetidine, anticonvulsant drug gabapentin, and a tumor necrosis factor (TNF) blocker used for rheumatoid arthritis like etanercept) will not cause serious drug interaction when taken with naproxen.
CN: Physiological Integrity; CNS: Pharmacological therapies; CL: Apply; DIFFICULTY: Difficult

46. A client is receiving 1 liter of 0.9% sodium chloride IV to be infused for 12 hours. The IV infusion set has a drop factor of 15 drops per milliliter. How many drops per minute should the nurse set the IV to infuse at? Record your answer using a whole number.

$= \dfrac{1\ liter \times .15}{12\,(60)}$

_____ gtts/min

46. 21.

$$\text{Drops per minute} = \frac{\text{mL/hr}}{60\,\text{mL/hr}} \times \text{Drop Factor}$$

$$1{,}000\,\text{mL} \times 12\,\text{hr} = 83\,\text{mL/hr}$$

$$\text{Drops per minute} = \frac{83\,\text{mL/hr}}{60\,\text{min/hr}} \times 15\,\text{gtts}$$

$$\text{Drops per minute} = 21\,\text{gtts/min}$$

CN: Physiological integrity; CNS: Pharmacological therapies; CL: Apply; DIFFICULTY: Difficult

47. A client undergoing colon cancer treatment has developed thrombocytopenia. The nurse should check the client for which manifestations? Select all that apply.
1. Diarrhea
2. Hematuria
3. Ecchymosis
4. Melena
5. Epistaxis

47. 2, 3, 4, 5. With thrombocytopenia, there's an abnormal decrease in the number of blood platelets, which can result in bleeding. Hematuria, ecchymosis, melena, and epistaxis are all signs of bleeding. The client may have constipation but usually not diarrhea.

CN: Physiological integrity; CNS: Reduction of risk potential; CL: Analyze; DIFFICULTY: Difficult

48. A client involved in a motor vehicle collision arrives in the emergency department with multiple fractures. The client is also unconscious and severely hypotensive. Which parenteral fluid would the nurse expect to administer to this client **first**?
1. Fresh-frozen plasma
2. Normal saline solution
3. Lactated Ringer solution
4. Packed red blood cells (RBCs)

48. 4. In a trauma situation, the first blood product given is unmatched (O negative) packed RBCs. Fresh frozen plasma is commonly used to replace clotting factors. Normal saline or lactated Ringer solution is used to increase volume and blood pressure, but too much colloid will hemodilute the blood and won't improve oxygen-carrying capacity as RBCs would.

CN: Physiological integrity; CNS: Physiological adaptation; CL: Apply; DIFFICULTY: Difficult

49. A nurse is monitoring a client who's receiving a blood transfusion for volume replacement. The client reports itching about 20 minutes after the infusion begins. What is the **priority** action by the nurse?
1. Report the symptom so that the infusion can be stopped immediately.
2. Call the health care provider immediately.
3. Give the client oral diphenhydramine and continue to monitor the client's symptoms.
4. Do nothing because itching is a normal response to a blood transfusion.

49. 1. Itching is a sign of an adverse reaction, so the nurse must report the symptom immediately so that the infusion can be stopped. The health care provider should be called but only after the infusion has been stopped and the client is assessed. No medications should be administered without first reporting the symptom and having the infusion stopped.

CN: Physiological integrity; CNS: Reduction of risk potential; CL: Apply; DIFFICULTY: Moderate

Any special requests for dinner? Halal it is!

50. A nurse is assigned to a practicing Muslim client. Which cultural considerations should the nurse expect in the care plan? Select all that apply.
1. Administration of blood and blood products is forbidden
2. Preference to be treated by health care worker of same sex
3. Meat products not ritually slaughtered are forbidden
4. Right hand should be used in handing over items
5. Any combination of meat and milk is forbidden
6. Organ donation and transplantation is not allowed

50. 2, 3, 4. Muslim clients prefer same-gender health care clients to take care of them. Muslims only eat "halal" meat or ritually slaughtered meat products. Eating pork is prohibited in Islam. Left hand is reserved for bodily hygiene and is considered unclean. The nurse should always use the right hand in handing over items. Organ donation is allowed for the purpose of saving life. Administration of blood and blood products is prohibited in Jehovah Witnesses. Eating meat with milk is prohibited in Judaism.

CN: Psychosocial integrity; CNS: None; CL: Analyze; DIFFICULTY: Difficult

CN: Client needs category   CNS: Client needs subcategory   CL: Cognitive level

51. A nurse is reviewing the laboratory results of a client with anemia and anticipates which lab value would be decreased?
  1. Erythrocyte count of $3.1 \times 10^6/\mu L$ ($3.10 \times 10^{12}/L$)
  2. Neutrophil count of $2,100/\mu L$ ($2.10 \times 10^9/L$)
  3. Leukocytes count of $2,300/\mu L$ ($2.30 \times 10^9/L$)
  4. Platelets count of $115,000/\mu L$ ($115 \times 10^9/L$)

52. A client who received massive packed red blood cell (PRBC) blood transfusions due to trauma has a potassium level of 7.1 mEq/L (7.1 mmol/L). Which medication should the nurse expect to administer?
  1. Insulin
  2. Potassium chloride
  3. Spironolactone
  4. Lisinopril

53. Which statement shows that a client needs more education about the cause of an exacerbation of systemic lupus erythematosus (SLE)?
  1. "I need to stay away from sunlight."
  2. "I don't have to worry if I get strep throat."
  3. "I need to work on managing stress in my life."
  4. "I don't have to worry about changing my diet."

54. Which sign or symptom reported by a client with systemic lupus erythematosus (SLE) alerts the nurse that the client may be experiencing a life-threatening complication?
  1. Joint pain
  2. Foamy urine
  3. Butterfly rash
  4. Fever

55. A nurse is reinforcing teaching instructions about the adverse reactions of kanamycin. What should the nurse include in the teaching? Select all that apply.
  1. Decreased urine output
  2. Bone damage
  3. Hearing loss
  4. Dry mouth
  5. Increased blood glucose

51. 1. Anemia is defined as a decreased number of erythrocytes (RBC). Leukopenia is a decreased number of leukocytes (WBC). Thrombocytopenia is a decreased number of thrombocytes (platelets). Neutropenia is a decreased number of neutrophils (a type of WBC).
CN: Physiological integrity; CNS: Reduction of risk potential; CL: Analyze; DIFFICULTY: Moderate

52. 1. The client is experiencing transfusion-associated hyperkalemia. Storing packed red blood cells increases the potassium concentration. IV regular insulin pushes potassium from the blood into the cell, decreasing the serum potassium level. Severe cases require hemodialysis. Potassium chloride and spironolactone, a potassium-sparing diuretic, will further increase the potassium. An Angiotensin-converting enzyme (ACE) inhibitors such as lisinopril cause hyperkalemia.
CN: Physiological integrity; CNS: Pharmacological therapies; CL: Analyze; DIFFICULTY: Difficult

53. 2. Infection may cause an exacerbation of SLE. Other factors that can precipitate an exacerbation are immunizations, sunlight exposure, and stress. A client's diet doesn't exacerbate SLE.
CN: Health promotion and maintenance; CNS: None; CL: Apply; DIFFICULTY: Moderate

54. 2. Foamy urine indicates proteinuria and is associated with kidney damage, which is a life-threatening complication of SLE. Joint pain, rashes, and fever are all common symptoms of SLE but aren't life-threatening.
CN: Physiological integrity; CNS: Physiological adaptation; CL: Apply; DIFFICULTY: Moderate

55. 1, 3. Kanamycin is an aminoglycoside antibiotic. Adverse reactions to kanamycin include ototoxicity and nephrotoxicity. Bone damage, dry mouth, and hyperglycemia are not considered adverse effects of this medication.
CN: Physiological integrity; CNS: Pharmacological therapies; CL: Analyze; DIFFICULTY: Challenge

56. The nurse is reinforcing teaching about what to expect during bone marrow aspiration. Place the following nursing actions in chronological order of how the nurse will assist the client during the procedure. Use all of the options.

| **1.** Apply direct pressure over the puncture site |
| **2.** Explain procedure and obtain consent |
| **3.** Monitor puncture site for bleeding |
| **4.** Help the client maintain position |
| **5.** Check coagulation studies |
| **6.** Position on lateral decubitus or prone |

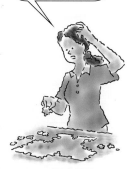

If I could just get these in the right order …

56. Ordered Response:

| **2.** Explain procedure and obtain consent |
| **5.** Check coagulation studies |
| **6.** Position on lateral decubitus or prone |
| **4.** Help the client maintain position |
| **1.** Apply direct pressure over the puncture site |
| **3.** Monitor puncture site for bleeding |

CN: Physiological integrity; CNS: Reduction of risk potential; CL: Apply; DIFFICULTY: Difficult

57. A client is receiving the drug epoetin alfa. Which findings would indicate the effectiveness of the drug?
1. Increase in white blood cells
2. Decrease in blood glucose
3. Increase in red blood cells
4. Decrease in blood coagulation

57. 3. Epoetin alfa is a synthetic form of protein human erythropoietin. It stimulates the bone marrow to produce more red blood cells (RBC). The drug is used to treat anemia caused by chronic kidney disease, chemotherapy, and zidovudine (AZT), which is a drug used to treat HIV infection.

CN: Physiological integrity; CNS: Pharmacological therapies; CL: Analyze; DIFFICULTY: Moderate

58. The nurse is reviewing laboratory results for a client suspected of having systemic lupus erythematosus (SLE). Which laboratory test results support the diagnosis of this disorder?
1. Elevated serum complement level
2. Thrombocytosis, elevated erythrocyte sedimentation rate (ESR)
3. Pancytopenia, positive antinuclear antibody (ANA) titer
4. Leukocytosis, elevated blood urea nitrogen (BUN) and creatinine levels

58. 3. Laboratory findings for clients with SLE usually show pancytopenia, positive ANA titer, and decreased serum complement levels. Clients may have elevated BUN and creatinine levels from nephritis, but the increase does *not* indicate SLE. Thrombocytosis and elevated sedimentation rate usually indicate polyarteritis nodosa, not SLE.

CN: Physiological integrity; CNS: Physiological adaptation; CL: Apply; DIFFICULTY: Moderate

59. An anemic client is admitted with pallor, fatigue, dry lips, and smooth, bright red tongue. Which diagnostic test should the nurse anticipate to confirm the client's specific type of anemia?
1. Bone marrow examination
2. Ventilation-perfusion scan
3. Schilling test
4. Tensilon test

59. 3. Smooth, bright red tongue is a sign of vitamin B_{12} deficiency. Schilling test is performed to evaluate vitamin B_{12} absorption. It is used to diagnose pernicious anemia. Pernicious anemia is caused by lack of intrinsic factor produced by gastric mucosa, which is necessary for vitamin B_{12} absorption. In Schilling test, a radioactive vitamin B_{12} is given PO and then urine is collected over the next 24 hours to measure whether vitamin B_{12} is normally absorbed. Bone marrow examination is used for aplastic anemia. Ventilation-perfusion scan is used to help diagnose a client with pulmonary embolism. Tensilon test is a test for myasthenia gravis.

CN: Physiological Integrity; CNS: Reduction of risk potential; CL: Apply; DIFFICULTY: Moderate

60. A nurse receives laboratory results for a hospitalized adult client who has acute leukemia. Referring to the provided laboratory slip, which result requires immediate reporting by the nurse?
1. RBC count
2. Hemoglobin
3. Hematocrit
4. Platelet count

60. 4. A platelet count below 20,000/uL (20 × 10⁹/L) is considered a life-threatening situation and generally requires medical treatment of immediate platelet transfusions. The RBC count, hemoglobin, and hematocrit levels are lower than normal but don't require immediate intervention if the client is asymptomatic. The WBC count is slightly elevated and would be expected in a client with leukemia.
CN: Physiological integrity; CNS: Physiological adaptation; CL: Analyze; DIFFICULTY: Moderate

61. Which signs and symptoms would indicate involvement of upper chest and neck lymph nodes in a client with Hodgkin lymphoma?
1. Fever, weight loss, and night sweats
2. Bone pain and jaundice
3. Cough, dysphagia, and stridor
4. Weight loss and malaise

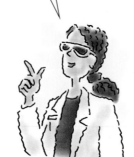

I love your swagger. Stay confident.

61. 3. Enlarged lymph nodes of the neck and upper chest can produce such symptoms as cough, dysphagia, and stridor due to pressure and obstruction of the structures of the respiratory system and esophagus. Although fever, weight loss, night sweats, and malaise are also seen with Hodgkin lymphoma, these symptoms aren't directly related to enlargement of neck and chest lymph nodes. Bone pain and jaundice may indicate bone and liver metastasis.
CN: Physiological integrity; CNS: Physiological adaptation; CL: Apply; DIFFICULTY: Moderate

62. A client is receiving aspirin. Which statement made by the client requires follow-up?
1. "I need to report if I have black stool."
2. "I'll take the medication after my meal."
3. "I can take Ginkgo biloba with aspirin."
4. "I need to report buzzing in my ears."

62. 3. Aspirin, also known as acetylsalicylic acid (ASA), is used for mild to moderate pain, fever, inflammation, and atrial fibrillation stroke prevention. Aspirin may increase the bleeding when taken with herbal supplement Ginkgo biloba. The medication can cause gastrointestinal bleeding and ototoxicity. It should be taken with food, especially if it causes stomach upset.
CN: Physiological integrity; CNS: Pharmacological therapies; CL: Analyze; DIFFICULTY: Moderate

63. When protective isolation isn't indicated, which activity is recommended for a client receiving chemotherapy?
1. Bed rest
2. Activity as tolerated
3. Walk to bathroom only
4. Out of bed for brief periods

63. 2. It's important that the client be able to engage in activities that are of interest and to maintain as much independence and autonomy as possible. Bed rest isn't necessary, nor is it necessary to limit the client's activity to just walks to the bathroom or brief periods out of the bed.
CN: Health promotion and maintenance; CNS: None; CL: Apply; DIFFICULTY: Easy

64. Which nursing intervention is **most** appropriate for a client with multiple myeloma?
1. Monitoring respiratory status
2. Balancing rest and activity
3. Restricting fluid intake
4. Preventing bone injury

64. 4. When caring for a client with multiple myeloma, the nurse should focus on relieving pain, preventing bone injury and infection, and maintaining hydration. Monitoring respiratory status and balancing rest and activity are appropriate interventions for any client. To prevent such complications as pyelonephritis and renal calculi, the nurse should keep the client well hydrated, not restrict the client's fluid intake.
CN: Safe, effective care environment; CNS: Safety and infection control; CL: Apply; DIFFICULTY: Challenge

65. A nurse is reinforcing discharge education to a client who had an anaphylactic reaction. Which recommendation is **most** appropriate for this client?
1. Dry-mop all hardwood floors.
2. Wear a medical identification bracelet at all times.
3. Have carpet installed in every room of the house.
4. Advise family and friends not to visit during the winter.

65. **2.** If the client becomes unconscious or can't report allergies, medical identification jewelry could provide that information and help health care providers intervene and treat anaphylaxis as soon as possible. The client should wet-mop hardwood floors because dry-mopping scatters dust, which can trigger allergies. The client should minimize the amount of carpet in the home because carpet traps allergens, such as dust and dirt. Unless the client is ill, the nurse may encourage visits by family and friends to promote healthy social interaction.
CN: Health promotion and maintenance; CNS: None; CL: Apply; DIFFICULTY: Easy

66. Which food should the nurse inform a client with a leukocyte (WBC) count of 2,500/μL (2.50 × 10⁹/L) to avoid?
1. White bread
2. Raw carrot sticks
3. Stewed apples
4. Well-done steak

66. **2.** The normal leukocyte (WBC) is 4.500/μL (4.50 × 10⁹/L) to 11,000/μL (11.00 × 10⁹/L). A WBC count of 2,500/μL (2.50 × 10⁹/L) is low, making the client prone to infection. A low-bacteria diet is indicated, which excludes raw fruits and vegetables.
CN: Health promotion and maintenance; CNS: None; CL: Apply; DIFFICULTY: Easy

67. A client with leukemia has neutropenia. Which function must be frequently monitored?
1. Blood pressure
2. Bowel sounds
3. Heart sounds
4. Breath sounds

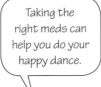

I'm feeling a little out of breath, here. Maybe I should get checked out.

67. **4.** Pneumonia—viral and fungal—is a common cause of death in clients with neutropenia, so frequent assessment of respiratory rate and breath sounds is required. Although assessing blood pressure, bowel sounds, and heart sounds is important, it won't help detect pneumonia.
CN: Physiological integrity; CNS: Physiological adaptation; CL: Apply; DIFFICULTY: Moderate

68. The nurse is gathering data on a client with pernicious anemia. Which data would support this diagnosis? Select all that apply.
1. Cracked corners of mouth
2. Smooth, bright red tongue
3. Hemoglobin of 14 g/dL (140 g/L)
4. Sensitivity to cold
5. Dyspnea on exertion

68. **1, 2, 4, 5.** Pernicious anemia is a vitamin B₁₂ deficiency due to a lack of the intrinsic factor produced by gastric mucosa. Intrinsic factor is necessary for the absorption of vitamin B₁₂. Clinical manifestations include pallor, fatigue, dyspnea on exertion, cheilosis (scaling of the surface of lips and fissures in the corner of the mouth), and sensitivity to cold. The client will also have a smooth, sore, bright red tongue because of the atrophy of the papillae of the tongue due to vitamin B₁₂ deficiency. Hemoglobin of 14 g/dL (140 g/L) is normal.
CN: Physiological integrity; CNS: Physiological adaptation; CL: Analyze; DIFFICULTY: Difficult

69. A nurse is reviewing the health care provider's prescription for a client who was admitted with fatigue, photosensitivity, and "butterfly" rash on face. Which medication would the nurse expect to find in the client's medication administration record?
1. Morphine
2. Ketoconazole
3. Hydroxychloroquine
4. Acyclovir

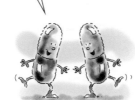

Taking the right meds can help you do your happy dance.

69. **3.** Fatigue, photosensitivity, and "butterfly" rash on face are all signs and symptoms of systemic lupus erythematosus (SLE). Hydroxychloroquine is used in the treatment of SLE to prevent inflammation. Pharmacologic treatment of SLE also involves nonsteroidal anti-inflammatory drugs (NSAIDs), corticosteroids, and immunosuppressive agents. Morphine is an opioid analgesic, ketoconazole is an antifungal agent, and acyclovir is an antiviral drug.
CN: Physiological Integrity; CNS: Pharmacological therapies; CL: Analyze; DIFFICULTY: Moderate

70. A client with multiple myeloma has developed hypercalcemia. Which nursing intervention has **priority**?
1. Protecting the client from trauma
2. Elevating the head of bed 45 degrees
3. Carefully monitoring fluid intake and output
4. Providing a quiet, darkened room

70. 3. Hypercalcemia may lead to renal dysfunction. By carefully monitoring fluid intake and output, the nurse would be alerted to decreased urine output. All clients should be protected from trauma. Elevating the head of the bed is an intervention for impaired ventilation, gastroesophageal reflux disease, and increased intracranial pressure. A quiet, dark room is commonly used to decrease sensory stimulus for clients who have meningitis or preeclampsia.
CN: Physiological integrity; CNS: Reduction of risk potential; CL: Apply; DIFFICULTY: Challenge

71. The nurse is caring for a client with multiple myeloma. Which condition should the client be closely monitored for?
1. Hypercalcemia
2. Hyperkalemia
3. Hypernatremia
4. Hypermagnesemia

71. 1. Calcium is released when bone is destroyed. This causes an increase in serum calcium levels. Multiple myeloma doesn't affect potassium, sodium, or magnesium levels.
CN: Physiological integrity; CNS: Physiological adaptation; CL: Apply; DIFFICULTY: Easy

72. A client is admitted with a serum calcium level of 6 mg/dL (1.5 mmol/L). Which signs and symptoms are associated with the result?
1. Fatigue, muscle weakness, confusion, constipation
2. Diarrhea, oliguria, headaches
3. Tremors, tetany, bradycardia, hypotension
4. Hallucinations, fainting, headaches, blurred vision

72. 1. The normal serum calcium level is 8.5 to 10.5 mg/dL (2.1 to 2.6 mmol/L). Common signs and symptoms of hypercalcemia include fatigue, muscle weakness, confusion, and constipation. Hallucinations, headaches, and hypertension are less common symptoms. Diarrhea, oliguria, fainting, and blurred vision aren't associated with hypercalcemia. Tremors, tetany, and cardiac arrhythmias are associated with hypocalcemia.
CN: Physiological integrity; CNS: Physiological adaptation; CL: Analyze; DIFFICULTY: Challenge

73. A client is admitted with multiple myeloma. Which sign or symptom should the nurse tell the client to immediately report?
1. Increased appetite
2. Back pain
3. Weight gain
4. Decreased thirst

73. 2. Back pain or paresthesia in the lower extremities may indicate impending spinal cord compression from a spinal tumor. This should be recognized and treated promptly because progression of the tumor may result in paraplegia. The other options are unrelated to multiple myeloma.
CN: Physiological integrity; CNS: Physiological adaptation; CL: Analyze; DIFFICULTY: Moderate

74. Although a client's physiologic response to a health crisis is important to the health outcome, which nursing intervention must also be addressed?
1. Educating the family on how to care for the client
2. Helping the client effectively cope with the crisis
3. Maintaining IV access, medications, and diet
4. Educating the client on basic information about the illness

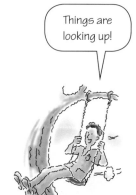

Things are looking up!

74. 2. Although all of the answers are important in the care of the client, if the individual can't cope with the emotional, spiritual, and psychological aspects of his crisis, the other components of care may be less effective as well.
CN: Psychosocial integrity; CNS: None; CL: Apply; DIFFICULTY: Moderate

75. The nurse is reinforcing client teaching about common physiologic changes of aging. Which information should the nurse include in the teaching? Select all that apply.
1. Decreased cardiac output
2. Deceased residual urine
3. Decreased elasticity of skin
4. Decreased visual acuity
5. Decreased resistance to infection

76. Which intervention should be stressed when reinforcing client education on multiple myeloma?
1. Maintaining bed rest
2. Enforcing fluid restriction
3. Drinking 3 qt (2.8 L) of fluid daily
4. Keeping the lower extremities elevated

77. A client is admitted with a serum potassium level of 6.5 mEq/L (6.5 mmol/L). Which medication should the nurse anticipate to administer?
1. Potassium chloride
2. Sodium polystyrene
3. Lisinopril
4. Spironolactone

78. An older adult client has a wound that is not healing normally. Interventions should be based on which factor?
1. Laboratory test results
2. Kidney function test results
3. Poor wound healing expected as part of the aging process
4. Diminished immune function interfering with ability to fight infection

79. A client is admitted with a platelet count of 98,000/μL (98 × 10⁹/L). Which instructions should the nurse reinforce during client education? Select all that apply.
1. Avoid using dental floss
2. Avoid using an electric razor
3. Avoid crowded places
4. Avoid eating crusty or rough foods
5. Avoid eating fresh vegetables

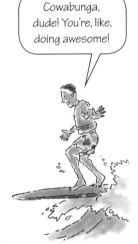

Cowabunga, dude! You're, like, doing awesome!

75. 1, 3, 4, 5. Decreased cardiac output, decreased skin turgor, decreased visual acuity, and decreased resistance to infection are all common physiologic changes of aging. There will be an *increase* in residual volume of the urine due to the decrease in muscle tone of bladder.
CN: Health promotion and maintenance; CNS: None; CL: Apply; DIFFICULTY: Difficult

76. 3. The client needs to drink 3 to 5 qt (2.8 to 4.7 L) of fluid each day to dilute calcium and uric acid and thereby reduce the risk of renal dysfunction. Walking is encouraged to prevent further bone demineralization. The lower extremities don't need to be elevated.
CN: Physiological integrity; CNS: Basic care and comfort; CL: Apply; DIFFICULTY: Moderate

77. 2. The client has an elevated serum potassium level. The normal serum potassium level is 3.5 to 5.3 mEq/L (3.5 to 5.3 mmol/L). Sodium polystyrene is used to lower serum potassium in clients with hyperkalemia. Giving potassium chloride, angiotensin-converting enzyme (ACE) inhibitor (such as lisinopril) and potassium-sparing diuretic (such as spironolactone) will further increase the serum potassium level.
CN: Physiological integrity; CNS: Pharmacological therapies; CL: Apply; DIFFICULTY: Difficult

78. 4. Immune function is important in the healing process, and diminished response may slow or prevent the healing process from taking place. Although immune function declines with age, there are healthy behaviors that will enhance the older adult's response to tissue trauma (e.g., nutrition, exercise). Kidney function and laboratory results are important but are *not solely* responsible for health outcomes.
CN: Physiological integrity; CNS: Physiological adaptation; CL: Analyze; DIFFICULTY: Moderate

79. 1, 4. The normal thrombocytes (platelet) count is 150,000/μL (150 × 10⁹/L) to 400,000/μL (400 × 10⁹/L). The client has thrombocytopenia or low platelet count, which will predispose the client to bleeding. The client should avoid using dental floss because it may injure the gums and cause bleeding. Eating crusty or rough foods like crackers, nuts, and chips may cut the inside of the mouth and cause bleeding. The use of an electric razor is recommended to avoid cuts. Avoiding crowded places and avoiding eating fresh vegetables are precautionary measures for a client with low white blood cell count.
CN: Physiological integrity; CNS: Reduction of risk potential; CL: Apply; DIFFICULTY: Challenge

80. Which intervention does the nurse determine has the **most** impact in delaying the development of acquired immunodeficiency syndrome (AIDS) once a client has been infected with human immunodeficiency virus (HIV)?

1. Monthly plasmapheresis
2. Eating a diet of balanced, nutritious foods
3. Compliance with the complete therapeutic regimen
4. Getting adequate rest and sleep

81. A client is receiving dabigatran. Which medication instruction should the nurse reinforce during client education?

1. Partial thromboplastin (PT) time and international normalize ratio (INR) will be monitored
2. Green leafy vegetables should be avoided
3. Stomach upset should be reported immediately
4. The medication should only be taken with food

82. A client is placed on neutropenic precaution. Which nursing action is appropriate?

1. Putting flowers in the room
2. Avoiding yogurt for breakfast
3. Adding fresh vegetables in the diet
4. Offering medium-rare cooked meat

83. Which additional health care provider order should a nurse anticipate for a client who has been prescribed corticosteroids?

1. Perform blood glucose checks every 6 hours.
2. Restrict fluids to 1,000 mL in 24 hours.
3. Administer lactulose 40 g in 4 oz of water daily.
4. Obtain complete blood count (CBC) every 12 hours.

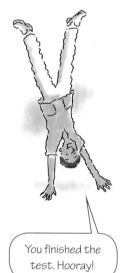

You finished the test. Hooray!

84. A nurse is assigned to a client experiencing hypovolemic shock. Which findings should the nurse expect to notice?

1. BP 132/85 mm Hg, HR 116, urine output of 45 mL/hour, warm skin
2. BP 149/92 mm Hg, HR 59, urine output of 57 mL/hour, cold skin
3. BP 87/58 mm Hg, HR 123, urine output of 20 mL/hour, clammy skin
4. BP 91/62 mm Hg, HR 99, urine output of 35 mL/hour, pale skin

80. 3. Compliance with the complete therapeutic regimen includes adhering to a healthy lifestyle, taking prescribed medications, and reducing risks from other infections. This is the most important intervention in delaying the onset of AIDS. Eating a balanced diet and getting adequate rest and sleep are part of the overall therapeutic regimen. Plasmapheresis isn't a treatment for HIV/AIDS.
CN: Health promotion and maintenance; CNS: None; CL: Analyze; DIFFICULTY: Easy

81. 3. Dabigatran is a direct thrombin inhibitor which reduces the risk of stroke, atrial fibrillation, deep vein thrombosis, and pulmonary embolism. The major side effect of this medication is bleeding. Stomach upset should be immediately reported because it may be a sign of gastric ulcer which would cause bleeding. Unlike warfarin, monitoring PT/INR and avoiding green leafy vegetables are not necessary while taking dabigatran. This medication can be taken with or without food.
CN: Physiological integrity; CNS: Pharmacological therapies; CL: Apply DIFFICULTY: Difficult

82. 2. Yogurt and yogurt products should be avoided because it has live and active cultures which may predispose a client with low white blood cells (WBC) to infection.
CN: Health Promotion and maintenance; CNS: None; CL: Apply; DIFFICULTY: Difficult

83. 1. Corticosteroids cause elevated blood glucose levels; insulin may be necessary to maintain normal blood glucose levels. Corticosteroids can cause edema, but fluid restrictions are generally unnecessary unless the client also has renal or cardiac disease. Lactulose is given for constipation and to treat hepatic encephalopathy. Hematologic studies, such as platelet counts, hemoglobin, and hematocrit levels, aren't usually necessary when monitoring clients undergoing corticosteroid therapy.
CN: Physiological integrity; CNS: Pharmacological therapies; CL: Apply; DIFFICULTY: Moderate

84. 3. Signs and symptoms of hypovolemic shock would include change in the level of consciousness; cool, clammy, and pale skin; hypotension; tachycardia; and tachypnea. The client will also have oliguria or decreased urine output because of decreased circulation of fluid volume. The normal urine output is between 30 to 50 mL/hour.
CN: Physiological integrity; CNS: Physiological adaptation; CL: Apply; DIFFICULTY: Easy

Chapter 5

Respiratory Disorders

Respiratory refresher

Acute respiratory distress syndrome

Sudden failure of the respiratory system, in which adequate oxygen is prevented from getting to the lungs or into blood

Key signs and symptoms
- Anxiety, restlessness
- Crackles, rhonchi, decreased breath sounds
- Dyspnea, tachypnea

Key test results
- Arterial blood gas (ABG) levels indicate:
  - respiratory acidosis
  - metabolic acidosis
  - hypoxemia that doesn't respond to increased fraction of inspired oxygen
- Chest x-ray indicates:
  - bilateral infiltrates (in early stages)
  - lung fields with a "ground-glass" appearance
  - (with irreversible hypoxemia) massive consolidation of both lung fields (in later stages)

Key treatments
- Intubation and mechanical ventilation using positive end-expiratory pressure (PEEP) or pressure-controlled inverse ratio ventilation
- Antibiotics most effective in treating causative organism
- Analgesic: morphine
- Neuromuscular blocking agents: pancuronium, vecuronium
- Steroids: hydrocortisone, methylprednisolone

Key interventions
- Monitor respiratory, cardiovascular, and neurologic status
- Monitor electrocardiogram (ECG)
- Maintain bed rest, with alternating supine and prone positioning if possible
- Perform turning, chest physiotherapy, and postural drainage

Acute respiratory failure

Inadequate gas exchange by the respiratory system, resulting in levels of arterial oxygen, carbon dioxide (or both) that cannot be maintained within normal limits

Key signs and symptoms
- Decreased respiratory excursion, accessory muscle use, retractions
- Difficulty breathing, dyspnea (shortness of breath), tachypnea, orthopnea
- Fatigue

Key test results
- ABG levels indicate:
  - hypoxemia
  - acidosis
  - alkalosis
  - hypercapnia

Key treatments
- Supplemental oxygen (O_2) therapy, intubation, and mechanical ventilation (possibly with PEEP)
- Analgesic: morphine
- Antianxiety agent: lorazepam
- Bronchodilators: terbutaline, theophylline; via nebulizer: albuterol, ipratropium bromide
- Neuromuscular blocking agents: pancuronium, vecuronium, atracurium besylate
- Steroids: hydrocortisone, methylprednisolone

Key interventions
- Monitor respiratory status
- Administer O_2
- Provide suctioning; assist with turning, coughing, and deep breathing; perform chest physiotherapy and postural drainage
- Maintain bed rest

Asbestosis

Serious and fatal lung disease resulting from inhaling, over time, a group of minerals with thin microscopic fibers

Key signs and symptoms
- Dry crackles at lung bases
- Dry cough

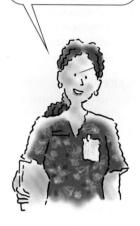

Looking for the latest information about respiratory disorders? Check out the American Association for Respiratory Care's Web site at www.aarc.org. It'll respire—er, inspire—you!

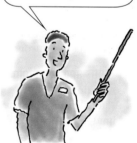

Quick—what are three key treatments for acute respiratory distress syndrome?

- Dyspnea on exertion (usually first symptom)
- Pleuritic chest pain

Key test results
- Chest x-rays:
  - show fine, irregular, and linear diffuse infiltrates; extensive fibrosis results in "honeycomb" or "ground-glass" appearance
  - show pleural thickening and calcification, with bilateral obliteration of costophrenic angles
  - in later stages, show an enlarged heart with a classic "shaggy" heart border
- Antibiotics most effective in treating causative organism

Key treatments
- Chest physiotherapy
- Fluid intake up to 3,000 mL/day
- O_2 therapy or mechanical ventilation (with advanced cases)
- Antibiotics most effective in treating causative organism (for treatment of respiratory tract infections)
- Mucolytic inhalation therapy: acetylcysteine

Key interventions
- Perform chest physiotherapy techniques (e.g., controlled coughing and segmental bronchial drainage) with chest percussion and vibration
- Administer O_2 by cannula or mask (1 to 2 L/minute); use mechanical ventilation if arterial oxygen saturation can't be maintained above 40 mm Hg

Asphyxia
Lack of oxygen or excess of carbon dioxide that results in state of unconsciousness or death

Key signs and symptoms
- Agitation
- Altered respiratory rate (apnea, bradypnea, occasionally tachypnea)
- Anxiety
- Central and peripheral cyanosis (cherry-red mucous membranes in late-stage carbon monoxide poisoning)
- Altered mental status
- Decreased breath sounds
- Dyspnea

Key test results
- Pulse oximetry reveals decreased oxygen saturation
- ABG measurement indicates:
  - decreased partial pressure of arterial oxygen (Pa_{O_2}) <60 mm Hg
  - increased partial pressure of arterial carbon dioxide (Pa_{CO_2}) >50 mm Hg

Key treatments
- O_2 therapy, which may include endotracheal (ET) intubation and mechanical ventilation
- Bronchoscopy (for extraction of a foreign body)
- Opioid antagonist: naloxone (for opioid overdose)

Key interventions
- Monitor cardiac and respiratory status
- Position the client upright, if tolerable
- Suction carefully, as needed, and encourage deep breathing

Asthma
Reactive airway disease in which airways narrow and swell, producing extra mucous and making breathing difficult

Key signs and symptoms
- Usually produces no symptoms between attacks
- Wheezing, primarily on expiration but sometimes on inspiration

Key test results
- Pulmonary function tests (PFTs) during attacks show:
  - decreased forced expiratory volumes that improve with therapy
  - increased residual volume
  - increased total lung capacity

Key treatments
- Fluid intake up to 3,000 mL/day as tolerated
- Beta-adrenergic drugs: epinephrine, salmeterol, formoterol
- Bronchodilators: terbutaline, theophylline; via nebulizer: albuterol, ipratropium bromide
- Mast cell stabilizer: cromolyn, nedocromil
- Anti-immunoglobulin E agent: omalizumab
- Inhaled corticosteroids: fluticasone, budesonide, mometasone, flunisolide

Key interventions
- Administer low-flow humidified O_2
- Monitor respiratory status and pulse oximetry values
- Keep the client in high Fowler position

Atelectasis
Collapse or closure of lung tissue, preventing normal oxygen absorption to healthy tissues

Key signs and symptoms
- Diminished or bronchial breath sounds
- Dyspnea

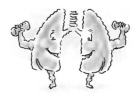

One! Two! Three! Four!" Physical exercise is a lifestyle factor that can affect oxygenation.

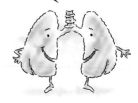

It feels great to breathe easy!

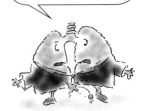

Relax or we'll start to come apart like a cheap suit!

- Low-grade fever
- In severe cases
  - anxiety
  - cyanosis
  - diaphoresis
  - severe dyspnea
  - substernal or intercostal retractions
  - tachycardia

Key test results
- Chest x-ray shows:
  - characteristic horizontal lines in the lower lung zones and, with segmental or lobar collapse, characteristic dense shadows often associated with hyper-inflation of neighboring lung zones (in widespread atelectasis)

Key treatments
- Bronchoscopy
- Chest physiotherapy
- Bronchodilators: albuterol
- Mucolytic inhalation therapy: acetylcysteine
- Pain control

Key interventions
- Encourage postoperative and other high-risk clients to cough and deep breathe every hour during their waking hours
- Postoperatively:
  - teach client to hold a pillow tightly over the incision while deep breathing or moving
  - gently reposition these clients often, and help them walk as soon as possible
- Administer adequate analgesics
- Teach client how to use an incentive spirometer and encourage him to use it hourly during waking hours
- Humidify inspired air
- Encourage adequate fluid intake
- Perform postural drainage and chest percussion
- Monitor breath sounds and ventilatory status frequently and be alert for any changes

Bronchiectasis
Condition in which lungs' airways are abnormally stretched and widened

Key signs and symptoms
- Chronic cough that produces copious, foul-smelling, mucopurulent secretions, possibly totaling several cupfuls daily
- Coarse crackles during inspiration over involved lobes or segments
- Dyspnea
- Hemoptysis
- Weight loss

Key test results
- Chest x-ray shows:
  - peribronchial thickening
  - areas of atelectasis
  - scattered cystic changes
- Sputum culture and Gram stain identify predominant organisms

Key treatments
- Bronchoscopy (to mobilize secretions)
- Chest physiotherapy
- O$_2$ therapy
- Antibiotics most effective in treating the causative organism
- Bronchodilator: albuterol

Key interventions
- Monitor respiratory status and pulse oximetry values
- Provide supportive care
- Help client adjust to permanent changes in lifestyle that irreversible lung damage makes necessary
- Perform chest physiotherapy, including postural drainage and chest percussion designed for involved lobes
  - Perform several times a day
  - Best times are early morning and just before bedtime
  - Instruct client to maintain each position for 10 minutes
  - Perform percussion and tell him to cough

Chronic bronchitis
Inflammation of bronchial tubes causing daily cough, which:
- produces mucous
- persists at least 3 months per year
- persists for at least 2 years consecutively

Key signs and symptoms
- Cyanosis
- Dyspnea
- Increased sputum production
- Productive cough

Key test results
- Chest x-ray shows:
  - Hyperinflation
  - Increased bronchovascular markings
- PFTs may reveal:
  - increased residual volume, decreased vital capacity and forced expiratory volumes, and normal static compliance and diffusion capacity

Key treatments
- Fluid intake up to 3,000 mL/day, if not contraindicated by other conditions

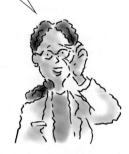

A client is suspected of having bronchiectasis. What signs should you look for?

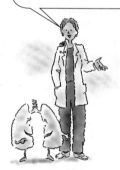

O$_2$ therapy is used to treat many respiratory disorders.

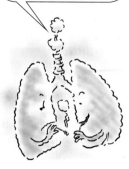

I wonder if there's any connection between this and our chronic bronchitis? Oh well—my turn.

- Intubation and mechanical ventilation, if respiratory status deteriorates
- Antibiotics most effective in treating causative organism
- Bronchodilators: terbutaline, theophylline; via nebulizer: albuterol, ipratropium bromide
- Influenza and pneumococcal vaccines
- Steroids: hydrocortisone, methylprednisolone
- Steroids (via nebulizer): beclomethasone, triamcinolone

Key interventions
- Administer low-flow O_2
- Monitor respiratory status and pulse oximetry values
- Assist with diaphragmatic and pursed-lip breathing
- Monitor and record the color, amount, and consistency of sputum
- Provide chest physiotherapy, postural drainage, incentive spirometry, and suction

Cor pulmonale
Increase in size of right ventricle caused by a disorder of the respiratory system

Key signs and symptoms
- Dyspnea on exertion
- Edema
- Fatigue
- Orthopnea
- Tachypnea
- Weakness

Key test results
- ABG analysis: decreased Pa_{O_2} (less than 70 mm Hg)
- Chest x-ray:
  - shows large central pulmonary arteries
  - suggests right ventricular enlargement by rightward enlargement of cardiac silhouette on an anterior chest film
- Pulmonary artery pressure measurements:
  - show increased right ventricular and pulmonary artery pressures because of increased pulmonary vascular resistance.

Key treatments
- O_2 therapy as necessary by mask or cannula in concentrations of 24% to 40%, depending on Pa_{O_2} and, in acute cases, mechanical ventilation
- Cardiac glycoside: digoxin
- Diuretic (to reduce edema): furosemide
- Vasodilators: hydralazine, nitroprusside, prostaglandins (in primary pulmonary hypertension)

- Calcium channel blocker: diltiazem
- Angiotensin-converting enzyme (ACE) inhibitor: captopril

Key interventions
- Monitor respiratory status and pulse oximetry values
- Monitor cardiovascular status
- Limit the client's fluid intake to 1,000 to 2,000 mL/day, and provide a low-sodium diet
- Reposition bedridden clients often
- Provide meticulous respiratory care, including O_2 therapy
- For clients with chronic obstructive pulmonary disease, teach pursed-lip breathing exercises
- Watch for signs of respiratory failure (e.g., change in pulse rate, increased fatigue from exertion, deep and labored respirations)

Emphysema
Long-term progressive disease of lungs, causing shortness of breath due to overinflation of the alveoli

Key signs and symptoms
- Barrel chest
- Dyspnea
- Pursed-lip breathing

Key test results
- Chest x-ray of clients in advanced disease stage reveals:
  - flattened diaphragm
  - reduced vascular markings in lung periphery
  - enlarged anteroposterior chest diameter
  - vertical heart
- PFTs show:
  - increased residual volume
  - total lung capacity and compliance
  - decreased vital capacity
  - diffusing capacity
  - expiratory volumes

Key treatments
- Chest physiotherapy, postural drainage, and incentive spirometry
- Fluid intake up to 3,000 mL/day, if not contraindicated by heart failure
- O_2 therapy at 2 to 3 L/minute, transtracheal therapy for home O_2 therapy
- Antibiotics most effective in treating causative organism
- Bronchodilators: terbutaline, theophylline; via nebulizer: albuterol, ipratropium bromide
- Influenza and pneumococcal vaccines

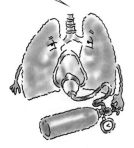

Just breathe.

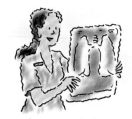

Hmm. I see some barrel chest here. Do you know what that means?

- Steroids: hydrocortisone, methylprednisolone
- Steroids (via nebulizer): beclomethasone, triamcinolone

Key interventions
- Monitor respiratory status, pulse oximetry values
- Assist with diaphragmatic and pursed-lip breathing
- Monitor and record color, amount, and consistency of sputum
- Perform chest physiotherapy, postural drainage, incentive spirometry, suction

Legionnaires disease
Serious type of lung infection or pneumonia caused by bacterium known as *Legionella*

Key signs and symptoms
- Cough, initially nonproductive, that eventually produces grayish, nonpurulent, blood-streaked sputum
- Fever
- Generalized weakness
- Malaise
- Recurrent chills

Key test results
- Chest x-ray shows patchy, localized infiltration, which progresses to multilobar consolidation (usually involving the lower lobes); pleural effusion; and, in fulminant disease, opacification of the entire lung
- Direct immunofluorescence of *Legionella pneumophila* and indirect fluorescent serum antibody testing compare findings from initial blood studies with findings from those done at least 3 weeks later; convalescent serum sample showing a 4-fold or greater rise in antibody titer for *L. pneumophila* confirms the diagnosis

Key treatments
- Antibiotics: erythromycin, rifampin, tetracycline
- Antipyretics: acetaminophen, aspirin

Key interventions
- Closely monitor client's respiratory status
- Evaluate chest wall expansion, depth and pattern of respirations, cough, and chest pain
- Monitor client's vital signs, pulse oximetry values, level of consciousness (LOC), and dryness and color of the lips and mucous membranes
- Watch for signs of shock (decreased blood pressure, thready pulse, diaphoresis, clammy skin)

- Administer IV fluids
- Provide respiratory therapy as needed
- Give antibiotics as necessary and observe carefully for adverse effects

Lung cancer
Carcinoma of the lung, characterized by uncontrollable cell growth in tissues of the lung

Key signs and symptoms
- Cough, hemoptysis
- Weight loss, anorexia

Key test results
- Chest x-ray shows lesion or mass

Key treatments
- Resection of the affected lobe (lobectomy) or lung (pneumonectomy)
- Antineoplastics: cyclophosphamide, doxorubicin, cisplatin, vincristine, vinorelbine, gemcitabine, paclitaxel, docetaxel, irinotecan

Key interventions
- Monitor client's pain level
- Administer analgesics as prescribed
- Perform suctioning and assist with turning, coughing, and deep breathing
- Monitor for bleeding, infection, and electrolyte imbalance caused by effects of chemotherapy

Pleural effusion and empyema
Excess fluid that accumulates in the pleural cavity (pleural effusion); accumulation of pus in the pleural cavity (empyema)

Key signs and symptoms
- Decreased breath sounds
- Dyspnea
- Fever
- Pleuritic chest pain

Key test results
- Chest x-ray shows radiopaque fluid in dependent regions.
- Thoracentesis results include:
  - lactate dehydrogenase (LD) levels less than 200 IU
  - protein levels less than 3 g/dL (in transudative effusions)
  - ratio of protein in pleural fluid to protein in serum greater than or equal to 0.5
  - LD in pleural fluid greater than or equal to 200 IU
  - ratio of LD in pleural fluid to LD in serum greater than 0.6 (in exudative effusions)
  - acute inflammatory white blood cells and microorganisms (in empyema)

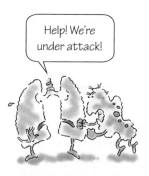

Help! We're under attack!

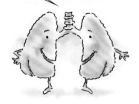

Keep us pink and healthy—put down that cigarette!

Key treatments
- Supplemental O_2 therapy
- Thoracentesis to remove fluid
- Thoracotomy if thoracentesis isn't effective
- Antibiotics most effective in treating the organism that causes empyema

Key interventions
- Explain thoracentesis to the client
- Before the procedure, tell the client to expect a stinging sensation from the local anesthetic and a feeling of pressure when the needle is inserted
- Instruct the client to tell you immediately if he feels uncomfortable or has trouble breathing during the procedure
- Administer O_2
- Administer antibiotics
- Use care when inspecting chest tube so as not to dislodge it
- Ensure chest tube patency by watching for bubbles in the underwater seal chamber
- Record amount, color, and consistency of any tube drainage

Pleurisy
Inflammation of the pleura (lining of the lungs)

Key signs and symptoms
- Pleural friction rub (a coarse, creaky sound heard during late inspiration and early expiration)
- Sharp, stabbing pain that increases with respiration

Key test results
- Diagnosis generally rests on client's history and respiratory assessment
- Diagnostic tests help rule out other causes and pinpoint underlying disorder

Key treatments
- Bed rest
- Analgesic: acetaminophen with oxycodone
- Anti-inflammatory: indomethacin

Key interventions
- Stress the importance of bed rest
- Allow client as much uninterrupted rest as possible
- Administer antitussives and pain medication as needed
- Encourage client to cough
- During coughing exercises, apply firm pressure at the pain site

Pneumocystitis pneumonia (PCP)
Form of pneumonia caused by the yeast-like fungus pneumocystis; usually found in those with weakened immune system

Key signs and symptoms
- Generalized fatigue
- Low-grade, intermittent fever
- Nonproductive cough
- Dyspnea
- Weight loss

Key test results
- Chest x-ray may show:
  - slowly progressing, fluffy infiltrates and occasionally nodular lesions or a spontaneous pneumothorax
- These findings must be differentiated from findings in other types of pneumonia or acute respiratory distress syndrome
- Histologic study results confirm *Pneumocystis jirovecii*. In clients with human immunodeficiency virus (HIV) infection, initial examination of a first morning sputum specimen (induced by inhaling an ultrasonically dispersed saline mist) may be sufficient; however, this technique is usually ineffective in clients without HIV infection

Key treatments
- O_2 therapy, which may include ET intubation and mechanical ventilation

Key interventions
- Monitor the client's respiratory status and pulse oximetry values
- Administer O_2 therapy as needed
- Encourage client to ambulate
- Encourage client to perform deep-breathing exercises and incentive spirometry
- Administer antipyretics as needed
- Monitor intake and output and weigh the client daily. Replace fluids as needed
- Administer antimicrobial drugs as ordered
  - Never give pentamidine IM
  - Administer the IV form slowly over 60 minutes
- Monitor the client for adverse reactions to antimicrobial drugs
  - If receiving sulfamethoxazole and trimethoprim, watch for nausea, vomiting, rash, bone marrow suppression, thrush, fever, hepatotoxicity, and anaphylaxis
  - If receiving pentamidine, watch for cardiac arrhythmias, hypotension, dizziness, azotemia, hypocalcemia, and hepatic disturbances
- Supply nutritional supplements as needed

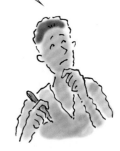

Let's see ... pleurisy is inflammation of the ...

- Encourage client to eat a high-calorie, protein-rich diet
- Offer small, frequent meals if client can't tolerate large amounts of food

Pneumonia

Lung infection that can be caused by bacteria, fungi or virus

Key signs and symptoms

- Chills, fever
- Crackles, rhonchi, and pleural friction rub on auscultation
- Dyspnea, tachypnea, and accessory muscle use
- Sputum that's rusty, green, or bloody with pneumococcal pneumonia and yellow-green with bronchopneumonia

Key test results

- Chest x-ray shows pulmonary infiltrates
- Sputum study identifies the causative organism

Key treatments

- Antibiotics most effective in treating causative organism
- Supplemental O_2 therapy; intubation and mechanical ventilation if condition deteriorates

Key interventions

- Monitor and record intake and output
- Monitor pulse oximetry values
- Monitor respiratory status
- Force fluids to 3 to 4 L/day and maintain IV fluids

Pneumothorax and hemothorax

Abnormal collection of air or gas in the pleural space (pneumothorax); pocket of blood in pleural space (hemothorax)

Key signs and symptoms

- Diminished or absent breath sounds unilaterally
- Dyspnea, tachypnea, subcutaneous emphysema, and cough
- Sharp chest pain that increases with exertion

Key test results

- Chest x-ray confirms diagnosis

Key treatments

- Chest tube to water-seal drainage

Key interventions

- Monitor and record vital signs
- Monitor respiratory status and pulse oximetry values

- Monitor chest tube site for subcutaneous emphysema
- Monitor chest tube drainage
- Evaluate cardiovascular status
- Maintain chest tube to water-seal drainage
  - the water seal chamber prevents air from entering the chest tube when the client inhales

Pulmonary embolism

Sudden blockage of a major blood vessel in the lung, usually by a blood clot

Key signs and symptoms

- Sudden onset of dyspnea, tachypnea, and crackles

Key test results

- ABG levels typically show decreased Pa_{O_2} and Pa_{CO_2}
- Lung scan shows ventilation-perfusion mismatch

Key treatments

- Vena cava filter insertion
- Anticoagulants: heparin (heparin sodium injection), warfarin
- Fibrinolytics: tissue plasminogen activator

Key interventions

- Monitor respiratory status and pulse oximetry values
- Evaluate cardiovascular status and monitor ECG
- Administer O_2

Respiratory acidosis

Inability of lungs to remove all of the carbon dioxide produced by body; usually accompanied by hypoventilation

Key signs and symptoms

- Cardiovascular abnormalities (e.g., tachycardia, hypertension, atrial and ventricular arrhythmias and, in severe acidosis, hypotension with vasodilation)

Key test results

- ABG measurements confirm presence of respiratory acidosis
  - Pa_{CO_2} exceeds the normal level of 45 mm Hg
  - pH is usually below the normal range of 7.35 to 7.45
  - client's bicarbonate level is normal in the acute stage and elevated in the chronic stage

Key treatments

- Correction of the underlying cause
- Sodium bicarbonate in severe cases

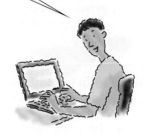

What actually causes pneumonia? My mom always said it was going outside without a coat on in winter.

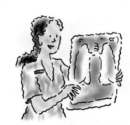

This x-ray confirms your diagnosis.

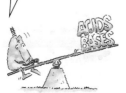

Keeping that acid-base balance in the lungs in critical.

Key interventions

- Closely monitor client's blood pH level
- Be alert for critical changes in the client's respiratory, central nervous system (CNS), and cardiovascular functions
- Maintain adequate hydration
- If acidosis requires mechanical ventilation:
  - maintain patent airway
  - provide adequate humidification
  - perform tracheal suctioning regularly and vigorous chest physiotherapy if needed

Respiratory alkalosis

Low levels of carbon dioxide due to hyperventilation

Key signs and symptoms

- Agitation
- Cardiac arrhythmias that fail to respond to conventional treatment (severe respiratory alkalosis)
- Circumoral or peripheral paresthesia (a prickling sensation around the mouth or extremities)
- Deep, rapid breathing, possibly exceeding 40 breaths/minute (cardinal sign)
- Light-headedness or dizziness (from decreased cerebral blood flow)

Key test results

- ABG analysis confirms respiratory alkalosis and rules out respiratory compensation for metabolic acidosis:
  - Pa_{CO_2} is below 35 mm Hg
  - pH is elevated in proportion to the fall in Pa_{CO_2} in acute stage
  - pH drops toward normal in chronic stage
  - bicarbonate level is normal in acute stage
  - bicarbonate level is below normal in chronic stage

Key treatments

- Instruct client to breathe into a paper bag:
  - helps relieve acute anxiety
  - increases CO_2 levels (for severe respiratory alkalosis)

Key interventions

- Watch for and report any changes in neurologic, neuromuscular, or cardiovascular function
- Monitor respiratory status

Sarcoidosis

Abnormal collection of inflammatory cells that form as nodules in different body organs

Key signs and symptoms

Initial
- Arthralgia in the wrists, ankles, and elbows
- Fatigue
- Malaise
- Weight loss

Respiratory
- Breathlessness
- Substernal pain

Cutaneous
- Erythema nodosum
- Subcutaneous skin nodules with maculo-papular eruptions

Ophthalmic
- Anterior uveitis (common)

Musculoskeletal
- Muscle weakness
- Pain

Hepatic
- Granulomatous hepatitis (usually produces no symptoms)

Genitourinary
- Hypercalciuria (excessive calcium in the urine)

Cardiovascular
- Arrhythmias (premature beats, bundle-branch block, or complete heart block)

Central nervous system
- Cranial or peripheral nerve palsies
- Basilar meningitis (inflammation of the meninges at the base of the brain)

Key test results

- Positive Kveim-Siltzbach skin test supports the diagnosis; in this test, client receives an intradermal injection of an antigen prepared from human sarcoidal spleen or lymph nodes from clients with sarcoidosis; if client has active sarcoidosis, granuloma develops at the injection site in 2 to 6 weeks; reaction is considered positive when biopsy of the skin at the injection site shows discrete epithelioid cell granuloma

Key treatments

- Low-calcium diet
- Avoidance of direct exposure to sunlight (in clients with hypercalcemia)
- O_2 therapy
- Corticosteroid: prednisone
- Cytotoxic agents: methotrexate, azathioprine

Key interventions

- Provide nutritious, high-calorie diet and plenty of fluids
- If client has hypercalcemia, suggest low-calcium diet
- Weigh client regularly

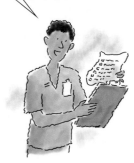

Your client is breathing at a rate of 45 breaths/minute. What respiratory condition will this lead to?

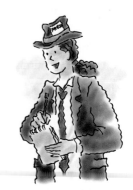

Word on the street is that sarcoidosis is a real pain in the joints. Care to comment on any other symptoms?

Severe acute respiratory syndrome (SARS)

Serious form of pneumonia caused by a virus

Key signs and symptoms
- High fever (usually greater than 100.4° F [38° C])
- Dry cough
- Dyspnea

Key test results
- History reveals recent travel to an area with documented SARS cases or close contact with a person suspected of having SARS
- Chest x-ray shows atypical pneumonia
- Reverse transcription polymerase chain reaction (RT-PCR) test detects ribonucleic acid of the SARS virus

Key treatments
- Supplemental O_2; may require ET intubation and mechanical ventilation
- Droplet precautions
- Antiviral agents: oseltamivir, ribavirin, interferon beta-1a

Key interventions
- Monitor respiratory status
- Administer supplemental O_2 as prescribed
- Maintain droplet precautions

Tuberculosis

Infection caused by mycobacterium that usually attacks the lungs but can spread to any part of the body

Key signs and symptoms
- Fever
- Night sweats

Key test results
- Mantoux skin test is positive
- Sputum study results are positive for:
  - acid-fast bacillus
  - *Mycobacterium tuberculosis*

Key treatments
- Standard and airborne precautions:
  - while client is contagious, everyone entering client's room must wear a respirator with a high-efficiency particulate air filter
- Antitubercular agents: isoniazid (INH), ethambutol, rifampin, pyrazinamide

Key interventions
- Monitor respiratory status and pulse oximetry values
- Maintain infection-control precautions
- Instruct the client to cover nose and mouth when sneezing
- Provide a room with negative-pressure ventilation

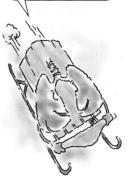

Hold on tight, partner, we're in this together!"

thePoint® You can download tables of drug information to help you prepare for the NCLEX®! View Generic Drug Names, Drug Classifications, Drug Actions, and Nursing Implications for the drugs discussed in this refresher at **http://thePoint.lww.com**.

Respiratory questions, answers, and rationales

1. Clients with chronic illnesses are more likely to get pneumonia when which situation is present?
1. Dehydration
2. Group living
3. Malnutrition
4. Severe periodontal disease

1. 2. Clients with chronic illness generally have poor immune systems. Typically, residing in group living situations increases the chance of disease transmission. Adequate fluid intake, adequate nutrition, and proper oral hygiene help maintain normal defenses and can reduce the incidence of getting such diseases as pneumonia.
CN: Physiological integrity; CNS: Physiological adaptation; CL: Understand; DIFFICULTY: Moderate

2. A client is admitted with signs and symptoms of early pneumonia. Which process should the nurse monitor the client for?
1. Atelectasis
2. Bronchiectasis
3. Effusion
4. Inflammation

2. 4. The common feature of all types of pneumonia is an inflammatory pulmonary response to the offending organism or agent. Atelectasis and bronchiectasis indicate a collapse of a portion of the airway that doesn't occur in pneumonia. An effusion is an accumulation of excess pleural fluid in the pleural space, which may be a secondary response to pneumonia.
CN: Physiological integrity; CNS: Physiological adaptation; CL: Apply; DIFFICULTY: Difficult

3. An older adult client has just been admitted with pneumonia. The client tells the nurse, "I have never had pneumonia before and nobody in my family has ever had pneumonia. I don't understand how I contracted this disease." Which statement by the nurse would be **most** appropriate?
1. "You should not worry about it."
2. "You could have had it in the past and did not know it."
3. "Advanced age is a risk factor for developing pneumonia."
4. "Immobility can help to prevent this disease."

4. The nurse is caring for an older adult client. Which commonly observed symptom should the nurse monitor this client for **first**?
1. Altered mental status and dehydration
2. Fever and chills
3. Hemoptysis and dyspnea
4. Pleuritic chest pain and cough

5. When auscultating the chest of a client with pneumonia, the nurse hears bronchial sounds. What does this sound indicate to the nurse?
1. Consolidation
2. Friction rub
3. Normal lung sound
4. Pus in lung

6. A client is admitted with symptoms of fever, cough with copious secretions, and chest pain. Which test should the nurse ensure is performed prior to giving an antibiotic?
1. Arterial blood gas (ABG) analysis
2. Chest x-ray
3. Blood cultures
4. Sputum culture and sensitivity

7. A client with pneumonia has a nonproductive cough and copious secretions. Which intervention would facilitate effective coughing in this client?
1. Lying in semi-Fowler position
2. Sipping water, hot tea, or coffee
3. Inhaling and exhaling from pursed lips
4. Using thoracic breathing

8. An older adult client with pneumonia has copious secretions but is having difficulty coughing them up. Which nursing action would be **most** appropriate?
1. Monitoring the need for suctioning every hour
2. Suctioning every hour
3. Suctioning once per shift
4. Asking the health care provider for an order to suction

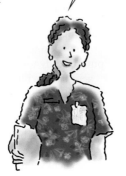

Answering your client's questions accurately is an important part of nursing.

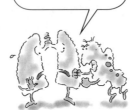

Don't let pneumonia pummel your client's lungs. Get that antibiotic started STAT!

3. 3. Advanced age, due to the possibility of a depressed cough and glottis reflexes, and nutritional depletion, is a risk factor for developing pneumonia. Telling the client not to worry is incorrect as it can be deadly. Telling the client he might have contracted pneumonia in the past is not really helpful or therapeutic. Immobility is a risk factor and not a factor that will prevent pneumonia.
CN: Physiological integrity; CNS: Reduction of risk potential;
CL: Apply; DIFFICULTY: Easy

4. 1. Fever, chills, hemoptysis, dyspnea, cough, and pleuritic chest pain are the common symptoms of pneumonia, but older adult clients may *first* exhibit only an altered mental status and dehydration due to a blunted immune response.
CN: Physiological integrity; CNS: Physiological adaptation;
CL: Apply; DIFFICULTY: Moderate

5. 1. Chest auscultation reveals bronchial breath sounds over areas of consolidation. It does not indicate a friction rub or normal lung sounds. Consolidation is not indicative of pus.
CN: Physiological integrity; CNS: Physiological adaptation;
CL: Apply; DIFFICULTY: Difficult

6. 4. Sputum culture and sensitivity will identify the organism causing the pneumonia and should be done prior to giving an antibiotic. A chest x-ray will show the presence of lung infiltrates, confirming the diagnosis, but can be done after starting an antibiotic. ABG analysis will determine the extent of hypoxia present due to the pneumonia, and blood cultures will help determine if the infection is systemic.
CN: Physiological integrity; CNS: Physiological adaptation;
CL: Apply; DIFFICULTY: Moderate

7. 2. Sips of water, hot tea, or coffee may stimulate coughing. The best position is sitting in a chair with the knees flexed and the feet placed firmly on the floor. The client should inhale through the nose and exhale through pursed lips. Diaphragmatic, not thoracic, breathing helps to facilitate coughing.
CN: Physiological integrity; CNS: Basic care and comfort;
CL: Apply; DIFFICULTY: Difficult

8. 1. Suctioning should be performed only when necessary, based on the client's condition at the time of assessment. Suctioning is a nursing procedure and doesn't require a health care provider's order.
CN: Physiological integrity; CNS: Basic care and comfort;
CL: Apply; DIFFICULTY: Easy

CN: Client needs category   CNS: Client needs subcategory   CL: Cognitive level

9. On entering the room of a client with chronic obstructive pulmonary disease (COPD), the nurse observes that the client is receiving oxygen at 4 L/minute by way of a nasal cannula. The nurse's next action should be based on which statement?
1. "The flow rate is too high."
2. "The flow rate is too low."
3. "The flow rate is correct."
4. "The client shouldn't receive oxygen."

10. A client has been treated with antibiotic therapy for right lower lobe pneumonia for 10 days and will be discharged today. Which physical finding would lead the nurse to believe it's appropriate to discharge this client?
1. Continued dyspnea
2. Fever of 102° F (38.9° C)
3. Respiratory rate of 32 breaths/minute
4. Normal vesicular breath sounds in right base

11. A client who is being treated for pneumonia has a persistent cough and reports severe pain on coughing. Which instruction should be given to help the client reduce the discomfort?
1. "Hold in your cough as much as possible."
2. "Place the head of your bed flat to help with coughing."
3. "Restrict fluids to help decrease the amount of sputum."
4. "Splint your chest wall with a pillow when you cough."

Brace yourself for the answer to question #11.

12. The right forearm of a client who had a purified protein derivative (PPD) test for tuberculosis (TB) is reddened and raised about 3 mm where the test was given. What should be the nurse's next action?
1. No action is required
2. Place the client on isolation
3. Check to see if client had an x-ray
4. Notify relatives about the result

13. A nurse working in a walk-in clinic has been alerted that there's an outbreak of tuberculosis (TB). Which client does the nurse identify as having the highest risk for developing TB?
1. A 16-year-old female high school student
2. A 33-year-old day care worker
3. A 43-year-old homeless man with a history of alcoholism
4. A 54-year-old businessman

9. 1. The administration of oxygen at 1 to 2 L/minute by way of a nasal cannula is recommended for clients with COPD; therefore, a rate of 4 L/minute is too high. The normal mechanism that stimulates breathing is a rise in blood carbon dioxide. Clients with COPD retain blood carbon dioxide, so their mechanism for stimulating breathing is a low blood oxygen level. High levels of oxygen may cause hypoventilation and apnea. Oxygen delivered at 1 to 2 L/minute should aid in oxygenation without causing hypoventilation. Oxygen therapy is the only therapy that has been demonstrated to be life-preserving for clients with COPD.
CN: Safe, effective care environment; CNS: Safety and infection control; CL: Apply; DIFFICULTY: Easy

10. 4. If the client still has pneumonia, the breath sounds in the right base will be bronchial, not the normal vesicular breath sounds. If the client still has dyspnea, fever, and increased respiratory rate, the client should be reexamined by the health care provider before discharge, as he may have another source of infection or still have pneumonia.
CN: Physiological integrity; CNS: Physiological adaptation; CL: Analyze; DIFFICULTY: Easy

11. 4. Showing this client how to splint his chest wall will help decrease discomfort when coughing. Holding in his coughs will only increase his pain. Placing the head of the bed flat may increase the frequency of his cough and require more respiratory effort; a 45-degree angle may help him cough more efficiently and with less pain. Increasing fluid intake will help thin his secretions, making it easier for him to clear them. Promoting fluid intake is appropriate in this situation.
CN: Physiological integrity; CNS: Basic care and comfort; CL: Apply; DIFFICULTY: Easy

12. 1. This test would be classed as negative; therefore, the nurse does not have to do anything. A 3-mm raised area would be a positive result if a client had recent close contact with someone diagnosed with, or suspected of having, infectious TB.
CN: Physiological integrity; CNS: Reduction of risk potential None; CL: Apply: DIFFICULTY: Challenge

13. 3. Clients who are economically disadvantaged, malnourished, and have reduced immunity, such as a client with a history of alcoholism, are at extremely high risk for developing TB. A high school student, a businessman, and a day care worker probably have a much lower risk of contracting TB.
CN: Physiological integrity; CNS: Physiological adaptation; CL: Apply; DIFFICULTY: Easy

14. A client comes to the clinic and is diagnosed with active tuberculosis (TB). Which medication does the nurse expect the health care provider to order initially for this client? Select all that apply.
1. Isoniazid
2. Ethambutol
3. Clindamycin
4. Rifampin
5. Pyrazinamide

15. A client is being screened in the clinic for tuberculosis. The client reports having negative purified protein derivative (PPD) tests results in the past. The nurse performs a PPD test on the right forearm. Which statement made by the client would indicate a need for further education?
1. "I need to return to clinic to assess the results."
2. "I should return in 48 hours for the results."
3. "I should return in 24 hours for the results."
4. "It's very important to have a health care worker read the results."

16. A client with a primary tuberculosis (TB) infection can expect to develop which condition?
1. Active TB within 2 weeks
2. Active TB within 1 month
3. A fever requiring hospitalization
4. A positive skin test

17. A client was infected with tuberculosis (TB) bacillus 10 years ago but never developed the disease. The client is now being treated for cancer and begins to develop signs of TB. Which statement by the nurse is **most** accurate?
1. "Some people carry dormant TB infections that may develop into active disease."
2. "You should be all right since 10 years ago is a long time."
3. "You might develop a superinfection from this."
4. "It is not unusual to develop another infection when you have cancer."

18. A client comes to the clinic with signs of chills, low grade fever, night sweats and hemoptysis. Which interventions should the nurse perform at this time? Select all that apply.
1. Promoting airway clearance
2. Advocating adherence to treatment regimen
3. Promoting activity and nutrition
4. Prescribing medications therapy
5. Preventing transmission

In question #15, timing is everything.

Stay focused. You're doing great!

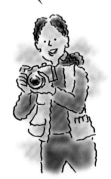

14. **1, 2, 4, 5.** The TB bacillus is airborne and carried in droplets exhaled by an infected person. Key treatments include the medications isoniazid, ethambutol, rifampin and pyrazinamide.
CN: Physiological integrity; CNS: Pharmacological therapies; CL: Apply; DIFFICULTY: Difficult

15. **3.** It's very important to have the results read accurately and clients should return to the clinic for this. PPD tests should be read in 48 to 72 hours. If read too early or too late, the results won't be accurate. It is also important that a health care worker read the results.
CN: Health promotion and maintenance; CNS: None; CL: Apply: DIFFICULTY: Easy

16. **4.** A primary TB infection occurs when the bacillus has successfully invaded the entire body after entering through the lungs. At this point, the bacilli are walled off and skin tests read positive. However, all but infants and immunosuppressed people will remain asymptomatic. The general population has a 10% risk of developing active TB over their lifetime often because of a break in the body's immune defenses. The active stage shows the classic symptoms of TB: fever, hemoptysis, and night sweats.
CN: Physiological integrity; CNS: Physiological adaptation; CL: Apply; DIFFICULTY: Easy

17. **1.** Some people carry dormant TB infections that may develop into active disease. In addition, primary sites of infection containing TB bacilli may remain latent for years and then activate when the client's resistance is lowered, as when a client is being treated for cancer. The nurse should not tell the client that he will be all right. Superinfection doesn't apply in this case. This is not a usual development for a client who has cancer.
CN: Physiological integrity; CNS: Physiological adaptation; CL: Apply; DIFFICULTY: Easy

18. **1, 2, 3, 5.** Typical signs and symptoms of active TB are chills, fever, night sweats, and hemoptysis. Clients with TB typically have low-grade fevers, not higher than 102° F (38.9° C). When active TB is diagnosed it is important for the nurse to help promote airway clearance, advocate for adherence to treatment regimen, promote the importance of good nutrition and activity, and instruct the client in ways to prevent transmission. The health care provider, not the nurse, will prescribe the necessary medications.
CN: Physiological integrity; CNS: Physiological adaptation; CL: Analyze ; DIFFICULTY: Difficult

CN: Client needs category   CNS: Client needs subcategory   CL: Cognitive level

19. A client who recently has been exposed to a family member diagnosed with active TB and has had several false positive skin tests in the past should undergo which test?
1. Chest x-ray
2. Mantoux skin test
3. Sputum culture
4. Tuberculin skin test

20. A client with a positive Mantoux skin test result will be sent for a chest x-ray. The client is confused and asks the nurse why the extra radiation is necessary. What would be the nurse's **best** explanation?
1. To confirm the diagnosis
2. To determine if a repeat skin test is needed
3. To determine the extent of lesions
4. To determine if this is a primary or secondary infection

21. A chest x-ray shows a client's lungs to be clear. The tuberculin Mantoux skin test is positive, with 10 mm of induration, but a previous test was negative. What is the **best** explanation for these results?
1. He had tuberculosis (TB) in the past and no longer has it.
2. He was successfully treated for TB but skin tests always stay positive.
3. He is a "seroconverter," meaning the TB has entered his bloodstream.
4. He is a "tuberculin converter," which means he has been infected with TB since his last skin test.

22. A client with a productive cough, chills, and night sweats is suspected of having active tuberculosis (TB). Which action should the nurse take **first**?
1. Admit him to the hospital in respiratory isolation.
2. Prescribe isoniazid and tell him to go home and rest.
3. Give a tuberculin skin test and tell him to come back in 48 hours to have it read.
4. Give a prescription for isoniazid, 300 mg daily for 2 weeks, and send him home.

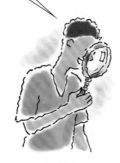

In question #22, look for the action the nurse should take first.

19. 3. Skin tests may be false positive or false negative. Lesions in the lung may not be big enough to be seen on x-ray. The sputum culture for *Mycobacterium tuberculosis* is the only method of confirming the diagnosis.
CN: Physiological integrity; CNS: Physiological adaptation; CL: Apply; DIFFICULTY: Difficult

20. 3. If the lesions are large enough, the chest x-ray will show their presence in the lungs. Sputum culture confirms the diagnosis. There can be false positive and false negative skin test results. A chest x-ray can't determine if this is a primary or secondary infection.
CN: Physiological integrity; CNS: Physiological adaptation; CL: Analyze; DIFFICULTY: Challenge

21. 4. A tuberculin converter's skin test will be positive, meaning he's been exposed to, and infected with, TB and now has a cell-mediated immune response to the skin test. The client's blood and x-ray results may stay negative. It doesn't mean the infection has advanced to the active stage. Because his x-ray is negative, he should be monitored every 6 months to see if he develops changes in his chest x-ray or pulmonary examination. Being a seroconverter doesn't mean the TB has entered his bloodstream; it means it can be detected by a blood test.
CN: Physiological integrity; CNS: Physiological adaptation; CL: Apply; DIFFICULTY: Moderate

22. 1. This client is showing signs and symptoms of active TB and, because of the productive cough, is highly contagious. He should be admitted to the hospital and placed in respiratory isolation, and three sputum cultures should be obtained to confirm the diagnosis. He would most likely be given isoniazid and two or three other antitubercular antibiotics until the diagnosis is confirmed, and then isolation and treatment would continue if the cultures were positive for TB. After 7 to 10 days, three more consecutive sputum cultures will be obtained. If they're negative, he would be considered non-contagious and may be sent home, although he'll continue to take the antitubercular drugs for 9 to 12 months.
CN: Physiological integrity; CNS: Physiological adaptation; CL: Analyze; DIFFICULTY: Easy

23. A client with a positive skin test for tuberculosis (TB) isn't showing signs of active disease. Still, the client is worried and asks the nurse what can be done to help prevent the development of active TB. Which therapy would be **best** for this client?
1. Metronidazole therapy for 10 to 14 days
2. Metronidazole therapy for 2 to 4 weeks
3. Isoniazid therapy for 3 to 6 months
4. Isoniazid therapy for 9 to 12 months

24. A client diagnosed with active tuberculosis is started on triple antibiotic therapy. Which signs and symptoms would indicate that the therapy is inadequate?
1. Decreased shortness of breath
2. Improved chest x-ray
3. Nonproductive cough
4. Positive acid-fast bacilli in a sputum sample after 2 months of treatment

25. Which instruction about therapy for active tuberculosis (TB) is **priority** for the nurse to give a client?
1. "It's okay to miss a dose every day or two."
2. "If adverse effects occur, stop taking the medication."
3. "Only take the medication until you feel better."
4. "You must comply with the medication regimen to treat TB."

26. A client diagnosed with active tuberculosis (TB) would be hospitalized **primarily** for which reason?
1. To evaluate the client's condition
2. To determine compliance
3. To prevent spread of the disease
4. To determine the need for antibiotic therapy

27. A client is admitted with chronic obstructive pulmonary disease (COPD). Which nursing actions should the nurse perform for this client? Select all that apply.
1. Maintain adequate airway for client
2. Educate client on smoking and other triggers
3. Teach pursed lips breathing technique to client
4. Decrease the calories in the diet
5. Assess pulse oximetry

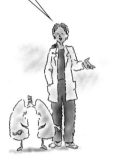

Which instruction is best to get rid of TB?

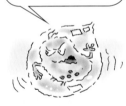

Watch out for those sneezes. TB germs like to travel by water droplets.

23. 4. Because of the increasing incidence of resistant strains of TB, the disease must be treated for up to 24 months in some cases, but treatment typically lasts from 9 to 12 months. Isoniazid is the most common medication used for the treatment of TB, but other antibiotics are added to the regimen to obtain the best results. Metronidazole is an antibiotic but is not normally used in the treatment of TB.
CN: Physiological integrity; CNS: Pharmacological therapies; CL: Apply; DIFFICULTY: Challenge

24. 4. Continuing to have acid-fast bacilli in the sputum after 2 months indicates continued infection. The other choices indicate improvement.
CN: Physiological integrity; CNS: Physiological adaptation; CL: Analyze; DIFFICULTY: Easy

25. 4. The treatment regimen for TB may last up to 24 months. It's essential that the client comply with therapy during that time or resistance will develop. At no time should the client stop taking the medications without the health care provider's approval.
CN: Physiological integrity; CNS: Physiological adaptation; CL: Analyze; DIFFICULTY: Easy

26. 3. The client with active TB is highly contagious until three consecutive sputum cultures are negative, so he's put in respiratory isolation in the hospital. Assessment of his physical condition, need for antibiotic therapy, and determinations of compliance aren't considered primary reasons for hospitalization in this case.
CN: Safe, effective care environment; CNS: Safely and infection control; CL: Apply; DIFFICULTY: Easy

27. 1, 2, 3, 5. Typical findings for clients with COPD include dyspnea on exertion, a barrel chest, and clubbed fingers and toes. Clients with COPD are usually tachypneic with a prolonged expiratory phase. It is important for the nurse to maintain an adequate airway and breathing pattern for this client as well as educate the client in the importance of avoiding any triggers that increase mucus production such as smoking. Pursed lips breathing technique helps the client in expelling carbon dioxide; because these clients expend many calories their diet should be increased and not decreased. Monitoring pulse oximetry is important to maintain a normal level of oxygen throughout the body.
CN: Physiological integrity; CNS: Physiological adaptation; CL: Apply; DIFFICULTY: Moderate

28. A child is exhibiting signs of asthma. Which finding by the nurse would assist with confirmation of this diagnosis? Select all that apply.
1. Circumoral cyanosis
2. Increased forced expiratory volume
3. Inspiratory wheezing
4. Normal breath sounds
5. Expiratory wheezing

28. 3, 5. Inspiratory and expiratory wheezes are typical findings in asthma. Circumoral cyanosis may be present in extreme cases of respiratory distress. The nurse would expect the client to have a decreased forced expiratory volume because asthma is an obstructive pulmonary disease. Breath sounds will be "tight" sounding or markedly decreased; they won't be normal.
CN: Physiological integrity; CNS: Physiological adaptation; CL: Analyze; DIFFICULTY: Challenge

29. A client is experiencing a new-onset asthma attack. Which position should the nurse encourage for this client to assist in improving air exchange?
1. High Fowler
2. Left side-lying
3. Right side-lying
4. Supine with pillows under each arm

29. 1. The best position is high Fowler, which helps lower the diaphragm and facilitates passive breathing and thereby improves air exchange. A side-lying position won't facilitate the client's breathing. A supine position increases the breathing difficulty of a client with asthma.
CN: Physiological integrity; CNS: Physiological adaptation; CL: Apply; DIFFICULTY: Easy

30. The nurse auscultates inspiratory and expiratory wheezes with a decreased forced expiratory volume in a client with asthma. Which class of medication would the nurse expect to administer **immediately**?
1. Beta-blockers
2. Bronchodilators
3. Inhaled steroids
4. Oral steroids

30. 2. Bronchodilators are the first line of treatment for asthma because bronchoconstriction is the cause of reduced airflow. Inhaled or oral steroids may be given to reduce the inflammation but aren't used for emergency relief. Beta-blockers aren't used to treat asthma and can cause bronchoconstriction.
CN: Physiological integrity; CNS: Pharmacological therapies; CL: Apply; DIFFICULTY: Easy

31. An adolescent client comes to the emergency department with acute asthma. The respiratory rate is 44 breaths/minute and the client is experiencing severe respiratory distress. What is the **priority** nursing action by the nurse?
1. Take a full medical history.
2. Give a bronchodilator by nebulizer.
3. Apply a cardiac monitor to the client.
4. Provide emotional support to the client.

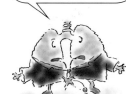

I feel anxious and can't breathe. What's wrong?

31. 2. The client having an acute asthma attack needs to increase oxygen delivery to the lung and body. Nebulized bronchodilators open airways and increase the amount of oxygen delivered. The priority at this time is the respiratory status and the client will be anxious until this is resolved. First, resolve the acute phase of the attack; afterward, obtain a full medical history to determine the cause of the attack and how to prevent attacks in the future. Application of a cardiac monitor is not a priority at this point in the treatment plan.
CN: Physiological integrity; CNS: Physiological adaptation; CL: Apply; DIFFICULTY: Easy

32. A client has symptoms of acute asthma every time the family eats at a Chinese restaurant. Which instruction should the nurse reinforce for this client to avoid complications?
1. "Only eat Chinese food once per month."
2. "Use your inhalers before eating Chinese food."
3. "Avoid Chinese food because it's a trigger for you."
4. "Determine other causes, because Chinese food wouldn't cause such a violent reaction."

32. 3. If the trigger of an acute asthma attack is known, this trigger should always be avoided. Food is typically a trigger for an acute asthma attack, and using an inhaler before eating wouldn't prevent an attack.
CN: Physiological integrity; CNS: Reduction of risk potential; CL: Apply; DIFFICULTY: Easy

33. Which nursing action requires greater caution when performed on a client with chronic obstructive pulmonary disease (COPD)?
1. Administering opioids for pain relief
2. Increasing the client's fluid intake
3. Monitoring the client's cardiac rhythm
4. Assisting the client with coughing and deep breathing

34. A client admitted with a diagnosis of pneumonia is known to be a "blue bloater." What would be the nurse's **best** explanation to the client for using this term?
1. Exhaling more carbon dioxide
2. Producing more sputum
3. Retaining more carbon dioxide
4. Coughing more frequently

35. A client with emphysema is considered a "pink puffer." Which symptom would this client exhibit? Select all that apply.
1. Increased residual lung capacity
2. Dyspnea and pink color
3. Prolonged expiratory time, causing client to puff
4. Decreased expiratory flow rate
5. Cyanosis

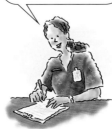

Why are clients with emphysema sometimes called "pink puffers"?

36. A client has marked dyspnea at rest, is thin, and uses accessory muscles to breathe. The client is tachypneic with a prolonged expiratory phase but has no cough. The nurse observes the client leaning forward with arms braced on the knees to support the chest and shoulders for breathing. What does this indicate to the nurse?
1. Acute respiratory distress syndrome (ARDS)
2. Asthma
3. Chronic obstructive bronchitis
4. Emphysema

33. 1. Opioids suppress the respiratory center in the medulla. Both COPD and pneumonia cause alterations in gas exchange; any further problems with oxygenation could result in respiratory failure and cardiac arrest. Increasing the fluid intake would help to thin the client's secretions. Although the nurse would need to monitor the intake and output and watch for signs of heart failure, this isn't as critical as administering opioids. The cardiac rhythm provides an indication of the client's myocardial oxygenation; it should be a part of the nurse's regular assessment. Assisting the client in coughing and with deep breathing should be included in the plan of care. The only caution would be to assess for possible rupture of emphysematous alveolar sacs and pneumothorax.
CN: Physiological integrity; CNS: Reduction of risk potential
CL: Apply; DIFFICULTY: Moderate

34. 3. Clients with chronic obstructive bronchitis appear bloated; they have large barrel chests and peripheral edema, cyanotic nail beds and, at times, circumoral cyanosis. Retaining more carbon dioxide, not exhaling more, is the reason for the blue color. Producing more sputum and coughing more frequently does not contribute to the overall color of the client. Clients with emphysema appear pink and cachectic.
CN: Physiological integrity; CNS: Physiological adaptation;
CL: Apply; DIFFICULTY: Easy

35. 1, 2, 4. Clients with emphysema usually have an increased residual lung capacity and volume, as well as decreased elastic recoil. They also have a decreased expiratory flow rate. Because of the large amount of energy it takes to breathe, clients with emphysema are usually pink and they usually breathe through pursed lips, hence the term "puffer." They also suffer from dyspnea.
CN: Physiological integrity; CNS: Physiological adaptation;
CL: Apply; DIFFICULTY: Challenge

36. 4. These are classic signs and symptoms of a client with emphysema. Clients with asthma are acutely short of breath during an attack and appear very frightened. Clients with bronchitis are bloated and cyanotic in appearance, and clients with ARDS are acutely short of breath and require emergency care.
CN: Physiological integrity; CNS: Physiological adaptation;
CL: Apply; DIFFICULTY: Moderate

37. An older adult client who has chronic respiratory disease comes to the clinic for a 6-month check. The nurse informs the client that it's time for the pneumococcal and flu vaccines. What would be the nurse's **best** explanation to the client for these injections?

1. All clients are recommended to have these vaccines.
2. These vaccines produce bronchodilation and improve oxygenation.
3. These vaccines help reduce the tachypnea these clients experience.
4. Respiratory infections can cause severe hypoxia and possibly death in clients with chronic respiratory diseases.

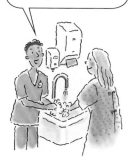

Always model excellent hand hygiene for your clients.

37. 4. It's highly recommended that clients with respiratory disorders be given vaccines to protect against respiratory infection. Infections can cause respiratory failure, and these clients may need to be intubated and mechanically ventilated. The vaccines have no effect on respiratory rate or bronchodilation.

CN: Health promotion and maintenance; CNS: None;

CL: Understand; DIFFICULTY: Easy

38. A client with chronic bronchitis asks the nurse about why it's important to exercise. What would be the nurse's **best** response?

1. "It enhances cardiovascular fitness."
2. "It improves respiratory muscle strength."
3. "It reduces the number of acute attacks."
4. "It worsens respiratory function and is discouraged."

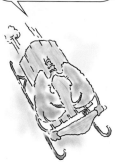

We love exercise. So get out there and get moving!

38. 1. Exercise can improve cardiovascular fitness and it helps the client to better tolerate periods of hypoxia, perhaps reducing the risk of heart attack. Most exercise has little effect on respiratory muscle strength, and these clients can't tolerate the type of exercise necessary to do this. Exercise won't reduce the number of acute attacks. In some instances, exercise may be contraindicated. The client should check with the health care provider before starting any exercise program.

CN: Health promotion and maintenance; CNS: None;

CL: Apply; DIFFICULTY: Challenge

39. A client who has chronic obstructive bronchitis is prescribed a diuretic. What would be the nurse's **best** explanation to the client for the rationale of this therapy?

1. Reducing fluid volume reduces oxygen demand.
2. Reducing fluid volume improves clients' mobility.
3. Reducing fluid volume reduces sputum production.
4. Reducing fluid volume improves respiratory function.

39. 1. Reducing fluid volume reduces the workload of the heart, which reduces oxygen demand and, in turn, reduces the respiratory rate. Sputum may get thicker and make it harder to clear airways. Reducing fluid volume won't improve respiratory function but may improve oxygenation. Reducing fluid volume may reduce edema and improve mobility slightly, but exercise tolerance will still be poor.

CN: Physiological integrity; CNS: Physiological adaptation;

CL: Apply; DIFFICULTY: Challenge

40. A client diagnosed with a pleural effusion has been on supplemental oxygen for 24 hours and is still having dyspnea with decreased breath sounds on the left. The client's condition is worsening. Which procedure will the nurse prepare the client for?

1. Thoracotomy
2. CT scan
3. Bronchoscopy
4. Thoracentesis

40. 4. Pleural fluid normally seeps continually into the pleural space from the capillaries, lining the parietal pleura; the fluid is reabsorbed by the visceral pleural capillaries and lymphatics. Any condition that interferes with either the secretion or drainage of this fluid will lead to a pleural effusion. Key treatments include supplemental oxygen, and a thoracentesis to remove the fluid. If this is not successful then a thoracotomy is performed. The client is also placed on antibiotics to treat the organism that causes empyema.

CN: Physiological integrity; CNS: Physiological adaptation;

CL: Apply; DIFFICULTY: Moderate

41. A client with emphysema should receive only enough supplemental oxygen to maintain a Pa_{O_2} at 60 mm Hg or higher, or the client may lose the hypoxic drive. When explaining the hypoxic drive to the client which statement by the nurse is **best**?
1. "This is when you do not notice you need to breathe."
2. "This is when you only breathe when your oxygen levels climb above a certain point."
3. "This is when you only breathe when your oxygen levels dip below a certain point."
4. "This is when you only breathe when your carbon dioxide level dips below a certain point."

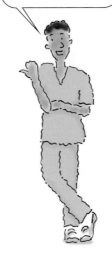

Hypoxic drive? This question sounds like it should be on a mechanic's exam.

41. 3. Clients with emphysema breathe when their oxygen levels drop to a certain level; this is known as the hypoxic drive. Clients with emphysema and chronic obstructive pulmonary disease take a breath when they've reached this low oxygen level. They don't take a breath when their levels of carbon dioxide are higher than normal, as do those with healthy respiratory physiology. If too much oxygen is given, the client has little stimulus to take another breath. His carbon dioxide levels climb, he loses consciousness, and respiratory arrest occurs.
CN: Physiological integrity; CNS: Physiological adaptation; CL: Apply; DIFFICULTY: Moderate

42. A client is diagnosed with chronic obstructive pulmonary disease (COPD). What education about the prevention of complications should the nurse reinforce?
1. Listen to lung sounds with a stethoscope
2. Decrease fluid intake
3. Treat respiratory infections with over the counter medications
4. Recognize the signs of an impending respiratory infection and report to health care provider.

42. 4. Respiratory infection in clients with a respiratory disorder can be fatal. It's important that the client understands how to recognize the signs and symptoms of an impending respiratory infection. The client can't listen to his own lungs effectively. The client should be taught to increase fluid intake to help thin secretions. If the client has signs and symptoms of an infection, contact the health care provider at once to obtain prompt treatment.
CN: Physiological integrity; CNS: Reduction of risk potential; CL: Apply; DIFFICULTY: Easy

43. A client underwent an open cholecystectomy. Which complication should the nurse monitor this client for over the next 24 hours?
1. Atelectasis
2. Bronchitis
3. Pneumonia
4. Pneumothorax

43. 1. Atelectasis develops when there's interference with the normal negative pressure that promotes lung expansion. Clients in the postoperative phase typically guard their breathing because of pain and positioning, which causes hypoxia. It's uncommon for any of the other respiratory disorders to develop after surgery.
CN: Physiological integrity; CNS: Physiological adaptation; CL: Apply ; DIFFICULTY: Challenge

44. A client returns to the acute care unit after abdominal surgery. Which measure should the nurse perform **first** that will help reduce or prevent the incidence of atelectasis?
1. Chest physiotherapy
2. Mechanical ventilation
3. Reducing oxygen requirements
4. Use of an incentive spirometer

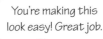
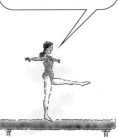

You're making this look easy! Great job.

44. 4. Using an incentive spirometer requires the client to take deep breaths and promotes lung expansion. Chest physiotherapy helps mobilize secretions but won't prevent atelectasis. Reducing oxygen requirements or placing someone on mechanical ventilation doesn't affect the development of atelectasis.
CN: Physiological integrity; CNS: Basic care and comfort; CL: Apply; DIFFICULTY: Easy

45. The nurse is caring for a client that begins experiencing status asthmaticus. Which medication does the nurse prepare to administer for this client?
1. Inhaled beta-adrenergic agents
2. Inhaled corticosteroids
3. IV beta-adrenergic agents
4. Oral corticosteroids

45. 1. Inhaled beta-adrenergic agents help promote bronchodilation, which improves oxygenation. IV beta-adrenergic agents can be used but have to be monitored because of their greater systemic effects. They're typically used when the inhaled beta-adrenergic agents don't work. Corticosteroids are slow-acting, so their use won't reduce hypoxia in the acute phase.
CN: Physiological integrity; CNS: Pharmacological therapies; CL: Understand; DIFFICULTY: Challenge

CN: Client needs category   CNS: Client needs subcategory   CL: Cognitive level

46. A client who is being treated in the emergency department with a diagnosis of status asthmaticus is prescribed beta-adrenergic agents and intravenous (IV) corticosteroids. What does the nurse identify as an indication that the treatment is not working?
1. The client needs to be intubated.
2. The client has reduced secretions.
3. The client has increased secretions.
4. The client can still speak.

47. A client was given morphine sulfate for pain as ordered. The client is sleeping and the respiratory rate is 4 breaths/ minute. The nurse needs to act quickly in order to prevent which complication?
1. Asthma attack
2. Respiratory arrest
3. Seizure
4. Hyperventilation

48. Which additional data should immediately be gathered to determine the status of a client with a respiratory rate of 4 breaths/minute?
1. Arterial blood gas (ABG) levels and breath sounds
2. Level of consciousness (LOC) and a pulse oximetry value
3. Breath sounds and reflexes
4. Pulse oximetry value and heart sounds

49. A client following the administration of an opioid analgesic has a Pa_{CO_2} value of 80 mm Hg upon drawing blood gases. What does this blood gas value indicate?
1. A mild case of hyperventilation
2. This value is perfectly normal
3. The possibility of developing a mild case of pneumonia
4. The danger of respiratory arrest

50. A client requires a chest tube to be inserted in the right upper chest. Which action is part of the nurse's role?
1. Injecting local anesthetic to prevent pain
2. Preparing the chest tube drainage system
3. Bringing the chest x-ray to the client's room
4. Inserting the chest tube

51. Which client is at the **highest** risk for respiratory failure?
1. A client with breast cancer
2. A client with a cervical sprain
3. A client with a fractured hip
4. A client with Guillain-Barré syndrome

46. 1. The client needs to be intubated. Inhaled beta-adrenergic agents, IV corticosteroids, and supplemental oxygen are used to reduce bronchospasm, improve oxygenation, and avoid intubation. Typically, secretions aren't a problem in status asthmaticus. If the client can still speak, adequate oxygen is being delivered and intubation is not normally needed.
CN: Physiological integrity; CNS: Pharmacological therapies; CL: Apply; DIFFICULTY: Moderate

47. 2. Opioids suppress the respiratory center in the medulla and can cause respiratory arrest if given in large quantities. It's unlikely this client will have an asthma attack, or a seizure. The client is currently experiencing hypoventilation and hyperventilation is not likely to occur.
CN: Physiological integrity; CNS: Pharmacological therapies; CL: Analyze; DIFFICULTY: Easy

48. 2. First, the nurse should attempt to rouse the client because this should increase the client's respiratory rate. Then a spot pulse oximetry check should be done and breath sounds should be checked. The health care provider should be notified immediately of the findings. He'll probably order an ABG to determine specific carbon dioxide and oxygen levels. Heart sounds and reflexes will be checked after these initial actions are completed.
CN: Physiological integrity; CNS: Physiological adaptation; CL: Analyze; DIFFICULTY: Moderate

49. 4. A client about to go into respiratory arrest will have inefficient ventilation and will be retaining carbon dioxide. The Pa_{CO_2} value expected would be around 80 mm Hg. It is not indicative of hyperventilation as the CO_2 is high and it does not rise in pneumonia.
CN: Physiological integrity; CNS: Physiological adaptation; CL: Analyze; DIFFICULTY: Moderate

50. 2. The nurse must anticipate that a drainage system is required and assemble it before the insertion, so that the tube can be directly connected to the drainage system. The chest x-ray doesn't need to be brought to the client's room. The health care provider will administer the local anesthetic and insert the chest tube.
CN: Physiological integrity; CNS: Physiological adaptation; CL: Apply; DIFFICULTY: Easy

51. 4. Guillain-Barré syndrome is a progressive neuromuscular disorder that can affect the respiratory muscles and cause ascending paralysis and potential for respiratory failure. The other conditions typically don't affect the respiratory system.
CN: Physiological integrity; CNS: Physiological adaptation; CL: Analyze; DIFFICULTY: Easy

Hey! You've made it through 50 questions. Way to go.

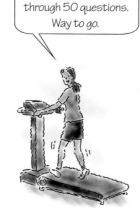

52. A client has been prescribed a new drug for hypertension. Thirty minutes after taking the drug, the client develops chest tightness, becomes short of breath and tachypneic, and exhibits an altered level of consciousness. What is the **best** explanation for these symptoms?
1. The client is having an asthma attack.
2. The client is having a pulmonary embolism.
3. The client is experiencing hypersensitivity to the medication.
4. The client is suffering from rheumatoid arthritis.

53. A client is suspected of impending anaphylaxis secondary to hypersensitivity to a medication. What is the **priority** action by the nurse?
1. Administer oxygen.
2. Insert an IV catheter.
3. Obtain a complete blood count (CBC).
4. Take vital signs.

54. The nurse is caring for a client with asthma and impending anaphylaxis from hypersensitivity to a drug. What is the **priority** action by the nurse?
1. Administer beta-blockers.
2. Administer bronchodilators.
3. Obtain serum electrolyte levels.
4. Lay the client flat on the bed.

55. The client went to a party, took "some pills," and drank beer. The client is brought to the emergency department because the client will not wake up. What reaction would the nurse expect to find when collecting data from the client?
1. Hyperreflexive reflexes
2. Muscle spasms
3. Shallow respirations
4. Tachypnea

56. An unconscious client has been diagnosed with a probable drug overdose complicated by alcohol ingestion. What should be the **priority** nursing intervention?
1. Administer IV fluids.
2. Administer IV naloxone.
3. Continue close monitoring of vital signs.
4. Draw blood for a drug screen.

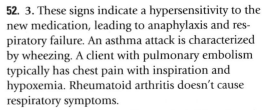

Here's a hint for question # 53.

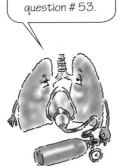

52. 3. These signs indicate a hypersensitivity to the new medication, leading to anaphylaxis and respiratory failure. An asthma attack is characterized by wheezing. A client with pulmonary embolism typically has chest pain with inspiration and hypoxemia. Rheumatoid arthritis doesn't cause respiratory symptoms.
CN: Physiological integrity; CNS: Pharmacological therapies; CL: Analyze; DIFFICULTY: Easy

53. 1. Giving oxygen would be the best first action in this case. Vital signs then should be checked and the health care provider immediately notified. If the client doesn't already have an IV catheter, one may be inserted now if anaphylactic shock is developing. Obtaining a CBC would not help the emergency situation.
CN: Physiological integrity; CNS: Pharmacological therapies; CL: Analyze; DIFFICULTY: Easy

54. 2. Bronchodilators would help open the client's airway and improve his oxygenation status. Beta-blockers aren't indicated in the management of asthma because they may cause bronchospasm. Obtaining laboratory values wouldn't be done on an emergency basis, and having the client lie flat in bed could worsen the client's ability to breathe.
CN: Physiological integrity; CNS: Physiological adaptation; CL: Apply; DIFFICULTY: Easy

55. 3. The client can't be roused from the combination of pills and alcohol taken. This has probably caused shallow breathing, which, if action isn't taken immediately, could lead to respiratory arrest. The nurse wouldn't expect to find tachypnea and doesn't have enough information about which drugs taken to expect muscle spasms or hyperreflexia.
CN: Physiological integrity; CNS: Physiological adaptation; CL: Apply; DIFFICULTY: Easy

56. 2. If the client took opioids, giving naloxone could reverse the effects and awaken the client. IV fluids will most likely be administered, and he'll be closely monitored over a period of several hours to several days. A drug screen should be drawn in the emergency department, but results may not come back for several hours.
CN: Physiological integrity; CNS: Physiological adaptation; CL: Analyze; DIFFICULTY: Moderate

57. An unconscious client who took an overdose of an opioid receives naloxone to reverse the effect of the opioid. After the client wakens, what is the **priority** action by the nurse?
1. Feed the client.
2. Educate the client on the effects of taking pills and alcohol together.
3. Discharge the client from the hospital.
4. Admit the client to a psychiatric facility.

58. A client arrives in the emergency department with smoke inhalation due to a house fire. What should be the nurse's **priority** action for this client?
1. Checking the oral mucous membranes
2. Checking for any burned areas
3. Obtaining a medical history
4. Ensuring a patent airway

59. The nurse is gathering data from a client with smoke inhalation. When auscultating the lungs, what breath sounds would the nurse expect to hear?
1. Crackles
2. Decreased breath sounds
3. Inspiratory and expiratory wheezing
4. Upper airway rhonchi

60. A client is receiving oxygen by way of a nasal cannula at a rate of 2 L/minute. How can the nurse promote oxygenation in this client? Select all that apply.
1. Position client in Fowler position.
2. Decrease anxiety in the client.
3. Set the line marked "2" so it cuts the ball in half.
4. Set any part of the ball so it touches the line marked "2."
5. Give the client an extra dose of a narcotic to allow for rest and sleep.

61. The client comes to the emergency department and the chest x-ray shows fluid in the alveolar spaces. Which disease should the nurse suspect this client to have?
1. Asthma
2. Bronchitis
3. Acute respiratory distress syndrome (ARDS)
4. TB

62. An older adult client postoperative for a fractured right femur develops acute shortness of breath and progressive hypoxia requiring mechanical ventilation. What is the **most** likely cause of this hypoxia?
1. Asthma attack
2. Atelectasis
3. Bronchitis
4. Fat embolism

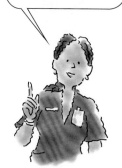

Snap, crackle, pop. Listening to breath sounds can tell you a lot about a client's respiratory function.

57. 2. This client needs information about the dangers of combining pills and alcohol. Discharge at this point is inappropriate. Unless the client was trying to commit suicide, admission to a psychiatric facility isn't necessary. It may not be advisable to feed the client at first; the level of consciousness could drop again, increasing the possibility of aspiration.
CN: Physiological integrity; CNS: Physiological adaptation; CL: Apply; DIFFICULTY: Moderate

58. 4. The nurse's priority is to make sure the airway is open and the client is breathing. Checking the mucous membranes and burned areas is important but not as vital as maintaining a patent airway. Obtaining a medical history can be pursued after ensuring a patent airway.
CN: Physiological integrity; CNS: Physiological adaptation; CL: Apply; DIFFICULTY: Easy

59. 1. When treating smoke inhalation, the most frequently heard sounds are crackles throughout the lung fields. Decreased breath sounds or inspiratory and expiratory wheezing are associated with asthma, and rhonchi are heard when there's sputum in the airways.
CN: Physiological integrity; CNS: Physiological adaptation; CL: Understand; DIFFICULTY: Challenge

60. 1, 2, 3. Positioning client in Fowler position will allow for maximum chest expansion that eases respirations. Decreasing anxiety in the client will also ease the respiratory effort. The oxygen flow rate is set by centering the indicator on the line marked "2." Having any part of the ball touching the line marked "2" is not the correct dose; giving a client an extra dose of narcotic is not safe and is considered to be a medication error.
CN: Safe, effective care environment; CNS: Safety and infection control; CL: Remember; DIFFICULTY: Challenge

61. 3. In ARDS, the alveolar membranes are more permeable and the spaces are filled with fluid. The fluid interferes with gas exchange and reduces perfusion. This is usually not seen in the other diseases listed.
CN: Physiological integrity; CNS: Physiological adaptation; CL: Understand; DIFFICULTY: Challenge

62. 4. Long bone fractures are correlated with fat emboli, which cause shortness of breath and hypoxia. It's unlikely the client has developed asthma or bronchitis without a previous history. He could develop atelectasis, but it typically doesn't produce progressive hypoxia.
CN: Physiological integrity; CNS: Physiological adaptation; CL: Apply; DIFFICULTY: Moderate

63. The nurse is caring for a client with a fracture of the right femur caused by a skiing accident. Which clinical manifestation should the nurse suspect is a complication of the fracture?
1. Abdominal cramping
2. Fatty stools
3. Confusion
4. Numbness in the right foot

64. The nurse is caring for a client with a fat embolism after a fractured femur. What is the **best** intervention by the nurse when the client continues to be hypoxic following respiratory therapy?
1. Administer diuretics.
2. Administer neuromuscular blockers.
3. Place the head of the bed flat.
4. Administer bronchodilators.

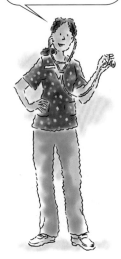

Don't be confused by question #63. I'm sure the answer will come to you.

65. A client arrives in the emergency department displaying apnea, altered mental status, and dyspnea and central cyanosis. The client was found inside a car by neighbors while the motor was still running. Which sign or symptom would the nurse expect to observe and is indicative of late-stage carbon monoxide poisoning?
1. Dilated pupils
2. Chest pains
3. Increased breath sounds
4. Cherry-red mucous membranes

66. A client suffering from acute respiratory distress is lying flat in bed. The nurse when entering the room suggests to the client that a change in position would be beneficial. Which position should the nurse recommend?
1. Prone
2. Side-lying on the left side
3. Side-lying on the right side
4. Alternating prone and supine

67. A nurse working in an emergency department correctly identifies which client to be at a high risk for developing ARDS and therefore should be assessed **first**?
1. A healthy 20-year-old in moderate pain due to probable appendicitis
2. A 55-year-old who has pneumonia and an unproductive cough
3. A client who just received conscious sedation for a minor procedure
4. A client who had massive trauma

63. 3. Confusion and irritability are signs of hypoxia, which is caused by the fat emboli traveling to the lungs and producing an inflammatory response in the lung tissue. Abdominal cramping may be a sign of abdominal distention and constipation caused by immobility. Fatty stools occur with pancreatitis. Numbness may be secondary to neurovascular impairment.
CN: Physiological integrity; CNS: Physiological adaptation; CL: Analyze; DIFFICULTY: Challenge

64. 2. Neuromuscular blockers cause skeletal muscle paralysis, reducing the amount of oxygen used by the restless skeletal muscles. This should improve oxygenation. Bronchodilators may be used, but they typically don't have enough of an effect to reduce the amount of hypoxia present. The head of the bed should be partially elevated to facilitate diaphragm movement, and diuretics can be administered to reduce pulmonary congestion. However, bronchodilators, diuretics, and head elevation would improve oxygen delivery, not reduce oxygen demand.
CN: Physiological integrity; CNS: Physiological adaptation; CL: Apply; DIFFICULTY: Challenge

65. 4. In late-stage carbon monoxide poisoning the nurse would see cherry-red mucous membranes. Key signs of asphyxia are agitation, altered respiratory rate, anxiety, altered mental status, decreased breath sounds, dyspnea, and central and peripheral cyanosis.
CN: Physiological integrity; CNS: Physiological adaptation; CL: Apply; DIFFICULTY: Moderate

66. 4. Alternating supine and prone positioning (if possible) is recommended for clients with acute respiratory distress. Turning the client to the prone position may recruit new alveoli in the posterior region of the lung and improve oxygenation status.
CN: Physiological integrity; CNS: Physiological adaptation; CL: Apply; DIFFICULTY: Challenge

67. 4. In a client with massive trauma, the tissues lining the alveoli and pulmonary capillaries are injured directly or indirectly, increasing the permeability of protein and fluid and leading to the development of hypoxemia and ARDS. Appendicitis, unless it causes overwhelming sepsis, won't lead to ARDS. Pneumonia and conscious sedation don't lead to ARDS.
CN: Physiological integrity; CNS: Physiological adaptation; CL: Analyze; DIFFICULTY: Easy

68. A nurse is monitoring the progress of a client with acute respiratory distress syndrome (ARDS). Which data **best** indicate that the client's condition is improving?
1. Arterial blood gas (ABG) values are normal.
2. The bronchoscopy results are negative.
3. The client's blood pressure has stabilized.
4. The sputum and sensitivity culture shows no growth in bacteria.

69. A nurse has advised a client's family that they shouldn't increase the oxygen flow rate. Which rationale is **most** correct for not increasing the oxygen level on a client when it isn't needed?
1. Extra oxygen may cause the client to breathe too rapidly.
2. Oxygen toxicity may reduce the amount of functional alveolar surface area.
3. Increased oxygen may decrease carbon dioxide levels and cause apnea.
4. Increasing the oxygen level may cause pulmonary barotrauma.

70. Which client is at **highest** risk for developing a problem with lung function?
1. Client scheduled for an appendectomy
2. Client with a meniscus tear
3. Client with sleep apnea
4. Client with thoracic kyphoscoliosis

71. A client arrives in the clinic reporting right-sided chest pain and shortness of breath which started suddenly. What should be the nurse's **first** action?
1. Auscultation of breath sounds
2. A chest x-ray
3. An echocardiogram
4. An electrocardiogram

72. After a motor vehicle crash, a client has a chest tube inserted that begins to drain a large amount of dark red fluid. Which explanation **best** describes what caused this type of drainage from the chest tube insertion?
1. The chest tube was inserted improperly.
2. It is normal for the drainage to be dark red.
3. An artery was nicked when the chest tube was inserted.
4. The client has experienced a hemothorax instead of a pneumothorax.

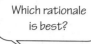

Which rationale is best?

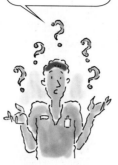

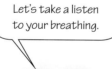

Let's take a listen to your breathing.

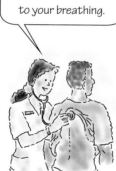

68. 1. Normal ABG values would indicate that the client's oxygenation has improved. ARDS is characterized by hypoxia, so the bronchoscopy and sputum culture results have no bearing on the improvement of ARDS. Increased blood pressure isn't relative to the client's respiratory condition.
CN: Physiological integrity; CNS: Physiological adaptation; CL: Analyze; DIFFICULTY: Easy

69. 2. Oxygen toxicity causes direct pulmonary trauma, reducing the amount of alveolar surface area available for gaseous exchange, which results in increased carbon dioxide levels and decreased oxygen uptake. Excessive oxygen therapy may eliminate hypoxic respiratory drive, causing the client to breathe too slowly or even to stop breathing. Pulmonary barotrauma is caused by high lung pressures, not excessive oxygenation.
CN: Physiological integrity; CNS: Physiological adaptation; CL: Apply; DIFFICULTY: Moderate

70. 4. Thoracic kyphoscoliosis causes lung compression, restricts lung expansion, and results in more rapid and shallow respiration. A healthy client who is scheduled for an appendectomy or has a meniscus tear will not see any problems with lung function due to their illnesses. Clients with sleep apnea also will not have problems with lung function normally.
CN: Physiological integrity; CNS: Physiological adaptation; CL: Analyze DIFFICULTY: Moderate

71. 1. Because the client is short of breath, auscultation of the lungs will indicate normal or abnormal breath sounds. The client may need a chest x-ray and an electrocardiogram, but require a health care provider's order. An echocardiogram also requires a health care provider's order and may be necessary if a pulmonary embolus is suspected.
CN: Physiological integrity; CNS: Physiological adaptation; CL: Apply; DIFFICULTY: Moderate

72. 4. Because of the traumatic cause of injury, the client has a hemothorax, in which blood collection causes the collapse of the lung. The placement of the chest tube will drain the blood from the space and reexpand the lung. There's a slight chance of nicking an intercostal artery during insertion, but it's fairly unlikely if the person placing the chest tube has been trained. The initial chest x-ray would help confirm whether there was blood in the pleural space or just air.
CN: Physiological integrity; CNS: Physiological adaptation; CL: Analyze; DIFFICULTY: Easy

73. A client is treated in the emergency department with reports of dyspnea, cough, and sharp pain that increases with exertion. The nurse auscultates diminished breath sounds and the health care provider prescribes a chest x-ray. What does the nurse suspect this will indicate?
1. Asthma
2. Pulmonary embolism
3. Spontaneous pneumothorax
4. Tuberculosis

74. A client is receiving emergency care following a motor vehicle collision. The health care provider has diagnosed a left pneumothorax. Which sign would typically be present upon auscultation of the client's lungs?
1. Absence of breath sounds over the left lung field
2. Crackles one-third up the posterior lung fields
3. Wheezing on expiration throughout the lung fields
4. Clear breath sounds bilaterally

75. A nurse is reviewing data on a client suspected of having a pneumothorax. Which intervention would **best** confirm the diagnosis?
1. Auscultation of breath sounds
2. Chest x-ray results
3. Client can't use incentive spirometer
4. Client is experiencing dyspnea

76. A client presents with shortness of breath and absent breath sounds on the right side, from the apex to the base. Which condition **best** explains these symptoms?
1. Acute asthma
2. Chronic bronchitis
3. Pneumonia
4. Spontaneous pneumothorax

77. A hospitalized client needs a central venous access device inserted. The health care provider places the device in the subclavian vein. Shortly afterward, the client develops shortness of breath and appears restless. Which action should the nurse take **first**?
1. Administer a sedative.
2. Advise the client to calm down.
3. Auscultate breath sounds.
4. Check to see if the client can have medication.

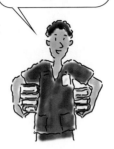

All your studying is paying off. This test is a breeze for you.

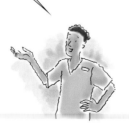

Which is the priority intervention in question #77?

73. 3. Spontaneous pneumothorax is characterized by diminished or absent breath sounds with dyspnea, a cough, and tachypnea. Sharp chest pain that increases with exertion is a Key sign of this process. Asthma is usually accompanied by wheezes and produces no symptoms between attacks. Pulmonary embolism will have sudden onset of dyspnea and crackles in the lungs. TB is demonstrated by fever, night sweats and at times a cough.
CN: Physiological integrity; CNS: Physiological adaptation; CL: Apply; DIFFICULTY: Challenge

74. 1. Pneumothorax can occur as a result of trauma where the pleurae separating the lung from the chest wall are damaged, allowing air to enter the pleural space. This air causes the lung to collapse, resulting in absent breath sounds.
CN: Physiological integrity; CNS: Physiological adaptation; CL: Apply; DIFFICULTY: Easy

75. 2. A chest x-ray will show the area of collapsed lung if pneumothorax is present, as well as the volume of air in the pleural space. Listening to breath sounds won't confirm a diagnosis. The client wouldn't do well with an incentive spirometer at this time. A client may experience dyspnea for many reasons besides a pneumothorax.
CN: Physiological integrity; CNS: Physiological adaptation; CL: Apply; DIFFICULTY: Easy

76. 4. Spontaneous pneumothorax occurs when the client's lung collapses, causing an acute decrease in the amount of functional lung used in oxygenation; this results in shortness of breath with absent breath sounds. A client with an asthma attack would present with wheezing breath sounds, and bronchitis would be indicated by auscultating rhonchi. Bronchial breath sounds over the area of consolidation would indicate pneumonia.
CN: Physiological integrity; CNS: Physiological adaptation; CL: Apply; DIFFICULTY: Easy

77. 3. Because this is an acute episode, listen to the client's lungs to see if anything has changed. Don't give this client medication, especially sedatives, if he's having trouble breathing; the medication may decrease respirations further. Give the client emotional support and contact the health care provider who placed the central venous access.
CN: Safe, effective care environment; CNS: Coordinated care; CL: Analyze; DIFFICULTY: Easy

78. Which intervention would be prescribed **first** for a client who recently had a central venous access device inserted and now appears short of breath and anxious?
1. Chest x-ray
2. Electrocardiogram
3. Laboratory tests
4. Sedation

79. A client with acute respiratory failure has just been admitted to the acute care unit. For which nursing actions does the nurse prepare the client? Select all that apply.
1. Administration of supplemental oxygen
2. Administration of an analgesic
3. Administration of a bronchodilator
4. Administration of an antibiotic
5. Administration of a steroid

80. When monitoring the closed-chest drainage system of a client who has just returned from a lobectomy, what should the nurse be sure is occurring?
1. The fluid in the water seal chamber rises from inspiration and falls with expiration.
2. The tubing remains looped below the level of the bed.
3. The drainage chamber doesn't drain more than 100 mL in 8 hours.
4. The suction-control chamber bubbles vigorously when connected to suction.

81. When a chest tube is inadvertently dislodged from a client, which should be the nurse's **first** action?
1. Notify the health care provider.
2. Wipe the chest tube with alcohol and reinsert.
3. Cover the chest tube insertion site opening with petroleum gauze and apply pressure.
4. Auscultate the lung fields for breath sounds.

82. Which intervention should be done before a chest tube is removed?
1. Provide the results of the most recent chest x-ray for the health care provider to review before removal.
2. Make sure that the health care provider orders arterial blood gas analysis before removal.
3. Disconnect the drainage system from the chest tube before the tube's removal.
4. Sedate the client; the health care provider will remove the tube without warning the client.

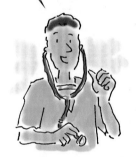

Congrats! You've finished 80 questions. You're over halfway done.

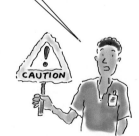

A dislodged chest tube is a serious concern. What should be the nurse's first response?

CAUTION

78. 1. Inserting an IV catheter in the subclavian vein can result in a pneumothorax, so a chest x-ray should be done. If it's negative, then other tests should be done, but they aren't appropriate as the first intervention.
CN: Physiological integrity; CNS: Reduction of risk potential;
CL: Apply; DIFFICULTY: Moderate

79. 1, 2, 3, 5. Key treatments for a client with acute respiratory failure include supplemental oxygen, an analgesic such as morphine, an antianxiety agent, a bronchodilator such as albuterol, and a steroid such as hydrocortisone. Antibiotics are not necessarily needed for this client.
CN: Physiological integrity; CNS: Physiological adaptation;
CL: Analyze; DIFFICULTY: Challenge

80. 1. Rise and fall of the water seal chamber immediately after surgery indicates patency of the chest tube drainage system. The tubing should be coiled on the bed, without dependent loops, to promote drainage. Up to 500 mL of drainage can occur in the first 24 hours after surgery. Gentle bubbling is indicated after surgery to prevent excessive evaporation.
CN: Physiological integrity; CNS: Physiological adaptation;
CL: Apply; DIFFICULTY: Moderate

81. 3. If a chest tube is unintentionally dislodged, immediately cover the insertion site opening with petroleum gauze and apply pressure in order to prevent air from entering the chest and causing tension pneumothorax. Next, notify the health care provider. It isn't appropriate to attempt to reinsert the chest tube. Auscultation of the lungs may be important but isn't the priority.
CN: Physiological integrity; CNS: Physiological adaptation;
CL: Apply; DIFFICULTY: Easy

82. 1. A chest x-ray should be done before chest tube removal to ensure that the client's lung has remained expanded after suction was discontinued. Pulse oximetry would be sufficient and is the more commonly used method to track oxygenation. Disconnecting the drainage system before the chest tube is removed could cause tension pneumothorax. Client cooperation is desirable; if the client can hold the breath while the chest tube is removed, there's less chance that air will be drawn back into the pleural space during removal.
CN: Physiological integrity; CNS: Reduction of risk potential;
CL: Apply; DIFFICULTY: Moderate

83. A client is placed on oxygen therapy via a nasal cannula. Which should be the **first** action by the nurse?
1. Make sure all electronic monitoring devices in use are properly grounded.
2. Know the location of O₂ turn-off valve on nursing unit.
3. Instruct the client and family, as well as visitors, not to smoke.
4. Confirm the health care provider's order for oxygen.

83. 4. The priority when administering oxygen is to check the health care provider's order, as this is considered a medication. The nurse also should make sure all electronic monitoring devices are grounded, instruct everyone not to smoke, and should know the location of the turn-off valve for the O₂.
CN: Safe, effective care environment; CNS: Safety and infection control; CL: Apply; DIFFICULTY: Moderate

84. A nurse is preparing to reinforce the education plan for a client who has recently been diagnosed with squamous cell carcinoma of the left lung. Which statement by the nurse is **best**?
1. "You have a slow-growing cancer that rarely spreads."
2. "In terms of prognosis, you may have only a few months to live."
3. "Squamous cell cancer is a very rapid-growing cancer."
4. "The cancer has generally metastasized by the time the diagnosis is made."

84. 1. Squamous cell carcinoma of the lung is a slow-growing, rarely metastasizing type of cancer. It has the best prognosis of all lung cancer types.
CN: Physiological integrity; CNS: Physiological adaptation; CL: Analyze; DIFFICULTY: Challenge

85. A client is admitted to the acute care unit due to a chronic cough with copious, foul-smelling secretions. The nurse identifies dyspnea, hemoptysis, and recent weight loss. What should be the **priority** independent action by the nurse for this client?
1. Monitor respiratory status and pulse oximetry values
2. Provide supportive care
3. Administer antibiotics
4. Administer a bronchodilator

The key word in question #85 is "independent."

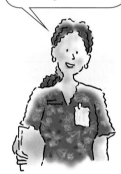

85. 1. The client is suffering from bronchiectasis. The priority intervention would be to monitor respiratory status and pulse oximetry. Providing supportive care is also important but values need to be monitored to ensure adequate oxygenation. Antibiotics and bronchodilators are part of the overall treatment but are not independent actions by the nurse.
CN: Physiological integrity; CNS: Physiological adaptation; CL: Apply; DIFFICULTY: Moderate

86. A client who is a longtime smoker receives lab results that indicate an elevated carcinoembryonic antigen level. How **best** should the nurse reinforce education to the client regarding these results?
1. Inform the client that it means that lung cancer is definitely present.
2. No action is needed; this level is usually elevated in a smoker.
3. Inform the client that cancer was present and now the cancer has spread to other organs.
4. Inform the client that he definitely will die from some cancer in the body.

86. 2. Because the level of carcinoembryonic antigen is elevated in clients who smoke, it can't be used as a general indicator of cancer. This test by itself cannot confirm cancer of any kind in a smoker. However, the carcinoembryonic antigen level is helpful in monitoring cancer treatment because it usually falls to normal within 1 month if treatment is successful.
CN: Physiological integrity; CNS: Physiological adaptation; CL: Analyze; DIFFICULTY: Moderate

87. A client arrives in the local clinic and reports a chronic cough and fatigue. The client admits to smoking two packs of cigarettes daily for 10 years and also informs the nurse of a 9 kg weight loss over the last 2 months. Which test, required for a definitive diagnosis of cancer, does the nurse prepare the client for?
1. Bronchoscopy
2. Chest x-ray
3. Computerized tomography of the chest
4. Surgical biopsy

87. 4. Only surgical biopsy with cytologic examination of the cells can give a definitive diagnosis of the type of cancer. Bronchoscopy gives positive results in only 30% of the cases. Chest x-ray and computerized tomography can identify location but don't diagnose the type of cancer.
CN: Physiological integrity; CNS: Physiological adaptation; CL: Apply; DIFFICULTY: Easy

CN: Client needs category   CNS: Client needs subcategory   CL: Cognitive level

88. The nurse is reinforcing education about the staging of a tumor to a client who is newly diagnosed with cancer. Which statement made by the client would indicate to the nurse a need for further teaching?
1. "Staging describes the severity of the cancer."
2. "Staging helps the health care provider plan appropriate treatment."
3. "Staging systems change over time."
4. "Surgical biopsy with cytologic cell examination is the only data collection method used to perform staging."

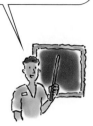

Question #88 sounds like an opportunity for some teaching.

88. 4. Staging describes the extent and severity of the cancer and helps the health care provider determine the most appropriate therapy. Staging systems continue to evolve as cancer is better understood. Multiple data collection methods, such as laboratory results, physical examinations, and imaging results, are used to determine the stage of a cancer.
CN: Physiological integrity; CNS: Physiological adaptation; CL: Analyze; DIFFICULTY: Moderate

89. Which intervention is **most** important for a client with lung cancer to perform in order to increase survival rate?
1. Early bronchoscopy
2. Early detection
3. High-dose chemotherapy
4. Smoking cessation

89. 2. Detecting cancer early when the cells may be premalignant and potentially curable would be most beneficial. However, a tumor must be 1 cm in diameter before it's detectable on a chest x-ray, so this is difficult. If the cancer is detected early, a bronchoscopy may help identify cell type. High-dose chemotherapy has minimal effect on long-term survival. Smoking cessation won't reverse the process but may prevent further decompensation.
CN: Health promotion and maintenance; CNS: None; CL: Apply; DIFFICULTY: Challenge

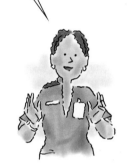

Bubbling is never a good thing when chest tubes are involved.

90. A nurse is assigned to care for a client with a chest tube and observes that there's constant bubbling in the water seal chamber of the closed drainage system. Which explanation **best** describes this observation?
1. Constant bubbling indicates that the tube is working correctly.
2. Constant bubbling indicates that there's a loose connection.
3. Constant bubbling indicates that the suction rate is too high.
4. Constant bubbling indicates that the suction rate is too low.

90. 2. Constant bubbling in the water seal chamber indicates that there's a leak or loose connection between the client and the water seal chamber. The amount of suction affects the suction control chamber, not the water seal chamber.
CN: Physiological integrity; CNS: Physiological adaptation; CL: Apply; DIFFICULTY: Moderate

91. A client has been diagnosed with lung cancer and is told that a wedge resection is required. The client appears confused and asks the nurse for an explanation. What would be the nurse's **best** response?
1. "One entire lung will be removed."
2. "The lobe of the lung involved will be removed."
3. "A small, localized area near the surface of the lung will be removed."
4. "A segment of the lung, including a bronchiole and its alveoli, will be removed."

91. 3. A very small area of tissue close to the surface of the lung is removed in a wedge resection. A segment of the lung is removed in a segmental resection, a lobe is removed in a lobectomy, and an entire lung is removed in a pneumonectomy.
CN: Physiological integrity; CNS: Physiological adaptation; CL: Apply; DIFFICULTY: Moderate

92. A client has been diagnosed with cor pulmonale. Which test results would the nurse expect to see in this client? Select all that apply.
1. Large central pulmonary arteries upon x-ray
2. Increased right pulmonary artery pressure
3. Decreased pulmonary vascular resistance
4. Decreased right ventricular pressure
5. Increased pulmonary vascular resistance

92. 1, 2, 5. The client with cor pulmonale will exhibit the following key test results: ABG analysis will show decreased Pa_{O_2}. Chest x-ray will show large central pulmonary arteries and suggest right ventricular enlargement by rightward enlargement of cardiac silhouette. Pulmonary artery pressure measurements show increased right ventricular and pulmonary artery pressures because of increased pulmonary vascular resistance.
CN: Physiological integrity; CNS: Physiological adaptation; CL: Analyze; DIFFICULTY: Difficult

93. A client has been admitted with an exacerbation of emphysema. Which classification of medications should the nurse expect to administer? Select all that apply.
1. Antibiotics
2. Bronchodilators
3. Steroids
4. Diuretics
5. Calcium channel blockers

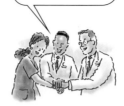

Health care is a team sport. Go team!

94. During a pneumonectomy, the phrenic nerve on the surgical side is typically cut to cause hemidiaphragm paralysis. What is the **best** explanation for the nurse to use when reinforcing teaching the client about this procedure?
1. Paralyzing the diaphragm reduces oxygen demand.
2. Cutting the phrenic nerve is a mistake during surgery.
3. The client isn't using that lung to breathe any longer.
4. Paralyzing the diaphragm reduces the space left by the pneumonectomy.

95. A client with lung cancer is experiencing excruciating pain due to the size of the tumor and is scheduled for a lung resection the next morning. What education should the nurse reinforce about the lung resection?
1. To explain that the surgery will remove the tumor and all surrounding tissue
2. To explain that the surgery will remove the tumor and as little surrounding tissue as possible
3. To explain that a biopsy of the tumor will be done as well as remove all of the tumor
4. To explain that a biopsy of several areas of the tumor will be done and half of the tumor will be removed

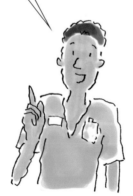

The answer to question #96 might be counterintuitive to you.

96. A client who has just undergone a pneumonectomy asks the nurse which position is **best** when lying in bed. What would be the nurse's best response?
1. Always lay on the non-operative site.
2. It doesn't matter. Any position is fine.
3. Always lay prone.
4. Lay on the operative side or on the back.

93. 1, 2, 3. Key treatments for the client with emphysema in regards to medications include antibiotics to treat the causative agent, bronchodilators to assist in ventilation, and steroids to decrease inflammation. Diuretics and calcium channel blockers are not ordered unless there is an underlying problem.
CN: Physiological integrity; CNS: Pharmacological Therapies; CL: Apply; DIFFICULTY: Difficult

94. 4. Because the hemidiaphragm is a muscle that doesn't contract when paralyzed, an uncontracted hemidiaphragm remains in an "up" position, which reduces the space left by the pneumonectomy. Serous fluid has less space to fill, thus reducing the extent and duration of mediastinal shift after surgery. Although it's true that the client no longer needs the hemidiaphragm on the operative side to breathe, this alone wouldn't be sufficient justification for cutting the phrenic nerve. Paralyzing the hemidiaphragm doesn't significantly decrease total-body oxygen demand.
CN: Physiological integrity; CNS: Physiological adaptation; CL: Apply; DIFFICULTY: Difficult

95. 2. The goal of surgical lung resection is to remove the cancerous lung tissue that has tumor in it while preserving as much surrounding tissue as possible. It may be necessary to remove alveoli and bronchioles, but care is taken to remove only what's absolutely necessary.
CN: Physiological integrity; CNS: Physiological adaptation; CL: Apply; DIFFICULTY: Moderate

96. 4. A client who has undergone a pneumonectomy doesn't have a chest tube in place; therefore, the client could lay on the operative side. In fact, the best position for this client is to lie on the operative side or on the back to prevent fluid from draining into the unaffected lung and to promote maximum ventilation. The client should not lie on the non-operative side, which would allow unwanted drainage.
CN: Physiological integrity; CNS: Reduction of risk potential; CL: Apply; DIFFICULTY: Challenge

97. What is the main purpose for the nurse reinforcing preoperative education for a client who will be undergoing surgery?
   1. Deciding if the client should have surgery
   2. Providing emotional support to the client and family
   3. Providing detailed explanations of the surgery to the client and family
   4. Providing general information, answering questions, and offering emotional support to the client and family

98. A client reporting no pain is diagnosed with a benign lung tumor. Which statement made by the client demonstrates an understanding of the reason for the procedure?
   1. "I am going to experience pain control."
   2. "It will prevent further compression of lung tissue."
   3. "It will help to prevent metastatic cancer."
   4. "It is for cosmetic purpose."

99. What is the **primary** intervention by the nurse while caring for a client with terminal lung cancer?
   1. Providing emotional support
   2. Providing nutritional support
   3. Providing pain control
   4. Preparing the client's will

100. A client has been diagnosed with a pulmonary embolism. When the nurse informs the family members, they become very upset and say they do not understand what that means. Which statement by the nurse to the family would be **most** effective?
   1. "It's a blood clot that originates in the lung."
   2. "It's a blood clot that has occluded an alveolus."
   3. "It's a blood clot that has occluded a bronchiole."
   4. "It's a blood clot that has occluded a pulmonary blood vessel."

101. A nurse reinforces education for a pregnant woman who is scheduled for a cesarean birth regarding prevention of complications that can develop after the birth. Which statement by the client indicates a need for further education?
   1. "At least one complication I don't have to worry about is blood clots."
   2. "I will be sure to drink plenty of fluids so my milk will come in."
   3. "I will cough and take deep breaths so I do not develop pneumonia."
   4. "I will need to be active as soon as possible so I do not get muscle atrophy."

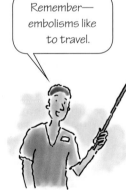

Remember—embolisms like to travel.

97. 4. The nurse's role is to provide general information about the client's surgery, explain his preoperative and postoperative care, and offer emotional support. The nurse's role isn't to decide whether the client should have surgery. Providing only emotional support isn't sufficient. If the client has questions that require detailed explanations of the surgery, he should be referred to his surgeon.
CN: Physiological integrity; CNS: Physiological adaptation; CL: Apply; DIFFICULTY: Easy

98. 2. The tumor is removed to prevent further compression of lung tissue as the tumor grows, which could lead to respiratory decompensation. If for some reason the tumor can't be removed, then chemotherapy or radiation may be used to try to shrink it. At this point pain is not a problem; preventing cancer and cosmetics is not an issue.
CN: Physiological integrity; CNS: Physiological adaptation; CL: Apply; DIFFICULTY: Challenge

99. 3. The client with terminal lung cancer may have extreme pleuritic pain and should be treated to reduce his discomfort. Preparing the client and his family for the impending death is also important but shouldn't be the primary focus until pain is under control. Nutritional support may be provided, but as the terminal phase advances, the client's nutritional needs greatly decrease. Nursing care doesn't focus on helping the client prepare a will.
CN: Physiological integrity; CNS: Basic care and comfort; CL: Apply; DIFFICULTY: Easy

100. 4. A pulmonary embolism is a blood clot (or some other material) that originated in one area of the body, traveled through the bloodstream, and lodged in the pulmonary arteries. It doesn't originate in a pulmonary artery. An embolism remains in the bloodstream and isn't in the bronchial tree, the "air side" of the lung architecture; therefore, it isn't in the bronchiole or the alveoli.
CN: Physiological integrity; CNS: Physiological adaptation; CL: Apply; DIFFICULTY: Easy

101. 1. Although venous thrombi in the thigh and pelvis are the most common sources for pulmonary emboli, clients who have undergone a cesarean birth are prone to develop clots in the amniotic fluid, leading to pulmonary embolus and possible death. Increasing fluids, coughing, and deep breathing—as well as being active—are all components that will help to prevent complications following a cesarean birth.
CN: Physiological integrity; CNS: Physiological adaptation; CL: Apply; DIFFICULTY: Easy

102. Which client is at **highest** risk for developing a pulmonary embolism?
 1. An ambulatory client with an inflammatory joint disease
 2. An ambulatory client who has type 1 diabetes
 3. A healthy client who's 6 months pregnant
 4. A client who has fractures of his pelvis and right femur

103. A client who has just had a right arthroscopy is back on the acute care unit. What action does the nurse identify as the **best** to prevent a pulmonary embolism in this client?
 1. Early ambulation
 2. Frequent chest x-rays to find a pulmonary embolism
 3. Frequent lower extremity venous scans
 4. Intubation of the client

104. At 8 a.m., the nurse gathers data from a client scheduled for surgery at 10 a.m. The nurse observes dyspnea, nonproductive cough, and back pain. What should be the nurse's **priority** action?
 1. Check to see that the chest x-ray was done yesterday, as ordered.
 2. Check the serum electrolyte levels and complete blood count (CBC).
 3. Make sure that the health care provider is immediately notified of these findings.
 4. Sign the preoperative checklist for this client.

105. When a client is placed on oxygen therapy the nurse should follow protocol. Place the following steps in the correct order.

1.	Attach flow meter to wall outlet, fill humidifier with water, attach the delivery system and tubing
2.	Explain procedure to client
3.	Check the health care provider's order
4.	Place the face mask or cannula on the client
5.	Re-assess client and document the procedure

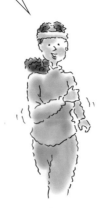

Taking the NCLEX is more like running a marathon than a sprint. Hang in there!

102. 4. Thrombosis formation is caused by abnormalities in blood flow, vein wall integrity, and blood coagulation. The client with pelvic and femur fractures will be immobilized and probably have edema, which leads to venous stasis and predisposes him to the development of deep vein thrombosis. A pulmonary embolus commonly arises from clots in the deep veins of the legs that break off and travel to the pulmonary arteries. The risk of developing venous thrombosis isn't as high with the other conditions.
CN: Physiological integrity; CNS: Physiological adaptation; CL: Apply; DIFFICULTY: Easy

103. 1. Early ambulation helps reduce pooling of blood, which reduces the tendency of the blood to form a clot that could then dislodge. None of the other measures will prevent pulmonary embolism from forming.
CN: Physiological integrity; CNS: Physiological adaptation; CL: Apply; DIFFICULTY: Easy

104. 3. The nurse should make sure that the health care provider is immediately notified of the findings because dyspnea, a nonproductive cough, and back pain may signal a change in the client's respiratory status. The nurse should check any ordered tests (such as chest x-ray, serum electrolyte levels, and CBC) after notifying the health care provider because they may help explain the change in the client's condition. The nurse should sign the preoperative checklist after notifying the health care provider of the client's condition and learning the health care provider's decision on whether to proceed with surgery.
CN: Safe, effective care environment; CNS: Coordinated care; CL: Apply; DIFFICULTY: Easy

105. Ordered Response:

3.	Check the health care provider's order
2.	Explain procedure to client
1.	Attach flow meter to wall outlet, fill humidifier with water, attach the delivery system and tubing
4.	Place the face mask or cannula on the client
5.	Re-assess client and document the procedure

CN: Safe, effective care environment; CNS: Safety and infection control; CL: Apply; DIFFICULTY: Easy

106. A client who has a pulmonary embolism has the potential to develop chest pain. What would be the nurse's **best** explanation for this when reinforcing education for the client?
1. It is the same as costochondritis.
2. It is a result of a myocardial infarction.
3. It is pleuritic pain due to inflammation.
4. It is caused by referred pain from the pelvis.

107. Which symptom would a nurse **most** likely observe first in a client with an acute pulmonary embolism?
1. Distended jugular veins
2. Bradycardia
3. Dyspnea
4. Nonproductive cough

108. The client who has a pulmonary embolus is also experiencing hemoptysis. What is the nurse's **best** explanation for this when reinforcing education for the client?
1. Alveolar damage in the infarcted area can cause this blood.
2. Involvement of major blood vessels in the occluded area can cause this.
3. Loss of lung parenchyma usually causes this.
4. Loss of massive lung tissue is the cause.

109. A client with a large pulmonary embolism has an arterial blood gas analysis indicating respiratory alkalosis. What does the nurse determine is the potential cause of this result?
1. Hypoventilation
2. Alveolar damage
3. Large amount of bloody sputum
4. Large region of lung tissue unavailable for perfusion

110. A ventilation-perfusion scan is frequently performed to help diagnose a pulmonary embolism. What other uses does the nurse correctly identify for this test? Select all that apply.
1. To detect poor blood flow in the lungs, blood vessels
2. To examine the lungs before different types of surgeries
3. To detect air trapping in the lungs
4. Location and size of the pulmonary embolism
5. Location of all the peripheral arteries

106. 3. Pleuritic pain is caused by the inflammatory reaction of the lung parenchyma to the pulmonary embolism. The pain isn't associated with myocardial infarction, costochondritis, or referred pain from the pelvis to the chest.
CN: Physiological integrity; CNS: Physiological adaptation; CL: Apply; DIFFICULTY: Challenge

107. 3. Dyspnea is usually the first symptom of pulmonary embolus because the thrombus prevents gas exchange in the pulmonary arterial bed. If the embolus is large enough, the client may then develop right ventricular failure with such symptoms as distended jugular veins, tachycardia, and circulatory collapse. He may also have hemoptysis.
CN: Physiological integrity; CNS: Physiological adaptation; CL: Analyze; DIFFICULTY: Easy

108. 1. The infarcted area produces alveolar damage that can lead to the production of bloody sputum, sometimes in large amounts. There's a loss of lung parenchyma and subsequent scar tissue formation; blood vessels may be involved, but these don't cause hemoptysis.
CN: Physiological integrity; CNS: Physiological adaptation; CL: Apply; DIFFICULTY: Challenge

109. 4. A client with a large pulmonary embolism will have a large region of lung tissue unavailable for perfusion. This causes the client to hyperventilate and blow off large amounts of carbon dioxide, which crosses the unaffected alveolar-capillary membrane more readily than does oxygen, resulting in respiratory alkalosis. A client with respiratory alkalosis will hyperventilate and not hypoventilate. Alveolar damage can be present with a pulmonary embolus, but it does not cause respiratory alkalosis or a large amount of bloody sputum.
CN: Physiological integrity; CNS: Physiological adaptation; CL: Apply; DIFFICULTY: Challenge

110. 1, 2, 3. The ventilation-perfusion scan provides information on the extent of occlusion caused by the pulmonary embolism and the amount of lung tissue involved in the area not perfused. It does not tell the size of the pulmonary embolism. There are others reasons for doing this test: to detect poor blood flow, to detect air trapping, and to examine the lungs before different surgeries.
CN: Physiological integrity; CNS: Reduction and risk potential; CL: Understand; DIFFICULTY: Challenge

111. A client is suspected of having a pulmonary embolus. Which test should the nurse prepare the client for that is definitive?
  1. Arterial blood gas (ABG) analysis
  2. Computed tomography scan
  3. Pulmonary angiogram
  4. Ventilation-perfusion scan

111. 3. Pulmonary angiogram is used to definitively diagnose a pulmonary embolism. A catheter is passed through the circulation to the region of the occlusion; the region can be outlined with an injection of contrast medium and viewed by fluoroscopy. This shows the location of the clot, as well as the extent of the perfusion defect. Computed tomography scan can show the location of infarcted or ischemic tissue. ABG levels can define the amount of hypoxia present. The ventilation-perfusion scan can report whether there's a ventilation-perfusion mismatch present and define the amount of tissue involved.
CN: Physiological integrity; CNS: Reduction of risk potential;
CL: Apply; DIFFICULTY: Moderate

112. A client with a pulmonary embolism has received a thrombolytic medication. What is the **most** important concept the nurse should reinforce with this client and family at this time?
  1. The medication was given to break apart the blood clot blocking the pulmonary artery.
  2. The medication is taken orally and will thin the blood.
  3. The medication will prevent future clots from forming.
  4. The medication will help the client to breathe by dilating bronchial tubes.

112. 1. A thrombolytic medication is given IV to break apart or dissolve blood clots. It isn't given orally, doesn't prevent future clots from forming, and has no effect on the bronchial tubes.
CN: Physiological integrity; CNS: Pharmacological therapies;
CL: Apply; DIFFICULTY: Moderate

113. Following a pulmonary embolism, a client is placed on IV heparin. The client asks the nurse about the purpose of the heparin. Which statement by the nurse is correct?
  1. "Heparin will dissolve the clot in your lungs."
  2. "Heparin will slow the development of any more clots."
  3. "Heparin will prevent pieces of the clot from breaking off and going to your lung."
  4. "Heparin will dissolve any circulating clots."

113. 2. Heparin is an anticoagulant and is administered to slow thrombus formation. Fibrinolytic medications dissolve clots. Heparin won't prevent clots from embolizing or dissolve circulating clots.
CN: Physiological integrity; CNS: Pharmacological therapies;
CL: Apply; DIFFICULTY: Moderate

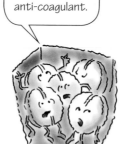

Remember— Warfarin is an anti-coagulant.

114. A client who was hospitalized for pulmonary embolism is being discharged on warfarin therapy. Which statement by the nurse about warfarin therapy is correct?
  1. It inhibits the formation of blood clots.
  2. It's given to continue to reduce the size of the pulmonary embolism.
  3. It will reduce blood pressure and prevent venous stasis.
  4. Coagulation studies to monitor bleeding times will be necessary every 6 months.

114. 1. Warfarin inhibits clot formation by interfering with clotting factors that are dependent on vitamin K. Warfarin doesn't dissolve clots and won't reduce the size of the pulmonary embolus. It doesn't reduce blood pressure and won't prevent venous stasis. Coagulation studies will be performed every 2 to 4 weeks while the client is receiving warfarin.
CN: Physiological integrity; CNS: Physiological adaptation;
CL: Apply; DIFFICULTY: Easy

115. A client suspected of having a pulmonary embolus is scheduled for a lung scan. What is the **most** important action for the nurse prior to the procedure?
  1. Explain the procedure to the client.
  2. Check all allergies of the client.
  3. Watch for radioactive gas leaks.
  4. Obtain the client's vital signs.

115. 2. The priority action for the nurse is checking to see if the client has any allergies, as lung scans are contraindicated in clients that have a hypersensitivity to the radiopharmaceutical dye. After that it is important to also explain the procedure, obtain the vital signs, and during the procedure watch for any gas leaks.
CN: Safe, effective care environment; CNS: Coordinated care;
CL: Apply; DIFFICULTY: Moderate

116. A client who has chronic bronchitis has asked the nurse to identify things that will help to promote better oxygenation. Which of the following lifestyle factors does the nurse identify as affecting a client's oxygenation? Select all that apply.
1. Nutrition
2. Physical exercise
3. Ethnicity
4. Genetics
5. Anxiety

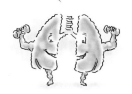

Exercise strengthens the lungs and improves oxygenation.

116. 1, 2, 5. Lifestyle factors that affect oxygenation are nutrition, physical exercise, smoking, substance abuse, and anxiety. Other factors may affect a client's oxygenation as well. Ethnicity and genetics are not lifestyle factors.
CN: Physiological integrity; CNS: Reduction of risk potential;
CL: Apply; DIFFICULTY: Challenge

117. What is the **priority** nursing intervention when caring for a client with a pulmonary embolism?
1. Assessing oxygenation status
2. Monitoring the oxygen delivery device
3. Monitoring for other sources of clots
4. Determining whether the client requires another ventilation-perfusion scan

117. 1. Nursing management of a client with a pulmonary embolism focuses on assessing oxygenation status and ensuring treatment is adequate. If the client's status begins to deteriorate, it's the nurse's responsibility to contact the health care provider and attempt to improve oxygenation. Monitoring for other clot sources and ensuring the oxygen delivery device is working properly are other nursing responsibilities, but they aren't the focus of care.
CN: Physiological integrity; CNS: Physiological adaptation;
CL: Apply; DIFFICULTY: Easy

118. A client with a pulmonary embolism is having a vena cava filter inserted. What would be the **best** explanation by the nurse for the filter?
1. The filter prevents further clot formation.
2. The filter collects clots so they don't go to the lung.
3. The filter breaks up clots into insignificantly small pieces.
4. The filter contains anticoagulants that are slowly released, dissolving any clots.

118. 3. The umbrella-like filter is placed in a client at high risk for the formation of more clots that could potentially become pulmonary emboli. The filter breaks the clots into small pieces that won't significantly occlude the pulmonary vasculature. The filter doesn't release anticoagulants and doesn't prevent further clot formation. The filter doesn't collect the clots; if it did, it would have to be emptied periodically, causing the client to require surgery in the future.
CN: Physiological integrity; CNS: Physiological adaptation;
CL: Apply; DIFFICULTY: Difficult

119. A client with a pulmonary embolism may need an embolectomy. Which statement by the nurse **most** accurately describes the procedure when teaching the client?
1. Removal of an embolism in the lower extremity
2. Extracting the embolism from the lung by bronchoscopy
3. Surgical removal of the embolism source in the pelvis
4. Surgical removal of the embolism in the pulmonary vasculature

119. 4. If the pulmonary embolism is large and doesn't respond to treatment, surgical removal may be necessary to restore perfusion to the area of the lung. This is rarely done because of the associated high-mortality risk. It's impossible to remove a pulmonary embolism through bronchoscopy because the defect isn't in the bronchial tree. A thrombectomy can be performed at other sources of clots, but when a pulmonary embolism has already occurred, it would have little effect on oxygenation.
CN: Physiological integrity; CNS: Physiological adaptation;
CL: Apply; DIFFICULTY: Moderate

120. A client placed on pulse oximetry monitoring asks the nurse to explain what that is. What would be the **best** explanation by the nurse?
1. It is the amount of carbon dioxide in the blood.
2. It is the amount of oxygen in the blood.
3. It is the percentage of hemoglobin carrying oxygen.
4. It is the respiratory rate.

120. 3. Pulse oximetry determines the percentage of hemoglobin carrying oxygen. This doesn't ensure that the oxygen being carried through the bloodstream is actually being taken up by the tissue. Pulse oximetry doesn't provide information about the amount of oxygen or carbon dioxide in the blood or the client's respiratory rate.
CN: Physiological integrity; CNS: Physiological adaptation;
CL: Apply; DIFFICULTY: Challenge

121. A client diagnosed with a pulmonary embolism is having chest pain and apprehension. What is an appropriate nursing intervention for this client?
1. Administering analgesics
2. Using guided imagery
3. Positioning the client on the left side
4. Providing emotional support

121. 1. After the pulmonary embolism has been diagnosed and the amount of hypoxia determined, chest pain and the accompanying apprehension can be treated with analgesics. The nurse must monitor respiratory status frequently. Guided imagery and providing emotional support can be used as alternatives. Positioning the client on the left side when a pulmonary embolism is suspected may prevent a clot that has extended through the capillaries and into the pulmonary veins from breaking off and traveling through the heart into the arterial circulation, leading to a massive stroke.
CN: Physiological integrity; CNS: Physiological adaptation; CL: Apply; DIFFICULTY: Moderate

122. When reinforcing education for the client about the importance of blood levels in relation to breathing, what would be the nurse's **best** explanation?
1. The level of hemoglobin has no effect on oxygenation.
2. The more hemoglobin you have the less oxygen in your body.
3. Low hemoglobin levels cause reduced oxygen-carrying capacity.
4. Low hemoglobin levels cause increased oxygen-carrying capacity.

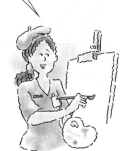

Looks like you've made test-taking into a fine art. Well done!

122. 3. The level of hemoglobin in one's body does have an effect on oxygenation. Hemoglobin carries oxygen to all tissues in the body. If the hemoglobin level is low, the amount of oxygen-carrying capacity is also low. More hemoglobin will increase oxygen-carrying capacity and thus increase the total amount of oxygen available in the blood.
CN: Physiological integrity; CNS: Physiological adaptation; CL: Apply; DIFFICULTY: Easy

123. A client with atelectasis is ordered oxygen therapy. What would the nurse expect the health care provider to order for this client?
1. Ventilation with CPAP (continuous positive airway pressure)
2. Ventilation with nasal cannula
3. Ventilation with PEEP (positive end-expiratory pressure)
4. Ventilation with a facemask only

123. 3. Positive end-expiratory pressure (PEEP) delivers positive pressure to the lung at the end of expiration. This helps open collapsed alveoli and helps them stay open so gas exchange can occur in these newly opened alveoli, improving oxygenation. CPAP, or continuous positive airway pressure, is a treatment that uses mild air pressure to keep the airways open CPAP typically is used by people who have breathing problems such as sleep apnea. A facemask or nasal cannula would not be helpful in this situation.
CN: Physiological integrity; CNS: Physiological adaptation; CL: Apply; DIFFICULTY: Difficult

124. A client who is having difficulty breathing is told by the health care provider that oxygen will be ordered due to collapsed alveoli. Which statement made by the nurse will **best** explain to the client how opening up collapsed alveoli improves oxygenation?
1. Alveoli need oxygen to live.
2. Alveoli have no effect on oxygenation.
3. Collapsed alveoli increase oxygen demand.
4. Gaseous exchange occurs in the alveolar membrane.

124. 4. Gaseous exchange occurs in the alveolar membrane, so if the alveoli collapse, no exchange occurs. Collapsed alveoli receive oxygen, as well as other nutrients, from the bloodstream. Collapsed alveoli have no effect on oxygen demand, although by decreasing the surface area available for gas exchange, they decrease oxygenation of the blood.
CN: Physiological integrity; CNS: Physiological adaptation; CL: Apply; DIFFICULTY: Easy

125. A client will need CPAP (Continuous positive airway pressure) and is told that an oxygen mask will be required. How can the nurse **best** explain why the mask is needed for CPAP?
1. The mask provides 100% oxygen to the client.
2. The mask provides continuous air that the client can breathe.
3. The mask provides pressurized oxygen so the client can breathe more easily.
4. The mask provides pressurized oxygen at the end of expiration to open collapsed alveoli.

126. The nurse is caring for a client with pneumonia. The health care provider orders 600 mg of ceftriaxone oral suspension to be given once per day. The medication label indicates that the strength is 125 mg/5 mL. How many milliliters of medication should the nurse pour to administer the correct dose? Record your answer using a whole number.

_____mL

127. The nurse is caring for a client who's scheduled for a bronchoscopy. Which interventions should the nurse perform to prepare the client for this procedure? Select all that apply.
1. Explain the procedure.
2. Withhold food and fluids for 2 hours before the test.
3. Provide a clear liquid diet for 6 to 12 hours before the test.
4. Confirm that a signed informed consent form has been obtained.
5. Ask the client to remove his dentures.
6. Administer a sedative.

128. A nurse is auscultating a client's lungs. Identify the area on the client's vertebrae, representing the base of the lungs, where the nurse expects the breath sounds to stop at the end of expiration.

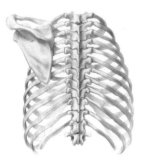

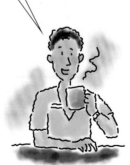

125. 3. The mask provides pressurized oxygen continuously through both inspiration and expiration. By providing a client with pressurized oxygen, the client has less resistance to overcome in taking in the next breath, making it easier to breathe. The mask can be set to deliver any amount of oxygen needed. Pressurized oxygen delivered at the end of expiration is positive end-expiratory pressure (PEEP), not continuous positive airway pressure.
CN: Physiological integrity; CNS: Physiological adaptation; CL: Apply; DIFFICULTY: Difficult

126. 24. To calculate drug dosages, use the formula:

Dose on hand/quantity on hand = Dose desired/X

In this case,

$$125 \text{ mg}/5 \text{ mL} = 600 \text{ mg}/X.$$

Therefore, X = 24 mL.
CN: Physiological integrity; CNS: Pharmacological therapies; CL: Analyze; DIFFICULTY: Easy

127. 1, 4, 5, 6. All procedures must be explained to the client in order to obtain informed consent and to reduce anxiety. A signed informed consent form is required for all invasive procedures. Dentures need to be removed for bronchoscopy because they may become dislodged during the procedure. A sedative is given to relax the client. Food and fluids are restricted for 6 to 12 hours before the test to avoid the risk of aspiration during the procedure.
CN: Physiological integrity; CNS: Reduction of risk potential; CL: Apply; DIFFICULTY: Difficult

128. Based on posterior land marks, the lungs extend from the cervical area to the level of the 10th thoracic vertebrae (T10) at the end of expiration.

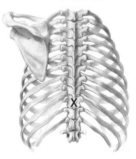

CN: Health promotion and maintenance; CNS: None; CL: Apply; DIFFICULTY: Moderate

Chapter 6

Neurosensory Disorders

Neurosensory refresher

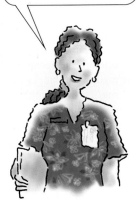

Stroke, subdural hematoma, laminectomy—they're all here in this comprehensive chapter on neurosensory disorders in adults. I've got a sixth sense you're going to do great!

Acute head injury

Trauma to the brain, skull, or scalp due to external mechanical force, causing brain damage

Key signs and symptoms
- Altered mental status
- Unequal pupil size, loss of pupillary reaction (late sign)

Key test results
- Computed tomography (CT) scan shows hemorrhage, cerebral edema, or shift of midline structures
- Magnetic resonance imaging (MRI) shows hemorrhage, cerebral edema, or shift of midline structures

Key treatments
- Cervical collar (until neck injury is ruled out)
- Anticonvulsant: phenytoin
- Barbiturate: pentobarbital if unable to control intracranial pressure (ICP) with diuresis
- Diuretics: mannitol, furosemide to combat cerebral edema
- Vasopressors: dopamine or phenylephrine to maintain cerebral perfusion pressure above 60 mm Hg (if blood pressure is low and ICP is elevated)
- Glucocorticoid: dexamethasone to reduce cerebral edema
- Histamine-2 (H_2) receptor antagonists: cimetidine, ranitidine, famotidine, nizatidine
- Mucosal barrier fortifier: sucralfate
- Posterior pituitary hormone: vasopressin, if client develops diabetes insipidus

Key interventions
- Monitor neurologic and respiratory status
- Keep client free from stimuli
- Monitor and record vital signs, intake and output, urine specific gravity, laboratory studies, and pulse oximetry values
- Check for signs of diabetes insipidus (low urine specific gravity, high urine output)
- Allow a rest period between nursing activities

Amyotrophic lateral sclerosis

Progressive, degenerative disorder that affects motor neurons

Key signs and symptoms
- Awkwardness of fine finger movements
- Muscle atrophy
- Dysphagia
- Fatigue
- Muscle weakness of hands and feet
- Fasciculations (twitching)

Key test results
- Creatine kinase level is elevated
- Electromyography (EMG) shows impaired impulse conduction in the muscles

Key treatments
- Symptomatic relief
- Neuroprotective agent: riluzole

Key interventions
- Monitor neurologic and respiratory status
- Evaluate swallow and gag reflexes
- Monitor and record vital signs and intake and output
- Devise an alternate method of communication when necessary
- Suction the oropharynx as necessary

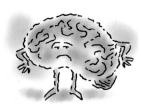

Ever since that car wreck, I've felt a little "altered."

Bell's palsy

Disorder of facial nerve (cranial nerve VII) causing paralysis of one side of face

Key signs and symptoms
- Inability to close eye completely on the affected side
- Pain around jaw or ear
- Unilateral facial weakness

Key test results
- EMG helps predict level of expected recovery by distinguishing temporary conduction defects from a pathologic interruption of nerve fibers

Key treatments
- Moist heat

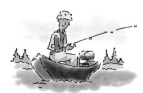

ALS is a degenerative disorder that affects motor neurons. Can you remember its symptoms?

- Corticosteroid: prednisone to reduce facial nerve edema and improve nerve conduction and blood flow
- Artificial tears to protect the cornea from injury

Key interventions
- During treatment with prednisone, watch for adverse reactions, especially GI distress and fluid retention
- Apply moist heat to affected side of face, taking care not to burn the skin
- Massage client's face with a gentle upward motion two or three times daily for 5 to 10 minutes, or have client massage face himself
- When ready for active facial exercises, teach client to grimace in front of mirror
- Arrange for privacy at mealtimes
- Offer psychological support; give reassurance that recovery is likely within 1 to 8 weeks

Brain abscess
Accumulation of pus within the brain following an infection

Key signs and symptoms
- Headache
- Chills
- Fever
- Confusion
- Drowsiness

Key test results
- Physical examination shows increased ICP
- Enhanced CT scan reveals abscess site
- CT-guided stereotactic biopsy may be performed to drain and culture the abscess

Key treatments
- Penicillinase-resistant antibiotics: nafcillin, methicillin
- Surgical aspiration or drainage of the abscess

Key interventions
- Frequently monitor neurologic status
- Monitor and record vital signs at least once every hour
- Monitor fluid intake and output carefully
- After surgery, monitor neurologic status; monitor vital signs and intake and output
- Watch for signs of meningitis (nuchal rigidity, headaches, chills, sweats)
- Change the dressing when damp; never allow bandages to remain damp
- Position the client on the operative side
- Measure drainage from a Jackson-Pratt drain or other type of drain as instructed by surgeon

Brain tumor
Benign or malignant tumor within the cranial cavity

Key signs or symptoms
- Various, depending on location of tumor

Key test results
- CT scan shows location and size of tumor.
- MRI shows location and size of tumor.

Key treatments
- Craniotomy
- Anticonvulsant: phenytoin
- Glucocorticoid: dexamethasone
- Histamine-2 (H_2) receptor antagonists: cimetidine, ranitidine, famotidine, nizatidine
- Mucosal barrier fortifier: sucralfate

Key interventions
- Monitor neurologic and respiratory status
- Evaluate pain
- Observe for signs and symptoms of increased ICP
- Monitor for signs and symptoms of syndrome of inappropriate antidiuretic hormone (edema, weight gain, positive fluid balance, high urine specific gravity)
- Encourage client to express feelings about changes in body image and fear of dying

Cataract
Opacity of the normally transparent lens

Key signs and symptoms
- Dimmed or blurred vision
- Poor night vision
- Yellow, gray, or white lens

Key test results
- Ophthalmoscopy or slit-lamp examination confirms diagnosis by revealing a dark area in the normally homogeneous red reflex

Key treatments
- Extracapsular cataract extraction
- Intracapsular lens implant

Key interventions
- Provide a safe environment for the client
- Modify environment to help client meet self-care needs (e.g., by placing items on the unaffected side)

Cerebral aneurysm
Protrusion or sac on a cerebral blood vessel due to weakness of the vessel wall

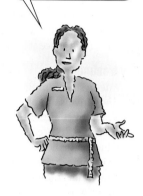
The good news about Bell palsy is that it typically only lasts 8 weeks, at most.

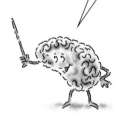
Stand back while I fight off this infection!

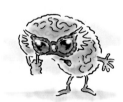
Sunglasses can help clients avoid bright lights that may exacerbate some disorders of the eye.

Key signs or symptoms
- Sudden headache (commonly described by the client as the worst he's ever experienced)

Key test results
- Cerebral angiogram identifies the aneurysm
- CT scan may show a shift of intracranial midline structures and blood in the sub-arachnoid space

Key treatments
- Aneurysm clipping
- Anticonvulsant: phenytoin
- Calcium channel blocker: nimodipine preferred to prevent cerebral vasospasm
- Glucocorticoid: dexamethasone
- Histamine-2 (H$_2$) receptor antagonists: cimetidine, ranitidine, famotidine, nizatidine
- Stool softener: docusate sodium

Key interventions
- Monitor neurologic status
- Maintain crystalloid solutions after aneurysm clipping
- Take vital signs every 1 to 2 hours initially and then every 4 hours when the client becomes stable
- Allow rest period between nursing activities

Conjunctivitis
Infection of the delicate membrane lining of the eyelid and the outer surface of the eye

Key signs and symptoms
- Excessive tearing
- Itching, burning
- Mucopurulent discharge

Key test results
- Culture and sensitivity tests:
  - identify causative bacterial organism
  - indicate appropriate antibiotic therapy

Key treatments
- Antiviral agents: oral acyclovir (if herpes simplex is cause)
- Corticosteroids: dexamethasone, fluorometholone (if cause is nonviral)
- Mast cell stabilizer: cromolyn for allergic conjunctivitis
- Topical antibiotics: according to the sensitivity of the infective organism (if bacterial)

Key interventions
- Teach proper hand-washing technique
- Stress risk of spreading infection to family members by sharing washcloths, towels, and pillows

- Warn against rubbing the infected eye (spreads infection to the other eye and to other persons)
- Apply warm compresses and therapeutic ointment or drops; don't irrigate the eye
- Instruct the client to wash hands before using medication
- Instruct client to use clean washcloths or towels frequently
- Teach client to instill eyedrops and ointments correctly—without touching the bottle tip to his eye or lashes

Corneal abrasion
Scrape on the outer, clear layer of the eye

Key signs and symptoms
- Burning
- Increased tearing
- Redness

Key test results
- Staining the cornea with fluorescein stain confirms diagnosis
  - injured area appears green when examined with a flashlight

Key treatments
- Cycloplegic agent: tropicamide
- Irrigation with saline solution
- Pressure patch (a tightly applied eye patch)
- Removal of a deeply embedded foreign body with a foreign body spud, using a topical anesthetic

Key interventions
- Assist with examination of the eye
- Check visual acuity before beginning treatment
- If foreign body is visible, carefully irrigate eye with normal saline solution
- Tell the client with an eye patch to leave patch in place for 6 to 8 hours
- Stress the importance of instilling prescribed antibiotic eyedrops

Encephalitis
Inflammation of the brain

Key signs and symptoms
- Meningeal irritation (stiff neck and back) and neuronal damage (drowsiness, coma, paralysis, seizures, ataxia, and organic psychoses)
- Sudden onset of fever
- Headache
- Vomiting

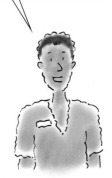

What key interventions should you undertake to assist a client with cerebral aneurysm?

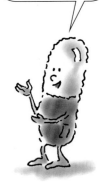

What meds are best for treating conjunctivitis?

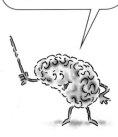

What's the condition called when I get inflamed? Can you remember?

Key test results
- Blood studies identify the virus and confirm diagnosis
- Cerebrospinal fluid (CSF) analysis identifies the virus

Key treatments
- Endotracheal (ET) intubation and mechanical ventilation
- Nasogastric (NG) tube feedings or total parenteral nutrition (if unable to use the GI tract)
- Anticonvulsants: phenytoin, phenobarbital
- Analgesics and antipyretics: aspirin, acetaminophen to relieve headache and reduce fever
- Diuretics: furosemide, mannitol to reduce cerebral swelling
- Corticosteroid: dexamethasone to reduce cerebral inflammation and edema

Key interventions
- Monitor neurologic function often
- Observe client's mental status and cognitive abilities
- Avoid fluid overload; measure and record intake and output accurately
- Carefully position client and turn him often
- Assist with range-of-motion exercises
- Maintain a quiet environment; darken the room

Glaucoma
Group of eye disorders that causes an increase in intraocular pressure

Key signs and symptoms
Chronic open-angle glaucoma
- Initially asymptomatic

Acute angle-closure glaucoma
- Acute ocular pain
- Blurred vision
- Dilated pupil
- Halo vision

Key test results
- Ophthalmoscopy shows atrophy and cupping of optic nerve head
- Tonometry shows increased intraocular pressure

Key treatments
Chronic open-angle glaucoma
- Alpha$_2$-agonist: brimonidine
- Beta-blocker: timolol

Acute angle-closure glaucoma
- Cholinergic: pilocarpine
- Laser iridectomy or surgical iridectomy (if pressure doesn't decrease with drug therapy)

Key interventions
- Monitor eye pain
- Administer medication as prescribed
- Modify the environment

Guillain-Barré syndrome
Progressive autoimmune response causing inflammation and demyelination of the peripheral nervous system

Key signs or symptoms
- Symmetrical muscle weakness (ascending from the legs to the arms)

Key test results
- History of preceding febrile illness (usually a respiratory tract infection) and typical clinical features
- CSF protein level begins to rise, peaking in 4 to 6 weeks
- CSF white blood cell count remains normal (in severe disease, CSF pressure may rise above normal)

Key treatments
- Anticoagulants: heparin, warfarin
- Corticosteroid: prednisone
- ET intubation or tracheotomy, possibly mechanical ventilation
- IV fluid therapy
- NG tube feedings or parenteral nutrition (if unable to use GI tract)
- Plasmapheresis

Key interventions
- Watch for ascending sensory loss, which precedes motor loss
- Monitor vital signs and level of consciousness
- Monitor and treat respiratory dysfunction
- Maintain respiratory support, if needed
- Reposition the client every 2 hours
- If aspiration can't be minimized by diet and position modification, expect to provide NG tube feeding
- Inspect client's legs regularly for signs of thrombophlebitis; apply antiembolism stockings and sequential compression devices; give prophylactic anticoagulants as needed
- Encourage adequate fluid intake (2,000 mL/day), unless contraindicated

Huntington disease
Rare, progressive, hereditary disorder that causes degeneration of basal ganglia and excess production of dopamine, leading to excessive involuntary movements and mental deterioration

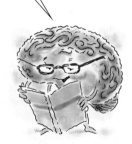

Blurred vision can be an indicator of various disorders.

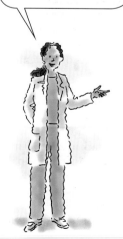

Which condition involves a progressive, autoimmune response causing inflammation and demyelination of the peripheral nervous system?

Key signs and symptoms
- Dementia (can be mild at first but eventually disrupts client's personality)
- Choreiform movements (abnormal and excessive involuntary movements)
- Gradual loss of musculoskeletal control (eventually leading to total dependence)

Key test results
- Positron emission tomography detects the disease.
- Deoxyribonucleic acid analysis detects the disease.

Key treatments
- Antidepressant: imipramine to alleviate depression
- Antipsychotics: chlorpromazine, haloperidol to help control choreic movements
- Supportive, protective treatment aimed at relieving symptoms (Huntington disease has no known cure)

Key interventions
- Provide physical support by attending to client's basic needs (e.g., hygiene, skin care, bowel and bladder care, nutrition)
- Increase this support as mental and physical deterioration makes client increasingly immobile
- Stay alert for possible suicide attempts
- Control client's environment to protect him from suicide or other self-inflicted injury
- Pad side rails of the bed but avoid restraints

Ménière disease
Disorder of the inner ear, resulting in excess production of endolymphatic fluid in the semicircular canals

Key signs and symptoms
- Sensorineural hearing loss
- Severe vertigo
- Tinnitus

Key test results
- Audiometric studies indicate:
  - sensorineural hearing loss
  - loss of discrimination and recruitment

Key treatments
- Restriction of sodium intake to less than 2 g/day
- Anticholinergic: atropine (may stop an attack in 20 to 30 minutes)
- Antihistamine: diphenhydramine for severe attack

Key interventions
- Advise client against reading and exposure to glaring lights during an attack
- Stress safety measures
- Instruct client not to get out of bed or walk without assistance during an attack
- Instruct client to avoid sudden position changes
- Instruct client to avoid tasks that vertigo makes hazardous
- Before surgery, if client is vomiting, record fluid intake and output and characteristics of vomitus
- Administer antiemetics as necessary
- Give small amounts of fluid frequently
- Tell client to expect dizziness and nausea for 1 or 2 days after surgery

Meningitis
Inflammation of the meninges covering the brain and spinal cord

Key signs and symptoms
- Chills
- Fever
- Headache
- Malaise
- Photophobia
- Positive Brudzinski sign (client flexes hips or knees when the nurse places her hands behind his neck and flexes it forward)—a sign of meningeal inflammation and irritation
- Positive Kernig sign (pain or resistance when the client's leg is flexed at the hip or knee while he's in a supine position)
- Stiff neck and back
- Vomiting

Key test results
- Lumbar puncture shows:
  - elevated CSF pressure
  - cloudy or milky white CSF
  - high protein level
  - positive Gram stain and culture that usually identifies the infecting organism (unless it's a virus)
  - depressed CSF glucose concentration

Key treatments
- Bed rest
- Hypothermia
- IV fluid administration
- Oxygen therapy, possibly with ET intubation and mechanical ventilation
- Antibiotics: penicillin G, ampicillin, or nafcillin; if allergic to penicillin, then tetracycline or chloramphenicol
- Diuretic: mannitol
- Anticonvulsants: phenytoin, phenobarbital
- Analgesics or antipyretics: acetaminophen, aspirin

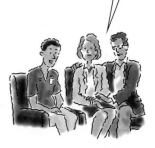

Clients diagnosed with Huntington disease may need extra care and support due to the degenerative nature of this condition.

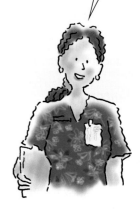

What safety measures are needed for a client with Ménière disease and why?

Key interventions

- Monitor neurologic function often
- Watch for deterioration in client's condition
- Monitor fluid balance; maintain adequate fluid intake
- Suction client only if necessary
- Limit suctioning to 10 to 15 seconds per pass of the catheter
- Hyperoxygenate the lungs with 100% oxygen for 1 minute before and after suctioning
- Position the client carefully
- Darken the room
- Relieve headache with a nonopioid analgesic (e.g., aspirin or acetaminophen, as needed)

Multiple sclerosis

Chronic, progressive, intermittent degenerative disorder that involves destruction of myelin sheath of the neurons in the brain and spinal cord

Key signs and symptoms

- Nystagmus, diplopia, blurred vision, optic neuritis
- Weakness, paresthesia, impaired sensation, paralysis

Key test results

- CT scan eliminates other diagnoses such as brain or spinal cord tumors
- MRI may reveal plaques associated with multiple sclerosis

Key treatments

- Plasmapheresis (for antibody removal)
- Cholinergic: bethanechol
- Glucocorticoids: prednisone, dexamethasone, corticotropin (ACTH)
- Immunosuppressants: interferon beta-1b, cyclophosphamide, methotrexate, glatiramer acetate
- Skeletal muscle relaxants: dantrolene, baclofen

Key interventions

- Monitor for changes in motor coordination, paralysis, or muscle weakness
- Encourage client to express feelings about changes in body image
- Establish a bowel and bladder program
- Maintain activity as tolerated (alternating rest and activity)

Myasthenia gravis

Neuromuscular disease characterized by deficiency of acetylcholine at the myoneural junction, causing extreme voluntary muscle weakness

Key signs and symptoms

- Dysphagia, drooling
- Ptosis or drooping of eyelids (early sign)
- Muscle weakness and fatigue (typically, muscles are strongest in the morning but weaken throughout the day, especially after exercise)
- Profuse sweating

Key test results

- EMG shows impaired impulse conduction in the muscles
- Edrophonium test relieves symptoms after medication administration—a positive indication of the disease

Key treatments

- Anticholinesterase inhibitors: pyridostigmine, neostigmine
- Glucocorticoids: prednisone, dexamethasone, corticotropin (ACTH)
- Immunosuppressants: azathioprine, cyclophosphamide
- Thymectomy

Key interventions

- Monitor neurologic and respiratory status
- Evaluate swallow and gag reflexes
- Watch client for choking while eating

Otosclerosis

Disease of the middle ear that involves progressive hardening of the ossicles

Key signs and symptoms

- Progressive hearing loss
- Tinnitus

Key test results

- Audiometric testing confirms hearing loss

Key treatments

- Stapedectomy and insertion of a prosthesis to restore partial or total hearing

Key interventions

- Develop alternative means of communication

Parkinson disease

Chronic, progressive, neurologic disease that involves a deficiency of dopamine production due to degeneration of substantia nigra

Key signs and symptoms

- "Pill-rolling" tremors, tremors at rest
- Masklike facial expression
- Shuffling gait, stiff joints, bradykinesia, "cogwheel" rigidity, stooped posture

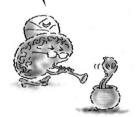

Charmed, I'm sure, but what's that ringing in my ears?

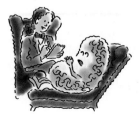

I haven't been feeling quite right lately.

Key test results

- EEG reveals minimal slowing of brain activity

Key treatments

- Antidepressant: amitriptyline
- Antiparkinson drugs: levodopa, levodopa-carbidopa, benztropine
- MAO-B inhibitors: selegiline, rasagiline
- COMT inhibitors: tolcapone, entacapone
- Dopamine agonist: ropinirole

Key interventions

- Monitor neurologic and respiratory status
- Reinforce gait training
- Reinforce independence in care

Retinal detachment

Separation of retina to the pigmented vascular layer of the eyeball

Key signs and symptoms

- Painless change in vision (floaters and flashes of light)
- Painless vision loss described as a "veil," "curtain," or "cobweb" that eliminates part of visual field (with progression of detachment)

Key test results

- Indirect ophthalmoscopy shows retinal tear or detachment
- Slit-lamp examination shows retinal tear or detachment

Key treatments

- Scleral buckling to reattach the retina

Key interventions

- Postoperatively, instruct client to lie on back or on unoperated side
- Discourage straining during defecation; bending down; and hard coughing, sneezing, or vomiting

Spinal cord injury

Damage to spinal cord due to traumatic or non-traumatic causes that may lead to loss of motor function, sensory function, reflexes, and control of elimination

Key signs and symptoms

- Loss of bowel and bladder control
- Paralysis below the level of the injury
- Paresthesia below the level of the injury

Key test results

- CT scan shows spinal cord edema, vertebral fracture, and spinal cord compression
- MRI shows spinal cord edema, vertebral fracture, and spinal cord compression

Key treatments

- Flat position, with neck immobilized in a cervical collar
- Maintenance of vertebral alignment through Crutchfield tongs, Gardner-Wells tongs, or Halo vest
- Surgery for stabilization of the upper spine, such as insertion of Harrington rods
- Antianxiety agent: lorazepam
- Glucocorticoid: methylprednisolone given as infusion immediately following injury (may improve neurologic recovery when administered within 8 hours of injury)
- Histamine-2 (H_2) receptor antagonists: cimetidine, ranitidine, famotidine, nizatidine
- Laxative: bisacodyl
- Mucosal barrier fortifier: sucralfate
- Muscle relaxant: dantrolene

Key interventions

- Monitor neurologic and respiratory status
- Observe for signs and symptoms of spinal shock
- Check for autonomic dysreflexia (sudden, extreme rise in blood pressure)
- Provide skin care

Cerebrovascular accident (stroke)

Destruction of brain cells due to a decrease in cerebral blood flow and oxygen. (two major types: ischemic stroke and hemorrhagic stroke)

Key signs and symptoms

- Garbled or impaired speech
- Inability to move, or difficulty moving, limbs on one side of the body
- Hemianopsia (loss of half of visual field)
- Headache
- Mental impairment
- Seizures
- Coma
- Vomiting

Key test results

- CT scan reveals intracranial bleeding, infarct (shows up 24 hours after the initial symptoms), or shift of midline structures
- Digital subtraction angiography reveals occlusion or narrowing of vessels
- MRI shows intracranial bleeding, infarct, or shift of midline structures

Key treatments

- Anticoagulants: heparin, warfarin, dabigatran, apixaban, rivaroxaban, edoxaban
- Anticonvulsant: phenytoin

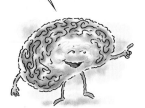

Healthy brain function is a beautiful thing.

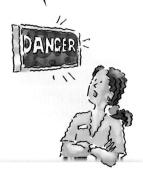

Strokes are life-threatening, and sudden symptoms of garbled or impaired speech, inability to move a limb, or loss of half the visual field should be taken seriously.

- Glucocorticoid: dexamethasone
- Thrombolytic therapy: tissue plasminogen activator given within first 3 hours of an ischemic stroke to:
  - restore circulation to the affected brain tissue
  - limit extent of brain injury upon review of CT scan (head)
- Antiplatelet aggregation agent: ticlopidine, clopidogrel

Key interventions
- Take vital signs every 1 to 2 hours initially and then every 4 hours when client becomes stable
- Elevate the head of the bed 30 degrees
- Conduct a neurologic assessment every 1 to 2 hours initially and then every 4 hours when client becomes stable

Trigeminal neuralgia
Disorder of trigeminal nerve (cranial nerve V) that causes severe stabbing pain on one side of the face

Key signs or symptoms
- Searing pain in the facial area

Key test results
- Observation during examination shows client favoring (splinting) affected area
- To ward off painful attack, client often holds face immobile when talking
- Client may leave affected side of face unwashed and unshaven

Key treatments
- Anticonvulsants: carbamazepine or phenytoin
- Microsurgery for vascular decompression

Key interventions
- Observe and record characteristics of each attack, including client's protective mechanisms
- Provide adequate nutrition in small, frequent meals at room temperature
- Advise client to place food in unaffected side of mouth when chewing,
- Advise client to brush teeth and rinse mouth often,
- Advise client to see dentist twice per year to detect cavities
- After surgical decompression of the root or partial nerve dissection, check neurologic and vital signs often
- Watch for adverse reactions to prescribed medications

West Nile encephalitis
Inflammation of the brain caused by a mosquito-borne virus

Key signs and symptoms
- Fever
- Headache
- Disorientation

Key test results
- Client history reveals recent mosquito bites

Key treatments
- Symptom control (e.g., IV fluids, respiratory support)
- Antipyretic: acetaminophen

Key interventions
- Monitor respiratory status
- Administer supplemental oxygen as prescribed
- Monitor neurologic status
- Administer medications, as prescribed
- Monitor pulse oximetry values

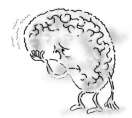

Many different disorders can cause headaches.

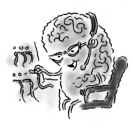

It is important to monitor neurologic status and function to ensure that all "connections" are up and running.

thePoint® You can download tables of drug information to help you prepare for the NCLEX®! View Generic Drug Names, Drug Classifications, Drug Actions, and Nursing Implications for the drugs discussed in this refresher at **http://thePoint.lww.com.**

Neurosensory questions, answers, and rationales

1. A client is admitted with homonymous hemianopsia. Which appropriate interventions should the nurse implement? Select all that apply.
1. Check gag reflex before feeding the client.
2. Approach client on the unaffected side.
3. Allow enough time for the client to answer.
4. Test bath water with the use of thermometer.
5. Gradually teach client to compensate by scanning.

1. **2, 5.** Homonymous hemianopsia is the loss of half of each visual field. This is usually seen in clients with cerebrovascular accident or stroke. The nurse should approach the client on the unaffected side and teach the client to compensate by scanning or turning the head to see things on the affected side. The other options are not related to homonymous hemianopsia.
CN: Safe, effective care environment; CNS: Safety and infection control; CL: Apply; DIFFICULTY: Difficult

2. A client is admitted with cardioembolic stroke. Which vital piece of information in the client's history is strongly associated with this type of stroke?
1. Atrial fibrillation
2. Bradycardia
3. Deep vein thrombosis (DVT)
4. Myocardial infarction (MI)

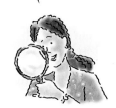

Look carefully in question #2 for the "vital" piece of information.

3. The health care provider prescribed t-PA, a thrombolytic agent. The order is for 0.9 mg/kg over 1 hour. The client weighs 110 lb (50 kg). What is the total dose in milligrams the client will receive? Record your answer using a whole number.

_____ mg

4. A client is receiving apixaban. Which medication instruction should the nurse reinforce during client teaching?
1. Avoid people with upper respiratory infections.
2. The medication will be discontinued before surgery.
3. Monitor for signs of deep vein thrombosis (DVT).
4. Administer the medication with urokinase.

5. The nurse is caring for a client with stroke in evolution. Which nursing intervention is **priority**?
1. Thicken all dietary liquids.
2. Restrict dietary and parenteral fluids.
3. Place the client in the supine position.
4. Have tracheal suction available at all times.

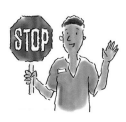

Read question #5 slowly. You are looking for the highest priority.

6. A client is receiving clopidogrel bisulfate. Which should the nurse closely monitor while the client is on this medication? Select all that apply.
1. Sepsis
2. Melena
3. Ecchymosis
4. Drowsiness
5. Hematuria
6. Petechiae

7. A client is admitted with myasthenia gravis. Which nursing intervention should be **priority**?
1. Observe for bleeding
2. Promote mobility
3. Monitor respiratory status
4. Prevent dehydration

2. 1. Cardioembolic strokes are associated with cardiac arrhythmias, usually atrial fibrillation. Atrial fibrillation occurs with the irregular and rapid discharge from multiple ectopic atrial foci that cause quivering of the atria without atrial systole. This asynchronous atrial contraction predisposes to mural thrombi, which may embolize, leading to a stroke. Bradycardia, past MI, or DVT don't lead to arterial embolization.
CN: Physiological integrity; CNS: Physiological adaptation; CL: Apply; DIFFICULTY: Difficult

3. 45.
$$0.9 \text{ mg/kg} \times 50 \text{ kg} = 45 \text{ mg.}$$
CN: Physiological integrity; CNS: Pharmacological therapies; CL: Apply; DIFFICULTY: Easy

4. 2. Apixaban is an anticoagulant used to reduce the risk of having stroke, atrial fibrillation, and pulmonary embolism. It should be discontinued at least 48 hours prior to elective surgery or invasive procedures because it would cause bleeding. Giving apixaban with antiplatelet agents, heparin, aspirin, NSAID, and fibrinolytic agent such as urokinase would cause further bleeding.
CN: Physiological integrity; CNS: Pharmacological therapies; CL: Apply; DIFFICULTY: Challenge

5. 4. Because of a potential loss of gag reflex and potential altered level of consciousness, the client should be kept in Fowler's or a semi-prone position with tracheal suction available at all times. Unless heart failure is present, restricting fluids isn't indicated. Thickening dietary liquids isn't done until the gag reflex returns or the stroke has evolved and the deficit can be assessed.
CN: Physiological integrity; CNS: Reduction of risk potential; CL: Apply; DIFFICULTY: Easy

6. 2, 3, 5, 6. Clopidogrel bisulfate is an antiplatelet agent. The client should be monitored for signs of bleeding like ecchymosis, melena, hematuria, and petechiae while on this medication. The other options are not related to signs of bleeding.
CN: Physiological integrity; CNS: Pharmacological therapies; CL: Apply; DIFFICULTY: Challenge

7. 3. Myasthenia gravis is a neuromuscular disorder that causes extreme muscle weakness because of the deficiency of acetylcholine at the myoneural junction. The nurse should monitor the respiratory status frequently because the respiratory muscles may also be involved. Airway is always the priority.
CN: Physiological integrity; CNS: Physiological adaptation; CL: Apply; DIFFICULTY: Easy

8. A client had a thrombotic right brain stroke with swelling of the left arm. Which condition does the nurse identify that can cause swelling after a stroke?
1. Elbow contracture
2. Loss of muscle contraction
3. Deep vein thrombosis (DVT)
4. Hypoalbuminemia

8. 2. In clients with hemiplegia or hemiparesis, loss of muscle contraction decreases venous return and may cause swelling of the affected extremity. Stroke isn't linked to protein loss. DVT may develop in clients with a stroke but is more likely in the lower extremities. Contractures, or bony calcifications, may occur with stroke but don't appear with swelling.
CN: Physiological integrity; CNS: Physiological adaptation; CL: Analyze; DIFFICULTY: Moderate

9. A client was diagnosed with a brain stem infarction. During data collection, the nurse should observe the client for which condition?
1. Aphasia
2. Bradypnea
3. Contralateral hemiplegia
4. Numbness of the face

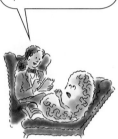

Assessing brain injuries and conditions requires patience and care.

9. 2. The brain stem contains the medulla and the vital cardiac, vasomotor, and respiratory centers. A brain stem infarction leads to vital sign changes such as bradypnea. Numbness, tingling in the face, contralateral hemiplegia, and aphasia may occur with a stroke.
CN: Physiological integrity; CNS: Physiological adaptation; CL: Apply; DIFFICULTY: Difficult

10. A client with cerebrovascular accident (CVA) is admitted with receptive aphasia. Which action by the nurse is appropriate?
1. Listen and watch carefully while the client is speaking.
2. Allow enough time for the client to answer questions.
3. Check the client's gag reflex.
4. Give client simple and slow instructions.

10. 4. Receptive aphasia means that the client is having difficulty in understanding spoken and written language. Giving simple and slow directions would help the client understand the message. Listening and watching carefully while the client is speaking, and giving enough time to answer questions, are appropriate nursing interventions for a client with expressive aphasia. Checking the gag reflex is necessary for a client with dysphagia or difficulty in swallowing.
CN: Physiological integrity; CNS: Basic care and comfort; CL: Apply DIFFICULTY: Difficult

11. A client had cataract surgery. Which sign or symptom should the nurse tell the client to report immediately to the health care provider?
1. Blurred vision
2. Eye pain
3. Glare
4. Itching

11. 2. Pain shouldn't be present after cataract surgery. Pain may be an indication of hyphema or clouding in the anterior chamber, and infection. The client should be told that the other symptoms might be present.
CN: Physiological integrity; CNS: Physiological adaptation; CL: Understand; DIFFICULTY: Moderate

12. The nurse observes clear fluid is draining from the nose of a client who had a head trauma 3 hours ago. Which condition does the nurse suspect from this observation?
1. Basilar skull fracture
2. Cerebral concussion
3. Cerebral palsy
4. Sinus infection

12. 1. Clear fluid draining from the ear or nose of a client may mean a cerebrospinal fluid leak, which is common in basilar skull fractures. Concussion is associated with a brief loss of consciousness; sinus infection is associated with facial pain and pressure with or without nasal drainage; and cerebral palsy is associated with nonprogressive paralysis present since birth.
CN: Physiological integrity; CNS: Physiological adaptation; CL: Analyze; DIFFICULTY: Challenge

13. A client with a mild concussion reports a headache. When offered acetaminophen, the client asks for a stronger pain medication. Which response by the nurse is appropriate?
1. "You have a mild concussion; acetaminophen is strong enough."
2. "Aspirin is avoided because of the danger of Reye syndrome in children or young adults."
3. "Opioids are avoided after a head injury because they may hide a worsening condition."
4. "Stronger medications may lead to vomiting, which increases intracranial pressure (ICP)."

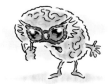

Be aware that opioids can mask changes in level of consciousness.

13. 3. Opioids may mask changes in the level of consciousness (LOC) that indicate increased ICP and shouldn't be given. Saying acetaminophen is strong enough ignores the client's question and therefore isn't appropriate. Aspirin is contraindicated in conditions that may cause bleeding, such as trauma, and for children or young adults with viral illnesses because of the danger of Reye syndrome. Stronger medications may not necessarily lead to vomiting but will sedate the client, thereby masking changes in his LOC.
CN: Physiological integrity; CNS: Reduction of risk potential; CL: Apply; DIFFICULTY: Moderate

14. A client admitted to the hospital with a subarachnoid hemorrhage (SAH) reports severe headache, nuchal rigidity, and projectile vomiting. The nurse suspects that lumbar puncture (LP) may be contraindicated due to which circumstance?
1. Continued vomiting
2. Increased intracranial pressure (ICP)
3. Mechanical ventilation needed
4. Anticipated blood in the cerebrospinal fluid

14. 2. Severe headache, nuchal rigidity, and projectile vomiting are signs of ICP. Sudden removal of cerebrospinal fluid results in pressures in the lumbar area lower than the brain and favors herniation of the brain; therefore, LP is contraindicated with increased ICP. Vomiting may be caused by reasons other than increased ICP; therefore, LP isn't strictly contraindicated. Blood in the cerebrospinal fluid is diagnostic for SAH and was obtained before signs and symptoms of increased ICP. An LP may be performed on clients needing mechanical ventilation.
CN: Physiological integrity; CNS: Physiological adaptation; CL: Apply; DIFFICULTY: Moderate

15. A client with head trauma develops a urine output of 300 mL/hour, dry skin, and dry mucous membranes. Which nursing intervention is **most** appropriate to perform immediately?
1. Check urine specific gravity.
2. Anticipate treatment for renal failure.
3. Apply emollients to the skin.
4. Decrease IV fluid rate.

15. 1. Urine output of 300 mL/hour may indicate diabetes insipidus, which is failure of the pituitary to produce antidiuretic hormone. This may occur with increased intracranial pressure and head trauma; the nurse evaluates for low urine specific gravity, increased serum osmolarity, and dehydration. There's no evidence that the client is experiencing renal failure. Providing emollients to prevent skin breakdown is important but doesn't need to be performed immediately. A health care provider's order is necessary to slow the IV rate, and lowering the rate would contribute to dehydration when polyuria is present.
CN: Physiological integrity; CNS: Physiological adaptation; CL: Analyze; DIFFICULTY: Moderate

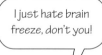

I just hate brain freeze, don't you!

16. A nurse is taking care of four clients. Which client should the nurse see **first**?
1. A client with meningitis reporting nuchal rigidity
2. A client with cerebrovascular accident with hemianopsia
3. A client with myasthenia gravis with flu-like symptoms
4. A client with trigeminal neuralgia with stabbing pain on the face

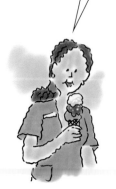

16. 3. A client with myasthenia gravis with flu-like symptoms should be checked first because infection may cause myasthenic crisis. The client may have an abrupt onset of extreme muscle weakness with inability to swallow, speak, and maintain respiration. Airway is always the priority. A client with meningitis is expected to have stiff neck or nuchal rigidity. Hemianopsia or loss of the half of visual field is usually seen in clients with stroke. A client with trigeminal neuralgia will usually report stabbing pain on one side of the face during acute episode.
CN: Safe, effective care environment; CNS: Coordinated care; CL: Apply; DIFFICULTY: Difficult

17. A client was admitted with a brain tumor. Which vital signs would the nurse expect to notice?
 1. T, 98 F; P, 108; R, 14; BP, 120/82
 2. T, 97 F; P, 60; R, 23; BP, 158/94
 3. T, 99 F; P, 52; R, 12; BP, 176/86
 4. T, 99 F; P, 82; R, 16; BP, 149/82

18. A client with a subdural hematoma was given mannitol. Which result would **best** show the effectiveness of the medication?
 1. Urine output of 65 mL/hour.
 2. Pupils are 8 mm and nonreactive.
 3. Systolic blood pressure of 150 mm Hg.
 4. Serum creatinine of 2.5 mg/dL (221 µmol/L).

19. When evaluating an arterial blood gas (ABG) from a client with a subdural hematoma, the nurse notes the Pa_{CO_2} is 30 mm Hg. Which response **best** describes this result?
 1. Appropriate; lowering carbon dioxide (CO_2) reduces intracranial pressure (ICP)
 2. Emergent; the client is poorly oxygenated
 3. Normal
 4. Significant; the client has alveolar hypoventilation

20. Which nursing intervention should be used to prevent footdrop and contractures in a client recovering from a subdural hematoma?
 1. High-top sneakers
 2. Low-dose heparin therapy
 3. Physical therapy consultation
 4. Sequential compression device

21. A client was diagnosed with having right subarachnoid hemorrhage. The nurse should plan to place the client in which position?
 1. With the head of the bed elevated
 2. On right side
 3. On left side
 4. Flat in bed

22. A client with a history of convulsions suddenly says to the nurse, "I see bright lights and zigzag lines." Which action should the nurse take **first**?
 1. Tell the client to ignore the bright lights.
 2. Place the client away from the nurses' station.
 3. Leave the room and inform the registered nurse.
 4. Pad side rails and lower the height of the bed.

17. 3. A client with brain tumor will experience an increase in intracranial pressure (ICP). One of the assessment findings in increased ICP is Cushing's triad, which includes hypertension, bradycardia, and widening pulse pressure.
CN: Physiological integrity; CNS: Physiological adaptation; CL: Apply; DIFFICULTY: Moderate

18. 1. Mannitol promotes osmotic diuresis by increasing the pressure gradient in the renal tubules. The normal urine output is 30 to 50 mL/hour. A urine output of 65 mL/hour means the client has an increase in urine output and therefore a sign of effectiveness of the medication. The normal serum creatinine is 0.6 to 1.2 mg/dL (53 to 106 µmol/L). Serum creatinine of 2.5 mg/dL (221 µmol/L) is not sign of effectiveness of the medication because the result is elevated. The systolic blood pressure should go down because of diuresis. Fixed and dilated pupils are symptoms of increased ICP or cranial nerve damage.
CN: Physiological integrity; CNS: Physiological adaptation; CL: Apply; DIFFICULTY: Moderate

19. 1. A normal Pa_{CO_2} value is 35 to 45 mm Hg. CO_2 has vasodilating properties; therefore, lowering Pa_{CO_2} through hyperventilation will lower ICP caused by dilated cerebral vessels. Alveolar hypoventilation would be reflected in an increased Pa_{CO_2}. Oxygenation is evaluated through Pa_{CO_2} and oxygen saturation.
CN: Physiological integrity; CNS: Physiological adaptation; CL: Analyze; DIFFICULTY: Moderate

20. 1. High-top sneakers are used to prevent footdrop and contractures in neurologic clients. Low-dose heparin therapy and sequential compression boots will prevent deep vein thrombosis. Although a consultation with physical therapy is important to prevent footdrop, a nurse may use high-top sneakers independently.
CN: Physiological integrity; CNS: Basic care and comfort; CL: Apply; DIFFICULTY: Moderate

21. 1. Elevating the head of the bed enhances cerebral venous return and thereby decreases intracranial pressure (ICP). The other positions wouldn't decrease ICP.
CN: Physiological integrity; CNS: Reduction of risk potential; CL: Apply; DIFFICULTY: Moderate

22. 4. The client is experiencing a visual aura, which is a warning sign of an impending seizure. The nurse should immediately institute seizure precautions such as padding the side rails and lowering the bed. All the other options are inappropriate.
CN: Safe, effective care environment; CNS: Safety an infection control; CL: Apply; DIFFICULTY: Easy

CN: Client needs category CNS: Client needs subcategory CL: Cognitive level

23. A client with Parkinson disease is receiving selegiline. Which foods should the nurse instruct the client to avoid while taking this medication? Select all that apply.
1. Salami
2. Eggs
3. Aged cheese
4. Soy sauce
5. Milk
6. Sauerkraut

23. 1, 3, 4, 6. Selegiline is a monoamine oxidase B (MAO-B) inhibitor used in clients with Parkinson disease. The nurse should tell the client to avoid foods with high tyramine content while on this medication because it would cause hypertensive crisis. Salami, aged cheese, soy sauce, and sauerkraut are foods with high tyramine content and therefore should be avoided. Milk and eggs can be safely given to the client while on selegiline.
CN: Physiological integrity; CNS: Pharmacological therapies; CL: Apply; DIFFICULTY: Difficult

24. A client undergoes an L4–L5 laminectomy. Which nursing action would be **best** to prevent postoperative complications?
1. Encourage the client to be out of bed the first postoperative day.
2. Maximize bracing while in bed.
3. Limit movement in bed and reposition only when necessary.
4. Use a soft mattress.

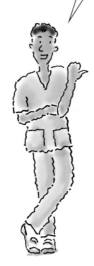

Looks like airborne precautions are needed. What should you do?

24. 1. In most cases, clients should be out of bed the first postoperative day. Frequent repositioning, use of a chair-like brace for the lower back when out of bed, and a firm mattress will help minimize complications.
CN: Physiological integrity; CNS: Reduction of risk potential; CL: Apply; DIFFICULTY: Challenge

25. A client was admitted with a diagnosis of meningitis. Which infection control measures should the nurse implement when caring for the client? Select all that apply.
1. Wear gloves
2. Wear gown
3. Wear mask
4. Wear goggles
5. Wash hands

25. 3, 5. A client with meningitis is placed on airborne precaution. The nurse should wear a mask when taking care of this client. The nurse should always wash hands before and after client care. Gloves and gown are both used for contact precaution. Goggles are used when there is any chance of splashing.
CN: Safe, effective care environment; CNS: Safety and infection control; CL: Apply; DIFFICULTY: Challenge

26. A client was admitted with amyotrophic lateral sclerosis (ALS). Which manifestations would the nurse observe during data collection? Select all that apply.
1. Muscle atrophy
2. Ascending paralysis
3. Memory loss
4. Drooping of eyelids
5. Dysphagia

26. 1, 5. Amyotrophic lateral sclerosis (ALS) or Lou Gehrig's disease is a progressive motor neuron disease that causes muscle wasting or atrophy. The client may also experience dysphagia. Ascending paralysis is a key sign of Guillain-Barré Syndrome (GBS). The intellectual functioning of a client with ALS is intact. Memory loss is a classic sign of Alzheimer's disease. Drooping of the eyelids or ptosis is seen in clients with myasthenia gravis.
CN: Physiological integrity; CNS: Physiological adaptation; CL: Apply; DIFFICULTY: Challenge

27. A nurse is preparing a client with suspected herniated nucleus pulposus (HNP) for myelography. Which nursing intervention should the nurse perform before the test?
1. Question the client about allergy to iodine.
2. Mark distal pulses on the foot in ink.
3. Check and document pain along the sciatic nerve.
4. Tell the client to cough or pant to clear the dye.

27. 1. A radiopaque dye, commonly iodine-based, is instilled into the spinal canal to outline structures during myelography; therefore, asking about iodine allergy is needed. Pain may be expected along the sciatic nerve with HNP. During cardiac catheterization, a client coughs or pants to clear the dye; before cardiac catheterization or arteriogram, the nurse marks pedal pulses in ink.
CN: Physiological integrity; CNS: Reduction of risk potential; CL: Apply; DIFFICULTY: Easy

28. A client recovering from a stroke has residual dysphagia. When assisting the client to eat, which educational points should the nurse reinforce? Select all that apply.
  1. "Look up at the ceiling when you swallow."
  2. "Tuck your chin in when you swallow."
  3. "Turn your head toward your weaker side when you swallow."
  4. "After you swallow food, wait a few seconds and then swallow again."
  5. "Swallow softly between each bite of food."

28. 2, 3, 4. Tucking the chin in reduces the size of the airway opening, which helps prevent aspiration, and a double swallow helps clear the pharynx between bites of food. Having the client turn the head toward his weaker side makes swallowing easier. Swallowing forcefully reduces the amount of residual food in the client's pharynx.
CN: Physiological integrity; CNS: Basic care and comfort;
CL: Apply; DIFFICULTY: Challenge

29. A nurse is taking care of four clients. Which client should the nurse see **first**?
  1. A 17-year-old client 24 hours postappendectomy
  2. A 33-year-old client with a recent diagnosis of Guillain-Barré syndrome
  3. A 50-year-old client 3 days post–myocardial infarction (MI)
  4. A 50-year-old client with diverticulitis

29. 2. Guillain-Barré syndrome is characterized by ascending paralysis and potential respiratory failure. The order of client assessment should follow client priorities, with disorders of airway, breathing, and then circulation. There's no information to suggest the post-MI client has an arrhythmia or other complication. There's no evidence to suggest hemorrhage or perforation for the remaining clients as a priority of care.
CN: Safe, effective care environment; CNS: Coordinated care;
CL: Analyze; DIFFICULTY: Moderate

30. A client is newly diagnosed with myasthenia gravis. When reinforcing education what should the nurse indicate as the cause of this disease?
  1. A postviral illness characterized by ascending paralysis.
  2. Loss of the myelin sheath surrounding peripheral nerves.
  3. Inability of basal ganglia to produce sufficient dopamine.
  4. Destruction of acetylcholine receptors, causing muscle weakness.

30. 4. Myasthenia gravis, an autoimmune disorder, is caused by the destruction of acetylcholine receptors. Multiple sclerosis is caused by loss of the myelin sheath. Guillain-Barré syndrome is a postviral illness characterized by ascending paralysis, and Parkinson disease is caused by the inability of basal ganglia to produce sufficient dopamine.
CN: Health promotion and maintenance; CNS: None;
CL: Understand; DIFFICULTY: Easy

31. A client is scheduled for electroencephalogram (EEG). Which nursing actions should be included in preparing the client before the procedure? Select all that apply.
  1. Ask client about allergy to iodine or shellfish.
  2. Advise client to shampoo hair before the procedure.
  3. Tell client to avoid caffeine 8 to 12 hours prior to the test.
  4. Instruct client not to eat or drink anything after midnight.
  5. Inform client that the procedure is painful.

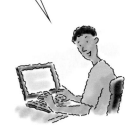
In question #31, remember to select all that apply.

31. 2, 3. Electroencephalogram (EEG) is a test that measures the electrical activity of the brain. The nurse should advise the client to shampoo hair and avoid using hairsprays or hair gels before the procedure because electrodes will be placed on the client's scalp. Caffeine should also be avoided 8 to 12 hours prior to the test. A dye or contrast medium is not injected during EEG, therefore asking client about allergy to iodine or shellfish is not necessary. The client should avoid fasting because hypoglycemia will alter the result of the test. EEG is a painless procedure.
CN: Physiological integrity; CNS: Reduction of risk potential;
CL: Apply; DIFFICULTY: Difficult

32. One hour after receiving pyridostigmine, a client reports difficulty swallowing and excessive respiratory secretions. The nurse notifies the health care provider and prepares to administer which medication?
1. Additional pyridostigmine
2. Atropine
3. Edrophonium
4. Acyclovir

33. A client is prescribed sumatriptan. Which conditions would cause the nurse to question this health care provider's order? Select all that apply.
1. Uncontrolled hypertension
2. Myocardial infarction
3. Hypersensitivity reaction
4. Cerebrovascular accident
5. Migraine headache

34. A client is admitted with Bell palsy. What should the nurse and health care team include in the plan of care?
1. Protect client's skin integrity
2. Prevent complications of immobility
3. Provide eye care
4. Maintain normal bowel elimination

35. When collecting data on a client with glaucoma, the nurse expects which finding? Select all that apply.
1. Reports of double vision
2. Reports of halos around lights
3. Loss of central vision
4. Soft globe on palpation
5. Decreased accommodation

36. A client at the eye clinic is newly diagnosed with glaucoma. What should the nurse inform the client might occur if administration of the medication is not closely adhered to?
1. Diplopia
2. Permanent vision loss
3. Loss of central vision
4. Pupillary constriction

32. 2. These symptoms suggest cholinergic crisis or excessive acetylcholinesterase medication, typically appearing 45 to 60 minutes after the last dose of acetylcholinesterase inhibitor. Atropine, an anticholinergic drug, is used to antagonize acetylcholinesterase inhibitors. The other drugs are acetylcholinesterase inhibitors. Edrophonium is used to diagnose myasthenia gravis, and pyridostigmine is used to treat the condition and would worsen the symptoms. Acyclovir is an antiviral and would not be used to treat the client's symptoms.
CN: Physiological integrity; CNS: Pharmacological therapies; CL: Analyze; DIFFICULTY: Easy

33. 1, 2, 3, 4. Sumatriptan is a selective serotonin receptor agonist used for the treatment of migraine headache. Sumatriptan is contraindicated in clients with myocardial infarction, hypersensitivity reaction, uncontrolled hypertension, and history of cerebrovascular accident (CVA).
CN: Physiological integrity; CNS: Pharmacological therapies; CL: Apply; DIFFICULTY: Difficult

34. 3. Bell palsy is the disorder of cranial nerve VII (facial nerve) that causes weakness or paralysis of one side of the face. The client will also have difficulty closing the eye of the affected side. The nurse should provide eye care by using eye drops and an eye patch to prevent corneal dryness and to protect the eye from irritation. The other options are not appropriate.
CN: Physiological integrity; CNS: Basic care and comfort; CL: Apply; DIFFICULTY: Difficult

35. 2, 5. Glaucoma is largely asymptomatic. Symptoms can include loss of peripheral vision or blind spots, reddened sclera, firm globe, decreased accommodation, halos around lights, and occasional eye pain. Loss of central vision is seen in clients with macular degeneration.
CN: Physiological integrity; CNS: Physiological adaptation; CL: Apply; DIFFICULTY: Challenge

36. 2. Without proper treatment, glaucoma may progress to irreversible blindness. Treatment won't restore visual damage but will halt disease progression. Miotics, which constrict the pupil, are used in the treatment of glaucoma to permit outflow of the aqueous humor. Loss of peripheral vision and blurred or foggy vision (not diplopia) are typical in glaucoma. Loss of central vision is common in clients with macular degeneration.
CN: Physiological integrity; CNS: Pharmacological therapies; CL: Apply; DIFFICULTY: Easy

37. The nurse is caring for a client with a cerebral injury who has impaired speech and hearing. Which part of the brain does the nurse suspect has been affected?
1. Frontal lobe
2. Parietal lobe
3. Occipital lobe
4. Temporal lobe

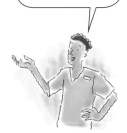

Which lobe is associated with speech and hearing?

38. The nurse is caring for a client with Parkinson disease. Which complication should the nurse observe for related to the decreased amount of dopamine?
1. Exophthalmos
2. Diminished distal extremity sensation
3. Excessive involuntary movements
4. Bradykinesia

39. A client is receiving neostigmine. Which side effects should the nurse monitor for in this client? Select all that apply.
1. Dry mouth
2. Abdominal cramps
3. Increased sweating
4. Tachycardia
5. Increased urination

40. Which client would be **most** at risk for secondary Parkinson disease caused by pharmacotherapy?
1. A 30-year-old client with schizophrenia taking chlorpromazine
2. A 50-year-old client taking nitroglycerin tablets for angina
3. A 60-year-old client taking prednisone for chronic obstructive pulmonary disease (COPD)
4. A 75-year-old client using naproxen for rheumatoid arthritis

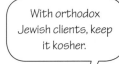

With orthodox Jewish clients, keep it kosher.

41. A nurse is assigned to care for an orthodox Jewish client. Which dietary instructions should the nurse be sure the team includes in the plan of care? Select all that apply.
1. Strictly adhere to lacto-ovo-vegetarian diet
2. Only fish that have scales and fins can be offered
3. Meat products not ritually slaughtered are forbidden
4. Fasting is observed during the month of Ramadan
5. Any combination of meat and milk is forbidden

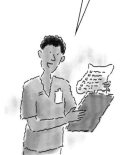

37. 4. The portion of the cerebrum that controls speech and hearing is the temporal lobe. Injury to the frontal lobe causes personality changes, difficulty speaking, and disturbances in memory, reasoning, and concentration. Injury to the parietal lobe causes sensory alterations and problems with spatial relationships. Damage to the occipital lobe causes vision disturbances.
CN: Physiological integrity; CNS: Physiological adaptation; CL: Understand; DIFFICULTY: Moderate

38. 4. Parkinson disease is characterized by the slowing of voluntary muscle movement (bradykinesia), muscular rigidity, and resting tremor. Dopamine is deficient in this disorder. Diminished distal extremity sensation doesn't occur in Parkinson disease. Bulging eyeballs (exophthalmos) occurs in Graves disease. Excessive involuntary movement is a sign of Huntington disease.
CN: Physiological integrity; CNS: Physiological adaptation; CL: Apply; DIFFICULTY: Challenge

39. 2, 3, 5. Neostigmine is an anticholinesterase drug used to improve muscle strength in clients with myasthenia gravis. It blocks the action of cholinesterase and increases the level of acetylcholine at the neuromuscular junction. Abdominal cramps, increased sweating, and increased urination are all side effects of neostigmine. This drug causes excessive salivation, not dry mouth. The client may also experience bradycardia, not tachycardia.
CN: Physiological integrity; CNS: Pharmacological therapies; CL: Analyze; DIFFICULTY: Difficult

40. 1. Phenothiazines, such as chlorpromazine, deplete dopamine, which may lead to tremor and rigidity (extrapyramidal effects). The other clients aren't at a greater risk for developing Parkinson disease caused by pharmacotherapy.
CN: Physiological integrity; CNS: Pharmacological therapies; CL: Apply; DIFFICULTY: Moderate

41. 2, 3, 5. Jewish dietary kosher laws include eating only fish that have scales and fins, prohibiting eating meat products not ritually slaughtered, and avoiding eating meat with milk products. Seventh Day Adventists and Buddhists follow a lacto-ovo-vegetarian diet. Muslims fast during the month of Ramadan.
CN: Psychosocial integrity; CNS: None; CL: Apply; DIFFICULTY: Difficult

42. To evaluate the effectiveness of levodopa-carbidopa in a client with Parkinson disease, the nurse would observe for which outcome?
1. Improved visual acuity
2. Increased dyskinesia
3. Reduced short-term memory
4. Lessened rigidity and tremor

42. 4. Levodopa-carbidopa increases the amount of dopamine in the central nervous system, allowing for smooth, purposeful movements. The drug doesn't affect visual acuity and should improve dyskinesia and short-term memory.
CN: Physiological integrity; CNS: Pharmacological therapies;
CL: Apply; DIFFICULTY: Easy

43. Two days after starting therapy with trihexyphenidyl, a client reports a dry mouth. Which nursing intervention would **best** relieve the client's dry mouth?
1. Offering the client ice chips and frequent sips of water
2. Withholding the drug and notifying the health care provider
3. Changing the client's diet to clear liquid until the symptoms subside
4. Encouraging the use of supplemental puddings and shakes to maintain weight

43. 1. Trihexyphenidyl is an anticholinergic agent that causes blurred vision, dry mouth, constipation, and urine retention. There's no need to withhold the drug unless hypotension or tachyarrhythmia occurs. Weight loss may occur with Parkinson disease; however, the question relates to the effects of trihexyphenidyl. A clear liquid diet doesn't provide adequate nutrition and may be more difficult to swallow than thickened liquids if dysphagia is present; it isn't indicated at this time.
CN: Physiological integrity; CNS: Pharmacological therapies;
CL: Apply; DIFFICULTY: Easy

44. A client with encephalitis is receiving acyclovir. Which laboratory tests should the nurse monitor during treatment with this medication? Select all that apply.
1. Blood urea nitrogen (BUN)
2. Aspartate aminotransferase (AST)
3. Alanine aminotransferase (ALT)
4. Amylase
5. Creatinine
6. Lipase

44. 1, 2, 3, 5. Acyclovir is antiviral medication. The nurse should monitor the BUN and creatinine because this drug is nephrotoxic. AST and ALT should also be monitored because acyclovir is hepatotoxic.
CN: Physiological integrity; CNS: Pharmacological therapies;
CL: Apply; DIFFICULTY: Difficult

45. A client is receiving levodopa-carbidopa. What should the nurse reinforce during client teaching? Select all that apply.
1. Avoid sudden changes in position
2. Always administer with grapefruit
3. Avoid eating high-protein foods
4. Encourage use of CNS depressants
5. Avoid large doses of pyridoxine

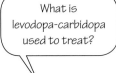

What is levodopa-carbidopa used to treat?

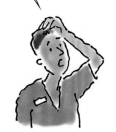

45. 1, 3, 5. Levodopa-carbidopa is used to treat symptoms of Parkinson disease. The client should avoid sudden changes in position because the medication will cause orthostatic hypotension. High-protein diet and large doses of pyridoxine (vitamin B$_6$) should be avoided because it will reduce the effectiveness of the levodopa-carbidopa. Since the medication will cause drowsiness, central nervous system (CNS) depressants should also be avoided. Grapefruit should be avoided because it will decrease the breakdown of the medication by the liver and cause increased drug level in the blood.
CN: Physiological integrity; CNS: Pharmacological therapies;
CL: Apply; DIFFICULTY: Moderate

46. A client with history of seizures is receiving gabapentin. Which side effects should the nurse monitor for in this client? Select all that apply.
1. Drowsiness
2. Dizziness
3. Increased salivation
4. Weight loss
5. Tremors

46. 1, 2, 5. Gabapentin is a medication used for seizures and neuropathic pain. The nurse should monitor for the side effects of this drug, which includes drowsiness, dizziness, and tremors. Gabapentin also causes weight gain and dry mouth.
CN: Physiological integrity; CNS: Pharmacological therapies;
CL: Analyze; DIFFICULTY: Difficult

47. An adult client was admitted with myasthenia gravis. While reviewing the client's chart, the licensed practical nurse (LPN)/licensed vocational nurse (LVN) noticed the medication administration record (MAR), noted below.

Progress notes

Medications
Furosemide 20 mg PO bid
Neostigmine 15 mg PO every 4 hours
Potassium chloride 20 mEq PO once a day
Morphine sulfate 10 mg IM every 4 hours
Docusate sodium 100 mg PO once a day

Based on the information, what should the nurse do next?
1. Always administer neostigmine and morphine together.
2. Administer the morphine sulfate and hold the neostigmine.
3. Notify the registered nurse and question the morphine sulfate.
4. Check the platelet count before administering neostigmine.

48. Which measure should the nurse emphasize when reinforcing education for a client with multiple sclerosis (MS) to avoid exacerbation of the disease?
1. Patch the affected eye.
2. Sleep 8 hours each night.
3. Take hot baths for relaxation.
4. Drink 1,500 to 2,000 mL of fluid daily.

49. A client is admitted with complications related to myasthenia gravis. Which medications should the nurse avoid administering to this client? Select all that apply.
1. Ciprofloxacin
2. Pyridostigmine
3. Propranolol
4. Ambenonium
5. Lithium

50. A client with suspected multiple sclerosis (MS) undergoes a lumbar puncture. When reviewing the results of the laboratory analysis of the cerebrospinal fluid (CSF), what does the nurse expect to find?
1. Blood or increased red blood cells
2. Elevated white blood cells (WBCs)
3. Increased glucose concentrations
4. Increased protein levels

47. 3. Myasthenia gravis is a neuromuscular disease characterized by deficiency of acetylcholine at the myoneural junction, causing extreme voluntary muscle weakness. Clients with myasthenia gravis are usually given an anticholinesterase drug like neostigmine to improve muscle strength. Anticholinesterase drugs may potentiate the effect of morphine. The LPN/LVN should inform the RN and question the medication because narcotic analgesic such as morphine may cause respiratory depression.
CN: Physiological integrity; CNS: Pharmacological therapies; CL: Understand; DIFFICULTY: Moderate

48. 2. MS is exacerbated by exposure to stress, fatigue, and heat. Clients should balance activity with rest. Patching the affected eye may result in improvement in vision and balance but won't prevent exacerbation of the disease. Adequate hydration will help prevent urinary tract infections secondary to a neurogenic bladder.
CN: Physiological integrity; CNS: Reduction of risk potential; CL: Apply; DIFFICULTY: Moderate

Caution! Some drugs can cause further muscle weakness in clients with myasthenia gravis.

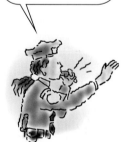

49. 1, 3, 5. The client with myasthenia gravis should avoid taking ciprofloxacin, propranolol, and lithium because these drugs will further cause muscle weakness. Pyridostigmine and ambenonium are anticholinesterase agents used in clients with myasthenia gravis.
CN: Physiological integrity; CNS: Pharmacological therapies; CL: Analyze; DIFFICULTY: Difficult

50. 4. Elevated gamma globulin fraction in CSF without an elevated level in the blood occurs in MS. Blood may be found with trauma or subarachnoid hemorrhage. Increased glucose concentration is a nonspecific finding indicating infection or subarachnoid hemorrhage. Elevated WBCs or pus indicate infection.
CN: Physiological integrity; CNS: Physiological adaptation; CL: Analyze; DIFFICULTY: Moderate

51. A client was admitted with meningitis. Which finding would support the diagnosis? Select all that apply.
1. Turner sign
2. Brudzinski sign
3. Murphy sign
4. Kernig sign
5. Cullen sign
6. Battle sign

51. 2, 4. A client with meningitis will experience signs of meningeal irritation which includes nuchal rigidity (stiff neck), Brudzinski sign, and Kernig sign. Brudzinski sign is the flexion at the hip and knee in response to forward flexion of the neck. Kernig sign is the severe stiffness and pain in the hamstring muscle when attempting to extend the leg when the hip is flexed. Turner sign and Cullen sign are both signs of retroperitoneal bleeding seen in clients with acute pancreatitis. Battle sign is the ecchymosis behind the ear, which is a sign of head injury.
CN: Physiological integrity; CNS: Physiological adaptation; CL: Apply; DIFFICULTY: Difficult

52. Which nursing intervention takes **priority** for the client having a tonic-clonic seizure?
1. Maintaining a patent airway
2. Timing the duration of the seizure
3. Noting the origin of seizure activity
4. Inserting tongue blade inside the mouth

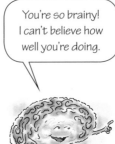

You're so brainy! I can't believe how well you're doing.

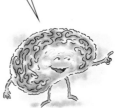

52. 1. The priority during and after a seizure is to maintain a patent airway. Nothing should be placed in the client's mouth during a seizure because teeth may be dislodged or the tongue pushed back, further obstructing the airway. Noting the origin of the seizure activity and the duration of the seizure are important, but they do not take priority over maintenance of a patent airway.
CN: Physiological integrity; CNS: Reduction of risk potential; CL: Apply; DIFFICULTY: Easy

53. A client is receiving dabigatran. Which medication instructions should the nurse reinforce during client teaching? Select all that apply.
1. Avoid eating green, leafy vegetables.
2. Prothrombin (PT) and international normalized ratio (INR) will be monitored.
3. Do not chew, break, or open capsules.
4. Immediately report signs of bleeding.
5. Take medication with a full glass of water.

53. 3, 4, 5. Dabigatran is a direct thrombin inhibitor that reduces the risk of cerebrovascular accident (stroke), atrial fibrillation, deep vein thrombosis (DVT), and pulmonary embolism. Unlike warfarin, there is no need to avoid foods high in vitamin K and it is not necessary to monitor the PT/INR while on this medication. Client should not chew, break, or open capsules while taking this drug. The medication should also be taken with full glass of water. Signs of bleeding should be immediately reported because of its anticoagulant effect.
CN: Physiological integrity; CNS: Pharmacological therapies; CL: Apply; DIFFICULTY: Difficult

54. A client with new-onset seizures of unknown cause is started on phenytoin, 750 mg IV now and 100 mg PO t.i.d. Which statement **best** describes the purpose of the loading dose?
1. To ensure that the drug reaches the cerebrospinal fluid
2. To prevent the need for surgical excision of the epileptic focus
3. To reduce secretions in case another seizure occurs
4. To more quickly attain therapeutic levels

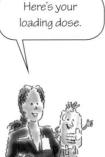

Here's your loading dose.

54. 4. A loading dose of phenytoin and other drugs is given to reach therapeutic levels more quickly; maintenance dosing follows. A loading dose of phenytoin can be oral or parenteral. Surgical excision of an epileptic focus is considered when seizures aren't controlled with anticonvulsant therapy. Phenytoin doesn't reduce secretions.
CN: Physiological integrity; CNS: Pharmacological therapies; CL: Apply; DIFFICULTY: Easy

55. A client with history of seizure disorder is receiving phenytoin. Which adverse effects should the nurse monitor during phenytoin therapy? Select all that apply.
1. Dry mouth
2. Furry tongue
3. Somnolence
4. Tachycardia
5. Drowsiness

55. 3, 5. Adverse effects of phenytoin include sedation, drowsiness, somnolence, gingival hyperplasia, blood dyscrasia, and toxicity. The other symptoms aren't adverse effects of phenytoin.
CN: Physiological integrity; CNS: Pharmacological therapies; CL: Analyze; DIFFICULTY: Challenge

CN: Client needs category   CNS: Client needs subcategory   CL: Cognitive level

56. A client has a phenytoin level of 32 mg/dL. Which symptoms should the nurse monitor based on the result?
1. Ataxia and confusion
2. Sodium depletion
3. Tonic-clonic seizure
4. Urinary incontinence

57. Which precaution must the nurse take when giving phenytoin to a client with a nasogastric (NG) tube for feeding?
1. Check the phenytoin level after giving the drug to check for toxicity.
2. Elevate the head of the bed before giving phenytoin through the NG tube.
3. Give phenytoin 1 hour before or 2 hours after NG tube feedings to ensure absorption.
4. Verify proper placement of the NG tube by placing the end of the tube in a glass of water and observing for bubbles.

58. The nurse is reinforcing education to a client taking phenytoin for the treatment of seizures. The client asks, "Can I still have my beer every day"? What is the **best** response by the nurse?
1. Alcohol increases phenytoin activity.
2. Alcohol raises the seizure threshold.
3. Alcohol impairs judgment and coordination.
4. Alcohol decreases the effectiveness of phenytoin.

59. The nurse is obtaining vital signs for a client with a seizure disorder. Which method would the nurse use to obtain the **most** accurate measure?
1. Check for a pulse deficit.
2. Check for pulsus paradoxus.
3. Take an axillary temperature instead of an oral temperature.
4. Check the blood pressure for an auscultatory gap.

60. A client with increased intracranial pressure has been exhibiting decorticate posturing. Which picture shows decorticate posturing?

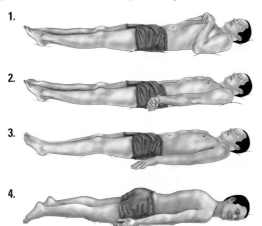

1.

2.

3.

4.

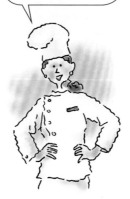

Be sure to time phenytoin administration around the client's feeding time.

56. **1.** A therapeutic phenytoin level is 10 to 20 mg/dL. A level of 32 mg/dL indicates phenytoin toxicity. Symptoms of toxicity include confusion and ataxia. Phenytoin doesn't cause hyponatremia, seizure, or urinary incontinence. Incontinence may occur during or after a seizure.
CN: Physiological integrity; CNS: Pharmacological therapies; CL: Analyze; DIFFICULTY: Moderate

57. **3.** Nutritional supplements and milk interfere with the absorption of phenytoin, decreasing its effectiveness. The nurse verifies NG tube placement by checking for stomach contents before giving drugs and feedings. The head of the bed is elevated when giving all drugs or solutions and isn't specific to phenytoin administration. Phenytoin levels are checked before giving the drug, and the drug is withheld for elevated levels to avoid compounding toxicity.
CN: Physiological integrity; CNS: Pharmacological therapies; CL: Apply; DIFFICULTY: Moderate

58. **4.** Although alcohol impairs judgment and coordination, the larger concern is a lowered phenytoin level and lower threshold for seizures.
CN: Physiological integrity; CNS: Pharmacological therapies; CL: Apply; DIFFICULTY: Moderate

59. **3.** To reduce the risk of injury, the nurse should take an axillary temperature, or the nurse should use a metal thermometer when taking an oral temperature to prevent injury if a seizure occurs. An auscultatory gap occurs in hypertension. Pulse deficit occurs in an arrhythmia. Pulsus paradoxus may occur with cardiac tamponade.
CN: Physiological integrity; CNS: Reduction of risk potential; CL: Apply; DIFFICULTY: Moderate

60. **1.** Decorticate posturing is characterized by rigidity, adduction and flexion of arms, with the wrists and fingers flexed on the chest. There is also extension and internal rotation of legs with plantar flexion of the feet. Decorticate posturing is seen in clients with damage in corticospinal tract. Picture 2 is decerebrate posturing. Picture 3 is flaccid paralysis. Picture 4 is a client in prone position.
CN: Physiological integrity; CNS: Physiological adaptation; CL: Analyze; DIFFICULTY: Easy

CN: Client needs category   CNS: Client needs subcategory   CL: Cognitive level

61. A client comes to the emergency department after hitting the head in a motor vehicle collision. The client is alert and oriented. Which nursing intervention should be done **first**?
1. Perform full range of motion (ROM).
2. Call for an immediate chest x-ray.
3. Immobilize the client's head and neck.
4. Open airway using head tilt/chin lift maneuver.

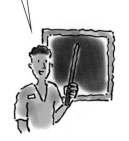

In question #61, focus on what should be done first.

61. 3. All clients with a head injury are treated as if a cervical spine injury is present until x-rays confirm their absence. Performing ROM would be contraindicated at this time. There's no indication the client needs a chest x-ray. The airway doesn't need to be opened because the client appears alert and not in respiratory distress. In addition, the head tilt/chin lift maneuver wouldn't be used until cervical spine injury is ruled out.
CN: Physiological integrity; CNS: Reduction of risk potential; CL: Apply; DIFFICULTY: Easy

62. A client sustained a C6 spinal injury when diving into a shallow lake. What residual effect does the nurse expect to observe?
1. Aphasia
2. Hemiparesis
3. Paraplegia
4. Quadriplegia

62. 4. Quadriplegia occurs as a result of cervical spine injuries. Paraplegia occurs as a result of injury to the thoracic cord and below. Hemiparesis describes weakness of one side of the body. Aphasia refers to difficulty expressing or understanding spoken words.
CN: Physiological integrity; CNS: Physiological adaptation; CL: Apply; DIFFICULTY: Moderate

63. A client has a spinal cord transection at the T4 level. The nurse can expect the client to have which symptom?
1. Paraplegia
2. Quadriplegia
3. Autonomic dysreflexia
4. No deficits

63. 1. Spinal cord injuries at the T4 level affect all motor and sensory nerves below the level of injury and result in dysfunction of legs, bowel, and bladder. Paraplegic injuries involve the thoracic, lumbar, or sacral region of the spinal cord. Quadriplegic injuries result from damage to the cervical region of the spine. Autonomic dysreflexia occurs because of a massive sympathetic discharge of stimuli from the autonomic nervous system.
CN: Physiological integrity; CNS: Physiological adaptation; CL: Apply; DIFFICULTY: Moderate

64. A client admitted with a spinal cord injury at the level of T12 reports loss of movement of lower extremities. Which medication would the nurse anticipate will be administered to control edema of the spinal cord?
1. Acetazolamide
2. Furosemide
3. Methylprednisolone
4. Sodium bicarbonate

64. 3. High doses of methylprednisolone are used within 24 hours of spinal cord injury to reduce cord swelling and limit neurologic deficits. The other drugs aren't indicated in this circumstance.
CN: Physiological integrity; CNS: Pharmacological therapies; CL: Apply; DIFFICULTY: Challenge

65. A client is admitted to the progressive care unit with a C5 fracture from a motorcycle collision. Which findings would take **priority**?
1. Bladder distention
2. Neurologic deficit
3. Pulse oximetry readings
4. The client's feelings about the injury

65. 3. After a spinal cord injury, ascending cord edema may cause a higher level of injury. The diaphragm is innervated at the level of C4, so assessment of adequate oxygenation and ventilation through pulse oximetry readings is necessary. Although the other options would be necessary at a later time, observation for respiratory failure is the priority.
CN: Safe, effective care environment; CNS: Coordinated care; CL: Apply; DIFFICULTY: Challenge

66. While in the emergency department, a client with C8 quadriplegia develops a blood pressure of 80/44 mm Hg, pulse of 48 beats/minute, and respiratory rate of 18 breaths/minute. The nurse suspects which condition?
1. Autonomic dysreflexia
2. Hemorrhagic shock
3. Neurogenic shock
4. Pulmonary embolism

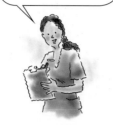

Wow—those are low numbers. Which condition is most likely to produce them?

66. 3. Symptoms of neurogenic shock include hypotension, bradycardia, and warm, dry skin due to loss of adrenergic stimulation below the level of the lesion. Hypertension, bradycardia, flushing, and sweating of the skin are seen with autonomic dysreflexia. Hemorrhagic shock presents with anxiety, tachycardia, and hypotension; this wouldn't be suspected without an injury. Pulmonary embolism presents with chest pain, hypotension, hypoxemia, tachycardia, and hemoptysis; this may be a later complication of spinal cord injury due to immobility.
CN: Health promotion and maintenance; CNS: None; CL: Analyze; DIFFICULTY: Moderate

67. A client with quadriplegia is apprehensive and flushed, with a blood pressure of 210/100 mm Hg and heart rate of 50 beats/minute. Which nursing intervention should be done **first**?
1. Place the client flat in bed.
2. Check patency of the indwelling urinary catheter.
3. Give one sublingual nitroglycerin tablet.
4. Raise the head of the bed immediately to 90 degrees.

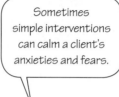

Sometimes simple interventions can calm a client's anxieties and fears.

67. 4. Anxiety, flushing above the level of the lesion, piloerection, hypertension, and bradycardia are symptoms of autonomic dysreflexia, typically caused by such noxious stimuli as a full bladder, fecal impaction, or pressure ulcer. The client is immediately placed in a sitting position to lower blood pressure. Placing the client flat will cause the blood pressure to increase. Nitroglycerin is given to relieve chest pain and reduce preload; it isn't used for hypertension or dysreflexia. The indwelling urinary catheter should be checked immediately after the head of the bed is raised.
CN: Physiological integrity; CNS: Physiological adaptation; CL: Analyze; DIFFICULTY: Moderate

68. A client with paraplegia from a T10 injury is getting ready to transfer to a rehabilitation hospital. When a nurse offers assistance, the client throws the suitcase on the floor and says, "You don't want to help me." Which response would be **most** appropriate for the nurse to give?
1. "You know I want to help you; I offered."
2. "I'll pick these things up for you and come back later."
3. "You seem angry today. How do you feel about your transfer to rehab?"
4. "When you get to rehab, they won't let you behave like a spoiled brat."

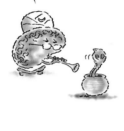

Impressive. You're already halfway done!

68. 3. The nurse should always focus on the feelings underlying a particular action. The nurse saying that she offered to help or calling the client a spoiled brat is confrontational. Offering to pick up the client's belongings doesn't deal with the situation and assumes he can't do it alone.
CN: Psychosocial integrity; CNS: None; CL: Apply; DIFFICULTY: Easy

69. A client with a cervical spine injury is placed in a Minerva body vest. The client is uncomfortable and would like to try a different device. Which information should the nurse explain to the client?
1. The vest protects the neck against excessive motion.
2. The vest will provide for immobilization of the mid-cervical segments.
3. The vest will provide significant immobilization, including lateral flexion.
4. There are other soft-type collars that can be used.

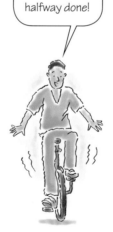

69. 3. The Minerva vest will provide significant immobilization, including lateral flexion. Most soft collars do not limit cervical motion but act as a reminder against excessive motion. More rigid devices such as the Philadelphia collar provide reasonable immobilization of the mid-cervical segments for flexion and extension but not for lateral flexion.
CN: Physiological integrity; CNS: Physiological adaptation; CL: Apply; DIFFICULTY: Difficult

70. When a client with a halo vest is discharged from the hospital, which instruction should the nurse reinforce to the client and family?
1. Don't use the wheelchair while the halo vest is in place.
2. Clean the pin sites every other day especially when there is abscess.
3. Keep the wrench that opens the vest attached to the client at all times.
4. Perform range-of-motion (ROM) exercises to the neck and shoulders four times daily.

71. A licensed practical nurse/licensed vocational nurse is caring for a client with trigeminal neuralgia who reports severe stabbing pain on one side of the face. Which action should the LPN/LVN perform **first**?
1. Divert the client's attention.
2. Medicate the client.
3. Inform the registered nurse.
4. Monitor pain scale.

72. Which early intervention describes an appropriate bladder program for a client in rehabilitation for spinal cord injury?
1. Insert an indwelling urinary catheter.
2. Schedule intermittent catheterization every 2 to 4 hours.
3. Perform a straight catheterization every 8 hours while awake.
4. Perform Credé maneuver to the lower abdomen before the client voids.

73. The nurse is caring for a client that underwent a stapedectomy. Which position would have the **greatest** benefit for prevention of complications and promotion of comfort?
1. On the affected side
2. On the unaffected side
3. Prone
4. Sims

74. A client with breast cancer reports back pain and difficulty in moving her legs. Which nursing intervention is **most** appropriate?
1. Notify the health care provider.
2. Position the client on her side, and prop her with a foam wedge.
3. Ask the health care provider for a physical therapy consultation.
4. Give acetaminophen, and reassure the client that the pain will resolve soon.

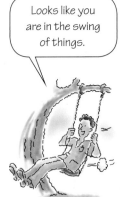

Looks like you are in the swing of things.

70. 3. The wrench must be attached at all times to remove the vest in case the client needs cardiopulmonary resuscitation. The vest is designed to improve mobility; the client may use a wheelchair. The pins are cleaned daily. The purpose of the vest is to immobilize the neck; ROM exercises to the neck are prohibited but should be performed to other areas.
CN: Physiological integrity; CNS: Reduction of risk potential; CL: Apply; DIFFICULTY: Moderate

71. 3. The LPN/LVN should inform the registered nurse (RN) first since an LPN/LVN works under the supervision of the RN. The LPN/LVN can administer the medication after informing the RN. Diverting the client's attention and monitoring pain scale are appropriate interventions but informing the RN should be the first step.
CN: Safe, effective care environment; CNS: Coordinated care; CL: Apply; DIFFICULTY: Challenge

72. 2. Intermittent catheterization should begin every 2 to 4 hours early in treatment. When residual volume is less than 400 mL, the schedule may advance to every 4 to 6 hours. Indwelling catheters may predispose the client to infection and are removed as soon as possible. Credé maneuver is applied after voiding to enhance bladder emptying.
CN: Physiological integrity; CNS: Basic care and comfort; CL: Apply; DIFFICULTY: Moderate

73. 2. The client should be positioned on the unaffected with the operative ear up. Although Sims position is a side-lying position, the option doesn't consider which side is best following ear surgery.
CN: Physiological integrity; CNS: Physiological adaptation; CL: Apply; DIFFICULTY: Moderate

74. 1. Symptoms of back pain and neurologic deficits may indicate metastasis; therefore, the health care provider should be notified. Repositioning the client, physical therapy, or acetaminophen may help the pain but may delay evaluation and treatment.
CN: Health promotion and maintenance; CNS: None; CL: Apply; DIFFICULTY: Easy

75. A client was admitted to the hospital because of a transient ischemic attack (TIA) secondary to atrial fibrillation. Which medication will the nurse administer to prevent further neurologic deficit?
1. Digoxin
2. Diltiazem
3. Heparin
4. Quinidine gluconate

76. A client is admitted with Ménière disease. Which condiments should the nurse tell the client to avoid? Select all that apply.
1. Soy sauce
2. Pepper
3. Vinegar
4. Olive oil
5. Ketchup

77. Which symptom would the nurse expect to find when collecting data from a client with Ménière disease?
1. Epistaxis
2. Facial pain
3. Ptosis
4. Tinnitus

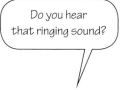

Do you hear that ringing sound?

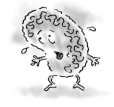

78. Which nursing intervention takes **priority** for a nurse treating a client with a foreign body protruding from the eye?
1. Irrigating the eye with sterile saline
2. Assessing visual acuity with a Snellen chart
3. Removing the foreign body with sterile forceps
4. Patching both eyes until seen by the ophthalmologist

79. The health care provider ordered a nasogastric (NG) tube insertion on a client with dysphagia. Place the following nursing actions in chronological order of how the nurse will perform the procedure. Use all of the options.

1. Instruct client to hyperextend the head
2. Advance tube 1 to 2 inches with each swallow
3. Instruct client to flex head forward
4. Position client on high Fowler's
5. Measure distance to insert tube
6. Pass lubricated tube along floor of nasal passage

75. 3. Atrial fibrillation may lead to the formation of mural thrombi, which may embolize to the brain. Heparin will prevent further clot formation and clot enlargement. The other drugs are used in the treatment and control of atrial fibrillation but won't affect clot formation.
CN: Physiological integrity; CNS: Pharmacological therapies; CL: Apply; DIFFICULTY: Difficult

76. 1, 5. Ménière disease is a disorder of the inner ear in which there is an excess production of endo-lymphatic fluid in the semicircular canals. The client's diet should be low in sodium. Both soy sauce and ketchup are high in sodium and should be avoided.
CN: Health promotion and maintenance; CNS: None; CL: Apply; DIFFICULTY: Challenge

77. 4. Tinnitus, dizziness, and vertigo occur in Ménière disease. Facial pain may occur with trigeminal neuralgia. Ptosis occurs with a variety of conditions, including myasthenia gravis. Epistaxis may occur with a variety of blood dyscrasias or local lesions.
CN: Physiological integrity; CNS: Physiological adaptation; CL: Apply; DIFFICULTY: Easy

78. 4. One or both eyes may be patched to prevent pain with extraocular movement or accommodation. Assessment of visual acuity isn't a priority, although it may be done after treatment. Chemicals or small foreign bodies may be irrigated. Protruding objects aren't removed by the nurse because the vitreous body may rupture.
CN: Safe, effective care environment; CNS: Coordinated care; CL: Apply; DIFFICULTY: Moderate

79. Ordered Response:

4. Position client on high Fowler's
5. Measure distance to insert tube
1. Instruct client to hyperextend the head
6. Pass lubricated tube along floor of nasal passage
3. Instruct client to flex head forward
2. Advance tube 1 to 2 inches with each swallow

CN: Physiological integrity; CNS: Reduction of risk potential; CL: Apply; DIFFICULTY: Difficult

80. A client with severe eye pain requests a prescription for the topical anesthetic that the ophthalmologist instilled. A nurse explains that these drugs shouldn't be used on an ongoing basis for which reason?
   1. They're a way for pathogens to enter the eye.
   2. They cause dependence and rebound pain.
   3. Damage could occur to the cornea because of lack of sensation.
   4. The resulting blurred vision from mydriasis makes activity hazardous.

81. An older adult client admitted to the hospital with chest pain has difficulty hearing. Which method should the nurse use when collecting data from this client?
   1. Obtain an ear wick.
   2. Shout into the better ear.
   3. Lower voice pitch while facing the client.
   4. Ask the family to go home and get the client's hearing aid.

82. A client is scheduled for magnetic resonance imaging (MRI) of the head. Which area is essential to check before the procedure? Select all that apply.
   1. Food or drink intake within the past 8 hours
   2. Metal fillings, prostheses, or a pacemaker
   3. The presence of carotid artery disease
   4. Voiding before the procedure
   5. History of claustrophobia

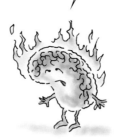

If your brain feels like it's on fire, you might want to take a break.

83. A client who has had cataract surgery on the right eye is being discharged. Which discharge instructions should the nurse reinforce to the client? Select all that apply.
   1. Avoid bending over at the waist.
   2. Reduce sodium intake to reduce intraocular pressure.
   3. When sleeping, lie on the same side as the surgery.
   4. Eye makeup can be applied tomorrow.
   5. Call your health care provider if you have vision loss or see flashing lights.
   6. When sleeping, lie on the side opposite to the surgery.

80. 3. Corneal damage may occur with the prolonged use of topical anesthetics. Dependence and rebound pain don't occur from topical anesthetics. Anesthetics don't cause mydriasis. If the bottle isn't touched to the eye or lashes, the entry of pathogens should be limited.
CN: Physiological integrity; CNS: Reduction of risk potential;
CL: Apply; DIFFICULTY: Moderate

81. 3. Hearing loss in the older adult typically involves the upper ranges; lowering the pitch of the voice and facing the client is essential for the client to use other means of understanding, such as lip reading, mood, and so on. Shouting is typically in the upper ranges and could increase anxiety in an already anxious client. An ear wick is used to allow medications to enter the ear canal. Alternate means of communication, such as writing, may also be used to assess chest pain while waiting for the family to bring the hearing aid from home.
CN: Physiological integrity; CNS: Basic care and comfort;
CL: Apply; DIFFICULTY: Easy

82. 2, 5. Strong magnetic waves may dislodge metal in the client's body, causing tissue injury. Although the client may be told to restrict food for 8 hours, particularly if contrast is used, metal is an absolute contraindication for this procedure. The client with history of claustrophobia should be evaluated because the client will be confined in a small, enclosed, tube-shaped machine during MRI. Voiding beforehand would make the client more comfortable and better able to remain still during the procedure, but it isn't essential for the test. Having carotid artery disease isn't a contraindication to having an MRI.
CN: Safe, effective care environment; CNS: Safety and infection control; CL: Apply; DIFFICULTY: Challenge

83. 1, 5, 6. Bending over may increase intraocular pressure and strain the sutures. Vision loss or seeing flashing lights may signal complications, such as retinal detachment or increased intraocular pressure, and should be reported. Intraocular pressure is reduced when sleeping on the nonsurgical side. Reducing sodium intake doesn't decrease intraocular pressure. Applying eye makeup may introduce infection and cause irritation.
CN: Physiological integrity; CNS: Reduction of risk potential;
CL: Apply; DIFFICULTY: Challenge

84. Which method should the nurse use to properly instill eardrops in an adult client with otitis externa?
1. Pull the pinna down and back.
2. Pull the pinna up and back.
3. Pull the tragus up and back.
4. Separate the palpebral fissures with a clean gauze pad.

85. The nurse is monitoring a client with a symptom of increased intracranial pressure (ICP) after head trauma. What observation does the nurse recognize as an early sign?
1. Bradycardia
2. Large amounts of very dilute urine
3. Restlessness and confusion
4. Widened pulse pressure

86. A client admitted to the emergency department for head trauma is diagnosed with an epidural hematoma from a skiing accident. What is the **priority** action by the nurse?
1. Emergently prepare the client for evacuation of the hematoma.
2. Monitor the client closely for 24 hours.
3. Apply direct pressure to the scalp.
4. Obtain vital signs every 2 hours.

87. A client has been hit on the head with a baseball bat. The nurse notes clear fluid draining from ears and nose. Which nursing intervention is appropriate?
1. Positioning the client flat in bed
2. Checking the fluid for glucose with a dipstick
3. Suctioning the nose to maintain airway patency
4. Inserting nasal and ear packing with sterile gauze

88. When observing a client in the emergency department after a head trauma, the nurse knows to monitor the client for a lucid interval. Which statement **best** describes a lucid interval?
1. An interval when the client's speech is garbled
2. An interval when the client is alert but can't recall recent events
3. An interval when the client is oriented but then becomes somnolent
4. An interval when the client has a "warning" symptom, such as an odor or visual disturbance

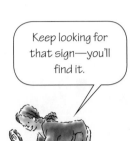

Keep looking for that sign—you'll find it.

84. 2. To straighten the ear canal of an adult, the pinna is pulled up and back. The palpebral fissures are in the eye. The other options aren't appropriate methods for preparing the ear to receive eardrops.
CN: Physiological integrity; CNS: Pharmacological therapies;
CL: Apply; DIFFICULTY: Easy

85. 3. The earliest symptom of increased ICP is a change in mental status. Bradycardia, widened pulse pressure, and bradypnea occur later. The client may void large amounts of very dilute urine if there's damage to the posterior pituitary.
CN: Physiological integrity; CNS: Physiological adaptation;
CL: Apply; DIFFICULTY: Easy

86. 1. Epidural hematoma or extradural hematoma is usually caused by laceration of the middle meningeal artery. This condition is emergent and requires immediate evacuation of the hematoma. Monitoring the client for 24 hours is not an appropriate action since the client will require emergency surgery to evacuate the hematoma. Applying direct pressure to the scalp is an ineffective treatment since the artery is ruptured and it is not a surface vessel that is ruptured. Vital signs will be obtained at least every 15 minutes prior to surgery.
CN: Physiological integrity; CNS: Physiological adaptation;
CL: Apply; DIFFICULTY: Moderate

87. 2. Clear liquid from the nose (rhinorrhea) or ear (otorrhea) can be determined to be cerebral spinal fluid or mucus by the presence of glucose. Glucose would be present in cerebral spinal fluid. Placing the client flat in bed may increase intracranial pressure and promote pulmonary aspiration. Nothing is inserted into the ears or nose of a client with a skull fracture because of the risk of infection. The nose wouldn't be suctioned because of the risk of suctioning brain tissue through the sinuses.
CN: Physiological integrity; CNS: Physiological adaptation;
CL: Analyze; DIFFICULTY: Easy

88. 3. A lucid interval is described as a brief period of unconsciousness at the time of the trauma followed by alertness; after several hours, the client deteriorates neurologically. Garbled speech is known as dysarthria. An interval in which the client is alert but can't recall recent events is known as amnesia. Warning symptoms or auras typically occur before seizures.
CN: Health promotion and maintenance; CNS: None;
CL: Understand; DIFFICULTY: Moderate

89. Which client on the rehabilitation unit is **most** likely to develop autonomic dysreflexia?
1. A client with brain injury
2. A client with herniated nucleus pulposus
3. A client with a high cervical spine injury
4. A client with a stroke

90. When assisting with the education of the family of a client with C4 quadriplegia on how to perform tracheostomy suctioning, which instruction should the nurse be sure to include?
1. Suction for 10 to 15 seconds at a time.
2. Regulate the suction machine to 300 cm suction.
3. Apply suction to the catheter during insertion only.
4. Pass the suction catheter into the opening of the tracheostomy tube 2 to 3 cm.

91. A client is diagnosed with a hemorrhagic stroke. Which risk factors are strongly associated with this condition? Select all that apply.
1. Coronary artery disease
2. Diabetes
3. Hypertension
4. Recent viral infection
5. Cerebral aneurysm

92. The nurse is assisting a client during lumbar puncture. In which position should the nurse place the client during the procedure?

1.
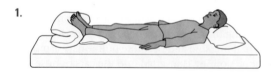

2.
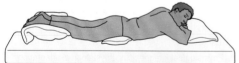

3.
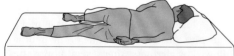

4.
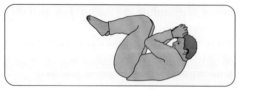

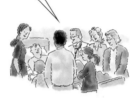
When possible, recruit family members to help provide basic comfort and care measures for the client.

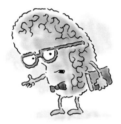
Hemorrhagic strokes are caused by bleeding from a ruptured blood vessel in the brain. What risk factors would contribute to this condition?

89. 3. Autonomic dysreflexia refers to uninhibited sympathetic outflow in clients with spinal cord injuries above the level of T10. The other clients aren't prone to dysreflexia.
CN: Physiological integrity; CNS: Physiological adaptation;
CL: Apply; DIFFICULTY: Moderate

90. 1. Suction should be applied for 10 to 15 seconds at a time. When suctioning the trachea, the catheter is inserted 4 to 6 inches or until resistance is felt. Suction should be applied only during withdrawal of the catheter. Suction is regulated to 80 to 120 cm.
CN: Physiological integrity; CNS: Reduction of risk potential;
CL: Apply; DIFFICULTY: Easy

91. 3, 5. Uncontrolled hypertension and cerebral aneurysm are major causes of hemorrhagic stroke. The other options are not directly linked to this problem.
CN: Physiological integrity; CNS: Reduction of risk potential;
CL: Analyze; DIFFICULTY: Challenge

92. 4. During lumbar puncture, the client will be placed on a lateral (side-lying) position to widen the intervertebral spaces for easy insertion of the spinal needle.
CN: Physiological integrity; CNS: Reduction of risk potential;
CL: Apply; DIFFICULTY: Moderate

93. What observation made by the nurse is an indication that spinal shock is resolving in a client with C7 quadriplegia?
  1. Absence of pain sensation in chest
  2. Spasticity
  3. Spontaneous respirations
  4. Urinary continence

94. When discharging a client from the hospital after a laminectomy, the nurse recognizes that further education is necessary when the client makes which statement?
  1. "I'll sleep on a firm mattress."
  2. "I won't drive for 2 to 4 weeks."
  3. "When I pick things up, I'll always bend my knees."
  4. "I can't wait to toss my granddaughter up in the air."

95. The nurse is collecting data on a client with herniated nucleus pulposus (HNP) of L4–L5. Which of the following sign or symptom would the nurse anticipate?
  1. Low back pain
  2. Pain radiating across the buttocks
  3. Positive Kernig sign
  4. Urinary incontinence

96. A nurse is collecting data on a client who has episodes of autonomic dysreflexia. Which condition does the nurse monitor for that can contribute to the development of autonomic dysreflexia?
  1. Headache
  2. Lumbar spinal cord injury
  3. Neurogenic shock
  4. Noxious stimuli

97. The nurse is reinforcing dietary instructions to a client with Parkinson disease. Which signs and symptoms would be **most** important for the nurse to address?
  1. Fluid overload and drooling
  2. Aspiration and anorexia
  3. Choking and diarrhea
  4. Dysphagia and constipation

98. A client recovering from a spinal cord injury has a great deal of spasticity. What medication administered by the nurse may be used to control spasticity?
  1. Hydralazine
  2. Baclofen
  3. Lidocaine
  4. Methylprednisolone

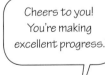

Cheers to you! You're making excellent progress.

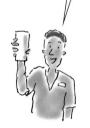

93. 2. Spasticity, the return of reflexes, is a sign of resolving shock. Spinal or neurogenic shock is characterized by hypotension, bradycardia, dry skin, flaccid paralysis, or the absence of reflexes below the level of injury. Slight muscle contraction at the bulbocavernosus reflex occurs but not enough for urinary continence. Spinal shock descends from the injury, and respiratory difficulties occur at C4 and above. The absence of pain sensation in the chest doesn't apply to spinal shock.
CN: Physiological integrity; CNS: Physiological adaptation; CL: Apply; DIFFICULTY: Difficult

94. 4. Lifting more than 10 lb (4.5 kg) for several weeks after surgery is contraindicated. The other responses are appropriate.
CN: Physiological integrity; CNS: Reduction of risk potential; CL: Analyze; DIFFICULTY: Easy

95. 4. Progressive neurologic deficits at L4–L5, including worsening muscle weakness, paresthesia, and loss of bowel and bladder control, are symptoms of spinal cord compression. The other symptoms usually occur in clients with HNP without spinal cord compression.
CN: Physiological integrity; CNS: Physiological adaptation; CL: Analyze; DIFFICULTY: Difficult

96. 4. Noxious stimuli, such as a full bladder, fecal impaction, or a pressure ulcer, may cause autonomic dysreflexia. Neurogenic shock isn't a cause of dysreflexia. Autonomic dysreflexia is most commonly seen with injuries at T10 or above. A headache is a symptom, not a cause, of autonomic dysreflexia.
CN: Physiological integrity; CNS: Physiological adaptation; CL: Apply; DIFFICULTY: Challenge

97. 4. The eating problems associated with Parkinson disease include dysphagia, risk of choking, aspiration, and constipation. Fluid overload, anorexia, and diarrhea aren't problems specifically related to Parkinson disease.
CN: Physiological integrity; CNS: Reduction of risk potential; CL: Analyze; DIFFICULTY: Challenge

98. 2. Baclofen is a skeletal muscle relaxant used to decrease spasms. Methylprednisolone, an anti-inflammatory drug, is used to decrease spinal cord edema. Hydralazine is an antihypertensive and afterload-reducing agent. Lidocaine is an antiarrhythmic and a local anesthetic agent.
CN: Physiological integrity; CNS: Pharmacological therapies; CL: Apply; DIFFICULTY: Moderate

99. A nurse performs a neurologic data collection on a client reporting headache and dizziness. Which data collection technique helps determine the motor function of cranial nerve VII?

1. Asking the client to clench his jaw
2. Testing the gag reflex by placing an applicator against the pharynx
3. Asking the client to frown, smile, and raise his eyebrows
4. Asking the client to swallow

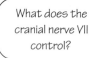

What does the cranial nerve VII control?

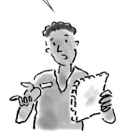

99. 3. To check the motor function of cranial nerve VII, the nurse should ask the client to frown, smile, and raise his eyebrows. If these facial expressions are symmetrical, motor function is intact. Jaw clenching is a test for cranial nerve V function. Testing the gag reflex by placing an applicator against the pharynx, and checking swallowing ability, are ways to evaluate cranial nerve IX function. Testing the gag reflex also helps evaluate cranial nerve X function.

CN: Health promotion and maintenance; CNS: None; CL: Apply; DIFFICULTY: Easy

100. A client with a T1 spinal cord injury arrives at the emergency department with a blood pressure of 82/40 mm Hg, pulse rate of 34 beats/minute, dry skin, and flaccid paralysis of the lower extremities. Which condition would **most** likely be suspected?

1. Autonomic dysreflexia
2. Hypervolemia
3. Neurogenic shock
4. Sepsis

100. 3. Loss of sympathetic control and unopposed vagal stimulation below the level of the injury typically cause hypotension, bradycardia, pallor, flaccid paralysis, and warm, dry skin in the client in neurogenic shock. Hypervolemia is indicated by a bounding and rapid pulse and edema. Autonomic dysreflexia occurs after neurogenic shock abates. Signs of sepsis would include elevated temperature, increased heart rate, and increased respiratory rate.

CN: Physiological integrity; CNS: Physiological adaptation; CL: Analyze; DIFFICULTY: Easy

101. A client with C7 quadriplegia is flushed and anxious and reports a pounding headache. Which symptom would also be anticipated?

1. Decreased urine output or oliguria
2. Hypertension and bradycardia
3. Respiratory depression
4. Symptoms of shock

101. 2. Hypertension, bradycardia, anxiety, blurred vision, and flushing above the lesion occur with autonomic dysreflexia due to uninhibited sympathetic nervous system discharge. The other options are incorrect.

CN: Physiological integrity; CNS: Physiological adaptation; CL: Analyze; DIFFICULTY: Moderate

102. A client has a cervical spinal cord injury at the level of C5. Which condition would the nurse anticipate during the acute phase?

1. Absent corneal reflex
2. Decerebrate posturing
3. Movement of only the right or left half of the body
4. The need for mechanical ventilation

102. 4. The diaphragm is stimulated by nerves at the level of C4. Initially, this client may need mechanical ventilation because of cord edema. This may resolve in time. Decerebrate posturing, hemiplegia, and absent corneal reflexes occur with brain injuries, not spinal cord injuries.

CN: Physiological integrity; CNS: Physiological adaptation; CL: Apply; DIFFICULTY: Moderate

103. When caring for a client with quadriplegia, which nursing intervention takes **priority**?

1. Forcing fluids to prevent renal calculi
2. Maintaining skin integrity
3. Obtaining adaptive devices for more independence
4. Preventing atelectasis

103. 4. Clients with quadriplegia have paralysis or weakness of the diaphragm, abdominal, or intercostal muscles. Maintenance of airway and breathing take top priority. Although forcing fluids, maintaining skin integrity, and obtaining adaptive devices for more independence are all important interventions, preventing atelectasis has more priority.

CN: Physiological integrity; CNS: Reduction of risk potential; CL: Apply; DIFFICULTY: Challenge

104. A client has a diagnosis of stroke versus transient ischemic attack (TIA). Which statement demonstrates the difference between a TIA and a stroke?
1. TIAs typically resolve in 24 hours.
2. TIAs may be hemorrhagic in origin.
3. TIAs may cause a permanent motor deficit.
4. TIAs may predispose the client to a myocardial infarction (MI).

105. A client with a right stroke has a flaccid left side. Which intervention would **best** prevent shoulder subluxation?
1. Splinting the wrist
2. Using an air splint
3. Putting the affected arm in a sling
4. Performing range-of-motion (ROM) exercises

106. A client with paraplegia must perform intermittent catheterization of the bladder. Which instruction should be given?
1. Clean the meatus from back to front.
2. Measure the quantity of urine.
3. Gently rotate the catheter during removal.
4. Clean the meatus with soap and water.

107. When obtaining data about pupillary responses, which method should the nurse use to evaluate pupil accommodation?
1. Check for peripheral vision.
2. Touch the cornea lightly with a wisp of cotton.
3. Have the client follow an object upward, downward, obliquely, and horizontally.
4. Observe for pupil constriction and convergence while focusing on an object coming toward the client.

108. A client at the eye clinic reports difficulty seeing at night. Which nutritional deficiency should the nurse be sure the client is monitored for?
1. Vitamin A
2. Vitamin B₆
3. Vitamin C
4. Vitamin K

109. A client with a spinal cord injury has a neurogenic bladder. When planning for discharge, the nurse anticipates that the client will need which procedure or program?
1. Intermittent catheterization
2. Kock pouch
3. Transurethral prostatectomy
4. Ureterostomy

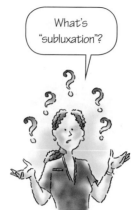

What's "subluxation"?

Which one of us should help?

104. 1. Symptoms of TIA result from a transient lack of oxygen to the brain and usually resolve within 24 hours. Hemorrhage into the brain has the worst neurologic outcome and isn't associated with a TIA. Permanent motor deficits don't result from TIA. Unstable angina, not a TIA, may predispose the client to a future MI.
CN: Physiological integrity; CNS: Physiological adaptation; CL: Understand; DIFFICULTY: Moderate

105. 3. Because of the weight of the flaccid extremity, the shoulder may disarticulate. A sling will support the extremity. The other options won't support the shoulder.
CN: Physiological integrity; CNS: Basic care and comfort; CL: Apply; DIFFICULTY: Challenge

106. 4. Intermittent catheterization may be performed chronically with clean technique, using soap and water to clean the urinary meatus. The meatus is always cleaned from front to back in a woman, or in expanding circles working outward from the meatus in a man. The catheter doesn't need to be rotated during removal. It isn't necessary to measure the urine.
CN: Physiological integrity; CNS: Basic care and comfort; CL: Apply; DIFFICULTY: Moderate

107. 4. Accommodation refers to convergence and constriction of the pupil while focusing on a nearing object. Touching the cornea lightly with a wisp of cotton describes evaluation of the corneal reflex. Having the client follow an object upward, downward, obliquely, and horizontally refers to cardinal fields of gaze. Checking for peripheral vision refers to visual fields.
CN: Health promotion and maintenance; CNS: None; CL: Apply; DIFFICULTY: Challenge

108. 1. Night blindness (nyctalopia) may be caused from a vitamin A deficiency or dysfunctional rod receptors. None of the other deficiencies leads to nyctalopia.
CN: Physiological integrity; CNS: Physiological adaptation; CL: Apply; DIFFICULTY: Easy

109. 1. Intermittent catheterization, starting with 2-hour intervals and increasing to 4- to 6-hour intervals, is used to manage neurogenic bladder. A Kock pouch is a continent ileostomy. An ileostomy or ureterostomy isn't necessary. Transurethral prostatectomy is indicated for obstruction to urinary outflow by benign prostatic hyperplasia or for the treatment of cancer.
CN: Physiological integrity; CNS: Basic care and comfort; CL: Apply; DIFFICULTY: Easy

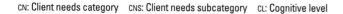

110. When using a Snellen alphabet chart, the nurse records the client's vision as 20/40. What does this evaluation determine for the client?
1. The client has alterations in near vision and is legally blind.
2. The client can see at 20 feet what the person with normal vision sees at 40 feet.
3. The client can see at 40 feet what the person with normal vision sees at 20 feet.
4. The client has a 20% decrease in acuity in one eye and a 40% decrease in the other eye.

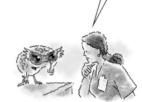

Sometimes neurosensory disorders can be difficult to identify.

110. 2. The numerator refers to the client's vision while comparing the normal vision in the denominator. Legal blindness refers to 20/150 or less. Alterations in near vision may be due to loss of accommodation caused by the aging process (presbyopia) or farsightedness.

CN: Physiological integrity; CNS: Physiological adaptation; CL: Analyze; DIFFICULTY: Moderate

111. The client is taking rivaroxaban. Which herb should the nurse tell the client to avoid while on this medication?
1. Bilberry
2. Kava
3. Goldenseal
4. Valerian

111. 3. Rivaroxaban is an anticoagulant that reduces the risk of CVA, atrial fibrillation, DVT, and pulmonary embolism. Goldenseal has an anticoagulant effect and could predispose the client to bleeding when given with rivaroxaban. Bilberry is used for improving eyesight. Kava and valerian are both used to decrease anxiety, stress, restlessness, and insomnia.

CN: Physiological integrity; CNS: Pharmacological therapies; CL: Apply; DIFFICULTY: Difficult

112. A nurse instills atropine drops on both eyes of a client undergoing an ophthalmic examination. Which instruction should the nurse reinforce after administering the medication?
1. Be careful because the blink reflex is paralyzed.
2. Avoid wearing regular glasses when driving.
3. It is normal to expect that the pupils may be unusually small.
4. Wear dark glasses in bright light because the pupils are dilated.

112. 4. Atropine, an anticholinergic drug, has mydriatic effects causing pupil dilation. This allows more light onto the retina and causes photophobia and blurred vision. Atropine doesn't paralyze the blink reflex or cause miosis (pupil constriction). Driving may be contraindicated because of blurred vision.

CN: Physiological integrity; CNS: Pharmacological therapies; CL: Apply; DIFFICULTY: Moderate

113. A client was admitted with right-sided paralysis. Which contributing factors are strongly associated with the development of stroke or cerebrovascular accident (CVA)? Select all that apply.
1. Hypotension
2. Diabetes insipidus
3. Oral contraceptive use
4. Atherosclerosis
5. Obesity

113. 3, 4, 5. Atherosclerosis, obesity, and use of oral contraceptives are all risk factors for the development of stroke or CVA. Hypertension is a risk factor, not hypotension. Diabetes mellitus is a risk factor, not diabetes insipidus.

CN: Health promotion and maintenance; CNS: None; CL: Analyze; DIFFICULTY: Difficult

114. A client is scheduled for an eye surgery. What nursing action should be included in preparing a client before the surgical procedure?
1. Clip the client's eyelashes.
2. Put a patch on the affected eye.
3. Keep the client on NPO.
4. Obtain informed consent.

114. 3. Maintaining nothing-by-mouth status for at least 8 hours before surgical procedures prevents vomiting and aspiration. The health care provider is responsible for obtaining informed consent; the nurse validates that the consent is obtained. There's no need to patch an eye before most surgeries or to clip the eyelashes unless specifically ordered by the health care provider.

CN: Physiological intergrity; CNS: Reduction of risk potential; CL: Apply; DIFFICULTY: Challenge

115. When contributing to the development of an education session on glaucoma for the community, which statement would the nurse emphasize?
1. Glaucoma is easily corrected with eyeglasses.
2. The disorder will not lead to complete loss of vision.
3. Yearly screening for people ages 20 to 40 is recommended.
4. Glaucoma can be painless with loss of peripheral vision.

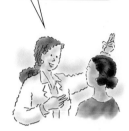

If glaucoma is suspected, be sure to check to check the client's vision.

115. 4. Open-angle glaucoma causes a painless increase in intraocular pressure with loss of peripheral vision. A variety of miotics and agents to decrease intraocular pressure (and occasionally surgery) are used to treat glaucoma. The other options are not correct.
CN: Health promotion and maintenance; CNS: None; CL: Apply; DIFFICULTY: Easy

116. Which statement indicates that a client needs additional education after cataract surgery?
1. "I'll avoid eating until the nausea subsides."
2. "I can't wait to pick up my granddaughter."
3. "I'll avoid bending over to tie my shoelaces."
4. "I'll wear an eye shield to protect the eye."

116. 2. Lifting, often involving the Valsalva maneuver, increases intraocular pressure and strain on the surgical site. Preventing nausea and subsequent vomiting will prevent increased intraocular pressure, as will avoiding bending or placing the head in a dependent position. The client will be wearing an eye shield to protect the affected eye.
CN: Physiological integrity; CNS: Reduction of risk potential; CL: Analyze; DIFFICULTY: Easy

117. A client is admitted because of an episode of acute angle-closure glaucoma. Which medication should the nurse expect to administer?
1. Acetazolamide
2. Atropine
3. Furosemide
4. Urokinase

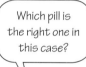

Which pill is the right one in this case?

117. 1. Acetazolamide, a carbonic anhydrase inhibitor, decreases intraocular pressure by decreasing the secretion of aqueous humor. Urokinase is a thrombolytic agent, and furosemide is a loop diuretic; these aren't used in the treatment of glaucoma. Atropine dilates the pupil and decreases outflow of aqueous humor, causing a further increase in intraocular pressure.
CN: Physiological integrity; CNS: Pharmacological therapies; CL: Apply; DIFFICULTY: Moderate

118. A client is admitted with retinal detachment. Which sign or symptom would the nurse anticipate during data collection?
1. Flashing lights and floaters
2. Homonymous hemianopia
3. Loss of central vision
4. Drooping of the eyelids

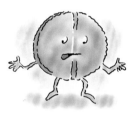

118. 1. Signs and symptoms of retinal detachment include abrupt flashing lights, floaters, and a sudden shadow or curtain in the vision. Occasionally, vision loss is gradual. Homonymous hemianopia is the loss of half of the visual field; it's seen in clients with CVA or stroke. Loss of central vision is for macular degeneration. Ptosis or drooping of the eyelid is an early sign of myasthenia gravis.
CN: Physiological integrity; CNS: Physiological adaptation; CL: Apply; DIFFICULTY: Easy

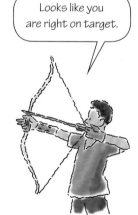

Looks like you are right on target.

119. A client is receiving pilocarpine eye drops. Which statement made by the client shows correct understanding about the medication?
1. "The medication will help dilate the pupils of my eyes."
2. "The medication will help decrease pressure in my eyes."
3. "The medication will prevent eye infection."
4. "The medication will prevent eye movement."

119. 2. Pilocarpine is a miotic drug that causes constriction of the pupils. It's given to a client with glaucoma to decrease the intraocular pressure. The other options are not associated with the use of pilocarpine.
CN: Physiological integrity; CNS: Pharmacological therapies; CL: Apply; DIFFICULTY: Easy

120. A client underwent an enucleation of the right eye for a malignancy. Which intervention will the nurse perform?

1. Instill miotics, as prescribed by the health care provider, to the affected eye.
2. Reinforce teaching the client to clean the prosthesis in soap and water.
3. Determine reactivity of the pupils to light and accommodation.
4. Teach the client to avoid straining at stool to prevent intraocular pressure.

121. The nurse is scheduled to administer an otic medication. Which action should the nurse perform **first**?

1. Check and verify the client's name.
2. Warm the solution to prevent dizziness.
3. Hold an emesis basin under the client's ear.
4. Place the client in the semi-Fowler's position.

122. A client is admitted with Ménière's disease. Which instruction should the nurse reinforce in client teaching?

1. Report dizziness at once.
2. Drive in daylight hours only.
3. Get up slowly, turning the entire body.
4. Use logrolling technique when moving.

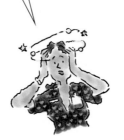

Ugghh. I think I got up too quickly. Everything is spinning.

123. A client is receiving phenytoin. Which response by a client **best** indicates an understanding of the adverse effects of the medication?

1. "I should take the medication without food."
2. "I can stop this medication if seizures stop."
3. "I need to see the dentist every 6 months."
4. "I should report drowsiness immediately."

124. The nurse is testing the client's extraocular eye movements. Which cranial nerves is the nurse checking? Select all that apply.

1. Optic (II)
2. Oculomotor (III)
3. Trochlear (IV)
4. Trigeminal (V)
5. Abducens (VI)

120. 2. Enucleation of the eye refers to surgical removal of the entire eye; therefore, the client needs instructions about the prosthesis. There are no activity restrictions or need for eyedrops; however, prophylactic antibiotics may be used in the immediate postoperative period.
CN: Physiological integrity; CNS: Physiological adaptation;
CL: Apply; DIFFICULTY: Difficult

121. 1. When giving medications, a nurse follows the 10 rights of medication administration: right client, right drug, right dose, right route, and right time, right documentation, right assessment, right to refuse, right evaluation, and right client education or information. Put the client in the lateral position, not semi-Fowler's position, for 5 minutes to prevent the drops from draining out. The drops may be warmed to prevent pain or dizziness, but this is not the first action. An emesis basin would be used for irrigation of the ear.
CN: Physiological integrity; CNS: Pharmacological therapies;
CL: Apply; DIFFICULTY: Moderate

122. 3. A client with Ménière's disease experiences dizziness, vertigo, and tinnitus. Turning the entire body, not the head, will prevent vertigo. Turning the client in bed slowly and smoothly will be helpful; logrolling isn't needed. The client shouldn't drive because he may reflexively turn the wheel to correct for vertigo. Dizziness is expected with Ménière's disease but can be prevented.
CN: Physiological integrity; CNS: Reduction of risk potential;
CL: Apply; DIFFICULTY: Easy

123. 3. Phenytoin can cause hypertrophy of the gums and gingivitis; therefore, regular dental checkups are essential. Phenytoin needs to be taken with food or after meals to decrease adverse GI reactions, and should never be discontinued unless ordered by the health care provider. Some drowsiness is expected initially; however, this usually decreases with continued use.
CN: Physiological therapy; CNS: Pharmacological therapies;
CL: Apply; DIFFICULTY: Moderate

124. 2, 3, 5. CN III (oculomotor), CN IV (trochlear), and CN VI (abducens) are all responsible for the movement of the eye. CN II is the optic nerve, which controls vision. CN V is the trigeminal nerve, which innervates the muscles of chewing.
CN: Health promotion and maintenance; CNS: None; CL: Apply;
DIFFICULTY: Challenge

125. A client is taking carbamazepine. The nurse should monitor the client for what potential complications? Select all that apply.
1. Acute respiratory distress syndrome (ARDS)
2. Elevated phenytoin serum level
3. Leukocytosis
4. Diplopia
5. Ataxia

126. The nurse is observing a client with cerebral edema for evidence of increasing intracranial pressure. The client's current blood pressure is 170/80 mm Hg. What's the client's pulse pressure? Record your answer using a whole number.

_____

127. A client was hit in the head with a baseball during practice. Which discharge instructions should the nurse reinforce?
1. Watch client for keyhole pupil for the next 24 hours.
2. Expect profuse vomiting for 24 hours after the injury.
3. Wake client every hour and check orientation to person, time, and place.
4. Notify health care provider immediately when experiencing headache.

128. A client was admitted with injury to the thalamus. Which manifestation would the nurse observe during data collection?
1. Aching sensation over one-half of the body
2. Seizure activity
3. Problems with initiating body movement
4. Memory lapses

129. The nurse is making assignments for the day. Which of the following tasks can be safely assigned to unlicensed assistive personnel (UAP)?
1. Performing assessment on a client with encephalitis
2. Feeding a client with stroke reporting dysphagia
3. Measuring the intake of a client with multiple sclerosis
4. Turning a client with fracture of cervical spine

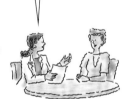

Be sure to cover all discharge instructions carefully with the client.

125. 4, 5. Carbamazepine is likely to cause diplopia, dizziness, ataxia, and a rash. Carbamazepine causes agranulocytosis because of the reduction in leukocytes. ARDS isn't a complication of carbamazepine. Carbamazepine decreases blood levels of phenytoin and oral contraceptives.
CN: Physiological integrity; CNS: Pharmacological therapies;
CL: Apply; DIFFICULTY: Difficult

126. 90.
Pulse pressure is the difference between the systolic blood pressure and the diastolic blood pressure. For this client:

$$170 \text{ mm Hg} - 80 \text{ mm Hg} = 90 \text{ mm Hg}.$$

CN: Physiological integrity; CNS: Reduction of risk potential;
CL: Apply; DIFFICULTY: Easy

127. 3. Changes in level of consciousness (LOC) may indicate expanding lesions such as subdural hematoma; orientation and LOC are assessed frequently for 24 hours. Profuse or projectile vomiting is a symptom of increased intracranial pressure and should be reported immediately. A slight headache may last for several days after concussion; severe or worsening headaches should be reported. A keyhole pupil is found after iridectomy.
CN: Physiological integrity; CNS: Physiological adaptation;
CL: Apply; DIFFICULTY: Moderate

128. 1. Damage to the thalamus may result in thalamic syndrome, which is characterized by pain, burning, or an aching sensation over one half of the body. It is often accompanied by mood swings. Problems initiating movement are associated with the basal ganglia and memory problems with the hippocampus. Seizures are not specific to thalamic injury.
CN: Physiological integrity; CNS: Physiological adaptation;
CL: Apply; DIFFICULTY: Difficult

129. 3. The unlicensed assistive personnel (UAP) can be assigned to perform a routine task such as measuring the intake of a client with multiple sclerosis. However, UAP cannot be assigned to a client who is not stable. A client with CVA may have dysphagia or difficulty swallowing. This client should not be assigned to a UAP because of risk of aspiration. A client with fracture of the cervical spine should not be assigned to UAP because the client is also unstable. Performing assessment is not within the scope of practice of UAP.
CN: Safe, effective care environment; CNS: Coordinated Care;
CL: Apply; DIFFICULTY: Easy

130. A client was admitted with an injury to the occipital lobe. Which nursing action should the nurse perform?
1. Test water temperature before bathing or showering.
2. Assist client while walking due to loss of balance.
3. Monitor client for visual disturbances.
4. Evaluate the client's hearing condition.

131. The nurse is caring for a client with multiple sclerosis (MS). Which problems should the nurse expect the client to experience? Select all that apply.
1. Vision disturbances
2. Coagulation abnormalities
3. Impaired motor function
4. Immunity compromise
5. Decreased sensation

132. The nurse is reinforcing teaching instructions to a client with trigeminal neuralgia on how to minimize pain episodes. Which comments by the client would indicate correct understanding of instructions? Select all that apply.
1. "I'll eat food that's very hot or cold."
2. "I'll chew food on the unaffected side."
3. "I can wash my face with icy water."
4. "I'll drink fluids at room temperature."
5. "I'll perform mouth care after meals."

133. A client is experiencing problems with balance and fine gross motor function. Identify the area of the client's brain that's malfunctioning.

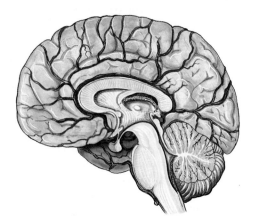

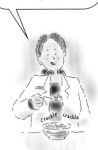

Yahoo! You're almost done. Keep going.

With trigeminal neuralgia, remember to chew on the good side.

130. **3.** The nurse should monitor client for visual disturbances since occipital lobe regulates vision. The parietal lobe primarily regulates sensory function. The cerebellum controls balance. The temporal lobe is involved in hearing.
CN: Physiological integrity; CNS: Basic care and comfort; CL: Apply; DIFFICULTY: Challenge

131. **1, 3, 5.** Multiple sclerosis, a neuromuscular disorder, may cause vision disturbances, impaired sensation, and impaired motor function. MS doesn't cause coagulation abnormalities or immunity problems.
CN: Physiological integrity; CNS: Reduction of risk potential; CL: Apply; DIFFICULTY: Challenge

132. **2, 4, 5.** The facial pain of trigeminal neuralgia is triggered by mechanical or thermal stimuli. Chewing food on the unaffected side and rinsing the mouth rather than brushing the teeth reduce mechanical stimulation. Drinking fluids at room temperature reduces thermal stimulation. Eating hot or cold food and washing the face with cold water are likely to trigger pain.
CN: Health promotion and maintenance; CNS: None; CL: Understand; DIFFICULTY: Moderate

133. The cerebellum is the portion of the brain that controls balance and fine and gross motor function.

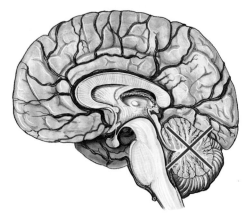

CN: Physiological integrity; CNS: Reduction of risk potential; CL: Understand; DIFFICULTY: Moderate

Chapter 7

Musculoskeletal Disorders

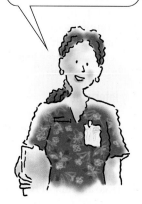

Here's a test that covers nursing care for clients with a disorder of the musculoskeletal system. So get moving and break a leg. Oh—I mean good luck!

Musculoskeletal refresher

Arm and leg fractures

Complete or incomplete break in a bone resulting from the application of excessive force

Key signs and symptoms
- Loss of limb function
- Pain
- Deformity

Key test results
- Anterior, posterior, and lateral x-rays of the suspected fracture as well as x-rays of the joints above and below it confirm diagnosis

Key treatments
- Closed reduction (restoring displaced bone segments to their normal position)
- Immobilization with a splint, cast, or traction
- Open reduction during surgery to reduce and immobilize the fracture with rods, plates, or screws when closed reduction is impossible, usually followed by application of a plaster cast
- Analgesics: morphine, acetaminophen, oxycodone, hydrocodone

Key interventions
- Monitor vital signs and be especially alert for rapid pulse, decreased blood pressure, pallor, and cool, clammy skin
- Maintain IV fluids as ordered
- Ease pain with analgesics as ordered
- Reposition the immobilized client often
- Assist with active range-of-motion (ROM) exercises to the unaffected extremities
- Encourage deep breathing and coughing
- Ensure that immobilized client receives adequate fluid intake
- Watch for signs of renal calculi, such as flank pain, nausea, and vomiting
- Provide cast care
- Encourage client to start moving around as soon as possible
- Assist with walking, keeping in mind that client who has been bedridden for some time may be dizzy at first
- Demonstrate how to use crutches properly

Carpal tunnel syndrome

Compression and irritation of the median nerve as it passes under the transverse carpal ligament in the wrist

Key signs and symptoms
- Numbness, burning, or tingling in arms
- Pain in arms and hands
- Weakness in arms and hands

Key test results
- Blood pressure cuff on the forearm (inflated above systolic pressure for 1 to 2 minutes) evokes pain and paresthesia along the distribution of median nerve
- Electromyography detects median nerve motor conduction delay of more than 5 milliseconds

Key treatments
- Resting the hands by splinting the wrist in neutral extension for 1 to 2 weeks
- Possibly changing occupations (if definite link has been established between client's occupation and development of carpal tunnel syndrome)
- Corticosteroid injections: betamethasone, hydrocortisone
- Nonsteroidal anti-inflammatory drugs (NSAIDs): indomethacin, ibuprofen, naproxen

Key interventions
- Administer NSAIDs as needed
- Assist with eating and bathing if client's dominant hand has been impaired
- Monitor vital signs and regularly check color, sensation, and motion of affected hand, if surgery is performed

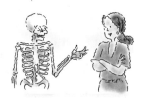

What could be causing this pain in my arms and hands?

Compartment syndrome

Serious condition that involves increased pressure in a muscle compartment

Key signs and symptoms
- Severe or increased pain that occurs when the affected muscle is stretched or elevated (pain is unrelieved by opioid analgesics)
- Loss of distal pulse

- Tense, swollen muscle
- Paresthesia

Key test results

- Intracompartmental pressure is elevated, as indicated by a blood pressure sphygmomanometer

Key treatments

- Fasciotomy
- Positioning the affected extremity lower than the heart
- Removal of dressings or constrictive coverings of the area

Key interventions

- Monitor the affected extremity
- Perform frequent neurovascular checks
- Perform dressing changes after fasciotomy, and reinforce dressings frequently; (expect a large amount of bloody drainage)

Gout

Disease in which defective metabolism of uric acid causes arthritis

Key signs or symptoms

- Inflamed, painful joints

Key test results

- Blood studies indicate:
  - serum uric acid level that's above normal
  - urine uric acid level usually higher in secondary gout than in primary gout

Key treatments

- Antigout drugs: colchicine, allopurinol
- Uricosuric drugs: probenecid, sulfinpyrazone
- Corticosteroids: betamethasone, hydrocortisone
- NSAIDs: ibuprofen, naproxen

Key interventions

- Encourage bed rest, and use a bed cradle to reduce discomfort
- Give analgesics, as needed, especially during acute attacks
- Apply hot or cold packs to inflamed joints
- Administer anti-inflammatory medication and other drugs
- Urge client to drink plenty of fluids (up to 2 L/day)
- When encouraging fluids, record intake and output accurately
- Alkalinize urine with sodium bicarbonate or another agent, as needed
- Ensure client understands importance of having serum uric acid levels checked periodically

Herniated nucleus pulposus

Disk is displaced from its normal position in between the vertebral bodies of spine

Key signs and symptoms

In lumbosacral area

- Acute pain in lower back that radiates across the buttock and down the leg
- Pain on ambulation
- Weakness, numbness, and tingling of foot and leg

In cervical area

- Neck pain that radiates down arm to the hand
- Neck stiffness
- Weakness of the affected upper extremities
- Weakness, numbness, and tingling of hand

Key test results

- Myelogram shows compression of the spinal cord
- X-ray shows narrowing of disk space
- Magnetic resonance imaging identifies the herniated disk

Key treatments

- Corticosteroid: cortisone
- NSAIDs: indomethacin, ibuprofen, sulindac, piroxicam, flurbiprofen, diclofenac sodium, naproxen, diflunisal

Key interventions

- Monitor neurovascular status
- Turn the client every 2 hours using the log-rolling technique

Hip fracture

Fracture of the femoral neck

Key signs and symptoms

- Shorter appearance and outward rotation of affected leg, resulting in limited or abnormal ROM
- Edema and discoloration of surrounding tissue

Key test results

- Computed tomography scan (for complicated fractures) pinpoints abnormalities
- X-ray reveals a break in the continuity of the bone

Key treatments

- Surgical immobilization or joint replacement
- Abductor splint or trochanter roll between legs to prevent loss of alignment (postoperatively)
- Anticoagulant: warfarin (postoperatively)

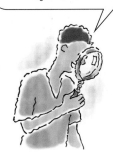

What signs should you look for in compartment syndrome?

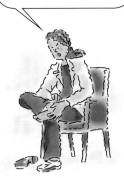

Arrgghh! My gout is acting up. I guess I need to drink more water.

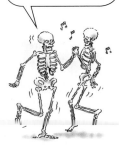

Shake those bones! Exercise helps keep bones and joints healthy.

Key interventions

- Monitor neurovascular and respiratory status
- Priority: check for compromised circulation, hemorrhage, and neurologic impairment in the affected extremity and pneumonia in the bedridden client
- Provide active and passive ROM and isometric exercises for unaffected limbs
- Provide a trapeze
- Maintain traction before surgery at all times, if using conservative treatment

Osteoarthritis

Type of arthritis caused by inflammation, breakdown, and eventual loss of cartilage in the joints

Key signs and symptoms

- Crepitation
- Joint stiffness
- Pain relieved by resting the joints

Key test results

- Arthroscopy reveals bone spurs and narrowing of joint space
- X-rays show joint deformity, narrowing of joint space, and bone spurs

Key treatments

- Exercise
- Application of warm, moist heat
- NSAIDs: indomethacin, ibuprofen, naproxen, diflunisal, celecoxib

Key interventions

- Evaluate musculoskeletal status
- Observe for increased bleeding or bruising tendency

Osteomyelitis

Bone infection caused by bacteria or other pathogens

Key signs and symptoms

- Pain
- Tenderness
- Swelling

Key test results

- Blood cultures identify causative organism
- Erythrocyte sedimentation rate and C-reactive protein (CRP) are elevated (CRP appears to be a better diagnostic tool)

Key treatments

- Immobilization of affected bone by plaster cast, traction, or bed rest
- Antibiotics: large doses of IV antibiotics after blood cultures are taken, usually:

  - penicillinase-resistant penicillin (e.g., nafcillin and oxacillin)
  - cephalosporin (e.g., cefazolin)

Key interventions

- Use strict aseptic technique when changing dressings and irrigating wounds
- Check vital signs and wound appearance daily, and monitor for new pain
- Check circulation and drainage; if wet spot appears on cast, circle it with a marking pen and note the time of appearance (on the cast); be aware of how much drainage is expected; check the circled spot at least every 4 hours; watch for any enlargement

Osteoporosis

Softening of the bones that gradually increases and makes them more fragile

Key signs and symptoms

- Deformity
- Kyphosis
- Pain

Key test results

- X-rays show typical degeneration in the lower thoracic and lumbar vertebrae
- Vertebral bodies may appear flattened and may look denser than normal
- Loss of bone mineral becomes evident in later stages
- Dual-energy x-ray absorptiometry (DXA) shows bone mineral density at the spine and hip

Key treatments

- Physical therapy consisting of weight-bearing exercise and activity
- Hormonal agents: conjugated estrogen, calcitonin, teriparatide
- Vitamin D supplements
- Antiosteoporotics: alendronate, risedronate, raloxifene, ibandronate
- Calcium supplements

Key interventions

- Check the client's skin daily for redness, warmth, and new sites of pain
- Encourage activity; help client walk several times daily
- Perform passive ROM exercises, or encourage the client to perform active exercises
- Encourage regular attendance at physical therapy sessions
- Provide a balanced diet high in vitamin D, calcium, and protein
- Administer analgesics and apply heat

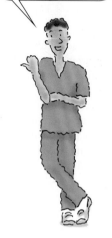

"Crepitation." That word gives me the creeps.

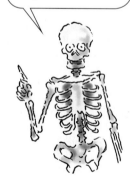

Make sure you're getting enough calcium and vitamin D, my friend. I need to stay strong and healthy for years to come.

Musculoskeletal questions, answers, and rationales

1. A nurse admits an older adult client with a history of osteoporosis experiencing a right wrist and hip fracture after a fall. Which intervention by the nurse is **priority**?
  1. Administer opioid analgesics as prescribed.
  2. Assist with activities of daily living.
  3. Give the client water as requested.
  4. Obtain data regarding skin integrity

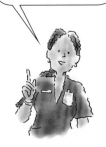

Remember— Priority means which intervention should you make first?

2. An older adult client reports pain in the lower back and is diagnosed with osteoporosis. What education should the nurse reinforce to prevent complications?
  1. Pain control
  2. Safety precautions to prevent fractures
  3. The bones will harden and become stiff
  4. An increase in the bone matrix and remineralization

3. The nurse is reinforcing education for a client on preventing complications of primary osteoporosis. Which statement made by the client indicates an understanding of the education provided?
  1. "I will refrain from drinking alcohol."
  2. "I will be sure to take my calcium supplements."
  3. "I must eat 3 meals a day."
  4. "I can't help it since I have rheumatoid arthritis."

4. A client recently had a total hysterectomy. Which response by the client indicates that education has been effective?
  1. "My risk for osteoporosis is low because I still have my thyroid gland."
  2. "Osteoporosis affects only women over 65 years old."
  3. "I'm still producing hormones, so I don't have to worry about osteoporosis."
  4. "I need to take precautions to protect myself from osteoporosis because I've had surgically induced menopause."

5. A nurse is providing nutritional information to a client with a diagnosis of gout. Which of the client's favorite foods should be limited?
  1. Blackberries
  2. Tofu
  3. Liver
  4. Tomatoes

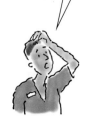

Let's see— which one of these contains a lot of purine?

1. 1. Relieving pain and making the client more comfortable should have priority. Water should not be administered unless cleared by the surgeon in case the client requires surgery. Obtaining data regarding skin integrity and assisting with activities of daily living are important but not the priority at this time.
CN: Safe, effective care environment;
CNS: Safety and infection control; CL: Analyze; DIFFICULTY: Moderate

2. 2. The primary complication of osteoporosis is fractures. Bones soften, and there's a decrease in bone matrix and remineralization. Pain may occur, but fractures can be life-threatening.
CN: Physiological integrity; CNS: Physiological adaptation;
CL: Apply; DIFFICULTY: Easy

3. 2. Hormonal imbalance, faulty metabolism, and poor dietary intake of calcium cause primary osteoporosis. Malnutrition, alcoholism, osteogenesis imperfecta, rheumatoid arthritis, liver disease, scurvy, lactose intolerance, hyperthyroidism, and trauma cause secondary osteoporosis.
CN: Physiological integrity; CNS: Physiological adaptation;
CL: Apply; DIFFICULTY: Challenge

4. 4. Menopause at any age puts women at risk for osteoporosis because of the associated hormonal imbalance. This client's thyroid gland won't protect her from menopause. With her ovaries removed, she's no longer producing the necessary hormones.
CN: Physiological integrity; CNS: Physiological adaptation;
CL: Analyze; DIFFICULTY: Easy

5. 3. A client with gout should reduce his intake of purine-rich food, such as liver. Blackberries, tofu, and tomatoes aren't rich in purine.
CN: Physiological integrity; CNS: Basic care and comfort;
CL: Apply; DIFFICULTY: Easy

6. A client is diagnosed with primary osteoporosis. Which nursing intervention should be included in the plan of care?
1. Placing items within reach of the client
2. Installing bars in the bathroom to prevent falls
3. Maintaining optimal calcium and vitamin D intake
4. Using a professional alert system in the home in case the client falls when alone

7. A nurse is providing care to a client with an acute attack of gout. Which action should the nurse provide **first**?
1. Force fluids.
2. Instruct the client on relaxation techniques.
3. Encourage bed rest.
4. Administer analgesics.

8. A client is experiencing nonchronic gout. Which clinical manifestation reported by the client would lead the nurse to suspect this form of gout?
1. Frequent painful attacks
2. Generally painful joints at all times
3. Painful attacks with pain-free periods
4. Painful attacks with less painful periods, but pain never subsides

9. A client has been prescribed a diet that limits purine-rich foods. Which foods should the nurse encourage the client to avoid? Select all that apply.
1. Bananas and dried fruits
2. Sweetbreads and lentils
3. Cheese, preserved fruits, meats, and vegetables
4. Anchovies, sardines, kidneys
5. Bacon and tuna

10. A client is recovering from an attack of gout. Client education should include the need to lose weight for which reason?
1. Weight loss will decrease purine levels.
2. Weight loss will decrease inflammation.
3. Weight loss will increase uric acid levels and decrease stress on joints.
4. Weight loss will decrease uric acid levels and decrease stress on joints.

11. The nurse is collecting a health history from a client who is exhibiting signs of gout. Which of the client's joints would the nurse expect to be **most** commonly affected?
1. Great toe
2. Wrist
3. Ankle
4. Knee

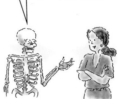

So, my gout has really been flaring up lately. What should I do about it?

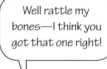

Well rattle my bones—I think you got that one right!

6. 3. Primary prevention of osteoporosis includes maintaining optimal calcium and vitamin D intake. Using a professional alert system in the home, installing bars in bathrooms to prevent falls, and placing items within reach of the client are all secondary and tertiary prevention methods.
CN: Health promotion and maintenance; CNS: None; CL: Apply; DIFFICULTY: Easy

7. 4. Administering analgesics to relieve the pain of gout should be the priority. The other actions are appropriate measures to institute but aren't the priority.
CN: Physiological integrity; CNS: Physiological adaptation; CL: Analyze; DIFFICULTY: Moderate

8. 3. The usual pattern of gout involves painful attacks with pain-free periods. Chronic gout may lead to frequent attacks with persistently painful joints.
CN: Physiological integrity; CNS: Physiological adaptation; CL: Apply; DIFFICULTY: Easy

9. 2, 4, 5. Anchovies, sardines, tuna, kidneys, sweetbreads, bacon, and lentils are high in purines. Bananas and dried fruits are high in potassium. Cheese, preserved fruits, meats, and vegetables contain tyramine.
CN: Health promotion and maintenance; CNS: None; CL: Apply; DIFFICULTY: Challenge

10. 4. Weight loss will decrease uric acid levels and decrease stress on joints. Weight loss won't decrease purine levels, increase uric acid levels, or decrease inflammation.
CN: Health promotion and maintenance; CNS: None; CL: Apply; DIFFICULTY: Easy

11. 1. The great toe is most commonly affected in clients with gout. Gout can affect any joint but most commonly affects the great toe.
CN: Physiological integrity; CNS: Reduction of risk potential; CL: Apply; DIFFICULTY: Easy

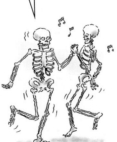

12. Which statement by a client diagnosed with gout indicates an understanding of the discharge instructions?
1. "I'll increase my fluids so that the inflammation will be reduced."
2. "Increasing fluid intake will increase the calcium my body absorbs."
3. "Increasing fluid intake will cause my body to excrete more uric acid."
4. "Increasing fluids will help provide a cushion for my bones."

12. 3. Fluids promote the excretion of uric acid. Fluids don't decrease inflammation, increase calcium absorption, or provide a cushion for bones.
CN: Physiological integrity; CNS: Physiological adaptation; CL: Apply; DIFFICULTY: Easy

13. A client who has been recently diagnosed with gout asks the nurse to explain why they need to take colchicine. What should the nurse base the response on?
1. Colchicine increases estrogen levels in the bloodstream.
2. Colchicine decreases the risk of infection.
3. Colchicine decreases inflammation.
4. Colchicine decreases bone demineralization.

13. 3. The action of colchicine is to decrease inflammation by reducing the migration of leukocytes to synovial fluid. Colchicine doesn't decrease the risk of infection, increase estrogen levels, or decrease bone demineralization.
CN: Physiological integrity; CNS: Pharmacological therapies; CL: Apply; DIFFICULTY: Easy

14. A nurse is gathering data from a client with osteoarthritis. Which findings should the nurse recognize correlate with this disease? Select all that apply.
1. Joint pain after exercise relieved by rest
2. Symmetrical swelling of the joints of both hands
3. Joint stiffness
4. Fever
5. Crepitation

14. 1, 3, 5. The symptoms of osteoarthritis are joint pain after exercise or weight-bearing (usually relieved by rest), joint stiffness, and crepitation. The other options are symptoms of rheumatoid arthritis.
CN: Physiological integrity; CNS: Physiological adaptation; CL: Apply; DIFFICULTY: Difficult

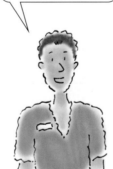

Great! I'm always looking for an excuse to eat.

15. A client with osteoarthritis is receiving ibuprofen for pain. Which instruction should the nurse give to a client taking nonsteroidal anti-inflammatory drugs (NSAIDs)?
1. Bleeding isn't a problem with NSAIDs.
2. Take NSAIDs with food to avoid an upset stomach.
3. Take NSAIDs on an empty stomach to increase absorption.
4. Don't take NSAIDs at bedtime because they may cause excitement.

15. 2. Ibuprofen, like other NSAIDs, should be taken with food because it can irritate the GI mucosa and lead to GI bleeding. It can cause drowsiness and complications from bleeding.
CN: Physiological integrity; CNS: Pharmacological therapies; CL: Apply; DIFFICULTY: Easy

16. A client asks for information about osteoarthritis. Which statement should the nurse include when reinforcing education for the client on this condition?
1. "Osteoarthritis is rarely debilitating."
2. "Osteoarthritis is a rare form of arthritis."
3. "Osteoarthritis is the most common form of arthritis."
4. "Osteoarthritis afflicts people older than age 60."

16. 3. Osteoarthritis is the most common form of arthritis. It can afflict people of any age, although most are older adults, and it can be extremely debilitating.
CN: Physiological integrity; CNS: Physiological adaptation; CL: Apply; DIFFICULTY: Easy

17. A client with a diagnosis of primary osteoarthritis asks the nurse what may have caused this disease. Which statements are appropriate responses by the nurse? Select all that apply.
1. "Overuse of joints can cause the disorder."
2. "Obesity can cause added weight on the joints causing primary osteoarthritis."
3. "Congenital abnormality"
4. "The process of aging"
5. "Diabetes mellitus"

17. 1, 2. 4. Primary osteoarthritis may be caused by the overuse of joints, aging, or obesity. Congenital abnormalities and diabetes mellitus can cause secondary osteoarthritis.
CN: Physiological integrity; CNS: Physiological adaptation;
CL: Apply; DIFFICULTY: Moderate

18. The nurse knows that a client with osteoarthritis of the knee understands the discharge instructions when the client makes which statement?
1. "I'll take my ibuprofen on an empty stomach."
2. "I'll try taking a warm shower in the morning."
3. "I'll wear my knee splint every night."
4. "I'll jog at least a mile every evening."

18. 2. A client with osteoarthritis has joint stiffness that may be partially relieved with a warm shower on arising in the morning. Ibuprofen should be taken with food, as should all nonsteroidal anti-inflammatory drugs (NSAIDs). Splints are usually used by clients with rheumatoid arthritis. Because osteoarthritis continually stresses the joint, exercise that puts less strain on the joint, such as swimming, may be a good choice.
CN: Physiological integrity; CNS: Basic care and comfort;
CL: Apply; DIFFICULTY: Challenge

19. A client is taking salicylates for osteoarthritis. What should the nurse carefully monitor the client for?
1. Hearing loss
2. Increased pain in joints
3. Decreased calcium absorption
4. Increased bone demineralization

19. 1. Many older adults already have diminished hearing, and salicylate use can lead to further or total hearing loss. Salicylates don't increase bone demineralization, decrease calcium absorption, or increase pain in joints.
CN: Physiological integrity; CNS: Pharmacological therapies;
CL: Apply; DIFFICULTY: Moderate

20. A client with osteoarthritis may be on bed rest for prolonged periods. Which nursing intervention would be appropriate for these clients?
1. Encouraging coughing and deep breathing, and limiting fluid intake
2. Providing only passive range of motion (ROM), and decreasing stimulation
3. Having the client lie as still as possible, and giving adequate pain medicine
4. Turning the client every 2 hours, and encouraging coughing and deep breathing

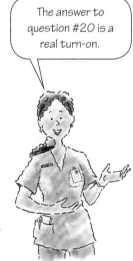

The answer to question #20 is a real turn-on.

20. 4. A bedridden client needs to be turned every 2 hours, have adequate nutrition, and cough and deep-breathe. Adequate pain medication, active *and* passive ROM, and hydration are also appropriate nursing measures. The client shouldn't lie as still as possible (to prevent contractures) or limit his fluid intake.
CN: Physiological integrity; CNS: Basic care and comfort;
CL: Apply; DIFFICULTY: Easy

21. Use of which types of clothing would help a client with osteoarthritis perform activities of daily living at home? Select all that apply.
1. Zippered clothing
2. Rubber grippers
3. Velcro clothing
4. Slip-on shoes
5. Tied shoes

21. 2, 3. 4. Velcro clothing, slip-on shoes, and rubber grippers make it easier for the client to dress and grip objects. Zippers and tied shoes may be difficult for the client to use.
CN: Physiological integrity; CNS: Basic care and comfort;
CL: Apply; DIFFICULTY: Moderate

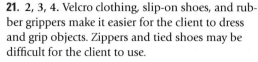

22. A client asks the nurse, "What's the difference between rheumatoid arthritis and osteoarthritis?" Which statement is the correct response?
1. "Osteoarthritis is gender-specific; rheumatoid arthritis isn't."
2. "Osteoarthritis is a localized disease; rheumatoid arthritis is systemic."
3. "Osteoarthritis is a systemic disease; rheumatoid arthritis is localized."
4. "Osteoarthritis has dislocations and subluxations; rheumatoid arthritis doesn't."

23. An older adult client is seen in the clinic with reports of right hip pain that worsens after activity, decreased range of motion (ROM) of the right hip, and difficulty getting up after sitting for long periods. The nurse hears crepitus in the right hip upon movement and determines that these symptoms are associated with which condition?
1. Gout
2. Osteoarthritis
3. Rheumatoid arthritis
4. Hip fracture

24. Which instruction by the nurse would be considered primary prevention of injury from osteoarthritis? Select all that apply.
1. Stay on bed rest.
2. Avoid physical activity.
3. Avoid repetitive tasks.
4. Warm up before exercise.
5. Perform only repetitive tasks

25. Which statement by the client indicates that client education regarding osteoarthritis has been effective?
1. "It's a systemic inflammatory disease of the joints."
2. "It involves fusing of the joints in the hand."
3. "It's an inflammatory joint disease that causes loss of articular cartilage in the synovial joint."
4. "It's a noninflammatory joint disease that causes degeneration of the joints."

26. A client with osteoarthritis is refusing to perform independent daily care. Which approach would be **most** appropriate to use with this client?
1. Perform the care for the client.
2. Explain that complete independence should be maintained
3. Encourage the client to perform as much care as pain will allow.
4. Inform the client that after care is completed, pain medication will be administered.

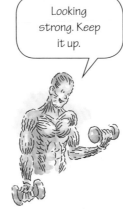

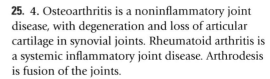
Looking strong. Keep it up.

22. 2. Osteoarthritis is a localized disease; rheumatoid arthritis is systemic. Osteoarthritis isn't gender-specific, but rheumatoid arthritis is, affecting twice as many women as men. Clients have dislocations and subluxations in both disorders.
CN: Physiological integrity; CNS: Physiological adaptation;
CL: Apply; DIFFICULTY: Easy

23. 2. Osteoarthritis of the hip is associated with joint pain that worsens with activity, diminished ROM, joint crepitus, and difficulty arising after long periods of rest. Gout is associated with intermittent periods of joint pain that resolve. Rheumatoid arthritis is a systemic disease that affects multiple joints. Clients with hip fractures have severe pain in the hip or groin and are unable to bear weight, and the leg may be externally rotated.
CN: Physiological integrity; CNS: Physiological adaptation;
CL: Analyze; DIFFICULTY: Moderate

24. 3, 4. Primary prevention of injury from osteoarthritis includes warming up and avoiding repetitive tasks. Physical activity is important to remain fit and healthy and to maintain joint function. Bed rest would contribute to many other systemic complications.
CN: Health promotion and maintenance; CNS: None; CL: Apply;
DIFFICULTY: Difficult

25. 4. Osteoarthritis is a noninflammatory joint disease, with degeneration and loss of articular cartilage in synovial joints. Rheumatoid arthritis is a systemic inflammatory joint disease. Arthrodesis is fusion of the joints.
CN: Physiological integrity; CNS: Physiological adaptation;
CL: Apply; DIFFICULTY: Moderate

26. 3. A client with osteoarthritis should be encouraged to perform as much of her care as possible. The nurse's goal should be to allow the client to maintain her self-care abilities with help as needed. It's never appropriate to use pain medication as a bargaining tool.
CN: Psychosocial integrity; CNS: None; CL: Apply; DIFFICULTY: Easy

CN: Client needs category   CNS: Client needs subcategory   CL: Cognitive level

27. The nurse is gathering data from a client in the late stage of osteoarthritis and asks the client to describe the pain. What description does the nurse anticipate the client will give?
1. Grating
2. Dull ache
3. Deep, aching pain
4. Deep aching, relieved with rest

27. 1. In the late stages of osteoarthritis, the client typically describes joint pain as grating. As the disease progresses, the cartilage covering the ends of bones is destroyed and bones rub against each other. Osteophytes, or bone spurs, may also form on the ends of bones. A dull ache and deep, aching pain that's relieved with or without rest is usually seen in the earlier stages of osteoarthritis.
CN: Physiological integrity; CNS: Physiological adaptation;
CL: Analyze; DIFFICULTY: Difficult

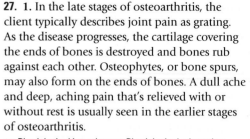

Now you're moving.

28. A client uses a cane for assistance in walking. Which instruction should be reinforced when the client is using assistive devices for ambulation?
1. "A walker is a better choice than a cane."
2. "The cane should be used on the affected side."
3. "The cane should be used on the unaffected side."
4. "A client with osteoarthritis should be encouraged to ambulate without the cane."

28. 3. A cane should be used on the unaffected side. A client with osteoarthritis should be encouraged to ambulate with a cane, walker, or other assistive device as needed; such use takes weight and stress off joints.
CN: Physiological integrity; CNS: Physiological adaptation;
CL: Apply; DIFFICULTY: Challenge

29. The nurse is preparing to reinforce discharge instructions for a client who was diagnosed with osteoarthritis. Which discharge instruction about home activity should be given to this client?
1. Learn to pace activity.
2. Remain as sedentary as possible.
3. Return to a normal level of activity.
4. Include vigorous exercise in daily routine.

29. 1. A client with osteoarthritis should pace his activities and avoid overexertion. Overexertion can increase degeneration and cause pain. The client shouldn't become sedentary because he'll have a high risk of pneumonia and contractures.
CN: Physiological integrity; CNS: Physiological adaptation;
CL: Apply; DIFFICULTY: Easy

30. A client has been prescribed an anti-inflammatory for osteoarthritis, and the nurse has reinforced educating the client about taking the medication. Which statement by the client indicates that the nurse's education has been effective?
1. "If I'm not free from pain in a week, I'll come back to the clinic."
2. "It can take up to 2 to 3 weeks for me to feel the full effects from the medication."
3. "I'll increase my dose if I'm not better in a few days."
4. "If I don't experience pain relief in a few days, I need to stop taking the medication."

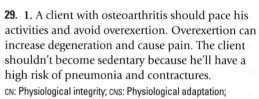

Patience. Sometimes it takes me a while to kick in.

30. 2. Anti-inflammatory drugs may take up to 2 to 3 weeks for full benefits to be appreciated. If the client can tolerate the pain, continue on the present dose and practice other pain reduction measures, such as rest, massage, heat, or cold. Clients should never adjust their dosage or discontinue a medication without consulting the health care provider.
CN: Physiological integrity; CNS: Pharmacological therapies;
CL: Apply; DIFFICULTY: Easy

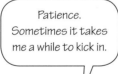

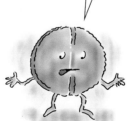

31. A client reports low back pain that radiates down the right leg, with numbness and weakness of the right leg. The nurse recognizes these symptoms as related to which disorder?
1. Herniated nucleus pulposus (HNP)
2. Muscular dystrophy
3. Parkinson disease
4. Osteoarthritis

31. 1. Compression of nerves by the HNP causes back pain that radiates into the leg, with numbness and weakness of the leg. Muscular dystrophy causes wasting of skeletal muscles. Parkinson disease is characterized by progressive muscle rigidity and tremors. Osteoarthritis causes deep, aching joint pain.
CN: Physiological integrity; CNS: Physiological adaptation;
CL: Analyze; DIFFICULTY: Moderate

32. A client is diagnosed with a herniated nucleus pulposus (HNP) or herniated disk. Which statement should the nurse include when reinforcing education about a herniated disk?
  1. The disk slips out of alignment.
  2. The disk shatters, and fragments place pressure on nerve roots.
  3. The nucleus tissue itself remains centralized, and the surrounding tissue is displaced.
  4. The nucleus of the disk puts pressure on the anulus, causing pressure on the nerve root.

32. 4. With a herniated nucleus pulposus, or herniated disk, the nucleus of the disk puts pressure on the anulus, causing pressure on the nerve root. The disk itself doesn't slip, rupture, or shatter. The nucleus tissue usually moves from the center of the disk.
CN: Physiological integrity; CNS: Physiological adaptation; CL: Apply; DIFFICULTY: Moderate

33. The client is being treated conservatively for a herniated nucleus pulposus (HNP). Which interventions should the nurse be sure the care team includes in the plan of care? Select all that apply.
  1. Pain medication
  2. Bone fusion
  3. Heat application
  4. Physiotherapy
  5. Surgery

33. 1, 3, 4. Conservative treatment of an HNP may include heat application, pain medication, and physiotherapy. Aggressive treatment may include surgery, such as a bone fusion.
CN: Physiological integrity; CNS: Reduction of risk potential; CL: Apply; DIFFICULTY: Moderate

34. A client is admitted for closed spine surgery to repair a herniated disk. The nurse is discussing the surgery with the client. Which instruction should the nurse reinforce in the preoperative education?
  1. "It's riskier than open spine surgery."
  2. "Intense physical therapy is needed after the procedure."
  3. "An endoscope is used to perform the surgery."
  4. "Recovery time is longer than with open spine surgery."

34. 3. Closed spine surgery uses endoscopy to fix a herniated disk. It's less risky than open surgery and has a shorter recovery time; it's commonly done as a same-day surgical procedure. Physical therapy may be less intensive or not needed at all.
CN: Physiological integrity; CNS: Reduction of risk potential; CL: Analyze; DIFFICULTY: Moderate

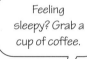

Feeling sleepy? Grab a cup of coffee.

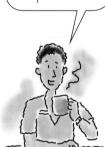

35. A client asks the nurse why he needs to apply a cold pack on a sprained ankle. Which response would be **most** appropriate?
  1. "It decreases pain and increases circulation."
  2. "It numbs the nerves and dilates the blood vessels."
  3. "It promotes circulation and reduces muscle spasm."
  4. "It constricts local blood vessels and decreases swelling."

35. 4. Application of a cold pack causes the blood vessels to constrict, which reduces the leakage of fluid into the tissues and prevents swelling. It may have an effect on muscle spasms. Cold therapy may reduce pain by numbing the nerves and tissues. Cold therapy doesn't promote circulation or dilate the blood vessels.
CN: Physiological integrity; CNS: Basic care and comfort; CL: Apply; DIFFICULTY: Easy

36. A client is admitted to the emergency department with severe lower back pain, weakness, and atrophy of leg muscles. For which diagnostic tests should the nurse prepare the client? Select all that apply.
  1. MRI
  2. CT scan
  3. Lumbar puncture
  4. Myelography
  5. Chest x-ray

36. 1, 2, 4. Tests used to diagnose a herniated nucleus pulposus (HNP) include myelography, MRI, and CT scan. Lumbar puncture and chest x-ray aren't conclusive tests for a herniated disk.
CN: Physiological integrity; CNS: Physiological adaptation; CL: Apply; DIFFICULTY: Moderate

37. The nurse is reinforcing education for a community class on back injuries. Which area should the nurse indicate is the **most** common area for vertebral herniation?
1. L1–L2, L4–L5 vertebrae
2. L1–L2, L5–S1 vertebrae
3. L4–L5, L5–S1 vertebrae
4. L5–S1, S2–S3 vertebrae

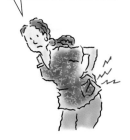

Ouch! I wonder which vertebra that was?

37. 3. The most common areas of herniation are L4–L5, L5–S1 vertebrae.
CN: Health promotion and maintenance; CNS: None; CL: Apply; DIFFICULTY: Moderate

38. Which response by the client indicates that the nurse's education regarding back safety has been effective?
1. "I'll start carrying objects at arm's length from my body."
2. "I'll sleep on my back at night."
3. "I'll carry objects close to my body."
4. "I'll lift items by bending over at my waist."

38. 3. Keeping objects close to the body's center of gravity by carrying them close to the body lessens strain on the back. Carrying objects away from the body, sleeping on the back, and bending over at the waist to lift objects all increase back strain.
CN: Health promotion and maintenance; CNS: None; CL: Apply; DIFFICULTY: Easy

39. A client has been prescribed a skeletal muscle relaxant to treat a herniated nucleus pulposus. After the nurse has instructed the client about taking the medication, which client statement indicates that further education is needed?
1. "I'll stand up slowly to avoid dizziness."
2. "If I miss a dose of the medicine, I'll take an extra pill at the next dose."
3. "I'll call my health care provider before taking over-the-counter medications."
4. "I'll avoid activities that require alertness while taking the medication."

39. 2. It isn't appropriate to take more than the prescribed dosage, as serious adverse effects can occur. Changing position slowly will help avoid dizziness. Over-the-counter medications may intensify adverse effects. Skeletal muscle relaxants can cause drowsiness.
CN: Physiological integrity; CNS: Pharmacological therapies; CL: Apply; DIFFICULTY: Easy

40. A client with a recent fracture is suspected of having compartment syndrome. Which findings does the nurse recognize correlate with this diagnosis?
1. Body wide decrease in bone mass
2. A growth in and around the bone tissue
3. Inability to perform active movement; pain with passive movement
4. Inability to perform passive movement; pain with active movement

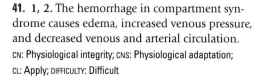

How do all of these symptoms fit together?

40. 3. With compartment syndrome, the client is unable to perform active movement and pain occurs with passive movement. A bone tumor shows growth in and around the bone tissue. Osteoporosis has a bodywide decrease in bone mass.
CN: Physiological integrity; CNS: Physiological adaptation; CL: Apply; DIFFICULTY: Moderate

41. The nurse is gathering data from a client with hemorrhage from compartment syndrome. Which symptoms would the nurse expect to find? Select all that apply.
1. Edema
2. Increased venous pressure
3. Increased venous circulation
4. Increased arterial circulation
5. Decreased venous pressure

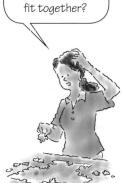

41. 1, 2. The hemorrhage in compartment syndrome causes edema, increased venous pressure, and decreased venous and arterial circulation.
CN: Physiological integrity; CNS: Physiological adaptation; CL: Apply; DIFFICULTY: Difficult

42. A client who was casted for a recent fracture of the right ulna reports severe pain, numbness, and tingling of the right arm. What would be the nurse's **most** appropriate response?
1. Administer acetaminophen as prescribed.
2. Lower the arm below the level of the heart.
3. Immediately report the client's symptoms.
4. Apply a heating pad to the area.

42. 3. Severe pain, numbness, and tingling are symptoms of impaired circulation due to compartment syndrome, which is a medical emergency. Don't give analgesics until the client has been assessed and treated. Lowering the arm below the level of the heart and applying heat will decrease venous outflow and impair the circulation even more.
CN: Physiological integrity; CNS: Physiological adaptation; CL: Apply; DIFFICULTY: Easy

43. A client has developed compartment syndrome from full thickness burns on both arms. What treatment will the nurse prepare the client for?
1. Amputation
2. Casting
3. Fasciotomy
4. Observation

44. A client is admitted to the emergency department with a foot fracture and the care provider is placing the foot in a brace. What education will the nurse reinforce as to the reason the brace is important to wear?
1. To act as a splint
2. To prevent infection
3. To allow for movement
4. To encourage direct contact

45. After treatment of compartment syndrome, a client reports experiencing paresthesia. Which symptoms should the nurse monitor?
1. Fever and chills
2. Change in range of motion (ROM)
3. Pain and blanching
4. Numbness and tingling

46. A nurse is reinforcing instruction for a client with a recent leg fracture and cast. Which statements by the client indicate that further education is needed? Select all that apply.
1. "I need to report any numbness or tingling in my leg at once."
2. "It's normal to have some numbness or tingling following a fracture."
3. "It's normal to have severe pain even after the cast is on."
4. "I need to keep my leg elevated as much as possible."
5. "The color and temperature of my toes will be checked frequently."
6. "It's normal to have swelling and for the cast to feel really tight."

47. Which characteristic of the fascia can cause it to develop compartment syndrome?
1. It is highly flexible.
2. It is fragile and weak.
3. It is unable to expand.
4. It is the only tissue within the compartment.

48. A client arrives in the emergency department reporting falling down the stairs and that feels as though the right leg may be broken. What data gathered by the nurse would indicate that the client might be correct in assumption?
1. Tingling, coolness, loss of pulses
2. Loss of sensation, redness, warmth
3. Coolness, redness, pain at the site of injury
4. Redness, warmth, pain at the site of injury

43. 3. Treatment of compartment syndrome includes fasciotomy. A fasciotomy involves cutting the fascia over the affected area to permit muscle expansion. Casting, observation, and amputation aren't treatments for compartment syndrome.
CN: Physiological integrity; CNS: Physiological adaptation; CL: Apply; DIFFICULTY: Moderate

44. 1. The purpose of the brace is to act as a splint, prevent direct contact, and maintain immobility. A brace doesn't prevent infection.
CN: Physiological integrity; CNS: Reduction of risk potential; CL: Apply; DIFFICULTY: Easy

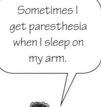

Sometimes I get paresthesia when I sleep on my arm.

45. 4. Paresthesia is described as numbness and tingling. It doesn't include pain or blanching, and isn't associated with fever and chills or change in ROM.
CN: Physiological integrity; CNS: Physiological adaptation; CL: Apply; DIFFICULTY: Easy

46. 2, 3, 6. Paresthesia (numbness or tingling) is the earliest sign, and severe pain is a later sign of compartment syndrome; they should be reported at once. Elevating the leg will help prevent venous stasis, edema, and impaired circulation. Circulation and limb sensation need to be monitored frequently.
CN: Physiological integrity; CNS: Physiological adaptation; CL: Analyze; DIFFICULTY: Moderate

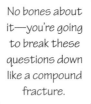

No bones about it—you're going to break these questions down like a compound fracture.

47. 3. Compartment syndrome occurs because the fascia can't expand. It isn't flexible or weak. The compartment contains blood vessels and nerves.
CN: Physiological integrity; CNS: Physiological adaptation; CL: Understand; DIFFICULTY: Moderate

48. 4. Signs of a fracture may include redness, warmth, and intense pain at the fracture site. Coolness, tingling, and loss of pulses are signs of arterial insufficiency.
CN: Physiological integrity; CNS: Physiological adaptation; CL: Apply; DIFFICULTY: Easy

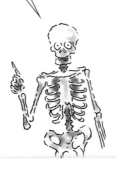

49. A client has a long leg cast applied for a tibia fracture. Which statement made by the client would indicate to the nurse that compartment syndrome may be developing?
1. "I have some discomfort when I try and move my foot around."
2. "My toenails are pink."
3. "My leg really itches."
4. "I am having a decrease in sensation of my toes."

49. 4. Compartment syndrome can occur from internal (bleeding) and external pressure (cast or dressing) and can cause a feeling similar to the foot "falling asleep" (related to a lack of sensation). Blood flow is impaired. The toenails should be pink and capillary refill less than 3 seconds. The leg will itch underneath the cast and it is important to reinforce that no objects should be placed under the cast to scratch the skin. This can damage skin integrity and predispose the client to infection.
CN: Physiological integrity; CNS: Physiological adaptation; CL: Analyze; DIFFICULTY: Easy

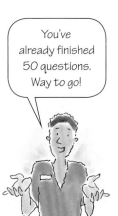

You've already finished 50 questions. Way to go!

50. The nurse is gathering data from a client who has the potential to have impaired neurovascular function from a cast application. What data is important for the nurse to gather to make sure there is not neurovascular impairment?
1. Orientation, movement, pulses, warmth
2. Capillary refill, movement, pulses, warmth
3. Orientation, pupillary response, temperature, pulses
4. Respiratory pattern, orientation, pulses, temperature

50. 2. A thorough neurovascular assessment should include checking capillary refill, movement, pulses, and warmth. Neurovascular assessment involves nerve and blood supply to an area. Respiratory pattern, orientation, temperature, and pupillary response aren't part of a neurovascular examination.
CN: Physiological integrity; CNS: Reduction of risk potential; CL: Apply; DIFFICULTY: Moderate

51. A nurse has reinforced instruction for a client to accurately measure the circumference of both calves each morning and to report any increase in circumference. Which client statement indicates that the education has been effective?
1. "I'll use a measuring tape to check circumference."
2. "I only have to call if one leg is significantly larger than the other."
3. "I can measure my calves either near the knee or closer to the ankle."
4. "I'll use the standardized chart for limb circumference."

51. 1. The correct method for measuring calf circumference is to use a measuring tape, place the tape at the level where the calf circumference is largest, and measure at this same place each time. The client was instructed to report any increase in circumference. A significant increase in calf circumference size might be unilateral or bilateral. There's no standardized chart for limb circumference.
CN: Health promotion and maintenance; CNS: None; CL: Apply; DIFFICULTY: Easy

52. The nurse is unable to detect a dorsalis pedis pulse on the left foot. What is the **priority** action by the nurse?
1. Check again in 1 hour.
2. Alert the nurse in charge immediately.
3. Verify the findings with a handheld Doppler.
4. Alert the health care provider immediately.

52. 3. If pulses aren't palpable, verify the observation with Doppler ultrasonography. If pulses can't be found with a handheld Doppler, immediately notify the health care provider.
CN: Physiological integrity; CNS: Physiological adaptation; CL: Apply; DIFFICULTY: Moderate

53. The client calls the nurse in the clinic and states that the cast feels very rough around the edges and is scratching the skin. What is the **best** response by the nurse?
1. Apply moleskin or pink tape around the edges.
2. Elevate the limb above the level of the heart.
3. Break off the rough area and file it down.
4. Distribute pressure evenly.

53. 1. To reduce the roughness of the cast, apply moleskin or pink tape around the rough edges. Elevating the limb will prevent swelling. Distributing pressure evenly will prevent pressure ulcers. Never break a rough area off the cast.
CN: Physiological integrity; CNS: Basic care and comfort; CL: Apply; DIFFICULTY: Easy

54. A client calls the clinic and informs the nurse that there is a foul odor coming from the cast. What is the **best** response by the nurse?
1. Tell the client to come to the clinic immediately since the foul odor may be a sign of infection.
2. Reinforce education for proper cast care, including hygiene measures.
3. Inform the client that odor is normal after the cast has been on for a while.
4. Inform the client that there may be some neurovascular compromise but it should resolve.

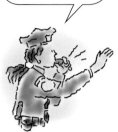

Foul odor coming from the cast?

54. 1. A foul odor from a cast may be a sign of infection. The nurse needs to monitor the client for fever, malaise, and possibly an elevation in white blood cells. Odor from a cast is never normal, and it isn't a sign of neurovascular compromise, which would include decreased pulses, coolness, and paresthesia.
CN: Physiological integrity; CNS: Reduction of risk potential;
CL: Analyze; DIFFICULTY: Challenge

55. The nurse is reinforcing education on cast care for a client with a cast on the arm. How should the nurse instruct the client to place the casted limb, if there is swelling?
1. Close to the body
2. At the level of the heart
3. Below the level of the heart
4. Above the level of the heart

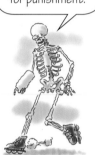

What can I say? I'm a glutton for punishment.

55. 4. To reduce swelling, place the limb with the cast above the level of the heart. Placing it below or at the level of the heart won't reduce swelling. To elevate a cast, the limb may need to be extended from the body.
CN: Physiological integrity; CNS: Physiological adaptation;
CL: Apply; DIFFICULTY: Easy

56. A client who's being discharged with an arm cast wants to shower at home. The nurse demonstrates how to shower without getting the cast wet. For which reason is this important?
1. A wet cast can cause a foul odor.
2. A wet cast will weaken or decompose.
3. A wet cast is heavy and difficult to maneuver.
4. It's all right to get the cast wet; just use a hair dryer to dry it off.

56. 2. A wet cast will weaken or decompose. A foul odor is a sign of infection. It's never appropriate to get a cast wet.
CN: Physiological integrity; CNS: Reduction of risk potential;
CL: Apply; DIFFICULTY: Easy

57. A client with a fractured femur is in Russell traction and asks the nurse to help with back care. Which nursing action is **most** appropriate?
1. Telling the client that back care cannot be performed while he's in traction
2. Removing the weight to give the client more slack to move
3. Supporting the weight to give the client more slack to move
4. Telling the client to use the trapeze to lift his back off the bed

57. 4. The traction must not be disturbed to maintain correct alignment. Therefore, the client should use the trapeze to lift his back off of the bed. The client can have back care as long as the trapeze is used and the alignment is not disturbed. The weight shouldn't be moved without a health care provider's order; it should hang freely without touching anything.
CN: Physiological integrity; CNS: Reduction of risk potential;
CL: Apply; DIFFICULTY: Easy

58. A client is involved in a motor vehicle crash and is being transferred to a trauma center. For which classic fractures that typically occur from trauma should the nurse gather data from?
1. Brachial and clavicle
2. Brachial and humerus
3. Humerus and clavicle
4. Occipital and humerus

58. 3. Classic fractures that occur with trauma are those of the humerus and clavicle. There are no brachial bones. Occipital bones aren't usually involved in a traumatic injury.
CN: Physiological integrity; CNS: Physiological adaptation;
CL: Analyze; DIFFICULTY: Moderate

59. A client comes to the emergency department reporting dull, deep bone pain unrelated to movement. Which statement is correct to determine if the bone pain is caused by a fracture?
1. These are classic symptoms of a fracture.
2. Fracture pain is sharp and related to movement.
3. Fracture pain is sharp and unrelated to movement.
4. Fracture pain is dull and deep and related to movement.

60. A client asks why he is being placed in traction prior to surgery. Which response by the nurse is **most** appropriate?
1. Traction will help prevent skin breakdown.
2. Traction helps with repositioning while in bed.
3. Traction allows for more activity.
4. Traction helps to prevent trauma and overcome muscle spasms.

61. A client with skeletal fracture to the right leg reports severe right leg pain. Which action should the nurse take **first**?
1. Call the health care provider.
2. Check the client's alignment in bed.
3. Remove the weights from the fracture.
4. Perform pin care.

62. The nurse is examining an older adult client with a fracture. Identify the location of the **most** common fracture in older adults to cause death within 1 year of sustaining the fracture.

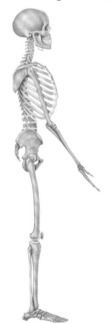
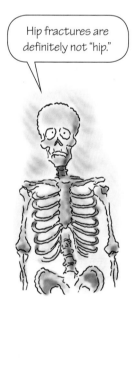

Tough break, kid.

Hip fractures are definitely not "hip."

59. 2. Fracture pain is sharp and related to movement. Pain that's dull and deep and unrelated to movement isn't typical of a fracture.
CN: Health promotion and maintenance; CNS: None; CL: Analyze; DIFFICULTY: Moderate

60. 4. Traction prevents trauma and overcomes muscle spasms. Traction doesn't help in preventing skin breakdown, repositioning the client, or allowing the client to become active.
CN: Physiological integrity; CNS: Basic care and comfort; CL: Apply; DIFFICULTY: Easy

61. 2. A client who reports severe leg pain may need realignment to ease some pressure on the fracture site. If this is ineffective, then the health care provider may need to be notified. The weights ordered may be too heavy, but the nurse can't remove them without a health care provider's order. Performing pin care isn't appropriate at this time.
CN: Safe, effective care environment; CNS: Coordinated care; CL: Apply; DIFFICULTY: Easy

62. Hip fracture is the most common injury in the older adult population and has a high rate of mortality due to complications of surgery, and prolonged immobility.

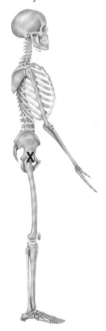

CN: Physiological integrity; CNS: Reduction of risk potential; CL: Understand; DIFFICULTY: Easy

63. An older adult client with Paget disease is undergoing tests for a suspected fracture. The nurse should expect to see which type of fracture?
1. Linear
2. Longitudinal
3. Oblique
4. Transverse

64. A client is reporting severe pain in the right upper arm. Which x-ray finding would indicate to the nurse that further investigation is required?
1. Longitudinal fracture
2. Oblique fracture
3. Spiral fracture
4. Transverse fracture

65. A client sustained a femur fracture while skiing. After the client undergoes surgery to stabilize the fracture, what does the nurse determine will assist with healing of this fracture?
1. The formation of scar tissue
2. Displacement of the fracture
3. The formation of necrotic tissue
4. Formation of new bone tissue

66. A client has just had a plaster cast applied to the right forearm following reduction of a closed radius fracture, the result of an inline skating accident. Which is **most** important for the nurse to check?
1. Whether the cast is completely dry
2. Sensation and movement of the fingers
3. Whether the client is having any pain
4. Whether the cast needs petaling

67. A client is diagnosed with a long bone fracture. What potential complication related to this form of fracture should the nurse carefully monitor?
1. Bone emboli
2. Fat emboli
3. Platelet emboli
4. Serous emboli

68. A client is diagnosed with a fat emboli. Which signs and symptoms would the nurse expect to find when gathering data from this client?
1. Tachypnea, tachycardia, shortness of breath, paresthesia
2. Paresthesia, bradypnea, bradycardia, petechial rash on chest and neck
3. Bradypnea, bradycardia, shortness of breath, petechial rash on chest and neck
4. Tachypnea, tachycardia, shortness of breath, petechial rash on chest and neck

63. 4. A transverse fracture commonly occurs with Paget disease. Linear, longitudinal, and oblique fractures generally occur with trauma.
CN: Physiological integrity; CNS: Physiological adaptation; CL: Apply; DIFFICULTY: Difficult

64. 3. Spiral fractures are commonly seen in the upper extremities and are related to physical abuse. Oblique and longitudinal fractures generally occur with trauma. A transverse fracture commonly occurs with such bone diseases as osteomalacia and Paget disease.
CN: Physiological integrity; CNS: Physiological adaptation; CL: Apply; DIFFICULTY: Moderate

65. 4. Healing of a fracture occurs by the formation of new bone tissue. Bone doesn't heal by forming scar tissue or necrotic tissue, or by displacement.
CN: Physiological integrity; CNS: Physiological adaptation; CL: Remember; DIFFICULTY: Easy

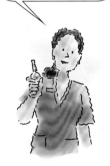

The key words in question #66 are "most important."

66. 2. Neurovascular checks are most important because they're used to determine if any impairment exists after cast application and reduction of the fracture. Checking to see if the cast is completely dry isn't the nurse's priority. Checking to see if the client has pain is important but not the priority. Petaling to smooth the cast edge is done when the cast is completely dry.
CN: Physiological integrity; CNS: Reduction of risk potential; CL: Apply; DIFFICULTY: Easy

67. 2. A serious complication of long bone fractures is the development of fat emboli. Platelet or bone emboli are rare occurrences. There aren't emboli known as *serous emboli*.
CN: Physiological integrity; CNS: Physiological adaptation; CL: Apply; DIFFICULTY: Easy

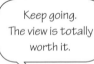

Keep going. The view is totally worth it.

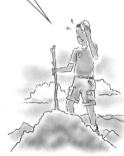

68. 4. Signs and symptoms of fat emboli include tachypnea, tachycardia, shortness of breath, and a petechial rash on the chest and neck. The fat molecules enter the venous circulation and travel to the lung, obstructing pulmonary circulation. Bradycardia, bradypnea, and paresthesia aren't usual symptoms.
CN: Health promotion and maintenance; CNS: None; CL: Analyze; DIFFICULTY: Moderate

69. The community health nurse found an older adult client lying in the snow, unable to move the right leg because of a suspected fracture. What's the nurse's **priority**?
1. Realign the fracture ends.
2. Reduce the fracture.
3. Immobilize the fracture in its present position.
4. Elevate the leg on whatever is available.

70. The client reports a flare-up of acute gout. Identify the location of the **most** common site of acute gout.

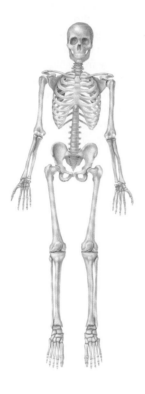

71. A high-protein diet is ordered for a client recovering from a fracture. High protein is ordered for which reason?
1. Protein promotes gluconeogenesis.
2. Protein has anti-inflammatory properties.
3. Protein promotes cell growth and bone union.
4. Protein decreases pain medication requirements.

72. The nurse is reinforcing instruction for a client on a 3-point gait using crutches. The client demonstrates an understanding when placing weight on what part of the body?
1. Feet
2. Axillary areas
3. Palms of the hands
4. Palms and axillary areas

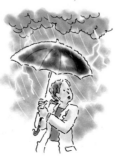

Feeling overwhelmed? Take a deep breath and keep on going. You'll ride out the storm.

69. 3. Initial treatment of obvious and suspected fractures includes immobilizing and splinting the limb. Any attempt to realign or rest the fracture at the site may cause further injury and complications. The leg may be elevated only after immobilization.
CN: Physiological integrity; CNS: Physiological adaptation;
CL: Apply; DIFFICULTY: Easy

70. Pain and inflammation of a gout attack usually occur in one or more small joints of the great toe; the metatarsophalangeal joint of the great toe is most common.

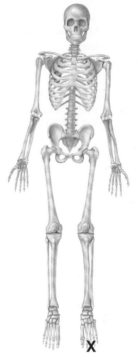

X

CN: Physiological integrity; CNS: Physiological adaptation;
CL: Understand; DIFFICULTY: Difficult

71. 3. High-protein intake promotes cell growth and bone union. Protein doesn't decrease pain medication requirements, exert anti-inflammatory properties, or promote gluconeogenesis.
CN: Physiological integrity; CNS: Basic care and comfort;
CL: Apply; DIFFICULTY: Easy

72. 3. To avoid damage to the brachial plexus nerves in the axilla, the palms of the hands should bear the client's weight. Minimal weight should be placed on the affected leg.
CN: Physiological integrity; CNS: Basic care and comfort;
CL: Apply; DIFFICULTY: Moderate

73. A client has undergone a total hip replacement on the right side. After surgery, how often should the nurse turn the client?
1. Every 1 to 2 hours, from the unaffected side to the back
2. Every 1 to 2 hours, from the affected side to the back
3. Every 4 to 6 hours, from the unaffected side to the back
4. Every 4 to 6 hours, from the affected side to the back

74. The nurse is instructing unlicensed assistive personnel (UAP) on the proper care of a client in Buck extension traction following a fracture of his left fibula. Which observation indicates that the education was effective?
1. The weights are allowed to hang freely over the end of the bed.
2. The UAP lifts the weights when assisting the client to move up in bed.
3. The leg in traction is kept externally rotated.
4. The UAP instructs the client to perform ankle rotation exercises.

75. A client is receiving nutritional counseling following application of a plaster cast for a fracture. Why would it be important for the nurse to promote the intake of Vitamin D?
1. Excretion of calcium and phosphorus
2. Excretion of potassium and calcium
3. Absorption and use of potassium and phosphorus
4. Absorption and use of calcium and phosphorus

76. The nurse is instructing unlicensed assistive personnel (UAP) on how to properly position a client who underwent total hip replacement. The nurse explains that the client's hip needs to be in which position?
1. Straight with the knee flexed
2. In an abducted position
3. In an adducted position
4. Externally rotated

77. A client underwent a bipolar hip replacement after a fracture. Which interventions would help prevent deep vein thrombosis (DVT) after surgery? Select all that apply.
1. Promote bed rest
2. Placing an egg crate mattress on the bed
3. Vigorous pulmonary care
4. Administration of subcutaneous heparin
5. Application of pneumatic compression boots

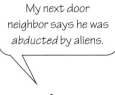
My next door neighbor says he was *abducted* by aliens.

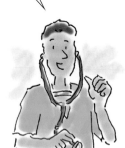

73. 1. The client should be turned at least every 2 hours and always from the unaffected side to the back. The client should never be placed on the affected side. Turning the client every 4 to 6 hours places her at greater risk for skin breakdown.
CN: Physiological integrity; CNS: Reduction of risk potential; CL: Apply; DIFFICULTY: Easy

74. 1. In Buck extension traction, the weights should hang freely without touching the bed or floor. Lifting the weights would break the traction. The client should be moved up in bed, allowing the weights to move freely along with the client. The leg should be kept in straight alignment. Performing ankle rotation exercises could cause the leg to go out of alignment.
CN: Physiological integrity; CNS: Basic care and comfort; CL: Remember; DIFFICULTY: Easy

75. 4. Vitamin D increases the absorption and use of calcium and phosphorus. It doesn't affect potassium, nor does it reduce the absorption or affect the excretion of calcium and phosphorus.
CN: Physiological integrity; CNS: Physiological adaptation; CL: Apply; DIFFICULTY: Easy

76. 2. An abducted position keeps the new joint from becoming displaced out of the socket. The client can keep the hip straight with the knee flexed as long as an abductor pillow is kept in place. Keeping the hip adducted or externally rotated can dislocate the hip joint.
CN: Physiological integrity; CNS: Basic care and comfort; CL: Apply; DIFFICULTY: Moderate

77. 4, 5. To prevent DVT after hip surgery, subcutaneous heparin and pneumatic compression boots are used. Egg crate mattresses and pulmonary care don't prevent DVT. Bed rest can *cause* DVT.
CN: Physiological integrity; CNS: Reduction of risk potential; CL: Apply; DIFFICULTY: Easy

78. The nurse is caring for a postoperative client. Identify the location of the **most** likely site of deep vein thrombosis for this client.

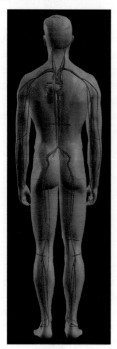

79. A client who had a recent total hip replacement is being seen by the home care nurse. When the nurse arrives, there are a large number of small carpets scattered throughout the client's home. Which action should the nurse take as a result of this finding?
1. Ask the client why there are so many scattered carpets throughout the home.
2. Collect the small carpets, and place them together near the main door of the home.
3. Review with the client the hazard small carpets play, especially for a person with musculoskeletal impairment.
4. Nothing; there's nothing wrong with having small carpets scattered throughout the home.

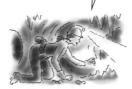

80. A client is in traction for a fracture. Which nursing intervention is appropriate for this client?
1. Assessing the pin sites every shift and as needed
2. Adding and removing weights as the client desires
3. Making sure the knots in the rope catch on the pulley
4. Giving range of motion (ROM) to all joints, including those immediately proximal and distal to the fracture, every shift

78. Deep vein thrombosis, or DVT, is a blood clot that forms in a vein deep in the body. Most deep vein blood clots occur in the lower leg.

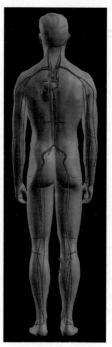

CN: Physiological integrity; CNS: Physiological adaptation; CL: Understand; DIFFICULTY: Easy

79. 3. Questioning the client about the small scattered carpets would only begin to help the client understand home injuries, especially for a person with an alteration in musculoskeletal status. Collecting the small carpets and doing nothing aren't appropriate actions for the nurse. The nurse should review the hazards of having small carpets on the floors so that the client can take the appropriate action and reduce the likelihood of injury by removing the carpets.
CN: Safe, effective care environment; CNS: Safety and infection control; CL: Apply; DIFFICULTY: Easy

80. 1. Nursing care for a client in traction may include assessing pin sites every shift (and as needed) and making sure the knots in the rope don't catch on the pulley. The nurse should add and remove weights only as the health care provider orders, and every shift the nurse should give ROM to all joints *except* those immediately proximal and distal to the fracture.
CN: Physiological integrity; CNS: Basic care and comfort; CL: Apply; DIFFICULTY: Moderate

81. A nurse reads the following Progress Notes entry on a client who has had surgical repair of a right hip fracture. The nurse knows these findings are consistent with which condition?

Progress notes	
4/30/17	Client reports new left calf pain (4/5)
1400	on pain scale, that worsens to touch and
	with dorsiflexion of left foot. +4 nonpitting
	edema left foot to knee noted. Prominent
	superficial veins notes on left leg. Dr. Smith
	notified.
	— Ann Jones, RN

1. Deep vein thrombosis (DVT)
2. Fat embolus
3. Infection
4. Pulmonary embolism

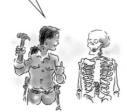

Progress notes are an important tool of the trade in nursing.

82. A client who fell while washing the outside windows has a fractured right ankle and is being fitted with a cast. After assisting with the cast application, what instructions should the nurse reinforce to the client?
1. Go home and stay in bed for about 5 days.
2. Keep the cast covered with plastic until it feels dry.
3. Move the right toes for several minutes every hour.
4. Expect some swelling and blueness of the toes.

83. The health care provider has just removed the cast from a client's lower leg. During the removal, a small superficial abrasion occurred over the ankle. Which statement by the client indicates the need for additional client education?
1. "I must use a moisturizing lotion on the dry areas."
2. "The dry, peeling skin will go away by itself."
3. "I can wash the abrasion on my ankle with soap and water."
4. "I'll wait until the abrasion is healed before I go swimming."

84. The nurse is reinforcing education for a client on a recently applied synthetic cast. The nurse informs the client that synthetic casts take approximately how long to set?
1. Immediately
2. 20 minutes
3. 45 minutes
4. 2 hours

81. 1. Unilateral leg pain and edema with a positive Homans sign (calf pain with dorsiflexion of the foot that isn't always present) might be symptoms of DVT. Tachycardia, chest pain, and shortness of breath may be symptoms of a pulmonary embolism. It's unlikely an infection would occur on the opposite side of the fracture without cause. Symptoms of fat emboli include restlessness, tachypnea, and tachycardia; they're more common in long-bone injuries.
CN: Physiological integrity; CNS: Reduction of risk potential; CL: Apply; DIFFICULTY: Moderate

82. 3. Moving the toes is encouraged to facilitate circulation and prevent swelling. By moving the toes, the client will be aware of any numbness or swelling and can take appropriate action, such as elevating the extremity and reporting the findings to her health care provider. Usually, clients are instructed to remain in bed for 24 hours while the cast dries. Prolonged immobility creates problems for the client. While the cast is still damp, the ankle should be elevated on a pillow that's protected with plastic; the cast itself should be left open to the air. Swelling and a bluish color of the toes aren't expected; they indicate compromised circulation and should be reported immediately.
CN: Physiological integrity; CNS: Reduction of risk potential; CL: Apply; DIFFICULTY: Easy

83. 1. The dry, peeling skin will heal in a few days with normal cleaning; therefore, lotions are unnecessary. Vigorous scrubbing isn't necessary. Washing the abrasion and delaying swimming until healing are correct procedures to follow after removal of a cast.
CN: Physiological integrity; CNS: Reduction of risk potential; CL: Apply; DIFFICULTY: Difficult

84. 2. Synthetic casts take about 20 minutes to set.
CN: Physiological integrity; CNS: Reduction of risk potential; CL: Apply; DIFFICULTY: Difficult

CN: Client needs category   CNS: Client needs subcategory   CL: Cognitive level

85. Which statement by a client who recently had a cast applied indicates that the nurse's education has been effective?
1. "The cast will need to be removed if I feel any heat."
2. "Heat is a normal sensation as a cast dries."
3. "The heat I feel is most likely caused by an infection."
4. "I'll call my health care provider if I feel any heat."

86. A nurse is providing care for a client with a leg cast. To help prevent footdrop, which action by the nurse is the **most** appropriate?
1. Encouraging bed rest
2. Supporting the foot with 45 degrees of flexion
3. Supporting the foot with 90 degrees of flexion
4. Placing a stocking on the foot to provide warmth

87. A client is diagnosed with gout. Which foods should the nurse instruct the client to avoid? Select all that apply.
1. Green leafy vegetables
2. Liver
3. Cod
4. Chocolate
5. Sardines
6. Eggs

88. A client developed osteomyelitis 2 weeks after a fishhook was removed from the foot. Which rationale **best** explains the expected long-term antibiotic therapy?
1. Bone has poor circulation.
2. Tissue trauma requires antibiotics.
3. Feet are normally difficult to treat.
4. Fishhook injuries are highly contaminated.

89. The nurse is reinforcing preoperative education for a client having a total hip arthroplasty and explaining which actions to avoid postoperatively. Which statements made by the client indicate the need for additional education? Select all that apply.
1. "I will keep my legs apart while lying in bed"
2. "I will periodically tighten my leg muscles."
3. "I will rotate my feet internally."
4. "I will bend from my waste to pick items up from the floor."
5. "I will sleep in a side-lying position on the unaffected side."

Looking good. Ride that wave all the way in, dude.

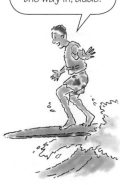

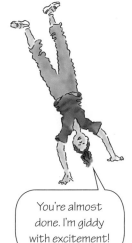

You're almost done. I'm giddy with excitement!

85. 2. Normally, as the cast dries, a client may report heat from the cast. Offer reassurance. The cast won't need to be removed and the health care provider doesn't need to be notified. Heat from the cast isn't a sign of infection.
CN: Physiological integrity; CNS: Reduction of risk potential; CL: Apply; DIFFICULTY: Moderate

86. 3. To prevent footdrop in a leg with a cast, the foot should be supported with 90 degrees of flexion. Bed rest can *cause* footdrop. Keeping the extremity warm won't prevent footdrop.
CN: Health promotion and maintenance; CNS: None; CL: Apply; DIFFICULTY: Challenge

87. 2, 3, 5. The client with gout should avoid foods that are high in purines, such as liver, cod, and sardines. Other foods that should be avoided include anchovies, kidneys, sweetbreads, lentils, and alcoholic beverages, especially beer and wine. Green leafy vegetables, chocolate, and eggs aren't high in purines and, therefore, aren't restricted in the diet of a client with gout.
CN: Physiological integrity; CNS: Basic care and comfort; CL: Apply; DIFFICULTY: Difficult

88. 1. Bone has poor circulation, making it difficult to treat an infection in the bone. This requires long-term use of IV antibiotics to make sure the infection is cleared. Tissue trauma doesn't always require antibiotics, at least not long term. Fishhooks may not be any more contaminated than another instrument that caused an injury. Feet aren't more difficult to treat than other parts of the body unless the client has a circulatory problem or diabetes.
CN: Physiological integrity; CNS: Pharmacological therapies; CL: Apply; DIFFICULTY: Difficult

89. 3, 4. After hip replacement surgery, the client should avoid internally rotating the feet and bending more than 90 degrees. These activities can compromise the hip joint. The client should lie with the legs abducted. Leg-strengthening exercises, such as periodically tightening the leg muscles, are recommended to maintain muscle strength and reduce the risk of thrombus formation. A side-lying position is acceptable; however, some health care providers restrict lying on the operative side.
CN: Physiological integrity; CNS: Reduction of risk potential; CL: Analyze; DIFFICULTY: Difficult

90. Which information is the **priority** to include in the discharge plan for a client leaving the hospital in a leg cast?
1. Cast care procedures and devices to relieve itching
2. Skin care, mouth care, and cast removal procedures
3. Cast care, neurovascular checks, and hygiene measures
4. Cast removal procedures, neurovascular checks, and devices to relieve itching

90. 3. Proper cast care procedures include observing the skin nearest the cast edges for signs of pressure ulcers, keeping the cast dry and intact, and avoiding the use of insertable devices (such as wire hangers or sticks) to relieve itching. Frequent neurovascular checks can reveal evidence of pressure or impaired circulation to the leg under the cast. This includes checking the toes frequently for discoloration, swelling, or lack of movement or sensation. Hygiene measures should focus on the client's normal elimination patterns and the importance of cleanliness after elimination, as well as on the need to maintain skin integrity by taking sponge baths and caring for dry skin. Devices should never be inserted between the cast and the skin. Although mouth care and cast removal are important issues, they aren't priority discharge instructions in this case.
CN: Physiological integrity; CNS: Physiological adaptation; CL: Apply; DIFFICULTY: Easy

91. A client has just returned from the postanesthesia care unit (PACU) after undergoing internal fixation of a left femoral neck fracture. The nurse should place the client in which position?
1. On the left side with the right knee bent
2. On the back with two pillows between the legs
3. On the right side with the left knee bent
4. Sitting at a 90-degree angle

91. 2. The operative leg must be kept abducted to prevent dislocation of the hip. Placing the client on the left or right side with knee bent doesn't promote abduction. Acute flexion of the operated hip may cause dislocation. The head of the bed may be raised 35 to 40 degrees.
CN: Physiological integrity; CNS: Reduction of risk potential; CL: Apply; DIFFICULTY: Moderate

92. A client has just had total hip replacement surgery. The health care provider orders heparin 8,000 units to be administered subcutaneously. The label on the heparin vial reads: heparin 10,000 units/mL. How many milliliters of heparin should the nurse draw up in the syringe to administer the correct dose? Record your answer using one decimal place.

_____mL

92. 0.8.
This formula is used to calculate drug dosages:

$$\text{Dose on hand} = \frac{\text{Dose desired}}{X}$$

In this example, the equation is as follows:

$$10,000 \text{ units}/\text{mL} = \frac{8,000 \text{ units}}{X}$$

$$X = 0.8 \text{ mL}.$$

CN: Physiological integrity; CNS: Pharmacological therapies; CL: Apply; DIFFICULTY: Easy

93. A client is 2 weeks post op from knee replacement surgery and has been on warfarin therapy. The client's most recent INR blood level was 5.6. What should the nurse prepare to administer to the client?
1. Vitamin K
2. Protamine sulfate
3. Acetylcysteine
4. Sodium polystyrene sulfonate

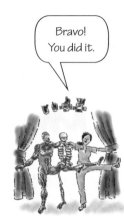

Bravo! You did it.

93. 1. The antidote for warfarin is Vitamin K. Protamine sulfate is the antidote for heparin toxicity. Acetylcysteine is the antidote for acetaminophen toxicity. Sodium polystyrene sulfonate is the antidote for potassium toxicity.
CN: Physiological integrity; CNS: Pharmacological therapies; CL: Apply; DIFFICULTY: Easy

Chapter 8

Gastrointestinal Disorders

Gastrointestinal refresher

Appendicitis

Inflammation of the appendix resulting from blockage of the organ, which causes infection, inflammation and pus accumulation

Key signs and symptoms
- Anorexia, nausea, and vomiting
- Abdominal pain that localizes in the right lower abdomen (McBurney point) or in the periumbilical area
- Sudden cessation of pain (indicates rupture)

Key test results
- Hematology shows moderately elevated white blood cell count

Key treatments
- Appendectomy

Key interventions
- Monitor vital signs, GI status, and pain
- Maintain nothing-by-mouth status until bowel sounds return postoperatively; advance diet as tolerated
- Monitor for signs of peritonitis (rigid abdomen and guarding)

Cancer of the gastrointestinal system

Colorectal
Abnormal growth (adenoma) occurring in the inner lining of the colon or rectum

Esophageal
Growth of cancer in the cells that line the inside of the esophagus

Gastric
Growth of cancer cells in the mucus-producing cells of the gastric lining

Pancreatic
Growth of cancer cells in the pancreas

Key signs and symptoms
Colorectal
- Change of bowel habits, abdominal pain, bloody stools, and rectal bleeding

Esophageal
- Nagging cough, dysphagia, hoarseness, and sub-sternal pain

Gastric
- Anorexia, epigastric fullness, and pain after eating not relieved by antacids
- Unexplained nausea, indigestion, and/or heartburn

Pancreatic
- Asymptomatic until late stages; may have jaundice and upper abdominal pain that radiates to the back

Key test results
Colorectal
- Colonoscopy identifies and locates a mass
- Digital rectal examination reveals a mass
- Fecal occult blood positive; (screen for fecal occult blood starting at age 50)

Esophageal
- Endoscopic examination of the esophagus, biopsies, and cytological test confirm esophageal tumors; CT and PET scans for tumor staging

Gastric
- Gastric analysis shows positive cancer cells and achlorhydria
- Gastric biopsy reveals cancer cells

Pancreatic
- Ultrasound, computerized tomography (CT) scan, and magnetic resonance imaging (MRI)

Key treatments
- Surgery to remove the tumor or resect the bowel depending on tumor location
- Radical surgery to excise the tumor and resect the esophagus or both the stomach and esophagus (gastroduodenostomy, gastrojejunostomy, partial gastric resection, total gastrectomy)
- Radiation to reduce tumor size
- Chemotherapy: 5-fluorouracil common use for each type along with doxorubicin for colorectal; cisplatin for esophageal; carmustine for gastric
- Palliative or hospice care referrals
- Support groups and organizations for emotional health

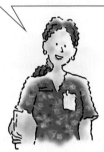

From hiatal hernia to diverticulitis to pancreatitis, this chapter covers all the GI disorders you could ask for, in one handy package. Are you ready to attack this chapter? Remember—no guts, no glory!

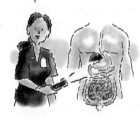

Uh oh. Looks like we have an inflamed appendix here. There's only one treatment for that.

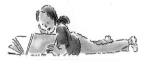

Wow. I never realized how many different types of GI cancer there are, all with different symptoms.

Key interventions

- Surgery: Preoperative:
  - answer client's questions
  - explain what to expect after surgery (gastrostomy tubes, closed chest drainage, and NG suctioning)
  - witness the consent
  - prep the skin and surgical region/area
  - maintain IV site access
  - monitor labs
  - administer pre-op meds
- Radiation therapy:
  - leave skin markings intact
  - avoid creams, lotions, deodorants, and perfumes
  - use lukewarm water to clean skin and assess skin for redness and cracking
  - teach client to wear loose fitting cloths
- Chemotherapy:
  - assess breath sounds, vital signs, cardiovascular system, renal, skin, hair, and lab results
  - monitor for signs of infection (fever, sore throat, elevated WBC)
  - assess for stomatitis (erythema, ulcers, and bleeding)
  - rinse the mouth with saline or chlorhexidine
  - avoid toothbrushes, lemon-glycerin swabs, dental floss, and hot or spicy foods
  - use topical anesthetics and antifungals (nystatin swish and swallow)
  - encourage deep breathing and meticulous hygiene
  - inspect IV site for infection
  - place in private room if possible and do not allow fresh salads, fruits, of flowers in room
  - perform meticulous hand hygiene and avoid contact with staff or visitors who have cold or flu-like symptoms
- Encourage participation in self-care and decision-making
- Provide referrals to support groups and organizations
- Maintain comfort and allow verbalization of feelings
- Provide supportive care for the client and family
- Encourage verbalization of feelings
- Promote adequate nutrition, and evaluate the client's nutritional and hydration status

Esophageal and gastric cancer

- Place the client in Fowler position for meals and allow plenty of time to eat
- Provide high-calorie, high-protein, pureed diet as needed
- Place client with esophageal anastomosis flat on back

- Gastrostomy tube:
  - administer feeding slowly
  - use gravity to adjust flow rate
  - offer something to chew before each feeding
  - provide mouth care.
- Esophageal and gastric surgery:
  - monitor for signs and symptoms of dumping syndrome (can occur after removal parts of the stomach or esophagus [diaphoresis, hypotension, tachycardia, and diarrhea])
  - teach client how to prevent dumping syndrome (restrict fluids 1 hour before meals or 1 hour after meals)
  - instruct client to eat sitting up semi-Fowler
  - instruct client to lie down 20 minutes after eating
  - instruct client to eat small, frequent meals
  - encourage a low carbohydrates and low fiber diet
  - take antispasmodics as ordered

Colorectal cancer

- Provide ostomy care as indicated

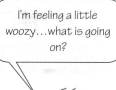

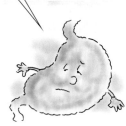

I'm feeling a little woozy...what is going on?

Cholecystitis

Inflammation of the gallbladder resulting from infection and by blockage of the common bowel duct by stones, problems with the duct, or tumors

Key signs and symptoms

- Episodic colicky pain in epigastric area, which radiates to the back and shoulder
- Indigestion or chest pain after eating fatty or fried foods
- Nausea, vomiting, and flatulence

Key test results

- Blood chemistry reveals increased alkaline phosphatase, bilirubin, direct bilirubin transaminase, amylase, lipase, aspartate aminotransferase (AST), and lactate dehydrogenase (LD) levels
- Cholangiogram shows stones in the biliary tree

Key treatments

- Cholecystostomy—opening the gallbladder and removing the stones
- Extracorporeal shock wave therapy (ESWL)—shock wave therapy to destroy the stones
- Cholecystectomy—removal of the gallbladder laparoscopically or by open abdominal incision

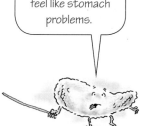

Remember, my stones could feel like stomach problems.

- Choledochostomy—opening the common bowel duct and removal of the stones with insertion of a drainage tube (T-tube) to a drainage device.
- Analgesic: morphine, hydromorphone, ketorolac
- Antibiotics: piperacillin/tazobactam, ceftriaxone
- Antiemetics: ondansetron, metoclopramide

Key interventions
- Assess abdominal status, color of stools, and pain
- Administer analgesics and antibiotics as ordered
- Monitor fluid and electrolyte balance.
- Provide postoperative care; if open cholecystectomy, monitor and record T-tube drainage-report > 1,000 mL/day
- Maintain the position, patency, and low suction of the nasogastric (NG) tube

Cirrhosis
Irreversible scarring of the liver that disrupts structure and functioning; causes include hepatitis, chronic alcohol abuse, biliary disease, or severe right-sided heart failure

Key signs and symptoms
- Abdominal pain (possibly because of an enlarged liver)
- Anorexia
- Ascites (which can cause dyspnea)
- Fatigue
- Jaundice
- Nausea and or vomiting
- Dark urine and clay colored stools
- Pruritus and easy bruising or bleeding

Key test results
- Liver biopsy—definitive test for cirrhosis; detects destruction and fibrosis of hepatic tissue
- Computed tomography (CT) scan with IV contrast reveals enlarged liver, identifies liver masses, and visualizes hepatic blood flow and obstruction, if present

Key treatments
- IV therapy using colloid volume expanders or crystalloids.
- Diuretics: furosemide, spironolactone for edema
- Lactulose to reduce ammonia levels
- Vitamin K: phytonadione for bleeding tendencies due to hypoprothrombinemia
- Vasopressin and sclerotherapy for esophageal varices
- Gastric intubation and esophageal balloon tamponade for bleeding esophageal varices

(Sengstaken-Blakemore-4 lumen tube and Minnesota-3 lumen tube)
- Blood transfusions to replace loss and shunt insertion to relieve portal hypertension

Key interventions
- Monitor cardiac status
- Monitor respiratory status
- Monitor level of consciousness (observe for behavioral or personality changes, increased confusion, stupor, lethargy, hallucinations, and neuromuscular dysfunction)
- Measure I&O
- Maintain fluid restriction (if indicated)
- Weigh daily
- Measure abdominal girth
- Check orders regarding T-tube clamping before/after meals
- Provide appropriate nutrition:
  - early stages: high protein and carbohydrates
  - advanced stages: high calorie, low protein, low fat, low sodium
- Provide skin care, avoid strong soaps
- Position frequently for comfort
- Provide pain medication as needed and promote rest
- Monitor for bleeding (check skin, gums, stool, and emesis) and monitor Na+, K+, ammonia level, platelets, PT/INR, CBC, WBC, and bilirubin
- Carefully evaluate before, during, and after paracentesis
- Administer diuretics and other medications as ordered

Crohn disease
Inflammation of the large or small intestine with ulcers that have a "cobblestone" appearance, separated by normal tissue; can affect areas from the mouth to the anus

Key signs and symptoms
- Abdominal pain (right lower quadrant): aggravated by eating
- Chronic diarrhea, mucus, pus and fat (steatorrhea) in stools
- Weight loss (emaciation can occur)

Key test results
- Upper GI series shows classic string sign: segments of stricture separated by normal bowel

Key treatments
- Hemicolectomy or ileostomy in clients with extensive disease of the large intestine and rectum
- Antibiotics: sulfasalazine, metronidazole

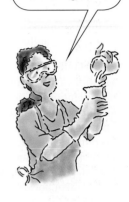

It is best to use precision when measuring fluids.

- Anticholinergics: propantheline, dicyclomine hydrochloride
- Antidiarrheal: diphenoxylate hydrochloride–atropine sulfate
- Corticosteroid: prednisone
- Immunosuppressants: mercaptopurine, azathioprine, infliximab

Key interventions
- Monitor GI status (note excessive abdominal distention)
- Monitor fluid balance
- Encourage rest
- Encourage client to minimize stress
- Promote verbalization of feelings
- Encourage maintenance of high calorie, high protein, low-fiber, low fat and dairy free diet
- Encourage client to avoid caffeine, alcohol, and smoking
- TPN for those on bowel rest is indicated in some cases
- Administer medications as ordered
- Encourage client to avoid foods and other things that produce flare-ups

Dental caries
Erosive process of the teeth caused by the action of bacteria, medications, or other substances or fermentables when acid if formed

Key signs and symptoms
- Halitosis, tooth discoloration, bleeding gums, pain, and tooth erosion

Key test results
- X-ray of teeth and gums reveals tooth destruction

Key treatments
- Extraction, filling, or deep scaling with antibiotic treatment
- Prevention: Dental hygiene and mouth care, especially for at-risk clients (those who are intubated, NPO, in septic shock, and multisystem organ failure)
- Fluoridation of water sources or supplementation with fluoride rinses

Key interventions
- Teach prevention measures:
  - brush after eating
  - floss regularly
  - consume a diet high in fresh fruits and vegetables, nuts, cheese, and plain yogurt
- If water is not fluoridated (well water), obtain fluoride from another source
- Encourage client to see a dentist regularly and consider sealants

- Provide meticulous mouth care for clients who are:
  - receiving gastric suctioning
  - receiving enteral or parenteral feedings
  - on ventilators
  - NPO and are not able to perform the care for themselves

Diverticular disease
Sacs or pouch-like projections in the wall of the intestine that can become infected, inflamed, or obstructed

Diverticulosis
- Pouch-like projections (sacs) along the wall of the intestine

Diverticulitis
- Inflammation of the one or more diverticula (sacs)

Key signs and symptoms
- Change in bowel habits (alternating diarrhea and constipation) and decreased bowel sounds
- Left lower quadrant pain or mid-abdominal pain (Colicky or cramping pain that radiates to the back)
- Fever and increased WBCs

Key test results
- Sigmoidoscopy shows a thickened wall in the diverticula

Key treatments
- Colon resection or temporary colostomy (for hemorrhage, abscess, perforation, peritonitis, obstruction, or fistula that accompanies diverticulitis)
- Liquid diet for mild diverticulitis or diverticulosis before pain subsides
- High-fiber, low-fat diet for mild diverticulitis or diverticulosis after pain subsides
- Analgesic: morphine
- Antibiotics: metronidazole, ciprofloxacin, sulfamethoxazole and trimethoprim for mild diverticulitis
- Anticholinergic: oxyphencyclimine or propantheline

Key interventions
- Monitor the following for complications:
  - abdominal distention
  - bowel sounds
  - bowel elimination patterns
- NPO to rest bowel then clear liquids; Increase fluid intake to 3 L/day
- Prepare the client for surgery, if indicated (administer cleansing enemas, osmotic purgative, oral and parenteral antibiotics)
- Postoperative care: see post op care

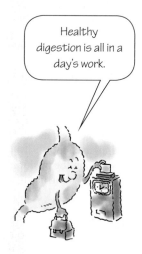

Healthy digestion is all in a day's work.

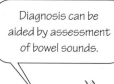

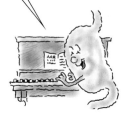

Diagnosis can be aided by assessment of bowel sounds.

Gastritis

Inflammation or irritation of the lining of the stomach caused by stress, medications, alcohol consumption or *Helicobacter pylori* bacteria

Key signs and symptoms
- Abdominal cramping and bloating
- Epigastric discomfort (burning between meals or at night)
- Hematemesis
- Indigestion

Key test results
- Upper GI endoscopy with biopsy confirms the diagnosis when performed within 24 hours of bleeding

Key treatments
- Histamine-2 (H_2) receptor antagonists: cimetidine, ranitidine, famotidine, nizatidine
- Proton pump inhibitors: omeprazole
- IV fluid therapy and NG lavage to control bleeding if present

Key interventions
- Administer antiemetic and IV fluids as ordered
- Monitor I&O and electrolytes
- NPO and progress to a bland diet
- Monitor the client for recurrent symptoms as food is reintroduced
- Offer small, frequent meals and eliminate foods that cause gastric upset
- Administer antacids and other prescribed medications
- Provide emotional support to the client and collaborate for referral for alcohol abuse if verified
- If surgery is necessary, prepare client preoperatively and provide appropriate postoperative care
- Teach client to avoid medications that may aggravate GI lining (e.g., NSAIDs)

Gastroenteritis

Inflammation of the stomach and intestines caused by an irritant, bacteria, parasite, or virus that produces vomiting and diarrhea

Key signs and symptoms
- Abdominal discomfort
- Diarrhea
- Nausea and vomiting

Key test results
- Stool culture identifies the causative bacteria, parasites, or amoebae

Key treatments
- IV fluid and electrolyte replacement
- Antidiarrheals: diphenoxylate hydrochloride–atropine sulfate, loperamide

Key interventions
- Collect stool specimens as ordered
- Administer medications
- Correlate dosages, routes, and times appropriately with the client's meals and activities
- Give antiemetics 30 to 60 minutes before meals
- If client is unable to tolerate food, replace lost fluids and electrolytes with clear liquids and sports drinks
- Record strict I&O
- Monitor for signs of dehydration (dry skin and mucous membranes, fever, and sunken eyes)
- Provide perineal care and wash hands thoroughly after providing care

Gastroesophageal reflux disease

Backup of stomach contents through the lower esophageal sphincter (LES) that does not close properly

Key signs and symptoms
- Dysphagia, dyspepsia, belching, and regurgitation of food
- Heartburn (burning sensation in the upper abdomen)

Key test results
- Barium swallow fluoroscopy indicates reflux
- Esophagoscopy shows reflux
- Endoscopy allows visualization and confirmation of pathologic changes in the mucosa

Key treatments
- Positional therapy to help relieve symptoms by decreasing intra-abdominal pressure:
- Histamine blockers: famotidine, ranitidine, cimetidine
- Proton pump inhibitors: omeprazole, esomeprazole, or pantoprazole may be given IV

Key interventions
- Dietary planning:
  - Take into account client's food preferences
  - Limit or eliminate chocolate, caffeine, fatty foods, alcohol, carbonated beverages, spicy and acidic foods (decrease LES pressure)
  - Encourage four to six small meals per day
- Encourage client to wear loose clothing

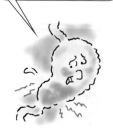

Stress is a real pain in the gut!

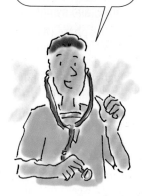

Gastroenteritis, eh? What lab test will help us figure out what's causing it?

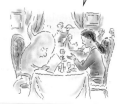

No caffeine, no chocolate, no alcohol, no fatty foods—GERD takes all the fun out of eating.

- Elevate the head of the bed 6″ to 12″ (15 to 30 cm) - reverse Trendelenburg position, and encourage client to sleep on right side
- Encourage smoking cessation, alcohol cessation, and weight reduction programs

Hepatitis

Inflammation of the liver caused by infectious organisms, toxins, or chemicals that invaded the organ

Hepatitis A
- Fecal-oral/person-person

Hepatitis B
- Blood and body fluids

Hepatitis C
- Blood borne and illicit IV drug sharing

Key signs and symptoms

Pre-icteric phase (usually 1 to 5 days)
- Clay-colored stools
- Fatigue
- Right upper quadrant pain
- Dark urine

Icteric phase (~1 to 2 weeks)
- Jaundice and yellow sclera
- Pruritus
- Weight loss

Post-icteric or recovery phase (~2 to 12 weeks or longer in clients with hepatitis B, C, or E)
- Decreased hepatomegaly
- Decreased jaundice
- Fatigue

Key test results
- Blood chemistry shows increased:
  - alanine aminotransferase (ALT)
  - aspartate aminotransferase (AST)
  - alkaline phosphatase (ALP)
  - lactate dehydrogenase (LD)
  - bilirubin
  - erythrocyte sedimentation rate (ESR)
- Serologic tests identify hepatitis A virus, hepatitis B virus, hepatitis C virus, and delta antigen, if present

Key treatments
- Vitamins and minerals: vitamin K, vitamin C (ascorbic acid), vitamin B-complex (mega-B)
- Antivirals: lamivudine, interferon, peginterferon-alfa 2b

Key interventions
- Monitor GI status
- Provide symptomatic care
- Watch for bleeding and fulminant hepatitis
- Provide for rest and maintain high carbohydrate, high protein, and low fat diet

- Avoid hepatotoxic OTC/prescription medications (acetaminophen and sedatives)
- Maintain standard and appropriate transmission based precautions

Hiatal hernia

Protrusion of a portion of the stomach through the esophageal hiatus of the diaphragm

Key signs and symptoms
- Regurgitation
- Persistent heartburn and dysphagia
- Sternal pain and breathlessness after eating

Key test results
- Barium swallow with fluoroscopy reveals protrusion of the hernia
- Chest x-ray shows protrusion of abdominal organs into the thorax
- Esophagoscopy shows incompetent cardiac sphincter

Key treatments
- Bland diet; small, frequent meals with decreased intake of caffeine and spicy foods
- Anticholinergic: propantheline
- Histamine-2 (H_2) receptor antagonists: cimetidine, ranitidine, famotidine
- Proton pump-inhibitors: omeprazole
- Surgery to tighten cardiac sphincter

Key interventions
- Obtain diet history
- Encourage small, frequent meals
- Have client sit up 1 to 2 hours after meals, and avoid eating 3 hours prior to bedtime
- Reinforce need to avoid tight clothing, straining, and flexion at the waist
- Encourage weight reduction for clients with BMI >25
- Monitor for respiratory:
  - aggravation of asthma
  - onset of pulmonary edema
  - chronic cough (this is reason to delay surgery)
- Monitor for GI complications:
  - esophageal ulcers or bleeding
- Provide pre-op and post-op care for abdominal surgery
- Remind client of no heavy lifting for 6 weeks after surgery

Intestinal obstruction

Partial or complete blockage of the lumen in the small or large intestine; small bowel obstruction (SBO) is the most common and serious

Key signs and symptoms
- Abdominal distention with cramping pain

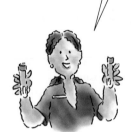

Blood test can really help diagnose the correct hepatitis virus.

- Vomiting with SBO
- Unable to pass gas or stool for >8 hours; leakage of loose stool if there is blockage of large intestine (sign of impaction)
- Bowel sounds:
  - hyperactive above the obstruction
  - hypoactive below the obstruction

Key test results
- Abdominal x-ray shows increased amount of gas in bowel
- Endoscopy and CT scan reveals a mass or obstruction and the location
- Barium enema: shows the flow of barium stops at area of obstruction

Key treatments
- Bowel resection with or without anastomosis
- GI decompression using NG, Miller-Abbott, or Cantor tube
- Fluid and electrolyte replacement

Key interventions
- Maintain NPO
- Assess bowel sounds
- Measure and record abdominal girth
- Monitor IV fluids and measure I&O
- Monitor for fluid and electrolyte deficits and imbalances
- Maintain the position, patency, and low intermittent suction of NG tubes
- Provide pre-op and post-op care if indicated

Irritable bowel syndrome

Chronic condition with recurrent diarrhea, constipation, and abdominal pain with bloating

Key signs and symptoms
- Erratic bowel patterns and bloating
- Abdominal pain (relieved by defecation)
- Constipation, diarrhea, or both
- Passage of mucus in stool

Key test results
- Sigmoidoscopy may disclose spastic contraction of the colon

Key treatments
- Dietary management
- Stress management
- Antispasmodic: propantheline
- Antidiarrheal: diphenoxylate hydrochloride–atropine sulfate

Key interventions
- Reinforce teaching:
  - eat slowly
  - eat at regular times
  - chew food thoroughly
  - drink adequate fluids

- Encourage a high fiber diet:
  - 15 to 20 g daily
  - maintain a food diary to identify triggers
  - avoid food intolerances
- Encourage regular exercise (walking and yoga)
- Assist client to deal with stress and warn against dependence on sedatives or antispasmodics

---

Pancreatitis

Acute
Inflammation of the pancreas by auto-digestion due to diminished functioning (life threatening)

Chronic
Progressive disease of the pancreas that is associated with remissions and exacerbations

Key signs and symptoms
- Abrupt onset of pain in the epigastric area that radiates to the shoulder, substernal area, back, and flank (intensifies after meals or lying down)
- Abdominal tenderness, nausea, vomiting, and fatty stools (steatorrhea)
- Positive Turner sign and Cullen sign

Key test results
- Elevated amylase, lipase, liver enzymes, lactate dehydrogenase (LD), glucose, aspartate aminotransferase (AST), and lipid levels; decreased calcium and potassium levels
- CT scan and ultrasonography reveal cysts, bile duct inflammation, and dilation

Key treatments
- IV fluids, antibiotic therapy, and TPN.
- Anticholinergics: Histamine-2 (H_2) receptor antagonists or proton pump inhibitors
- Opioid analgesic: morphine or hydromorphone; meperidine contraindicated
- Blood sugar control: insulin and pancreatic enzymes
- Potassium supplement: IV potassium chloride
- Surgery:
  - ERCP to create an opening in the sphincter of Oddi
  - Cholecystectomy
  - Pancreaticojejunostomy (Roux-en-Y) to reroute pancreatic enzymes to the jejunum

Key interventions
- Maintain NPO; after 24 to 48 hours start jejunal feedings; when food is tolerated advance to small, frequent meals (moderate to high carbohydrate, high-protein, and low-fat meals)

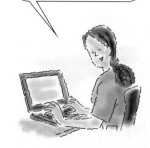

What tests are used to determine the cause of an intestinal obstruction?

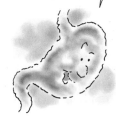

You'd be irritable, too, if you had recurrent diarrhea, constipation, and abdominal pain.

- Maintain patency of NG tube
- Monitor abdominal, cardiac, and respiratory status (watch for respiratory failure and tachycardia—signs of hypocalcemia and hypomagnesemia)
- Maintain IV fluids and monitor I&O
- Monitor blood glucose, laboratory results
- Position for comfort (knee chest, sitting up, leaning forward)
- Administer pain medications
- Reassure client and explain procedures to reduce anxiety

Peptic ulcer disease

Ulceration of the stomach or duodenal lining that is caused by destruction of the mucosal tissue

Key signs and symptoms
- Anorexia
- Hematemesis
- Left epigastric pain 1 to 2 hours after eating
- Relief of pain after administration of antacids

Key test results
- Urea breath test to detect presence of *Helicobacter pylori*
- Barium swallow shows ulceration of the gastric mucosa
- Upper GI endoscopy shows the location of the ulcer

Key treatments
- If GI hemorrhage: gastric surgery that may include gastroduodenostomy, gastrojejunostomy, partial gastric resection, and total gastrectomy
- Saline lavage by NG tube until return is clear (if bleeding is present)
- Antibiotic if *Helicobacter pylori* is present
- Histamine-2 (H$_2$)receptor antagonists: cimetidine, ranitidine, nizatidine, famotidine
- Mucosal barrier fortifier: sucralfate

Key interventions
- Teach client to eat small, frequent meals three times a day (not necessary if on histamine-2 [H$_2$] receptor antagonist)
- Teach client to avoid caffeine, alcohol, spicy foods, milk and cream
- Teach client to reduce stress and take medications as ordered
- Post-op care for gastric resection, total or partial gastrectomy with esophageal anastomosis:
  - administer B$_{12}$ supplementation via parenteral route
  - maintain NG tube
  - auscultate bowel sounds and when able to eat again teach preventive measures for "dumping syndrome" (rapid passage of food to stomach, causing diaphoresis, tachycardia, diarrhea, and hypotension) usually 15 minutes after eating
  - restrict fluids with meals
  - avoid stress after eating
  - eat smaller, frequent meals
  - lie down 20 minutes after eating

Peritonitis

Inflammation of the peritoneal membrane that covers the abdominal organs

Key signs and symptoms
- Abdominal rigidity and muscle guarding
- Constant, intense abdominal pain
- Decreased or absent bowel sounds
- Shock (weak rapid pulse, pallor, diaphoresis) and elevated temperature

Key test results
- Abdominal x-ray shows free air in the abdomen under the diaphragm

Key treatments
- IV fluids and antibiotics
- Gastric decompression: NG tube to low intermittent suction
- Surgical intervention when the client's condition has stabilized (to treat the cause [e.g., if client has a perforated appendix, then an appendectomy is indicated]; drains will also be placed for drainage of infected material)

Key interventions
- Monitor abdominal, cardiovascular, and respiratory status
- Watch for fluid and electrolyte imbalance
- Monitor and record vital signs, intake and output, laboratory studies, daily weight, and urine specific gravity
- Administer IV fluids and antibiotics
- Maintain NPO and NG tube to low-intermittent suction
- Provide postoperative care as indicated
- Salivary, oral, and pharyngeal disorders

Oral candidiasis (thrush), parotitis, sialadenitis, sialolithiasis, stomatitis, esophageal cancer

Disorders that affect lubrication, protection from harmful bacteria, and digestion

Key signs and symptoms
- Pain, inflammation, and redness

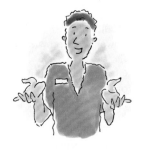

What's that bacterium that causes ulcers? Helicopter pie?

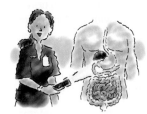

Now, this is my kind of x-ray.

- Cheesy white plaque on the tongue (oral candidiasis)
- Persistent, painless lesion the does not heal (cancer)
- Xerostomia (dry mouth), sticky and stringy saliva, change in taste

Key test results
- Biopsy of cells of the lips to rule out Sjögren syndrome (autoimmune disease in which the WBCs attack the moisture-producing glands)
- Oral examination, tissue scraping and brushing

Key treatments
- Preventative: regular dental and oral screenings
- Pilocarpine or cevimeline to stimulate saliva production
- Mycostatin to treat candidiasis

Key interventions
- Monitor nutritional status, chewing and swallowing ability, and ensure adequate food intake
- Provide support to client and family and encourage verbalization of feelings (cancer)
- Provide mouth care and teach regular and thorough oral hygiene
- Administer pain medication and monitor for infection
- Encourage a positive self-image
- Maintain methods of alternative communication when needed

Ulcerative colitis

Inflammation of the colon characterized by eroded areas of the mucous membrane and underlying tissue

Key signs and symptoms
- Abdominal cramping and fecal incontinence
- Bloody, purulent, mucoid, watery stools (10 to 20 per day)
- Hyperactive bowel sounds
- Weight loss (unintentional)

Key test results
- Barium enema shows ulcerations
- Sigmoidoscopy shows ulceration and hyperemia

Key treatments
- Colectomy or pouch ileostomy
- Total parenteral nutrition (TPN) if necessary to rest the GI tract
- Antibiotic: sulfasalazine
- Anticholinergics: propantheline, dicyclomine hydrochloride
- Antidiarrheals: diphenoxylate hydrochloride–atropine sulfate, loperamide

- Antiemetic: prochlorperazine
- Corticosteroid: hydrocortisone
- Immunosuppressants: azathioprine, cyclophosphamide

Key interventions
- Monitor GI and cardiovascular status (irregular pulse) and for edema
- Monitor I&O (especially number, amount, and character of stools) and for fluid and electrolyte imbalance
- Maintain IV fluids, TPN or enteral feedings for nutritional support
- Maintain the position, patency, and low suction of NG tube
- Provide skin care, perineal care, and observe for vitamin and mineral deficiency
- Postoperative: Provide ostomy care if indicated

Postoperative care for abdominal surgery

- Postoperative care interventions: assess neuro, heart, lungs, GI focused assessment (assess abdomen: bowel sounds, passage of flatus or stool, distention, bruising, tone, etc.), pain, and renal systems
- Monitor vital signs and I&O
- Maintain NG tube patency, do not reposition the NG tube:
  - irrigate NG tube gently if ordered
  - lubricate nares with water soluble lubricant
  - perform meticulous mouth care
  - monitor NG output
- Maintain IV fluids and TPN if ordered
- Administer pain medications as ordered
- Reinforce teaching that encourages use of patient-controlled anesthesia (PCA) pump
- Monitor dressings and drains (note the size of any drainage or blood on dressings)
- Monitor ostomy drainage and perform ostomy care as needed
- Apply sequential compression device (SCD) while on bed rest
- Turn and reposition client for comfort
- Encourage deep breathing, coughing, and use of incentive spirometer
- Get client out of bed as soon as ordered
- Teach client to splint the incision and to change positions slowly
- Monitor lab results (CBC with differential, chemistry or metabolic panel, coagulation panel if liver involvement or on anticoagulants, liver panel if indicated)
- Monitor for signs and symptoms of:
  - atelectasis (dyspnea, cyanosis)
  - bleeding/hemorrhage (decreased blood pressure, increased pulse rate, cool, clammy skin)

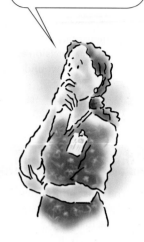

What interventions are needed for a client with ulcerative colitis?

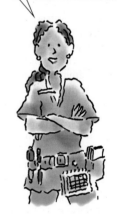

Make sure you have all the tools you need before assessing your client.

- ○ peritonitis (rigid abdomen and guarding)
- ○ fluid and electrolyte disturbances
- ○ infection
- ○ paralytic ileus (absence of bowel sounds, inability to pass gas or stool, and abdominal distention)
- ○ dehiscence (unexpected opening of surgical incision caused by infection or improper wound healing)
- ○ wound evisceration (care for organ protrusion through the wound: use moist, sterile, saline gauze to cover the organs/wound and notify the health care provider immediately; if client is at home instruct to cover with wax paper and call 911)

thePoint® You can download tables of drug information to help you prepare for the NCLEX®! View Generic Drug Names, Drug Classifications, Drug Actions, and Nursing Implications for the drugs discussed in this refresher at **http://thePoint.lww.com.**

Gastrointestinal questions, answers, and rationales

1. The nurse administers lactulose to a client with cirrhosis. Which assessment finding indicates to the nurse that the medication has been effective?
1. Four or more loose stools in 24 hours
2. Serum sodium level 135 mEq/L
3. Improvement in mental status
4. Reduction in abdominal ascites

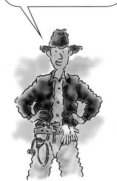

Ready to wrangle up some multiple choice answers? Let's roll.

1. 2. Lactulose, used to treat portal-systemic encephalopathy in clients with cirrhosis, works by acidifying colonic contents and trapping ammonia in the colon. The laxative action of lactulose assists in expelling the ammonia from the colon. This leads to a reduction in serum ammonia levels and improvements in mental and cardiac status. Lactulose causes diarrhea as a side effect and is expected—but it is not the intended effect of the medication. Adverse effects of lactulose are increased serum sodium and decreased serum potassium levels. Abdominal ascites is not affected by this medication.
CN: Physiologic integrity; CNS: Pharmacological therapies; CL: Analyze; DIFFICULTY: Challenge

2. The nurse reinforces home care instructions given to a client with a diagnosis of hiatal hernia. Which statement made by the client indicates an understanding of the instructions?
1. "I'll drink carbonated cola beverages with my meals."
2. "I'll be sure to lie down immediately after eating."
3. "I should eat three large, high-carbohydrate meals each day."
4. "I'll sleep with my head elevated about 3 to 4 inches."

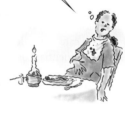

Uggh. I need to work on my portion control.

2. 4. With a hiatal hernia, sleeping with the head of the bed elevated 30 degrees (about 3 to 4 inches [7.5 to 10 cm]) prevents stomach acids from refluxing into the esophagus. Carbonated beverages would create gas and belching (eructation), causing an increase in intra-abdominal pressure, which will irritate the herniated area. Lying down immediately after eating leads to the reflux of stomach acids, causing irritation. Clients with hiatal hernia should eat small meals.
CN: Physiological integrity; CNS: Reduction of risk potential; CL: Analyze; DIFFICULTY: Easy

3. The nurse interviews a client presenting to the clinic with reports of nausea, dark urine, weight loss, and fatigue for the past 2 weeks. Which additional information should the nurse gather from this client related to the presenting symptoms?
1. Presence of anorexia
2. 24-hour dietary history
3. Number and color of stools
4. Use of over-the-counter medications

3. 3. Weight loss, nausea, fatigue, and dark urine lasting 2 weeks or more are signs of hepatitis. The nurse should question the client about the presence of clay-colored stools. This additional symptom would prompt the nurse to look at the eyes for the presence of a yellow sclera (jaundice). A 24-hour diet history is not appropriate in a case where the nausea has been ongoing for 2 weeks but is useful in cases where nausea and vomiting have just started. A client who has nausea will not eat as much as he normally would if he were not nauseated. Asking about loss of appetite does not add to what the nurse already knows in the presenting report.
CN: Physiological integrity; CNS: Physiological adaptation; CL: Analyze; DIFFICULTY: Difficult

---

CN: Client needs category   CNS: Client needs subcategory   CL: Cognitive level

4. A nurse would expect to prepare a client for which test to aid in diagnosing a hiatal hernia?
1. Colonoscopy
2. Lower GI series
3. Barium swallow
4. Abdominal x-ray series

5. A client with acute pancreatitis is admitted to the acute care facility. Which health care provider order should the nurse question?
1. Start normal saline (0.9% NaCl) IV to run at 100 mL/hour.
2. Give meperidine 4 mg IM every 6 hours p.r.n. for pain.
3. Monitor blood glucose levels every 6 hours
4. Connect NG tube to low intermittent suction.

6. Which findings should the nurse expect when gathering data from a client admitted with suspected appendicitis? Select all that apply.
1. Loss of appetite
2. Nausea and vomiting
3. Sudden cessation of pain
4. Yellow pigment to the skin
5. Right lower quadrant pain
6. Abdominal rigidity and tenderness

Stay focused. You can do it!

7. The nurse should place a client with appendicitis in which position to help relieve pain?

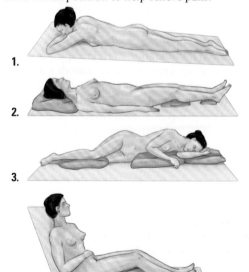

1.

2.

3.

4.

4. 3. A barium swallow with fluoroscopy shows the position of the stomach in relation to the diaphragm. A colonoscopy and a lower GI series show disorders of the intestine. An abdominal x-ray series will show structural defects but not necessarily a hiatal hernia, unless it's sliding or rolling at the time of the x-ray.
CN: Physiological integrity; CNS: Reduction of risk potential; CL: Apply; DIFFICULTY: Difficult

5. 2. The use of meperidine in the treatment of clients with pancreatitis and other biliary disorders is contraindicated because it causes spasm of the sphincter of Oddi. Morphine is one of the medications of choice used to treat pain associated with biliary disorders. IV fluids are given to prevent fluid volume deficit. Blood glucose monitoring is indicated because the pancreas is responsible for the release of insulin that is needed for glucose metabolism; when inflamed the organ does not function normally. Connecting the NG tube to low intermittent suction is indicated for very ill clients or for those with vomiting that is intractable.
CN: Safe, effective care environment; CNS: Coordinated care; CL: Apply; DIFFICULTY: Difficult

6. 1, 2, 5. The pain begins in the periumbilical region, then shifts to the right lower quadrant (McBurney point) and becomes steady. The pain may be moderate to severe. Other signs and symptoms include anorexia, nausea, and vomiting. Sudden cessation of the pain indicates rupture of the appendix and requires surgery. Yellow-pigmented skin (jaundice) is a sign of hepatitis or liver failure/cirrhosis. Abdominal rigidity and tenderness are signs of peritonitis.
CN: Physiological integrity; CNS: Physiological adaptation; CL: Understand; DIFFICULTY: Challenge

7. 4. The nurse should sit the client in the Fowler position with a pillow at the knees. Lying still with the legs drawn up toward the chest helps relieve tension on the abdominal muscles, which helps to reduce the amount of discomfort felt. Lying flat or sitting may increase the amount of pain experienced.
CN: Physiological integrity; CNS: Basic care and comfort; CL: Apply; DIFFICULTY: Challenge

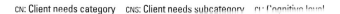

8. Which **priority** nursing intervention should the nurse perform when providing care for a client with appendicitis?
1. Monitoring for pain
2. Encouraging rest periods
3. Providing discharge education
4. Monitoring for signs of peritonitis

8. **4.** The priority of care is to monitor for peritonitis, or inflammation of the peritoneal cavity. Peritonitis is caused by appendix rupture and invasion of bacteria, which could be lethal. The client with appendicitis receives pain medication after confirmation of the diagnosis of appendicitis. This prevents masking of symptoms. The nurse should prevent oral intake in preparation for surgery. Discharge education is important; however, in the acute phase, management should focus on minimizing preoperative complications and recognizing when they may be occurring.
CN: Safe, effective care environment; CNS: Coordinated care;
CL: Apply; DIFFICULTY: Easy

9. Which intervention should the nurse expect to perform when caring for a client with acute pancreatitis?
1. Institute transmission-based precautions
2. Administer sedatives to control anxiety
3. Withhold oral intake as ordered
4. Encourage the client to ambulate

9. **3.** Clients admitted with pancreatitis are acutely ill and will be NPO on admission. Maintain NPO status as ordered by the health care provider. Transmission based precautions are not indicated because this is not an infectious process spread by contact with body fluids, airborne, or contact modes. Administer morphine or hydromorphone for pain relief, not sedatives. During acute pancreatitis, the client is on bed rest and not encouraged to ambulate.
CN: Physiological integrity; CNS: Physiological adaptation;
CL: Apply; DIFFICULTY: Moderate

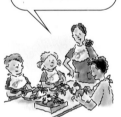

No, Brian. Eating it with the shell on will give you serious GI issues.

10. A client is brought to the emergency room with suspected cholecystitis. Which findings are characteristic of this diagnosis? Select all that apply.
1. Epigastric pain radiating to the back
2. Indigestion after eating fatty foods
3. Blood tinged emesis
4. Abdominal distention
5. Itching and dry skin

10. **1, 2.** Cholecystitis has characteristic symptoms of epigastric pain radiating to the back and indigestion after eating fatty foods. Eating foods high in fat is associated with nausea and indigestion. Itching and dry skin are associated with pancreatic cancer. Abdominal bloating is associated with irritable bowel syndrome.
CN: Physiological integrity; CNS: Physiological adaptation;
CL: Apply; DIFFICULTY: Challenge

11. Which nursing intervention would be the **priority** in the immediate postoperative care of a client who has undergone gastric surgery?
1. Monitoring gastric pH
2. Assessing bowel sounds
3. Providing nutritional support
4. Monitoring for symptoms of hemorrhage

11. **4.** Hemorrhage is a post-op complication detected by monitoring vital signs, abdominal dressings, and NG tube drainage for bleeding. Monitor the post-op client closely for signs and symptoms of hemorrhage, such as bright red blood in the nasogastric tube suction, tachycardia, or a drop in blood pressure. Gastric pH helps to evaluate the need for histamine-2 (H_2) receptor antagonists but is not a priority. Bowel sounds may not return for up to 72 hours postoperatively. Providing nutritional support is not an immediate priority.
CN: Physiological integrity; CNS: Reduction of risk potential;
CL: Apply; DIFFICULTY: Moderate

12. The nurse receives a shift report on a client who is 2 days postoperative bowel resection and reports the sudden onset of pain unrelieved by pain medication. The abdomen is rigid and bowel sounds are absent. Which action should the nurse take next?
1. Administer a dose of pain medication
2. Perform an abdominal assessment
3. Obtain a complete set of vital signs
4. Notify the health care provider

12. **3.** The client is exhibiting signs of peritonitis. The nurse needs a set of vital signs to make sure that the client is not going into shock from hidden bleeding before calling the provider. The abdominal assessment has been completed—there are not bowel sounds. Once the vital signs are gathered then the health care provider should be notified.
CN: Safe, effective care environment; CNS: Coordinated care;
CL: Analyze; DIFFICULTY: Challenge

CN: Client needs category   CNS: Client needs subcategory   CL: Cognitive level

13. Which interventions should the nurse perform when caring for a client with acute gastritis? Select all that apply.
1. Maintaining the client on bed rest
2. Preparing for gastric resection
3. Monitoring laboratory values
4. Administering parenteral nutrition
5. Assess for changes in abdominal status
6. Administer antispasmodics as ordered

14. When reviewing the medical record of a client, which factor leads the nurse to suspect that the client is at risk for chronic gastritis?
1. Consumes an occasional glass of wine with dinner
2. Finishing a 7-day course of amoxicillin for an infection
3. 28-years old with a history of gallbladder disease
4. Taking naproxen three times a day for a sports injury

> Remember to carefully review your client's history, multiple factors can contribute to gastrointestinal disorders.

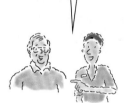

15. Which instruction is **most** appropriate for the nurse to give to a client who reports cramping abdominal pain, vomiting, and inability to pass gas and stool 5 days after undergoing open abdominal surgery to remove an intestinal mass?
1. "Add additional fiber and fluids to your diet."
2. "Eat dried prunes to help you pass a stool."
3. "Sip on clear liquids until the vomiting subsides."
4. "Go to the emergency department for evaluation."

16. A client was hospitalized and treated for acute diverticulitis. The nurse has reinforced discharge education. Which statement by the client indicates that the client understands the discharge instructions?
1. "I'll reduce my fluid intake."
2. "I'll decrease the fiber in my diet."
3. "I'll take all of my antibiotics."
4. "I'll exercise to increase my intra-abdominal pressure."

13. 3, 5. Monitor lab values for changes in hematocrit, hemoglobin, and electrolytes. Assess for changes in abdominal status, which includes increased tenderness, distention, pain, bowel sounds, etc. Gastric resection is an option only when serious erosion has occurred. Antispasmodics are for irritable bowel syndrome. Bed rest is not necessary unless the client is unstable and neither is parenteral nutrition.
CN: Safe, effective care environment; CNS: Coordinated care; CL: Understand; DIFFICULTY: Challenge

14. 4. Risk factors for acute and chronic gastritis include overuse of nonsteroidal anti-inflammatory drugs (NSAIDs), alcohol overuse, and bacterial colonization with *H. pylori* infection in the GI tract can lead to chronic atrophic gastritis. Conditions that allow reflux of bile acids into the stomach can also cause gastritis. Chronic gastritis can occur at any age but is more common in older adults; antibiotics and gallbladder disease are not causes of gastritis.
CN: Physiological integrity; CNS: Physiological adaptation; CL: Analyze; DIFFICULTY: Moderate

15. 4. The client is exhibiting symptoms of an intestinal obstruction. The nurse should advise the client to go to the ED for evaluation of the symptoms, especially when this occurs after open abdominal surgery (inflammation of the colon and scar tissue development are causes of intestinal obstruction). Signs and symptoms of an intestinal obstruction include abdominal distention, nausea, vomiting, diarrhea, crampy abdominal pain, and inability to pass gas and stool. Consuming foods that are high in indigestible fiber (such as bran cereal, lettuce, apricots, raisins, dried prunes, brown rice, and fresh peeled apples) promotes regular bowel movements and the passage of gas. The client in this case is vomiting; therefore, offering this advice is not appropriate at this time.
CN: Physiological integrity; CNS: Reduction of risk potential; CL: Apply; DIFFICULTY: Moderate

16. 3. Antibiotics are used to reduce inflammation. The client with acute diverticulitis typically isn't allowed anything orally until the acute episode subsides. Parenteral fluids are given until the client feels better; then it's recommended that the client drink eight 8-oz (237-mL) glasses of water per day and gradually increase fiber in the diet to improve intestinal motility. During the acute phase, activities that increase intra-abdominal pressure should be avoided to decrease pain and the chance of intestinal obstruction.
CN: Physiological integrity; CNS: Reduction of risk potential; CL: Apply; DIFFICULTY: Easy

17. The nurse has reinforced education for a teenage client and the parents about Crohn disease and the dietary changes needed to manage it. Which statement made to the nurse by the parents indicates an accurate understanding of the child's dietary needs?
1. "We'll need to include plenty of calories in our child's diet."
2. "We'll need to make certain that our child's food is gluten-free."
3. "We'll only give our child foods that are low in sodium."
4. "We'll be sure to provide foods that are high in fiber for our child."

18. The nurse reinforces discharge education for a client with Crohn disease. Which long-term symptom management instruction should the nurse reinforce to this client?
1. Increase your intake of fiber and take a probiotic daily.
2. Join a support group and exercise three times a day.
3. Take your multivitamin and corticosteroid for a year.
4. Keep a food diary and eat small, frequent meals.

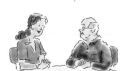

Take time to carefully explain any needed dietary changes to clients.

19. The nurse admits a client with Crohn disease who is experiencing an exacerbation. Which intervention should the nurse make a **priority** of care?
1. Maintaining current weight
1. Encouraging ambulation
2. Promoting bowel rest
3. Providing mouth care

20. A client with irritable bowel syndrome (IBS) is reporting pain. The nurse should expect to administer which medication to help alleviate the underlying cause of the client's pain?
1. Acetaminophen
2. Opiates
3. Steroids
4. Stool softeners

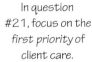

In question #21, focus on the first priority of client care.

21. During the first few days of recovery from ostomy surgery for ulcerative colitis, what should be the **priority** of client care?
1. Body image
2. Ostomy care
3. Sexual concerns
4. Skin care

17. 1. Crohn disease is an inflammatory bowel disease that causes diarrhea with subsequent weight loss and malnutrition. A high-calorie, nutritious diet helps replenish nutrients that are lost through the affected bowel. A gluten-free diet is appropriate for a client with celiac disease, not Crohn disease. A client with Crohn disease doesn't need to restrict dietary sodium but should avoid high-fiber foods during a flare-up of the disease, because these foods can contribute to bowel irritation.
CN: Physiological integrity; CNS: Basic care and comfort; CL: Apply; DIFFICULTY: Difficult

18. 4. Keeping a food diary to determine foods that produce or aggravate symptoms and eating small, frequent meals will help to manage symptom flare-ups long term. Managing stress with exercise can increase the time between flare-ups; however, joining a support group may not help to manage symptoms. Increased fiber, fatty foods, dairy products, alcohol, smoking, and caffeine can aggravate symptoms. Probiotics have not shown any benefit with the management of Crohn disease symptoms. Steroids are not for long-term use. Short-term (3 to 4 months) steroid therapy is used with immune suppressants to induce disease remission until immune suppressant therapy can maintain the disease in remission. A multivitamin does not help to manage symptoms.
CN: Health promotion and maintenance; CNS: None; CL: Apply; DIFFICULTY: Challenge

19. 3. Promoting bowel rest is the priority during an acute exacerbation. This is accomplished by decreasing activity and initially putting the client on nothing-by-mouth (NPO) status. Weight loss may occur, but the priority is bowel rest.
CN: Safe, effective care environment; CNS: Coordinated care; CL: Analyze; DIFFICULTY: Moderate

20. 3. The pain of IBS is caused by inflammation, which steroids can reduce. Acetaminophen has little effect on the pain, and opiates won't treat its underlying cause. Stool softeners aren't necessary.
CN: Physiological integrity; CNS: Pharmacological therapies; CL: Apply; DIFFICULTY: Difficult

21. 2. Although all of these are concerns the nurse should address, it is crucial that the client is able to safely manage the ostomy before discharge.
CN: Safe, effective care environment; CNS: Coordinated care; CL: Apply; DIFFICULTY: Easy

CN: Client needs category   CNS: Client needs subcategory   CL: Cognitive level

22. The nurse receives a client who has undergone an open surgical procedure for hiatal hernia repair. Which nursing intervention is a priority?
1. Turning and repositioning for comfort
2. Encouraging incentive spirometer use
3. Palpating the bladder for distention
4. Administering pain medications

23. A client with gastric cancer is scheduled for a gastric resection. What is the preoperative **priority** nursing care for this client?
1. Discharge planning
2. Correction of nutritional deficits
3. Prevention of deep vein thrombosis
4. Instruction regarding radiation treatment

24. The nurse is reviewing laboratory results for a client with peritonitis. Which results would the nurse expect to observe?
1. Partial thromboplastin time (PTT) longer than 100 seconds
2. Hemoglobin (Hb) level below 10 mg/dL
3. Potassium level above 5.5 mEq/L
4. White blood cell (WBC) count above 15,000/μL

25. A recently admitted client suspected of having peritonitis is requesting a glass of water to drink. What is the **best** response by the nurse?
1. "I can give you small amounts of water frequently."
2. "You're getting your fluids intravenously."
3. "I'll check with the health care provider."
4. "It wouldn't be safe to give you anything to drink."

26. A nurse is caring for a client with acute pancreatitis. The nurse knows that it is **most** important to monitor the client closely for which sign or symptom?
1. Increased appetite
2. Vomiting
3. Hypoglycemia
4. Pain

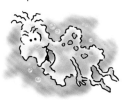

I don't exactly get along with white blood cells.

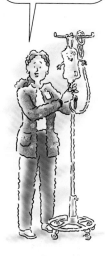

For clients with peritonitis, is drinking a glass of water a good idea?

22. 2. Although all of these are concerns the nurse should address, it is crucial that the client utilize the incentive spirometer to maintain lung expansion and prevent atelectasis.
CN: Safe, effective care environment; CNS: Coordinated care; CL: Apply; DIFFICULTY: Challenge

23. 2. Clients with gastric cancer commonly have nutritional deficits and may be cachectic. Discharge planning before surgery is important, but correcting the nutritional deficit is the priority. Prevention of deep vein thrombosis also isn't the priority before surgery, though it assumes greater importance after surgery. At present, radiation therapy hasn't been proven effective for gastric cancer, and teaching about it preoperatively wouldn't be appropriate.
CN: Physiological integrity; CNS: Reduction of risk potential; CL: Apply; DIFFICULTY: Moderate

24. 4. Because of infection, the client's WBC count will be elevated. A PTT longer than 100 seconds may suggest disseminated intravascular coagulation (DIC), a serious complication of septic shock. A hemoglobin level below 10 mg/dL may occur from hemorrhage. A potassium level above 5.5 mEq/L may suggest renal failure.
CN: Physiological integrity; CNS: Reduction of risk potential; CL: Apply; DIFFICULTY: Easy

25. 4. The client with peritonitis commonly isn't allowed anything orally until the source of the peritonitis is confirmed and treated. IV fluids are given to maintain hydration and hemodynamic stability and to replace electrolytes; however, saying, "You're getting your fluids intravenously" doesn't explain to the client why he can't have fluids orally. Checking with the health care provider isn't necessary.
CN: Physiological integrity; CNS: Physiological adaptation; CL: Apply; DIFFICULTY: Moderate

26. 2. Acute pancreatitis is commonly associated with fluid isolation and accumulation in the bowel secondary to ileus or peripancreatic edema. Fluid and electrolyte loss from vomiting is the primary concern. A client with acute pancreatitis may have increased pain on eating and is unlikely to demonstrate an increased appetite. A client with acute pancreatitis is at risk for hyperglycemia, not hypoglycemia. Although pain is an important concern, it's less significant than vomiting.
CN: Physiological integrity; CNS: Physiological adaptation; CL: Apply; DIFFICULTY: Difficult

27. A client had a gastroscopy while under local anesthesia. Before resuming the client's oral fluid intake, which action should the nurse take **first**?
1. Listen for bowel sounds.
2. Determine whether the client can talk.
3. Check for a gag reflex.
4. Determine the client's mental status.

27. 3. After a gastroscopy, the nurse should check for the presence of a gag reflex before giving oral fluids. This step is essential to prevent aspiration. The presence of bowel sounds, the ability to speak, and mental status within normal limits wouldn't ensure the presence of a gag reflex.
CN: Physiological integrity; CNS: Reduction of risk potential; CL: Apply; DIFFICULTY: Easy

28. A nurse is completing the intake record for a client with chronic pancreatitis. The client has had the following intake during the previous 8 hours. How many milliliters should the nurse record as the client's intake? Record your answer using a whole number.

Intake:

4 oz apple juice
½ cup fruit-flavored gelatin
6 oz water
500 mL 0.45% sodium chloride IV

_____ mL

28. 920. Fluid intake for this client includes 4 oz (120 mL) apple juice, 1/2 cup (120 mL) fruit-flavored gelatin, 6 oz (180 mL) water, and 500 mL 0.45% sodium chloride IV for a total of 920 mL.
CN: Physiological integrity; CNS: Basic care and comfort; CL: Apply; DIFFICULTY: Moderate

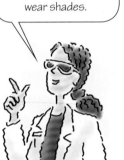

Your future's so bright, you have to wear shades.

29. Several children at a day care center have been infected with hepatitis A virus. Which instruction by the nurse would reduce the risk of spreading hepatitis A to other children and staff members?
1. Hand washing after diaper changes
2. Isolation of the sick children
3. Using masks during contact with children
4. Sterilization of all eating utensils

29. 1. Children in day care centers are at risk of hepatitis A infection, which is transmitted via the fecal-oral route due to poor hand hygiene practices and poor sanitation. Isolation of sick children, use of masks during contact, and sterilization of all eating utensils would not be useful in breaking the chain of infection.
CN: Safe, effective care environment; CNS: Safety and infection control; CL: Apply; DIFFICULTY: Easy

30. Which client statement indicates that the nurse's education about hepatitis A has been effective?
1. "I'll wear a mask all of the time."
2. "I should keep my door closed."
3. "I should wash my hands frequently."
4. "I'm allowed to save part of my sandwich to give to my wife."

30. 3. Hepatitis A is transmitted through the fecal-oral route, so frequent hand washing, especially after elimination, will help prevent transmission. It isn't necessary to wear a mask or keep the door closed. Sharing food allows for viral transmission.
CN: Safe, effective care environment; CNS: Safety and infection control; CL: Apply; DIFFICULTY: Easy

31. A client with a liver disorder is having an invasive procedure. The nurse helps ensure safety by reviewing the results of which test?
1. Coagulation studies
2. Liver enzyme levels
3. Serum chemistries
4. White blood cell count

31. 1. The liver produces coagulation factors. If the liver is affected negatively, production of these factors may be altered, placing the client at risk for hemorrhage. The other laboratory tests should be monitored as well, but the results may not necessarily relate to the safety of the procedure.
CN: Physiological integrity; CNS: Reduction of risk potential; CL: Analyze; DIFFICULTY: Challenge

32. The nurse is reinforcing discharge instructions to a client with chronic cholecystitis. Which response by the client indicates the education has been effective?
1. "I need to rest more."
2. "I should avoid taking antacids."
3. "I should increase the fat in my diet."
4. "I will take my anticholinergic medications as prescribed."

32. 4. Conservative therapy for chronic cholecystitis includes weight reduction by increasing physical activity, a low-fat diet, antacid use to treat dyspepsia, and anticholinergic use to relax smooth muscles and reduce ductal tone and spasm, thereby reducing pain.
CN: Physiological integrity; CNS: Pharmacological therapies; CL: Apply; DIFFICULTY: Moderate

33. Which instruction should the nurse reinforce to a client with pancreatitis during discharge education?
1. Consume high-fat meals.
2. Consume low-calorie meals.
3. Limit daily intake of alcohol.
4. Avoid beverages that contain caffeine.

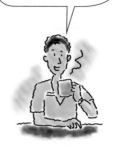

Don't panic. You're doing fine. Keep on trucking.

34. After laparoscopic cholecystectomy, a client reports abdominal pain. The nurse prepares morphine 2 mg. If the label on the morphine reads 10 mg/mL, how many milliliters should the nurse have in the syringe after the correct dose is drawn up? Record your answer using one decimal place.

_____ mL

35. A client with osteoarthritis is admitted to the hospital with peptic ulcer disease. Which findings are commonly associated with peptic ulcer disease? Select all that apply.
1. Localized, colicky periumbilical pain
2. History of nonsteroidal anti-inflammatory drug (NSAID) use
3. Epigastric pain that's relieved by antacids
4. Tachycardia
5. Nausea and weight loss
6. Low-grade fever

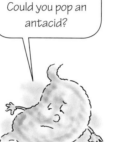

I'm feeling a little nausea and stomach pain. Could you pop an antacid?

36. A client undergoes a barium swallow fluoroscopy that confirms gastroesophageal reflux disease (GERD). Based on this diagnosis, the nurse should instruct the client to take which actions? Select all that apply.
1. Follow a high-fat, low-fiber diet.
2. Avoid caffeine and carbonated beverages.
3. Sleep with the head of the bed flat.
4. Stop smoking.
5. Take antacids 1 hour and 3 hours after meals.
6. Limit alcohol consumption to one drink per day.

37. A nurse is assigned to care for a client with peptic ulcer disease. Which finding will the nurse report immediately to the health care provider?
1. Black, tarry stools
2. Abdominal pain
3. Loss of appetite
4. Tachycardia

33. 4. Caffeine must be avoided because it is a stimulant that will further irritate the pancreas. A client with pancreatitis must avoid all alcohol because chronic alcohol use is one of the causes of pancreatitis. The diet should be low in fat and high in calories, especially carbohydrates.
CN: Physiological integrity; CNS: Reduction of risk potential; CL: Apply; DIFFICULTY: Challenge

34. 0.2. This formula is used to calculate drug dosages:

$$\frac{\text{Dose on hand}}{\text{Quantity on hand}} = \frac{\text{Dose desired}}{X}$$

In this example, the formula for calculating the amount of Morphine is as follows:

$$\frac{10\,\text{mg}}{\text{mL}} = \frac{2\,\text{mg}}{X}$$

$$X = 0.2 \text{ mL.}$$

CN: Physiological integrity; CNS: Pharmacological therapies; CL: Apply; DIFFICULTY: Easy

35. 2, 3, 5. Peptic ulcer disease is characterized by nausea, hematemesis, melena, weight loss, and left-sided epigastric pain—occurring 1 to 2 hours after eating—that's relieved with antacids. NSAID use is also associated with peptic ulcer disease. Appendicitis begins with generalized or localized colicky periumbilical or epigastric pain, followed by anorexia, nausea, a few episodes of vomiting, low-grade fever, and tachycardia.
CN: Physiological integrity; CNS: Physiological adaptation; CL: Understand; DIFFICULTY: Difficult

36. 2, 4, 5. The nurse should instruct the client with GERD to follow a low-fat, high-fiber diet. Caffeine, carbonated beverages, alcohol, and smoking should be avoided because they aggravate GERD. In addition, the client should take antacids as prescribed (typically 1 hour and 3 hours after meals and at bedtime). Lying down with the head of the bed elevated, not flat, reduces intra-abdominal pressure, thereby reducing the symptoms of GERD.
CN: Health promotion and maintenance; CNS: None; CL: Apply; DIFFICULTY: Challenge

37. 4. Pulse rate is a cardiovascular system assessment and tachycardia is an indicator of hidden bleeding, as well as a compensatory mechanism when a client is in the early stage of shock. Loss of appetite can occur from a number of factors and is not something to be alarmed about. Abdominal pain and black, tarry stools are expected with peptic ulcer disease. As blood from the GI tract passes through the intestines, bacterial action causes it to become black and tarry colored.
CN: Physiological integrity; CNS: Physiological adaptation; CL: Apply; DIFFICULTY: Challenge

38. A client is ordered to receive 1 g of neomycin sulfate orally every hour × 4 doses followed by 1 g orally every 4 hours for the remaining balance of the 24 days. Neomycin sulfate tablets are available in 500 mg per tablet. How many tablets should the nurse administer for each dose? Record your answer using a whole number.

_____ tablets

38. 2.
First, convert from g to mg.

1 g to mg: 1,000 mg = 1 g, therefore the order is for 1000 mg of neomycin.

Then use this formula for calculating the number of tablets to administer:

$$\frac{\text{Desired}}{\text{Form on hand}} = \text{Dose}$$

$$\frac{1,000\,\text{g}}{500\,\text{mg}} = 2\,\text{tablets}$$

CN: Physiological integrity; CNS: Pharmacological therapies; CL: Apply; DIFFICULTY: Easy

39. The nurse obtains data from a client admitted with a diagnosis of cirrhosis and ascites. The client is lethargic and confused. Which action should the nurse take?
1. Elevate the head of the bed
2. Notify the health care provider
3. Reorient to time, place, and circumstance.
4. Supply 2 L of oxygen via nasal cannula

39. 2. Notify the provider for changes in the level of consciousness (observe for behavioral or personality changes, increased confusion, stupor, lethargy, hallucinations, and neuromuscular dysfunction) which indicate hepatic encephalopathy due to increased ammonia levels. Ammonia is a byproduct of the metabolism of nitrogen-containing compounds and is neurotoxic. Elevating the head of the bed will not improve confusion and lethargy and may be appropriate if the client was semi-conscious. Reorientation will not improve the confusion, and although O_2 is a choice it does not fix the problem (elevated ammonia and possible swollen brain).

CN: Physiological integrity; CNS: Physiologic adaptation; CL: Analyze; DIFFICULTY: Difficult

40. While caring for a client with cirrhosis, the nurse reviews the laboratory data in the client's chart. Which data should the nurse report immediately?
1. White blood cells (WBC) 3.8 × 10⁹/L
2. Red blood cells (RBC) 5.03 × 10¹²/L
3. Prothrombin time (PT) 18 seconds
4. Total bilirubin (T. Bili) 0.2 mg/dL

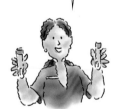

Do you choose the results of test tube A or test tube B?

40. 3. Clotting factors may not be produced normally when a client has cirrhosis, increasing the potential for bleeding. PT measures the time required for a fibrin clot to form. There's no associated change in carbon dioxide level or pH unless the client is developing other comorbidities such as metabolic alkalosis. The WBC count can be elevated in acute cirrhosis but isn't always altered. The total bilirubin level will be elevated in cirrhosis of the liver. The elevation in bilirubin levels is what causes jaundice. The RBC count is not abnormal.

CN: Physiological integrity; CNS: Reduction of risk potential; CL: Analyze; DIFFICULTY: Challenge

41. When counseling a client in the ways to prevent cholecystitis, which guideline is **most** important for the nurse to include?
1. Eat low-protein foods.
2. Eat high-fat, high-cholesterol foods.
3. Limit exercise to 10 minutes per day.
4. Keep weight proportional to height.

41. 4. Obesity is a known cause of gallstones, and maintaining a recommended weight will help to protect against cholecystitis. Excessive dietary intake of cholesterol is associated with the development of gallstones in many people. Dietary protein isn't implicated in cholecystitis. Liquid protein and low-calorie diets (with rapid weight loss of more than 5 lb [2.3 kg] per week) are implicated as the cause of some cases of cholecystitis. Regular exercise (30 minutes/three times per week) may help to reduce weight and improve fat metabolism.

CN: Health promotion and maintenance; CNS: None; CL: Apply; DIFFICULTY: Moderate

42. The nurse prepares to administer care for a client with gastroenteritis who has nausea, vomiting and diarrhea. Which action should the nurse take **first** to maintain the client's nutritional status?
1. Administer loperamide 10 mg orally for loose stools.
2. Encourage sips of Gatorade to prevent dehydration.
3. Administer promethazine 25 mg orally before meals.
4. Offer the snacks appropriate for the client's dietary orders.

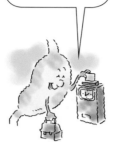

Your stomach works hard for you every day. Treat it well.

42. 3. Offer the client an antiemetic 30 minutes to 1 hour prior to meals to control nausea and vomiting so that the client is able to tolerate oral fluids and food. Give the loperamide next to slow the frequency of diarrheal stools. Offer sips of Gatorade after the antiemetic to increase the chances of the client keeping the fluids down. If the Gatorade is tolerated then offer snacks that are appropriate for the client's dietary orders.
CN: Safe, effective care environment; CNS: Coordinated care; CL: Apply; DIFFICULTY: Challenge

43. A client with cirrhosis is prescribed lactulose 2 tablespoons orally every day, to start if indicated by the client's lab results or signs and symptoms. Which finding indicates to the nurse a need to administer the medication?
1. Serum potassium level 5.6 mEq/dL
2. Blood pressure 158/94
3. Increasing confusion
4. Increase in ascites

43. 3. Lactulose is given when the client's ammonia level is elevated. The only sign of elevation in the ammonia levels is increasing confusion, which can indicate hepatic encephalopathy. Elevation in blood pressure and potassium level is not an indicator of elevated ammonia, nor is an increase in ascites.
CN: Physiological integrity; CNS: Pharmacological therapies; CL: Apply; DIFFICULTY: Difficult

44. The nurse receives a client into the medical unit immediately after a liver biopsy. Which finding indicates to the nurse that the client is experiencing a post-procedure complication?
1. Abdominal cramping
2. Weak, rapid pulse
3. Onset of vomiting
4. Temp 100.1° F (37.8° C)

44. 2. The liver is so vascular that taking a biopsy could cause the client to hemorrhage. Hemorrhage may be hidden, frank, or slow, therefore monitor dressing for visible bleeding and monitor client's vital signs (changes in pulse rate, quality, and rhythm and a drop in blood pressure). The client may experience some discomfort but typically not cramping. Nausea and vomiting may be present and infection may occur, but not immediately after the procedure.
CN: Physiological integrity; CNS: Reduction of risk potential; CL: Apply; DIFFICULTY: Moderate

45. A client has just been given a prescription for diphenoxylate hydrochloride–atropine sulfate. Which information should the nurse reinforce about the use of this medication?
1. Drooling is a side effect of this medication.
2. Irritability is an adverse effect of the medication.
3. Diphenoxylate hydrochloride–atropine sulfate is habit-forming.
4. Finish all of the medication as it is prescribed.

45. 3. Diphenoxylate hydrochloride–atropine sulfate is an antidiarrheal. The client should not exceed the recommended dose of this medication because it may be habit-forming. Since this medication is an antidiarrheal, it should not be taken until it is finished. Side effects of the medication include dry mouth and drowsiness.
CN: Physiological integrity; CNS: Pharmacological therapies; CL: Apply; DIFFICULTY: Moderate

46. Which symptoms, if reported by a client, should lead the nurse to suspect Crohn disease affecting the small intestine?
1. Nausea accompanied by vomiting
2. Weight gain and fluid retention
3. Diarrhea alternating with constipation
4. Stools that have an oily consistency

46. 4. Excessive amounts of fat in the feces due to malabsorption can occur with Crohn disease. Weight loss (not weight gain) due to malabsorption is common. Nausea and vomiting are symptoms of many different GI disorders. Fluid loss (not fluid retention) occurs with Crohn disease due to diarrhea.
CN: Health promotion and maintenance; CNS: None; CL: Understand; DIFFICULTY: Difficult

47. Oral lactulose is prescribed for the client with a hepatic disorder and the nurse provides instructions to the client regarding this medication. Which statement by the client indicates an understanding of the instructions?
1. "Increasing my fluid intake will make the medication work better."
2. "I should remain close to the restroom when I take the medication."
3. "I need to include more high fiber foods in my diet."
4. "I should call the health care provider immediately if I start having nausea."

48. The nurse cares for a client who is post-op bowel resection and has a nasogastric (NG) tube to low intermittent suction. Which care intervention should the nurse administer that is included in the plan of care?
1. Flush the NG with saline once per shift.
2. Offer ice chips to moisturize the mouth.
3. Secure the suction tubing to the bed rail.
4. Provide meticulous mouth care as needed.

49. The nurse prepares to administer morning medications to a client with hepatitis. The client's medications are listed below. Which medication should the nurse withhold?
1. Lamivudine 150 mg orally twice daily
2. Acetaminophen 650 mg orally every day
3. Vitamin B$_{12}$ one capsule twice daily
4. Phytonadione 5 mg IM once daily

50. The nurse collects data from a client with ascites from liver cirrhosis who is taking spironolactone. Which finding indicates to the nurse that the client is responding well to the medication?
1. Decrease in abdominal circumference
2. Urine output increases to 50 mL/hour
3. Serum potassium level 5.8 mg/dL
4. Improvement in breathing pattern

Which medication is hardest on the liver?

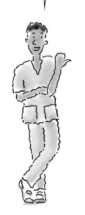

47. 3. Lactulose retains ammonia in the colon, and promotes increased peristalsis and bowel evacuation, expelling ammonia from the colon. It should be taken with water or juice to aid in softening the stool. An increased fluid intake and a high-fiber diet will promote defecation but is unrelated to the medication and why it is being given to this client. Nausea is a side effect and the client should be instructed to drink cola, eat unsalted crackers, or dry toast. It is not necessary to notify the health care provider.
CN: Physiological integrity; CNS: Pharmacological therapies; CL: Apply; DIFFICULTY: Difficult

48. 4. Provide mouth care for clients who are receiving enteral or parenteral feedings or NPO and are not able to perform for themselves. The NG tube should not be flushed once per shift; the health care provider's orders will determine the frequency of flushing if ordered. A client who is on gastric suctioning will be NPO. Avoid securing the suction tubing to the bed rail; doing so may cause the NG tube to become dislodged if the bedrail is let down, which can inadvertently dislodge the NG tube.
CN: Physiological integrity; CNS: Basic care and comfort; CL: Apply; DIFFICULTY: Moderate

49. 2. Acetaminophen is contraindicated in clients with liver disorders. The medication should be withheld and the health care provider should be contacted regarding this medication. Lamivudine is an antiviral used to treat Hepatitis B, B$_{12}$ is a vitamin supplement used to treat anemia associated with hepatitis, and phytonadione a form of vitamin K is used to prevent bleeding when the liver is not functioning properly and does not produce adequate amounts to support clotting.
CN: Physiological integrity; CNS: Pharmacological therapies; CL: Analyze; DIFFICULTY: Moderate

50. 1. In clients with ascites, spironolactone is used to reduce ascites and portal hypertension that causes the ascites. The medication will help to reduce the accumulation of fluid in the abdominal region and other regions of the body. Spironolactone is a potassium-sparing diuretic which can cause potassium levels to rise dramatically in clients, so this should be monitored. Elevation of serum potassium levels above the normal range should be reported. Increased urine output is an expected finding but does not indicate how well the client's ascites is responding to the medication (think about what the medication is being used for in the specific client... what is being treated?).
CN: Physiological integrity; CNS: Pharmacological therapies; CL: Analyze; DIFFICULTY: Moderate

51. A client who takes famotidine for gastritis asks the home care nurse which medication is **best** to take for a headache. Which over the counter medication should the nurse suggest for this client?
  1. Acetylsalicylic acid
  2. Acetaminophen
  3. Ibuprofen
  4. Naproxen

52. The nurse gathers data for a client with colon cancer. Which finding should the nurse anticipate? Select all that apply:
  1. Change in bowel habits
  2. A palpable abdominal mass
  3. Fecal smears in client's underwear.
  4. Reports of rectal bleeding
  5. Diarrhea and constipation
  6. Abdominal swelling and tenderness.

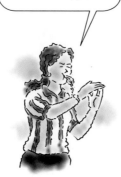

Time out! Take a careful look at all the options in question #52 and then select all that apply.

53. When reinforcing discharge education for a client with ulcerative colitis, the nurse emphasizes the importance of regular examinations. Which statement by the client indicates an understanding of the instructions?
  1. "People who have ulcerative colitis tend to have more problems with their teeth than those with other GI problems."
  2. "I should report any rectal bleeding to the health care provider because this could indicate that I have developed an ulcer."
  3. "The health care provider needs to see me frequently because my chance of developing appendicitis is higher.
  4. "I will need to have routine screenings because having ulcerative colitis places me at risk for colon cancer."

54. Which nursing intervention should be provided for a client admitted with a perforated gastric ulcer?
  1. Administration of antacids
  2. Fluid and electrolyte replacement
  3. Removal of nasogastric (NG) tube
  4. Histamine-2 (H$_2$) receptor antagonist administration

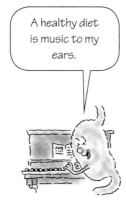

A healthy diet is music to my ears.

55. A nurse is caring for a client with chronic pancreatitis. Which response by the client indicates that discharge education has been effective?
  1. "I'll eat a low-carbohydrate diet."
  2. "I can have an occasional glass of wine."
  3. "I'll take pancreatic enzymes with each meal."
  4. "I'll take pancreatic enzymes before breakfast and at bedtime."

51. 2. The client is taking famotidine, a histamine-2 (H$_2$) receptor antagonist. This implies that the client has a disorder characterized by gastrointestinal (GI) irritation. The only medication among the answer choices that is not irritating to the GI tract is acetaminophen. The other medications could aggravate an already existing GI problem. CN: Physiological integrity; CNS: Pharmacological therapies; CL: Analyze; DIFFICULTY: Challenge

52. 1, 4, 5. The key signs and symptoms of colon cancer are: change in bowel habits and shape of stools; abdominal pain (bloating, gas, cramps), diarrhea and constipation; bloody stools or rectal bleeding; weight loss from (GI) irritation. A mass is not usually palpable in the abdomen unless this is an advanced case. The fecal smearing is a sign of incontinence caused by loss of sphincter control/tone or diarrhea. Abdominal pain and swelling may be the cause of something else going on with the abdomen since these are common signs of a GI problem. CN: Physiological integrity; CNS: Physiological adaptation; CL: Analyze; DIFFICULTY: Difficult

53. 4. Clients with chronic ulcerative colitis, granulomas, and familial polyposis have an increased risk of developing colon cancer. Clients with ulcerative colitis don't have an increased risk of developing the other disorders. CN: Health promotion and maintenance; CNS: None; CL: Apply; DIFFICULTY: Challenge

54. 2. The client should be treated with fluid and electrolyte replacement, blood products, and antibiotics. NG tube suctioning may also be performed to prevent further spillage of stomach contents into the peritoneal cavity. Antacids and histamine-2 (H$_2$) receptor antagonists aren't helpful in this situation. CN: Physiological integrity; CNS: Physiological adaptation; CL: Apply; DIFFICULTY: Difficult

55. 3. Oral pancreatic enzymes are taken with each meal to aid digestion and control steatorrhea. The client should adhere to a low-fat (not low-carbohydrate) diet. The client should eliminate alcohol from the diet completely as it will continue to cause pancreatic damage. CN: Physiological integrity; CNS: Physiological adaptation; CL: Apply; DIFFICULTY: Moderate

CN: Client needs category   CNS: Client needs subcategory   CL: Cognitive level

56. The nurse is caring for a client with alcohol-related acute pancreatitis. Which intervention is **most** appropriate to reduce the exacerbation of pain?
1. Lying supine
2. Taking aspirin
3. Eating low-fat foods
4. Abstaining from alcohol

56. 4. Abstaining from alcohol is imperative to reduce injury to the pancreas; in fact, it may be enough to completely control pain. Lying supine usually aggravates the pain because it stretches the abdominal muscles. Taking aspirin can cause bleeding in hemorrhagic pancreatitis. During an attack of acute pancreatitis, the client usually isn't allowed to ingest anything orally.
CN: Physiological integrity; CNS: Reduction of risk potential;
CL: Apply; DIFFICULTY: Easy

57. Which nursing intervention is a **priority** when caring for the client with esophageal varices?
1. Recognizing hemorrhage
2. Controlling blood pressure
3. Encouraging nutritional intake
4. Reinforcing education to the client about varices

57. 1. Recognizing the rupture of esophageal varices, or hemorrhage, is the focus of nursing care because the client could succumb to this quickly. Controlling blood pressure is also important because it helps reduce the risk of variceal rupture. It's also important to educate the client on what varices are and what foods to avoid, such as spicy foods.
CN: Physiological integrity; CNS: Physiological adaptation;
CL: Apply; DIFFICULTY: Moderate

58. Which process **best** describes the mode of action of medications such as ranitidine, which are used in the treatment of peptic ulcer disease?
1. Neutralize acid
2. Reduce acid secretions
3. Stimulate gastrin release
4. Protect the mucosal barrier

58. 2. Ranitidine is a histamine-2 (H_2) receptor antagonist that reduces acid secretion by inhibiting gastrin secretion. Antacids neutralize acid, and mucosal barrier fortifiers protect the mucosal barrier.
CN: Physiological integrity; CNS: Pharmacological therapies;
CL: Understand; DIFFICULTY: Moderate

59. A nurse is reviewing data in a client's chart to determine confirmation of the diagnosis of cholecystitis. Which data would help confirm a diagnosis of cholecystitis?
1. Results of a colonoscopy
2. Results of an abdominal ultrasound
3. Results of barium swallow
4. Results of endoscopy

59. 2. An abdominal ultrasound can show if the gallbladder is enlarged, if gallstones are present, if the gallbladder wall is thickened, or if distention of the gallbladder lumen is present. A colonoscopy looks at the inner surface of the colon. A barium swallow looks at the stomach and the duodenum. Endoscopy looks at the esophagus, stomach, and duodenum.
CN: Health promotion and maintenance; CNS: None;
CL: Understand; DIFFICULTY: Difficult

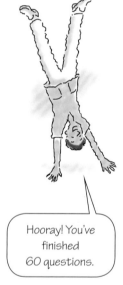

Hooray! You've finished 60 questions.

60. The nurse receives a client at the clinic for follow-up after being treated in the hospital for pancreatitis. When gathering data from the client, which finding should immediately be reported to the health care provider?
1. Dry, itchy, and scaly skin
2. Abdomen bloated but non-tender
3. Greenish-yellow bruise over the IV site
4. Shortness of breath with minimal exertion

60. 4. In pancreatitis, the nurse should watch for signs and symptoms of worsening of the condition: shortness of breath with minimal exertion; respiratory failure and tachycardia (signs of hypocalcemia and hypomagnesemia); and acute changes in abdominal symptoms/size. The other findings are expected and are not a reason to be alarmed.
CN: Physiological integrity; CNS: Physiological adaptation;
CL: Analyze; DIFFICULTY: Moderate

61. Which symptom, if reported by a client, would lead the nurse to suspect possible gastric cancer?
1. Abdominal cramping
2. Constant hunger
3. Feeling of fullness
4. Weight gain

61. 3. The client with gastric cancer may report a feeling of fullness in the stomach but not enough to cause him to seek medical care. Abdominal cramping isn't associated with gastric cancer. Anorexia and weight loss (not increased hunger or weight gain) are common symptoms of gastric cancer.
CN: Physiological integrity; CNS: Physiological adaptation;
CL: Understand; DIFFICULTY: Challenge

62. A nurse is preparing to obtain a stool sample from a client admitted with suspected hepatitis. Which precautions should the nurse take to reduce the possible transmission of this virus? Select all that apply.

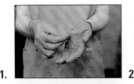
1.

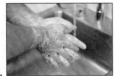
2.

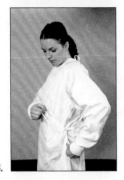
3.

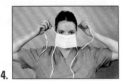
4.

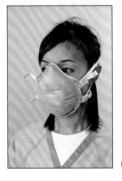
5.

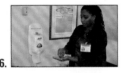
6.

62. **1, 2. 3, 6.** Hepatitis transmission occurs via the fecal-oral route, exposure to infected blood feces and urine, and through the ingestion of contaminated food or liquids. To collect a specimen when the type of hepatitis in unknown, the nurse should take these precautions: wear gloves and a gown, perform meticulous handwashing, and use an alcohol-based hand sanitizer help to reduce the possibility of spreading infection. A mask and goggles are not needed unless there is the possibility of splashing (e.g., when performing gastric lavage; flushing G-tubes or catheters; suctioning; and when working with clients who are vomiting, have explosive diarrhea, or are vomiting/coughing up blood).

CN: Safe, effective care environment; CNS: Safety and infection control; CL: Apply; DIFFICULTY: Moderate

63. A nurse is educating a 52-year-old client on cancer screening. The nurse emphasizes that which diagnostic test should be performed annually after age 50 to screen for colon cancer?
1. Abdominal computed tomography (CT) scan
2. Abdominal x-ray
3. Colonoscopy
4. Fecal occult blood test

63. **4.** The American Cancer Society guidelines include annual screenings for colon cancer using fecal occult blood tests beginning at age 50. Surface blood vessels of polyps and cancers are fragile and often bleed with the passage of stools, so a fecal occult blood test should be performed annually. CT scan and abdominal x-ray can help establish tumor size and metastasis. A colonoscopy can help locate a tumor as well as polyps, and can be used for screening every 10 years.

CN: Health promotion and maintenance; CNS: None; CL: Apply; DIFFICULTY: Challenge

Puzzled by a question? Try to eliminate as many wrong answers as you can before answering.

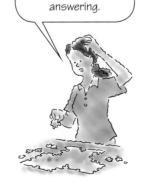

64. A client with gastric cancer can expect to have surgery for resection. Which intervention is a **priority** for the preoperative client with gastric cancer?
1. Discharge planning
2. Correction of nutritional deficits
3. Prevention of deep vein thrombosis
4. Instruction regarding radiation treatment

64. **2.** Clients with gastric cancer commonly have nutritional deficits and may be cachectic. Discharge planning before surgery is important, but correcting the nutritional deficit is the priority. Prevention of deep vein thrombosis also isn't the priority before surgery, though it assumes greater importance *after* surgery. At present, radiation therapy hasn't been proven effective for gastric cancer, and teaching about it preoperatively wouldn't be appropriate.

CN: Physiological integrity; CNS: Reduction of risk potential; CL: Apply; DIFFICULTY: Challenge

CN: Client needs category   CNS: Client needs subcategory   CL: Cognitive level

65. A client with colon cancer asks the nurse why he is getting radiation therapy before surgery. Which response would be **most** appropriate?

1. "It helps reduce the size of the tumor."
2. "It eliminates the malignant cells."
3. "The chances of curing the cancer are improved."
4. "The therapy helps to heal the bowel after surgery."

65. 1. Radiation therapy is used to treat colon cancer before surgery to reduce the size of the tumor, making it easier to resect. Radiation therapy can't eliminate the malignant cells (though it helps to define tumor margins), isn't curative, and could slow postoperative healing.

CN: Physiological integrity; CNS: Physiological adaptation;
CL: Apply; DIFFICULTY: Moderate

66. A client is suspected of having gastric cancer. The nurse expects to prepare the client for which diagnostic test that will aid in confirming the diagnosis of gastric cancer?

1. Barium enema
2. Colonoscopy
3. Gastroscopy
4. Serum chemistry levels

66. 3. A gastroscopy will allow direct visualization of the tumor. A barium enema or colonoscopy would help to diagnose colon cancer. Serum chemistry levels don't contribute data useful to the assessment of gastric cancer.

CN: Health promotion and maintenance; CNS: None;
CL: Understand; DIFFICULTY: Moderate

67. When assisting with development of a postoperative care plan for a client after gastric resection, which would be the **priority**?

1. Body image
2. Nutritional needs
3. Skin care
4. Spiritual needs

67. 2. After gastric resection, a client may require total parenteral nutrition or jejunostomy tube feedings to maintain adequate nutritional status. Body image isn't much of a problem for this client because clothing can cover the incision site. Wound care of the incision site is necessary to prevent infection; otherwise, the skin shouldn't be affected. Spiritual needs may be a concern, depending on the client, and should be addressed as the client demonstrates readiness to share concerns.

CN: Physiological integrity; CNS: Reduction of risk potential;
CL: Apply; DIFFICULTY: Easy

68. A client recently diagnosed with colon cancer tells the nurse that he is having trouble sleeping because of thoughts of how life will change after surgery. Which action should the nurse take in this situation?

1. Request a chaplain to come and talk to the client
2. Refer the client to a cancer support group
3. Discuss the client's remarks with the charge nurse
4. Encourage the client to discuss feelings

68. 3. The client is having trouble sleeping because of concerns about life changes. The client may be experiencing anxiety and powerlessness. Encouraging the client to verbalize feelings will help the nurse to determine how to assist the client and may reduce the client's anxiety. The other options do not directly address the client's comments and concerns.

CN: Psychosocial integrity; CNS: None; CL: Apply;
DIFFICULTY: Challenge

> A bath is a great way to engage your parasympathetic (rest-and-digest) system.

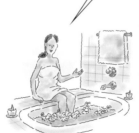

69. To reduce occurrence of dumping syndrome, which action should the nurse instruct a client to take?

1. Sip fluids with meals.
2. Eat three meals daily.
3. Rest after meals for 20 to 30 minutes.
4. Eat high-carbohydrate, low-fat foods.

69. 3. To reduce occurrences of dumping syndrome, clients should be taught to lie down for 20 to 30 minutes after eating; take fluids between meals only; eat smaller amounts more frequently in a semi-recumbent position; and follow a low-carbohydrate diet, with high-protein and moderate-fat-foods, and avoid sweets.

CN: Physiological integrity; CNS: Reduction of risk potential;
CL: Apply; DIFFICULTY: Challenge

70. Which findings in a client with Crohn disease indicate early signs of dehydration? Select all that apply.
1. Poor skin turgor
2. Decreased creatinine
3. Low specific gravity
4. Elevated blood pressure
5. Increased heart rate
6. Bradypnea

71. Which nursing intervention would be the **priority** in the immediate postoperative care of a client who has undergone gastric resection?
1. Monitoring gastric pH to detect complications
2. Assessing bowel sounds
3. Providing nutritional support
4. Monitoring for symptoms of hemorrhage

72. A client who is 1-week post-op colon resection calls the nurse and says, "My incision is wide open on one side and something is poking out of it." Which **priority** instruction should the nurse give to this client?
1. "Drive to the nearest emergency department to be evaluated by a health care provider."
2. "Wrap an ace bandage around your abdomen and monitor for bleeding."
3. "Place wax paper over the wound and call an ambulance."
4. "Apply Vaseline gauze over the wound and come to the office."

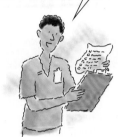

Dehydration is serious business. Remember to stay well hydrated.

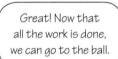

Great! Now that all the work is done, we can go to the ball.

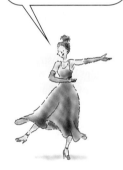

70. 1, 5. Signs and symptoms of dehydration include poor skin turgor, increased heart rate, concentrated urine, and decreased blood pressure. Other signs are dry skin and mouth, sunken eyes, and lethargy.
CN: Physiological integrity; CNS: Physiological adaptation; CL: Understand; DIFFICULTY: Difficult

71. 4. The client should be monitored closely for signs and symptoms of hemorrhage, such as bright red blood in the nasogastric tube suction, tachycardia, or a drop in blood pressure. Gastric pH may be monitored to evaluate the need for histamine-2 (H_2) receptor antagonists. Bowel sounds may not return for up to 72 hours postoperatively. Nutritional needs should be addressed soon after surgery.
CN: Physiological integrity; CNS: Reduction of risk potential; CL: Apply; DIFFICULTY: Moderate

72. 3. The client is experiencing wound evisceration (occurs 5 to 7 days post-op). The client should be instructed to cover the wound with wax paper to maintain moisture of the internal organs and call 911 for ambulance transport to the hospital. Petroleum products, an elastic bandage, and driving to the hospital are contraindicated in the care of this client.
CN: Physiological integrity; CNS: Physiological adaptation; CL: Apply; DIFFICULTY: Difficult

Chapter 9

Endocrine Disorders

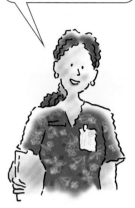

Time to get all hormonal ... this chapter covers diabetes and other endocrine disorders, typically a difficult area for nursing students. Don't worry, though, I'll help you through all the tough spots.

Endocrine refresher

Acromegaly and gigantism (hyperpituitarism)

Acromegaly
Oversecretion of growth hormone (GH) by the pituitary gland in adulthood (after closure of the epiphyseal plates)

Gigantism
Oversecretion of growth hormone (GH) prior to puberty (before closure of the epiphyseal plates)

Key signs and symptoms

Acromegaly
- Enlarged supraorbital ridge
- Thickened ears and nose
- Thickening of the tongue

Gigantism
- Excessive growth in all parts of the body

Key test results
- Plasma human growth hormone (HGH) levels measured by radioimmunoassay typically are elevated. However, because HGH secretion is pulsatile, the results of random sampling may be misleading. IGF-1 (somatomedin-C) levels offer a better screening alternative.

Key treatments
- Surgery to remove the affecting tumor (transsphenoidal hypophysectomy)
- Thyroid hormone replacement therapy after surgery: levothyroxine
- Inhibitor of HGH release: bromocriptine, pegvisomant
- Somatotropic hormone: octreotide

Key interventions
- Provide the client with emotional support
- Perform or assist with range-of-motion (ROM) exercises
- Keep in mind that this disease can also cause inexplicable mood changes; reassure the family that these mood changes result from the disease and can be modified with treatment
- After surgery, monitor vital signs and neurologic status; be alert for any alterations in level of consciousness, pupil equality,

or visual acuity as well as vomiting, falling pulse rate, and rising blood pressure
- Check blood glucose levels
- Measure intake and output hourly, watching for large increases
- Encourage the client to ambulate on the first or second day after surgery

Diabetes insipidus

Insufficient antidiuretic hormone (ADH) secreted by the pituitary gland resulting in excretion of copious volumes of urine

Key signs and symptoms
- Polydipsia (consumption of 4 to 40 L/day)
- Polyuria (greater than 5 L/day of dilute urine)

Key test results
- Urine chemistry shows urine specific gravity less than 1.005, osmolality 50 to 200 mOsm/kg, decreased urine pH, and decreased sodium and potassium levels

Key treatments
- IV therapy: hydration (when first diagnosed, intake and output must be matched milliliter to milliliter to prevent dehydration), electrolyte replacement
- Control excess production of cortisol; ketoconazole, mitotane, and metyrapone

Key interventions
- Monitor fluid balance and daily weight
- Monitor and record vital signs, intake and output (urine output should be measured every hour when first diagnosed), urine specific gravity (check every 1 to 2 hours when first diagnosed), and laboratory studies
- Maintain IV fluid

Syndrome of inappropriate antidiuretic hormone secretion (SIADH)

Posterior pituitary gland disorder in which there is a continued release of ADH that results in renal reabsorption of water rather than its normal excretion

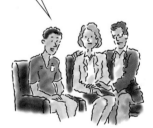

Acromegaly can affect both the client's appearance and mood, so be prepared to provide emotional support.

Key signs and symptoms

- Water retention, edema, weight gain
- Oliguria
- Headache
- Muscle cramps
- Anorexia
- With worsening of condition: nausea, vomiting, muscle twitching, and changes in level of consciousness (LOC)

Key test results

- Decreased serum sodium levels
- Decreased serum osmolality
- Increased urine sodium and osmolality

Key treatments

- Eliminate underlying cause
- Osmotic diuretics (mannitol)
- Loop diuretics (furosemide)
- IV administration of a 3% hypertonic sodium chloride solution for severe hyponatremia

Key interventions

- Monitor intake and output
- Assess LOC frequently
- Monitor for signs and symptoms of fluid overload and hyponatremia

Addison disease (primary adrenal insufficiency)

Disorder that results from destruction of the adrenal cortex by disease; this results in decreased adrenal cortical function

Key signs and symptoms

- Orthostatic hypotension
- Weakness and lethargy
- Weight loss

Key test results

- Blood chemistry reveals decreased cortisol, glucose, sodium, chloride, and aldosterone levels; and increased blood urea nitrogen (BUN), potassium level, and plasma ACTH
- Hematology tests reveal elevated hematocrit and decreased hemoglobin
- Blood or capillary glucose levels reveal hypoglycemia
- Urine chemistry shows decreased 17-ketosteroids and hydroxycorticosteroids (17-OHCS)

Key treatments

- With adrenal crisis, IV hydrocortisone given promptly along with 3 to 5 L of normal saline solution
- Glucocorticoids: hydrocortisone
- Mineralocorticoid: fludrocortisone

Key interventions

- Administer appropriate medications
- Maintain IV fluids
- Don't allow the client to sit up or stand quickly

Cushing syndrome (adrenocortical hyperfunction)

Excessive secretion of hormones by the adrenal cortex.

Key signs and symptoms

- History of amenorrhea
- History of mood swings
- Hypertension
- Muscle wasting
- Weight gain, especially truncal obesity, buffalo hump, and moonface

Key test results

- Blood chemistry shows increased cortisol, aldosterone, sodium, corticotropin, and glucose levels, and a decreased potassium level
- Dexamethasone suppression test shows no decrease in 17-OHCS
- Magnetic resonance imaging shows pituitary or adrenal tumors

Key treatments

- Hypophysectomy or bilateral adrenalectomy
- Antidiabetic agents: insulin or oral agents such as glyburide, glipizide, metformin

Key interventions

- Perform postoperative care
- Observe for edema
- Limit water intake
- Weigh the client daily

Diabetes mellitus

Metabolic disorder of the pancreas that affects carbohydrate, fat, and protein metabolism

- Type 1 is characterized by no insulin production by the pancreas; onset most likely to occur in childhood and adolescence
- Type 2 is characterized by insulin resistance or insufficient insulin production; more common in aging adults

Key signs and symptoms

- Polydipsia
- Polyphagia
- Polyuria
- Weight loss (with type 1)

Key test results

- Fasting blood glucose level is increased (greater than or equal to 126 mg/dL)

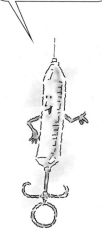

Diuretics are the "appropriate" treatment for the syndrome of inappropriate ADH.

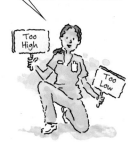

Cushing syndrome is characterized by adrenocortical hyperfunction. You remember what "hyper" means, don't you?

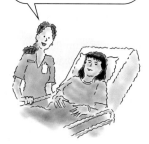

When assessing for diabetes mellitus, remember the three "polys": -dipsia, -phagia, and –uria.

- Glycosylated hemoglobin assay is increased to 7 or above
- 2-hour postprandial blood glucose level shows hyperglycemia (greater than 200 mg/dL)

Key treatments

- Antidiabetic agents: insulin or oral agents, such as glimepiride, glyburide, glipizide, metformin

Key interventions

- Monitor acid-base and fluid balance
- Monitor for signs of hypoglycemia (altered mental status, dizziness, weakness, pallor, tachycardia, diaphoresis, seizures, and coma), ketoacidosis (acetone breath, dehydration, weak or rapid pulse, Kussmaul respirations), and hyperosmolar coma (polyuria, thirst, neurologic abnormalities, stupor)
- Be prepared to treat hypoglycemia; immediately give carbohydrates in the form of fruit juice, hard candy, or honey. If the client is unconscious, maintain safety until glucagon or dextrose is administered IV
- Be prepared to maintain IV fluid; administer insulin and, usually, potassium replacement for ketoacidosis or hyperosmolar coma
- Monitor wound healing
- Maintain the client's diet
- Provide meticulous skin and foot care; clients with diabetes are at increased risk for infection from impaired leukocyte activity
- Foster independence

Goiter

Enlarged thyroid gland; endemic goiter is caused by dietary deficiency of iodine or the inability of the thyroid gland to utilize iodine

Key signs and symptoms

- Single or multinodular, firm, irregular enlargement of the thyroid gland
- Dizziness or syncope when the client raises his arms above his head (Pemberton sign)
- Dysphagia

Key test results

- Laboratory tests reveal high or normal thyroid-stimulating hormone (TSH), low serum thyroxine (T4) concentrations, and increased iodine-131 uptake

Key treatments

- Subtotal thyroidectomy
- Thyroid hormone replacement: levothyroxine

Key interventions

- Measure the client's neck circumference. Also check for the development of hard nodules in the gland
- Provide preoperative teaching and postoperative care if subtotal thyroidectomy is indicated

Hyperthyroidism

Hypersecretion of thyroid hormones (T3, T4) that results in an increased metabolic rate

Key signs and symptoms

- Atrial fibrillation
- Bruit or thrill over thyroid
- Diaphoresis
- Palpitations
- Tachycardia

Key test results

- Blood chemistry shows increased triiodothyronine (T3), T4, and free thyroxine levels; also shows decreased TSH and cholesterol levels
- Radioactive iodine uptake (RAIU) is increased

Key treatments

- Radiation therapy
- Thyroidectomy
- Iodine preparations: potassium iodide (SSKI), radioactive iodine

Key interventions

- Monitor cardiovascular status
- Avoid stimulants, such as caffeine-containing drugs and foods
- Maintain IV fluids
- Weigh the client daily
- Provide postoperative care

Hypothyroidism

Thyroid gland fails to secrete adequate amounts of thyroid hormones; this results in slowing of all metabolic processes

Key signs and symptoms

- Dry, flaky skin and thinning nails
- Fatigue
- Hypothermia
- Menstrual disorders
- Mental sluggishness
- Weight gain or anorexia

Key test results

- Blood chemistry shows decreased T3, T4, free thyroxine, and sodium levels; TSH levels are increased with thyroid insufficiency and decreased with hypothalamic or pituitary insufficiency
- RAIU is decreased

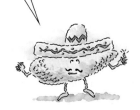

Hey, everybody—the insulin has arrived. Let's get this party started!

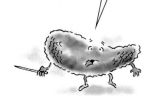

Producing insulin is usually as easy for me as waving a magic wand!

Key treatments
- Thyroid hormone replacement: levothyroxine, liothyronine

Key interventions
- Avoid sedation; administer one-half to one-third the normal dose of sedatives or opioids.
- Check for constipation and edema
- Encourage fluids

Thyroid cancer
Growth of malignant cells in the thyroid gland

Key signs and symptoms
- Enlarged thyroid gland
- Painless, firm, irregular, and enlarged thyroid nodule or mass

Key test results
- Blood chemistry shows increased calcitonin, serotonin, and prostaglandin levels
- RAIU shows a "cold," or nonfunctioning, nodule
- Thyroid biopsy shows cytology positive for cancer cells

Key treatments
- Radiation therapy
- Thyroidectomy (total or subtotal); with or without radical neck excision

Key interventions
- Monitor respiratory status for signs of airway obstruction
- Evaluate ability to swallow
- Provide postoperative thyroidectomy care

Thyroiditis
Inflammation of the thyroid gland that involves release of excessive amounts of thyroid hormones; this results in thyroid dysfunction from hyperactivity to eventual hypoactivity as the stores of thyroid hormones in the gland are depleted. Hashimoto thyroiditis (an autoimmune disorder) is the most common form

Key signs and symptoms
- Thyroid enlargement
- Fever
- Pain
- Tenderness and reddened skin over the gland

Key test results
- Precise diagnosis depends on the type of thyroiditis:
  - With autoimmune thyroiditis, high titers of thyroglobulin and microsomal antibodies may be present in serum
  - With subacute granulomatous thyroiditis, tests may reveal elevated erythrocyte sedimentation rate, increased thyroid hormone levels, and decreased thyroidal RAIU
  - With chronic infective and noninfective thyroiditis, varied findings occur, depending on underlying infection or other disease

Key treatments
- Partial thyroidectomy to relieve tracheal or esophageal compression in Riedel thyroiditis
- Thyroid hormone replacement: levothyroxine for accompanying hypothyroidism

Key interventions
- Check vital signs and examine the client's neck for unusual swelling, enlargement, or redness
- If the neck is swollen, measure and record the circumference daily
- After thyroidectomy:
  - Check vital signs every 15 to 30 minutes until the client's condition stabilizes. Stay alert for signs of tetany secondary to unintentional parathyroid injury during surgery. Keep 10% calcium gluconate available for IM use if needed.
  - Check dressings frequently for excessive bleeding
  - Keep the head of the client's bed elevated
  - Watch for signs of airway obstruction, such as difficulty talking and increased swallowing; keep tracheotomy equipment handy.

Hyperparathyroidism
Excessive secretion of parathormone (parathyroid hormone) which results in increased urinary excretion of phosphorus and loss of calcium from the bones

Key signs and symptoms
- Fatigue and muscle weakness
- Bone pain, especially on weight bearing
- Pathologic fractures
- Calcium renal calculi (stones)

Key test results
- Increased serum calcium levels
- Decreased serum phosphorus levels
- Elevated urine calcium levels in a 24-hour collection

Key treatments
Primary hyperparathyroidism
- Surgical excision of the hypertrophied glandular tissue or adenoma

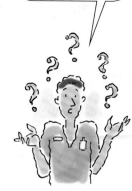

Can you remember the signs and symptoms of thyroiditis?

Secondary hyperparathyroidism

- Correct the underlying cause (vitamin D therapy, management of renal failure, calcium restricted diet)

Key interventions

- Measure intake and output
- Observe for development of renal calculi (flank pain, increased serum calcium, decreased urine output)
- Increase PO fluid intake
- Frequent rest periods
- Postoperative care: similar to care after thyroidectomy

Hypoparathyroidism

Insufficient secretion of parathormone due to trauma or inadvertent removal of all (or nearly all) of the glands during thyroidectomy

Key signs and symptoms

- Tetany
- Numbness in fingers, toes, or around the lips
- Positive Chvostek sign, Trousseau sign
- Laryngeal spasm

Key test results

- Elevated serum phosphorus level
- Decreased serum calcium level
- Decreased urinary calcium and phosphorus levels

Key treatments

- Administration of an IV calcium salt
- Intubation and mechanical ventilation for acute respiratory distress
- Long-term treatment: oral calcium supplements, vitamin D or D2, and a high calcium, low phosphorus diet

Key interventions

- Observe for tetany and assess Chvostek and Trousseau signs
- Insert IV line for emergency administration of calcium
- Observe during calcium administration for adverse effects (bradycardia, flushing, tingling in the arms and legs, metallic taste)
- Observe for respiratory distress and keep emergency equipment for intubation/tracheostomy/mechanical ventilation at the bedside
- To prevent muscle contractions and convulsions, keep noise, movement, and other environmental triggers to a minimum

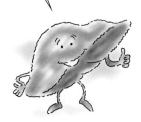

Detoxification gets a thumbs up.

thePoint® You can download tables of drug information to help you prepare for the NCLEX®! View Generic Drug Names, Drug Classifications, Drug Actions, and Nursing Implications for the drugs discussed in this refresher at **http://thePoint.lww.com.**

Endocrine system questions, answers, and rationales

1. After reviewing a client's history and physical examination, which symptoms would lead the nurse to suspect hyperglycemia?
1. Polydipsia, polyuria, and polyphagia
2. Weight gain, tiredness, and bradycardia
3. Irritability, diaphoresis, and tachycardia
4. Diarrhea, abdominal pain, and weight loss

1. **1.** Symptoms of hyperglycemia include polydipsia, polyuria, and polyphagia. Weight gain, tiredness, and bradycardia are symptoms of hypothyroidism. Irritability, diaphoresis, and tachycardia are symptoms of hypoglycemia. Symptoms of Crohn disease include diarrhea, abdominal pain, and weight loss.
CN: Physiological integrity; CNS: Reduction of risk potential; CL: Analyze; DIFFICULTY: Easy

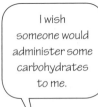

I wish someone would administer some carbohydrates to me.

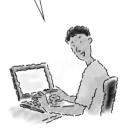

2. A client presents with diaphoresis, palpitations, jitters, and tachycardia approximately 4 hours after taking the prescribed usual morning insulin. What is the nurse's **priority** action?
1. Check blood glucose level, and administer carbohydrates.
2. Give nitroglycerin, and perform an electrocardiogram (ECG).
3. Check pulse oximetry, and administer oxygen therapy.
4. Restrict salt, administer diuretics, and perform paracentesis.

2. **1.** The client is experiencing symptoms of hypoglycemia. Checking the blood glucose level and administering carbohydrates will elevate blood glucose. ECG and nitroglycerin are treatments for myocardial infarction. Administering oxygen won't help correct the low blood glucose level. Restricting salt, administering diuretics, and performing paracentesis are treatments for ascites.
CN: Physiological integrity; CNS: Physiological adaptation; CL: Apply; DIFFICULTY: Easy

CN: Client needs category   CNS: Client needs subcategory   CL: Cognitive level

3. The nurse is monitoring a client receiving iso-phane insulin suspension. Which data obtained by the nurse would cause suspicion that the client is experiencing hypoglycemia? Select all that apply.
1. Diaphoresis
2. Hunger
3. Polyuria
4. Excessive thirst
5. Confusion

4. The nurse is caring for a client who vomits 1 hour after taking a morning glyburide? What is the **priority** nursing action?
1. Give glyburide again.
2. Give subcutaneous insulin and monitor blood glucose.
3. Monitor blood glucose closely and look for signs of hypoglycemia.
4. Monitor blood glucose and assess for symptoms of hyperglycemia.

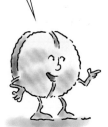

Vomiting may be a sign that I'm working a little too well.

5. A health care provider prescribes diet, exercise, and oral antidiabetic agents for a client with diabetes. Which type of diabetes will the nurse reinforce educating the client about?
1. Diabetes insipidus
2. Diabetic ketoacidosis
3. Type 1 diabetes
4. Type 2 diabetes

6. The nurse is caring for a client with new-onset type 2 diabetes mellitus. Which statement by the client indicates that additional education regarding the relationship between diabetes and exercise is required?
1. "I need to carry candy or juice when I go jogging."
2. "I should wait to eat until after I have finished exercising."
3. "I should give my insulin in my abdomen."
4. "I should warm up before my aerobic exercise."

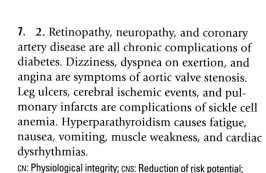

Pace yourself. The NCLEX is more like a marathon than a sprint.

7. A client with diabetes is being taught about possible complications. The nurse should include which conditions in the discussion with the client?
1. Dizziness, dyspnea on exertion, and angina
2. Retinopathy, neuropathy, and coronary artery disease
3. Leg ulcers, cerebral ischemic events, and pulmonary infarcts
4. Fatigue, nausea, vomiting, muscle weakness, and cardiac dysrhythmias

3. 1, 2, 5. Signs and symptoms of hypoglycemia include: diaphoresis, weakness, headache, nausea, drowsiness, nervousness, hunger, tremors, malaise, characteristic behavioral changes, confusion, and dizziness. Excessive thirst and polyuria suggest *hyper*glycemia rather than hypoglycemia.
CN: Physiological integrity; CNS: Physiological adaptation; CL: Analyze; DIFFICULTY: Challenge

4. 3. When a client who has taken an oral anti-diabetic agent vomits, the nurse should monitor glucose and assess frequently for signs of hypoglycemia. Most of the medication has probably been absorbed. Therefore, repeating the dose would further lower glucose levels later in the day. Giving insulin will also lower glucose levels, causing hypoglycemia. The client wouldn't have hyperglycemia if the glyburide had been absorbed.
CN: Physiological integrity; CNS: Pharmacological therapies; CL: Analyze; DIFFICULTY: Challenge

5. 4. Type 2 diabetes is controlled primarily through diet, exercise, and oral antidiabetic agents. Desmopressin acetate, a long-acting vasopressin given intranasally, is the treatment of choice for diabetes insipidus. Treatment for diabetic ketoaci-dosis includes restoration of fluid volume, electro-lyte management, reversal of acidosis, and control of blood glucose. Diet and exercise are important in type 1 diabetes, but blood glucose levels are controlled by insulin injections in that disorder.
CN: Physiological integrity; CNS: Reduction of risk potential; CL: Apply; DIFFICULTY: Easy

6. 2. The client should eat before exercising to prevent hypoglycemia. Carbohydrate snacking may be necessary with prolonged exercise. Insulin should be given in the abdomen before exercise because it's more rapidly absorbed. Warming up is effective in any exercise plan.
CN: Physiological integrity; CNS: Physiological adaptation; CL: Apply; DIFFICULTY: Challenge

7. 2. Retinopathy, neuropathy, and coronary artery disease are all chronic complications of diabetes. Dizziness, dyspnea on exertion, and angina are symptoms of aortic valve stenosis. Leg ulcers, cerebral ischemic events, and pul-monary infarcts are complications of sickle cell anemia. Hyperparathyroidism causes fatigue, nausea, vomiting, muscle weakness, and cardiac dysrhythmias.
CN: Physiological integrity; CNS: Reduction of risk potential; CL: Apply; DIFFICULTY: Easy

8. When caring for a client with a diagnosis of type 2 diabetes mellitus, which diagnostic test(s) would the nurse anticipate being performed? Select all that apply.
1. Fasting blood glucose
2. Glycosylated hemoglobin
3. Pancreatic CT scan
4. Postprandial glucose
5. Cardiac catheterization

8. **1, 2, 4.** Screening for diabetes mellitus is relatively simple. Insulin resistance or insufficient insulin production is reflected in faulty glucose metabolism. Fasting blood glucose and postprandial glucose reflect current glucose levels. Glycosylated hemoglobin reflects average glucose levels over the preceding 120 days. Pancreatic CT scan does not assess diabetes mellitus. Cardiovascular complications may eventually necessitate cardiac catheterization; however, it is not a diagnostic test for diabetes mellitus.
CN: Physiological integrity; CNS: Reduction of risk potential; CL: Apply; DIFFICULTY: Challenge

9. After reinforcing education with a client about types of insulin, the nurse determines the teaching was successful when the client identifies which product as a long-acting insulin? Select all that apply.
1. Insulin aspart
2. Insulin glargine
3. Insulin detemir
4. Isophane insulin suspension
5. Insulin lispro

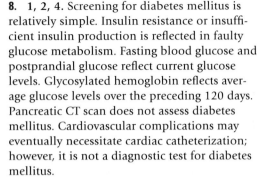

Does "hypo-" or "hyper-" thyroidism lead to weight gain?

9. **2, 3.** Insulin glargine and insulin detemir are long-acting insulins. Insulins aspart and lispro are rapid-acting insulins. Isophane insulin suspension is an intermediate-acting insulin.
CN: Physiological integrity; CNS: Pharmacological therapies; CL: Analyze; DIFFICULTY: Difficult

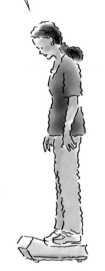

10. A client reports weight gain and tiredness. The nurse obtains data that reveal the following: blood pressure 120/74 mm Hg, pulse rate 52 beats/minute, respiratory rate 20 breaths/minute, and temperature 98° F. Laboratory results show low thyroxine (T4) and triiodothyronine (T3) levels. The nurse determines these symptoms are associated with which condition?
1. Tetany
2. Hypothyroidism
3. Hyperthyroidism
4. Hypokalemia

10. **2.** Weight gain, lethargy, and slow pulse rate along with decreased T3 and T4 levels indicate hypothyroidism. T3 and T4 are thyroid hormones that affect growth and development as well as metabolic rate. Tetany is related to low calcium levels. Hypokalemia is a low potassium level.
CN: Physiological integrity; CNS: Physiological adaptation; CL: Analyze; DIFFICULTY: Easy

11. A client is receiving isophane insulin suspension every morning. When would the nurse expect the client to possibly develop hypoglycemia?
1. 15 minutes to 1 hour
2. 2 to 6 hours
3. 4 to 12 hours
4. 14 to 26 hours

11. **3.** Isophane insulin suspension is an intermediate-acting insulin with a peak (when hypoglycemia is most likely to occur) of 4 to 12 hours. The onset of rapid-acting insulin is 15 minutes to 1 hour. The peak effect of rapid-acting insulin is 2 to 6 hours. Long-acting insulin has a peak effect of 14 to 26 hours.
CN: Physiological integrity; CNS: Pharmacological therapies; CL: Apply; DIFFICULTY: Difficult

12. Which medication would a nurse expect the health care provider to prescribe for a client with hypothyroidism?
1. Dexamethasone
2. Lactulose
3. Levothyroxine
4. Lidocaine

12. **3.** Levothyroxine, a synthetic form of the thyroid hormone thyroxine, is the medication of choice for treating hypothyroidism. Dexamethasone is a steroid and an antithyroid medication. Lactulose is a laxative used to treat constipation. Lidocaine is used to treat ventricular dysrhythmias.
CN: Physiological integrity; CNS: Pharmacological therapies; CL: Understand; DIFFICULTY: Easy

13. The nurse and a client have just discussed the client's recent diagnosis of hypothyroidism and its causes and effects. Which statement indicates that the client needs further instruction?
1. "Now I see. My clumsiness is caused by a hormone problem."
2. "I just eat too much. That's why I'm depressed and overweight."
3. "No wonder I'm constipated. I'm predisposed to it no matter what I eat."
4. "I'm not cold all the time because I'm getting older. I'm cold because of a metabolic problem."

14. A client with hypothyroidism who experiences trauma, emergency surgery, or severe infection is at risk for developing which condition?
1. Hepatitis B
2. Malignant hyperthermia
3. Myxedema coma
4. Thyroid storm

15. When caring for a client with hypothyroidism, what potentially serious complication should the nurse monitor the client for?
1. Acute hemolytic reaction
2. Angina or cardiac dysrhythmia
3. Retinopathy
4. Thrombocytopenia

16. A client is suspected of having hypothyroidism. Which diagnostic test would be **most** appropriate for the nurse to monitor?
1. Liver function studies
2. Hemoglobin A1c
3. Thyroxine (T4) and thyroid-stimulating hormone (TSH)
4. 24-hour urine for cortisol

17. The nurse is caring for a client with hypothyroidism. Which client data would the nurse expect to collect?
1. Polyuria, polydipsia, and weight loss
2. Heat intolerance, nervousness, weight loss, and hair loss
3. Coarsening of facial features and extremity enlargement
4. Tiredness, cold intolerance, weight gain, and constipation

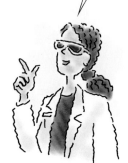

Keep your cool. You're doing just fine.

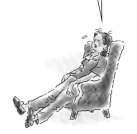

Uggh! I feel so "hypo" today. Maybe I should have my hormone levels checked out.

13. 2. Hypothyroidism results from an inadequate secretion of thyroid hormones, which slows metabolic processes and can cause depression and weight gain. A client with hypothyroidism who insists that overeating has caused depression and obesity needs further instruction about the effects of the disease. The other statements reflect an accurate understanding that hypothyroidism can cause clumsiness, constipation, and a feeling of coldness.
CN: Physiological integrity; CNS: Reduction of risk potential;
CL: Analyze; DIFFICULTY: Moderate

14. 3. Myxedema coma represents the most severe form of hypothyroidism. The client develops severe hypothermia and hypoglycemia and becomes comatose. Myxedema coma can be precipitated by opioids, stress (such as surgery), trauma, and infections. Hepatitis B is a virus and isn't caused by thyroid disorders. The client would be *hypo*thermic, not hyperthermic. Thyroid storm is a complication of hyperthyroidism.
CN: Physiological integrity; CNS: Reduction of risk potential;
CL: Apply; DIFFICULTY: Challenge

15. 2. Precipitation of angina or cardiac dysrhythmia is a potentially serious complication of hypothyroidism treatment, especially for older adult clients or those with underlying heart disease. Acute hemolytic reaction is a complication of blood transfusions. Retinopathy is usually a complication of diabetes. Thrombocytopenia is defined as a platelet count of less than 150,000/μL and doesn't result from treating hypothyroidism.
CN: Physiological integrity; CNS: Reduction of risk potential;
CL: Apply; DIFFICULTY: Moderate

16. 3. T4 and TSH are diagnostic tests for hypothyroidism. Liver function studies are indicated in many disorders to check for liver damage. Hemoglobin A1c measurement is used to assess hyperglycemia. Cortisol levels would be checked if adrenal insufficiency is suspected.
CN: Physiological integrity; CNS: Physiological adaptation;
CL: Analyze; DIFFICULTY: Easy

17. 4. Tiredness, cold intolerance, weight gain, and constipation are symptoms of hypothyroidism, secondary to a decrease in cellular metabolism. Polyuria, polydipsia, and weight loss are symptoms of type 1 diabetes. Hyperthyroidism has symptoms of heat intolerance, nervousness, weight loss, and hair loss. Coarsening of facial features and extremity enlargement are symptoms of acromegaly.
CN: Physiological integrity; CNS: Physiological adaptation;
CL: Understand; DIFFICULTY: Easy

18. After a client is admitted with an adrenal malfunction, the nurse demonstrates an understanding of the function of the adrenal gland by identifying which hormones as being released by the adrenal medulla?
1. Epinephrine and norepinephrine
2. Glucocorticoids, mineralocorticoids, and androgens
3. Thyroxine (T4), triiodothyronine (T3), and calcitonin
4. Insulin, glucagon, and somatostatin

19. When preparing a client scheduled for a thyroid function test, the nurse questions the client about medications. Which medications contain iodine and could alter the results?
1. Acetaminophen and aspirin
2. Estrogen and amphetamines
3. Insulin and oral antidiabetic agents
4. Topical antiseptics and multivitamins

20. While monitoring a client with hypothyroidism, which symptoms would the nurse anticipate observing?
1. Hypoactive bowel sounds
2. Hypertension
3. Photophobia
4. Flushed skin

21. A client with Cushing syndrome is admitted to the medical-surgical unit. When gathering data, the nurse notes that the client is agitated and irritable, has poor memory, reports loss of appetite, and is disheveled. The nurse recognizes that these signs and symptoms are associated with which condition?
1. Depression
2. Neuropathy
3. Hypoglycemia
4. Hyperthyroidism

22. After reinforcing education to a client on how to correctly self-administer daily maintenance dose of 3 units of regular insulin and 4 units of NPH insulin, which client statement demonstrates that the education has been successful?
1. "I'll check my blood sugar after breakfast and give myself shots in my stomach."
2. "After taking my insulin out of the refrigerator, I'll draw up the clear insulin first to the line for 3 units and then cloudy insulin until there's a total of 7 units in the syringe."
3. "First, I'll check my blood sugar; then I'll get the insulin from the refrigerator and withdraw 7 units."
4. "I should inject the insulin into a different site each time and then put it back in the pantry for safekeeping."

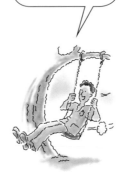

Looks like your knowledge is on the upswing. Well done!

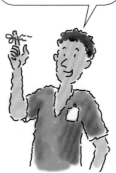

Hmm. What condition is associated with poor memory? I forget.

18. 1. The medulla of the adrenal gland causes the release of epinephrine and norepinephrine. Glucocorticoids, mineralocorticoids, and androgens are released from the adrenal cortex. T4, T3, and calcitonin are secreted by the thyroid gland. The islet cells of the pancreas secrete insulin, glucagon, and somatostatin.
CN: Physiological integrity; CNS: Physiological adaptation; CL: Understand; DIFFICULTY: Moderate

19. 4. Topical antiseptics and multivitamins contain iodine and can alter thyroid function test results. Estrogen and amphetamines don't contain iodine but may alter thyroid function test results. Insulin, oral antidiabetic agents, acetaminophen, and aspirin won't affect a thyroid test.
CN: Physiological integrity; CNS: Pharmacological therapies; CL: Analyze; DIFFICULTY: Moderate

20. 1. Hypothyroidism is associated with a general slowing of the body systems as indicated by hypoactive bowel sounds. The nurse would expect to find the client hypotensive, not hypertensive. Photophobia and flushed skin are symptoms associated with hyperthyroidism.
CN: Physiological integrity; CNS: Physiological adaptation; CL: Apply; DIFFICULTY: Moderate

21. 1. Agitation, irritability, poor memory, loss of appetite, and neglect of one's appearance may signal depression, which is common in clients with Cushing syndrome. Neuropathy affects clients with diabetes, not Cushing syndrome. Although hypoglycemia can cause irritability, it also produces increased appetite, rather than loss of appetite. Hyperthyroidism typically causes such signs as goiter, nervousness, heat intolerance, and weight loss despite increased appetite.
CN: Psychosocial integrity; CNS: None; CL: Analyze; DIFFICULTY: Difficult

22. 2. By indicating the proper dosage and order in which the insulin should be drawn, the client reveals a higher level of knowledge and demonstrates greater readiness to manage his care alone. The next step would be to ask him to demonstrate how an actual injection would be given. Blood sugar should be checked before meals, and insulin should be kept refrigerated. The statement by the client which indicates checking the blood sugar, then getting the insulin and withdrawing 7 units suggest that the client doesn't demonstrate an understanding of how the insulin is drawn into the syringe.
CN: Physiological integrity; CNS: Pharmacological therapies; CL: Analyze; DIFFICULTY: Easy

23. A client reports muscle weakness, anorexia, and darkening of the skin. The nurse reviews laboratory data and notes findings of low serum sodium and high serum potassium levels. The nurse recognizes these signs and symptoms as associated with which condition?
1. Addison disease
2. Cushing syndrome
3. Diabetes insipidus
4. Thyrotoxic crisis

24. A nurse is caring for a client following surgical ablation of the pituitary gland. Which condition must the nurse be alert for?
1. Addison disease
2. Cushing syndrome
3. Diabetes insipidus
4. Hypothyroidism

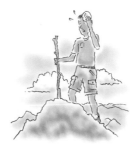

Keep on truckin'. The view from the top is worth it.

25. A client with diabetes insipidus has had limited fluid intake over the past 12 hours. Which complications should the nurse monitor the client for?
1. Hypertension and bradycardia
2. Glucosuria and weight gain
3. Peripheral edema and hyperglycemia
4. Severe dehydration and hypernatremia

Clients with diabetes insipidus have to pee a lot, which puts them at risk of dehydration. So, what should you encourage them to do?

26. When caring for a client with a diagnosis of diabetes insipidus, which nursing intervention should be the nurse's **priority**?
1. Watch for signs and symptoms of septic shock.
2. Maintain adequate fluid intake.
3. Check weight every 3 days.
4. Monitor urine for specific gravity greater than 1.030.

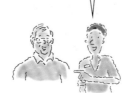

27. A client experiences polydipsia and voiding large amounts of waterlike urine with a specific gravity of 1.003. What do these clinical manifestations indicate to the nurse?
1. Diabetes
2. Diabetes insipidus
3. Diabetic ketoacidosis
4. Syndrome of inappropriate antidiuretic hormone (SIADH) secretion

23. 1. The clinical picture of Addison disease includes muscle weakness, anorexia, darkening of the skin's pigmentation, low sodium level, and high potassium level. Cushing syndrome involves obesity, "buffalo hump," "moonface," and thin extremities. Symptoms of diabetes insipidus include excretion of large volumes of dilute urine. Thyrotoxic crisis can occur with severe hyperthyroidism.
CN: Physiological integrity; CNS: Physiological adaptation; CL: Analyze; DIFFICULTY: Moderate

24. 3. The cause of diabetes insipidus is unknown, but it may be secondary to head trauma, brain tumors, or surgical ablation of the pituitary gland. Addison disease is caused by a deficiency of cortical hormones, whereas Cushing syndrome is an excess of cortical hormones. Hypothyroidism occurs when the thyroid gland secretes low levels of thyroid hormone.
CN: Physiological integrity; CNS: Physiological adaptation; CL: Analyze; DIFFICULTY: Difficult

25. 4. A client with diabetes insipidus has high volumes of urine, even without fluid replacement. Therefore, limiting fluid intake will cause severe dehydration and hypernatremia. A client undergoing a fluid deprivation test may experience tachycardia and hypotension. A client with diabetes insipidus will usually experience weight loss, and his urine won't contain glucose. Diabetes insipidus has no effect on blood glucose; therefore, the client wouldn't suffer from hyperglycemia. Peripheral edema isn't a symptom of diabetes insipidus.
CN: Physiological integrity; CNS: Physiological adaptation; CL: Analyze; DIFFICULTY: Easy

26. 2. In a client with diabetes insipidus, maintaining fluid intake is essential to prevent severe dehydration. The client is at risk for developing hypovolemic shock because of increased urine output. Weight should be measured on a daily basis to check for adequate fluid balance. Urine specific gravity should be monitored for low osmolality, generally less than 1.005, due to the body's inability to concentrate urine.
CN: Safe, effective care environment; CNS: Coordinated care; CL: Apply; DIFFICULTY: Moderate

27. 2. Diabetes insipidus is characterized by a great thirst (polydipsia) and large amounts of waterlike urine, which has a specific gravity of 1.001 to 1.005. Diabetes involves polydipsia, polyuria, and polyphagia, but the client also has hyperglycemia. Diabetic ketoacidosis involves weight loss, polyuria, and polydipsia, and the client has severe acidosis. A client with SIADH secretion can't excrete a dilute urine; he retains fluid and develops a sodium deficiency.
CN: Physiological integrity; CNS: Physiological adaptation; CL: Analyze; DIFFICULTY: Moderate

28. A client with a diagnosis of diabetes insipidus is being treated with desmopressin acetate. The client asks, "What is this medication?". What is the best response by the nurse?
1. A synthetic vasopressin
2. A hormone secreted by the adrenal gland
3. An antidiabetic agent
4. A type of insulin

29. The nurse is caring for a client with syndrome of inappropriate antidiuretic hormone secretion (SIADH). Which data would the nurse expect to collect? Select all that apply.
1. History of a head injury
2. Water retention
3. Excessive thirst
4. Weight loss
5. Oliguria

30. A client is diagnosed with diabetes insipidus. The nurse assists with the development of a care plan based on the understanding that which hormone is deficient?
1. Androgen
2. Epinephrine
3. Norepinephrine
4. Vasopressin

31. A client is suspected of having diabetes insipidus. For which diagnostic test should the nurse prepare the client?
1. Capillary blood glucose test
2. Fluid deprivation test
3. Serum ketone test
4. Urine glucose test

32. A nurse is reviewing data in the progress notes entry of a client with adrenocortical insufficiency (Addison disease). The client reports difficulties in the work environment and a recent upper respiratory infection. The nurse identifies the client as at risk for which condition?
1. Adrenal crisis
2. Diabetic ketoacidosis
3. Myxedema
4. Thyrotoxic crisis

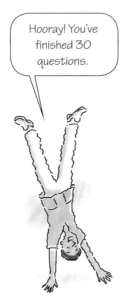

Hooray! You've finished 30 questions.

28. 1. Diabetes insipidus results from a deficiency of circulating antidiuretic hormone (vasopressin). Desmopressin acetate, a synthetic vasopressin, is the medication of choice for treating diabetes insipidus. Glucocorticoids are hormones secreted by the adrenal gland, which isn't involved with diabetes insipidus. Insulin and oral antidiabetic agents are used to treat diabetes, a disorder of glucose metabolism.
CN: Physiological integrity; CNS: Pharmacological therapies; CL: Apply; DIFFICULTY: Easy

29. 1, 2, 5. SIADH is a disorder of excessive antidiuretic hormone secretion by the posterior pituitary gland. Causes include lung tumors, CNS disorders, CVA, head trauma, and drugs such as vasopressin, general anesthetics, oral hypoglycemic, and tricyclic antidepressants. It is manifested by water retention, edema, and weight gain, not weight loss. Excessive thirst is a symptom of diabetes insipidus (DI), a disorder of insufficient ADH secretion.
CN: Physiological integrity; CNS: Physiological adaptation; CL: Analyze; DIFFICULTY: Challenge

30. 4. Clients with diabetes insipidus have a deficiency of vasopressin, the antidiuretic hormone. Androgen, epinephrine, and norepinephrine are hormones secreted by the adrenal gland and aren't related to diabetes insipidus.
CN: Physiological integrity; CNS: Physiological adaptation; CL: Apply; DIFFICULTY: Easy

31. 2. The fluid deprivation test involves withholding water for 4 to 18 hours and checking urine osmolality periodically. Plasma osmolality is also checked. A client with diabetes insipidus will have an increased serum osmolality (of less than 300 mOsm/kg). Urine osmolality won't increase. The capillary blood glucose test allows a rapid measurement of glucose in whole blood. The serum ketone test documents diabetic ketoacidosis. The urine glucose test monitors glucose levels in urine, but diabetes insipidus doesn't affect urine glucose levels.
CN: Physiological integrity; CNS: Reduction of risk potential; CL: Analyze; DIFFICULTY: Difficult

32. 1. As Addison disease progresses, the client may develop a life-threatening emergency—adrenal crisis, which is related to insufficient levels of cortisol, a hormone produced by the adrenal glands. The crisis occurs as a result of deterioration of the adrenal gland or inadequate treatment of adrenal insufficiency. Stress and infection can both necessitate a dose adjustment in corticosteroid therapy to prevent adrenal insufficiency and the development of adrenal crisis. Diabetic ketoacidosis is a form of hyperglycemia. Myxedema is a form of severe hypothyroidism. Thyrotoxic crisis is a form of severe hyperthyroidism.
CN: Physiological integrity; CNS: Physiological adaptation; CL: Analyze; DIFFICULTY: Easy

33. A client's laboratory findings indicating a deficiency of cortical hormones would correlate with which disease?
1. Addison disease
2. Cushing syndrome
3. Diabetes
4. Diabetic ketoacidosis

34. The nurse is caring for a client undergoing evaluation of endocrine function, and laboratory findings indicate excessive levels of adrenocortical hormones. This would correlate with which disease?
1. Addison disease
2. Cushing syndrome
3. Diabetes
4. Hypothyroidism

35. A nurse reviews the laboratory data of a client. The data reveals increased blood and urine levels of triiodothyronine (T3) and thyroxine (T4). The nurse determines these values are associated with which condition?
1. Addison disease
2. Cushing syndrome
3. Hyperthyroidism
4. Hypopituitarism

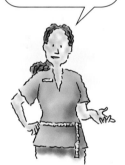

T3 and T4 are hormones secreted by the thyroid. So, increased levels would point to what condition?

36. The health care provider prescribes an oral antidiabetic medication and weekly glucose monitoring for a client who is overweight with a poor diet and stressful job, recently diagnosed with type 2 diabetes. The client asks the nurse how this will impact life. Which response is **most** appropriate?
1. "The medication will help maintain a steady glucose level, but you need to cut back on snacking."
2. "Type 2 diabetes is common and easily treated. You don't have to make changes."
3. "I'll refer you to a diabetes nurse specialist. She'll help you develop a plan."
4. "You may want to change careers because your job takes so much of your energy."

37. A nurse is caring for a client with syndrome of inappropriate antidiuretic hormone secretion (SIADH). The client becomes confused and develops crackles and dyspnea. What is the **priority** action of the nurse?
1. Administer an IV a diuretic.
2. Notify the health care provider.
3. Monitor serum sodium level.
4. Weigh the client.

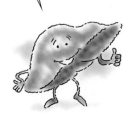

Great job answering these questions. You really know how to de-liver.

33. 1. Addison disease is caused by a deficiency of cortical hormones. Cushing syndrome is the opposite of Addison disease and includes excessive adrenocortical activity. Diabetes is an insulin deficiency. Diabetic ketoacidosis is severe hyperglycemia, causing acidosis.
CN: Physiological integrity; CNS: Physiological adaptation;
CL: Apply; DIFFICULTY: Moderate

34. 2. Cushing syndrome is indicated by excessive levels of adrenocortical hormones. Low levels of glucose and sodium, along with high levels of potassium and white blood cells, are diagnostic of Addison disease. Diabetes causes increased blood glucose levels. Hypothyroidism results in low levels of thyroid hormone.
CN: Physiological integrity; CNS: Physiological adaptation;
CL: Apply; DIFFICULTY: Challenge

35. 3. Hyperthyroidism causes high levels of T3 and T4. A definitive diagnosis of Addison disease must reflect low levels of adrenocortical hormones. Cushing syndrome manifests as excessive amounts of adrenocortical hormones. Lower pituitary hormone secretion levels are consistent with hypopituitarism.
CN: Physiological integrity; CNS: Physiological adaptation;
CL: Analyze; DIFFICULTY: Easy

36. 3. A referral to a nurse specialist who can develop an ongoing relationship with the client, spend more time assessing personal needs, and develop a workable plan would be most appropriate. Although the medication does help to maintain steady glucose levels, this response ignores the other factors contributing to the client's poor health habits. Telling the client that there will not be lifestyle changes is inappropriate, as is suggesting the client change careers.
CN: Health promotion and maintenance; CNS: None; CL: Apply;
DIFFICULTY: Easy

37. 2. Confusion and respiratory distress are indicators of fluid overload which can be a life-threatening complication of SIADH. The nurse notifies the health care provider immediately of a change in level of consciousness (LOC). The nurse cannot administer a diuretic without a health care provider's order. Weighing the client is not a priority. Hyponatremia does not manifest with these symptoms.
CN: Physiological integrity; CNS: Physiological adaptation;
CL: Analyze; DIFFICULTY: Moderate

38. The nurse is caring for a client admitted with a diagnosis of Addison disease. Which nursing intervention is most appropriate?
  1. Provide frequent rest periods.
  2. Administer diuretics.
  3. Encourage a high-potassium diet.
  4. Maintain fluid restrictions.

38. **1.** A client with Addison disease is dehydrated, hypotensive, and very weak. Frequent rest periods are needed to prevent exhausting the client. Diuretics would cause further dehydration and are contraindicated in a client with Addison disease. Potassium levels are usually elevated in Addison disease because aldosterone secretion is decreased, resulting in decreased sodium and increased potassium. Fluid intake would be encouraged, not restricted, in a dehydrated client.
CN: Physiological integrity; CNS: Physiological adaptation; CL: Analyze; DIFFICULTY: Moderate

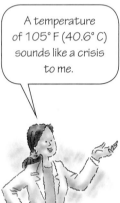

A temperature of 105° F (40.6° C) sounds like a crisis to me.

39. A client had a subtotal thyroidectomy in the early morning. During evening rounds, the nurse obtains data from the client, who now has nausea, a temperature of 105° F (40.6° C), tachycardia, and extreme restlessness. What's the **most** likely cause of these signs and symptoms?
  1. Diabetic ketoacidosis
  2. Thyroid crisis
  3. Hypoglycemia
  4. Tetany

39. **2.** Thyroid crisis usually occurs in the first 12 hours after thyroidectomy and causes exaggerated signs of hyperthyroidism, such as high fever, tachycardia, and extreme restlessness. Diabetic ketoacidosis is more likely to produce polyuria, polydipsia, and polyphagia. Hypoglycemia typically produces weakness, tremors, profuse perspiration, and hunger. Tetany typically causes uncontrollable muscle spasms, stridor, cyanosis, and possibly asphyxia.
CN: Physiological integrity; CNS: Physiological adaptation; CL: Apply; DIFFICULTY: Easy

40. A nurse can expect to see which signs and symptoms when a client overproduces adrenocortical hormone?
  1. Slow growth rate in children and obesity
  2. Weight loss and heat intolerance
  3. Changes in skin texture and low body temperature
  4. Polyuria and dehydration

40. **1.** Overproduction of adrenocortical hormone results in slow growth rate in children and obesity. Weight loss and heat intolerance indicate thyroid hormone overproduction. Changes in skin texture and low body temperature indicate thyroid hormone underproduction. Polyuria and dehydration indicate diabetic ketoacidosis.
CN: Physiological integrity; CNS: Physiological adaptation; CL: Apply; DIFFICULTY: Difficult

41. Observation of a client reveals thin extremities but an obese truncal area and a "buffalo hump" at the shoulder area with reports of weakness and disturbed sleep. The nurse interprets this data as indicating which disorder?
  1. Addison disease
  2. Cushing syndrome
  3. Graves disease
  4. Hyperparathyroidism

41. **2.** Clients with Cushing syndrome have truncal obesity with thin extremities and a fatty "buffalo hump" at the back of the neck. Clients with Addison disease show signs of weakness, anorexia, and dark pigmentation of the skin. Clients with Graves disease (hyperthyroidism) have symptoms of heat intolerance, irritability, and bulging eyes. Hyperparathyroidism is characterized by osteopenia and renal calculi.
CN: Physiological integrity; CNS: Physiological adaptation; CL: Analyze; DIFFICULTY: Easy

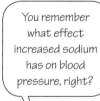

You remember what effect increased sodium has on blood pressure, right?

42. Sodium and water retention in a client with Cushing syndrome contributes to which commonly seen disorders?
  1. Hypoglycemia and dehydration
  2. Hypotension and hyperglycemia
  3. Pulmonary edema and dehydration
  4. Hypertension and heart failure

42. **4.** Increased mineralocorticoid activity in a client with Cushing syndrome commonly contributes to hypertension and heart failure. Hypoglycemia and dehydration are uncommon in a client with Cushing syndrome. Diabetes may develop, but hypotension isn't part of the disease process. Pulmonary edema and dehydration also aren't complications of Cushing syndrome.
CN: Physiological integrity; CNS: Physiological adaptation; CL: Analyze; DIFFICULTY: Moderate

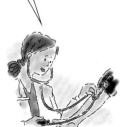

43. High serum sodium and glucose levels, low potassium level and eosinophil count, and disappearance of lymphoid tissue are associated with which disease process?
   1. Addison disease
   2. Cushing syndrome
   3. Graves disease
   4. Myxedema

43. 2. Test results in Cushing syndrome include high serum sodium and glucose levels, low potassium level, reduction of eosinophils, and disappearance of lymphoid tissue. Addison disease is the opposite of Cushing syndrome, with low serum sodium and glucose levels and a high potassium level. Graves disease causes increased thyroid hormone levels. Myxedema results in low levels of thyroid hormones.
CN: Physiological integrity; CNS: Physiological adaptation; CL: Analyze; DIFFICULTY: Moderate

44. A client presents with a "buffalo hump" at the shoulder area and an obese truncal area with thin extremities. Which test should the nurse anticipate?
   1. Fluid deprivation test
   2. Glucose tolerance test
   3. Low-dose dexamethasone suppression test
   4. Thallium stress test

44. 3. A low-dose dexamethasone suppression test is used to detect changes in plasma cortisol levels. A fluid deprivation test is used to diagnosis diabetes insipidus. The glucose tolerance test is used to determine gestational diabetes in pregnant women. A thallium stress test is used to monitor heart function under stress.
CN: Physiological integrity; CNS: Physiological adaptation; CL: Analyze; DIFFICULTY: Moderate

45. A client with adrenocortical hyperfunction has returned to the nursing unit after bilateral adrenalectomy. What are the nurse's priorities when caring for this client? Select all that apply.
   1. Administer prescribed corticosteroids as ordered.
   2. Observe closely for signs and symptoms of acute adrenal crisis.
   3. Maintain strict aseptic technique during dressing changes.
   4. Weigh the client prior to administering corticosteroids.
   5. Administer analgesics only for severe pain.

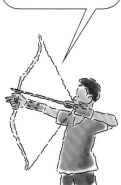

Aim for success ... it makes it a lot easier to hit it.

45. 1, 2, 3. Bilateral adrenalectomy results in acute adrenal insufficiency that is treated by corticosteroid replacement. It is critical that supplemental corticosteroids be administered in the right dose and time. The client needs to be monitored closely for signs and symptoms of adrenal crisis, which may occur if the prescribed corticosteroid dose is inadequate or the prescribed dose is not administered. Aseptic technique is critical due to immunosuppression secondary to steroid therapy. Weighing the client before a corticosteroid dose is not necessary. Pain management before it becomes severe is indicated.
CN: Physiological integrity; CNS: Reduction of risk potential; CL: Analyze; DIFFICULTY: Difficult

46. The nurse is caring for a client with hypoparathyroidism. During data collection, the nurse taps the client's face 2 cm anterior to the earlobe. The nurse is attempting to elicit which of the following?
   1. Trousseau sign
   2. Chadwick sign
   3. Hegar sign
   4. Chvostek sign

46. 4. Spasms of the facial nerve when tapped (positive Chvostek sign) is indication of hypocalcemia, which is a component of hypoparathyroidism. Trousseau sign is also indicative of hypocalcemia, but is not assessed in this manner. Chadwick sign and Hegar sign are changes to the cervix and vagina noted in pregnancy.
CN: Physiological integrity; CNS: Reduction of risk potential; CL: Analyze; DIFFICULTY: Easy

47. Which nursing intervention should be performed for a client with Cushing syndrome?
   1. Suggest clothing or bedding that feel cool and comfortable.
   2. Suggest consumption of high-carbohydrate and low-protein foods.
   3. Explain that physical changes are a result of excessive corticosteroids.
   4. Explain the rationale for increasing salt and fluid intake in times of illness, increased stress, and very hot weather.

47. 3. Clients with Cushing syndrome have physical changes related to excessive corticosteroids. Clients with hyperthyroidism are heat intolerant and must have comfortable, cool clothing and bedding. Clients with Cushing syndrome should eat a high-protein, not a low-protein, diet. Clients with Addison disease must increase sodium intake and fluid intake in times of stress to prevent hypotension.
CN: Physiological integrity; CNS: Physiological adaptation; CL: Apply; DIFFICULTY: Moderate

48. A client was recently admitted with a diagnosis of diabetes. The nurse observes that the client has acetone breath, a weak and rapid pulse, and Kussmaul respirations. The nurse recognizes that interventions should be provided for what condition?
1. Hypoglycemia
2. Diabetes insipidus
3. Diabetic ketoacidosis
4. Hyperosmolar hyperglycemic nonketotic syndrome (HHNS)

49. The nurse is caring for a client with type 1 diabetes who does not adhere to an insulin regimen regularly. The nurse identifies that the client is at risk for which complication?
1. Diabetic ketoacidosis
2. Hypoglycemia
3. Pancreatitis
4. Respiratory failure

50. A client with diabetes exhibits polyphagia, polydipsia, and oliguria; and also reports headache, malaise, and some vision changes with signs of dehydration present. Which condition does the nurse determine correlates with these symptoms?
1. Diabetes insipidus
2. Diabetic ketoacidosis
3. Hypoglycemia
4. Syndrome of inappropriate antidiuretic hormone (SIADH) secretion

51. The nurse is caring for a client with a history of hypothyroidism. Which clinical manifestations would indicate to the nurse the progression to myxedemic crisis? Select all that apply.
1. Hypothermia
2. Hypoglycemia
3. Hypotension
4. Hypoventilation
5. Irritability

52. The nurse is collecting data from an older adult client being screened for hypothyroidism. Which statement by the nurse demonstrates understanding of the effects of aging?
1. "Thyroid disorders are rare in the older adult population."
2. "Hypothyroidism can be difficult to diagnose in older adults because symptoms may resemble normal aging."
3. "Older adults diagnosed with hypothyroidism require larger doses of thyroid replacement."
4. "Older adults receiving thyroid replacement drugs have a decreased risk of adverse reactions."

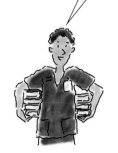
Looks like I need to read up on the symptoms described in question #48.

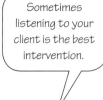
Sometimes listening to your client is the best intervention.

48. 3. Diabetic ketoacidosis is caused by inadequate amounts of insulin or absence of insulin, and leads to a series of biochemical disorders. Dizziness, slow cerebration, and tachycardia are signs and symptoms of hypoglycemia; extreme polyuria and dehydration indicate diabetes insipidus; and polyuria, thirst, neurologic abnormalities, and stupor are signs and symptoms of HHNS.
CN: Physiological integrity; CNS: Physiological adaptation; CL: Apply; DIFFICULTY: Easy

49. 1. A client with type I diabetes who fails to regularly take his insulin is at risk for hyperglycemia, which could lead to diabetic ketoacidosis. Hypoglycemia wouldn't occur because the lack of insulin would lead to increased levels of sugar in the blood. A client with chronic pancreatitis may develop diabetes (secondary to the pancreatitis), but insulin-dependent diabetes doesn't lead to pancreatitis. Respiratory failure isn't related to insulin levels.
CN: Physiological integrity; CNS: Physiological adaptation; CL: Apply; DIFFICULTY: Easy

50. 2. Early manifestations of diabetic ketoacidosis include polydipsia, polyphagia, and polyuria. As the client dehydrates and loses electrolytes, this condition commonly leads to oliguria, malaise, vision changes, and headache. Diabetes insipidus may result in dehydration but not in polyphagia and polydipsia. Symptoms of hypoglycemia include diaphoresis, tachycardia, and nervousness. A client with SIADH secretion can't excrete a dilute urine, causing hypernatremia.
CN: Physiological integrity; CNS: Physiological adaptation; CL: Apply; DIFFICULTY: Moderate

51. 1, 2, 3, 4. Myxedemic crisis or coma is a life-threatening event of severe hypothyroidism. Signs are hypothermia, hypotension, hypoglycemia, and hypoventilation. Irritability is seen in *hyper*thyroidism.
CN: Physiological integrity; CNS: Reduction of risk potential; CL: Apply; DIFFICULTY: Difficult

52. 2. Hypothyroidism is more difficult to diagnose in the aging population because many of the symptoms closely resemble normal aging and other chronic diseases. Dosages of thyroid replacement drugs are lower in older adults. Therapy is initiated more slowly and doses are increased with caution. Older adults have an increased risk of adverse reactions associated with cardiac function.
CN: Health promotion and maintenance; CNS: None; CL: Analyze; DIFFICULTY: Easy

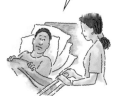

53. The nurse is reinforcing education with a client who has hypothyroidism about the thyroid gland. Which statement by the nurse would be **most** accurate about which gland controls the secretion of thyroid hormone?
1. Adrenal gland
2. Parathyroid gland
3. Pituitary gland
4. Thyroid gland

54. When assisting with the development of a care plan for a client with hyperthyroidism, the nurse would anticipate which treatment?
1. Cholelithotomy
2. Irradiation of the thyroid
3. Administration of oral thyroid hormones
4. Whipple procedure

55. The nurse is gathering data from an older adult client. Which symptoms of hyperthyroidism does the nurse determine will be found?
1. Depression, apathy, and weight loss
2. Palpitations, irritability, and heat intolerance
3. Cold intolerance, weight gain, and thinning hair
4. Numbness, tingling, and cramping of extremities

56. A client with hyperthyroidism develops high fever, extreme tachycardia, and altered mental status. Which condition does the nurse suspect is developing?
1. Hepatic coma
2. Thyroid storm
3. Myxedema coma
4. Hyperosmolar hyperglycemic nonketotic syndrome (HHNS)

57. A client is admitted with Graves disease. Which laboratory test should the nurse expect to be ordered?
1. Serum glucose
2. Serum calcium
3. Lipid panel
4. Thyroid panel

53. 3. By secreting TSH, the pituitary gland controls the rate of thyroid hormone released. The adrenal gland isn't involved in the release of thyroid hormone. The parathyroid gland secretes parathyroid hormones, depending on the levels of calcium and phosphorus in the blood. The thyroid gland secretes thyroid hormone but doesn't control how much is released.
CN: Physiological integrity; CNS: Physiological adaptation; CL: Apply; DIFFICULTY: Challenge

54. 2. Irradiation, involving the administration of 131I, destroys the thyroid gland, thereby treating hyperthyroidism. Cholelithotomy is used to treat gallstones. Oral thyroid hormones are the treatment for hypothyroidism. The Whipple procedure is a surgical treatment for pancreatic cancer.
CN: Physiological integrity; CNS: Pharmacological therapies; CL: Apply; DIFFICULTY: Challenge

55. 1. Most older adult clients demonstrate depression, apathy, and weight loss, which are typical signs and symptoms of hyperthyroidism. Palpitations, irritability, and heat intolerance can be present with hyperthyroidism, but these aren't typical symptoms in older adult clients. Cold intolerance, weight gain, and thinning hair are some of the signs of hypothyroidism. Numbness, tingling, and cramping of extremities are symptoms of hypocalcemia, which may be a symptom of hypoparathyroidism.
CN: Physiological integrity; CNS: Physiological adaptation; CL: Remember; DIFFICULTY: Challenge

56. 2. Thyroid storm is a form of severe hyperthyroidism that can be precipitated by stress, injury, or infection. Hepatic coma occurs in clients with profound liver failure. Myxedema coma is a rare disorder characterized by hypoventilation, hypotension, hypoglycemia, and hypothyroidism. HHNS occurs in clients with type 2 diabetes who are dehydrated and have severe hyperglycemia.
CN: Physiological integrity; CNS: Physiological adaptation; CL: Analyze; DIFFICULTY: Easy

57. 4. Graves disease is also known as hyperthyroidism. The nurse should expect a thyroid panel to be ordered.
CN: Physiological integrity; CNS: Physiological adaptation; CL: Apply; DIFFICULTY: Easy

58. The nurse is caring for a client receiving radio-active iodine (I-131) treatment for thyroid cancer. Which teaching should the nurse reinforce with this client to reduce exposure of family members? Select all that apply.
1. Wash hands carefully after using the bathroom.
2. Wear clothing that covers the throat.
3. Prepare food separately from family members.
4. Flush the toilet several times after use.
5. Avoid sexual contact and kissing.

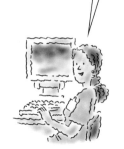

Remember to "select all that apply" in question #58.

58. 1, 4, 5. Radioactive iodine (I-131) is a form of systemic internal radiation therapy that is primarily excreted in urine, but also in saliva, sweat, and feces. I-131 has a half-life of approximately 8 days, so precautions should be followed for that period of time. Precautions include: washing hands after using the toilet, flushing the toilet at least twice after use, and avoiding kissing and sexual contact. Food does not need to be prepared separately, but separate utensils should be used. Covering the throat with clothing does not reduce exposure because effects are systemic.
CN: Safe, effective care environment; CNS: Safety and infection control; CL: Apply; DIFFICULTY: Difficult

59. A client has flushed skin, bulging eyes, and perspiration, and states he has been "irritable" and having palpitations. Which interpretation of these findings might the nurse suspect?
1. Hyperthyroidism
2. Myocardial infarction (MI)
3. Pancreatitis
4. Type 1 diabetes

59. 1. Signs and symptoms of hyperthyroidism include nervousness, palpitations, irritability, bulging eyes, heat intolerance, weight loss, and weakness. MI usually involves chest pain, which may radiate to the arms, back, or neck, and shortness of breath. Pancreatitis involves severe abdominal pain and back tenderness. Type 1 diabetes involves polyuria, polydipsia, and weight loss.
CN: Physiological integrity; CNS: Physiological adaptation; CL: Analyze; DIFFICULTY: Easy

60. Which technique should the nurse use to prevent the development of lipodystrophy when administering insulin to a client with diabetes?
1. Grasp the skin tightly.
2. Rotate injection sites.
3. Massage the site vigorously.
4. Inject into the deltoid muscle.

60. 2. The nurse should rotate insulin injection sites systematically to minimize tissue damage, promote absorption, avoid discomfort, and prevent lipodystrophy. Grasping the skin tightly can traumatize the skin; therefore, the nurse should hold it gently but firmly when giving an injection. Massaging the site vigorously is contraindicated because it hastens insulin absorption, which isn't recommended. Usually, insulin is administered subcutaneously, rather than into a muscle, because muscular activity increases insulin absorption.
CN: Physiological integrity; CNS: Pharmacological therapies; CL: Apply; DIFFICULTY: Easy

61. A client is brought into the emergency department with a brain stem contusion. Two days after admission, the client has a large amount of urine output and a serum sodium level of 155 mEq/dL. Which condition does the nurse suspect may be developing?
1. Myxedema coma
2. Diabetes insipidus
3. Type 1 diabetes
4. Syndrome of inappropriate antidiuretic hormone (SIADH) secretion

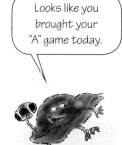

Looks like you brought your "A" game today.

61. 2. Two leading causes of diabetes insipidus are hypothalamic or pituitary tumors and closed-head injuries. Myxedema coma is a form of hypothyroidism. Type 1 diabetes isn't caused by a brain injury. A client with SIADH secretion would have symptoms of hyponatremia; this client's sodium level was 155 mEq/dL, which is above the normal levels of 135 to 145 mEq/dL.
CN: Physiological integrity; CNS: Physiological adaptation; CL: Apply; DIFFICULTY: Challenge

62. A client with a history of diabetes has serum ketones and a serum glucose level above 300 mg/dL. Which condition does the nurse expect is the cause?
1. Diabetes insipidus
2. Diabetic ketoacidosis
3. Hypoglycemia
4. Somogyi phenomenon

62. 2. Clients with serum ketones and serum glucose levels above 300 mg/dL could be diagnosed with diabetic ketoacidosis. Diabetes insipidus is an overproduction of antidiuretic hormone and doesn't create ketones in the blood. Hypoglycemia causes low blood glucose levels. The Somogyi phenomenon is rebound hyperglycemia following an episode of hypoglycemia.
CN: Physiological integrity; CNS: Physiological adaptation; CL: Analyze; DIFFICULTY: Easy

63. The nurse is caring for a client that developed ketoacidosis. Which prescribed treatment does the nurse anticipate administering?
1. Glucagon
2. Blood products
3. Glucocorticoids
4. Insulin and IV fluids

63. 4. A client with diabetic ketoacidosis would receive insulin to lower glucose and would receive IV fluids to correct hypotension. Glucagon is given to treat hypoglycemia; diabetic ketoacidosis involves hyperglycemia. Blood products aren't needed to correct diabetic ketoacidosis. Glucocorticoids are unnecessary because the adrenal glands aren't involved.
CN: Physiological integrity; CNS: Pharmacological therapies; CL: Apply; DIFFICULTY: Easy

64. Which method of insulin administration would a nurse expect to be used in the initial treatment of hyperglycemia in a client with diabetic ketoacidosis?
1. Subcutaneous
2. IM
3. IV bolus only
4. IV bolus, followed by continuous infusion

64. 4. An IV bolus of insulin is given initially to control the hyperglycemia, followed by a continuous infusion, titrated to control blood glucose. After the client is stabilized, subcutaneous insulin is given. Insulin is never given IM.
CN: Physiological integrity; CNS: Pharmacological therapies; CL: Apply; DIFFICULTY: Moderate

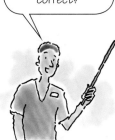

In other words, which statement by the client in question #65 is correct?

65. The health care provider has ordered a check of glycosylated hemoglobin (HbA1c) levels for a client with diabetes. Which statement by the client regarding this test indicates that education has been effective?
1. "It's used to monitor the control of my disease."
2. "It's used to diagnose diabetes."
3. "It's useful in determining if I have anemia."
4. "It reflects the average blood glucose level for the previous 3 weeks."

65. 1. The HbA1c test is used to gather data and to monitor progress of diabetes control. It isn't used to diagnose diabetes or anemia. Red blood cells live in the body for about 3 months. When the glucose that's attached to the hemoglobin is measured, it reflects the average blood glucose level for the previous 2 to 3 months.
CN: Physiological integrity; CNS: Physiological adaptation; CL: Apply; DIFFICULTY: Moderate

66. Which combination of adverse effects should the nurse carefully monitor when administering IV insulin to a client diagnosed with diabetic ketoacidosis?
1. Hypokalemia and hypoglycemia
2. Hypocalcemia and hyperkalemia
3. Hyperkalemia and hyperglycemia
4. Hypernatremia and hypercalcemia

66. 1. Blood glucose must be monitored because there's a chance for hypokalemia or hypoglycemia. Hypokalemia might occur because IV insulin forces potassium into cells, thereby lowering the plasma levels of potassium. Hypoglycemia might occur if too much insulin is administered. The client with diabetic ketoacidosis wouldn't have hyperkalemia. Calcium and sodium levels aren't affected.
CN: Physiological integrity; CNS: Pharmacological therapies; CL: Apply; DIFFICULTY: Moderate

67. The nurse is caring for a client with acromegaly. The client asks the nurse to explain the difference between acromegaly and gigantism. The nurse differentiates between the two with what statement?
1. "Acromegaly is an endocrine disorder of the pituitary gland and gigantism is a disorder of the musculoskeletal system."
2. "Acromegaly affects primarily children and young adults and gigantism affects the aging population."
3. "Both are characterized by excessive growth hormone production; acromegaly occurs after puberty and gigantism before puberty."
4. "Acromegaly and gigantism are actually terms that are used interchangeably to refer to the same condition of excessive growth hormone secretion."

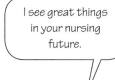

I see great things in your nursing future.

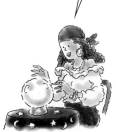

67. 3. Acromegaly and gigantism are both pituitary disorders characterized by excessive production of growth hormone (GH). Acromegaly is the excessive production of GH after the epiphyseal plates have closed (after puberty) and gigantism is excessive production of growth hormone prior to closure of the epiphyseal plates. The terms are not interchangeable.
CN: Physiological integrity; CNS: Physiological adaptation; CL: Apply; DIFFICULTY: Moderate

68. The nurse is caring for a client with diabetes. Which statement by the client demonstrates an understanding of foot care education instructions related to his diabetes? Select all that apply.
1. "I should cut my toenails once a week."
2. "I should never go barefoot."
3. "I should wash with very hot water and dry my feet well."
4. "I should inspect the skin on my feet every week for open areas."
5. "I should apply moisturizer to my feet every day."
6. "I should wear cotton socks."

69. A client with diabetes who had a stroke has right-sided paralysis and incontinence and is in the rehabilitation center. Which action should be the nurse's **priority** in caring for the client?
1. Apply body powder every 4 hours to keep the client dry.
2. To conserve energy, maintain bed rest when the client isn't in therapy.
3. Insert an indwelling urinary catheter to keep the client continent.
4. Wash the client's skin with soap and water, gently patting it dry.

70. An older adult client who has been on long-term steroid therapy now has drug-induced Cushing syndrome. Which condition does the nurse determine closely relates to chronic steroid use?
1. Periods of hypoglycemia
2. Periods of euphoria
3. Thin, easily damaged skin
4. Weight loss

71. A nurse is collecting data on a client with possible hyperaldosteronism. Which nursing intervention is the **priority**?
1. Monitoring blood glucose levels
2. Auscultating for breath sounds
3. Monitoring arterial blood gas (ABG) levels
4. Weighing the client weekly

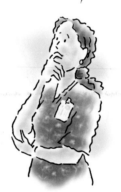

Let's see. A diabetic client who is confined to bed and incontinent would be at risk for skin breakdown and infection. Which intervention would best prevent this?

68. 2, 5, 6. The client with diabetes is prone to the development of foot problems, such as ulcers and infection, due to the combination of vascular disease and neuropathy. Daily moisturizer should be applied to prevent drying and cracking. Going barefoot subjects the feet to potential injury. Cotton socks worn with leather shoes keep the feet dry and protected from injury. A podiatrist should routinely examine the feet, and cut the nails as needed. Washing with hot water can result in burns; using lukewarm water is recommended. Visual inspection of the feet should be performed daily.
CN: Physiological integrity; CNS: Reduction of risk potential; CL: Apply; DIFFICULTY: Challenge

69. 4. The skin of a diabetic client should be kept dry to prevent breakdown and infection. The nurse should avoid excessive use of powders, which can cake with perspiration and cause irritation. Clients undergoing rehabilitation should be upright in a chair, except for short rest periods during the day, to promote optimal recovery. Clients with diabetes are especially prone to infections. Urinary tract infections are commonly caused by the use of indwelling catheters. Other methods should be used to encourage continence.
CN: Safe, effective care environment; CNS: Coordinated care; CL: Apply; DIFFICULTY: Moderate

70. 3. Clients taking steroids on a long-term basis lose subcutaneous fat under the skin and are especially vulnerable to skin breakdown and bruising. Such clients should take great care when performing tasks that may injure the skin, and should anticipate delayed healing when injuries occur. Clients taking long-term steroids are likely to have hyperglycemia. Prolonged steroid use can cause depression. Clients who experience weight loss should be monitored for weight gain and edema.
CN: Physiological integrity; CNS: Pharmacological therapies; CL: Apply; DIFFICULTY: Moderate

71. 2. Aldosterone is secreted by the adrenal cortex. One of its major functions is causing the kidneys to retain saline in the body. A client with hyperaldosteronism should be observed for signs of respiratory distress, crackles, and the use of accessory muscles. Blood glucose and ABG levels aren't immediate priorities when assessing a client with hyperaldosteronism. Rapid weight gain can indicate fluid volume excess, but the client should be weighed *daily*, not weekly.
CN: Safe, effective care environment; CNS: Coordinated care; CL: Apply; DIFFICULTY: Difficult

72. The nurse is caring for a client with acute hypoparathyroidism. What are the priority nursing interventions for this client? Select all that apply.
1. Keep noise and movement to a minimum.
2. Assess Trousseau sign.
3. Observe for development of renal calculi by straining the urine.
4. Insert an IV line for emergency administration of calcium.
5. Keep emergency intubation equipment at the bedside.

> Emergencies are the mother of all priorities.

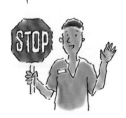

72. 1, 2, 4, 5. In acute hypoparathyroidism there is decreased serum calcium levels that put the client at risk for tetany, convulsions, and laryngeal spasms. The nurse observes for neuromuscular irritability by assessing Chvostek and Trousseau signs. The environment must be kept quiet and nondisruptive to prevent convulsions. Emergency intubation/mechanical ventilation equipment should be kept at the bedside in case laryngeal spasms occur and the client's respiratory status is compromised. An IV line needs to be in place for the emergency administration of a calcium salt. Renal calculi may develop in *hyper*parathyroidism, not hypoparathyroidism.
CN: Physiological integrity; CNS: Physiological adaptation; CL: Analyze; DIFFICULTY: Difficult

73. A client with hyperparathyroidism develops renal calculi. The nurse should expect to see which electrolyte levels?
1. Decreased calcium levels
2. Increased calcium levels
3. Increased potassium levels
4. Increased magnesium levels

73. 2. Renal calculi usually consist of calcium and phosphorus. In hyperparathyroidism, serum calcium levels are high, leading to renal calculi formation. Potassium and magnesium don't form renal calculi, and levels of these minerals aren't high in clients with hyperparathyroidism.
CN: Physiological integrity; CNS: Physiological adaptation; CL: Apply; DIFFICULTY: Easy

74. The nurse is caring for a client with suspected parathyroid dysfunction. Which laboratory results support a diagnosis of primary hyperparathyroidism?
1. High parathyroid hormone and high calcium levels
2. High magnesium and high thyroid hormone levels
3. Low parathyroid hormone and low potassium levels
4. Low thyroid-stimulating hormone (TSH) and high phosphorus levels

74. 1. A diagnosis of primary hyperparathyroidism is established based on increased serum calcium levels and elevated parathyroid hormone levels. Potassium, magnesium, TSH, and thyroid hormone levels aren't used to diagnose hyperparathyroidism.
CN: Physiological integrity; CNS: Physiological adaptation; CL: Apply; DIFFICULTY: Easy

> Which drug class in question #75 might actually worsen the effects of hyperparathyroidism?

75. The nurse is caring for a client with hyperparathyroidism. Which classification of drug, if prescribed for this client, would the nurse question prior to administration?
1. Nonsteroidal anti-inflammatory drugs (NSAIDs)
2. Salicylates
3. Potassium-wasting diuretics
4. Thiazide diuretics

75. 4. Thiazide diuretics shouldn't be used because they decrease renal excretion of calcium, thereby raising serum calcium levels even higher. There are no contraindications to NSAIDs or salicylates for clients with hyperparathyroidism. Potassium loss isn't an issue for clients with hyperparathyroidism.
CN: Physiological integrity; CNS: Pharmacological therapies; CL: Apply; DIFFICULTY: Difficult

76. In clients with hyperparathyroidism, which calcium level would indicate to the nurse an acute hypercalcemic crisis?
1. 2 mg/dL
2. 4 mg/dL
3. 10.5 mg/dL
4. 15 mg/dL

76. 4. Normal calcium levels are 8.5 to 10.5 mg/dL, so a level of 15 mg/dL is dangerously high.
CN: Physiological integrity; CNS: Physiological adaptation; CL: Remember; DIFFICULTY: Easy

77. A nurse reviewing the laboratory results on a client's chart notes findings of increased serum phosphate levels and decreased serum calcium levels. These findings indicate which condition?
1. Cushing syndrome
2. Graves disease
3. Hypoparathyroidism
4. Hypothyroidism

78. A client is admitted with hypoparathyroidism. When collecting data on the client, the nurse should expect to see which sign or symptom?
1. Chest pain
2. Exophthalmos
3. Shortness of breath
4. Hand twitching

79. A client is receiving oral calcium supplements. Which additional vitamin would the nurse encourage the client to consume to enhance absorption of calcium from the GI tract?
1. Vitamin A
2. Vitamin C
3. Vitamin D
4. Vitamin E

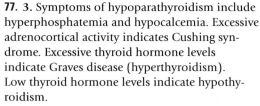

Which vitamin is calcium's best buddy?

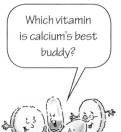

80. A nurse is caring for a client who had a subtotal thyroidectomy to treat hyperthyroidism. Which sign or symptom could indicate bleeding at the incision site?
1. Hoarseness
2. Severe stridor
3. Client reports a tight dressing.
4. Difficulty swallowing

81. A client is diagnosed with pituitary gigantism. Hypersecretion of which hormone would cause this condition?
1. Follicle-stimulating hormone (FSH)
2. Growth hormone (GH)
3. Parathyroid hormone (PTH)
4. Thyroid-stimulating hormone (TSH)

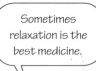

Sometimes relaxation is the best medicine.

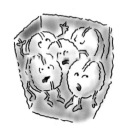

82. The nurse is caring for a client diagnosed with hyperthyroidism. Which nursing intervention should be the **priority** to decrease the client's anxiety?
1. Keeping the client warm
2. Encouraging the client to increase activity
3. Providing a calm, restful environment
4. Placing the client in semi-Fowler position

77. 3. Symptoms of hypoparathyroidism include hyperphosphatemia and hypocalcemia. Excessive adrenocortical activity indicates Cushing syndrome. Excessive thyroid hormone levels indicate Graves disease (hyperthyroidism). Low thyroid hormone levels indicate hypothyroidism.
CN: Physiological integrity; CNS: Physiological adaptation; CL: Analyze; DIFFICULTY: Moderate

78. 4. Tetany, which is manifested by muscle twitching or spasms, is the chief symptom of hypoparathyroidism. Chest pain and shortness of breath aren't usually symptoms of hypoparathyroidism. Exophthalmos, or bulging eyes, is a common symptom of hyperthyroidism.
CN: Physiological integrity; CNS: Physiological adaptation; CL: Apply; DIFFICULTY: Moderate

79. 3. Variable doses of vitamin D preparations enhance the absorption of calcium from the GI tract. Vitamins A, C, and E aren't involved in this process.
CN: Physiological integrity; CNS: Pharmacological therapies; CL: Apply; DIFFICULTY: Easy

80. 3. Reports of a tight dressing indicate postoperative bleeding. Hoarseness or severe stridor indicates damage to the laryngeal nerve. Difficulty swallowing doesn't indicate postoperative bleeding.
CN: Physiological integrity; CNS: Physiological adaptation; CL: Apply; DIFFICULTY: Difficult

81. 2. Hypersecretion of growth hormone causes pituitary gigantism. FSH is involved in the development of ovaries and sperm. Hypersecretion of parathyroid hormone would cause hyperparathyroidism. Hypersecretion of TSH would cause hyperthyroidism.
CN: Physiological integrity; CNS: Physiological adaptation; CL: Understand; DIFFICULTY: Easy

82. 3. Clients with hyperthyroidism are typically anxious, diaphoretic, nervous, and fatigued; they need a calm, restful environment in which to relax and get adequate rest. Clients with hyperthyroidism are usually warm and need a cool environment. Activity shouldn't be increased. If a client is exhibiting dyspnea, he would benefit from high Fowler position.
CN: Safe, effective care environment; CNS: Coordinated care; CL: Apply; DIFFICULTY: Easy

83. A nurse is reinforcing education with a client about insulin. The health care provider has ordered "Regular insulin 6 units U100." Which statement by the client indicates that the education has been effective? Select all that apply.
1. "The insulin is cloudy."
2. "The insulin vial should be shaken vigorously before drawing it into the syringe."
3. "'U100' means that there are 100 units in each milliliter of the insulin and that 6 units are to be administered."
4. "I should rotate my injection sites to prevent damage to the tissue and poor absorption of the insulin."
5. "The insulin should be drawn up in a tuberculin syringe."

83. 3, 4. There are 100 units of insulin in each milliliter of U100 insulin, and it should be drawn up in a U100 syringe (orange needle cap). Six units are to be administered. Subcutaneous injection sites require rotation to avoid breakdown and/or buildup of subcutaneous fat, either of which can interfere with insulin absorption in the tissue. Regular insulin is clear. Cloudy insulin has a zinc precipitate that must be evenly distributed in the solution. Insulin vials should be rolled in the hands to mix, not shaken vigorously. Insulin syringes are the only type of syringe used for drawing up insulin.
CN: Physiological integrity; CNS: Pharmacological therapies; CL: Apply; DIFFICULTY: Moderate

84. After undergoing a thyroidectomy, a client develops hypocalcemia and tetany. Which medication should the nurse anticipate administering?
1. Calcium gluconate
2. Potassium chloride
3. Sodium bicarbonate
4. Sodium phosphorus

84. 1. Immediate treatment for a client who develops hypocalcemia and tetany after thyroidectomy is calcium gluconate. Potassium chloride and sodium bicarbonate aren't indicated. Sodium phosphorus wouldn't be given because phosphorus levels are already elevated.
CN: Physiological integrity; CNS: Pharmacological therapies; CL: Apply; DIFFICULTY: Easy

85. The nurse is reinforcing dietary teaching for a client with an endemic goiter. The nurse identifies that the education has been successful when the client selects the following foods as good sources of iodine. Select all that apply.
1. Spinach
2. Cod fish
3. Shrimp
4. Peanut butter
5. Eggs
6. Oranges

Remember to "select all that apply" in question #85.

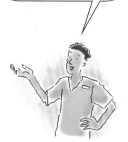

85. 1, 2, 3, 5. Natural iodine content is highest in seafood and shellfish. It is also found in smaller amounts in bread, milk, eggs, meat and spinach. Fruit and peanut butter are not good sources of iodine.
CN: Physiological integrity; CNS: Basic care and comfort; CL: Apply; DIFFICULTY: Challenge

86. The nurse is caring for a postpartum client with Hashimoto thyroiditis. While reinforcing education with the client the nurse identifies which of the following as the cause of the condition?
1. A long-term lack of iodine in the diet
2. A malfunction of the immune system in which antibodies attack the thyroid gland
3. Overproduction of the thyroid stimulating hormone (TSH) by the pituitary gland
4. An upper respiratory infection that extends to the thyroid gland

86. 2. Hashimoto thyroiditis is the most common form of thyroiditis. It is believed to be an autoimmune disorder that develops in response to some stressor. Lack of iodine in the diet and overproduction of FSH are not causes. Hashimoto thyroiditis is a noninfective form of thyroiditis.
CN: Physiological integrity; CNS: Physiological adaptation; CL: Apply; DIFFICULTY: Challenge

87. In caring for a client with insulin-dependent diabetes mellitus, the nurse identifies that the client may require which change to daily routine during periods of infection?
1. No changes
2. Less insulin
3. More insulin
4. Oral antidiabetic agents

87. 3. During periods of infection or illness, insulin-dependent clients may need even more insulin, rather than reducing the levels or not making any changes in their daily insulin routines, to compensate for increased blood glucose levels. Clients usually aren't switched from injectable insulin to oral antidiabetic agents during periods of infection.
CN: Physiological integrity; CNS: Pharmacological therapies; CL: Apply; DIFFICULTY: Easy

88. A well 50-year-old client with a history of diabetes mellitus type 2 has gone to the immunization clinic at the local health department. The client reports no known allergies and no immunizations for the last 5 years. Which vaccine would the nurse administer to the client? Select all that apply.
1. Influenza vaccine
2. Human papillomavirus vaccine
3. Rotavirus vaccine
4. Pneumococcal polyvalent vaccine
5. Respiratory syncytial virus immune globulin

89. A nonpregnant client tells the nurse that two recent, fasting blood glucose results were 132 mg/dL and 146 mg/dL. The nurse should expect which actions to occur?
1. These are normal results; no further action is needed.
2. These results indicate diabetes; further follow-up is needed.
3. The fasting blood glucose tests should be repeated two more times.
4. The client should be scheduled for an HbA1C test.

90. A client has diabetic ketoacidosis secondary to infection. As the condition progresses, which signs and symptoms might the nurse see?
1. Kussmaul respirations and a fruity odor on the breath
2. Shallow respirations and severe abdominal pain
3. Decreased respirations and increased urine output
4. Cheyne-Stokes respirations and foul-smelling urine

91. A nurse is preparing to administer regular insulin 4 units subcutaneously to a client with type 1 diabetes. Which equipment does the nurse need to perform the injection? Select all that apply.
1. Medication administration record
2. Nursing assessment sheet
3. 27-gauge, 1/2-inch needle
4. 22-gauge, 1/2-inch needle
5. 27-gauge, 1-inch needle
6. 22-gauge, 1-inch needle

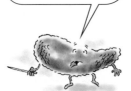

High blood glucose means something's out of whack with production of or sensitivity to insulin—what condition does that remind you of?

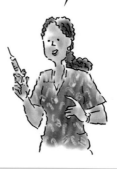

Sometimes nursing requires you to take your best shot.

88. 1, 4. Influenza vaccine is recommended annually for all people older than 6 months of age. Pneumococcal polyvalent vaccine is recommended for people over age 65 and people 2 to 64 years who have chronic conditions such as diabetes. Human papillomavirus vaccine is not recommended after 26 years of age. Rotavirus vaccine and respiratory syncytial virus immune globulin are recommended for infants.
CN: Health promotion and maintenance; CNS: None; CL: Analyze; DIFFICULTY: Difficult

89. 2. Based on American Diabetes Association guidelines, fasting blood glucose of 126 mg/dL or more, on at least two occasions, is indicative of diabetes. These are not normal results. Further tests to make a definitive diagnosis of diabetes should be random blood glucose or glucose tolerance tests, not a fasting blood glucose or HbA1C.
CN: Physiological integrity; CNS: Reduction of risk potential; CL: Analyze; DIFFICULTY: Challenge

90. 1. Coma and severe acidosis are ushered in with Kussmaul respirations (very deep but not labored respirations) and a fruity odor on the breath (acidemia). Shallow respirations and severe abdominal pain may be symptoms of pancreatitis. Decreased respirations and increased urine output aren't symptoms related to diabetic ketoacidosis. Cheyne-Stokes respirations and foul-smelling urine don't result from diabetic ketoacidosis.
CN: Physiological integrity; CNS: Physiological adaptation; CL: Apply; DIFFICULTY: Easy

91. 1, 3. To administer medication, the nurse needs the medication administration record to verify the correct client, medication, dose, time, and route. A subcutaneous injection, such as insulin, is administered with a 25-gauge to 27-gauge, 5/8-inch to 1/2-inch needle. The nursing assessment sheet isn't necessary for administering insulin. A 22-gauge needle is too large for a subcutaneous injection. A 1-inch needle will deliver the medication into muscle rather than subcutaneous tissue.
CN: Physiological integrity; CNS: Pharmacological therapies; CL: Apply; DIFFICULTY: Difficult

92. After falling off a ladder and suffering a brain injury, a client develops syndrome of inappropriate antidiuretic hormone (SIADH). Which findings indicate to the nurse the effectiveness of the treatment he's receiving? Select all that apply.
1. Decrease in body weight
2. Rise in blood pressure and drop in heart rate
3. Absence of wheezes in the lungs
4. Increased urine output
5. Decreased urine osmolarity

92. **1, 4, 5.** SIADH is an abnormality in which there's an abundance of antidiuretic hormone. The predominant feature is water retention, accompanied by oliguria, edema, and weight gain. Evidence of successful treatment includes a reduction in weight, an increase in urine output, and a decrease in the urine's concentration (urine osmolarity). SIADH doesn't manifest as symptoms associated with blood pressure, heart rate, or abnormal breath sounds.
CN: Physiological integrity; CNS: Physiological adaptation; CL: Analyze; DIFFICULTY: Difficult

93. A client is admitted with a diagnosis of diabetic ketoacidosis. An insulin drip is initiated with 50 units of insulin in 100 mL of normal saline solution. The IV is being infused via an infusion pump and the pump is correctly set at 10 mL/hour. The nurse determines that the client is receiving how many units of insulin each hour? Record your answer using a whole number.

_____ units

93. **5.** To determine the number of insulin units the client is receiving per hour, the nurse must first calculate the number of units in each mL of fluid (50 units ÷ 100 mL = 0.5 units/mL). Next, multiply the units/mL by the rate of mL/hour (0.5 units × 10 mL/hour = 5 units).
Dimensional analysis

$$\frac{\text{units}}{\text{hour}} = \frac{50 \text{ units}}{100 \text{ mL}} \times \frac{10 \text{ mL}}{\text{hr}} = \frac{500}{100} = 5 \text{ units/hr}$$

CN: Physiological integrity; CNS: Pharmacological therapies; CL: Apply; DIFFICULTY: Moderate

94. A client is seen in the clinic with suspected parathyroid hormone (PTH) deficiency. Part of the diagnosis of this condition includes the analysis of serum electrolyte levels. Which electrolyte levels would the nurse expect to be abnormal in a client with PTH deficiency? Select all that apply.
1. Sodium
2. Potassium
3. Calcium
4. Chloride
5. Phosphorus

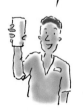

Cheers to you! You finished the chapter.

94. **3, 5.** A client with PTH deficiency has abnormal serum calcium and phosphorus levels because PTH regulates these two electrolytes. PTH deficiency doesn't affect sodium, potassium, or chloride.
CN: Physiological integrity; CNS: Physiological adaptation; CL: Analyze; DIFFICULTY: Difficult

Chapter 10

Genitourinary Disorders

Genitourinary refresher

Acute poststreptococcal glomerulonephritis

Inflammation of the kidney tubules (glomeruli) that occurs after infection with certain strains of *Streptococcus* bacteria

Key signs and symptoms
- Azotemia
- Fatigue
- Oliguria
- Edema

Key test results
- Blood tests show elevated serum creatinine and potassium levels
- 24-hour urine sample shows low creatinine clearance and impaired glomerular filtration
- Urinalysis typically reveals proteinuria and hematuria; red blood cells (RBCs), white blood cells, and mixed cell casts are common findings in urinary sediment
- Kidney-ureter-bladder (KUB) x-rays show bilateral kidney enlargement

Key treatments
- Bed rest
- Diuretics: metolazone, furosemide
- Antihypertensive: hydralazine
- Fluid restriction
- High-calorie, low-sodium, low-potassium, low-protein diet

Key interventions
- Check vital signs
- Monitor intake and output and daily weight
- Watch for signs of acute renal failure (oliguria, azotemia, and acidosis)
- Provide good nutrition, use good hygienic technique, and prevent contact with infected people
- Encourage necessary bed rest during the acute phase
- Encourage client to gradually resume normal activities as symptoms subside

Acute renal failure

Sudden loss of kidney function

Key signs and symptoms
- Urine output less than 400 mL/day for 1 to 2 weeks followed by diuresis (3 to 5 L/day) for 2 to 3 weeks
- Weight gain

Key test results
- Creatinine clearance is low
- Glomerular filtration rate is:
  - 20 to 40 mL/minute (renal insufficiency)
  - 10 to 20 mL/minute (renal failure)
  - less than 10 mL/minute (end-stage renal disease)

Key treatments
- Continuous renal replacement therapy or hemodialysis
- Low-protein; high-carbohydrate; moderate-fat; and moderate-calorie diet with potassium, sodium, and phosphorus intake regulated according to serum levels
- Inotropic agent: dopamine, initially low-dose to improve renal perfusion
- Diuretics: furosemide, metolazone, bumetanide

Key interventions
- Monitor fluid balance, respiratory, cardio-vascular, and neurologic status
- Monitor and record vital signs, intake and output, and daily weight
- Maintain the client's diet

Benign prostatic hyperplasia

Noncancerous enlargement of the prostate gland

Key signs and symptoms
- Decreased force and amount of urine
- Nocturia
- Urgency, frequency, and burning on urination

Key test results
- Cystoscopy shows enlarged prostate gland, obstructed urine flow, and urinary stasis
- Digital rectal examination shows enlarged prostate gland

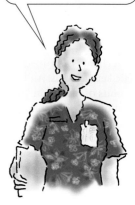

For more information about genitourinary system disorders, visit the Web site of the National Institute of Diabetes and Digestive and Kidney Diseases at www.niddk.nih.gov/.

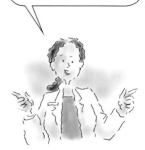

Reduced urine output is a key sign of acute renal failure.

Key treatments
- Forcing fluids
- Transurethral resection of the prostate (TURP) or prostatectomy

Key interventions
- Force fluids
- Provide postoperative care

Bladder cancer
Malignancy of the bladder

Key signs and symptoms
- Frequent urination
- Painless hematuria
- Urgency of urination
- Urinary obstruction
- Urinary retention

Key test results
- Biopsy and cytology examination are positive for malignant cells
- Cystoscopy reveals a bladder mass

Key treatments
- Surgery, depending on the location and progress of the tumor

Key interventions
- Provide postoperative care:
  - closely monitor urine output
  - observe for hematuria (reddish tint to gross bloodiness) or infection (cloudy, foul smelling, with sediment)
  - maintain continuous bladder irrigation, if indicated
  - assist with turning, coughing, deep breathing, and incentive spirometry
  - apply a sequential compression device while client is on bed rest
- Force fluids

Breast cancer
Malignancy involving the breast

Key signs and symptoms
- Cervical, supraclavicular, or axillary lymph node lump or enlargement on palpation
- Painless lump or mass in the breast or thickening of breast tissue
- Skin changes of the breast

Key test results
- Breast self-examination reveals a lump or mass in the breast or thickening of breast tissue
- Fine-needle aspiration and excisional biopsy provide histologic cells that confirm diagnosis
- Mammography and MRI detect a tumor

Key treatments
- Bone marrow and peripheral stem cell therapy for advanced breast cancer
- Surgery: lumpectomy, skin-sparing mastectomy, partial mastectomy, total mastectomy, modified radical mastectomy, and quandrantectomy
- Chemotherapy: cyclophosphamide, methotrexate, fluorouracil, doxorubicin
- Hormonal therapy: tamoxifen, raloxifene, fulvestrant, toremifene, megestrol

Key interventions
- Note the client's feelings about her illness, and determine what she knows about breast cancer and her expectations
- Provide routine postoperative care
- Perform comfort measures
- Administer analgesics as ordered and monitor their effectiveness
- Watch for treatment-related complications, such as nausea, vomiting, anorexia, leukopenia, thrombocytopenia, GI ulceration, and bleeding

Cervical cancer
Malignancy of the cervix

Key signs and symptoms
- Preinvasive: absence of symptoms
- Invasive: abnormal vaginal discharge (yellowish, blood-tinged, and foul-smelling)
- Postcoital pain and bleeding

Key test results
- Colposcopy determines the source of the abnormal cells seen on Papanicolaou (Pap) test
- Cone biopsy identifies malignant cells

Key treatments
- Preinvasive: cryosurgery
- Invasive: radiation therapy (internal, external, or both), radical hysterectomy

Key interventions
- Encourage client to use relaxation techniques
- Watch for complications related to therapy
- Provide postoperative care

Chlamydia
Sexually transmitted infection caused by the bacteria *Chlamydia trachomatis*

Key signs and symptoms
In women
- Dyspareunia
- Mucopurulent discharge
- Pelvic pain

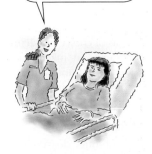

For any client with a urinary disorder, monitoring of fluid intake and output is essential.

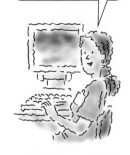

What key signs of cervical cancer should you instruct your client to look for?

In men
- Dysuria
- Erythema
- Tenderness of the meatus
- Urethral discharge
- Urinary frequency

Key test results
- Antigen detection methods are diagnostic tests of choice for identifying chlamydia:
  - enzyme-linked immunosorbent assay
  - direct fluorescent antibody test
- Tissue cell cultures are more sensitive and specific than antigen detection methods

Key treatments
- Antibiotics: doxycycline, azithromycin
- For pregnant women with chlamydial infections, azithromycin, in a single 1-g dose

Key interventions
- Practice standard and contact precautions when caring for a client with a chlamydial infection
- Make sure client fully understands dosage requirements of any prescribed medications for this infection
- Obtain appropriate specimens for diagnostic testing

Chronic glomerulonephritis
Long-standing kidney disease affecting the glomeruli

Key signs and symptoms
- Edema
- Hematuria
- Hypertension

Key test results
- Kidney biopsy identifies the underlying disease and provides data needed to guide therapy
- Blood studies reveal rising blood urea nitrogen (BUN) and serum creatinine levels, which indicate advanced renal insufficiency
- Urinalysis reveals proteinuria, hematuria, cylindruria, and RBC casts

Key treatments
- Dialysis
- Kidney transplant

Key interventions
- Client care is primarily supportive, focusing on continual observation and sound client teaching
- Accurately monitor vital signs, intake and output, and daily weight
- Observe for signs of fluid and electrolyte imbalances

- Administer medications
- Provide good skin care

Chronic renal failure
Long-standing damage to kidneys, preventing them from removing wastes from the body

Key signs and symptoms
- Azotemia
- Decreased urine output
- Indications of heart failure
- Lethargy
- Pruritus
- Weight gain

Key test results
- Blood chemistry shows:
  - increased BUN, creatinine, potassium, phosphorus, and lipid levels
  - decreased calcium, carbon dioxide, and albumin levels

Key treatments
- Limited fluids
- Low-protein, low-sodium, low-potassium, low-phosphorus, high-calorie, and high-carbohydrate diet
- Peritoneal dialysis or hemodialysis
- Antacid: aluminum hydroxide gel
- Antiemetic: prochlorperazine, metoclopramide
- Calcium supplement: calcium carbonate
- Cation exchange resin: sodium polystyrene sulfonate
- Diuretics: furosemide, bumetanide

Key interventions
- Monitor renal, respiratory, and cardiovascular status and fluid balance
- Check dialysis access for bruit and thrill
- Follow standard precautions
- Restrict fluids

Cystitis
Inflammation of the bladder usually caused by infection

Key signs and symptoms
- Dark, odoriferous urine
- Frequency of urination
- Urgency of urination

Key test results
- Urine culture and sensitivity positively identifies organisms (*Escherichia coli*, *Proteus vulgaris*, and *Streptococcus faecalis*)

Key treatments
- Diet: increased intake of fluids and vitamin C

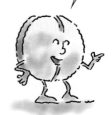

Many sexually transmitted infections, including chlamydia, respond well to antibiotics.

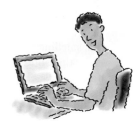

Hematuria is a key sign of chronic glomerulonephritis. Do you remember what this term means?

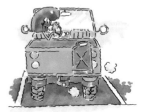

I prefer to keep things moving along!

Key interventions

- Monitor vital signs
- Monitor intake and output
- Force fluids (cranberry or orange juice) to 3 qt (2.8 L)/day
- Instruct client to decrease intake of carbonated beverages
- Instruct client to avoid coffee, tea, and alcohol

Gonorrhea

Sexually transmitted infection caused by *Neisseria gonorrhoeae*

Key signs and symptoms

- Dysuria
- Purulent urethral or cervical discharge
- Itching, burning, and pain

Key test results

- A culture from site of infection (urethra, cervix, rectum, or pharynx) is used to establish diagnosis by isolating the organism

Key treatments

- Antibiotics: ceftriaxone, doxycycline, erythromycin
- Prophylactic antibiotic: 1% silver nitrate or erythromycin eye drops to prevent infection in neonates

Key interventions

- Before treatment, establish whether client has any drug sensitivities
- Follow standard and contact precautions

Herpes simplex

Vesicular skin rash caused by herpes virus

Key signs and symptoms

- Blisters, which may form on any part of the mouth
- Dysuria (genital herpes)
- Erythema
- Flulike symptoms
- Fluid-filled blisters (genital herpes)

Key test results

- Confirmation requires:
  - isolation of the virus from local lesions
  - histologic biopsy

Key treatments

- Antiviral agents: idoxuridine, trifluridine, or vidarabine
- 5% acyclovir ointment (possible relief to clients with genital herpes or to immunosuppressed clients with *Herpesvirus hominis* skin infections; IV acyclovir to help treat more severe infections)

Key interventions

- Follow standard and contact precautions; for clients with extensive cutaneous, oral, or genital lesions, institute contact precautions
- Administer pain medication and prescribed antiviral agents as ordered
- Provide supportive care, as indicated, (e.g., oral hygiene, nutritional supplementation, antipyretics for fever)

Neurogenic bladder

Lack of bladder control due to a brain or spinal cord injury

Key symptoms

- Altered micturition

Key test results

- Voiding cystourethrography evaluates bladder neck function, vesicoureteral reflux, and continence

Key treatments

- Indwelling urinary catheter insertion (including teaching client self-catheterization techniques)

Key interventions

- Use strict sterile technique during insertion of an indwelling urinary catheter (a temporary measure to drain the incontinent client's bladder); don't interrupt the closed drainage system for any reason
- Clean catheter insertion site with soap and water at least twice a day
- Clamp tubing or empty the catheter bag before transferring client to a wheelchair or stretcher
- Watch for signs of infection (fever, cloudy or foul-smelling urine)

Ovarian cancer

Malignancy of the ovary(ies)

Key signs and symptoms

- Abdominal distention
- Pelvic discomfort
- Urinary frequency
- Weight loss

Key test results

- Abdominal ultrasonography, computed tomography (CT) scan, or x-ray may delineate tumor size

Key treatments

- Resection of the involved ovary
- Total abdominal hysterectomy and bilateral salpingo-oophorectomy with tumor resection, omentectomy, and appendectomy

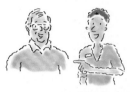

Be sure to check with your client about any drug sensitivities before administering medications.

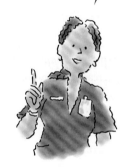

Neurogenic bladder typically occurs as a result of an injury to which part of the body?

- Antineoplastics: carboplatin, chlorambucil, cyclophosphamide, dactinomycin, doxorubicin, fluorouracil, cisplatin, paclitaxel, topotecan
- Analgesics: morphine, fentanyl

Key interventions

Before surgery

- Thoroughly explain:
  - all preoperative tests
  - expected course of treatment
  - surgical and postoperative procedures

After surgery

- Monitor vital signs frequently
- Monitor intake and output while maintaining good catheter care
- Check dressing regularly for excessive drainage or bleeding
- Watch for signs of infection
- Encourage coughing, deep breathing, and incentive spirometry hourly during the waking hours
- Reposition client often
- Encourage client to walk shortly after surgery

Prostate cancer

Malignancy of the prostate gland

Key signs and symptoms

- Decreased size and force of urinary stream
- Difficulty and frequency of urination
- Hematuria
- Urine retention

Key test results

- Carcinoembryonic antigen is elevated
- Digital rectal examination reveals palpable firm nodule in gland or diffuse induration in posterior lobe
- Prostatic-specific antigen (PSA) is increased

Key treatments

- Radiation implant
- Radical prostatectomy (for localized tumors without metastasis)
- Transurethral resection of the prostate (TURP) (to relieve obstruction in metastatic disease)
- Luteinizing hormone-releasing hormone agonists: goserelin acetate, leuprolide acetate
- Antiandrogens: bicalutamide, flutamide, nilutamide

Key interventions

- Monitor and record vital signs
- Monitor intake and output
- Check for signs of infection
- Monitor the client's pain and note the effectiveness of analgesia

---

- Maintain the client's diet
- Maintain the patency of the urinary catheter and note drainage

Renal calculi

Solid piece or pieces of material that form in the kidney from substances in the urine, known as kidney stones

Key signs and symptoms

- Flank pain

Key test results

- Excretory urography reveals stones
- KUB x-ray reveals stones

Key treatments

- Diet:
  - for calcium stones, acid-ash with limited intake of calcium and milk products
  - for oxalate stones, alkaline-ash with limited intake of foods high in oxalate (cola, tea)
  - for uric acid stones, alkaline-ash with limited intake of foods high in purine
- Extracorporeal shock wave therapy (ESWL)
- Surgery to remove the stone if other measures aren't effective (type of surgery depends on location of the stone)

Key interventions

- Monitor the client's urine for evidence of renal calculi
- Strain all urine and save all solid material for analysis
- Force fluids to 3 qt (2.8 L)/day
- If surgery was performed:
  - check dressings regularly for bloody drainage and report excessive amounts of bloody drainage to health care provider
  - use sterile technique to change dressing
  - maintain nephrostomy tube or indwelling urinary catheter if indicated
  - monitor incision site for signs of infection

Syphilis

Chronic infection caused by a spirochete, *Treponema pallidum*. Most commonly transmitted through sexual contact but can also be transmitted congenitally

Key signs and symptoms

Primary syphilis

- Chancres on the genitalia, anus, fingers, lips, tongue, nipples, tonsils, or eyelids

Secondary syphilis

- Symmetrical mucocutaneous lesions
- Malaise
- Anorexia

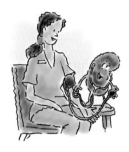

Don't forget to monitor those vital signs.

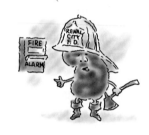

Flank pain is an alarm that often means you have kidney stones.

- Weight loss
- Slight fever

Key test results
- Fluorescent treponemal antibody-absorption test:
  - identifies antigens of *T. pallidum* in tissue, ocular fluid, cerebrospinal fluid, tracheobronchial secretions, and exudates from lesions
  - most sensitive test available for detecting syphilis in all stages
  - once reactive, it remains so permanently
- Venereal Disease Research Laboratory (VDRL) slide test and rapid plasma reagin test:
  - both tests detect nonspecific antibodies
  - both tests, if positive, become reactive within 1 to 2 weeks after the primary lesion appears or 4 to 5 weeks after infection begins

Key treatments
- Antibiotics: penicillin G benzathine; if allergic to penicillin, erythromycin or tetracycline

Key interventions
- Check for a history of drug sensitivity before administering first dose of penicillin
- Urge the client to seek VDRL testing after 3, 6, 12, and 24 months
- Client treated for latent or late syphilis should receive blood tests at 6-month intervals for 2 years

---

Testicular cancer
Malignancy of the testicle(s)

Key signs and symptoms
- Firm, painless, smooth testicular mass varying in size (sometimes producing a sense of testicular heaviness)

In advanced stages
- Ureteral obstruction
- Abdominal mass
- Weight loss
- Fatigue
- Back pain
- Pallor

Key test results
- Regular self-examinations and testicular palpation during routine physical examination may detect testicular tumors
- Surgical excision and biopsy of the tumor and testes permits histologic verification of the tumor cell types

Key treatments
- Surgery: orchiectomy (testicle removal; most surgeons remove the testicle but not the scrotum to allow for a prosthetic implant)
- High-calorie diet provided in small, frequent feedings
- IV fluid therapy
- Antineoplastics: bleomycin, carboplatin, cisplatin, dactinomycin, etoposide, ifosfamide, plicamycin, vinblastine
- Analgesics: morphine, fentanyl
- Antiemetics: trimethobenzamide, metoclopramide, ondansetron

Key interventions
- Develop a treatment plan that addresses the client's psychological and physical needs
- After orchiectomy:
  - for first day after surgery, apply an ice pack to the scrotum and provide an analgesic
  - check for excessive bleeding, swelling, and signs of infection
  - give an antiemetic, as needed
  - encourage small, frequent meals

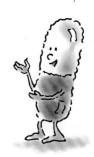

If syphilis is your villain, try killin it with penicillin.

the Point® You can download tables of drug information to help you prepare for the NCLEX®! View Generic Drug Names, Drug Classifications, Drug Actions, and Nursing Implications for the drugs discussed in this refresher at **http://thePoint.lww.com.**

Genitourinary questions, answers, and rationales

1. To treat cervical cancer, a client has had an applicator of radioactive material placed in her vagina. Which observation by the nurse indicates a radiation hazard?
1. The client is on strict bed rest.
2. The head of the bed is set at a 15-degree angle.
3. The client receives a complete bed bath each morning.
4. The nurse checks the applicator's position every 4 hours.

1. 3. The client shouldn't receive a complete bed bath while the applicator is in place. In fact, she shouldn't be bathed below the waist because of the risk of radiation exposure to the nurse. During this treatment, the client should remain on strict bed rest with the head of the bed raised no higher than a 15-degree angle. The nurse should check the applicator's position every 4 hours to ensure that it remains in the proper place.
CN: Safe, effective care environment; CNS: Safety and infection control; CL: Apply; DIFFICULTY: Moderate

2. A health care provider tells a client to return 1 week after treatment to have a repeat culture done to verify the cure. This order would be appropriate for a woman with which condition?
1. Genital warts
2. Genital herpes
3. Gonorrhea
4. Syphilis

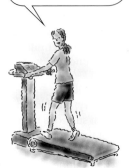

Keep it up. Remember: slow and steady wins the race.

3. A nurse is caring for a client in the clinic. Which sign or symptom may indicate that the client has gonorrhea? Select all that apply.
1. Burning on urination
2. Green vaginal discharge
3. Diffuse skin rash
4. Painless chancre
5. Vesicular rash

4. Which statement made by a client with a chlamydial infection indicates understanding of the potential complications?
1. "I'm glad I'm not pregnant; I'd hate to have a malformed baby from this disease."
2. "I hope this medicine works before this disease gets into my urine and destroys my kidneys."
3. "If I had known a diaphragm would put me at risk for this, I would have taken birth control pills."
4. "I need to treat this infection so it doesn't spread into my pelvis because I want to have children someday."

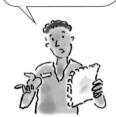

In other words, in question #5, which statement by the client is true?

5. A nurse is teaching comfort measures to a client with genital herpes. Which statement by the client indicates the education has been effective?
1. "I will wear loose cotton underwear."
2. "I will apply a water-based lubricant to my lesions."
3. "I should rub rather than scratch in response to itching."
4. "I can pour hydrogen peroxide and water over my lesions."

6. A nurse is examining the following laboratory values in the chart of a client with chronic renal failure. Which value indicates that hemodialysis is an effective treatment for this client?
1. Red blood cells (RBCs)
2. White blood cells (WBCs)
3. Calcium
4. Blood urea nitrogen (BUN)

2. 3. Gonococcal infections can be completely eliminated by drug therapy. This cure is documented by a negative culture 4 to 7 days after therapy is finished. Genital warts aren't curable and are identified by appearance, not culture. Genital herpes isn't curable and is identified by the appearance of the lesions or by cytologic studies. The diagnosis of syphilis is done using dark-field microscopy or serologic tests.
CN: Physiological integrity; CNS: Physiological adaptation; CL: Apply; DIFFICULTY: Moderate

3. 1, 2. Burning on urination may be a symptom of gonorrhea or urinary tract infection. A purulent discharge may be a sign of gonorrhea. A diffuse rash may indicate secondary stage syphilis. A painless chancre is the hallmark of primary syphilis. It appears wherever the organisms enter the body, such as on the genitalia, anus, or lips. A vesicular rash may indicate Herpes simplex virus (HSV).
CN: Physiological integrity; CNS: Physiological adaptation; CL: Analyze; DIFFICULTY: Moderate

4. 4. Chlamydia is a common cause of pelvic inflammatory disease and infertility. It doesn't affect the kidneys or cause birth defects. It can cause conjunctivitis and respiratory infection in neonates exposed to infected cervicovaginal secretions during birth. Use of a diaphragm isn't a risk factor.
CN: Physiological integrity; CNS: Reduction of risk potential; CL: Apply; DIFFICULTY: Easy

5. 1. Wearing loose cotton underwear promotes drying and helps avoid irritation of the lesions. The use of lubricants is contraindicated because they can prolong healing time and increase the risk of secondary infection. Lesions shouldn't be rubbed or scratched because of the risk of tissue damage and additional infection. Cool, wet compresses can be used to soothe the itch. The use of hydrogen peroxide and water on lesions isn't recommended.
CN: Physiological integrity; CNS: Basic care and comfort; CL: Analyze; DIFFICULTY: Moderate

6. 4. The BUN level reflects the amount of urea and nitrogenous waste products in the blood. Dialysis removes excess amounts of these elements from the blood, which is reflected in a lower BUN level. Hemodialysis doesn't affect the RBC or WBC count. Calcium levels are usually low in clients with chronic renal failure. These levels are corrected by giving calcium supplements, not through hemodialysis.
CN: Physiological integrity; CNS: Physiological adaptation; CL: Analyze; DIFFICULTY: Easy

---

7. A client with nephritis is taking the diuretic furosemide as prescribed. To avoid potassium depletion, the nurse reinforces education on prevention techniques. Which client statement indicates an accurate understanding of this education?
1. "I'll avoid consuming magnesium-rich foods."
2. "I'll watch for, and report signs of, hypercalcemia."
3. "I'll eat such foods as apricots, dates, and citrus fruits."
4. "I'll take furosemide with the usual dose of my antihypertensive drug."

7. **3.** Because furosemide is a potassium-wasting diuretic, the client should eat potassium-rich foods, such as apricots, dates, and citrus fruits, to prevent potassium depletion. The other client statements have no relationship to potassium balance. The client may consume magnesium-rich foods as desired. The client should watch for signs of adverse reactions to furosemide such as hypocalcemia—not hypercalcemia. The client should take furosemide with an antihypertensive drug only if prescribed; the combination may produce hypotension but doesn't cause potassium depletion.
CN: Health promotion and maintenance; CNS: None; CL: Apply; DIFFICULTY: Easy

8. A nurse reinforced disease prevention education with a female client who has genital herpes. Which client behavior indicates that the education has been successful?
1. The client keeps the affected area moist.
2. The client keeps her fingernails long.
3. The client wears tight-fitting jeans.
4. The client washes her hands before and after touching lesions.

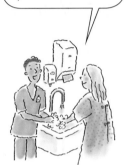

Frequent hand hygiene is the number-one way to prevent infections.

8. **4.** Because hand-to-body contact is a common method of transmitting the herpes simplex virus, the client should wash her hands before and after touching the lesions to prevent the spread of the disease. To promote lesion healing and client comfort, the client should keep the affected area dry. To prevent scratching of the lesions, the client should keep her fingernails short, instead of long. Because tight-fitting clothes retain heat and moisture, which can delay healing and cause discomfort, the client should wear loose-fitting garments.
CN: Safe, effective care environment; CNS: Safety and infection control; CL: Apply; DIFFICULTY: Easy

9. In which group is it **most** important for the client to understand the importance of an annual Papanicolaou (Pap) test?
1. Clients with a history of recurrent candidiasis
2. Clients with a pregnancy before age 20
3. Clients infected with the human papillomavirus (HPV)
4. Clients with a long history of oral contraceptive use

9. **3.** HPV causes genital warts, which are associated with an increased incidence of cervical cancer. Recurrent candidiasis, pregnancy before age 20, and use of oral contraceptives don't increase the risk of cervical cancer.
CN: Health promotion and maintenance; CNS: None; CL: Apply; DIFFICULTY: Easy

10. A nurse is caring for a client with candidiasis. What information should the nurse obtain from the client? Select all that apply.
1. Recent antibiotic use
2. Menopause
3. Use of corticosteroids
4. Use of oral contraceptives
5. Use of over the counter herbal medications

10. **1, 3, 4.** The use of antibiotics increases the risk of candidiasis. Small numbers of the fungus *Candida albicans* commonly inhabit the vagina. Because corticosteroids decrease host defense, they increase the risk of candidiasis. Candidiasis is rare before menarche and after menopause. The use of hormonal contraceptives increases the risk of candidiasis. OTC herbal medications do not increase the incidence of candidiasis.
CN: Health promotion and maintenance; CNS: None; CL: Apply; DIFFICULTY: Difficult

11. A nurse is caring for a client diagnosed with gonorrhea. Which treatment plan should the nurse anticipate? Select all that apply.
1. Ceftriaxone
2. Doxycycline
3. Amoxicillin
4. Ampicillin
5. Sulfamethoxazole-trimethoprim

11. **1, 2.** Treatment for gonorrhea includes ceftriaxone and doxycycline to prophylactically treat for chlamydia. Amoxicillin, ampicillin and sulfamethoxazole-trimethoprim are not recommended in the treatment of gonorrhea.
CN: Physiological integrity; CNS: Physiological adaptation; CL: Apply; DIFFICULTY: Difficult

12. A client reports an intermittent, milky vaginal discharge. The client isn't sexually active and doesn't report itching or burning. Which factor is the **most** likely cause of the milky discharge?
1. Inadequate cleaning of the perineal area
2. Sensitivity to a feminine hygiene product
3. Normal fluctuation in estrogen and progesterone levels
4. Reaction to heat and moisture from wearing tight clothing

13. A client underwent a left mastectomy yesterday and has a saline lock for intermittent IV access in her lower right arm. Which technique for obtaining a blood pressure reading would be **most** appropriate for this client?
1. Using the right arm, and placing the cuff above the saline lock insertion site
2. Using the left arm, and pumping the cuff only as necessary
3. Using the leg, and placing the cuff on the client's thigh
4. Using the right arm, and placing the cuff below the saline lock insertion site

14. A nurse must administer an antiseptic douche to a client scheduled for a vaginal hysterectomy. Place the steps in the correct order.

| 1. Clean the vaginal orifice |
| 2. Insert the douche nozzle 2 in (5 cm) |
| 3. Separate the labia |
| 4. Administer 100°F (37.7°C) solution 2 in (5 cm) above the client's hip level. |

15. A nurse enters the room of a client who had a left modified mastectomy 8 hours earlier. Which observation indicates that the unlicensed assistive personnel (UAP) assigned to the client needs further instruction and guidance?
1. The client is squeezing a ball in her left hand.
2. The client is wearing a robe with elastic cuffs.
3. The client's affected arm is elevated on a pillow.
4. A blood pressure cuff is on the client's right arm.

16. For which signs and symptoms should a client at risk for evisceration be monitored after an abdominal hysterectomy?
1. Tachycardia accompanied by a weak, thready pulse
2. Hypotension with a decreased level of consciousness (LOC)
3. Shallow, rapid respirations and increasing vaginal drainage
4. Low-grade fever with increasing serosanguineous incisional drainage

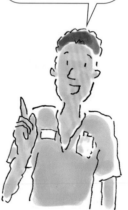

Question #13 is tricky. What's the most important consideration when taking a blood pressure reading for this client?

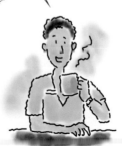

Stay focused and keep moving. You've got this.

12. 3. Vaginal fluid is clear, milky, or cloudy, depending on the fluctuating levels of estrogen and progesterone. A milky vaginal discharge is normal and isn't associated with sensitivity, reaction to heat or moisture, or inadequate cleaning.
CN: Health promotion and maintenance; CNS: None; CL: Apply; DIFFICULTY: Easy

13. 1. To obtain a blood pressure reading, the nurse should always use the arm opposite the side of the mastectomy. Never take a blood pressure reading in the arm on the affected side without a health care provider's order. Blood pressure readings may be taken in the leg in some cases, but doing so isn't necessary in this case. It isn't necessary to place the cuff below the saline lock to obtain a blood pressure reading.
CN: Health promotion and maintenance; CNS: None; CL: Apply; DIFFICULTY: Difficult

14. Ordered Response:

| 3. Separate the labia |
| 1. Clean the vaginal orifice |
| 2. Insert the douche nozzle 2 in (5 cm) |
| 4. Administer 100°F (37.7°C) solution 2 in (5 cm) above the client's hip level |

CN: Safe, effective care environment; CNS: Safety and infection control; CL: Apply; DIFFICULTY: Challenge

15. 2. Elastic cuffs can contribute to the development of lymphedema and should be avoided. Simple exercises such as squeezing a ball help promote circulation and should be started as soon as possible after surgery. Elevation of the affected arm promotes venous and lymphatic return from the extremity. Blood pressure measurements in the affected arm should be avoided.
CN: Safe, effective care environment; CNS: Coordinated care; CL: Analyze; DIFFICULTY: Moderate

16. 4. Signs of impending evisceration are low-grade fever and increasing serosanguineous incisional drainage. Tachycardia; weak, thready pulse; shallow, rapid respirations; hypotension; decreased LOC; and vaginal drainage after abdominal hysterectomy are all unrelated to impending evisceration, although they may be associated with other serious problems such as shock.
CN: Physiological integrity; CNS: Reduction of risk potential; CL: Apply; DIFFICULTY: Moderate

17. Which finding indicates that oxycodone given to a client with breast cancer that has metastasized to the bone is exerting the desired effect?
1. Bone density is increased.
2. Pain is 0 to 2 on a 10-point scale.
3. Alpha-fetoprotein level is decreased.
4. Serum calcium level is within normal range.

17. 2. Oxycodone is an opioid analgesic used for alleviating severe pain, especially in terminal illness. If a client's pain has decreased to 0 to 2 on a 10-point scale (where 0 is no pain and 10 is the worst pain), the medication is working as desired. The drug doesn't directly affect bone density, alpha-fetoprotein level, or serum calcium level.
CN: Physiological integrity; CNS: Pharmacological therapies; CL: Analyze; DIFFICULTY: Easy

18. A nurse is reinforcing education to a client with prostatitis who is receiving co-trimoxazole double strength. Which education is appropriate for this client?
1. Don't expect improvement of symptoms for 7 to 10 days.
2. Drink six to eight glasses of fluid daily while taking this medication.
3. If a sore mouth or throat develops, take the medication with milk or an antacid.
4. Use a sunscreen of at least SPF-15 with PABA to protect against drug-induced photosensitivity.

18. 2. Six to eight glasses of fluid daily are needed to prevent renal problems, such as crystalluria and calculi formation. The prostatitis symptoms should improve in a few days if the drug is effective. Sore throat and sore mouth are adverse effects that should be reported right away. The drug causes photosensitivity, but a PABA-free sunscreen should be used because PABA can interfere with the drug's action.
CN: Physiological integrity; CNS: Pharmacological therapies; CL: Apply; DIFFICULTY: Moderate

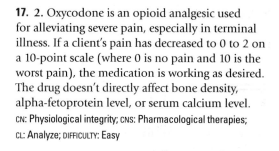

I just know there's a pattern here somewhere.

19. Which factor should the nurse evaluate when determining the effectiveness of an alpha-adrenergic blocker given to a client with benign prostatic hyperplasia (BPH)?
1. Voiding pattern
2. Size of the prostate
3. Creatinine clearance
4. Serum testosterone level

19. 1. The prostate gland has alpha-adrenergic receptors. Thus, alpha-adrenergic blockers relax the smooth muscle of the bladder neck and prostate, so the urinary symptoms of BPH (frequency, urgency, hesitancy) are reduced in many clients. These drugs don't affect the size of the prostate, renal function, or production or metabolism of testosterone.
CN: Physiological integrity; CNS: Pharmacological therapies; CL: Apply; DIFFICULTY: Moderate

20. A nurse is reinforcing education to a client diagnosed with renal calculi. Which statement by the client suggests further instruction is indicated?
1. "I should contact my health care provider if I develop flank pain again."
2. "I should contact my health care provider if I see blood in my urine."
3. "I should avoid foods that are high in calcium."
4. "I do not need to limit my intake of tea or cola."

20. 4. A client with a history of kidney stones should notify the health care provider if he develops flank pain or blood in the urine. Foods high in calcium can cause calcium stones. Cola and teas can cause oxalate stones and should be avoided.
CN: Physiological integrity; CNS: Reduction of risk potential; CL: Analyze; DIFFICULTY: Easy

21. A health care provider has ordered a condom catheter for a client. The nurse cleans the client's perineal area before application of the condom catheter and sees irritation, excoriation, and swelling of the penis. Which nursing intervention should be the nurse's **priority**?
1. Twisting the condom after application
2. Applying the condom with adhesive tape
3. Informing the charge nurse of the findings
4. Rolling the condom down securely over the tip of the penis

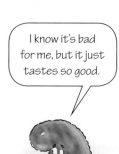

I know it's bad for me, but it just tastes so good.

21. 3. The nurse should inform the charge nurse of the baseline data because a condom catheter shouldn't be used on a client with penile irritation, excoriation, swelling, or discoloration. Further inflammation and ulceration may occur. A condom catheter shouldn't be twisted because twisting can obstruct urine flow. It should be secured with elastic tape or Velcro rather than adhesive tape, which is inflexible and can stop blood flow. It should have a 1-in (2.5-cm) gap between the tip of the penis and the connecting tube to prevent penile irritation and allow complete urine drainage.
CN: Safe, effective care environment; CNS: Coordinated care; CL: Apply; DIFFICULTY: Easy

22. The nurse is discussing prevention of toxic shock syndrome in a group of adolescent females. Which instruction is the **most** important to this group?
1. Avoid douching.
2. Wear loose, cotton underwear.
3. Use pads, not tampons, overnight.
4. Avoid sexual intercourse during menses.

22. 3. The cause of toxic shock syndrome is a toxin produced by *Staphylococcus aureus* bacteria. It is most common in menstruating women using tampons. Tampons, particularly when left in place for more than 8 hours (such as overnight), are believed to provide a good environment for growth of the bacteria, which then enter the bloodstream through breaks in the vaginal mucosa. Douching, use of loose cotton underwear, and sexual intercourse during menstruation have no direct association with toxic shock syndrome.
CN: Health promotion and maintenance; CNS: None; CL: Apply;
DIFFICULTY: Easy

23. Which response is the **most** appropriate when a client asks what activity limitations are necessary after a dilation and curettage (D & C) procedure?
1. Tampons may be used during exercise.
2. Avoid strenuous work and sexual intercourse for at least 2 weeks.
3. Stay on bed rest for 3 days, then gradually resume normal activity.
4. Engage in activity as tolerated, and take a soaking tub bath each day to promote relaxation.

23. 2. Strenuous work, which can result in increased bleeding, should be avoided for 2 weeks to allow time for healing. Sexual intercourse should also be avoided for 2 weeks to allow healing and decrease the risk of infection. Overall activity should be gradually resumed, reaching preoperative levels in the 2-week period, but bed rest isn't necessary. Tampons and tub baths should be avoided for 1 week. No other restrictions are routinely necessary.
CN: Physiological integrity; CNS: Reduction of risk potential;
CL: Apply; DIFFICULTY: Easy

24. A nurse is caring for an older adult male client. Which age-related changes are expected in this client? Select all that apply.
1. Decreased sperm count
2. Small, firm testes on palpation
3. History of slowed sexual response
4. Decreased plasma testosterone level
5. Thick brittle hair.

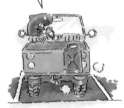

Don't forget to stop for potty breaks.

24. 2, 3, 4. Normal sperm production continues despite the age-related degenerative changes that occur in the male reproductive system. Among the normal age-related changes are decreased size and increased firmness of the testes, a decrease in sexual potency, and decreased production of testosterone and progesterone. Hair often thins with age.
CN: Physiological integrity; CNS: Physiological adaptation;
CL: Apply; DIFFICULTY: Challenge

25. After having transurethral resection of the prostate (TURP), a client returns to the unit with a three-way indwelling urinary catheter and continuous closed bladder irrigation. Which finding suggests that the client's catheter is occluded?
1. The urine in the drainage bag appears red to pink.
2. The client reports bladder spasms and the urge to void.
3. The normal saline irrigation is infusing at the rate of 50 gtt/minute.
4. About 1,000 mL of irrigant have been instilled, and 1,200 mL of drainage have been returned.

In other words, in question #26, which client statement shows that he does not understand his condition?

25. 2. Reports of bladder spasms and the urge to void suggest that a blood clot may be occluding the catheter. After TURP, urine normally appears red to pink, and normal saline irrigant is usually infused at a rate of 40 to 60 gtt/minute or according to facility protocol. The amount of returned fluid (1,200 mL) should correspond to the amount of instilled fluid, plus the client's urine output (1,000 mL + 200 mL), which reflects catheter patency.
CN: Physiological integrity; CNS: Basic care and comfort;
CL: Apply; DIFFICULTY: Easy

26. Which comment made by a client being treated for chronic prostatitis indicates that self-care instructions should be clarified?
1. "I miss not being able to have sex."
2. "I enjoy frequent soaking in a hot tub of water."
3. "Cutting down on coffee hasn't been as hard as I expected."
4. "I'm used to getting up and moving."

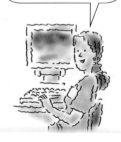

26. 1. Ejaculation can aid in the treatment of chronic prostatitis by decreasing the retention of prostatic fluid. Coffee should be eliminated from the diet because it can increase prostate secretion. Warm sitz baths and not sitting for too long at a time promote comfort.
CN: Physiological integrity; CNS: Physiological adaptation;
CL: Apply; DIFFICULTY: Challenge

27. A nurse is caring for a client with reports of abdominal pain. Which differential diagnosis should the nurse anticipate for this client? Select all that apply.
1. Urinary tract infection (UTI)
2. Internal hemorrhoids
3. Appendicitis
4. Renal calculi
5. Bronchitis

27. 1, 3, 4. Hemorrhoids cause rectal pain and pressure. Renal calculi typically produce flank pain but can also cause abdominal pain. Appendicitis often causes right lower quadrant (RLQ) abdominal pain. UTI often causes lower abdominal pain.
CN: Health promotion and maintenance; CNS: None;
CL: Understand; DIFFICULTY: Challenge

28. Which finding observed in a client taking finasteride should the nurse immediately report to the health care provider?
1. Azotemia
2. Breast enlargement
3. Decreased prostate size
4. Flushing

28. 1. Azotemia, a buildup of nitrogenous waste products in the blood, indicates impaired renal function. Finasteride is prescribed for chronic urine retention with large residual volumes secondary to benign prostatic hyperplasia (BPH). Azotemia in a client on finasteride therapy can indicate the drug isn't effective in relieving the urinary symptoms associated with BPH, or that an unrelated renal problem has occurred. Breast enlargement, decrease in prostate size, and flushing are expected effects of finasteride, an antiandrogenic agent.
CN: Physiological integrity; CNS: Pharmacological therapies;
CL: Apply; DIFFICULTY: Moderate

29. A nurse is caring for a client with cervical polyps being treated with cryosurgery. Which discharge instructions should the nurse reinforce to the client? Select all that apply.
1. Avoid douching for 2 weeks.
2. Complete all antibiotics as ordered.
3. Use intravaginal antibiotic cream.
4. Use of tampons for 72 hours
5. Avoid sexual intercourse for 24 hours.

29. 1, 2, 3. Intravaginal antibiotic cream is commonly used to aid healing and prevent infection. Oral antibiotics are used for clients with acute cervicitis or perimetritis. Douching and sexual intercourse are generally avoided for 2 weeks, as is the use of tampons.
CN: Physiological integrity; CNS: Reduction of risk potential;
CL: Apply; DIFFICULTY: Challenge

30. A nurse is caring for a female client having intracavitary radiation for cancer of the cervix. Which nursing intervention is **most** important for this client?
1. Ensure the client receives a high-residue diet.
2. Maintain Fowler position when in bed.
3. Intermittent urinary catheterization
4. Maintain the client on strict bed rest.

30. 4. Clients having intracavitary radiation therapy are on strict bed rest, with the head of the bed elevated no more than 15 degrees to avoid displacing the radiation source. A low-residue diet is used to prevent diarrhea during treatment. An order for Fowler position when in bed is incorrect. An indwelling urinary catheter is used to prevent urine from distending the bladder and changing the position of tissues relative to the radiation source.
CN: Physiological integrity; CNS: Reduction of risk potential;
CL: Analyze; DIFFICULTY: Moderate

31. Which condition of the female reproductive system does the nurse prepare to report for identification and treatment of sexual partners? Select all that apply.
1. Bartholinitis
2. Candidiasis
3. Chlamydia
4. Trichomoniasis
5. Herpes simplex virus

Remember—more than one answer can be right here.

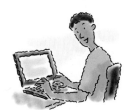

31. 3, 4. Chlamydia and trichomoniasis are common sexually transmitted diseases (STD) requiring the treatment of all current sexual partners to prevent reinfection. Bartholinitis results from obstruction of a duct and is not transmitted sexually. Candidiasis is a yeast infection that commonly occurs as a result of antibiotic use. Sexual partners may become infected, although men can usually be treated with over-the-counter products. HSV does not require identification of the sexual partner, although clients are encouraged to notify their sexual partners.
CN: Health promotion and maintenance; CNS: None; CL: Apply;
DIFFICULTY: Challenge

32. A nurse is reinforcing education for a client on metronidazole. What information should the nurse be sure is included? Select all that apply.
1. Breathlessness and cough are common adverse effects.
2. Urine may develop a greenish tinge while the client is taking this drug.
3. Mixing this drug with alcohol causes severe nausea and vomiting.
4. Complete all of the medication as ordered even if symptoms disappear.
5. Avoid using mouthwash or cough medication while taking this medication.

33. The nurse is reinforcing education to a client with metastatic prostate cancer about taking hydrocodone with acetaminophen. Which symptom should the nurse encourage the client to immediately report to the health care provider? Select all that apply.
1. Urine output less than 30 cc/hr
2. Diarrhea
3. Unusual dreams
4. Vomiting
5. Temperature of 98.9°F

34. A nurse is preparing a client for a hysterosalpingography. Which education should the nurse reinforce for this client? Select all that apply.
1. You will need to wear a perineal pad after the procedure.
2. Do not drink anything by mouth after midnight the night before the procedure.
3. You will be in the knee-chest position during the procedure.
4. You will be in a dorsal recumbent position for 4 hours after the procedure.
5. You will need to douche 24 hours after the procedure.

35. An adult man who has never had mumps reports that he was just notified that a child of a family with whom he stayed recently has been diagnosed with mumps. Which treatment should the man receive?
1. IV antibiotics
2. Ice packs to the scrotum
3. Application of a scrotal support
4. Administration of gamma globulin

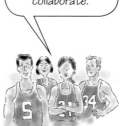

Providing excellent care requires teamwork; so don't forget to collaborate.

32. 3, 4, 5. When mixed with alcohol, metronidazole causes a disulfiram-like effect involving nausea, vomiting, and other unpleasant symptoms. Urine may turn reddish brown, not greenish, from use of the drug. Respiratory effects are not associated with this drug. Client should complete all medication as ordered. Mouthwash and cough medications may contain small amounts of alcohol, inducing nausea, vomiting and other unpleasant symptoms.
CN: Physiological integrity; CNS: Pharmacological therapies; CL: Apply; DIFFICULTY: Moderate

33. 1, 4. Vomiting is an adverse reaction to the drug that should be reported because it impairs the client's quality of life and places him at risk for dehydration. Decrease in urine output (less than 30cc/hr) should be reported to a health care provider. Taking the medication with food may prevent vomiting. If not, other opiate analgesics may be better tolerated. Blurred vision and diarrhea aren't associated with the use of hydrocodone with acetaminophen. Unusual dreams are a common adverse effect but don't need to be reported unless bothersome to the client. Clients should report temperature over 100.4°F.
CN: Physiological integrity; CNS: Pharmacological therapies; CL: Apply; DIFFICULTY: Challenge

34. 1, 3. A perineal pad is needed after hysterosalpingography because the contrast medium may leak from the vagina for several hours and stain the clothing. The bowel must be cleaned before the procedure, but the client doesn't have to refrain from having anything by mouth after midnight. The procedure is performed with the client in the lithotomy position, and no special positioning is required after the procedure. Douching is not recommended 24 hours after the procedure.
CN: Physiological integrity; CNS: Basic care and comfort; CL: Apply; DIFFICULTY: Challenge

35. 4. Gamma globulin provides passive immunity to mumps. Antibiotic therapy is used in the treatment of bacterial orchitis. Ice and a scrotal support are used as comfort measures in the treatment of orchitis.
CN: Health promotion and maintenance; CNS: None; CL: Apply; DIFFICULTY: Easy

36. The nurse is preparing to discuss administration of a vaginal irrigation with a client. Which step would be appropriate to have the client perform?
1. Insert the nozzle about 3 in (7.6 cm) into the vagina.
2. Direct the tip of the nozzle toward the sacrum.
3. Instill the solution in a constant flow over 5 to 10 minutes.
4. Raise the solution at least 24 in (61 cm) above the client's hip level.

36. 2. The normal position of the vagina slants up and back toward the sacrum. Directing the tip of the nozzle toward the sacrum allows it to follow the normal slant of the vagina and minimizes tissue trauma. The nozzle should be inserted about 2 in (5.1 cm). The fluid can be instilled intermittently and, for best therapeutic results, over 20 to 30 minutes. The container should be no higher than 24 in (61 cm) above the client's hip level to avoid forcing fluid and bacteria through the cervical os into the uterus.
CN: Safe, effective care environment; CNS: Safety and infection control; CL: Understand; DIFFICULTY: Challenge

37. Which statement by a man scheduled for a vasectomy indicates he needs further education about the procedure?
1. "If I decide I want a child, I'll just get a reversal."
2. "Amazing! I can make sperm but classify as sterile."
3. "I'm sure glad I made some deposits in the sperm bank."
4. "I can't believe I still have to worry about contraception after this surgery."

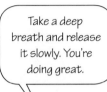

Take a deep breath and release it slowly. You're doing great.

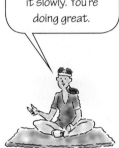

37. 1. Vasectomy procedures can be reversed but with varying degrees of success. Because of the variable success, a client can't be sure of reversibility and needs to consider vasectomy a permanent sterilization procedure when deciding to have it done. After vasectomy, the client remains fertile until sperm stored distal to the severed vas are evacuated. Once this occurs, sperm are still produced, but they don't enter the ejaculate and are absorbed by the body.
CN: Physiological integrity; CNS: Physiological adaptation; CL: Apply; DIFFICULTY: Moderate

38. A nurse is reinforcing education to a client on how to prevent the development of phimosis. What is the **priority** education for this client?
1. Proper cleaning of the prepuce
2. Importance of regular ejaculation
3. Technique of testicular self-examination
4. Proper hand washing before touching the genitals

38. 1. Proper cleaning of the preputial area to remove secretions is critical to the prevention of noncongenital phimosis. Regular ejaculation can decrease the symptoms of chronic prostatitis, but it has no effect on the development of phimosis. Testicular self-examination is important in the early detection and treatment of testicular cancer. Hand washing is important in preventing the spread of infection.
CN: Health promotion and maintenance; CNS: None; CL: Apply; DIFFICULTY: Easy

39. A nurse is caring for a client who has recently been diagnosed with testicular cancer. What information is **most** important to provide to this client?
1. Testicular cancer isn't responsive to chemotherapy, but it's highly curative with surgery.
2. Radiation therapy is never used, so the unaffected testicle remains healthy.
3. Testicular self-examination is still important because there's an increased risk of a second tumor.
4. Taking testosterone after orchiectomy prevents changes in appearance and sexual function.

39. 3. A history of a testicular malignancy puts the client at increased risk for a second tumor. Testicular self-examination enables early detection and treatment and is critical. Chemotherapy is added for clients who have evidence of metastasis after irradiation. Radiation therapy is used on the retroperitoneal lymph nodes. Testosterone isn't usually needed because the unaffected testis usually produces sufficient hormone.
CN: Physiological integrity; CNS: Reduction of risk potential; CL: Apply; DIFFICULTY: Easy

40. A nurse is caring for a client treated for testicular cancer who is returning for an alpha-fetoprotein (AFP) test. What would the nurse anticipate if the level is elevated?
1. Fertility is maintained.
2. The cancer has recurred.
3. There's metastatic disease.
4. Testosterone levels are low.

40. 3. AFP is a tumor marker elevated in nonseminomatous malignancies of the testicle. After the tumor is removed, the level should decrease. A persistent elevation after orchiectomy indicates tumor is present someplace outside the testicle that was removed. A recurrence of the cancer is indicated by a postsurgical decrease in AFP level, followed by an elevation as a new tumor starts to grow. The level of AFP isn't related to fertility or testosterone level.
CN: Physiological integrity; CNS: Physiological adaptation; CL: Analyze; DIFFICULTY: Difficult

41. A nurse is reinforcing instructions to a client who had a prostatectomy. What education is appropriate for this client? Select all that apply.
1. Avoid straining at stool.
2. Report large clots in the urine right away.
3. Soak in a warm tub daily for comfort.
4. Return to sexual activity in 3 weeks.
5. Return to work in 1 week.

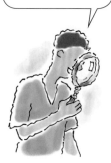

Check out these symptoms carefully. Which would be abnormal and concerning in this situation?

42. A nurse is caring for a client that has had a biopsy of the prostate. The nurse should advise the client to report which symptom(s) to the health care provider right away. Select all that apply.
1. Pain on the following day
2. Discolored semen
3. Difficulty urinating
4. Temperature of 101°F (38.3°C)
5. Urine output of 50 cc/hr

43. Two days after a transrectal biopsy of the prostate, a client calls the clinic to report his stools are streaked with blood. Which response by the nurse is appropriate?
1. Tell the client to take a laxative.
2. Tell the client to come in for examination.
3. Reassure the client that this is an expected occurrence.
4. Ask the client to collect a stool specimen for testing.

44. A nurse is caring for the following clients who have a history of genital herpes infection. Which client is **most** at risk for an outbreak of genital herpes?
1. A client who reports a headache and fever
2. A client who reports vaginal and urethral discharge
3. A client who reports dysuria and lymphadenopathy
4. A client who reports genital pruritus and paresthesia

45. A client has been admitted to the clinic with primary syphilis. Which signs or symptoms should the nurse expect to see with this diagnosis?
1. A painless genital ulcer that appeared about 3 weeks after unprotected sex
2. Copper-colored macules on the palms and soles that appeared after a brief fever
3. Patchy hair loss and red, broken skin involving the scalp, eyebrows, and beard areas
4. One or more flat, wartlike papules in the genital area that are sensitive to touch

41. 1, 2, 4. Straining at stool after prostatectomy can cause bleeding. Small blood clots or pieces of tissue commonly are passed in the urine for up to 2 weeks postoperatively. Large blood clots should be reported to the health care provider. Tub baths are prohibited because they cause dilation of pelvic blood vessels. Other activities are resumed based on the guidance of the health care provider. Sexual intercourse and driving are usually prohibited for about 3 weeks. Exercising and returning to work are usually prohibited for about 6 weeks.
CN: Physiological integrity; CNS: Reduction of risk potential; CL: Apply; DIFFICULTY: Difficult

42. 3, 4. Difficulty urinating suggests urethral obstruction. Mild pain is expected for 1 to 3 days after biopsy. Semen may be discolored for up to a month after the biopsy. Temperature of more than 101°F (38.3°C) should be reported because it suggests infection. Urine output of 50 cc/hr is normal and does not need to be reported.
CN: Physiological integrity; CNS: Reduction of risk potential; CL: Analyze; DIFFICULTY: Challenge

43. 3. After a transrectal prostatic biopsy, blood in the stools is expected for a number of days. Stool softeners are prescribed if the client reports constipation; straining at stool can precipitate bleeding, but laxatives generally aren't necessary. Because blood in the stools is expected, testing the stools or examining the client isn't necessary.
CN: Physiological integrity; CNS: Reduction of risk potential; CL: Apply; DIFFICULTY: Moderate

44. 4. Pruritus and paresthesia, as well as redness of the genital area, are prodromal symptoms of recurrent herpes infection. These symptoms occur 30 minutes to 48 hours before the lesions appear. Headache and fever are symptoms of viremia associated with the primary infection. Vaginal and urethral discharge are also local signs of primary infection. Dysuria and lymphadenopathy are local symptoms of primary infection that may also occur with recurrent infection.
CN: Physiological integrity; CNS: Physiological adaptation; CL: Analyze; DIFFICULTY: Moderate

45. 1. A painless genital ulcer is a symptom of primary syphilis. Macules on the palms and soles after fever are indicative of secondary syphilis, as is patchy hair loss. Wartlike papules are indicative of genital warts.
CN: Physiological integrity; CNS: Physiological adaptation; CL: Analyze; DIFFICULTY: Moderate

46. A nurse is caring for a woman newly diagnosed with genital herpes. What information should the nurse provide? Select all that apply.
1. Obtain a Papanicolaou (Pap) test every year.
2. Be sure your partner uses a condom.
3. Use a water-soluble lubricant for relief of pruritus.
4. Limit stress and emotional upset as much as possible.
5. Taking antiviral medications will cure the virus.

46. 1, 2, 4. Stress, anxiety, and emotional upset seem to predispose a client to recurrent outbreaks of genital herpes. Sexual intercourse and all genital contact should be avoided during outbreaks, and a condom should be used between outbreaks; it isn't known whether the virus can be transmitted at this time. During an outbreak, creams and lubricants should be avoided because they may delay healing. Because a relationship has been found between genital herpes and cervical cancer, a Pap test is recommended every year. There is no present cure for genital herpes but the antiviral medications may help decrease the outbreaks.
CN: Physiological integrity; CNS: Physiological adaptation; CL: Apply; DIFFICULTY: Challenge

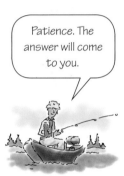

Patience. The answer will come to you.

47. During a routine physical examination, a firm mass is palpated in the right breast of a client. Which finding or client history would suggest cancer of the breast as opposed to fibrocystic disease?
1. Mass located in upper, outer quadrant
2. Cyclic change in mass size
3. History of anovulatory cycles
4. Increased vascularity of the breast

47. 4. Increase in breast size or vascularity is consistent with breast cancer. Masses associated with fibrocystic disease of the breast are firm, are most commonly located in the upper, outer quadrant of the breast, and increase in size before menstruation. They may be bilateral in a mirror image and are typically well demarcated and freely movable.
CN: Health promotion and maintenance; CNS: None; CL: Apply; DIFFICULTY: Difficult

48. After which procedure is the use of sterile technique in the provision of client hygiene **most** critical?
1. Radical prostatectomy
2. Perineal prostatectomy
3. Suprapubic prostatectomy
4. Transurethral resection of the prostate (TURP)

48. 2. The incision in a perineal prostatectomy is close to the rectum, which normally contains gram-negative organisms that can cause infection if introduced into other areas of the body. The use of proper sterile technique, including washing front to back, in providing hygiene is more critical to these clients than those with either no external incision, as with TURP, or abdominal incisions, as with radical or suprapubic prostatectomy.
CN: Physiological integrity; CNS: Reduction of risk potential; CL: Understand; DIFFICULTY: Challenge

49. The nurse is caring for a client that is suspected of having prerenal acute renal failure. Which finding in the client's history and physical would the nurse recognize as a potential cause?
1. Atherosclerosis
2. Decreased cardiac output
3. Prostatic hyperplasia
4. Rhabdomyolysis

49. 2. Prerenal acute renal failure refers to renal failure due to an interference with renal perfusion. Decreased cardiac output causes a decrease in renal perfusion, which leads to a lower glomerular filtration rate. Atherosclerosis and rhabdomyolysis are renal causes of acute renal failure. Prostatic hyperplasia would be an example of a postrenal cause of acute renal failure.
CN: Physiological integrity; CNS: Physiological adaptation; CL: Apply; DIFFICULTY: Moderate

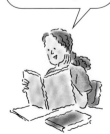

Acute pyelonephritis. What is that condition again?

50. A client admitted for acute pyelonephritis is about to start antibiotic therapy. Which symptom would the nurse expect to find in this client?
1. Hypertension
2. Flank pain on the affected side
3. Pain that radiates toward the unaffected side
4. No tenderness with deep palpation over the costovertebral angle

50. 2. The client may report flank pain on the affected side because the kidney is enlarged and might have formed an abscess. Hypertension is associated with chronic pyelonephritis. The client would have tenderness with deep palpation over the costovertebral angle. Pain may radiate down the ureters or to the epigastrium.
CN: Physiological integrity; CNS: Physiological adaptation; CL: Apply; DIFFICULTY: Easy

51. A client is reporting severe flank, abdominal pain and is diagnosed with urolithiasis. Which intervention should the nurse instruct the client to perform?
  1. Strain all urine.
  2. Limit fluid intake.
  3. Enforce strict bed rest.
  4. Encourage a high-calcium diet.

51. 1. Urine should be strained for calculi and sent to the laboratory for analysis. Fluid intake of 3 to 4 L/day is encouraged to flush the urinary tract and prevent further calculi formation. Ambulation is encouraged to help pass the calculi through gravity. A low-calcium diet is recommended to help prevent the formation of calcium calculi.
CN: Physiological integrity; CNS: Reduction of risk potential; CL: Apply; DIFFICULTY: Easy

52. The nurse is assisting with the discharge of a client with acute pyelonephritis. What should the nurse be sure to include in the client instructions?
  1. Avoid taking any dairy products.
  2. Return for follow-up urine cultures.
  3. Stop taking the prescribed antibiotics when the symptoms subside.
  4. Recurrence is unlikely because of treatment with antibiotics.

52. 2. The client needs to return for follow-up urine cultures because bacteriuria may be present but may not produce symptoms. Intake of dairy products won't contribute to pyelonephritis. Antibiotics must be taken for the full course of therapy regardless of symptoms. Pyelonephritis commonly recurs as a relapse or new infection, usually within 2 weeks of completing therapy.
CN: Health promotion and maintenance; CNS: None; CL: Apply; DIFFICULTY: Easy

53. A client has undergone a radical cystectomy and has an ileal conduit for the treatment of bladder cancer. Which postoperative assessment finding must be reported to the health care provider immediately?
  1. A red, moist stoma
  2. A dusky-colored stoma
  3. Urine output more than 30 mL/hour
  4. Slight bleeding from the stoma when changing the appliance

53. 2. The stoma should be red and moist, indicating adequate blood flow. A dusky or cyanotic stoma indicates insufficient blood supply and is an emergency needing prompt intervention. Urine output less than 30 mL/hr or no urine output for more than 15 minutes should be reported. Slight bleeding from the stoma when changing the appliance may occur because the intestinal mucosa is very fragile.
CN: Physiological integrity; CNS: Reduction of risk potential; CL: Apply; DIFFICULTY: Easy

54. A nurse is caring for a client diagnosed with cystitis. What information should the nurse include? Select all that apply
  1. Bathe in a tub.
  2. Wear cotton underpants.
  3. Use a feminine hygiene spray.
  4. Encourage intake of cranberry juice.
  5. Douche once a week.

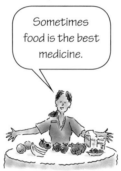

Sometimes food is the best medicine.

54. 2, 4. Cotton underpants prevent infection because they allow air to flow to the perineum. Cranberry juice helps prevent cystitis because it increases urine acidity and prevents *E. coli* from sticking to the urinary tract; alkaline urine supports bacterial growth. Women should shower instead of taking a tub bath to prevent infection. Feminine hygiene spray can act as an irritant. Douching is not recommended in women unless recommended by a health care provider.
CN: Health promotion and maintenance; CNS: None; CL: Apply; DIFFICULTY: Moderate

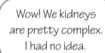

Wow! We kidneys are pretty complex. I had no idea.

55. A client with a history of chronic renal failure is admitted with pulmonary edema following a missed dialysis treatment yesterday. The laboratory results are: serum potassium 6.0 mEq/L, serum sodium 130 mEq/L, and serum bicarbonate 18 mEq/L. The nurse interprets that the client has which condition?
  1. Alkalemia
  2. Hyperkalemia
  3. Hypernatremia
  4. Hypokalemia

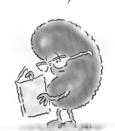

55. 2. The kidneys are responsible for excreting potassium. In renal failure, the kidneys can no longer excrete potassium, resulting in hyperkalemia. The kidneys are responsible for regulating the acid-base balance; in renal failure, acidemia, not alkalemia, would be likely. Generally, hyponatremia, not hypernatremia, would occur because of the dilutional effect of water retention. Hypokalemia is generally seen in clients undergoing diuresis.
CN: Physiological integrity; CNS: Physiological adaptation; CL: Analyze; DIFFICULTY: Easy

56. Which condition(s) makes an older adult client more prone to urinary tract infections (UTIs)? Select all that apply.
1. Incomplete emptying of the bladder
2. Increase in urine acidity
3. Fecal incontinence with perineal soiling
4. Shortening of the urethra
5. Increase in urine alkalinity

57. A client has just received a renal transplant and has started cyclosporine therapy to prevent graft rejection. Which condition indicates to the nurse that the client is experiencing a major adverse effect related to the medication?
1. Depression
2. Hemorrhage
3. Infection
4. Peptic ulcer disease

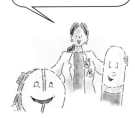

Drugs are great, but sometimes they have unintended effects.

58. A client received a kidney transplant 2 months ago and is admitted to the hospital with the diagnosis of acute rejection. Which finding would be expected? Select all that apply.
1. Hypertension
2. Temperature of 101°F
3. Decreased white blood cell (WBC) counts
4. Elevated blood urea nitrogen (BUN) and creatinine levels
5. Elevated hemoglobin

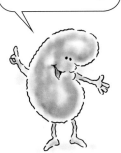

Your kidneys work hard every day for you. Have you thanked them lately?

59. A client with renal insufficiency is admitted with a diagnosis of pneumonia, episodes of hypotension, and is receiving intravenous antibiotics. Which laboratory value should the nurse monitor?
1. Blood urea nitrogen (BUN) and creatinine levels
2. Arterial blood gas (ABG) levels
3. Platelet count
4. Potassium level

60. A client had a transurethral prostatectomy for benign prostatic hyperplasia (BPH). He's currently being treated with continuous bladder irrigation and is reporting an increase in severity of bladder spasms. What should the nurse do **first** for this client?
1. Administer an oral analgesic.
2. Stop the irrigation and call the health care provider.
3. Administer a belladonna and opium suppository as ordered by the health care provider.
4. Check for the presence of clots, and make sure the catheter is draining properly.

56. 1, 3, 5. Incomplete emptying of the bladder predisposes a client to cystitis. Perineal soiling allows infectious organisms to remain near the urethral meatus, increasing the likelihood of migration into the urinary tract. Acidic urine impedes bacterial growth. The urethra does not shorten with age.
CN: Physiological integrity; CNS: Physiological adaptation; CL: Analyze; DIFFICULTY: Difficult

57. 3. Infection is the major complication to watch for in clients on cyclosporine therapy because cyclosporine is an immunosuppressive drug. Depression may occur posttransplantation but not because of cyclosporine. Hemorrhage is a complication associated with anticoagulant therapy. Peptic ulcer disease is a complication of steroid therapy.
CN: Physiological integrity; CNS: Pharmacological therapies; CL: Analyze; DIFFICULTY: Moderate

58. 1, 2, 4. In a client with acute renal graft rejection, evidence of deteriorating renal function, including elevated BUN and creatinine levels, is expected. The client would most likely have acute hypertension. The nurse would see elevated, not decreased, WBC counts as well as fever because the body is recognizing the graft as foreign and is attempting to fight it. Hemoglobin would be decreased in this client.
CN: Physiological integrity; CNS: Reduction of risk potential; CL: Analyze; DIFFICULTY: Moderate

59. 1. BUN and creatinine levels are used to monitor renal function. Because the client is receiving IV antibiotics, which can be nephrotoxic, these tests would be used to closely monitor renal function. The client is also hypotensive, which is a prerenal cause of acute renal failure. ABG determinations are inappropriate for this situation. Platelet and potassium levels should be monitored according to routine.
CN: Physiological integrity; CNS: Reduction of risk potential; CL: Analyze; DIFFICULTY: Moderate

60. 4. Blood clots and blocked outflow of the urine can increase spasms. The irrigation shouldn't be stopped as long as the catheter is draining because clots will form. A belladonna and opium suppository should be given to relieve spasms but only *after* assessment of the drainage. Oral analgesics should be given if the spasms are unrelieved by the belladonna and opium suppositories.
CN: Physiological integrity; CNS: Physiological adaptation; CL: Analyze; DIFFICULTY: Easy

61. A client with bladder cancer had his bladder removed and an ileal conduit created for urine diversion. While changing this client's pouch, the nurse observes that the area around the stoma is red, weeping, and painful. What should the nurse conclude?
1. The skin wasn't lubricated before the pouch was applied.
2. The pouch faceplate doesn't fit the stoma.
3. A skin barrier was applied properly.
4. Stoma dilation wasn't performed.

62. A client has an indwelling urinary catheter, and urine is leaking from a hole in the collection bag. Which nursing intervention would be **most** appropriate?
1. Cover the hole with tape.
2. Remove the catheter, and insert a new one using sterile technique.
3. Disconnect the drainage bag from the catheter, and replace it with a new bag.
4. Place a towel under the bag to prevent spillage of urine on the floor, which could cause the client to slip and fall.

63. When obtaining data from a client, which statement indicates a risk of renal calculi?
1. "I've been drinking a lot of cola soft drinks lately."
2. "I've been jogging more than usual."
3. "I've had more stress since we adopted a child last year."
4. "I'm a vegetarian and eat cheese two or three times each day."

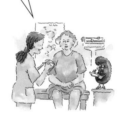

If you think your client may have renal calculi, don't forget to ask about her diet.

64. The nurse is gathering information on a client reporting painful urination during and after voiding. The nurse suspects the client may have a problem with which area of the urinary system?
1. Bladder
2. Kidneys
3. Ureters
4. Urethra

65. A nurse is reinforcing instructions for a client taking furosemide. Which education should the nurse reinforce? Select all that apply.
1. Take your medication every morning as instructed.
2. High doses of this medication can cause hearing loss.
3. Notify your health care provider if you are unable to void.
4. Drink grapefruit juice once a day.
5. Eating foods high in potassium is recommended while taking this medicine.

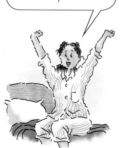

Yay! I slept through the whole night without having to get up to pee.

61. 2. If the pouch faceplate doesn't fit the stoma properly, the skin around the stoma will be exposed to continuous urine flow from the stoma, causing excoriation and red, weeping, painful skin. A lubricant shouldn't be used because it would prevent the pouch from adhering to the skin. When properly applied, a skin barrier prevents skin excoriation. Stoma dilation isn't performed with an ileal conduit, although it may be done with a colostomy, if ordered.
CN: Physiological integrity; CNS: Basic care and comfort; CL: Analyze; DIFFICULTY: Moderate

62. 2. The system is no longer a closed system, and bacteria might have been introduced into the system, so a new sterile catheter should be inserted. Placing a towel under the bag and taping up the hole leaves the system open, which increases the risk of infection. Replacing the drainage bag by disconnecting the old one from the catheter opens up the entire system and isn't recommended because of the increased risk of infection.
CN: Safe, effective care environment; CNS: Safety and infection control; CL: Analyze; DIFFICULTY: Challenge

63. 4. Renal calculi are commonly composed of calcium. Diets high in calcium may predispose a person to renal calculi. Milk and milk products are high in calcium. Cola soft drinks don't contain ingredients that would increase the risk of renal calculi. Jogging and increased stress aren't considered risk factors for renal calculi formation.
CN: Health promotion and maintenance; CNS: None; CL: Analyze; DIFFICULTY: Challenge

64. 1. Pain during or after voiding indicates a bladder problem, usually infection. Kidney and ureter pain would be in the flank area, and problems of the urethra would cause pain at the external orifice commonly felt at the start of voiding.
CN: Health promotion and maintenance; CNS: None; CL: Apply; DIFFICULTY: Challenge

65. 1, 2, 3. A diuretic such as furosemide given in the morning has time to work throughout the day. Diuretics given at nighttime will cause the client to get up to go to the bathroom frequently, interrupting sleep. High doses of furosemide can cause hearing loss. Clients should notify their health care provider if they are unable to void. Clients should avoid grapefruit and foods high in potassium while on this medication.
CN: Physiological integrity; CNS: Pharmacological therapies; CL: Apply; DIFFICULTY: Challenge

66. The nurse is caring for a client with postoperative urine retention. Which intervention should the nurse provide **first**?
1. Administer furosemide.
2. Pour warm water over the perineum.
3. Consider inserting a bladder catheter.
4. Lay the client flat in bed.

66. 2. Urine retention reflects bladder distention from urine. Sitting upright and pouring water over the perineum may help the client void. A diuretic isn't necessary. If these measures aren't successful, the nurse should consider inserting a bladder catheter to drain the bladder, which requires an order from the health care provider.
CN: Physiological integrity; CNS: Basic care and comfort; CL: Apply; DIFFICULTY: Challenge

67. A client has not voided for 10 hours following an inguinal hernia repair. Which factor may place a surgical client at risk for urine retention?
1. Dehydration
2. History of smoking
3. Duration of surgery
4. Anticholinergic medication before surgery

67. 4. Anticholinergic medications such as atropine may cause urine retention, particularly for the client who has had surgery in the pelvic area (inguinal hernia, hysterectomy). Dehydration, smoking, and duration of surgery aren't risk factors for urine retention.
CN: Physiological integrity; CNS: Reduction of risk potential; CL: Apply; DIFFICULTY: Moderate

68. The nurse is caring for a client with urinary retention. Which catheter should the nurse obtain for insertion for this client?
1. Coudé
2. Indwelling urinary
3. Straight
4. Three-way

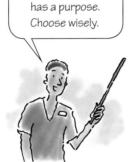

Each catheter has a purpose. Choose wisely.

68. 3. Urine retention is usually a temporary problem. A straight catheter is generally used for the client with urine retention. The three-way catheter is used for clients who need bladder irrigation, such as after a prostate resection. A Coudé catheter is used only when it's difficult to insert a standard catheter, usually because of an enlarged prostate. The other catheters are used for longer-term bladder problems.
CN: Physiological integrity; CNS: Basic care and comfort; CL: Apply; DIFFICULTY: Challenge

69. An older adult man reports urine retention. Which factor does the nurse discuss with the client that may be contributing to the problem?
1. Benign prostatic hyperplasia
2. Diabetes
3. Diet
4. Hypertension

69. 1. Benign prostatic hyperplasia is common among older adult men and generally results in urine retention, frequency, dribbling, and difficulty starting the urine stream. Diabetes, diet, and hypertension usually don't affect urine retention. Diabetes can cause renal failure.
CN: Physiological integrity; CNS: Reduction of risk potential; CL: Apply; DIFFICULTY: Easy

70. The nurse is educating a client on self-breast examination (SBE). Which pattern of palpation would the nurse encourage based on the American Cancer Society's (ACS) recommendations?

70. 3. The ACS recommends an up-and-down vertical pattern as the most effective pattern for covering the whole breast. Option 1 (circular pattern) and option 2 (wedged pattern) are alternative methods but may not be as effective. Option 4 (horizontal pattern) isn't a recognized method used in SBE.
CN: Physiological integrity; CNS: Reduction of risk potential; CL: Apply; DIFFICULTY: Challenge

1.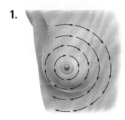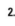

2.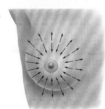

3.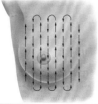

4.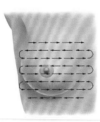

71. A client is injected with radiographic contrast medium and immediately shows signs of dyspnea, flushing, and pruritus. Which intervention should take **priority**?
1. Check vital signs.
2. Make sure the airway is patent.
3. Apply a cold pack to the IV site.
4. Call the health care provider.

72. A nurse is reinforcing information to a client who is scheduled for a biopsy of the bladder. Which medication(s) should the nurse anticipate the client will discontinue taking for 3 to 5 days prior to the procedure? Select all that apply.
1. Coumadin
2. Antibiotic
3. Aspirin
4. Lisinopril
5. Furosemide

73. A nurse is caring for a client with renal failure who is reporting nausea. Which factor **best** explains how nausea is related to renal failure?
1. Oliguria
2. Gastric ulcer
3. Electrolyte imbalance
4. Accumulation of metabolic wastes

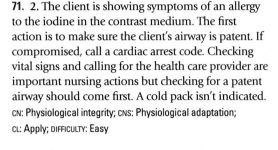

All this waste is starting to make me feel a little nauseated.

74. Which client is at **greatest** risk for developing acute renal failure?
1. A client on dialysis who gets influenza
2. A teenager who has an appendectomy
3. A pregnant woman who has a fractured femur
4. A client with diabetes who has a heart catheterization

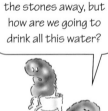

I know it's supposed to keep the stones away, but how are we going to drink all this water?

75. A nurse is caring for a client with urinary calculus. What information should the nurse provide to this client?
1. Save any stone larger than 0.25 cm.
2. Strain the urine, limit oral fluids, and give pain medications.
3. Encourage fluid intake, strain the urine, and give pain medications.
4. Insert an indwelling urinary catheter, check intake and output, and give pain medications.

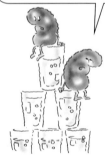

71. 2. The client is showing symptoms of an allergy to the iodine in the contrast medium. The first action is to make sure the client's airway is patent. If compromised, call a cardiac arrest code. Checking vital signs and calling for the health care provider are important nursing actions but checking for a patent airway should come first. A cold pack isn't indicated.
CN: Physiological integrity; CNS: Physiological adaptation; CL: Apply; DIFFICULTY: Easy

72. 1, 3. The client needs to take his antibiotic as ordered. Anticoagulants and aspirin should be discontinued for 3 to 5 days before the procedure due to the risk of increased bleeding. Lisinopril does not interfere with this procedure. Furosemide does not interfere with this procedure and should be taken as ordered.
CN: Physiological integrity; CNS: Reduction of risk potential; CL: Analyze; DIFFICULTY: Moderate

73. 4. Although a client with renal failure can develop stress ulcers, nausea is usually related to the poisons of metabolic wastes that accumulate when the kidneys can't eliminate them. The client may have electrolyte imbalances and oliguria, but these conditions don't directly cause nausea.
CN: Physiological integrity; CNS: Physiological adaptation; CL: Analyze; DIFFICULTY: Moderate

74. 4. Diabetes can damage the smaller arteries of the kidneys, and clients with diabetes are prone to renal insufficiency and renal failure. The contrast used for heart catheterization must be eliminated by the kidneys, which further stresses them and may produce acute renal failure. A dialysis client already has end-stage renal disease and wouldn't develop acute renal failure. A teenager who has an appendectomy and a pregnant woman who fractures a femur aren't at increased risk for renal failure.
CN: Health promotion and maintenance; CNS: None; CL: Analyze; DIFFICULTY: Challenge

75. 3. Encouraging fluids and straining all urine, saving all calculi, including "flecks," is the appropriate intervention. Give pain medications because renal calculi are extremely painful. Indwelling urinary catheters usually aren't needed.
CN: Physiological integrity; CNS: Basic care and comfort; CL: Apply; DIFFICULTY: Easy

76. A nurse is obtaining data from a client with a urinary tract infection (UTI). Which statement should the nurse expect the client to make? Select all that apply:
1. "I urinate large amounts."
2. "I need to urinate frequently."
3. "It burns when I urinate."
4. "My urine smells sweet."
5. "I need to urinate urgently."

77. A nurse is collecting a sterile urine specimen for culture and sensitivity from an indwelling urinary catheter. Identify the area on the indwelling urinary catheter where the nurse should insert the sterile syringe to obtain the urine specimen.

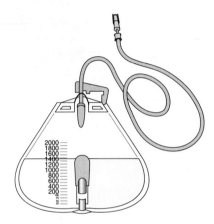

78. A nurse is completing an intake and output record for a client who's receiving continuous bladder irrigation after transurethral resection of the prostate (TURP). How many milliliters of urine should the nurse record as output for her shift if the client received 1,800 mL of normal saline irrigating solution and the output in the urine drainage bag is 2,400 mL? Record your answer as a whole number.

_____ mL

79. A client with chronic renal failure plans to receive a kidney transplant. Recently, the health care provider told the client that he is a poor candidate for transplant because of chronic uncontrolled hypertension and diabetes. Now, the client tells the nurse, "I want to go off dialysis. I'd rather not live than be on this treatment for the rest of my life." Which response is appropriate? Select all that apply.
1. Take a seat next to the client and sit quietly.
2. Say to the client, "We all have days when we don't feel like going on."
3. Leave the room to allow the client to collect his thoughts.
4. Say to the client, "You're feeling upset about the news you got about the transplant."
5. Say to the client, "The treatments are only 3 days a week. You can live with that."

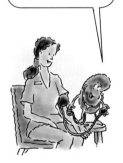

Your blood pressure is 118/73—that's good news for both of us!

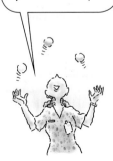

Congratulations! You juggled those questions like a pro.

76. 2, 3, 5. Typical assessment findings for a client with a UTI include urinary frequency, burning on urination, and urinary urgency. The client with a UTI typically reports that he voids frequently in small amounts, not large amounts. The client with a UTI reports foul-smelling, not sweet-smelling, urine.
CN: Physiological integrity; CNS: Physiological adaptation; CL: Apply; DIFFICULTY: Easy

77. A sterile urine specimen is obtained from an indwelling urinary catheter by clamping the catheter briefly, cleaning the rubber port with an alcohol wipe, and using a sterile syringe to withdraw the urine.

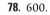

CN: Physiological integrity; CNS: Reduction of risk potential; CL: Apply; DIFFICULTY: Moderate

78. 600.
To calculate urine output, subtract the amount of irrigation solution infused into the bladder from the total amount of fluid in the drainage bag. For this client:

$$2,400 \text{ mL} - 1,800 \text{ mL} = 600 \text{ mL}.$$

CN: Physiological integrity; CNS: Reduction of risk potential; CL: Apply; DIFFICULTY: Moderate

79. 1, 4. Silence is a therapeutic communication technique that allows the nurse and client to reflect on what has been said or taken place. By waiting quietly and attentively, the nurse encourages the client to initiate and maintain conversation. By reflecting the client's implied feelings, the nurse promotes communication. Using such platitudes as "We all have days when we don't feel like going on" fails to address the client's needs. The nurse shouldn't leave the client alone because of the risk of harm to self. Minimizing the treatment frequency doesn't address the client's feelings.
CN: Psychosocial integrity; CNS: None; CL: Analyze; DIFFICULTY: Moderate

CN: Client needs category   CNS: Client needs subcategory   CL: Cognitive level

Chapter 11

Integumentary Disorders

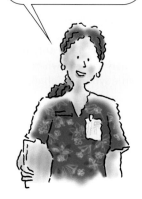

So, you think caring for a client with a skin disorder isn't your strong suit, eh? Check out this Web site before taking on this chapter: www.aad.org. Enjoy!

Integumentary refresher

Atopic dermatitis

Itchy skin that is warm, red, and tender

Key signs and symptoms

- Erythematous lesions that eventually become scaly and lichenified
- Excessively dry skin
- Hyperpigmentation
- Skin eruptions

Key test results

- Serum immunoglobulin E levels are commonly elevated (not a confirmation that client has atopic dermatitis)

Key treatments

- Antihistamines: diphenhydramine
- Corticosteroid: hydrocortisone

Key interventions

- Help client set up an individual schedule and plan for daily skin care
- Instruct client to bathe in plain water (bathing may have to be limited, according to severity of lesions)
- Instruct client to bathe with special nonfatty soap and tepid water (96° F [35.6° C])
- Instruct client to avoid using any soap when lesions are acutely inflamed
- Instruct client to limit baths and showers to 5 to 7 minutes
- For scalp involvement, advise client to shampoo frequently and to apply corticosteroid solution to scalp afterward
- Lubricate skin after a shower or bath

Burn

Injury caused by exposure to heat, flame or electricity

Key signs and symptoms

- Superficial partial-thickness burn
  - erythema, edema, pain, blanching
- Deep dermal partial-thickness burn
  - pain, oozing, fluid-filled vesicles
  - erythema
  - shiny and wet subcutaneous layer after vesicles rupture

- Full-thickness burn
  - eschar, edema, little or no pain

Key test results

- Visual inspection allows examiner to estimate extent of the burn (determined by the Rule of Nines and the Lund and Browder chart)

Key treatments

- IV therapy: hydration and electrolyte replacement using a fluid replacement formula such as the Parkland formula
- Skin grafts
- Analgesic: morphine
- Antianxiety agent: lorazepam
- Antibiotic: gentamicin
- Anti-infectives: mafenide, silver sulfadiazine, silver nitrate
- Antitetanus: tetanus toxoid
- Colloid: albumin 5%

Key interventions

- Monitor respiratory status
- Monitor fluid status
- Maintain IV fluids
- Administer oxygen
- Monitor total parenteral or enteral feedings
- Maintain protective precautions

Herpes zoster

Vesicular rash caused by herpesvirus, also known as shingles

Key signs and symptoms

- Neuralgia
- Severe, deep pain
- Unilaterally clustered skin vesicles along peripheral sensory nerves on the trunk, thorax, or face

Key test results

- A skin study identifies the organism
- Visual inspection identifies vesicles along the peripheral sensory nerves

Key treatments

- Analgesics: acetaminophen, codeine
- Antianxiety agents: lorazepam, hydroxyzine

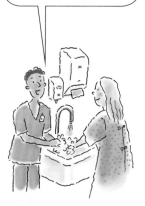

Clients with dermatitis may need to lay off the soap to prevent skin irritation.

- Antipruritic: diphenhydramine
- Antiviral agents: acyclovir, valacyclovir, famciclovir
- Vaccine: zoster vaccine, live

Key interventions
- Monitor neurologic status
- Monitor pain and note the effectiveness of analgesics
- Prevent scratching and rubbing of affected areas

Pressure ulcer
Injury to the skin caused by prolonged pressure

Key signs and symptoms
- Signs are determined by stage of ulceration

Key treatments
- High-protein, high-calorie diet in small, frequent feedings
- Parenteral or enteral feedings if client is unable or unwilling to take adequate nutrients orally
- Topical wound care according to facility protocol
- Wound debridement; tissue flap

Key interventions
- Monitor skin integrity and watch for signs of infection
- Monitor any bedridden client for possible changes in skin color, turgor, temperature, and sensation
- Reposition client every 1 to 2 hours
- Provide meticulous skin care and check bony prominences
- Maintain client's diet and encourage oral fluid intake

Psoriasis
Autoimmune disease characterized by itchy, red, scaly patches on the skin

Key signs and symptoms
- Itching
- Lesions (red and usually well-defined patches)
- Pustules (with secondary infection)

Key test results
- Skin biopsy is positive for the disorder

Key treatments
- Antipsoriatic agents: calcipotriene
- Corticosteroid ointments: hydrocortisone, clobetasol propionate

- Topical retinoids: tazarotene
- Ultraviolet light to retard cell production; may be used in conjunction with psoralens (psoralen plus ultraviolet A [PUVA] therapy)

Key interventions
- Make sure client understands prescribed therapy
- Provide written instructions
- Watch for adverse reactions, especially:
  - allergic reactions to anthralin
  - atrophy and acne from steroids
  - burning, itching, nausea, and squamous cell epitheliomas from PUVA therapy
- Caution client receiving PUVA therapy to:
  - stay out of the sun on day of treatment
  - protect eyes with sunglasses that screen UVA for 24 hours after treatment
  - wear goggles during any exposure to this light

Skin cancer
Malignancy involving any layer of the skin

Key signs and symptoms
- Change in color, size, or shape of preexisting lesion
- Irregular, circular bordered lesion with hues of tan, black, or blue (melanoma)
- Small, red, nodular lesion that begins as an erythematous macule or plaque with indistinct margins (squamous cell carcinoma)
- Waxy nodule with telangiectasis (basal cell epithelioma)

Key test results
- A skin biopsy shows cytology positive for cancer cells

Key treatments
- Chemosurgery with zinc chloride
- Cryosurgery with liquid nitrogen
- Curettage and electrodesiccation
- Antimetabolite: fluorouracil

Key interventions
- Monitor treated lesion sites
- Administer medications as prescribed
- Provide postchemotherapy and postradiation nursing care

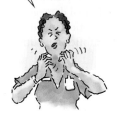

What could be causing this itching?

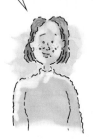

Great. I've got zits. Aren't I too old for this?

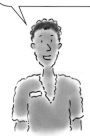

Your client comes in concerned that a skin lesion might be cancerous. What signs should you look for?

Integumentary questions, answers, and rationales

1. A client reports being exposed to lice and thinks they are on the scalp. Which observations made by the nurse would indicate the client's report is correct?
1. Diffuse, pruritic wheals
2. Oval, white dots stuck to the hair shafts
3. Pain, redness, and edema with an embedded stinger
4. Pruritic nodules and linear burrows of the finger and toe webs

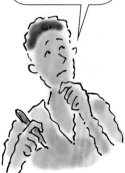

What you're looking for are the lice's eggs. Hmm. What would tiny eggs look like?

1. 2. Nits, the eggs of lice, are seen as white, oval dots. Diffuse, itchy wheals indicate an allergy. Bites from honeybees are associated with a stinger, pain, and redness. Pruritic nodules and linear burrows are diagnostic of scabies.
CN: Physiological integrity; CNS: Physiological adaptation;
CL: Apply; DIFFICULTY: Easy

2. A client is admitted to the emergency department with a deep partial-thickness burn on the arm after a fire in the workplace. Which signs and symptoms should the nurse expect to see?
1. Pain and redness
2. Minimal damage to the epidermis
3. Necrotic tissue through all layers of skin
4. Necrotic tissue through most of the dermis

2. 4. A deep, partial-thickness burn causes necrosis of the epidermal and dermal layers. Redness and pain are characteristics of a superficial injury. Superficial burns cause slight epidermal damage. With deep burns, the nerve fibers are destroyed and the client doesn't feel pain in the affected area. Necrosis through all skin layers is seen with full-thickness injuries.
CN: Physiological integrity; CNS: Physiological adaptation;
CL: Apply; DIFFICULTY: Moderate

3. The nurse is admitting a client who states, "I was bit by a brown recluse spider." Which observations made by the nurse would indicate the client's report is accurate?
1. Bull's-eye rash
2. Painful rash around a necrotic lesion
3. Herald patch of oval lesions
4. Line of papules and vesicles that appear 1 to 3 days after exposure

3. 2. Necrotic, painful rashes are associated with the bite of a brown recluse spider. A bull's-eye rash located primarily at the site of the bite is a classic sign of Lyme disease. A herald patch—a slightly raised, oval lesion about 2 to 6 cm in diameter that appears anywhere on the body—is indicative of pityriasis rosea. A linear, papular, vesicular rash is characteristic of exposure to poison ivy.
CN: Physiological integrity; CNS: Physiological adaptation;
CL: Analyze; DIFFICULTY: Moderate

4. The nurse is instructing a client after the administration of a Mantoux test. Which statement from the client indicates an understanding of the information given by the nurse?
1. "A Mantoux test is a screening for tuberculosis."
2. "I must return to the office in 24 hours to read the results."
3. "If the site itches, I should apply an anti-itch cream directly to the site."
4. "I should rub the area for 10 seconds after it is injected."

4. 1. The results of a Mantoux test are administered as a screening for tuberculosis and should be read 48 to 72 hours after placement by measuring the diameter of the induration that develops at the site. The purified protein derivative test is injected intradermally on the volar surface of the forearm, not into the deltoid. Rubbing the site of an intradermal injection could cause leakage from the injection site. Avoid applying anti-itch creams directly to the site.
CN: Physiological integrity; CNS: Reduction of risk potential;
CL: Apply; DIFFICULTY: Easy

5. A client is brought to the emergency department with partial-thickness and full-thickness burns on the left arm, left anterior leg, and anterior trunk. Using the Rule of Nines, what percentage of the total body surface area has been burned?
1. 9%
2. 18%
3. 34%
4. 36%

5. 4. The Rule of Nines divides body surface into percentages that, when totaled, equal 100%. According to the Rule of Nines, the arms account for 9% each, the anterior legs account for 9% each, and the anterior trunk accounts for 18%. Therefore, this client's burns cover 36% of his body surface area.
CN: Physiological integrity; CNS: Physiological adaptation;
CL: Analyze; DIFFICULTY: Moderate

CN: Client needs category   CNS: Client needs subcategory   CL: Cognitive level

6. A nurse is caring for a client with a burn injury. Which statement **best** describes the client's nutritional needs?
1. The client needs 100 cal/kg throughout hospitalization.
2. The hypermetabolic state after a burn injury leads to poor healing.
3. Controlling the temperature of the environment decreases caloric demands.
4. Maintaining a hypermetabolic rate decreases the client's risk of infection.

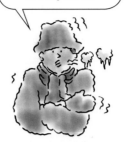

Make sure that the client doesn't expend energy trying to stay warm.

6. 2. A burn injury causes a hypermetabolic state resulting in protein and lipid catabolism that affects wound healing adversely. Caloric intake must be 1½ to 2 times the basal metabolic rate, with at least 1.5 to 2 g of protein per kg of body weight daily. An environmental temperature within normal range lets the body function efficiently and devote caloric expenditure to healing and normal physiologic processes. If the temperature is too warm or too cold, the body devotes energy to warming or cooling, which takes away from energy used for tissue repair. High metabolic rates increase the risk of infection.
CN: Physiological integrity; CNS: Basic care and comfort; CL: Apply; DIFFICULTY: Difficult

7. A client comes to the clinic with itching, dark red lesions on the hands, wrist, and waistline that are bleeding. The nurse instructs the client to try pressing on the itchy lesions. What is the rationale for this intervention?
1. Pressing the skin spreads beneficial microorganisms.
2. Pressing is suggested before scratching.
3. Pressing the skin promotes breaks in the skin.
4. Pressing the skin stimulates nerve endings.

Ugh! My foot is itching like crazy. How can I make it stop?

7. 4. Pressing the skin stimulates nerve endings and can reduce the sensation of itching. Scratching (not pressing) the skin spreads microorganisms and opens portals of entry for bacteria. Scratching isn't recommended at all. Pressing the skin doesn't promote breaks in the skin.
CN: Physiological integrity; CNS: Physiological adaptation; CL: Apply; DIFFICULTY: Challenge

8. A client arrives to the clinic with reports of a rash. The nurse observes the client and documents the lesion as a papule. What is the **best** way for the nurse to document this finding?
1. A 0.5-cm fluid filled lesion
2. A 0.5-cm red, flat pinpoint rash
3. A 0.5-cm elevated area
4. A 0.5-cm wheal

8. 3. Papules are elevated up to 0.5 cm, and nodules and tumors are masses elevated more than 0.5 cm. Erosions are characterized by loss of the epidermal layer. Macules and patches are nonpalpable, flat changes in skin color. Fluid-filled lesions are vesicles and pustules.
CN: Health promotion and maintenance; CNS: None; CL: Apply; DIFFICULTY: Moderate

9. The nurse is caring for a female client who is planning to start isotretinoin in 3 months. What should the nurse be sure to include in the instructions for the administration of this medication?
1. The need to begin contraceptive precautions.
2. Now is a good time to get pregnant if she is planning to have a baby.
3. Isotretinoin is safe in pregnancy.
4. Isotretinoin can cause women to become infertile.

9. 1. Even small amounts of isotretinoin are associated with severe birth defects. Most female clients are also prescribed oral contraceptives to prevent pregnancy. Isotretinoin does not cause infertility in women.
CN: Physiological integrity; CNS: Pharmacological therapies; CL: Apply; DIFFICULTY: Easy

10. A nurse is assisting in developing a plan of care for a pediatric client with a diagnosis of atopic dermatitis. Which actions would the nurse **most** likely include in the plan? Select all that apply.
1. Help the client develop a daily skin care schedule.
2. Lubricate the skin after bathing.
3. Scrub the areas for 10 minutes when acutely inflamed.
4. Shampoo often if the scalp is involved.
5. Take frequent showers in hot water every day.

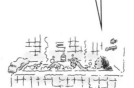

A long soak followed by some moisturizing lotion is a great way to care for your integument.

10. 1, 2, 4. Tepid baths and moisturizers are indicated for eczema to keep the infected areas clean and to minimize itching. Clients should lubricate the skin directly after bathing to reduce dryness and pruritus. Clients should shampoo their scalp frequently. Hot baths can exacerbate the condition and increase itching. Tepid baths are indicated for these clients, not hot showers.
CN: Physiological integrity; CNS: Physiological adaptation; CL: Apply; DIFFICULTY: Moderate

11. A nurse is caring for a client with thrush. Which instructions would be anticipated for treatment of this disorder?
1. Take the drug right after meals.
2. Take the drug right before meals.
3. Mix the drug with small amounts of food.
4. Take half the dose before and half after meals.

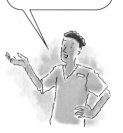

Timing matters when taking medication for thrush.

11. 1. Nystatin oral solution should be swished around the mouth after eating for the best contact with mucous membranes. Taking the drug before or with meals doesn't allow for the best contact with the mucous membranes.
CN: Physiological integrity; CNS: Pharmacological therapies; CL: Apply; DIFFICULTY: Challenge

12. A client is examined and found to have pinpoint, pink-to-purple, nonblanching macular lesions 1 to 3 mm in diameter. How should the nurse document the findings?
1. Ecchymosis
2. Hematoma
3. Petechiae
4. Purpura

12. 3. Petechiae are small macular lesions 1 to 3 mm in diameter. Ecchymosis is a purple-to-brown bruise, macular or papular, that varies in size. A hematoma is a collection of blood from ruptured blood vessels that's more than 1 cm in diameter. Purpura are purple macular lesions larger than 1 cm.
CN: Physiological integrity; CNS: Physiological adaptation; CL: Apply; DIFFICULTY: Moderate

13. The nurse observes several areas of ecchymosis on a client's arms and is informed by the client that she is being abused by her partner. What's the **most** appropriate nursing intervention?
1. Immediately inform the health care provider about the physical violence.
2. Tell the client that the health care provider will be contacted to obtain referrals for personal counseling.
3. Tell the client that the local police will need to be called.
4. Make sure the client has a safe place to go if needed.

13. 4. Because there are physical indicators of violence, ensuring the client's safety is a priority. Therefore, the nurse should make sure the client has a safe place to go if needed. Calling the local police or the health care provider right away are inappropriate options because they undermine the trust the client has placed in the nurse; safety could be jeopardized if the secret is revealed to the health care provider or legal authorities without permission.
CN: Psychosocial integrity; CNS: None; CL: Analyze; DIFFICULTY: Moderate

14. A nurse is caring for a client diagnosed with herpes zoster. What does the nurse anticipate observing on this client? Select all that apply.
1. Nontender vesicular lesions
2. A clustered rash following the sensory nerves
3. Lesions noted bilaterally on the inner aspect of the client's thighs
4. Severe, deep pain at the site of the rash
5. Pruritus

14. 2, 4. Herpes zoster causes a painful vesicular rash that follows a sensory nerve. The rash is unilateral and clustered. Clients often report itching at the site.
CN: Physiological integrity; CNS: Physiological adaptation; CL: Apply; DIFFICULTY: Difficult

15. A nurse is assisting with the development of a care plan to maintain skin integrity in an adult client. Which nursing intervention would **best** meet the client's needs?
1. Applying a pleasantly scented dusting powder to the axillae and groin, beneath the breasts, and between the toes
2. Applying a deodorant or antiperspirant immediately after shaving under the arms
3. Trying to keep skin intact because healthy skin is the body's first line of defense
4. Always using alcohol for back rubs instead of lotion

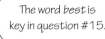

The word *best* is key in question #15.

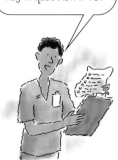

15. 3. Because healthy skin is the body's first line of defense, a key nursing goal is to keep the skin intact. To reduce moisture, the nurse can apply a nonirritating dusting powder, such as cornstarch, to the client's axillae and groin, beneath the breasts, and between the toes after those areas are dry. However, scented powder shouldn't be used because it can irritate the skin. Deodorants and antiperspirants shouldn't be applied to the skin immediately after shaving because they may cause irritation. The nurse should use lotion for back rubs because alcohol dries the skin and can irritate it.
CN: Physiological integrity; CNS: Basic care and comfort; CL: Apply; DIFFICULTY: Easy

16. A nurse is assisting with the preparation of a plan of care for a client with psoriasis. What should the nurse prepare the client for? Select all that apply.
1. Red, well-defined lesions
2. Preparing the client for a skin biopsy
3. Giving the client information on the use of antivirals
4. Caution the client on the use of corticosteroid ointments for long periods of time
5. PUVA therapy

17. A nurse is assisting with the development of a plan of care for a client diagnosed with ringworm. Which medication should the nurse anticipate discussing with this client?
1. Antibiotic
2. Corticosteroid cream
3. No medication treatment is required
4. Antifungal

18. A client has thick, discolored nails with splintered hemorrhages, easily separated from the nail bed. There are also "ice pick" pits and ridges. What does the nurse suspect is occurring with this client?
1. Paronychia
2. Psoriasis
3. Seborrhea
4. Scabies

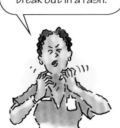

Grrr! All this stress is making me break out in a rash.

19. A client is diagnosed with a fungal infection of the scalp. The nurse knows the client understands the treatment plan when which statement is made? Select all that apply.
1. "I should throw away my combs and hats."
2. "I will need to take all of my medication even if the rash gets better."
3. "I can stop the medication once the rash is gone."
4. "The rash is not contagious."
5. "I should apply over the counter steroid cream if the rash begins to itch."

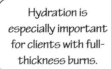

Hydration is especially important for clients with full-thickness burns.

20. A client has just arrived at the emergency department after sustaining both full-thickness and partial-thickness burns. What does the nurse anticipate administering to this client? Select all that apply.
1. IV therapy
2. Morphine
3. Tdap injection
4. IV antibiotic therapy
5. Oxygen

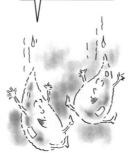

16. 1, 2, 4, 5. Psoriasis causes well-defined patches on the skin. Skin biopsy is positive for the disorder. The use of corticosteroids for long periods of time can cause thinning of the client's skin, increasing the risk for infection. PUVA therapy may be used as a treatment.
CN: Physiological integrity; CNS: Physiological adaptation; CL: Apply; DIFFICULTY: Difficult

17. 4. Antifungals are the treatment of choice for clients diagnosed with ringworm (fungal rash). Antibiotics and corticosteroids will not treat fungal infections and will often make them worse.
CN: Physiological integrity; CNS: Physiological adaptation; CL: Analyze; DIFFICULTY: Easy

18. 2. Psoriasis, a chronic skin disorder with an unknown cause, can make fingernails thick and discolored with splintered hemorrhages, and the nails can become easily separated from the nail bed with pits and ridges. A paronychia is a bacterial infection of the nail bed. Seborrhea is a chronic inflammatory dermatitis known as *cradle cap*. Scabies are mites that burrow under the skin, generally between the webbing of the fingers and toes.
CN: Physiological integrity; CNS: Physiological adaptation; CL: Apply; DIFFICULTY: Challenge

19. 1, 2. Tinea capitis is a fungal infection of the scalp. Tinea corporis describes fungal infections of the body. Tinea cruris describes fungal infections of the inner thigh and inguinal creases. Tinea pedis is the term for fungal infections of the foot. Over the counter steroid cream is not an appropriate treatment for fungal rashes. Fungal infections can be spread via a fomite transmission, so combs and hats should be discarded. Medications should be taken as ordered even if the rash is gone. Steroid cream will make fungal rashes worse.
CN: Physiological integrity; CNS: Physiological adaptation; CL: Apply; DIFFICULTY: Moderate

20. 1, 2, 5. Administering and maintaining fluid status are imperative for clients suffering from full-thickness burns. IV antibiotics may be ordered if a secondary infection develops but should not be anticipated as an initial treatment. Oxygen should be administered to this client to maintain oxygenation and tissue perfusion.
CN: Physiological integrity; CNS: Physiological adaptation; CL: Analyze; DIFFICULTY: Challenge

21. A nurse is reviewing a newly admitted client's chart. Based on this progress note entry, the nurse knows the data are consistent with which condition?

Progress notes	
10/04/17 1830	Client admitted from ED after having been found unconscious at home. Client is unresponsive to painful stimuli. Blood pressure 90/60 mm Hg. Heart rate 110 in sinus rhythm. Respiratory rate 14 breaths/ minute. Nail beds and all mucous membranes appear cherry red.
	— Barbara Smith, LPN

1. Spider bite
2. Aspirin ingestion overdose
3. Hydrocarbon ingestion
4. Carbon monoxide poisoning

22. A client has been admitted with burns on both legs. Which nursing intervention is **most** important to help prevent contractures?
1. Applying knee splints
2. Elevating the foot of the bed
3. Hyperextending the client's palms
4. Performing shoulder range-of-motion (ROM) exercises

23. A nurse is caring for a client with a third-degree burn. What should the nurse anticipate administering to this client? Select all that apply.
1. IV Therapy
2. Morphine
3. Mafenide
4. Malathion
5. Aspirin

24. A nurse is caring for an older adult client who is bedridden from a recent stroke. The nurse assists the team in the development of a care plan using the nursing diagnosis of Impaired Skin Integrity. Which interventions are appropriate for this diagnosis? Select all that apply.
1. Turn the client every 1 to 2 hours.
2. Encourage a diet high in protein.
3. Recommend an air mattress.
4. Splint the affected extremities.
5. Apply lotion during a.m. care.

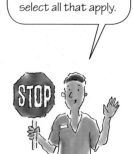

Remember to select all that apply.

21. 4. Cherry-red skin indicates exposure to high levels of carbon monoxide. Spider bite reactions are usually localized to the area of the bite. Nausea and vomiting and pale skin are symptoms of aspirin ingestion overdose. Hydrocarbon or petroleum ingestion usually causes respiratory symptoms and tachycardia.
CN: Physiological integrity; CNS: Physiological adaptation; CL: Analyze; DIFFICULTY: Moderate

22. 1. Applying knee splints prevents leg contractures by holding the joints in a position of function. Elevating the foot of the bed can't prevent contractures because this action doesn't hold the joints in a position of function. Hyperextending a body part for an extended time is inappropriate because it can cause contractures. Performing shoulder ROM exercises can prevent contractures in the shoulders, but not in the legs.
CN: Physiological integrity; CNS: Reduction of risk potential; CL: Apply; DIFFICULTY: Moderate

23. 1, 2, 3. IV therapy is a priority in clients with burns to replace fluid loss. The topical antibiotic mafenide is prescribed to prevent infection in clients with second- and third-degree burns. Malathion is a pediculicide used to treat lice infestation. The opioid analgesic morphine is used to help control pain in clients with burns. Aspirin is not routinely prescribed to burn clients.
CN: Physiological integrity; CNS: Pharmacological therapies; CL: Understand; DIFFICULTY: Difficult

24. 1, 2, 3, 5. Turning the client every 1 to 2 hours is a priority nursing intervention to prevent skin breakdown over bony prominences. A high-protein diet will help promote healing and blood supply. An air mattress will provide movement to promote blood supply and movement of the client when turning is not performed. Applying lotion will keep the skin moist and reduce the risk of skin breakdown.
CN: Physiological integrity; CNS: Basic care and comfort; CL: Apply; DIFFICULTY: Difficult

25. The nurse is caring for a postoperative client and finds that the dressing has not been changed from the previous shift. Which action can the nurse take to ensure the client receives necessary dressing changes?
1. Write the order in the client's care plan.
2. Put a sign above the head of the client's bed.
3. Tell the nurse on the upcoming shift about the treatment in the report.
4. Document the dressing change in the narrative note.

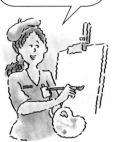

Beautiful work! Keep it up.

25. 1. Writing the order in the client's care plan notifies every one of the treatment. Posting a sign above the head of the bed is a good reminder but doesn't ensure that the treatment will be performed. Verbally reporting to the nurse on the upcoming shift doesn't ensure the dressing change will be done. Although the intervention should be documented in the narrative note, this doesn't guarantee that the next nurse will provide the treatment.
CN: Safe, effective care environment; CNS: Coordinated care; CL: Apply; DIFFICULTY: Moderate

26. A postoperative client has just been admitted to a unit from the postanesthesia care unit (PACU). When should the nurse change the dressing for the first time?
1. 2 hours after admission
2. When it becomes saturated
3. Based on written orders for dressing changes
4. The surgeon changes the first dressing; after that, the nurse follows written orders.

26. 4. The surgeon always performs the first postoperative dressing change. Generally, the surgeon will change the dressing and assess the wound the next morning during rounds. The dressing shouldn't need to be changed 2 hours after the procedure. If the first dressing becomes saturated, it may be secured with additional tape or bandages. If the nurse sees hemorrhage or excessive amount of drainage, the surgeon should be notified.
CN: Physiological integrity; CNS: Basic care and comfort; CL: Apply; DIFFICULTY: Easy

27. A nurse is assisting with the development of a care plan for a client with impaired wound healing. Which client would be a risk factor for this diagnosis? Select all that apply.
1. A 65-year-old client with hypertension
2. A 60-year-old client with impaired mobility secondary to a CVA
3. A 78-year-old client in good health
4. A 75-year-old client with poorly controlled diabetes
5. A 60-year-old client with elevated cholesterol

27. 2, 4. Poorly controlled diabetes is a serious risk factor for impaired wound healing. Other factors that impair wound healing include advanced age, inadequate blood supply, nutritional deficiencies, and obesity. Impaired mobility increases the risk for impaired wound healing. Elevated cholesterol does not impair wound healing.
CN: Physiological integrity; CNS: Physiological adaptation; CL: Analyze; DIFFICULTY: Moderate

28. A client has a possible postoperative wound infection. In which order should the nurse collect the wound culture?

1.	Properly label the collection tube.

2.	Gently roll the sterile swab in the center of the wound.

3.	Properly identify the client.

4.	Wash hands thoroughly.

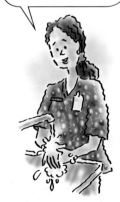

Washing your hands after working with an infected wound helps prevent spreading disease.

28. Ordered Response:

4.	Wash hands thoroughly.

3.	Properly identify the client.

1.	Properly label the collection tube.

2.	Gently roll the sterile swab in the center of the wound.

CN: Safe, effective care environment; CNS: Safety and infection control; CL: Apply; DIFFICULTY: Moderate

29. The nurse who is assessing a client with an abdominal incision suspects there is a potential for **delayed** wound healing. Which observation **most** likely supports this finding?
1. Sutures dry and intact
2. Wound edges in close approximation
3. Purulent drainage on a soiled wound dressing
4. Sanguineous drainage in a wound collection drainage bag

29. 3. Purulent drainage contains white blood cells, which fight infection. The sutures from a wound that is draining purulent secretions would pull away with an infection. Wound edges can't approximate in an infected wound. Sanguineous drainage indicates bleeding, not infection.
CN: Physiological integrity; CNS: Physiological adaptation; CL: Analyze; DIFFICULTY: Easy

30. A nurse is working with a kidney transplant client with herpes zoster. Which precautions should the nurse anticipate for this client? Select all that apply.

1. Shoe covers
2. Gown
3. Gloves
4. Mask
5. No precautions are needed

31. A nurse is caring for a client with a pressure ulcer. Which nursing interventions are appropriate for this client? Select all that apply.

1. Slide the client, instead of lifting, when turning him.
2. Turn and reposition the client at least every 2 hours.
3. Apply lotion after bathing the client and vigorously massage the skin.
4. Post a turning schedule at the client's bedside and adapt position changes to the client's situation.
5. Turning is required once a shift if an eggcrate mattress is used.

32. A nurse is caring for a client who recently had a skin graft. Which information is **most** important for the nurse to reinforce to the client?

1. Continue physical therapy.
2. Protect the graft from direct sunlight.
3. Use cosmetic camouflage techniques.
4. Apply lubricating lotion to the graft site.

33. The nurse is reinforcing prior education for a client on how to prevent development of basal cell epithelioma. Which information is **most** important for the nurse to tell the client?

1. Avoid thermal burns.
2. Avoid exposure to sun.
3. Avoid immunosuppression.
4. Avoid exposure to radiation.

34. The nurse observes an older adult client's skin turgor and finds inelasticity present. What is the nurse's **most** accurate interpretation of this finding?

1. The client is overhydrated.
2. The skin is considered to be normal skin turgor.
3. The skin is considered to be a normal part of the aging process.
4. The client is dehydrated.

35. A client received burns to the entire back and left arm. Using the Rule of Nines, the nurse calculates the client has sustained burns to which percentage of the body? Record your answer using a whole number.

_____ %

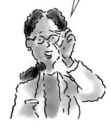

Stay focused. You're over halfway done.

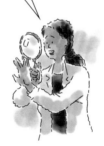

Routine self-checks can help detect skin irregularities.

30. 2, 3, 4. Immunocompromised clients with herpes zoster require health care professionals to use standard precautions, contact precautions and airborne precautions until the lesions are crusted over.
CN: Safe, effective care environment; CNS: Safety and infection control; CL: Analyze; DIFFICULTY: Challenge

31. 2, 4. A turning schedule with a signing sheet will ensure that the client gets turned. When moving a client, lift, rather than slide, to avoid shearing. A client in bed for prolonged periods should be turned every 1 to 2 hours. Apply lotion to keep the skin moist, but refrain from vigorous massage to avoid damaging capillaries. Eggcrate mattresses help to reduce pressure ulcers but turning is required every 1 to 2 hours.
CN: Safe, effective care environment; CNS: Safety and infection control; CL: Analyze; DIFFICULTY: Moderate

32. 2. To avoid burning and sloughing, the client must protect the graft from direct sunlight. The other three interventions are all helpful to the client and his recovery but aren't as important.
CN: Physiological integrity; CNS: Physiological adaptation; CL: Analyze; DIFFICULTY: Easy

33. 2. The sun is the best known and most common cause of basal cell epithelioma. Thermal burns, immunosuppression, and radiation are less common causes.
CN: Physiological integrity; CNS: Reduction of risk potential; CL: Analyze; DIFFICULTY: Easy

34. 3. Inelastic skin turgor is a normal part of aging. Overhydration causes the skin to appear edematous and spongy. Normal skin turgor is dry and firm. Dehydration causes inelastic skin with tenting.
CN: Physiological integrity; CNS: Basic care and comfort; CL: Apply; DIFFICULTY: Challenge

35. 27. According to the Rule of Nines, the posterior trunk, anterior trunk, and legs are each 18% of the total body surface. The head, neck, and arms are each 9% of total body surface, and the perineum is 1%. In this case, the client received burns to the back (18%) and one arm (9%), totaling 27% of the body.
CN: Physiological integrity; CNS: Reduction of risk potential; CL: Apply; DIFFICULTY: Moderate

36. The nurse is caring for a client receiving PUVA treatment. Which statement by the client indicates understanding?
1. "On the day of treatment, I need to stay out of the sun."
2. "I do not need to wear any protective eyewear during the UV light treatment."
3. "I need to wear sunglasses for 24 hours after the treatment."
4. "PUVA therapy is the use of UV light with topical ointments."

36. 1. On the day of treatment, the client should stay out of the sun. Clients should wear sunglasses for 24 hours after treatment. The client should wear goggles during any exposure to UV light. PUVA therapy is UV light used with psoralens.
CN: Physiological integrity; CNS: Basic care and comfort;
CL: Apply; DIFFICULTY: Moderate

37. A nurse is caring for a client with a pressure ulcer on the sacrum. When educating the client about dietary intake, which foods should the nurse plan to emphasize?
1. Legumes and cheese
2. Whole-grain products
3. Fruits and vegetables
4. Lean meats and low-fat milk

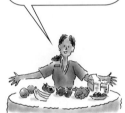

When it comes to healing ulcers, proteins are the name of the game.

37. 4. Although the client should eat a balanced diet with foods from all food groups, the diet should emphasize foods that supply complete protein, such as lean meats and low-fat milk. Protein helps build and repair body tissue, which promotes healing. Legumes provide incomplete protein. Cheese contains complete protein but also fat, which should be limited to 30% or less of caloric intake. Whole-grain products supply incomplete proteins and carbohydrates. Fruits and vegetables provide mainly carbohydrates.
CN: Physiological integrity; CNS: Basic care and comfort;
CL: Apply; DIFFICULTY: Easy

38. The nurse is examining the back of a client who was admitted with stage III pressure ulcers on his sacral area. Which illustration shows a stage III pressure ulcer?

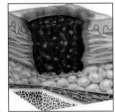
1.

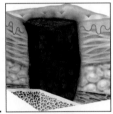
2.

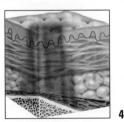
3.

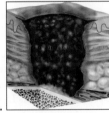
4.

This question is all about putting the steps in the right order.

38. 1. In a stage III pressure ulcer, there is full-thickness skin loss along with damage or necrosis of the subcutaneous tissue. It may or may not extend down to (but not through) the fascia. Undermining may be present. Option 2 shows an unstageable pressure ulcer. In an unstageable pressure ulcer, the true stage of the ulcer can't be determined until the base of the wound is exposed. Options 3 shows suspected deep tissue injury, which presents as a purple or maroon localized area of intact skin or blood-filled blister. Option 4 shows a stage IV pressure ulcer. In a stage IV pressure ulcer, there is full-thickness skin loss with extensive tissue destruction, tissue necrosis, or damage to the muscle, bone, or support structures.
CN: Physiological integrity; CNS: Physiological adaptation;
CL: Apply; DIFFICULTY: Moderate

39. A nurse is preparing to perform a dressing change on a client with a Stage III decubitus ulcer. Put the following interventions in order (first to last).

| 1. Put on gloves. |
| 2. Wash hands thoroughly. |
| 3. Slowly remove the soiled dressing. |
| 4. Observe the dressing for the amount, type, and odor of drainage. |

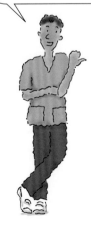

39. Ordered Response:

| 2. Wash hands thoroughly. |
| 3. Slowly remove the soiled dressing. |
| 4. Observe the dressing for the amount, type, and odor of drainage. |
| 1. Put on gloves. |

CN: Physiological integrity; CNS: Basic care and comfort;
CL: Apply; DIFFICULTY: Challenge

40. A client develops wound evisceration following abdominal surgery. Which intervention should be the nurse's **priority** for this client?
1. Giving prophylactic antibiotics as ordered
2. Giving the client as much fluid to drink as possible
3. Explaining to the client what's happening and giving support
4. Covering the protruding internal organs with sterile gauze moistened with sterile saline

40. 4. Evisceration requires emergency surgical repair. Covering the wound with sterile gauze moistened with sterile saline is essential to prevent the organs from drying. The gauze and saline must be sterile to reduce the risk of infection. Antibiotics will usually be ordered and started as soon as possible but aren't the priority. The nurse should place the client on nothing-by-mouth status immediately, but covering the wound takes priority. While the nurse works quickly to prepare the client for surgery, providing emotional support will help reduce the client's anxiety, but it isn't the priority for this client.
CN: Physiological integrity; CNS: Physiological adaptation; CL: Apply; DIFFICULTY: Easy

41. The nurse is assisting with the development of a plan of care for an immobile client. Which nursing action is a **priority** to prevent complications?
1. Turn every 30 minutes.
2. Turn every 1 to 2 hours.
3. Turn once every 8 hours.
4. Keep the client on his back as much as possible.

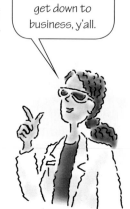

Alright. Let's get down to business, y'all.

41. 2. Turning the client every 1 to 2 hours will prevent pressure areas from developing and help prevent atelectasis and other pulmonary complications. Turning every half-hour is too frequent; every 8 hours is too infrequent and would make the client vulnerable to the development of complications. The client should spend time on his back according to the turning schedule. During that period, the head of the bed should be raised to prevent the client from aspirating.
CN: Physiological integrity; CNS: Basic care and comfort; CL: Apply; DIFFICULTY: Easy

42. The nurse is instructing a client regarding hypersensitivity after administering a skin test. Which instruction is **most** important for the nurse to include when discussing the skin test?
1. Wash the sites daily with a mild soap.
2. Read the sites on the correct date.
3. Keep the skin test areas moist with a mild lotion.
4. Stay out of direct sunlight until the tests are read.

42. 2. An important facet of evaluating skin tests is to read the skin test results at the proper time. Evaluating the skin test too late or too early will give inaccurate, unreliable results. There's no need to wash the test sites with soap. The sites should be kept dry. Direct sunlight isn't prohibited.
CN: Health promotion and maintenance; CNS: None; CL: Apply; DIFFICULTY: Challenge

43. A client is brought to the emergency department with partial-thickness and full-thickness burns over 15% of the body. Admission vital signs are as follows: blood pressure, 100/50 mm Hg; heart rate, 130 beats/minute; respiratory rate, 26 breaths/minute. Which nursing interventions are appropriate for this client? Select all that apply:
1. Clean the burns with hydrogen peroxide.
2. Cover the burns with saline-soaked towels.
3. Begin an IV infusion of lactated Ringer solution.
4. Place ice directly on the burn areas.
5. Administer 6 mg of morphine IV.
6. Administer tetanus prophylaxis, as ordered.

43. 3, 5, 6. Immediate interventions for this client should aim to stop the burning and relieve the pain. The nurse should begin IV therapy with a crystalloid, such as lactated Ringer solution, to prevent hypovolemic shock and to maintain cardiac output. Typically, 2 to 25 mg of morphine are administered IV in small increments to treat pain. Tetanus prophylaxis should also be administered, as ordered. Hydrogen peroxide and povidone-iodine solution could further damage tissue, and saline-soaked towels could lead to hypothermia. Ice placed directly on burn wounds could cause further thermal damage.
CN: Physiological integrity; CNS: Physiological adaptation; CL: Apply; DIFFICULTY: Challenge

44. A client is prescribed methotrexate 25 mg by mouth as a single weekly dose. The pharmacy dispenses 2.5-mg scored tablets. How many tablets should the nurse instruct the client to consume to achieve the prescribed dose? Record your answer using a whole number.

_____ tablets

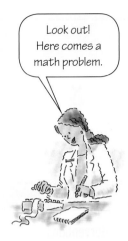

Look out! Here comes a math problem.

44. 10.
The correct formula to calculate a drug dose is:

$$\frac{\text{Dose on hand}}{\text{Quantity on hand}} = \frac{\text{Dose desired}}{X}$$

The health care provider prescribes 25 mg, which is the dose desired. The pharmacy dispenses 2.5-mg tablets, which is the dose on hand.

$$\frac{2.5\,\text{mg}}{1\,\text{tablet}} = \frac{25\,\text{mg}}{X}$$

$$X = 10\,\text{tablets}$$

CN: Physiological integrity; CNS: Pharmacological therapies; CL: Apply; DIFFICULTY: Easy

45. A client who's 5 ft 4 in (1.63 m) and weighs 145 lb (66 kg) is admitted to the long-term care facility. The admitting nurse takes this report: "The client sits for long periods in his wheelchair and has bowel and bladder incontinence. He has a fair appetite, eating best at breakfast, and is often observed to be crying and depressed. Medications include daily use of sedatives." Which factors place the client at risk for developing a pressure ulcer? Select all that apply.
1. Weight
2. Incontinence
3. Sitting for long periods
4. Sedation
5. Crying and depression
6. Decreased Appetite

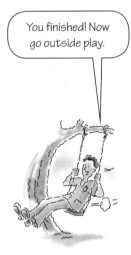

You finished! Now go outside play.

45. 2, 3, 4. Inactivity, immobility, incontinence, and sedation are all risk factors for developing pressure ulcers. The client's weight and poor eating habits at lunch and dinner aren't directly related to the risk of developing pressure ulcers, but a calorie count should be taken to see if the client is getting adequate calories and fluids because poor nutrition can contribute to pressure ulcers. The fact that the client cries and is depressed has no direct bearing on this client's risk for developing a pressure ulcer. However, clients with depression are commonly not as active, so his activity levels should be monitored closely to minimize inactivity.

CN: Physiological integrity; CNS: Reduction of risk potential; CL: Analyze; DIFFICULTY: Challenge

CN: Client needs category   CNS: Client needs subcategory   CL: Cognitive level

Somatic Symptom & Related Disorders

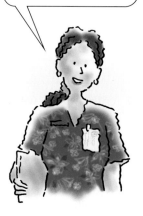

Somatic symptom & related disorders refresher

Conversion disorder (functional neurologic symptoms disorder)

When physiologic symptoms appear as a result of a psychological condition

Key signs and symptoms

- La belle indifference (a lack of concern about the symptoms or limitation on functioning)

Key test results

- Absence of expected diagnostic findings can confirm the disorder

Key treatments

- Individual therapy

Key interventions

- Establish supportive relationship that communicates acceptance of the client but keeps focus away from symptoms
- Review all laboratory and diagnostic study results
- Neurologic examination

Pain disorder

Presence of chronic or severe pain that is not supported by a physiologic condition

Key signs and symptoms

- May be attributed to a combination of factors
- Anger, frustration, and depression
- Drug-seeking behavior in an attempt to relieve pain
- History of frequent visits to multiple health care providers to seek pain relief
- Insomnia

Key test results

- Test results don't support client reports

Key treatments

- Individual therapy
- Tricyclic antidepressants: amitriptyline, imipramine, doxepin

Key interventions

- Acknowledge client's pain
- Encourage client to recognize situations that precipitate pain

Sleep-wake disorders

Characterized by impaired sleep quality or quantity

Key signs and symptoms

Insomnia disorder

- History of light or easily disturbed sleep, or difficulty falling asleep
- Insomnia

Breathing-related sleep disorder

- Obstructive sleep apnea hypopnea
- Central sleep apnea
- Sleep-related hypoventilation

Narcolepsy

- Cataplexy (bilateral loss of muscle tone triggered by strong emotion)
- Generalized daytime sleepiness
- Hypnagogic hallucination (intense dream-like images)
- Irresistible attacks of refreshing sleep
- Hypocretin deficiency

Key test results

- Polysomnography is diagnostic for individual sleep disorder

Key treatments

- Hypnotic: zolpidem

Key interventions

Insomnia disorder and circadian rhythm disturbance

- Encourage client to discuss concerns that may be preventing sleep
- Schedule regular sleep and awakening times

Breathing-related sleep disorder

- Administer continuous positive airway pressure (CPAP)

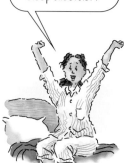

Neurodevelopmental disorders

Characterized by developmental delays in personal, social, academic or occupational functioning

Key signs and symptoms

Autism spectrum disorder
- Impaired social interaction skills
- Communication impairment
- Stereotypical behavioral patterns
- Little eye contact
- Few facial expressions to others

Tic disorders
- Rapid, recurring motor movement or vocal sounds
- Blinking, clearing the throat, sniffing, snorting, barking
- Repetition of words, coprolalia (use of socially inappropriate words)
- Palilalia (repeating one's own sounds or words)
- Echolalia (repeating last word or phrase said)

Key test results

Autism spectrum disorder
- Identified by 18 months of age and no later than 3 years of age
- Behavioral testing for definitive diagnosis

Tic disorders
- Magnetic resonance imaging
- Behavioral observation

Key treatments

Autism spectrum disorder
- Individualized treatment
- Special education and language therapy
- Cognitive behavioral therapy
- Antipsychotics: haloperidol, risperidone

Tic disorders
- Antipsychotics: risperidone, olanzapine

Key interventions

Autism spectrum disorder
- Prevent injury
- Promote learning and development

Tic disorders
- Encourage client to get plenty of rest
- Stress management

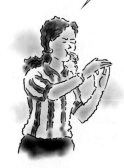

Time out! Can you list some of the key signs and symptoms of tic disorders?

Attention deficit hyperactivity disorder (ADHD)

Neurobehavioral disorder that interferes with a person's ability to stay on task and to exercise age-appropriate inhibition (cognitive alone or both cognitive and behavioral)

Key signs and symptoms
- Inability to sit still
- Difficult for child to carry on a conversation
- Behavioral immaturity
- Labile mood with temper tantrums
- Poor judgment and decision making

Key test results
- Behavioral observation

Key treatments
- Stimulants such as methylphenidate
- Amphetamines: adderall
- Antidepressants such as atomoxetine
- Antihypertensives such as clonidine

Key interventions
- Ensure safety
- Structure the daily routine
- Support for family members

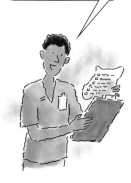

Can you name some of the common medications used to treat ADHD?

thePoint® You can download tables of drug information to help you prepare for the NCLEX®! View Generic Drug Names, Drug Classifications, Drug Actions, and Nursing Implications for the drugs discussed in this refresher at **http://thePoint.lww.com**.

Somatic symptom & related disorders questions, answers, and rationales

1. Which statement is correct about clients who have somatic symptom disorder?
1. They usually seek medical attention.
2. They have organic pathologic disorders.
3. They regularly attend psychotherapy sessions without encouragement.
4. They're eager to discover the true reasons for their physical symptoms.

1. **1.** A client with a somatic symptom disorder usually seeks medical attention. These clients have a history of reporting multiple physiologic symptoms without associated demonstrable, organic pathologic causes. The expected behavior for this type of disorder is to seek treatment from several medical health care providers for somatic symptoms, not psychiatric evaluation.
CN: Psychosocial integrity; CNS: None; CL: Apply; DIFFICULTY: Moderate

CN: Client needs category   CNS: Client needs subcategory   CL: Cognitive level

2. The health care provider has prescribed methylphenidate. Which findings in the client's medical history would warrant concern about this therapy? Select all that apply.
1. The client has a history of alcoholism.
2. The client has a familial history of hypoglycemia.
3. The client has type 1 diabetes mellitus.
4. The client has a history of gallbladder disease.
5. The client's history indicates a recent myocardial infarction.

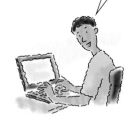

Remember to "select all that apply" in question #2.

2. 1, 5. Methylphenidate is addictive. Any history of alcohol or drug use past or current would warrant concern for the administration of this medication. The medication may be contraindicated in the presence of cardiac disorders. Health concerns such as hypoglycemia, diabetes and gallbladder disease are not contraindications for the use of methylphenidate.
CN: Physiological integrity; CNS: Pharmacological therapies; CL: Apply; DIFFICULTY: Difficult

3. Which reason **best** accounts for the physical symptoms in a client with a somatic symptom disorder?
1. To cope with delusional thinking
2. To provide attention for the individual
3. To prevent or relieve symptoms of anxiety
4. To protect the client from family conflict

3. 3. Anxiety and depression commonly occur in somatic symptom disorders. The client prevents or relieves symptoms of anxiety by focusing on physical symptoms. Somatic delusions occur in schizophrenia. The symptoms allow the client to avoid unpleasant activity, not to seek individual attention. Somatization in dysfunctional families shifts the open conflict to the client's illness, thus providing some stability for the family, not the client.
CN: Psychosocial integrity; CNS: None; CL: Analyze; DIFFICULTY: Moderate

4. The nurse is talking with a client who has been taking amphetamine salt combo for the past 3 weeks. Which statements by the client indicate the medication is having the desired effects? Select all that apply.
1. "I feel jittery in the morning."
2. "I have been sleeping well at night."
3. "My appetite is somewhat reduced."
4. "I feel increasingly focused when I am working."
5. "I am feeling less depressed."

4. 2, 4. Amphetamine salt combo is used to treat attention deficit hyperactivity disorder (ADHD). Individuals with this condition experience difficulty focusing on tasks. Amphetamine salt combo will modify the brain's chemistry and promote increased abilities to focus on tasks. Improvements in sleep patterns may also be noted with this medication. Feeling jittery may occur with the medication and is considered a side effect, not a desired effect. Appetite changes may occur but are not associated with the desired effects of the medication. Mood alteration is not the intended outcome of medication therapy with this drug.
CN: Physiological integrity; CNS: Pharmacological therapies; CL: Apply; DIFFICULTY: Challenge

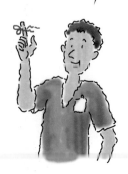

Remember: If physiological evidence for pain is present, it's not pain disorder.

5. A client comes to the health care provider's office with reports of chronic pain. The client's history reflects numerous visits to the health care provider for pain relief. Which therapies will be effective in caring for this client? Select all that apply.
1. Low-dose narcotic analgesics to be taken at bedtime
2. Behavioral therapy
3. Relaxation techniques
4. Hypnosis
5. Tricyclic antidepressants

5. 2, 3, 4, 5. When caring for the client with chronic pain the focus should be on promoting skills to improve the client's coping with regard to the discomfort. The use of narcotic medications should be avoided. They are habit forming and problematic when managing chronic pain disorders. Behavioral therapies focusing on stress reduction and coping are recommended. Relaxation techniques should be taught to the client. Hypnosis may also be employed. Pharmacologic therapies may include tricyclic antidepressants.
CN: Physiological integrity; CNS: Reduction of risk potential; CL: Apply; DIFFICULTY: Difficult

6. Parents of an 8-year-old child inform the school nurse that they believe their child has attention deficit hyperactivity disorder (ADHD). Which observations reported by the parents are consistent with this disorder? Select all that apply.
1. Child appears sad and withdrawn.
2. Child frequently does not want to go to school.
3. Child constantly fidgets.
4. Child reports nausea and stomachaches.
5. Child is outgoing and talkative.

7. The nurse observes a child with autism banging the head against the floor repetitively. Which nursing action is **priority**?
1. Apply a helmet on the child.
2. Administer sedation.
3. Restrain the child.
4. Allow the child to continue the repetitive behavior.

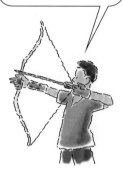

Looks like you're right on target. Keep up the good work.

8. A parent of a child with autism asks the nurse, "Will my child ever get better?" Which statements should be included in the response by the nurse? Select all that apply.
1. "Most likely, your child will always be like this."
2. "This is chronic, and your child's behavior will get worse."
3. "With behavioral therapy, your child's symptoms may get better."
4. "Since your child cannot recover institutionalization will likely be needed".
5. "Medication therapies may help to improve your child's condition."

9. A client is exhibiting anxiety, which is evidenced by muscle tension, distractibility, and increased heart rate and blood pressure. Which nursing intervention has **priority**?
1. Remain with the client and use a soft voice and reassuring approach.
2. Assist the client to identify factors that contribute to anxiety.
3. Educate the client on relaxation techniques, such as deep breathing and muscle relaxation.
4. Administer antianxiety medications as appropriate.

10. A client has been diagnosed with a tic disorder. Which information can the nurse provide to help the client reduce the frequency of the tics? Select all that apply.
1. Increase prescribed medications after tics are experienced.
2. Get plenty of rest.
3. Avoid extremes in temperature.
4. Decrease the amount of protein in the diet.
5. Reduce stress.

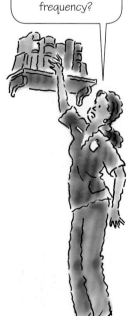

Hmm. What was that I read about reducing tic frequency?

6. 3. One of the characteristic behaviors of a child with ADHD is that the child has difficulty sitting or standing still. This behavior makes it difficult for the child to succeed in school. The child is not usually sad or withdrawn and may generally be outgoing and talkative. It is not a characteristic of ADHD for children to state they don't want to go to school. Nausea and stomachaches are not symptoms of the disorder.
CN: Physiological integrity; CNS: Physiological adaptation; CL: Remember; DIFFICULTY: Difficult

7. 1. The priority for all clients is their safety. A helmet should be applied to this child with autistic disorder so that the child will not sustain a head injury. It is not necessary to administer a sedative to the child. Restraining the child will increase the behavior and cause more anxiety and stress reactions. The child may continue the behavior but should be protected.
CN: Safe, effective care environment; CNS: Safety and infection control; CL: Apply; DIFFICULTY: Easy

8. 3, 5. Autism may improve when children begin to use speech to communicate. It will require a considerable commitment from the parents to assist the child with improving behaviors and, in some instances, special programs and schools. Medication therapies are commonly incorporated into the plan of care. The behavior usually does not get worse unless these programs are not utilized. There is no reason that the child will require institutionalization.
CN: Health promotion and maintenance; CNS: None; CL: Apply; DIFFICULTY: Easy

9. 1. The priority nursing intervention is to remain with the client and use a soft voice and reassuring approach. Remaining with the client provides for his safety, and a soft voice is calming and reassuring, which will add to feelings of safety and protection. Interventions such as identifying factors that contribute to anxiety, teaching relaxation techniques, and administering antianxiety medications are included in the client's care plan but should be addressed later.
CN: Safe, effective care environment; CNS: Coordinated care; CL: Apply; DIFFICULTY: Challenge

10. 2, 5. It is important that the client gets ample rest and uses stress reduction techniques in order to control the tics or motor responses. Stress and fatigue are shown to increase these symptoms. The client should not increase any medication without a health care provider's order. Extreme temperatures and decreasing the amount of protein in the diet will not have any effect on the tics.
CN: Physiological integrity; CNS: Physiological adaptation; CL: Apply; DIFFICULTY: Challenge

11. A client is given triazolam (Halcion) for a sleep disorder. The nurse is reinforcing some teaching precautions concerning the medication. Which statements by the client indicate an understanding of the information provided?
1. "I should take the medication with citrus juice."
2. "I shouldn't confuse this medication with Haldol."
3. "It's okay to take a short drive after taking the medication."
4. "It's okay to smoke while I take this medication."

12. Which measure should be included when educating a client on strategies to help promote sleep?
1. Keep the room warm.
2. Eat a large meal before bedtime.
3. Schedule bedtime when feeling tired.
4. Avoid caffeine, excessive fluid intake, alcohol, and stimulating drugs before bedtime.

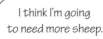

I think I'm going to need more sheep.

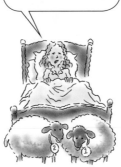

13. A client has been diagnosed with a conversion disorder after presenting with reports of new onset paralysis in a lower extremity. When providing education about this phenomena to a group of nurses, what information should be included? Select all that apply.
1. The onset of these symptoms may be attributed to psychological stressors.
2. The onset of the symptoms is normally gradual.
3. After an initial recovery, most clients will experience a reoccurrence of symptomology within a year.
4. Most symptoms will resolve.
5. Ignoring the manifestations is recommended.

14. A client reports having difficulty falling and staying asleep. Which suggestion for treatment should the nurse offer the client?
1. Behavior therapy
2. Biofeedback
3. Group therapy
4. Insight-oriented psychotherapy

15. The nurse is reviewing a nursing care plan for a client with a psychophysiologic disorder. Nursing interventions should address which symptoms?
1. Only the physical symptoms that are life-threatening
2. Only the physical symptoms that are distressing the client
3. Physical symptoms as well as psychosocial and spiritual problems
4. Only psychosocial symptoms

11. 2. Haldol is an antipsychotic that has a spelling similar to Halcion and is used for clients with psychoses, Tourette syndrome, severe behavioral problems in children, and emergency sedation of severely agitated, psychotic clients. Halcion is one of a group of sedative-hypnotic medications that can be used only for a limited time because of the risk of dependency. Grapefruit and grapefruit juices can alter the absorption of Halcion. The client should avoid driving and tasks that require alertness or motor skills because the medication may cause drowsiness. Smoking reduces drug effectiveness.
CN: Physiological integrity; CNS: Pharmacological therapies; CL: Analyze; DIFFICULTY: Easy

12. 4. Caffeine, excessive fluid intake, alcohol, and stimulating drugs act as stimulants; avoiding them should promote sleep. Maintaining a cool temperature in the room will better facilitate sleeping. Excessive fullness or hunger may interfere with sleep. Setting a regular bedtime and wake-up time facilitates physiologic patterns.
CN: Health promotion and maintenance; CNS: None; CL: Apply; DIFFICULTY: Easy

13. 1, 4. A conversion disorder results in the manifestation of physiologic symptoms that have developed in response to psychological stressors. The disorder usually suddenly occurs. A full recovery is normal. Approximately 25% of those affected will experience a reoccurrence of symptomology. Ignoring the physical manifestations is not recommended.
CN: Physiological integrity; CNS: Physiological adaptation; CL: Apply; DIFFICULTY: Challenge

14. 2. Biofeedback, relaxation therapy, and psychopharmacology are appropriate treatments for sleep disorders. Behavior therapy, group therapy, and insight-oriented psychotherapy are treatments related to somatic symptom disorders.
CN: Physiological integrity; CNS: Basic care and comfort; CL: Apply; DIFFICULTY: Moderate

15. 3. Physical, psychosocial, and spiritual problems are thoroughly and continuously assessed with each client. The nurse must include all symptoms, even those that aren't life-threatening, and consider all physical symptoms, even those the client doesn't find distressing. Psychosocial symptoms should be considered, but all three areas must be assessed to provide a thorough care plan.
CN: Psychosocial integrity; CNS: None; CL: Apply; DIFFICULTY: Easy

CN: Client needs category   CNS: Client needs subcategory   CL: Cognitive level

16. Which nursing intervention would be **most** appropriate for a depressed client with disturbed sleep patterns related to external factors?
1. Consult the health care provider about prescribing a bedtime sleep medication.
2. Allow the client to sit at the nurses' station for comfort.
3. Allow the client to watch television until sleepy.
4. Encourage the client to take a warm bath before retiring.

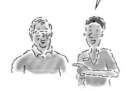

Which answer in question #16 will best help to engage your client's parasympathetic nervous system?

16. **4.** Sleep-inducing activities, such as a warm bath, help promote relaxation and sleep. Although consulting a health care provider about prescribing a bedtime sleep medication is possible, it wouldn't be the best nursing intervention for this client. Encouraging the client to watch television or sit at the nurses' station wouldn't necessarily promote sleep. In fact, these activities may provide too much stimulation, further delaying sleep.
CN: Physiological integrity; CNS: Basic care and comfort; CL: Apply; DIFFICULTY: Moderate

17. A nurse is instructing a client undergoing treatment for anxiety and insomnia. The practitioner has prescribed lorazepam 1 mg by mouth three times per day. The nurse determines that the education regarding the client's diagnosis and medication has been effective when the client gives which response?
1. "I'll avoid caffeine."
2. "I'll avoid aged cheese."
3. "I'll avoid sunlight."
4. "I'll maintain adequate salt intake."

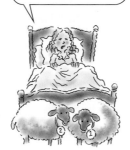

How many sheep do I have to count to fall asleep? Curse you, mocha latte!

17. **1.** Lorazepam is a benzodiazepine used to treat various forms of anxiety and insomnia. Caffeine is contraindicated because it's a stimulant and increases anxiety. A client on a monoamine oxidase inhibitor should avoid aged cheeses. Clients taking certain antipsychotic medications should avoid sunlight. Salt intake has no effect on lorazepam.
CN: Physiological integrity; CNS: Pharmacological therapies; CL: Analyze; DIFFICULTY: Easy

18. A home health nurse is caring for a client diagnosed with a conversion disorder manifested by paralysis in the left arm. An organic cause for the deficit has been ruled out. Which nursing intervention is **most** appropriate for this client?
1. Perform all physical tasks for the client to foster dependence.
2. Allot an hour each day to discuss the paralysis and its cause.
3. Identify primary or secondary gains that the physical symptom provides.
4. Allow the client to withdraw from all physical activities.

18. **3.** Primary or secondary gains should be identified because they're etiologic factors that can be used in problem resolution. The nurse should encourage the client to be as independent as possible and intervene only when the client requires assistance. The nurse shouldn't focus on the disability. The nurse should encourage the client to perform physical activities to the greatest extent possible.
CN: Psychosocial integrity; CNS: None; CL: Apply; DIFFICULTY: Easy

19. A client is diagnosed with conversion disorder with paralysis of the legs. What's the **best** nursing intervention for the nurse to use?
1. Discuss with the client ways to live with the paralysis.
2. Focus interactions on results of medical tests.
3. Encourage the client to move the legs as much as possible.
4. Avoid focusing on the client's physical limitations.

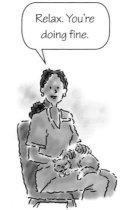

Relax. You're doing fine.

19. **4.** The paralysis is used as an unhealthy way of expressing unmet psychological needs. The nurse should avoid speaking about the paralysis to shift the client's attention to the mental aspect of the disorder. The other options focus too much on the paralysis, instead of recognizing the underlying psychological motivations.
CN: Psychosocial integrity; CNS: None; CL: Apply; DIFFICULTY: Challenge

20. Which outcome is **most** appropriate for a teenager who's irritable, hasn't slept well in 6 months, and has dropped out of social activities?
1. The client will sleep well at night.
2. The parents will stop worrying about the client.
3. The client will obtain appropriate mental health services.
4. The parents will impose strict behavior guidelines for the client to follow.

20. **3.** Mental health services can protect the client and offer the best means of regaining mental health. The client could reestablish a healthy sleeping pattern without addressing underlying issues. The parents' worry is unrelated to the child's immediate need for help. The child's behavior suggests the need for professional mental health services, not disciplinary measures.
CN: Psychosocial integrity; CNS: None; CL: Apply; DIFFICULTY: Challenge

21. The parent of a client approaches the nurses' station in tears and states, "I am upset about my child's diagnosis of conversion disorder." Which response is **best**?
1. "What is it that upsets you the most?"
2. "Are you afraid your child will never get well?"
3. "Her behavior is typical of someone with conversion disorder."
4. "Let me give you some information about the illness."

22. Which intervention would **most** likely be found in an education plan for an anxious client who reports difficulty settling down for sleep?
1. Educate the client on time management skills.
2. Educate the client on conflict resolution skills.
3. Educate the client on progressive muscle relaxation.
4. Educate the client about the adverse effects of antipsychotic medication.

23. A client is diagnosed with a conversion disorder. Which characteristic of the disorder does the nurse recognize is occurring?
1. The symptoms can be controlled.
2. The psychological conflict is repressed.
3. The client is aware of the psychological conflict.
4. The client shouldn't be made aware of the conflicts underlying the symptoms.

24. A client is admitted for abrupt onset of paralysis in the left arm. Although no physiologic cause has been found, the symptoms are exacerbated when the client speaks about losing custody of children in a recent divorce. The nurse determines these findings are characteristic of what disorder?
1. Body dysmorphic disorder
2. Conversion disorder
3. Delusional disorder
4. Factitious disease

25. The nurse is talking with a client who has a conversion disorder. When speaking with the client which statements will be **most** helpful? Select all that apply.
1. "Why do you think you are having vision trouble?"
2. "I'm going to sit here with you while you are watching television."
3. "How are you feeling today?"
4. "Let's focus on how you are going to live by yourself if you can't feel your left leg."
5. "I know you don't want to talk about the accident but if you don't, you will never feel better."

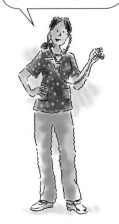

When your client is upset, practice your listening skills.

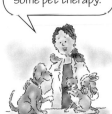

Feeling stressed? Take a break and try some pet therapy.

21. 1. Asking the parent an open-ended question permits the nurse to collect data reported in the parent's own words. The other options narrow the data collection process prematurely. Also, it's important to hear what the parent has to say without planting suggestions about the child's condition.
CN: Psychosocial integrity; CNS: None; CL: Apply; DIFFICULTY: Easy

22. 3. Progressive muscle relaxation is a systematic tensing and relaxing of separate muscle groups. As the technique is mastered, relaxation results. Time management skills and conflict resolution skills are helpful in an overall effort to reduce stress and anxiety, but don't provide immediate relief in an effort to sleep. Antipsychotic medications aren't usually used to treat anxiety or difficulty with sleep.
CN: Psychosocial integrity; CNS: None; CL: Apply; DIFFICULTY: Easy

23. 2. In conversion disorders, the client isn't conscious of intentionally producing symptoms that can't be self-controlled. The symptoms are characterized by one or more neurologic symptoms. Understanding the principles and conflicts behind the symptoms can prove helpful during a client's therapy.
CN: Psychosocial integrity; CNS: None; CL: Analyze; DIFFICULTY: Difficult

24. 2. Conversion disorders are characterized by one or more neurologic symptoms associated with psychological conflict. Body dysmorphic disorder is an imagined belief that there's a defect in the appearance of all or part of the body. The client isn't experiencing a delusion, which would be the criteria for a delusional disorder. Factitious disease is the intentional production of symptoms to avoid obligations or obtain rewards.
CN: Physiological integrity; CNS: Physiological adaptation; CL: Analyze; DIFFICULTY: Moderate

25. 2, 3. Establishing a supportive relationship that communicates acceptance of the client but keeps the focus away from symptoms is key in working with clients with conversion disorder. Using therapeutic communication techniques such as offering self and using open ended questions are ways to establish a supportive relationship. Requesting an explanation, such as asking why and probing, are both nontherapeutic communication techniques. The focus of the care is not on the loss of independence. This line of communication would not be therapeutic.
CN: Psychosocial integrity; CNS: None; CL: Apply; DIFFICULTY: Difficult

26. A client has been diagnosed with conversion-disorder blindness. The client shows "la belle indifference." Which statement **best** describes this term?

1. The client is suppressing true feelings.
2. The client's anxiety has been relieved through physical symptoms.
3. The client is acting indifferent because of not wanting to show actual fear.
4. The client's needs are being met, so she doesn't need to be anxious.

27. The parents of a child with attention deficit hyperactivity disorder (ADHD) say they are concerned because the child is losing weight. Which suggestions can the nurse give to the parents regarding the weight loss? Select all that apply.

1. Have high-calorie finger foods available for the child to eat.
2. Decrease the amount of medications being taken.
3. Force the child to sit for three meals a day with the family.
4. Administer an appetite stimulant.
5. Encourage small, frequent meals.

28. Which action by the nurse would help a client with conversion-disorder blindness to eat?

1. Direct the client to independently locate items on the tray and feed himself.
2. See to the needs of the other clients in the dining room, then feed this client last.
3. Establish a "buddy" system with other clients who can feed the client at each meal.
4. Expect the client to feed himself after explaining the location of food on the tray.

29. The nurse is caring for a client with a diagnosis of conversion disorder. Which clinical symptoms does the client demonstrate that correlate with this diagnosis?

1. Delusions of grandeur
2. Feelings of depression or euphoria
3. A feeling of dread accompanied by somatic signs
4. Neurologic symptoms associated with psychological conflict or need

30. A client has been diagnosed with conversion disorder and this has interrupted the family dynamic. Which goal will be appropriate for this client?

1. The client will resume former roles and tasks.
2. The client will take over roles of other family members.
3. The client will rely on family members to meet all client needs.
4. The client will focus energy on problems occurring in the family.

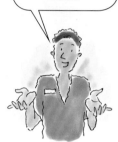

Sometimes lifestyle changes are the best way to meet a client's needs.

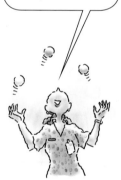

You're juggling these questions like a pro. Well done.

26. 2. Conversion accomplishes anxiety reduction through the production of a physical symptom symbolically linked to an underlying conflict. The client isn't aware of the internal conflict. Hospitalization doesn't remove the source of the conflict.
CN: Psychosocial integrity; CNS: None; CL: Analyze;
DIFFICULTY: Easy

27. 1, 5. Because it is difficult for children with ADHD to sit still while eating, it is acceptable to keep high-calorie finger foods available to avoid the weight loss that can accompany this disorder. Small, frequent meals will promote continuous intake throughout the day. The medication should not be decreased without a health care provider's order. The child should not be forced to sit at the table. An appetite stimulant is not necessary if foods are offered.
CN: Health Promotion and Maintenance; CNS: None; CL: Apply;
DIFFICULTY: Moderate

28. 4. The client is expected to maintain some level of independence by feeding himself. At the same time, the nurse should be supportive in a matter-of-fact way. Feeding the client leads to dependence.
CN: Physiological integrity; CNS: Basic care and comfort;
CL: Apply; DIFFICULTY: Challenge

29. 4. Symptoms of conversion disorders are neurologic in nature (paralysis, blindness). Delusional disorders are characterized by delusions. Mood disorders are characterized by abnormal feelings of depression or euphoria. Anxiety is characterized by a feeling of dread.
CN: Health promotion and maintenance; CNS: None; CL: Apply;
DIFFICULTY: Moderate

30. 1. The client who uses somatization has typically adopted a sick role in the family, characterized by dependence. Increasing independence and resumption of former roles are necessary to change this pattern. The client shouldn't be expected to take on the roles or responsibilities of other family members.
CN: Psychosocial integrity; CNS: None; CL: Apply;
DIFFICULTY: Moderate

31. The nurse is reviewing the medical record of a client who is hospitalized with a conversion disorder. Which findings are associated with this condition? Select all that apply.
1. A history of being treated for depression
2. A history of sexual abuse
3. Frequent use of marijuana
4. A history of hypothyroidism
5. Obesity

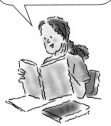

In conversion disorder, psychological concerns are "converted" to physical symptoms such as paralysis and blindness.

32. The nurse is preparing an educational program for new staff members. Which information about conversion disorder should the nurse include? Select all that apply.
1. Work to establish a therapeutic relationship with the client.
2. Set limits on time spent discussing the client's symptoms.
3. *La belle indifference* is a key symptom in conversion disorder.
4. Provide care focused on the client's symptoms.
5. Individualized therapy is the key treatment for this disorder.

33. A new client admitted to a psychiatric unit is diagnosed with conversion disorder. The client shows a lack of concern for his sudden paralysis, though athletic abilities have always been a source of pride. The nurse understands that the client is demonstrating which condition?
1. Acute dystonia
2. La belle indifference
3. Malingering
4. Secondary gain

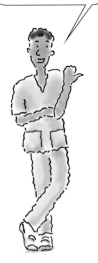

In conversion disorder, is it better to distract from or emphasize symptoms?

34. Which nursing intervention is the **most** appropriate for a client who had pseudoseizures and is diagnosed with conversion disorder?
1. Explain that the pseudoseizures are imaginary.
2. Promote dependence so that unfilled dependency needs are met.
3. Encourage the client to discuss feelings about the pseudoseizures.
4. Promote independence and withdraw attention from the pseudoseizures.

35. Which statement made by a client shows the nurse that the goal of stress management was attained?
1. "My arm hurts."
2. "I enjoy being dependent on others."
3. "I don't really understand why I'm here."
4. "My muscles feel relaxed after that progressive relaxation exercise."

31. 1, 2. A conversion disorder is a neurologic disorder in which psychological stressors are manifested with the display of physical disorders for which there is not a related cause. Conversion disorders are more common in those with a history of psychological disorders, including mood disorders. A history of neglect or sexual abuse may be noted in the medical record. Drug use is not tied to conversion disorders. Hypothyroidism and obesity disorders are not associated with conversion disorders.
CN: Psychosocial integrity; CNS: None; CL: Apply; DIFFICULTY: Difficult

32. 1, 2, 3, 5. Establishing a therapeutic relationship and focusing on the client as a whole, not on the symptoms, are key elements to working with clients with this disorder. La belle indifference is the key symptom and individualized therapy is the key treatment for this disorder.
CN: Psychosocial integrity; CNS: None; CL: Apply; DIFFICULTY: Difficult

33. 2. La belle indifference is a lack of concern about the present illness in some clients. Acute dystonia refers to muscle spasms. Malingering is voluntary production of symptoms. Secondary gain refers to the benefits of illness.
CN: Psychosocial integrity; CNS: None; CL: Apply; DIFFICULTY: Moderate

34. 4. Successful performance of independent activities enhances self-esteem. Stating that the symptoms are imaginary may jeopardize a long-term relationship with the client. Positive reinforcement encourages the continual use of the maladaptive responses. Discussing feelings about the disability may provide nontherapeutic positive gains for the client.
CN: Psychosocial integrity; CNS: None; CL: Apply; DIFFICULTY: Challenge

35. 4. The client is experiencing positive results from learning the relaxation exercise. The other responses alert the nurse that the client needs further interventions.
CN: Physiological integrity; CNS: Basic care and comfort; CL: Analyze; DIFFICULTY: Easy

36. Which intervention can the nurse discuss with the parents of a child with attention deficit hyperactivity disorder (ADHD) to help their child to achieve daily tasks?

1. Make sure to change the routine of the child daily to avoid repetition.
2. Repeat information to the child several times during the day.
3. Give general direction for the task to be completed.
4. Break up the task into smaller steps.

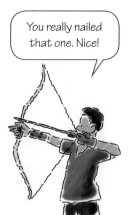

You really nailed that one. Nice!

36. 4. For the child to be able to complete daily tasks, it helps to break the task into smaller steps. This action should make it easier for the child to focus. The parents should provide specific, not general, directions and describe exactly what needs to be done. They do not need to be repetitive with information. The child should respond more effectively to a routine than to change.
CN: Physiological integrity; CNS: Physiological adaptation;
CL: Apply; DIFFICULTY: Easy

37. A nurse is teaching the family of a client diagnosed with a pain disorder. Which statement by the nurse **most** accurately describes this disorder?

1. A preoccupation with pain in the absence of physical disease
2. A report of physical or somatic symptoms without any demonstrable organic findings
3. One or more neurologic symptoms associated with psychological conflict or need
4. Anxiety related to health issues that have no physical cause

37. 1. Pain disorder is a preoccupation with pain in the absence of physical disease. A physical or somatic symptom refers to somatic symptom disorders in general. Neurologic symptoms are associated with conversion disorders. Anxiety related to health issues that have no physical cause is illness anxiety disorder.
CN: Psychosocial integrity; CNS: None; CL: Apply;
DIFFICULTY: Difficult

38. The nurse is caring for a client diagnosed with pain disorder. When reviewing the chart, which finding would cause the nurse to question this diagnosis?

1. Reports of back pain with spinal x-ray showing no significant findings
2. Narcotic medications ordered by three different health care providers
3. Twenty-two emergency department visits in the past 60 days
4. Client reports right hip pain with CT scan showing significant degenerative changes to the joint

38. 4. Pain disorder is the presence of chronic or severe pain that is not supported by a physiologic condition. A CT scan showing degenerative changes to the site of pain may not support the diagnosis of pain disorder. A report of back pain with no underlying physiologic condition, seeking medications from multiple health care providers and multiple visits to health care facilities **do** support the diagnosis of pain disorder.
CN: Physiological integrity; CNS: Physiological adaptation;
CL: Apply; DIFFICULTY: Challenge

39. A client with a tic disorder has tried to use stress reduction techniques without success. Which medication does the nurse anticipate the client may be prescribed for treatment?

1. Methylphenidate
2. Clonidine
3. Atomoxetine
4. Risperidone

39. 4. The atypical antipsychotic drug risperidone is effective in reducing the tics. The other medications are not effective for this disorder.
CN: Physiological integrity; CNS: Pharmacological therapies;
CL: Remember; DIFFICULTY: Moderate

40. A client informs the nurse that he has difficulty sleeping. About which conditions does the nurse question the client to determine factors that inhibit adequate sleep patterns? Select all that apply.

1. Shift work
2. Sleep apnea
3. Reduction of external stimuli
4. Caffeine intake in the evening
5. Consistent bedtime routine
6. Excessive worry or anxiety

40. 1, 2, 4, 6. Shift work can disrupt the circadian rhythm. Sleep apnea can cause a reduction in oxygen to the brain, which can reduce the quality of rest. Caffeine is a stimulant and, if taken too close to bedtime, it can interfere with falling asleep. Excessive worry or anxiety causes an increase in adrenaline, which enhances alertness and reduces sleepiness. A consistent bedtime routine and reduction of external stimuli promote good sleep.
CN: Health promotion and maintenance; CNS: None; CL: Analyze;
DIFFICULTY: Easy

CN: Client needs category   CNS: Client needs subcategory   CL: Cognitive level

41. The nurse is caring for a client who has been diagnosed with narcolepsy. Which actions may assist the client in managing this condition? Select all that apply.
1. Drink a small glass of red wine prior to retiring for the evening
2. Limit caffeine intake
3. Avoid smoking
4. Participate in vigorous exercise within 60 to 90 minutes of bedtime
5. Follow a regular schedule for sleep and rest

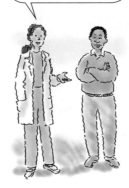

Don't forget to educate your client on lifestyle changes that can improve his condition.

42. The nurse is caring for a 3-year-old diagnosed with autism spectrum disorder. Which behaviors observed by the nurse support this diagnosis? Select all that apply.
1. Becomes easily upset with changes to routine
2. Rocking back and forth while sitting
3. Does not make eye contact when held
4. Speaks in short two- to three-word sentences
5. Smiles when parent walks into the room

43. A client has insomnia disorder and requires pharmaceutical assistance to sleep. The health care provider orders secobarbital sodium 75 mg by mouth at bedtime. The nurse has secobarbital sodium 25-mg tablets on hand. How many tablets should the nurse administer to the client? Record your answer using a whole number.

_____ tablets

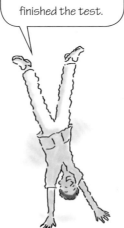

Woo hoo! You finished the test.

41. 2, 3, 5. Narcolepsy is a chronic sleep disorder. Individuals having this disorder experience excessive sleepiness. They may find themselves falling asleep without warning and at frequent intervals. Caffeine intake and smoking have simulating effects and can disrupt sleep. It is important that individuals with narcolepsy have activities that promote quality rest and sleep periods. A regular schedule of sleep and rest are important to ensure obtaining adequate rest. Exercise is recommended in the management of narcolepsy but it should be completed about 4 to 5 hours prior to bedtime.
CN: Health promotion and maintenance; CNS: None;
CL: Apply; DIFFICULTY: Easy

42. 1, 2, 3. Common symptoms of autism spectrum disorder include an inability to "handle" changes in routines or schedules. These individuals may become extremely agitated when these changes occur. Rocking back and forth is also often noted. Social skill impairments are common with the disorder. These impairments may include an inability to make eye contact. Other symptoms include limited to no verbal interaction; two-to three-word sentences would not be common in this disorder at this age. Limited facial expressions are also common. The client smiling at a parent would not be common either.
CN: Physiological integrity; CNS: Physiological adaptation;
CL: Apply; DIFFICULTY: Challenge

43. 3.
Each tablet contains 25 mg of the medication. The correct formula to calculate this drug dose is:

Dose of each tablet × X = Prescribed dose,

where X is the number of tablets.

$$25 \text{ mg/tablet} \times X = 75 \text{ mg.}$$

$$X = 75 \text{ mg} \div 25 \text{ mg/tablet.}$$

$$X = 3 \text{ tablets.}$$

CN: Physiological integrity; CNS: Pharmacological therapies;
CL: Analyze; DIFFICULTY: Easy

Chapter 13

Anxiety, Obsessive-Compulsive, Stress-Related, & Mood Disorders

Want more information on anxiety, obsessive-compulsive, stress-related, and mood disorders to help you prepare for the NCLEX®? Check out the Web site of the National Alliance for the Mentally Ill at www.nami.org/.

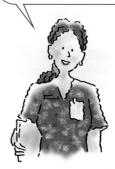

Anxiety, obsessive-compulsive, stress-related, & mood disorders refresher

Bipolar disorder
Manic and depressive episodes

Key signs and symptoms
During periods of mania
- Euphoria and hostility
- Feelings of grandiosity
- Inflated sense of self-worth
- Increased energy (feeling of being charged up)

During periods of depression
- Altered sleep patterns
- Anorexia and weight loss
- Helplessness
- Irritability
- Lack of motivation
- Low self-esteem
- Sadness and crying

Key test results
- EEG is abnormal during:
  - depressive episodes of bipolar I disorder
  - major depression

Key treatments
- Individual therapy
- Family therapy
- Antimanic agents: lithium carbonate, lithium citrate
- Antipsychotic agents: risperidone
- Anticonvulsants: valproic acid, divalproex, lamotrigine

Key interventions
Manic phase
- Decrease environmental stimuli by behaving consistently and supplying external controls
- Ensure a safe and supportive environment
- Define and explain acceptable behaviors and then set limits
- Monitor drug levels, especially lithium

Depressive phase
- Ensure a safe and supportive environment for the client

- Evaluate the risk of suicide and formulate a safety contract with the client, as appropriate
- Observe the client for medication compliance and adverse effects
- Encourage the client to identify current problems and stressors

Generalized anxiety disorder
Excessive or disproportionate anxiety about several aspects of life, such as work, social relationships, or financial matters

Key signs and symptoms
- Easy startle reflex
- Excessive worry and anxiety
- Fatigue
- Fears of grave misfortune or death
- Motor tension
- Muscle tension

Key test results
- Laboratory tests rule out physiologic causes

Key treatments
- Individual therapy focusing on coping skills
- Anxiolytics: alprazolam, lorazepam, clonazepam, buspirone

Key interventions
- Help the client identify and explore coping mechanisms used in the past
- Observe for signs of mounting anxiety

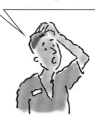

Some days I feel like the king of the world; other days I feel worthless. What's wrong with me?

Major depression
Persistent feeling of sadness and loss of interest

Key signs and symptoms
- Altered sleep patterns
- Anorexia and weight loss
- Helplessness
- Irritability
- Lack of motivation
- Low self-esteem
- Sadness and crying

Compliance is key. Medications should only be used as directed.

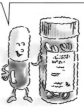

Key test results

- Beck Depression Inventory indicates depression

Key treatments

- Selective serotonin reuptake inhibitors (SSRIs): paroxetine, fluoxetine, sertraline, escitalopram, bupropion, citalopram, venlafaxine
- Tricyclic antidepressants (TCAs): imipramine, desipramine, amitriptyline, clomipramine, doxepin, nortriptyline
- Other antidepressants: mirtazapine, nefazodone

Key interventions

- Ensure safe, supportive environment for the client
- Evaluate the risk of suicide and formulate a safety contract with client
- Observe client for medication compliance and adverse effects

Obsessive-compulsive disorder

Unreasonable thoughts and fears (obsessions) that lead to repetitive behaviors (compulsions)

Key signs and symptoms

- Compulsive behavior
  - repetitive touching or counting
  - doing and undoing small tasks
  - any other repetitive activity
- Obsessive thoughts
  - thoughts of contamination
  - repetitive worries about impending tragedy
  - repeating and counting images or words

Key test results

- Positron emission tomography shows increased activity in the frontal lobe of the cerebral cortex

Key treatments

- Behavioral therapy
- Individual therapy
- Anxiolytics: alprazolam, lorazepam, clonazepam
- SSRIs: fluoxetine, fluvoxamine, paroxetine, sertraline

Key interventions

- Encourage client to express feelings
- Encourage client to identify situations that produce anxiety and precipitate obsessive-compulsive behavior
- Work with client to develop appropriate coping skills

Panic disorder

Debilitating anxiety and fear arising frequently and without reasonable cause

Key signs and symptoms

- Diminished ability to focus, even with direction from others
- Edginess or impatience
- Loss of objectivity
- Severely impaired rational thought
- Uneasiness and tension

Key test results

- Medical tests rule out physiologic causes

Key treatments

- Individual therapy
- Anxiolytics: alprazolam, lorazepam, clonazepam

Key interventions

- During panic attacks:
  - Distract the client from the attack
  - Approach the client calmly and unemotionally
  - Use short, simple sentences

Phobia

Extreme or irrational fear of, or aversion to, something

Key signs and symptoms

- Panic when confronted with the feared object
- Persistent fear of specific thing, place, or situation

Key test results

- No specific test is available to diagnose a phobia

Key treatments

- Family therapy
- Supportive therapy
- Benzodiazepines: alprazolam, lorazepam, clonazepam

Key interventions

- Provide a safe and supportive environment
- Collaborate with client to identify the feared object or situation
- Assist in desensitizing the client

Posttraumatic stress disorder (PTSD)

Persistent mental and emotional stress occurring as a result of injury or severe psychological shock, typically involving disturbance of sleep and constant vivid recall of the experience, with dulled responses to others and to the outside world

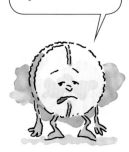

I just feel so sad.

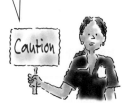

True panic attacks occur without reasonable cause, but life-threatening conditions, such as heart attack, can also cause panic and should be ruled out.

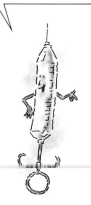

A lot of people have a phobia of me.

Key signs and symptoms

- Anxiety
- Flashbacks of the client's traumatic experience
- Nightmares about the traumatic experience
- Poor impulse control
- Social isolation
- Survivor guilt

Key test results

- No specific tests are available to identify or confirm posttraumatic stress disorder

Key treatments

- Individual therapy
- Group therapy
- Systematic desensitization
- Benzodiazepines: alprazolam, lorazepam, clonazepam
- Tricyclic antidepressants (TCAs): imipramine, amitriptyline
- SSRIS: Sertraline, paroxetine

Key interventions

- Work with client to identify stressors
- Provide safe, supportive environment
- Encourage client to explore the traumatic event and the meaning of the event
- Assist client with problem solving and resolving guilt

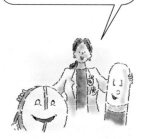

All together, now! Medication and therapy can work together to treat anxiety and related disorders.

thePoint® You can download tables of drug information to help you prepare for the NCLEX®! View Generic Drug Names, Drug Classifications, Drug Actions, and Nursing Implications for the drugs discussed in this refresher at **http://thePoint.lww.com**.

Anxiety, obsessive-compulsive, stress-related, & mood disorders questions, answers, and rationales

1. A client has been taking lithium carbonate for 6 months and recently developed symptoms of arthritis. The client asks the nurse for ibuprofen for pain. What is the **best** response by the nurse?
1. "Ibuprofen will cause lithium level to drop very low and arthritis symptoms may return."
2. "Let me assess your pain level, then I will administer your ibuprofen."
3. "Aspirin would be best for you, because ibuprofen can elevate your lithium blood level."
4. "You will have to stop taking the lithium if you take any pain medication."

2. A nurse caring for a client with panic disorder would identify which behavior experienced by the client?
1. Physiologic changes and sensations during the attacks
2. Advance warning "aura" symptoms prior to an attack
3. Little or no residual anxiety between attacks
4. Slight psychological distress during the attacks

3. A client sees a spider while raking leaves. Immediately, the client's heart begins beating rapidly and he breaks into a sweat. To which condition is the client's response related?
1. Anxiety triggered by sustained physical exertion
2. Fear triggered by an attempt to go outside into a public place
3. Anxiety triggered by reexperiencing a previously frightening event
4. Fear triggered by a known, specific object or event

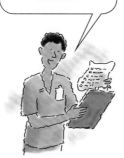

To answer question #2, you need to remember the difference between panic disorder and generalized anxiety disorder.

1. 2. Ibuprofen is an NSAID, which will increase renal lithium carbonate reabsorption; aspirin is also a NSAID, and does not increase lithium carbonate levels. Stronger analgesics are not necessary for mild arthritis. Not all pain medications are contraindicated while on lithium. However, ibuprofen will not cause the lithium level to fall too low.
CN: Physiological integrity; CNS: Pharmacological therapies; CL: Apply; DIFFICULTY: Difficult

2. 3. Most people who experience panic attacks have little or no residual anxiety between attacks. In some individuals, the panic attacks are reproducibly provoked by exposure to certain stimuli. In others, they appear unexpectedly or are most likely to occur in specific settings.
CN: Psychosocial integrity; CNS: None; CL: Apply; DIFFICULTY: Challenge

3. 4. The client's response is an example of fear because it is triggered by a known, specific object, the scorpion. The autonomic responses of the pounding heart and hair standing on end are directly related to the sight of the scorpion. A person experiencing anxiety would have a sense of dread without having a specific source or reason for the emotion.
CN: Psychosocial integrity; CNS: None; CL: Apply; DIFFICULTY: Easy

CN: Client needs category   CNS: Client needs subcategory   CL: Cognitive level

4. A nurse is reinforcing education for a client prescribed lamotrigine. Which adverse effects should the nurse instruct the client to watch for and report to the health care provider? Select all that apply.
1. Muscle weakness
2. Insomnia
3. Blurred vision
4. Skin rashes
5. Headache

5. A client informs the nurse of living alone and never leaving the bedroom because it creates a calm and relaxed environment. If the client leaves the room, extreme panic occurs. Which rationale would **best** explain this client's behavior?
1. The client is manifesting this disorder based on fear of becoming helpless and incurring a panic attack.
2. The client is manifesting this disorder based on unreasonable fear of specific objects and feeling an overwhelming need to perform ritualistic behaviors.
3. This client is not manifesting any anxiety disorder. This behavior is within the range of cultural norms.
4. This client is manifesting agoraphobia and generalized anxiety disorder.

6. A nurse is reinforcing education for a client who has been prescribed buspirone for long-term treatment of anxiety. The nurse determines that the education has been effective when which statement is made by the client?
1. "I will take the medicine only when I feel an anxiety attack coming on."
2. "I will not take the medicine with my meals."
3. "I will not stop the medicine if I become pregnant."
4. "I will not take the medicine with grapefruit juice."

7. A nurse is caring for a client experiencing a panic attack. Which intervention by the nurse would be **most** appropriate?
1. Tell the client to take deep breaths.
2. Tell the client to talk about the anxiety.
3. Encourage the client to verbalize feelings.
4. Ask the client about the cause of the attack.

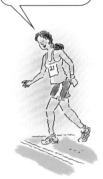

Here we go. Remember to pace yourself.

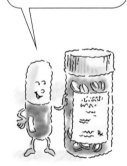

Careful what you mix us drugs with … sometimes we don't get along well with other substances.

4. 3, 4, 5. Blurred vision, headache, and skin rashes are common adverse effects of lamotrigine. The client will not develop insomnia or muscle weakness as a result of taking the medication.
CN: Physiological integrity; CNS: Pharmacological therapies; CL: Apply; DIFFICULTY: Challenge

5. 1. Nursing interventions would be based on the fact that the client is manifesting this disorder on fear of becoming helpless and incurring a panic attack; this disorder is not from fear of specific objects; this behavior is not normal and the client is not experiencing agoraphobia.
CN: Psychosocial integrity; CNS: None; CL: Analyze; DIFFICULTY: Challenge

6. 4. Clients who are taking buspirone should be instructed to avoid grapefruit juice. It can increase the effects of buspirone. Instruct clients to take buspirone with food to decrease nausea, to avoid during pregnancy, and to take on a regular basis—not "as needed."
CN: Physiological integrity; CNS: Pharmacological therapies; CL: Apply; DIFFICULTY: Easy

7. 1. During a panic attack, a client may experience symptoms of dizziness, shortness of breath, and feelings of suffocation. The nurse should remain with the client and direct any statements toward changing the physiologic response, such as taking deep breaths. During an attack, the client is unable to talk about anxious situations and isn't able to address feelings, especially uncomfortable feelings and frustrations. While having a panic attack, the client is also unable to focus on anything other than the symptoms, so the client won't be able to discuss the cause of the attack.
CN: Safe, effective care environment; CNS: Coordinated care; CL: Analyze; DIFFICULTY: Easy

8. The nurse is discussing the incidence of obsessive-compulsive disorder (OCD) with a client. Which statement made by the client demonstrates an understanding of the education?
1. OCD is extremely rare.
2. OCD seldom occurs in women.
3. OCD is as common as diabetes and asthma.
4. OCD only occurs among alcoholics and drug abusers.

9. A client asks about how various medications are prescribed to treat anxiety disorders. What is the **best** response by the nurse?
1. Benzodiazepines are the treatment of choice for short-term management of acute anxiety.
2. Selective serotonin reuptake inhibitor antidepressants are used primarily for acute management of panic attacks.
3. Beta-blockers are usually prescribed on a regularly scheduled daily basis for long-term treatment to manage generalized anxiety disorder.
4. Buspirone is the medication of choice to treat obsessive-compulsive disorder.

10. A client is diagnosed with generalized anxiety disorder. Which nursing intervention would **best** meet the needs of this client?
1. Conducting individual psychotherapy
2. Administering antianxiety medications p.r.n.
3. Reinforcing education about newly prescribed antianxiety medications
4. Conducting exposure therapy

11. The nurse is caring for a client who's in the panic level of anxiety. Which action is the nurse's **highest priority**?
1. Encourage the client to discuss feelings.
2. Provide for the client's safety needs.
3. Decrease environmental stimuli.
4. Respect the client's personal space.

12. Which nursing intervention is appropriate to include when assisting with the plan of care for a client with panic disorder?
1. Identify childhood trauma.
2. Monitor nutritional intake.
3. Institute suicide precautions.
4. Decrease episodes of disorientation.

8. 3. Obsessive-compulsive disorder is said to occur about as commonly as diabetes and asthma, and yet clients frequently hide their symptoms from family and health care providers. Most cases of this disorder begin in at a young age, often during young adulthood or before.
CN: Psychosocial integrity; CNS: None; CL: Analyze; DIFFICULTY: Moderate

9. 1. Benzodiazepines have established short-term effectiveness in the control of anxiety symptoms. They are the treatment choice for acute episodes of anxiety, such as during crises.
CN: Psychosocial integrity; CNS: None; CL: Analyze; DIFFICULTY: Moderate

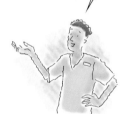

Don't miss out on opportunities to teach your clients.

10. 3. Teaching the client about antianxiety medications would be an important part of a nursing intervention. In addition, the nurse could also assess the level of anxiety and the degree of interference with normal nursing activities. Teaching the client skills dealing with cognitive restructuring and initiating supportive therapy are good options for the nurse to implement.
CN: Psychosocial integrity; CNS: None; CL: Analyze; DIFFICULTY: Moderate

11. 2. A client in the panic level of anxiety doesn't comprehend and can't follow instructions or care for his own basic needs. The client is unable to express feelings due to the level of anxiety. Decreased environmental stimulus is needed but only after the client's safety needs and other basic needs are met. The nurse must enter the client's personal space to provide personal care because a client in panic can't do so.
CN: Safe, effective care environment; CNS: Coordinated care; CL: Analyze; DIFFICULTY: Moderate

12. 3. Clients with panic disorder are at risk for suicide. Childhood trauma is associated with posttraumatic stress disorder, not panic disorder. Nutritional problems don't typically accompany panic disorder. Clients with panic disorder aren't typically disoriented; they may have a temporarily altered sense of reality, but that lasts only for the duration of the attack.
CN: Psychosocial integrity; CNS: None; CL: Apply; DIFFICULTY: Challenge

13. The nurse is assisting with the development of a treatment plan for a client with a specific phobia. Which intervention should the nurse prepare the client for?
  1. Behavioral therapy
  2. A neurological surgical procedure
  3. A large dose of various medications
  4. There is no known effective treatment for specific phobias

14. Which group therapy intervention would be of primary importance to a client with panic disorder?
  1. Explore how secondary gains are derived from the disorder.
  2. Discuss new ways of thinking and feeling about panic attacks.
  3. Work to eliminate manipulative behavior used for meeting needs.
  4. Learn the risk factors and other demographics associated with panic disorder.

15. The nurse is assigned to reinforce insulin administration for a client with diabetes who is anxious. During which stage should the nurse reinforce education for the client?
  1. In the mild stage of anxiety
  2. In the moderate stage of anxiety
  3. In the severe stage of anxiety
  4. In the panic stage of anxiety

16. A client diagnosed with panic disorder and agoraphobia is talking with the nurse about the progress made in treatment. Which statement indicates a positive client response?
  1. "I went to the mall with my friend last Saturday."
  2. "I'm hyperventilating only when I have a panic attack."
  3. "Today, I decided that I can stop taking my medication."
  4. "Last night, I decided to eat more than a bowl of cereal."

17. Which intervention by the nurse would be **most** appropriate when caring for a client newly diagnosed with insulin-dependent diabetes who also has blood-injection-injury phobia?
  1. Teach the client to avoid fainting by tensing the muscles of the legs and abdomen.
  2. Quickly expose the client to feared situations.
  3. Have the client avoid as much medical care as possible.
  4. Focus on treating the symptoms with antianxiety medication.

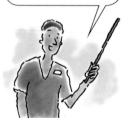

The timing of your teaching can be just as important as the content.

13. 1. Behavioral therapy has been shown to be the best treatment for specific phobias. In particular, some form of controlled exposure therapy has proven to be very effective. Medications, unless being used to treat a related illness such as depression, have not been conclusively shown to be effective.
CN: Psychosocial integrity; CNS: None; CL: Apply; DIFFICULTY: Challenge

14. 2. Discussion of new ways of thinking and feeling about panic attacks can enable others to learn and benefit from a variety of intervention strategies. There are usually no secondary gains obtained from having a panic disorder. People with panic disorder aren't using the disorder as a way to manipulate others. Learning the risk factors could be accomplished in another format such as a psychoeducational program.
CN: Psychosocial integrity; CNS: None; CL: Analyze; DIFFICULTY: Moderate

15. 1. The client will best pay attention to instructions if the client is experiencing mild anxiety. With mild anxiety, the client is alert and there is an increase in the perceptual field.
CN: Psychosocial integrity; CNS: None; CL: Analyze; DIFFICULTY: Easy

16. 1. Clients with panic disorder tend to be socially withdrawn. Going to the mall is a sign of working on avoidance behaviors. Hyperventilation is a key symptom of panic disorder. Teaching breathing control is a major intervention for clients with panic disorder. The client taking medications for panic disorder, such as tricyclic antidepressants and benzodiazepines, must be weaned off these drugs. Most clients with panic disorder and agoraphobia don't have nutritional problems.
CN: Psychosocial integrity; CNS: None; CL: Analyze; DIFFICULTY: Easy

17. 1. The client may be able to avoid fainting and relieve hypotension by tensing the large muscle groups. Desensitization by slowly, not quickly, exposing the client to blood injection is indicated to reduce fear. Clients with blood-injection-injury phobia may avoid *all* medical care, which is dangerous to their health. Antianxiety medications may help on a short-term basis only.
CN: Psychosocial integrity; CNS: None; CL: Apply; DIFFICULTY: Challenge

---

CN: Client needs category   CNS: Client needs subcategory   CL: Cognitive level

18. The nurse is caring for a client who has been diagnosed as having social anxiety disorder. Which intervention would be appropriate for the nurse to encourage the client to develop?
1. Being in situations where the client is alone
2. Speaking or performing in public
3. Being surrounded by other people in crowded places
4. Having to shake hands and be exposed to others' germs

19. A client on the sixth floor of a psychiatric unit has a morbid fear of elevators. The client is scheduled to attend occupational therapy, which is located on the ground floor of the hospital. However, the client refuses to take the elevator, insisting that the stairs are safer. Which nursing action would be **best** given the client's refusal to use the elevator?
1. Insist the client take the elevator.
2. Offer a special reward if the client rides the elevator.
3. Withhold occupational therapy privileges until the client is able to ride the elevator.
4. Allow the client to use the stairs.

20. The nurse is caring for a client experiencing dreams and flashbacks related to past experiences of sexual abuse and feelings of isolation. What does this behavior indicate to the nurse?
1. Panic disorder
2. Phobia
3. Posttraumatic stress disorder (PTSD)
4. Obsessive-compulsive disorder

21. Which statement made by the nurse would be useful when reinforcing education for the client and family about phobias and the need for a strong support system?
1. The use of a family support system is only temporary.
2. The need to be assertive can be reinforced by the family.
3. The family must set limits on inappropriate behaviors.
4. The family plays a role in promoting client independence.

22. The nurse is obtaining data from a client who reports not getting much sleep at night. The client checks the door to see if it is locked up to 300 times before going to bed. What does the nurse suspect is occurring with this client based on the data?
1. Panic disorder
2. Phobia
3. Posttraumatic stress disorder (PTSD)
4. Obsessive-compulsive disorder

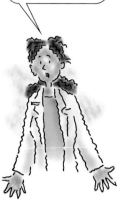

Sometimes it's best to just face your fears.

Educating the family can be just as important as educating the client when it comes to phobias.

18. 2. The client experiencing a social anxiety disorder is suffering from a social phobia. This type of phobia is a profound fear of public speaking. The nursing care plan would focus on social skills training and exposure to social situations. Interventions would be directed toward assisting the client with developing skills related to speaking or performing in public, meeting new people, or taking tests.
CN: Psychosocial integrity; CNS: None; CL: Apply;
DIFFICULTY: Challenge

19. 4. This client has a phobia and must not be forced to ride the elevator because of the risk of panic-level anxiety, which can occur if forced to contact the phobic object. This client can't control the fear; therefore, stating that the client must take the elevator or promising a reward won't work. Occupational therapy is a treatment the client needs, not a reward.
CN: Psychosocial integrity; CNS: None; CL: Apply; DIFFICULTY: Easy

20. 3. The client is most likely suffering from posttraumatic stress disorder. Individuals with this disorder have been exposed to an event that threatened the person's physical integrity. In this situation, the experience of sexual abuse was seen as a threat to the client's physical integrity. Flashbacks are often experienced when an individual suffers from this disorder.
CN: Psychosocial integrity; CNS: None; CL: Apply; DIFFICULTY: Easy

21. 4. The family plays a vital role in supporting the client in treatment and preventing the client from using the phobia to obtain secondary gains. Family support must be ongoing, not temporary. The family can be more helpful by focusing on effective handling of anxiety rather than focusing energy on developing assertiveness skills. People with phobias are already restrictive in their behavior; more restrictions aren't necessary.
CN: Psychosocial integrity; CNS: None; CL: Analyze;
DIFFICULTY: Moderate

22. 4. The client is most likely suffering from an obsessive-compulsive disorder. The act of checking the door to see if it is locked up to 300 times before going to bed is considered the compulsive act. Compulsive acts are an attempt to reduce anxiety related to some obsessive thought.
CN: Psychosocial integrity; CNS: None; CL: Analyze;
DIFFICULTY: Easy

23. Which nursing interventions would be **most** appropriate in assisting a client to cope with stress? Select all that apply.
1. Teach relaxation exercises.
2. Plan care for client.
3. Minimize environmental stimuli.
4. Encourage verbalization of feelings.
5. Encourage increase in workload.
6. Establish a trusting relationship.

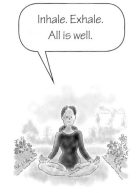

Inhale. Exhale. All is well.

23. 1, 3, 5, 6. Factors that affect a person's ability to cope with stress include immediate individual needs, individual perception of danger, amount of support from others, personal belief in ability to handle stress, and the number of concurrent or cumulative stressors with which the person is dealing. People use adaptive measures to deal directly with a stressful situation or the symptoms the situation produces; these measures require minimal expenditure of energy and include relaxation, behavioral changes, and support networks.
CN: Psychosocial integrity; CNS: None; CL: Analyze; DIFFICULTY: Challenge

24. A client is diagnosed with severe posttraumatic stress disorder (PTSD) and is prescribed a tricyclic antidepressant. Which outcome does the nurse observe for to determine success with the prescribed regimen?
1. The client will not have hyperactivity and purposeless movements.
2. The client will have an increase in the ability to concentrate.
3. The client will not experience the reenactment of the trauma.
4. The client will suspend the grieving process.

24. 3. Tricyclic antidepressant medication decreases the frequency of reenactment of the trauma for the client. It helps memory problems and sleeping difficulties and decreases numbing. The medication won't prevent hyperactivity and purposeless movements nor increase the client's concentration. No medication facilitates the grieving process.
CN: Physiological integrity; CNS: Pharmacological therapies; CL: Apply; DIFFICULTY: Easy

25. Which nursing action would be included in a care plan for a client with posttraumatic stress disorder (PTSD) who states that the experience was "bad luck"?
1. Encourage the client to verbalize the experience.
2. Assist the client in defining the experience as a trauma.
3. Work with the client to take steps to move on with life.
4. Help the client accept positive and negative feelings.

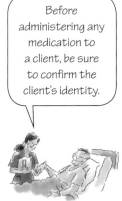

Before administering any medication to a client, be sure to confirm the client's identity.

25. 2. The client must define the experience as traumatic to realize the situation wasn't under personal control. Encouraging the client to verbalize the experience without first addressing the denial isn't a useful strategy. The client can move on with life only after acknowledging the trauma and processing the experience. Acknowledgment of the actual trauma and verbalization of the event should come before the acceptance of feelings.
CN: Psychosocial integrity; CNS: None; CL: Analyze; DIFFICULTY: Challenge

26. The nurse is reinforcing education for a client taking isocarboxazid. Which medication should the nurse have the client avoid while taking isocarboxazid?
1. Acetaminophen
2. Ibuprofen
3. Guaifenesin
4. Meperidine

26. 3. Clients taking monoamine oxidase inhibitors should avoid meperidine. Other medications to avoid include tricyclic antidepressants, fluoxetine, amphetamines, and amphetamine-like medications, including all sympathomimetics.
CN: Physiological integrity; CNS: Pharmacological therapies; CL: Apply; DIFFICULTY: Difficult

27. The nurse is obtaining data from a group of clients with depression. Which client would the nurse recognize would **most** benefit from electroconvulsive therapy (ECT)?
1. Clients who are suicidal or homicidal
2. Clients who are aggressive or acting out and depressed
3. Clients with physical problems resulting in depression
4. Clients who are severely depressed and do not respond to medication trials

27. 4. Electroconvulsive therapy (ECT) is highly effective in helping clients who are severely depressed and do not respond to medication trials. Many studies on ECT and depression produces rates as high as 90%, in comparison to medications (tricyclic antidepressants and monoamine oxidase inhibitors).
CN: Psychosocial integrity; CNS: None; CL: Apply; DIFFICULTY: Easy

28. A client with bipolar disorder is experiencing mania with labile mood changes. The client is threatening to hit staff members and other clients. What is the **best** response by the nurse?
1. "That will only make things worse. Why would you want to hit someone?"
2. "You will be put in seclusion and kept there if you threaten anyone else."
3. "Do not hit any of the other clients or me. If you cannot control your behavior, we will help you."
4. "That's enough! You know we do not tolerate this type of behavior."

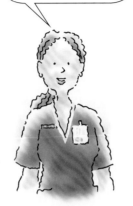

Clients with bipolar disorder may need help establishing appropriate boundaries.

28. 3. The correct response is to set limits in a simple, concrete sentence in order to de-escalate the situation. Asking the client why he would want to hit someone asks a question that the client cannot answer. Telling the client he will be put in seclusion threatens the client and that is assault. Yelling at the client that the behavior will not be tolerated does not help the client stop the behavior.
CN: Psychosocial Integrity; CNS: None; CL: Apply; DIFFICULTY: Difficult

29. The nurse is caring for a client with posttraumatic stress disorder (PTSD) and the family informs the nurse that loud noises cause a serious anxiety response. Which explanation by the nurse would help the family understand the client's response?
1. Environmental triggers can cause the client to react emotionally.
2. Clients commonly experience extreme fear of normal environmental stimuli.
3. After a trauma, the client can't respond to stimuli in an appropriate manner.
4. The response indicates another emotional problem needs investigation.

29. 1. Repeated exposure to environmental triggers can cause the client to experience a hyperarousal state because there's a loss of physiologic control of incoming stimuli. After experiencing a trauma, the client may have strong reactions to stimuli similar to those that occurred during the traumatic event. However, not all stimuli cause an anxiety response. The client's anxiety response is typically seen after a traumatic experience and doesn't indicate the presence of another problem.
CN: Psychosocial integrity; CNS: None; CL: Apply; DIFFICULTY: Easy

30. A client was the lone survivor of a train crash 6 months ago. Which statement by the client would indicate a maladaptive response to the trauma?
1. "I don't want to talk about it."
2. "I'm able to concentrate on reading a book."
3. "I've started to sleep through the night."
4. "I jump when I hear a train whistle because it reminds me of the wreck."

30. 1. Denial is used as a protective response to posttraumatic stress. Concentration and sleeping through the night indicate resolution of conflicts. Startling sounds can provoke anxiety in a client with posttraumatic stress disorder, but this client expresses understanding of why this is happening.
CN: Psychosocial integrity; CNS: None; CL: Apply; DIFFICULTY: Challenge

31. The nurse is reinforcing education for a client taking a monoamine oxidase inhibitor (MAOI). Which foods should the nurse make sure the client avoids? Select all that apply.
1. Smoked fish
2. A ripe avocado
3. Wine
4. Cottage cheese
5. Grilled chicken

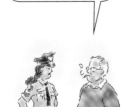

Seriously? In the hospital?

31. 1, 2, 3. Foods to be avoided are those containing tyramine and alcohol, such as smoked fish, ripe avocados, and wine. A client taking monoamine oxidase inhibitors should consider cottage cheese and chicken safe foods.
CN: Psychosocial integrity; CNS: None; CL: Apply; DIFFICULTY: Challenge

32. The nurse is obtaining a health history from a client with depression and determines the client is taking St. John's wort (hypericum). Which information should the nurse include when discussing this medication with the client?
1. Nonstandard preparation, so the amount of hypericum may vary among manufacturers
2. Much more expensive cost of preparation than other commonly prescribed drugs.
3. Blood testing required every week for dyscrasias
4. Purchase amounts limited to a 2-week supply

32. 1. St. John's wort (hypericum), which is an over-the-counter medication for depression, may have a nonstandard preparation and the amount of hypericum may vary among manufacturers. Other disadvantages of St. John's wort include reduced effectiveness compared to prescription drug therapy or cognitive therapy. In addition, drug interactions can occur and may be significant.
CN: Psychosocial integrity; CNS: None; CL: Apply; DIFFICULTY: Challenge

33. A nurse is obtaining data from a client diagnosed with major depression and observes that the client is unable to perform activities of daily living (ADL) independently. The nurse would assume which role?
1. Self-care agency
2. Nursing agency
3. Self-care deficit
4. Independent agency

34. The nurse obtaining data from a client on admission suspects this client may be depressed. Which self-rating scale should the nurse have the client complete?
1. Stanford and the WISC
2. Beck and Zung
3. Miller and GRE
4. Rorschach and MMPI

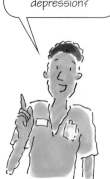

What key test is used to assess for depression?

35. The nurse is monitoring a client who is diagnosed with depression for signs of urinary retention and constipation. Which education should the nurse reinforce in order to prevent these complications?
1. Side effects of the medication
2. Lack of exercise
3. Avoidance of dehydration
4. Poor dietary choices

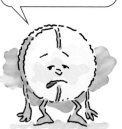

Sometimes we drugs have negative unintended effects … sorry about that.

36. Which principles should be kept in mind when the nurse evaluates the client's progress in managing depression?
1. Grieving resulting from significant loss should never exceed 2 months.
2. To be considered successful, all the identified outcomes should show progress.
3. The client's view of the changes since the beginning of therapy is not objective.
4. Significant energy and a conscious effort are required by the client to maintain perspective.

37. The nurse is providing group therapy for a group of adolescents who witnessed the violent death of a peer. Which outcome would **best** meet the needs of the students?
1. To learn violence prevention strategies
2. To talk about appropriate expression of anger
3. To discuss the effect of the trauma on their lives
4. To develop trusting relationships among their peers

33. 3. When the client begins to be able to care for basic physical and personal needs, the nurse will move to a supportive-educative role. This type of role focuses on enhancing the client's ability to carry on effectively without nursing support and to rise above the feelings of depression that brought on the initial deficit in self-care.
CN: Psychosocial integrity; CNS: None; CL: Analyze; DIFFICULTY: Moderate

34. 2. The two most common self-rating scales used with clients who may be depressed are the Beck Depression Inventory and the Zung Self-Rating Depression Scale. The Beck Depression Inventory is a 21-item scale used with individuals age 13 and older. It measures the severity of depression. The Zung Self-Rating Depression Scale is a 20-item scale that measures four common characteristics of depression.
CN: Psychosocial integrity; CNS: None; CL: Apply; DIFFICULTY: Difficult

35. 1. In this client's situation, urinary retention is most likely caused by medications. Educating the client on side effects of the medication addresses both constipation and urinary retention. Constipation can be related to inadequate food intake, poor diet, and lack of exercise.
CN: Physiological integrity; CNS: None; CL: Analyze; DIFFICULTY: Challenge

36. 4. When evaluating, the nurse needs to remind the client that managing depression often requires significant energy, and a conscious effort on the client's part to balance emotions and maintain perspective. It is also important to remember that depression resulting from a significant loss, such as loss of a loved one, may take many weeks or months to overcome; the client will need sensitive nursing care to adapt to the new situations and roles that accompany such a loss.
CN: Psychosocial integrity; CNS: None; CL: Apply; DIFFICULTY: Challenge

37. 3. By discussing the effect of the trauma on their lives, the adolescents can grieve and develop effective coping strategies. Learning violence prevention strategies isn't the most immediate concern after a trauma occurs, nor is working on developing healthy relationships. It's appropriate to talk about expressing anger after the trauma is addressed.
CN: Psychosocial integrity; CNS: None; CL: Apply; DIFFICULTY: Easy

38. The nurse is caring for a client with post-traumatic stress disorder (PTSD) experiencing a frightening flashback. The nurse can **best** offer reassurance of safety and security through which nursing action?
1. Encouraging the client to talk about the traumatic event
2. Assessing for maladaptive and coping strategies
3. Staying with the client
4. Acknowledging feelings of guilt or self-blame

39. Which behavior by the nurse would demonstrate caring to a client with a diagnosis of anxiety disorder?
1. Verbalize concern about the client.
2. Arrange group activities for clients.
3. Ask the client to sign the treatment plan.
4. Arrange for a psychoeducational group on medications.

40. Which finding should the nurse expect when talking about school to a child diagnosed with a generalized anxiety disorder (GAD)?
1. The child has been fighting with peers for the past month.
2. The child can't stop lying to parents and teachers.
3. The child has gained 15 lb (6.8 kg) in the past month.
4. The child expresses concerns about grades.

41. The nurse is caring for a client with generalized anxiety disorder (GAD). Which concurrent diagnosis should the nurse monitor for?
1. Bipolar disorder
2. Gender identity disorder
3. Panic disorder
4. Schizoaffective disorder

42. Which statement indicates a positive response from a client with generalized anxiety disorder (GAD) to a nurse's reinforcement of education about nutrition?
1. "I've stopped drinking so much diet cola."
2. "I've reduced my intake of carbohydrates."
3. "I now eat less at dinner and before bedtime."
4. "I've cut back on my use of dairy products."

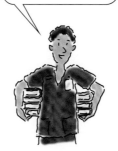

School can be a big source of anxiety for everyone.

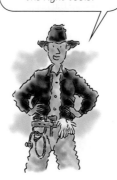

Working with clients with mood disorders can be a real adventure. Make sure you're armed with all the right tools.

38. 3. The nurse should stay with the client during periods of flashbacks and nightmares, offer reassurance of safety and security, and assure the client that these symptoms aren't uncommon following a severe trauma. Encouraging the client to talk about the traumatic event, observing for maladaptive and coping strategies, and acknowledging feelings of guilt or self-blame may be carried out in the future. The nurse's top priority during the flashback is to stay with the client.
CN: Psychosocial integrity; CNS: None; CL: Apply; DIFFICULTY: Moderate

39. 1. The nurse who verbally expresses concern about a client's well-being is acting in a caring and supportive manner. Arranging for group activities may be an action where the nurse has no direct client contact and therefore can't demonstrate caring to clients. Asking a client to sign the treatment plan may not be viewed as a sign of caring. A psychoeducational group on medications may be viewed by clients as an educational experience, as opposed to a sign of caring, because the nurse may have limited interaction with them.
CN: Health promotion and maintenance; CNS: None; CL: Apply; DIFFICULTY: Challenge

40. 4. Children with GAD will worry about how well they're performing in school. Children with GAD don't tend to be involved in conflict. They're more oriented toward good behavior. Children with GAD don't tend to lie to others. They would want to do their best and try to please others. A weight gain of 15 lb (6.8 kg) isn't a typical characteristic of a child with anxiety disorder.
CN: Psychosocial integrity; CNS: None; CL: Analyze; DIFFICULTY: Moderate

41. 3. Approximately 75% of clients with GAD may also have a diagnosis of phobia, panic disorder, or substance abuse. Clients with GAD don't tend to have a coexisting diagnosis of bipolar disorder, gender identity disorder, or schizoaffective disorder.
CN: Psychosocial integrity; CNS: None; CL: Apply; DIFFICULTY: Easy

42. 1. Clients with GAD can decrease anxiety by eliminating caffeine from their diets. It isn't necessary for clients with generalized anxiety to decrease their carbohydrate intake, eat less at dinner or before bedtime (unless there are other compelling health reasons), or cut back on their use of dairy products.
CN: Physiological integrity; CNS: Basic care and comfort; CL: Apply; DIFFICULTY: Moderate

43. A nurse assesses a client with depression who reports fatigue, sadness, insomnia, powerlessness and social isolation. What is the **priority** area of focus to meet the needs of the client?
1. Fatigue, so that the client can experience enough energy to work on other symptoms
2. Sadness, in order to reduce or eliminate the need for suicide precautions
3. The symptoms that the client identifies as the most urgent need
4. All of the identified symptoms simultaneously in a coordinated manner

43. 3. The nurse knows that the best practice is to focus on the symptoms that the client identifies as the most urgent. This approach would indicate to the client that the nurse cares about the client's feelings and perception of the problem. By focusing on the symptoms that the client feels are most urgent, the nurse can build a trusting relationship with the client.
CN: Psychosocial integrity; CNS: None; CL: Analyze;
DIFFICULTY: Challenge

44. A client describes unpredictable episodes of acute anxiety as "just awful" and feels as though they are about to die and can hardly breathe. The nurse recognizes that the symptoms described by the client are associated with which condition?
1. Agoraphobia
2. Dissociative disorder
3. Posttraumatic stress disorder (PTSD)
4. Panic disorder

44. 4. This client is describing the characteristics of someone with panic disorder. Agoraphobia is characterized by fear of public places; dissociative disorder, by lost periods of time; and PTSD, by hypervigilance and sleep disturbance.
CN: Psychosocial integrity; CNS: None; CL: Apply; DIFFICULTY: Easy

45. Which statement by a client with a diagnosis of generalized anxiety disorder (GAD) would convince the nurse that anxiety has been a long-standing problem?
1. "I was, and still am, an impulsive person."
2. "I've always been hyperactive but not in useful ways."
3. "When I was in college, I never thought I would finish."
4. "All my life, I've had intrusive dreams and scary nightmares."

45. 3. For many people who have GAD, the age of onset is during young adulthood. The symptoms of impulsiveness and hyperactivity aren't commonly associated with a diagnosis of GAD. The symptom of intrusive dreams and nightmares is associated with posttraumatic stress disorder (PTSD) rather than GAD.
CN: Psychosocial integrity; CNS: None; CL: Understand;
DIFFICULTY: Challenge

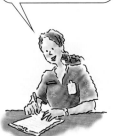

Don't get restless. You'll figure this one out.

46. Which symptom would the client with generalized anxiety disorder (GAD) **most** likely display when assessed for muscle tension?
1. Difficulty sleeping
2. Restlessness
3. Strong startle response
4. Tachycardia

46. 2. Restlessness is a symptom associated with muscle tension. Difficulty sleeping and a strong startle response are considered symptoms of vigilance and scanning of the environment, not muscle tension. Tachycardia is classified as a symptom of autonomic hyperactivity, not muscle tension.
CN: Physiological integrity; CNS: Physiological adaptation;
CL: Remember; DIFFICULTY: Moderate

47. When planning the care of a client with generalized anxiety disorder, which intervention is **most** important to include?
1. Encourage the client to engage in activities that increase feelings of power and self-esteem.
2. Promote the client's interaction and socialization with others.
3. Assist the client to make plans for regular periods of leisure time.
4. Encourage the client to use a diary to record when anxiety occurred, its cause, and which interventions may have helped.

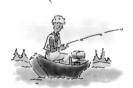

Being outdoors helps me keep my stress under control.

47. 4. One of the nurse's goals is to help the client with generalized anxiety disorder associate symptoms with an event, thereby beginning to learn appropriate ways to eliminate or reduce distress. A diary can be a beneficial tool for this purpose. Although encouraging the client to engage in activities that increase feelings of power and self-esteem, promoting interaction and socialization with others, and assisting the client to make plans for regular periods of leisure time may be appropriate, they aren't the priority.
CN: Psychosocial integrity; CNS: None; CL: Apply;
DIFFICULTY: Moderate

48. The nurse is obtaining data of the early life of a client with borderline personality disorder (BPD). Which statement made by the client would correlate with this diagnosis?
1. "I had an overprotective, ever-present mother."
2. "I had a violent, chaotic family life."
3. "I have a rigid, consistent daily schedule of activities."
4. "I had an intact family whose members were stoic and emotionally reserved."

48. **2.** When obtaining a history about the early life of individuals with BPD, one would most likely find a violent, chaotic family. One author describes the family history of the borderline personality as a "disaster a day" and likens the resultant family life to the plot of a television soap opera. Individuals with BPD have some history of feeling abandoned, fearful, and unprotected as children.
CN: Psychosocial integrity; CNS: None; CL: Apply; DIFFICULTY: Moderate

49. The nurse is educating a client that is demonstrating considerable anxiety about an impending surgical procedure. Which nursing intervention is **most** appropriate?
1. Reassure the client that there are many treatments for the problem.
2. Calmly ask the client to describe the procedure that is to be done.
3. Tell the client that the nursing staff will help in any way they can.
4. Tell the client not to keep feelings to themself.

49. **2.** An appropriate nursing intervention in this case is to ask the client to repeat to the nurse the major points of the procedure. By asking the client to describe the procedure, the nurse can assess the level of understanding and address anxiety by providing necessary education. Reassuring the client that there are many treatments; informing the client that the nursing staff will help; and saying not to keep feelings to themself don't address the client's anxiety or lack of knowledge about the procedure.
CN: Psychosocial integrity; CNS: None; CL: Understand; DIFFICULTY: Moderate

50. A client with a diagnosis of generalized anxiety disorder (GAD) wants to stop taking lorazepam. Which important fact should the nurse discuss with the client about discontinuing the medication?
1. Stopping the drug may cause depression.
2. Stopping the drug increases cognitive abilities.
3. Stopping the drug decreases sleeping difficulties.
4. Stopping the drug can cause withdrawal symptoms.

50. **4.** Stopping antianxiety drugs such as benzodiazepines can cause the client to have withdrawal symptoms. Stopping a benzodiazepine doesn't tend to cause depression, increase cognitive abilities, or decrease sleeping difficulties.
CN: Physiological integrity; CNS: Pharmacological therapies; CL: Apply; DIFFICULTY: Easy

51. During a conversation with a client, the nurse recognizes a delusion of persecution. What is the **priority** action by the nurse?
1. Ask the client to expand on the comment.
2. Redirect the conversation back to reality.
3. Engage the client and enter into the delusion.
4. Argue with the client over the reality of the delusion.

51. **2.** The priority action is for the nurse to redirect the conversation back to reality. The nurse should never ask the client to expand on the comment, enter into the delusion, or argue with the client over the reality of the delusion.
CN: Psychosocial integrity; CNS: None; CL: Understand; DIFFICULTY: Easy

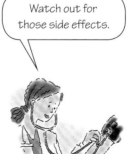

Watch out for those side effects.

52. A client taking alprazolam reports light-headedness and nausea every day while getting out of bed. Which action should the nurse take to objectively validate this client's problem?
1. Take the client's blood pressure.
2. Monitor body temperature.
3. Teach Valsalva maneuver.
4. Obtain a blood chemical profile.

52. **1.** The nurse should take a blood pressure reading to monitor for orthostatic hypotension. A body temperature reading or chemistry profile won't yield useful information about hypotension. Valsalva maneuver is performed to lower the heart rate and isn't an appropriate intervention.
CN: Physiological integrity; CNS: Reduction of risk potential; CL: Apply; DIFFICULTY: Easy

53. A client with chronic anxiety disorder reports chest pain. Which nursing intervention is **most** appropriate?
1. Reassure the client that the episode will pass.
2. Stay with the client.
3. Obtain vital signs.
4. Administer prescribed antianxiety medication.

54. Which communication guideline should the nurse use when talking with a client who is experiencing mania?
1. Address the client in a light and joking manner.
2. Focus and redirect the conversation as necessary.
3. Allow the client to talk about several different topics.
4. Ask only open-ended questions to facilitate conversation.

55. The client has been scheduled for electroconvulsive therapy (ECT). The health care provider has discussed the procedure with the client. The client says to the nurse, "My health care provider has discussed ECT with me, but could you remind me of some of the side effects I may experience?" Select all that apply.
1. Headache
2. Confusion
3. Dementia
4. Muscle pain
5. Short-term memory loss

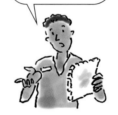

Be prepared to review the side effects of a medication with your client.

56. A client who has just had electroconvulsive therapy (ECT) asks for a drink of water. Which intervention would be the nurse's **priority**?
1. Check the client's blood pressure.
2. Assess the gag reflex.
3. Obtain a body temperature.
4. Determine level of consciousness.

57. A client experiencing paranoid delusions states, "They are conspiring against me; they're after me all night." Which response by the nurse would be the **most** empathic?
1. "That sounds frightening."
2. "You can't sleep?"
3. "This cannot be true."
4. "You are having a delusion."

53. 3. Although the client with chronic anxiety disorder may have somatic symptoms, physiologic causes for chest pain must be thoroughly assessed. Reassuring the client would be acceptable only after ruling out a physiologic cause for the symptoms. Staying with the client may be therapeutic, but obtaining vital signs would take precedence. Administering antianxiety agents might mask signs of cardiac problems.
CN: Psychosocial integrity; CNS: None; CL: Analyze; DIFFICULTY: Moderate

54. 2. To decrease stimulation, the nurse should attempt to redirect and focus the conversation, not allow the client to talk about different topics. Addressing the client in a light and joking manner may contribute to the client feeling out of control. It's best to ask a manic client closed questions because open-ended questions enable the client to talk endlessly, possibly contributing to the client feeling out of control.
CN: Psychosocial integrity; CNS: None; CL: Understand; DIFFICULTY: Easy

55. 1, 2, 4, 5. A client may temporarily experience headache, confusion, muscle pain, and short-term memory loss. Dementia is not a side effect of ECT; dementia would signal a long-term, irreversible condition.
CN: Physiological integrity; CNS: Physiological adaptation; CL: Apply; DIFFICULTY: Difficult

56. 2. The nurse must check the client's gag reflex before allowing the client to have a drink after an ECT procedure. Blood pressure and body temperature don't influence whether the client may have a drink after the procedure. The client would obviously be conscious if he's requesting a glass of water.
CN: Physiological integrity; CNS: Physiological adaptation; CL: Apply; DIFFICULTY: Easy

57. 1. The most empathic response would be to acknowledge that the delusion sounds frightening. This response would address the client's feelings. The other three options do not address feelings or demonstrate that the nurse is caring.
CN: Psychosocial integrity; CNS: None; CL: Apply; DIFFICULTY: Easy

58. A client with bipolar disorder reports headache, agitation, and indigestion. Which behavior does the nurse suspect this client is experiencing?
1. Depression
2. Cyclothymia
3. Hypomania
4. Mania

59. A client with bipolar disorder has abruptly stopped taking prescribed medication. Which behavior would indicate the client has experienced a manic episode?
1. Binge eating
2. Relationship avoidance
3. Sudden relocation
4. Thoughtless spending

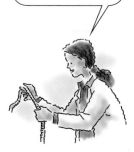

60. What nursing intervention would help the client with bipolar disorder to maintain adequate nutrition?
1. Determine the client's metabolic rate.
2. Instruct the client to sit down for each meal and snack.
3. Give the client foods to be eaten while active.
4. Allow the client to interact with a dietitian twice a week.

61. A nurse is providing education to a client being discharged on lithium. What should the nurse be sure to have the client report?
1. Black tongue
2. Increased lacrimation
3. Periods of disorientation
4. Persistent gastrointestinal (GI) upset

62. Which activity should the nurse encourage for a client with a diagnosis of bipolar disorder in the manic phase?
1. Playing a card game
2. Playing a vigorous basketball game
3. Playing a board game
4. Painting

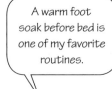

63. A client with bipolar disorder is having difficulty sleeping. Which behavior modification technique should the nurse reinforce with the client?
1. Use a sleep medication.
2. Work on solving a problem.
3. Exercise before bedtime.
4. Develop a sleep ritual.

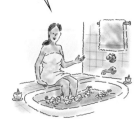

58. 4. Headache, agitation, and indigestion are symptoms that suggest mania in a client with a history of bipolar disorder. These symptoms aren't suggestive of depression, cyclothymia, or hypomania.
CN: Physiological integrity; CNS: Physiological adaptation;
CL: Analyze; DIFFICULTY: Moderate

59. 4. Thoughtless or reckless spending is a common symptom of a manic episode. Binge eating isn't a behavior that's characteristic of a client during a manic episode. Relationship avoidance doesn't occur in a client experiencing a manic episode. During episodes of mania, a client may, in fact, interact with many people and participate in unsafe sexual behavior. Sudden relocation isn't a characteristic of impulsive behavior demonstrated by a client with bipolar disorder.
CN: Psychosocial integrity; CNS: None; CL: Apply;
DIFFICULTY: Moderate

60. 3. By giving the client high-calorie foods that can be eaten while active, the nurse facilitates the client's nutritional intake. Determining the client's metabolic rate isn't useful information when the client is experiencing mania. During a manic episode, the client can't be still or focused long enough to interact with a dietitian or sit still long enough to eat.
CN: Psychosocial integrity; CNS: None; CL: Understand;
DIFFICULTY: Moderate

61. 4. Persistent GI upset indicates a mild-to-moderate toxic reaction. Black tongue is an adverse reaction of mirtazapine, not lithium. Increased lacrimation isn't an adverse effect of lithium. Periods of disorientation don't tend to occur with the use of lithium.
CN: Physiological integrity; CNS: Pharmacological therapies;
CL: Apply; DIFFICULTY: Challenge

62. 4. An activity that promotes minimal stimulation, such as painting, is the best choice. Activities such as cards, basketball, or a board game may escalate hyperactivity and should be avoided.
CN: Psychosocial integrity; CNS: None; CL: Apply; DIFFICULTY:
Moderate

63. 4. A sleep ritual or nighttime routine helps the client to relax and prepare for sleep. Obtaining sleep medication is a temporary solution. Working on problem solving may excite the client rather than tire him. Exercise before retiring is stimulating and not conducive to sleep.
CN: Physiological integrity; CNS: Reduction of risk potential;
CL: Apply; DIFFICULTY: Easy

64. Which explanation should the nurse give to a client newly diagnosed with bipolar disorder who doesn't understand why frequent blood work is necessary while taking lithium?
 1. Frequent measurement of lithium levels helps the health care provider to spot liver and renal damage early.
 2. Frequent measurement of lithium levels demonstrates whether the client is taking a high enough dosage.
 3. Frequent measurement of lithium levels indicates whether the drug passes through the blood-brain barrier.
 4. Frequent measurement of lithium levels is unnecessary if the client takes the drug as ordered.

65. The nurse is reinforcing education for a client with bipolar disorder. Which statement by the client indicates that the nurse's education on coping strategies was effective?
 1. "I can decide what to do to prevent family conflict."
 2. "I can handle problems without asking for any help."
 3. "I can stay away from my friends when I feel distressed."
 4. "I can ignore things that go wrong instead of getting upset."

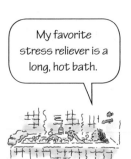

My favorite stress reliever is a long, hot bath.

66. The client is prescribed alprazolam 0.5 mg orally three times a day for panic disorder. The nurse has 0.25 mg tablets available. How many tablets will the nurse administer per dose? Record your answer using a whole number.

_____ tablets

67. The nurse obtains data from a client who reports insomnia, fatigue, and depression every day. "It has been like this since I was a child," said the client. Which behaviors demonstrated by the client would indicate to the nurse that the client has dysthymic disorder?
 1. Insomnia for several years—more days having problems sleeping than not having problems sleeping
 2. The triad of insomnia, fatigue, and depression over several continuous years
 3. Depressed mood for at least 2 years—more days depressed than not depressed
 4. Episodes of depression over time with no evidence of suicidal ideation

64. 2. Measurement of lithium levels in the blood determines whether an effective dose of lithium is being given to maintain a therapeutic level of the drug. The drug is contraindicated for clients with renal, cardiac, or liver disease. Lithium levels aren't measured to determine if the drug passes through the blood-brain barrier. Taking the drug as ordered doesn't eliminate the need for blood work.
CN: Physiological integrity; CNS: Pharmacological therapies; CL: Understand; DIFFICULTY: Challenge

65. 1. The client should be focusing on strengths and abilities to prevent family conflict. Not asking for help is problematic and not a good coping strategy. Avoiding problems also isn't a good coping strategy. It's better to identify and handle problems as they arise. Ignoring situations that cause discomfort won't facilitate solutions or allow the client to demonstrate effective coping skills.
CN: Psychosocial integrity; CNS: None; CL: Analyze; DIFFICULTY: Moderate

66. 2.
The correct formula to calculate a drug dose is:

$$\frac{\text{Dose on hand}}{\text{Quantity on hand}} = \frac{\text{Dose desired}}{X}$$

For this situation, the nurse should calculate:

$$\frac{0.25\,\text{mg}}{1\,\text{tablet}} = \frac{0.5\,\text{mg}}{X}$$

$$X = 2\,\text{tablets}$$

CN: Physiological integrity; CNS: Pharmacological therapies; CL: Apply; DIFFICULTY: Easy

67. 3. To be diagnosed with a dysthymic disorder, a person must experience a depressed mood for at least 2 years. The individual feels depressed nearly all of the time. The depressed mood is experienced most of the day, for more days than not. A person with dysthymic disorder must also have at least two of the following symptoms: appetite disturbances, sleep disturbances, fatigue, low self-esteem, poor concentration or difficulty making decisions, and feelings of hopelessness.
CN: Psychosocial integrity; CNS: None; CL: Apply; DIFFICULTY: Challenge

68. Which short-term goal should the nurse focus on for a client who makes statements about not deserving things?
1. Identify distorted thoughts.
2. Describe self-care patterns.
3. Discuss family relationships.
4. Explore communications skills.

69. The nurse is obtaining data when the postpartum client comes for follow-up visits at 2, 4, and 6 weeks. When would be the **best** time for the client to have postpartum depression screenings?
1. Using the Edinburgh Postnatal Depression Scale during each of the three visits
2. Through general conversation and observation beginning 4 weeks after birth
3. Beginning 6 weeks after birth using the Beck Depression Inventory
4. By interviewing the father of the child during each of the three visits

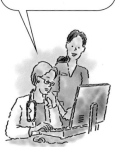

Frequent depression screenings in the postpartum period are key in detecting this disorder.

70. A client is diagnosed with postpartum depression. What does the nurse determine the outcome of this disorder to be?
1. It should self-correct without specific intervention.
2. It signals inadequate maternal instincts in the mother.
3. It may result in psychosis or infanticide.
4. It is a strong indicator of spousal abuse by the father of the child toward the new mother.

71. An adolescent who's depressed and reported by the parents as having difficulty in school is brought to the community mental health center to be evaluated. Which other health problem would the nurse suspect?
1. Anxiety disorder
2. Behavioral difficulties
3. Cognitive impairment
4. Labile moods

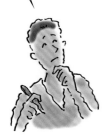

In other words, which statement by the client should cause the most concern?

72. The nurse is instructing a client about using the antianxiety medication lorazepam. Which statement by the client indicates a need for further education?
1. "I should get up slowly from a sitting or lying position."
2. "I shouldn't stop taking this medicine abruptly."
3. "I usually drink a beer every night to help me sleep."
4. "If I have a sore throat, I should report it to the health care provider."

68. 1. It's important to identify distorted thinking such as self-deprecating thoughts because they can lead to depression. Self-care patterns don't necessarily reflect distorted thinking. Family relationships might not influence distorted thinking patterns. A form of communication called negative self-talk would be explored only after distorted thinking patterns were identified.
CN: Psychosocial integrity; CNS: None; CL: Apply; DIFFICULTY: Easy

69. 1. The nurse midwife would best assess for postpartum depression using the Edinburgh Postnatal Depression Scale during each of the three visits. This scale is a commonly used short screening instrument that has been shown to perform well in detecting postpartum depression.
CN: Psychosocial integrity; CNS: None; CL: Analyze; DIFFICULTY: Moderate

70. 3. Undetected postpartum depression may lead to serious disturbances in mother-infant bonding, breastfeeding effectiveness, and family functioning. In rare circumstances postpartum depression may result in psychosis, infanticide, or both. Postpartum depression is a true form of depression that requires interventions. It does not indicate inadequate maternal instincts or spousal abuse.
CN: Psychosocial integrity; CNS: None; CL: Apply; DIFFICULTY: Moderate

71. 2. Adolescents tend to demonstrate severe irritability and behavioral problems rather than simply a depressed mood. Anxiety disorder is more commonly associated with small children rather than adolescents. Cognitive impairment is typically associated with delirium or dementia. Labile mood is more characteristic of a client with cognitive impairment or bipolar disorder.
CN: Psychosocial integrity; CNS: None; CL: Analyze; DIFFICULTY: Moderate

72. 3. The client shouldn't consume alcohol or any other central nervous system depressant while taking this drug. All of the other statements indicate that the client understands the nurse's instructions.
CN: Physiological integrity; CNS: Pharmacological therapies; CL: Apply; DIFFICULTY: Easy

73. A nurse is reinforcing education for the parents of a teenage client about the warning signs of potential adolescent suicide. Which signs should the nurse be sure to include?
1. Withdrawal
2. Reclaiming of possessions and gifts previously bestowed upon friends and loved ones
3. Statements such as not being around much longer
4. Increased interest in personal appearance and hygiene

73. 3. The warning signs of potential adolescent suicide include statements such as not being around much longer, restlessness, pacing, poor impulse control, making arrangements for putting personal affairs in order, and giving away personal possessions, especially treasured items.
CN: Psychosocial integrity; CNS: None; CL: Analyze;
DIFFICULTY: Moderate

74. A client has been receiving treatment for depression for 3 weeks. Which behavior suggests that the client's treatment is having a positive effect?
1. Talking about the difficulties of returning to college after discharge
2. Spending most of the day sitting alone in the corner of the room
3. Wearing a hospital gown instead of street clothes
4. Showing no emotion when visitors leave

74. 1. By talking about returning to college, the client is demonstrating an interest in making plans for the future, which is a sign of beginning recovery from depression. Decreased socialization, lack of interest in personal appearance, and lack of emotion are all symptoms of depression.
CN: Physiological integrity; CNS: Reduction of risk potential;
CL: Apply; DIFFICULTY: Easy

75. The nurse is reinforcing education for a client about nutrition and lithium medication. The nurse instructs the client that a lack of dietary salt intake can have which effect on lithium levels?
1. Decrease
2. Increase
3. Increase then decrease
4. No effect at all

75. 2. There's a direct relationship between the amount of salt and the plasma levels of lithium. Lithium plasma levels increase when there's a decrease in dietary salt. An increase in dietary salt causes the opposite effect of decreasing lithium plasma levels. It's important that the nurse monitors adequate dietary sodium.
CN: Physiological integrity; CNS: Pharmacological therapies;
CL: Apply; DIFFICULTY: Moderate

76. A client with bipolar disorder has been taking lithium, as prescribed, for the past 3 years. Today, family members brought this client to the hospital because the client hasn't slept, bathed, or changed clothes for 4 days; has lost 10 lb (4.5 kg) in the past month; and woke the entire family at 4 a.m. with plans to fly them to Hawaii for a vacation. What does the nurse suspect has occurred?
1. The family isn't supportive of the client.
2. The client has stopped taking the prescribed medication.
3. The client hasn't accepted the diagnosis of bipolar disorder.
4. The lithium level should be measured before the client receives the next lithium dose.

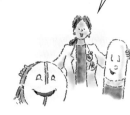

With any drug, it's all about finding the right level.

76. 4. Measuring the lithium level is the best way to evaluate the effectiveness of lithium therapy and begin to assess the client's current status. The client's unsupportive family, stopping the medication, and not accepting the diagnosis may all have contributed to the manic episode, but the nurse can't assume anything until after assessing the client and family more fully.
CN: Physiological Integrity; CNS: Reduction of risk potential;
CL: Apply; DIFFICULTY: Challenge

77. A client taking antidepressants for major depression for about 3 weeks is expressing feeling better. Which complication should the client now be monitored for?
1. Manic depression
2. Potential for violence
3. Substance abuse
4. Suicidal ideation

77. 4. After a client has been on antidepressants and is feeling better, he commonly then has the energy for self-harm. Manic depression isn't treated with antidepressants. Nothing in the client's history suggests a potential for violence. There are no signs or symptoms suggesting substance abuse.
CN: Psychosocial integrity; CNS: None; CL: Analyze;
DIFFICULTY: Easy

78. The nurse is caring for a client with paranoid personality disorder. Which therapeutic approach would have the **best** outcome?
1. Use a strict tone of voice to enforce limit setting.
2. Avoid giving the client any choices.
3. Employ a teaching manner to provide information.
4. Maintain a nonemotional and matter-of-fact manner.

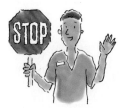

Check out that word "best" in question #78. It's kind of important.

78. 4. Maintaining a nonemotional, matter-of-fact manner with the client would be the most therapeutic approach when dealing with a client with paranoid personality disorder. The nurse should not attempt to talk to the client out of unfounded fears as this will merely lead to the client becoming more defensive. The nurse should provide feedback to the client's behaviors, as often the client does not realize how he comes across to others.
CN: Psychosocial integrity; CNS: None; CL: Apply; DIFFICULTY: Moderate

79. A client on the psychiatric unit is receiving lithium therapy and has a lithium level of 1 mEq/L. The nurse notes that the client has fine tremors of the hands. What is the **priority** action by the nurse?
1. Withhold the client's next lithium dose.
2. Notify the health care provider immediately.
3. Repeat the lithium level measurement.
4. Realize that a fine tremor is expected.

79. 4. Fine tremors of the hands are considered normal with lithium therapy. The lithium level is within normal limits so there's no need to withhold a dose, notify the health care provider, or repeat the blood work.
CN: Psychosocial integrity; CNS: None; CL: Apply; DIFFICULTY: Challenge

80. A rape victim is being prepared for discharge. The nurse is aware that the client is at risk for posttraumatic stress disorder (PTSD) and instructs the client that it's important that she report which symptoms associated with PTSD? Select all that apply.
1. Recurrent, intrusive recollections or nightmares
2. Gingival and dental problems
3. Sleep disturbances
4. Flight of ideas
5. Unusual talkativeness
6. Difficulty concentrating

80. 1, 3, 6. Clients diagnosed with PTSD typically experience recurrent, intrusive recollections or nightmares, sleep disturbances, difficulty concentrating, chronic anxiety or panic attacks, memory impairment, and feelings of detachment or estrangement that destroy interpersonal relationships. Gingival and dental problems are associated with bulimia. Flight of ideas and unusual talkativeness are characteristic of the acute manic phase of bipolar affective disorder.
CN: Psychosocial integrity; CNS: None; CL: Apply; DIFFICULTY: Difficult

81. The nurse is caring for a client that reports feeling very "stressed." When obtaining data from this client, which physiologic correlating manifestations does the nurse document? Select all that apply.
1. Irritability
2. Nausea
3. Increased breathing
4. Confusion
5. Insomnia
6. Headache

81. 2, 3, 6. Nausea, increased breathing, and headache are physiologic signs and symptoms of stress. Insomnia is a behavioral sign and symptom of stress, confusion is a cognitive sign and symptom of stress, and irritability is a psychological sign and symptom of stress.
CN: Psychosocial integrity; CNS: None; CL: Analyze; DIFFICULTY: Challenge

82. A client arrives to the health care clinic and informs the nurse they have been doubling the daily dose of bupropion to get better faster. For which complication should the nurse closely monitor the client?
1. Orthostatic hypotension
2. Weight gain
3. Seizure activity
4. Insomnia

82. 3. Bupropion is an atypical antidepressant and does not cause orthostatic hypotension. However, seizure activity is common is dosages greater than 450 mg daily. It frequently causes weight loss. Insomnia is a side effect, but seizure activity causes a greater client risk.
CN: Physiological Integrity; CNS: None; CL: Apply; DIFFICULTY: Challenge

83. The nurse interviews the family of a client who's hospitalized with severe depression and suicidal ideation. Which information about the family is essential for the nurse to obtain so as to assist in formulating an effective care plan? Select all that apply.
1. Physical pain
2. Personal responsibilities
3. Employment skills
4. Communication patterns
5. Role expectations
6. Current family stressors

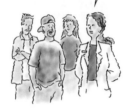

Family members can be a valuable source of information about a client with depression.

83. 4, 5, 6. When working with the family of a depressed client, it's helpful for the nurse to be aware of the family's communication style, the role expectations for its members, and current family stressors. This information can help identify family difficulties and teaching points that could benefit the client and the family. Information concerning physical pain, personal responsibilities, and employment skills isn't directly related to the experience of having a depressed family member.
CN: Psychosocial integrity; CNS: None; CL: Analyze;
DIFFICULTY: Challenge

84. A nurse is assisting with discharge instructions for a client who is prescribed sertraline. The nurse should monitor the client for which adverse drug effects? Select all that apply.
1. Agitation
2. Agranulocytosis
3. Sleep disturbance
4. Intermittent tachycardia
5. Dry mouth
6. Seizure

84. 1, 3, 5. Common adverse effects of sertraline include agitation, sleep disturbance, and dry mouth. Agranulocytosis, intermittent tachycardia, and seizures are adverse effects of clozapine.
CN: Physiological integrity; CNS: Pharmacological therapies;
CL: Apply; DIFFICULTY: Difficult

85. The health care provider orders olanzapine 15 mg orally once per day for bipolar mania. Available is olanzapine 7.5 mg. How many tablets will the nurse administer? Record your answer using a whole number.

_____ tablets

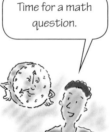

Time for a math question.

85. 2.
The correct formula to calculate a drug dose is:

$$\frac{\text{Dose on hand}}{\text{Quantity on hand}} = \frac{\text{Dose desired}}{X}$$

For this situation, the nurse should calculate:

$$\frac{15 \text{ mg}}{1 \text{ tablet}} = \frac{7.5 \text{ mg}}{X}$$

$$X = 2 \text{ tablets}$$

CN: Physiological integrity; CNS: Pharmacological therapies;
CL: Apply; DIFFICULTY: Easy

86. When a nurse is assisting with the development of a no-suicide contract with a client, what should be considered?
1. To increase client accountability, ask the client to promise the nurse or significant friend or family member to avoid self-harm.
2. Communicate belief in the client and establish a minimum time frame of at least 1 week for the first contract.
3. Make the agreement official and binding, have the document typed, signed by the client, and notarized.
4. Include a detailed plan of action with the names and phone numbers of persons to call and the number of the local suicide crisis hotline to call if experiencing suicidal thoughts.

86. 4. A no-suicide contract should include a promise that no harm will be self-inflicted, to maintain the contract no matter what happens, and to talk to someone if thoughts of suicide return. In addition there should be a detailed plan of action with the names and phone numbers of persons to call and the number of the local suicide crisis hotline to call if experiencing suicidal thoughts.
CN: Psychosocial integrity; CNS: None; CL: Analyze;
DIFFICULTY: Moderate

87. An adolescent client is diagnosed with attention deficit hyperactivity disorder (ADHD). What statement made by the client demonstrates an understanding of the disorder?
1. "I must have it because I was neglected as a young child."
2. "I will outgrow it."
3. "It increases sensitivity to the environment and surroundings."
4. "You can tell I have it because I don't always pay attention."

88. A client insists that the nurse place four sheets of newspaper beneath the nursing bag and that all supplies be returned to their original place after being counted three times. This behavior would **most** likely suggest which disorder?
1. Bipolar disorder
2. Depression
3. Schizophrenia
4. Obsessive-compulsive disorder

89. A client informs the nurse that last week he felt sad, had no appetite, and didn't want to go out, but this week felt better because their child asked to come to dinner. What does this behavior indicate to the nurse?
1. Normal fluctuation
2. Part of clinical depression
3. Predisposition to psychotic depression
4. Precursor to bipolar disorder

90. A student nurse is preparing to administer an injection to a client. The instructor asked the student questions related to the administration of the injection. The student did not hear the questions, muscles became tense, and hands sweaty. The student nurse may be experiencing which level of anxiety?
1. Mild
2. Moderate
3. Severe
4. Panic

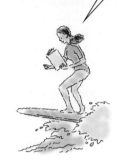

Some people think I'm obsessive-compulsive about studying.

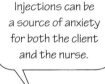

Injections can be a source of anxiety for both the client and the nurse.

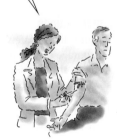

87. 3. Individuals with ADHD are extremely sensitive to their environment and surroundings and respond immediately to any type of stimuli or distraction that most individuals would not even notice. Neglect is not a cause of this disorder. Clients may go undiagnosed for many years and may continue into adulthood. Not paying attention is not the only indication that the client has ADHD.
CN: Psychosocial integrity; CNS: None; CL: Apply;
DIFFICULTY: Challenge

88. 4. The client's insistence indicates a compulsive behavior (which may include repetitive touching or counting, doing and undoing small tasks, or any other repetitive behavior).
CN: Psychosocial integrity; CNS: None; CL: Apply;
DIFFICULTY: Easy

89. 1. Feelings of sadness are normal for most individuals at some time. Losses and stresses far less profound than death can make an individual sad, but the feelings are usually fleeting, lasting a few hours to a few days. Even though the client felt fatigue, felt sadness, and did not eat, the mood changed when the child invited the client to dinner. This behavior does not indicate psychotic behavior, clinical depression, or bipolar disorder.
CN: Psychosocial integrity; CNS: None; CL: Analyze;
DIFFICULTY: Difficult

90. 2. Experiencing moderate anxiety is demonstrated by selective inattention. Perceptual field has narrowed, causing the inability to focus on what the instructor is saying.
CN: Psychosocial integrity; CNS: None; CL: Analyze;
DIFFICULTY: Moderate

Chapter 14

Cognitive Disorders

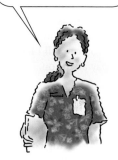

This chapter covers a host of cognitive disorders. Are your own cognitive powers ready? OK, let's go!

Cognitive disorders refresher

Alzheimer disease

Progressive, non-curable disorder characterized by memory loss, decline of cognitive function and eventual loss of motor skills

Key signs and symptoms

Stage 1 (mild symptoms)
- Confusion and short-term memory loss
- Disorientation to time and place
- Difficulty performing routine tasks
- Changes in personality and judgment

Stage 2 (moderate symptoms)
- Anxiety
- Obvious memory loss
- Suspicion
- Agitation
- Wandering
- Difficulty recognizing family members

Stage 3 (moderate to severe symptoms)
- Increasing loss of expressive language skills
- Loss of reasoning ability
- Loss of ability to perform activities of daily living

Stage 4 (severe symptoms)
- Absent cognitive abilities
- Disorientation to time and place
- Impaired or absent motor skills
- Bowel and bladder incontinence

Key test results
- Cognitive assessment scale demonstrates cognitive impairment
- Functional dementia scale shows the degree of the dementia
- Magnetic resonance imaging (MRI) shows apparent structural and neurologic changes
- The Mini-Mental State Examination reveals disorientation and cognitive impairment

Key treatments
- Group therapy
- Anticholinesterase agents: donepezil, rivastigmine, galantamine
- N-methyl-D-aspartate receptor: memantine

Key interventions
- Remove hazardous items or potential obstacles from client's environment
- Communicate verbally and nonverbally with the client in a consistent, structured way
- Increase client's social interaction
- Encourage the use of community resources

Amnesic disorder

Group of disorders characterized by impairments in memory in the absence of other cognitive dysfunction

Key signs and symptoms
- Confusion, disorientation, and lack of insight
- Inability to learn and retain new information
- Tendency to remember the remote past better than more recent events

Key test results
- The Mini-Mental State Examination shows:
  - client is disoriented
  - client has difficulty recalling events and information

Key treatments
- Correction of the underlying medical cause
- Group therapy
- Family therapy

Key interventions
- Ensure client's safety
- Encourage exploration of feelings
- Provide simple, clear medical information

Delirium

Presents with a loss of mental clarity; may be associated with physical or psychological causative factors

Key signs and symptoms
- Altered psychomotor activity (e.g., apathy, withdrawal, agitation)

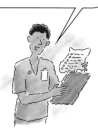

What are the key signs and symptoms of Stage 3 Alzheimer-type dementia?

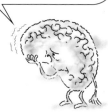

"Where did I leave my keys?" Persistent memory loss can be an indicator of cognitive disorder.

- Bizarre, destructive behavior that's worse at night
- Disorganized thinking
- Distractibility
- Impaired decision making
- Inability to complete tasks
- Insomnia or daytime sleepiness
- Poor impulse control
- Rambling, bizarre, or incoherent speech

Key test results
- Laboratory results indicate that the delirium is a result of :
  - physiologic condition
  - intoxication
  - substance withdrawal
  - toxic exposure
  - prescribed medicines
  - combination of these factors
- The Mini-Mental Status Examination shows that the client has difficulty with:
  - attention
  - cognition
  - awareness

Key treatments
- Correction of the underlying physiologic problem
- Antipsychotic agent: risperidone

Key interventions
- Minimize excessive sensory stimuli
- Create a structured, safe, and supportive environment
- Keep a light on in client's room

Vascular dementia
Loss of cognitive function associated with a reduction in blood perfusion to the brain

Key signs and symptoms
- Depression
- Difficulty following instructions
- Emotional lability
- Inappropriate emotional reactions
- Memory loss
- Wandering and getting lost in familiar places

Key test results
- Cognitive assessment scale shows a deterioration in cognitive ability
- Global Deterioration Scale signifies degenerative dementia
- The Mini-Mental Status Examination reveals that the client is:
  - disoriented
  - has difficulty recalling information

Key treatments
- Carotid endarterectomy to remove blockages in the carotid artery
- Treatment of the underlying condition (hypertension, high cholesterol, or diabetes)
- Antiplatelet aggregate drugs: aspirin, ticlopidine

Key interventions
- Orient client to surroundings
- Monitor client's environment
- Encourage client to express feelings of sadness and loss

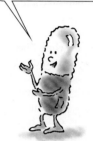

I'm an antipsychotic agent that is used to treat delirium. Do you know my name?

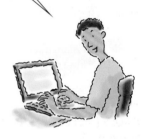

Can you remember what the key signs and symptoms of vascular dementia are?

thePoint® You can download tables of drug information to help you prepare for the NCLEX®! View Generic Drug Names, Drug Classifications, Drug Actions, and Nursing Implications for the drugs discussed in this refresher at **http://thePoint.lww.com**.

Cognitive disorders questions, answers, and rationales

1. A client is being seen for a routine physical exam. When asked about any concerns, the client reports her parent has been diagnosed with dementia and the client fears "getting it" when getting older. Which response by the nurse is **most** appropriate?
  1. "Dementia is a concern for all of us as we age."
  2. "Since there are not known familial factors you have no reason for alarm."
  3. "Although getting older and a family history elevate your risk there is no guarantee that you will develop dementia."
  4. "Your worries should be limited because most dementia occurs because of a history of head injury."

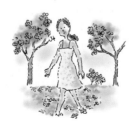

Take a deep breath and stretch your legs. You'll be done with this test before you know it.

1. 3. Dementia has risk factors, which include a family history and aging. Although aging is a risk factor this is not the best response by the nurse. This response does not address the concerns being voiced by the client. While family history is a risk factor it does not mean it will be "passed down" to the client. Dementia is not linked to a single incidence of head injury. If the trauma is severe, the client is diagnosed with traumatic brain injury, not dementia.

CN: Health Promotion and Maintenance; CNS: None; CL: Apply; DIFFICULTY: Easy

CN: Client needs category   CNS: Client needs subcategory   CL: Cognitive level

2. A client has been prescribed donepezil. Which statements by the client and family indicate an understanding of the medication? Select all that apply.
1. "This medication will halt the progression of Alzheimer's disease."
2. "It will take a few weeks for this medication to begin improving my condition."
3. "Some nausea and vomiting may be experienced when I begin this medication."
4. "If the medication impacts my ability to rest at night I can confer with my health care provider about changing the timing of my doses."
5. "This medication will likely only work for about a year before I will need to change to another medication."

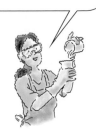

Hard work and a positive attitude are the perfect formula for success. Now let's get down to business.

2. 2, 3, 4. Donepezil is prescribed for Alzheimer's disease (AD). The medication is used to reduce confusion and may also aid in improved memory by the client. The medication does not halt the progression or cure Alzheimer's disease. The medication will take a few weeks to begin to work. Some gastrointestinal symptoms may be noted. These symptoms will gradually subside. The medication is normally prescribed to be taken at bedtime. If this impacts the ability to obtain rest the client may confer with the prescriber to review the timing of dosages. This medication will be effective for individualized periods of time.
CN: Physiological integrity; CNS: Pharmacological therapies; CL: Analyze; DIFFICULTY: Moderate

3. A health care provider is discussing a recent diagnosis of Alzheimer disease (AD) with a client and immediate family. Which statements by the family to the nurse concerning the condition indicate the need for further instruction? Select all that apply.
1. "Alzheimer disease is commonly caused by cerebral abscesses."
2. "Chronic alcohol abuse plays a significant role in the development of Alzheimer disease."
3. "Multiple small brain infarctions typically lead to Alzheimer disease."
4. "The cause of Alzheimer disease is currently unknown."
5. "Not all causes of memory losses and dementia are the result of Alzheimer disease."

3. 1, 2, 3. Several hypotheses suggest genetic factors, trauma, accumulation of aluminum, alterations in the immune system, or alterations in acetylcholine as contributing to the development of Alzheimer disease, but the exact cause is unknown. Chronic alcohol abuse hasn't been associated with the development of Alzheimer disease, nor has the presence of cerebral abscess or small brain infarction. Alzheimer disease is not the lone cause of dementia or memory loss.
CN: Health promotion and maintenance; CNS: None; CL: Apply; DIFFICULTY: Difficult

4. A client exhibits signs of recent dementia. Which condition that can cause a dementia similar to Alzheimer disease (AD) is reversible?
1. Multiple sclerosis
2. Electrolyte imbalance
3. Multiple small brain infarctions
4. Human immunodeficiency virus (HIV) infection

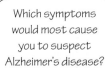

Which symptoms would most cause you to suspect Alzheimer's disease?

4. 2. Electrolyte imbalance is a correctable metabolic abnormality that may present with dementia type symptomology. Multiple sclerosis presents with neuromuscular changes, not dementia. Small brain infarctions do not present with dementia-like symptoms. HIV does not present with dementia.
CN: Physiological integrity; CNS: Physiological adaptation; CL: Apply; DIFFICULTY: Easy

5. A client is suspected of experiencing early stage Alzheimer disease (AD). Which symptoms does the nurse document that correlate with this suspicion? Select all that apply.
1. Dilated pupils
2. Rambling speech
3. Elevated blood pressure
4. Significant recent memory impairment
5. Experiencing difficulty grocery shopping.

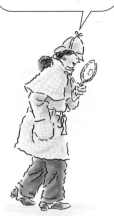

5. 4, 5. Significant recent memory impairment, indicated by the inability to verbalize remembrances after several minutes to an hour, can be assessed in the early stages of AD. Dilated pupils, elevated blood pressure, and rambling speech are expected symptoms of delirium. During the early stages of Alzheimer disease there is increasing difficulty performing simple tasks such as shopping or dressing.
CN: Physiological integrity; CNS: Physiological adaptation; CL: Apply; DIFFICULTY: Challenge

6. A nurse is caring for a client with delirium. Which nursing intervention is **priority**?
1. Providing a safe environment
2. Offering recreational activities
3. Providing a structured environment
4. Instituting measures to promote sleep

6. 1. The nurse's priority when caring for a client with delirium is to ensure client safety. Offering recreational activities, providing a structured environment, and promoting sleep are all appropriate interventions after safety measures are in place.
CN: Safe, effective care environment; CNS: Coordinated care; CL: Analyze; DIFFICULTY: Easy

7. Which data obtained by the nurse demonstrates that a client is exhibiting impairment in abstract thinking and reasoning? Select all that apply.
1. The client can't repeat a sentence.
2. The client has difficulty calculating simple problems.
3. The client doesn't know the name of the president of the United States.
4. The client can't find similarities between a group of geometric shapes.
5. When shown a grouping of words the client cannot determine which word does not belong.

7. **4, 5.** Abstract thinking is assessed by noting similarities and differences between related words or objects. Not being able to do a simple calculation or repeat a sentence shows a client's inability to concentrate and focus on thoughts. Not knowing the name of the president of the United States is a deficiency in general knowledge.
CN: Psychosocial integrity; CNS: None; CL: Analyze;
DIFFICULTY: Difficult

8. A Mini-Mental State Examination has been scheduled for a client who has been experiencing episodes of memory impairment. What information can be provided to the client and family about this test? Select all that apply.
1. The level of a client's education can impact overall scoring.
2. The test results will decline as a normal part of aging.
3. Lower scores are associated with dementia.
4. The test will be completed over several appointments with the clinician.
5. The test is used to diagnose Alzheimer disease.

8. **1, 3.** The Mini-Mental State Examination is used to assess cognition. Areas assessed include global cognition, orientation, and visuospatial ability. The assessment does not provide a definitive diagnosis but is a tool in the process. Clients with higher levels of education may score higher on the test. Test results do not decline with aging. The test is able to be completed in a short period of time and does not take multiple appointments. Lower scores are consistent with cognitive impairment.
CN: Health Promotion and Maintenance; CNS: None; CL: Analyze;
DIFFICULTY: Difficult

9. When assisting the team with planning care for the client with Alzheimer disease, what is the **priority**?
1. Provide a list of activities that the client will be expected to complete for the period of care.
2. Assist the client to establish routines.
3. Encourage placement of pictures of family and friends in the care environment.
4. Review safeguards that will limit wandering by the client.

9. **4.** Each of the activities listed would be beneficial to the client with Alzheimer disease. Protection of the client is the priority.
CN: Safe, effective care environment; CNS: Safety and infection control; CL: Apply; DIFFICULTY: Moderate

10. Which nursing interventions would help a client diagnosed with Alzheimer disease (AD) perform activities of daily living?
1. Urge the client to perform all basic care without help.
2. Tell the client that morning care must be done by 9 a.m.
3. Give the client a written list of activities he's expected to do.
4. Provide ample time for the client to complete basic tasks.

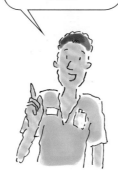

Don't rush clients with Alzheimer's disease. They just take a little longer to complete common tasks.

10. **4.** Clients with AD respond to the affect of those around them. A gentle, calm approach is comforting and nonthreatening, while a tense, hurried approach may agitate the client. The client has problems performing independently; expecting the client to perform self-care independently may lead to frustration.
CN: Physiological integrity; CNS: Basic care and comfort; CL: Apply; DIFFICULTY: Easy

11. The nurse is caring for a client with Alzheimer disease. Which medication does the nurse prepare to administer that will improve cognition and functional autonomy?
1. Bupropion
2. Haloperidol
3. Donepezil
4. Triazolam

11. **3.** Donepezil is used to improve cognition and functional autonomy in mild to moderate dementia of the Alzheimer type. Bupropion is used for depression. Haloperidol is used for agitation, aggression, hallucinations, thought disturbances, and wandering. Triazolam is used for sleep disturbances.
CN: Physiological integrity; CNS: Pharmacological therapies; CL: Apply; DIFFICULTY: Moderate

12. A nurse places an object in the hand of a client with Alzheimer disease (AD) and asks the client to identify the object. Which term represents the client's inability to name the object?
1. Agnosia
2. Aphasia
3. Apraxia
4. Perseveration

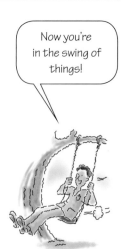

Now you're in the swing of things!

13. Which nursing intervention will help a client with progressive memory deficit function in the environment?
1. Help the client do simple tasks by giving step-by-step directions.
2. Avoid frustrating the client by performing basic care routines for the client.
3. Stimulate the client's intellectual functioning by bringing new topics to the client's attention.
4. Promote the use of the client's sense of humor by telling jokes or riddles and discussing cartoons.

14. When caring for a client diagnosed with Alzheimer's disease (AD), which nursing intervention is **priority**?
1. Avoid physical contact.
2. Apply wrist and ankle restraints.
3. Provide a high level of sensory stimulation.
4. Monitor the client carefully.

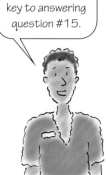

The word "priority" is the key to answering question #15.

15. Which nursing intervention is **priority** in caring for a client diagnosed with Alzheimer disease (AD)?
1. Make sure the environment is safe to prevent injury.
2. Make sure the client receives food they like to prevent hunger.
3. Make sure the client meets other clients to prevent social isolation.
4. Make sure the client takes care of daily physical care to prevent dependence.

16. The nurse is caring for a client with dementia who is agitated, violent, and having bizarre thoughts. Which medication does the nurse administer to the client to alleviate these symptoms?
1. Diazepam
2. Ergoloid
3. Haloperidol
4. Donepezil

12. 1. Agnosia is the inability to recognize familiar objects. Aphasia is characterized by an impaired ability to speak. Apraxia refers to the client's inability to use objects properly. All three impairments usually occur in stage 3 of AD. Perseveration is continued repetition of a meaningless word or phrase that occurs in stage 2 of Alzheimer disease.
CN: Health promotion and maintenance; CNS: None; CL: Apply; DIFFICULTY: Easy

13. 1. Clients with cognitive impairment should do all the tasks they can. By giving simple directions in a step-by-step fashion, the client can better process information and perform tasks. Clients with cognitive impairment may not be able to understand a joke or riddle, and cartoons may add to their confusion. Stimulation of intellect can be accomplished by discussing familiar topics with them; changes in topics may add to their confusion.
CN: Safe, effective care environment; CNS: Safety and infection Control; CL: Apply; DIFFICULTY: Easy

14. 4. Whenever client safety is at risk, careful observation and supervision are of ultimate importance in avoiding injury. Physical contact is implemented during basic care. Applying restraints may cause agitation and combativeness. A high level of sensory stimulation may be too stimulating and distracting.
CN: Safe, effective care environment; CNS: Coordinated care; CL: Apply; DIFFICULTY: Easy

15. 1. Providing for client safety is the number one priority when caring for any client, but particularly when a client is already compromised and at greater risk for injury. Promoting adequate nutrition, socialization, and self-care are important, but they are not the priority nursing interventions.
CN: Safe, effective care environment; CNS: Safety and infection control; CL: Apply; DIFFICULTY: Easy

16. 3. Haloperidol is an antipsychotic that decreases the symptoms of agitation, violence, and bizarre thoughts. Diazepam is used for anxiety and muscle relaxation. Ergoloid is an adrenergic blocker used to block vascular headaches. Donepezil is used for improvement of cognition.
CN: Physiological integrity; CNS: Reduction of risk potential; CL: Apply; DIFFICULTY: Moderate

17. A client diagnosed with Alzheimer disease (AD) tells the nurse that today they have a luncheon date with their child. The nurse knows that the child isn't visiting that day. Which response by the nurse would be **most** appropriate for this situation?
1. "Where are you planning to have your lunch?"
2. "You're confused and don't know what you're saying."
3. "I think you need some more medication, and I'll bring it to you."
4. "Today is Monday, March 8, and we'll be eating lunch in the dining room."

17. 4. The best nursing response is to reorient the client to the date and environment. Confrontation can provoke an outburst. Medication won't provide immediate relief for memory impairment.
CN: Psychosocial integrity; CNS: None; CL: Apply;
DIFFICULTY: Challenge

18. The nurse is caring for a client with a cognitive disorder. Which characteristic does the nurse determine correlates with a cognitive disorder?
1. Catatonia
2. Depression
3. Feeling of dread
4. Deficit in memory

18. 4. Cognitive disorders represent a significant change in cognition or memory from a previous level of functioning. Catatonia is a type of schizophrenia characterized by periods of physical rigidity, negativism, excitement, and stupor. Depression is a feeling of sadness and apathy and is part of major depressive and other mood disorders. A feeling of dread is characteristic of an anxiety disorder.
CN: Physiological integrity; CNS: Physiological adaptation;
CL: Apply; DIFFICULTY: Easy

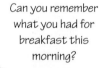

The word "degenerative" is key to answering question #19 correctly.

19. A nurse is obtaining data from an older adult client who is admitted with progressive deterioration in cognition. Which degenerative disorder does the nurse suspect the client is exhibiting?
1. Delirium
2. Dementia
3. Neurosis
4. Psychosis

19. 2. Dementia is progressive and commonly associated with aging or underlying metabolic or organic deterioration. Delirium is characterized by abrupt, spontaneous cognitive dysfunction with an underlying organic mental disorder. Neurosis and psychosis are psychological diagnoses.
CN: Physiological integrity; CNS: Physiological adaptation;
CL: Apply; DIFFICULTY: Easy

20. A nurse is assisting with the education for the family of a client with dementia. Which response by the nurse would be the **most** accurate definition of dementia?
1. Personal neglect in self-care
2. Poor judgment, especially in social situations
3. Memory loss occurring as a natural consequence of aging
4. Loss of intellectual abilities that impairs the ability to perform basic care

20. 4. The ability to perform self-care is an important measure of the progression of dementia. Personal neglect and poor judgment typically occur in dementia but aren't considered defining characteristics. Memory loss reflects underlying physical, metabolic, and pathologic processes.
CN: Physiological integrity; CNS: Physiological adaptation;
CL: Apply; DIFFICULTY: Moderate

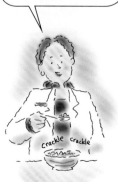

Can you remember what you had for breakfast this morning?

21. The nurse asks a client with a suspected dementia disorder to recall what was eaten for breakfast. What data is the nurse gathering from this client?
1. Food preferences
2. Recent memory
3. Remote memory
4. Speech capacity

21. 2. Persons with dementia have difficulty with recent memory or learning, which may be a key to early detection. Assessing food preferences may be helpful in determining what the client likes to eat, but this assessment has no direct correlation in assessing dementia. Speech difficulties, such as rambling, irrelevance, and incoherence, may be related to delirium.
CN: Health promotion and maintenance; CNS: None; CL: Apply;
DIFFICULTY: Easy

22. The nurse is collecting data for a client diagnosed with a dementia disorder. Which factor is **most** important for the nurse to determine when collecting data for this diagnosis?
1. Prognosis
2. Genetic information
3. Degree of impairment
4. Implications for treatment

22. 4. The progression of biological impairment in the central nervous system is a function of the underlying pathologic states, so it's important to collect data and treat the underlying cause. Prognosis isn't the most important factor when making a diagnosis. Genetic information isn't relevant. The degree of impairment is necessary information for developing a care plan.
CN: Health promotion and maintenance; CNS: None; CL: Analyze; DIFFICULTY: Challenge

23. The nurse is reviewing the client's medical record. The nurse notes that the health care provider has listed vascular dementia as a primary diagnosis. Which factors may be found in the medical record that are supportive of this diagnosis? Select all that apply.
1. History of diabetes with minimal compliance to the prescribed treatment regimen
2. History of hypotension
3. Obesity
4. History of mitral valve prolapse
5. History of addiction to opiates

23. 1, 3. Vascular dementia is an impairment in brain function that results from an alteration in perfusion to the organ. Risk factors for vascular edema include diabetes and obesity. Elevation in blood pressure, not hypotension, is a risk factor. Cardiovascular rhythm disorders, not mitral valve prolapse, are associated with this condition. The use or misuse of opiates is not associated with vascular dementia.
CN: Physiological integrity; CNS: Physiological adaptation; CL: Apply; DIFFICULTY: Difficult

24. A client has been prescribed donepezil. Which instruction should be included in the nurse's plans for administration?
1. Administer the medication in the morning upon awakening.
2. Administer the medication with milk.
3. Administer the medication in the evening.
4. Crush the medication and administer with pudding or applesauce.

24. 3. Donepezil is a medication used in the treatment of Alzheimer's disease. The medication should be administered in the evening close to bedtime. It is administered whole and with a glass of water.
CN: Physiological integrity; CNS: Pharmacological therapies; CL: Apply; DIFFICULTY: Challenge

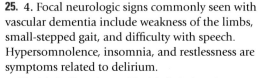
Once you answer question #25, you'll be one small step closer to finishing the test.

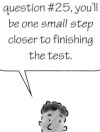

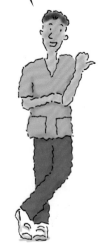

25. The nurse is gathering data for a client with vascular dementia. Which finding that correlates with this diagnosis does the nurse anticipate obtaining?
1. Hypersomnolence
2. Insomnia
3. Restlessness
4. Small-stepped gait

25. 4. Focal neurologic signs commonly seen with vascular dementia include weakness of the limbs, small-stepped gait, and difficulty with speech. Hypersomnolence, insomnia, and restlessness are symptoms related to delirium.
CN: Physiological integrity; CNS: Physiological adaptation; CL: Apply; DIFFICULTY: Difficult

26. The spouse of a client diagnosed with vascular dementia asks the nurse if this is the same as having Alzheimer disease. Which response by the nurse is **most** appropriate?
1. "Vascular dementia is another term for Alzheimer disease."
2. "There are similarities in the conditions but they are not the same condition."
3. "Vascular dementia is much more severe than Alzheimer disease."
4. "No, they are not the same condition as Alzheimer disease can be treated more successfully."

26. 2. Vascular dementia differs from AD in that it has a more abrupt onset and runs a highly variable course. Both conditions are characterized by losses in cognitive function. Both are severe conditions. Although treatments are available, neither condition can be cured nor can the damages be reversed.
CN: Physiological integrity; CNS: Physiological adaptation; CL: Apply; DIFFICULTY: Easy

27. A client is brought to the emergency department by the spouse, who reports the client has become increasingly confused over a period of 3 to 4 days. When questioned, the spouse reports there has never been a history of confusion before. Which initial question by the nurse is **most** appropriate?
1. "Is there a family history of dementia-related conditions?"
2. "What medications and supplements are being taken?"
3. "Is your spouse sleeping well?"
4. "Have there been any recent stressors at home?"

28. Memantine has been prescribed to a client. When discussing the planned therapy with the client's spouse, which statements indicate understanding of actions that can be used to prevent problems related to side effects of the medication? Select all that apply.
1. "I plan to add fiber-rich snacks to the daily menu."
2. "I may need to help my spouse get up."
3. "This medication will need to be administered with milk."
4. "Monitoring my spouse's weight will be necessary."
5. "Maintaining a routine with regard to sleep and nap periods will be important."

29. The nurse is preparing to administer ticlopidine to a client hospitalized with vascular dementia. The client questions the nurse about how this medication will help his condition. Which information should be included in the nurse's response? Select all that apply.
1. "This medication will promote the blood flow to your brain."
2. "This medication will reduce the blockages caused by a group of blood cells called platelets."
3. "Enzymes that are responsible for impulse controls in your brain will be increased by this medication."
4. "Plaques that are responsible for the confusion you are feeling will be lessened by this medication."
5. "Transmitters of impulses in your brain will be made more effective by this medication."

30. Memantine has been prescribed to a client to manage the symptoms associated with Alzheimer's disease. Which side effects if reported are consistent with overdose? Select all that apply.
1. Weakness
2. Bradycardia
3. Dizziness
4. Hallucinations
5. Tachycardia

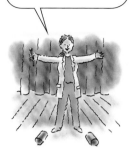

You really perform well under pressure. Bravo!

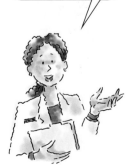

In question #30, keep in mind that "bradycardia" and "tachycardia" are opposites, so only one can be correct. Which is it?

27. 2. Delirium refers to a rapid onset of a loss of cognitive abilities. There are a variety of potential causative factors. Obtaining a history is the most important action. Many cases of delirium can be attributed to medication therapies. Rest and sleep can play a factor, but not with delirium of a period of nearly a week. Stress at home may intensify conditions but is not the underlying cause. Dementia and delirium are not the same condition so this question has no bearing on the determination of causes.
CN: Physiological Integrity; CNS: Physiological adaptation; CL: Apply; DIFFICULTY: Easy

28. 1, 2, 4, 5. Memantine is a medication used in the treatment of Alzheimer disease. The medication may result in constipation. Fiber-rich snacks will be helpful in preventing this side effect. The medication is associated with dizziness. Assistance with position changes will be beneficial in preventing falls. Weight gain is a side effect of the medication, so it's important to monitor weight. Sleeplessness may result, making so it's important to maintain organized sleep periods. There is no need to administer this medication with milk.
CN: Physiological integrity; CNS: Pharmacological therapies; CL: Evaluation; DIFFICULTY: Difficult

29. 1, 2. Ticlopidine is used to reduce platelet aggregation. This will promote increased perfusion to the brain. Enzymes and neurotransmitters are not impacted by ticlopidine. Plaques that are associated with Alzheimer disease are not impacted by this medication.
CN: Physiological Integrity; CNS: Pharmacological Therapies; CL: Analyze; DIFFICULTY: Difficult

30. 1, 2, 3, 4. Memantine is used in the treatment of Alzheimer's disease. The medication will typically be initiated and then increases in dosages will be made as needed. Manifestations associated with overdose include slowed movements, weakness, bradycardia, dizziness, and hallucinations. Tachycardia is not associated with an overdosage of this medication.
CN: Physiological integrity; CNS: Pharmacological therapies; CL: Apply; DIFFICULTY: Difficult

31. The nurse is caring for a client with a cognitive disorder. Which nursing action is **priority**?
1. Promote socialization.
2. Maintain optimal physical health.
3. Provide frequent changes in personnel.
4. Provide an overstimulating environment.

31. 2. A client's cognitive impairment may hinder self-care abilities. More socialization, frequent changes in staff members, and an overstimulating environment would only increase anxiety and confusion.
CN: Health promotion and maintenance; CNS: None; CL: Apply; DIFFICULTY: Challenge

32. During a routine physical exam the client reports concerns about getting older and losing cognitive abilities. Which response by the nurse is **most** appropriate?
1. "Aging does increase the risk for these changes in ability but they are not an absolute."
2. "Age has no bearing on mental function."
3. "There is nothing that can be done about this concern."
4. "It is unwise to worry about these changes before they occur."

32. 1. Aging is a risk factor for the loss of cognitive function and related disease processes. Not all older adults will experience delirium or dementia-related conditions. So the risk, while present, is not absolute. There are recommended steps an individual can take to reduce losses in cognitive function. These include activities that challenge the mind and promote memory. Concern for and prevention of health problems is wise for all individuals.
CN: Health promotion and maintenance; CNS: none; CL: Apply; DIFFICULTY: Easy

33. The nurse is assigned to care for a client with amnesia. When preparing to deliver care, which action will **best** meet the needs of this client?
1. Provide the client with lots of space to test independence.
2. Promote activities to keep the client busy on the care unit with group meetings, and assist client with tasks as able.
3. Use short, simple commands when providing instruction.
4. Spend time with the client, asking questions about recent life.

33. 3. Disruptions in the ability to perform basic care, along with confusion and anxiety, are commonly apparent in clients with amnesia. Offering simple directions to promote daily functions and reduce confusion helps increase feelings of safety and security. Giving this client lots of space may cause feelings of insecurity. There's no significant rationale for keeping the client busy all day with no rest periods; the client may become more tired and less functional at other basic tasks. Asking many questions that the client won't be able to answer would just intensify her anxiety level.
CN: Safe, effective care environment; CNS: Coordinated care; CL: Apply; DIFFICULTY: Moderate

34. A client has been diagnosed with an amnesic disorder. Which changes should the nurse anticipate with this condition? Select all that apply.
1. Speech patterns will be impaired or slurred.
2. The client will be easily distracted from the task at hand.
3. The client's ability to complete word games will be diminished.
4. The client will have an inability to recall recent activities from earlier in the day.
5. The client will display lapses of memory from periods of time in the past.

34. 4, 5. The primary area affected in amnesia is memory. This includes both short term and long term memory. Other areas of cognition are not impacted.
CN: Physiological integrity; CNS: Physiological adaptation; CL: Apply; DIFFICULTY: Difficult

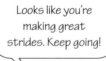

Looks like you're making great strides. Keep going!

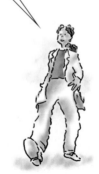

35. Which nursing action is the **best** way to help a client with mild Alzheimer's disease (AD) remain functional?
1. Obtain a health care provider's order for a mild anxiolytic to control behavior.
2. Call attention to all mistakes so the client can be quickly corrected.
3. Advise the client to move into a retirement center.
4. Maintain a stable, predictable environment and daily routine.

35. 4. Clients in the early stages of AD remain fairly functional with familiar surroundings and a predictable routine. They become easily disoriented with surprises and social overstimulation. Anxiolytics can impair memory and worsen function. Calling attention to all of the client's mistakes is nonproductive and serves to lower self-esteem. Moving the client to an unfamiliar environment will heighten agitation and confusion.
CN: Psychosocial integrity; CNS: None; CL: Apply; DIFFICULTY: Easy

CN: Client needs category   CNS: Client needs subcategory   CL: Cognitive level

36. The nurse is providing care to a client with Alzheimer's disease (AD). Which nursing intervention takes **priority**?
1. Establish a routine that supports former habits.
2. Maintain physical surroundings that are cheerful and pleasant.
3. Maintain an exact routine from day to day.
4. Control the environment by providing structure, boundaries, and safety.

36. 4. By controlling the environment and providing structure and boundaries, the nurse is helping to keep the client safe and secure, which is a priority nursing measure. Establishing a routine that supports former habits and maintaining cheerful, pleasant surroundings and an exact routine foster a supportive environment; however, keeping the client safe and secure takes priority.
CN: Safe, effective care environment; CNS: Coordinated care; CL: Apply; DIFFICULTY: Easy

37. The nurse finds a client with Alzheimer's disease wandering in the hall at 3 a.m. The client has removed the clothing and says to the nurse, "I'm just taking a stroll through the park." What's the **priority** action by the nurse?
1. Immediately help the client back to the room and into some clothing.
2. Tell the client that such behavior won't be tolerated.
3. Tell the client it's too early in the morning to be taking a stroll.
4. Ask the client if he would like to go back to his room.

37. 1. The nurse shouldn't allow the client to be embarrased in front of others, regardless of the time of day. Intervene as soon as the behavior is observed. Scolding the client isn't helpful because it isn't something the client can understand. Don't engage the client in social chatter; the interaction should be concrete and specific. Don't ask the client to choose unnecessarily. The client may not be able to make appropriate choices.
CN: Psychosocial integrity; CNS: None; CL: Apply; DIFFICULTY: Easy

38. Rivastigmine has been prescribed to a client. When reviewing home administration with the client and spouse, which response indicates the need for further instruction?
1. "If I miss a dose by more than an hour I should wait until the next day to take it."
2. "This medication should be taken at the same time each day."
3. "I can take this medication diluted in a beverage of choice."
4. "This medication can be taken without diluting it in a beverage."

38. 1. Rivastigmine is used to promote improved cognition in affected clients. The medication slows the breakdown of neurotransmitters in the brain. When taking the medication, a missed dose may be taken when noted unless it is almost time for the next dose. An hour is not an excessive amount of time. The medication is a liquid and may be taken with our without a beverage. Taking the medication at the same time each day is recommended.
CN: Physiological integrity; CNS: Pharmacological therapies; CL: Evaluation; DIFFICULTY: Difficult

39. The nurse is assisting with a care plan for a client admitted with Alzheimer dementia. The family reports that the client has to be watched closely for wandering behavior at night. Which nursing action will be of the **greatest** importance?
1. Use of a bed check monitor device to alert the nursing staff in the event the client gets up.
2. Use restraints as needed.
3. Place the call light in reach of the client.
4. Utilize a sitter to remain with the client during the night hours.

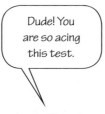

Dude! You are so acing this test.

39. 4. Providing a safe, effective care environment takes priority in this case. A sitter can remain with the client to limit the opportunities for him to get up unattended. Monitors are useful but do not prevent the client from getting up. The use of the call light is important but will not stop the client from getting out of bed unattended. If the client has a history of wandering this will not halt the behavior. Restraints are to be avoided.
CN: Safe, effective care environment; CNS: Coordinated care; CL: Apply; DIFFICULTY: Challenge

40. A client is admitted to the acute care facility with an amnesic disorder. Which condition should the nurse carefully monitor the client for that is associated with this disorder?
1. Drug overdose
2. Cerebral anoxia
3. Medications (anticonvulsants)
4. Lead, mercury, and carbon dioxide toxins

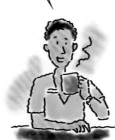

40. 2. A variety of medical conditions are related to amnesic disorders, such as head trauma, stroke, cerebral neoplastic disease, herpes simplex, encephalitis, poorly controlled insulin-dependent diabetes, and cerebral anoxia. Drug overdose, medications, and toxins cause substance-induced amnesia and aren't medical conditions.
CN: Physiological integrity; CNS: Physiological adaptation; CL: Apply; DIFFICULTY: Moderate

CN: Client needs category   CNS: Client needs subcategory   CL: Cognitive level

41. For which laboratory evaluation should the nurse prepare a client with amnesic disorder?
1. Angiography
2. Cardiac catheterization
3. Electrocardiography
4. Metabolic and endocrine tests

41. 4. An amnesic disorder is characterized by impairment in memory from direct physiologic effects of a medical condition or effects of a substance, medication, or toxin. Metabolic and endocrine tests will identify such causes. Angiography, cardiac catheterization, and electrocardiography are diagnostic tests related to the cardiovascular system.
CN: Health promotion and maintenance; CNS: None; CL: Apply; DIFFICULTY: Moderate

42. A nurse is working with the family of a client who has Alzheimer disease (AD). The nurse notes that the client's spouse is too exhausted to continue providing care all alone. The adult children live too far away to provide relief on a weekly basis. Which nursing intervention would be **most** helpful? Select all that apply.
1. Tell the absent children that they must participate in helping the client.
2. Suggest the spouse seek counseling to help cope with exhaustion.
3. Recommend community resources for adult day care and respite care.
4. Encourage the spouse to talk about the difficulties involved in caring for a loved one with Alzheimer's disease.
5. Ask whether friends or church members can help with errands or provide short periods of relief.
6. Recommend that the client be placed in a long-term care facility.

42. 3, 4, 5. Many community services exist for clients with Alzheimer disease and their families. Encouraging use of these resources may make it possible for the client to stay at home and alleviate the spouse's exhaustion. The nurse can also support the caregiver by urging conversation about the difficulties in caring for a spouse with AD. Friends and church members may be able to help provide care to the client, allowing the caregiver time for rest, exercise, or an enjoyable activity. Telling the children to participate more would probably be ineffective and may evoke anger or guilt. Counseling may be helpful, but it wouldn't alleviate the caregiver's physical exhaustion and wouldn't address the client's immediate needs. A long-term care facility isn't an option until the family is ready to make that decision.
CN: Psychosocial integrity; CNS: None; CL: Analyze; DIFFICULTY: Difficult

43. The nurse is assigned to care for a client with early-stage Alzheimer disease (AD). Which nursing interventions should be included in the client's care plan? Select all that apply.
1. Change the client's routine often.
2. Engage the client in complex discussions to improve memory.
3. Furnish the client's environment with familiar possessions.
4. Assist the client with activities of daily living (ADLs) as necessary.
5. Assign tasks in simple steps.

43. 3, 4, 5. A client with AD experiences progressive deterioration in cognitive functioning. Familiar possessions may help to orient the client. The client should be encouraged to perform ADLs but may need assistance with certain activities. Using a step-by-step approach helps the client complete tasks independently. A client with AD functions best with consistent routines. Complex discussions don't improve the memory of a client with Alzheimer disease.
CN: Psychosocial integrity; CNS: None; CL: Apply; DIFFICULTY: Easy

> Congratulations! You did it.

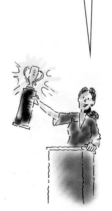

44. The nurse is obtaining data from a client to determine whether dementia or depression is present. Which information helps the nurse suspect dementia rather than depression? Select all that apply.
1. The progression of symptoms is slow.
2. The client answers questions with, "I don't know."
3. The client acts apathetic and pessimistic.
4. The family can't identify when the symptoms first appeared.
5. The client's personality has changed.
6. The client has great difficulty paying attention to others.

44. 1, 4, 5, 6. Common characteristics of dementia include a slow onset of symptoms, difficulty identifying when the symptoms first occurred, noticeable changes in the client's personality, and impaired ability to pay attention to other people. Answering questions with "I don't know" and displays of pessimism and apathy are symptoms of depression, not dementia.
CN: Psychosocial integrity; CNS: None; CL: Analyze; DIFFICULTY: Challenge

Chapter 15

Personality Disorders

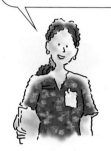

No, this chapter doesn't cover quirks of the rich and famous. It's all about mental disorders affecting the personality. Have a blast!

Personality disorders refresher

Antisocial personality disorder

Disregard to the needs or well-being of others

Key signs and symptoms
- Destructive tendencies
- General disregard for the rights and feelings of others
- Lack of remorse
- Sudden or frequent changes in job, residence, or relationships

Key test results
- The Minnesota Multiphasic Personality Inventory–2 reveals an antisocial personality disorder

Key treatments
- Behavioral therapy
- Antimanic agent: lithium carbonate
- beta-blocker: propranolol for controlling aggressive outbursts
- Selective serotonin reuptake inhibitor (SSRI): paroxetine

Key interventions
- Help the client to identify manipulative behaviors
- Establish a behavioral contract with the client
- Hold the client responsible for behavior

Borderline personality disorder

Erratic, unstable emotions and difficulty maintaining relationships

Key signs and symptoms
- Destructive behavior
- Impulsive behavior
- Inability to develop a healthy sense of self
- Inability to maintain relationships
- Moodiness
- Self-mutilation

Key test results
- Standard psychological tests reveal a high degree of dissociation

Key treatments
- Individual therapy
- Antimanic medications: valproate sodium, lithium carbonate
- Anxiolytic: buspirone
- SSRIs: paroxetine, fluoxetine, sertraline

Key interventions
- Recognize the behaviors that the client uses to manipulate others
- Set limits on behavior
- Provide a positive role model

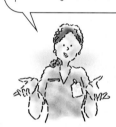

Finally, a chapter with personality! Let's dive in?

Dependent personality disorder

Abnormal and excessive need to be dependent/reliant on others

Key signs and symptoms
- Clinging, demanding behavior
- Fear and anxiety about losing the people on which the client is dependent
- Hypersensitivity to potential rejection and decision making
- Inability to make decisions
- Low self-esteem

Key test results
- Laboratory tests rule out any underlying medical condition

Key treatments
- Behavior modification through assertiveness training
- Individual therapy
- Benzodiazepines: alprazolam, lorazepam, clonazepam
- SSRIs: paroxetine, sertraline

Key interventions
- Support the client in accepting increased decision making (e.g., balancing a checkbook, planning meals, paying bills)
- Help client to identify manipulative behaviors, focusing on specific examples

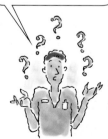

Your client has just been diagnosed with borderline personality disorder. What behavior should you expect to see?

Paranoid personality disorder
Distrust in others

Key signs and symptoms
- Feelings of being deceived
- Hostility
- Major distortions of reality
- Social isolation
- Suspicion and mistrust of friends and relatives

Key treatments
- Possible drug-free treatment to reduce the chance of causing increased paranoia
- Individual therapy
- Antipsychotic agents: olanzapine, risperidone, chlorpromazine, haloperidol, quetiapine

Key interventions
- Establish a therapeutic relationship by listening and responding to the client
- Instruct the client in, and help to practice, strategies that facilitate the development of social skills

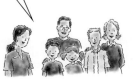

Personality disorders can make it challenging to maintain healthy relationships.

thePoint® You can download tables of drug information to help you prepare for the NCLEX®! View Generic Drug Names, Drug Classifications, Drug Actions, and Nursing Implications for the drugs discussed in this refresher at **http://thePoint.lww.com**.

Personality disorders questions, answers, and rationales

1. A client tells the nurse that coworkers are sabotaging the client's computer. When the nurse asks questions, the client becomes argumentative. Which intervention would be **most** appropriate for the nurse to implement?
   1. Encourage the client to vent anger about coworkers.
   2. Tell the client that coworkers haven't touched the computer.
   3. Talk with the client about the realistic situations.
   4. Ask the client what has been done about the reported violation.

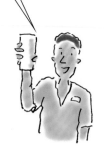

Cheers! You're off to a great start.

2. A nurse observes that a client is mistrustful and shows hostile behavior. Which type of personality disorder is associated with these characteristics?
   1. Antisocial
   2. Avoidant
   3. Borderline
   4. Paranoid

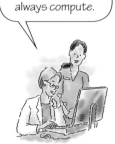

The behavior of clients with personality disorders doesn't always compute.

3. The nurse is caring for a client with paranoid personality disorder. Which behavior observed by the nurse is documented as a sign of this disorder?
   1. The client can't follow limits set on behavior.
   2. The client is afraid another person will inflict harm.
   3. The client avoids responsibility for health care.
   4. The client depends on others to make important decisions.

1. **3.** Establishing a therapeutic relationship with a client experiencing paranoid delusions is priority. Using clear and consistent speech when talking with the client helps focus on reality and fosters a therapeutic relationship. Encouraging the client to vent anger at coworkers validates suspicious thoughts and may cause more arguments and aggression. Trying to convince the client that coworkers haven't touched the computer or telling the client to go to the room may make the client more defensive.
CN: Psychosocial integrity; CNS: None; CL: Analyze; DIFFICULTY: Easy

2. **4.** Paranoid individuals have a need to constantly scan the environment for signs of betrayal, deception, and ridicule, appearing mistrustful and hostile. They expect to be tricked or deceived by others. The extreme suspiciousness is lacking in antisocial personalities, who tend to be more arrogant and self-assured despite their vigilance and mistrust. Individuals with avoidant personality disorders are guarded, fearing interpersonal rejection and humiliation. Clients with borderline personality disorders behave impulsively and tend to manipulate others.
CN: Psychosocial integrity; CNS: None; CL: Apply; DIFFICULTY: Moderate

3. **2.** A client with paranoid personality disorder is afraid others will inflict harm. A client with antisocial personality disorder won't be able to follow the limits set on behavior. A client with an avoidant personality might avoid responsibility for health care because of the tendency to scan the environment for threatening things. A client with dependent personality disorder is likely to want others to make important decisions for him.
CN: Psychosocial integrity; CNS: None; CL: Analyze; DIFFICULTY: Easy

CN: Client needs category   CNS: Client needs subcategory   CL: Cognitive level

4. Which statement made by a client to the nurse is typical of a diagnosis of paranoid personality disorder?
1. "I understand you're to blame."
2. "I must be seen first; it's not negotiable."
3. "I see nothing humorous in this situation."
4. "I wish someone would select the outfit for me."

5. The nurse is caring for a client diagnosed with borderline personality disorder. The nurse tells the client that they will be meeting for 1 hour every week on Monday at 1 p.m. Which statement **best** describes the rationale for setting limits for a client with borderline personality disorder?
1. It helps the client clarify limits.
2. It encourages the client to be manipulative.
3. It provides the nurse with leverage against unacceptable behavior.
4. It provides an opportunity for the client to assess the situation.

6. A nurse is caring for a client with paranoid personality disorder. The nurse would expect to observe which condition?
1. Exhibitionism
2. Impulsiveness
3. Secretiveness
4. Self-destructiveness

7. The nurse is talking with the family members of a client diagnosed with a paranoid personality disorder. Which statement by a family member is supportive of the diagnosis? Select all that apply.
1. "My spouse is so forgetful."
2. "Whenever possible, my spouse seems to take advantage of others."
3. "My parent is always thinking about something negative happening."
4. "Establishing friendships is hard for my spouse because of the lack of trust in others."
5. "My spouse is so flirtatious."

8. Which short-term goal is **most** appropriate for the client with paranoid personality disorder who has impaired social skills?
1. Obtain feedback from other people.
2. Discuss anxiety-provoking situations.
3. Address positive and negative feelings about self.
4. Identify personal feelings that hinder social interaction.

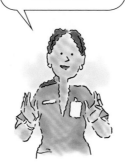

> Clients with borderline personality disorder often need help in establishing boundaries.

> Clients with paranoid personality disorder need help discovering the source of their problematic social interactions.

4. 3. Clients with paranoid personality disorder tend to be extremely serious and lack a sense of humor. Clients with borderline personality disorder tend to blame others for their problems. Clients with narcissistic personality disorders have a sense of self-importance and entitlement. Clients with dependent personality disorder want others to make their decisions.
CN: Psychosocial integrity; CNS: None; CL: Analyze; DIFFICULTY: Difficult

5. 1. Clarifying limits and making clear what may be unclear to the client helps the client establish boundaries independantly, which fosters a therapeutic, trusting relationship between the nurse and the client. The nurse should never encourage manipulation or attempt to gather leverage against the client, which would be unprofessional. The client must understand behavior patterns before starting to assess the situation.
CN: Psychosocial integrity; CNS: None; CL: Apply; DIFFICULTY: Moderate

6. 3. Clients with paranoid personality disorder tend to be secretive. Clients with histrionic personality disorder tend to be exhibitionists, and those with borderline personality disorder tend to be impulsive and self-destructive.
CN: Psychosocial integrity; CNS: None; CL: Apply; DIFFICULTY: Moderate

7. 3, 4. People with paranoid personality disorders are hypersensitive to perceived threats. This can be demonstrated by reports that something bad has happened or will happen. This can impair the ability to establish trusting relationships. There is not a loss of cognitive abilities so forgetfulness is not supportive of this diagnosis. Clients with narcissistic personality disorder are interpersonally exploitative to enhance themselves or to indulge their own desires. A client with histrionic personality disorder can be extremely seductive when in search of stimulation and approval.
CN: Psychosocial integrity; CNS: None; CL: Analyze; DIFFICULTY: Difficult

8. 4. The client must address the feelings that impede social interactions before developing ways to address impaired social skills. Feedback can be obtained only after action is taken to improve or change the situation. Discussion of anxiety-provoking situations is important but doesn't help the client with impaired social skills. Addressing the client's positive and negative feelings about themselves won't directly influence impaired social skills.
CN: Psychosocial integrity; CNS: None; CL: Apply; DIFFICULTY: Moderate

9. A client with paranoid personality disorder is discussing current problems with a nurse. Which nursing interventions are appropriate for inclusion in the care plan? Select all that apply.
   1. Encourage the client to look at sources of frustration.
   2. Ask the client to focus on ways to interact with others.
   3. Urge the client to discuss the use of defense mechanisms.
   4. Suggest the client clarify thoughts and beliefs about an event.
   5. Discuss with the client actions that could be taken to promote a better outcome with these problematic situations.

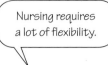

Nursing requires a lot of flexibility.

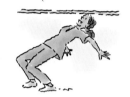

10. A client with a paranoid personality disorder makes an inappropriate and unreasonable report to a nurse. Which principle of good communication skills is important to use?
   1. Use logic to address the client's concern.
   2. Confront the client about the stated misperception.
   3. Use nonverbal communication to address the issue.
   4. The nurse should tell the client matter-of-factly that she does not agree with the client's interpretation.

11. The nurse is caring for a client diagnosed with histrionic personality disorder. The client is observed tearing pages out of the books in the unit library and putting them into the ventilation system. Which nursing interventions are appropriate for inclusion in the plan of care? Select all that apply.
   1. Place the client in a safe, secluded environment.
   2. Help the client develop more acceptable methods of seeking attention.
   3. Withdraw attention from the client at this time.
   4. Identify inappropriate behaviors to the client in a matter-of-fact manner.
   5. Discuss the client's sources of frustration.

12. The nurse is caring for a client with a paranoid personality disorder. The client has had several confrontations with the nursing staff as a result of misinterpretation of events on the unit. Which actions by the nurse to manage this client will be therapeutic? Select all that apply.
   1. Limit interaction between the client and staff to activities of daily living
   2. Address only problems and causes of distress.
   3. Explore anxious situations and offer reassurance.
   4. Speak in simple messages without details.
   5. Allow the client the opportunity to ask questions.

9. 4, 5. Clarifying thoughts and beliefs helps the client avoid misinterpretations. Clients with a paranoid personality disorder tend to be aggressive and argumentative rather than frustrated. They tend to mistrust people and don't see interacting with others as a way to handle problems. The client's priority must be to interpret thoughts and beliefs realistically, rather than discuss defense mechanisms. A paranoid client will focus on defending himself rather than acknowledging the use of defense mechanisms.
CN: Psychosocial integrity; CNS: None; CL: Analyze; DIFFICULTY: Challenge

10. 4. When the nurse tells the client that he/she doesn't agree with his interpretation, it helps the client differentiate between realistic and emotional thoughts and conclusions. When the nurse uses logic to respond to a client's inappropriate statement, the nurse risks creating a power struggle with the client. It's unwise to confront a client with a paranoid personality disorder because the client will immediately become defensive. The use of nonverbal communication would probably be misinterpreted and arouse the client's suspicion.
CN: Psychosocial integrity; CNS: None; CL: Analyze; DIFFICULTY: Challenge

11. 1, 4, 5. If the client begins destroying property or presenting potential harm to self or others, it may be necessary to immediately place the client in a safe, secluded environment. When the client regains control and ceases the behavior, then the nurse can attempt a conversation to explore more acceptable ways of handling frustration and expressing feelings. Lack of attention from the nurse wouldn't reduce the client's attention-seeking behaviors. When the client regains control and ceases the behavior, the nurse must make it clear which behaviors are inappropriate.
CN: Safe, effective care environment; CNS: Safety and infection Control; CL: Apply; DIFFICULTY: Challenge

12. 4, 5. The nurse who speaks to the client using clear, simple messages lessens the chance that information will be misinterpreted. Allowing the client time to ask questions will promote understanding of information provided. Interaction can't be limited because it will interfere with working on identified treatment goals. Discussing complex topics creates additional information for the client to misinterpret. The nurse who addresses only problems and specific stressors makes it difficult to establish a trusting relationship.
CN: Psychosocial integrity; CNS: None; CL: Apply; DIFFICULTY: Challenge

CN: Client needs category   CNS: Client needs subcategory   CL: Cognitive level

13. A client with paranoid personality disorder responds aggressively to something another client said during a psychoeducational group session. Which rationale explains the likely underlying cause of the client's response to the interaction?
1. The client doesn't want to participate in the group.
2. The client took the statement as a personal criticism.
3. The client is impulsive and was acting out frustrations.
4. The client was attempting to handle emotional distress.

14. A client has been prescribed lithium carbonate, extended release tablets. Which statements indicate an understanding of information provided? Select all that apply.
1. "I should take this medication at the same times each day."
2. "Since I have trouble swallowing pills it is fine to crush the tablet and add it to applesauce or pudding."
3. "It will take a few weeks for this medication to begin to help me feel calmer."
4. "Muscle tremors and weakness are common side effects and will resolve after a few weeks of taking the medication."
5. "Taking this medication with a citrus beverage will promote its absorption."

15. Which characteristic of a client with a paranoid personality disorder makes it difficult for a nurse to establish an interpersonal relationship?
1. Dysphoria
2. Hypervigilance
3. Indifference
4. Promiscuity

16. The health care provider has prescribed olanzapine for a client. Which statement from the client would indicate the medication is having the desired effect?
1. "I am feeling rested when I wake up in the morning."
2. "My appetite is getting better."
3. "I am feeling more comfortable talking with others."
4. "It is getting easier to rest at night."

17. A client with antisocial personality disorder tells a nurse, "Life has been full of problems since childhood." Which situation or condition would the nurse explore in the assessment?
1. Birth defects
2. Easy distractibility
3. Hypoactive behavior
4. Substance abuse

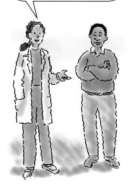

You're making this look easy.

SNAP

Getting your client with paranoid personality disorder to drop his guard is a key first step.

13. **2.** Clients with paranoid personality disorder tend to be hypersensitive and take what other people say as a personal attack on their character. The client is driven by the suspicion that others will inflict harm. The client's participation in group therapy would be minimal because the client is directing energy toward emotional self-protection. Clients with a paranoid personality disorder tend to be rigid and guarded rather than impulsive and rebellious. The client with a paranoid personality disorder is acting to defend himself or herself, not handle emotional distress.
CN: Psychosocial integrity; CNS: None; CL: Analyze; DIFFICULTY: Easy

14. **1, 3.** Lithium carbonate is prescribed to manage manic behaviors. Extended release tablets cannot be chewed or crushed. Taking the medication at the same time each day is important to maintain therapeutic medication levels. It will take 1 to 3 weeks for the client to begin to experience a relief of symptomology. Muscle tremors and weakness are not normal side effects and may signal a problem. If they occur the medication should be held and the health care provider contacted. Taking the medication with a citrus beverage will not impact the absorption of the drug.
CN: Physiological integrity; CNS: Pharmacological therapies; CL: evaluation; DIFFICULTY: Challenge

15. **2.** Clients with paranoid personality disorder think others will harm, deceive, or exploit them in some way, and they're commonly guarded and ready to defend themselves from actual or perceived attacks. They don't tend to be dysphoric, indifferent, or promiscuous.
CN: Psychosocial integrity; CNS: None; CL: Apply; DIFFICULTY: Moderate

16. **3.** Olanzapine is used in the treatment of paranoid personality disorders. If effective, the medication will help the client have control of symptoms, such as paranoia, that impair interactions with others. Restful sleep is not a goal of this medication. Appetite changes do not reflect that the medication is therapeutic.
CN: Physiological integrity; CNS: Pharmacological therapies; CL: Apply; DIFFICULTY: Moderate

17. **4.** Clients with antisocial personality disorder commonly engage in substance abuse during childhood. They don't have a higher incidence of birth defects than other people. Clients with antisocial personality disorder are commonly manipulative and are no more distracted from issues than others. They tend to be *hyperactive*, not hypoactive.
CN: Psychosocial integrity; CNS: None; CL: Apply; DIFFICULTY: Moderate

18. A client with a paranoid personality disorder tells a nurse, "That other nurse is out to get me." Which actions by the nurse may cause distress for this paranoid client? Select all that apply.
  1. Giving as-needed medication to another client
  2. Laughing and smiling with a group of clients
  3. Checking vital signs of each person on the unit
  4. Talking to another client in the corner of the lounge
  5. Conferring with the nurse in question in front of the client

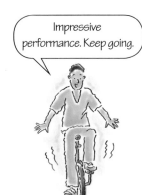

Impressive performance. Keep going.

18. 2, 4, 5. Clients with paranoid personality disorder tend to interpret any discussion that doesn't include them as evidence of a plot against them. Laughing and smiling with a group, talking with the nurse in question, or interacting with others in what appears to be a secretive manner can increase feelings of paranoia in this client. Giving medication to another client wouldn't alarm the client with paranoid personality disorder. Checking vital signs of each client on the unit wouldn't alarm the client with paranoid personality disorder.
CN: Psychosocial integrity; CNS: None; CL: Apply; DIFFICULTY: Moderate

19. Which statement made by a client with paranoid personality disorder shows that education about social relationships is effective?
  1. "As long as I live, I won't abide by social rules."
  2. "Sometimes I can see what causes relationship problems."
  3. "I'll find out what problems others have so I won't repeat them."
  4. "I don't have problems in social relationships; I never really did."

19. 2. Progress is shown when the client addresses behaviors that negatively affect relationships. Clients with paranoid personality disorder struggle to understand and express their feelings about social rules. Knowing other people's problems isn't useful; the client must focus on his own issues. Clients with paranoid personality disorder tend to have impaired social relationships and are very uncomfortable in social settings. By not recognizing the problem, the client indicates that he is in denial.
CN: Psychosocial integrity; CNS: None; CL: Apply; DIFFICULTY: Easy

20. Which long-term goal is appropriate for a client with paranoid personality disorder who's trying to improve peer relationships?
  1. The client will verbalize a realistic view of self.
  2. The client will take steps to address disorganized thinking.
  3. The client will become appropriately interdependent on others.
  4. The client will become involved in activities that foster social relationships.

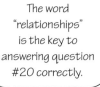
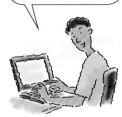

The word "relationships" is the key to answering question #20 correctly.

20. 4. An appropriate long-term goal is for the client with paranoid personality disorder to increase interactions, social skills, and make the commitment to become involved with others on a long-term basis. To verbalize a realistic view of self is a short-term goal. The client with a paranoid personality disorder doesn't tend to have disorganized thinking. A client with paranoid personality disorder won't allow himself to be interdependent on others.
CN: Psychosocial integrity; CNS: None; CL: Analyze; DIFFICULTY: Easy

21. A family of a client with paranoid personality disorder is trying to understand the client's behavior. Which intervention would help the family?
  1. Help the family find ways to handle stress.
  2. Explore the possibility of finding respite care.
  3. Help the family manage the client's eccentric actions.
  4. Encourage the family to focus on the client's strengths.

21. 3. The family needs to know how to handle the client's symptoms and eccentric behaviors. All people need to learn strategies for handling stress, but the focus must be on helping the family learn how to handle symptoms. There's no need to find respite care for a client with a paranoid personality disorder. Focusing on the client's strengths is a positive action, but the family in this situation must learn how to manage the client's eccentric behavior.
CN: Psychosocial integrity; CNS: None; CL: Apply; DIFFICULTY: Difficult

22. A client with antisocial personality disorder is trying to convince a nurse that he deserves special privileges and that an exception to the rules should be made. Which response by the nurse is appropriate?
  1. "I believe we need to sit down and talk about this."
  2. "Don't you know better than to try to bend the rules?"
  3. "What you're asking me to do for you is unacceptable."
  4. "Why don't you bring this request to the community meeting?"

23. Which behavior by a client with antisocial personality disorder alerts a nurse to the need for education related to interaction skills?
  1. Frequent crying
  2. Panic attacks
  3. Avoidance of social activities
  4. Failure to follow social norms

24. Which intervention should be done **first** for a client who has an antisocial personality disorder and a history of polysubstance use?
  1. Human immunodeficiency virus (HIV) testing
  2. Electrolyte profile
  3. Anxiety screening
  4. Psychological testing

Hint: a history of polysubstance use means the client probably engages in other high-risk behaviors

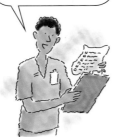

25. Which short-term goal is appropriate for a client with an antisocial personality disorder who acts out when distressed?
  1. Develop goals for personal improvement.
  2. Identify situations that are out of the client's control.
  3. Encourage the client to identify traumatic life events.
  4. Educate the client about expressing feelings in a nondestructive manner.

Keep calm and carry on.

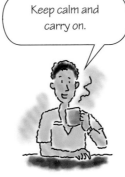

26. A nurse notices other clients on the unit avoiding a client diagnosed with antisocial personality disorder. When discussing appropriate behavior in group therapy, which comment made by his peers about this client is expected?
  1. "He's never honest."
  2. "He's superstitious."
  3. "He has temper tantrums."
  4. "He constantly needs attention."

22. 3. Clients with antisocial personality disorder commonly try to manipulate the nurse to get special privileges or make exceptions to the rules on their behalf. By informing the client directly when actions are inappropriate, the nurse helps the client learn to control unacceptable behaviors by setting limits. By sitting down to talk about the request, the nurse is telling the client there's room for negotiation when there isn't. Implying that the client wants to bend the rules is humiliating to the client. The client's request is unacceptable and shouldn't be brought to a community meeting.
CN: Psychosocial integrity; CNS: None; CL: Apply; DIFFICULTY: Challenge

23. 4. Failure to abide by social norms influences the client's ability to interact in a healthy manner with peers. Clients with antisocial personality disorders don't have frequent crying episodes or panic attacks. Avoiding social activities is more likely observed in an avoidance personality type.
CN: Psychosocial integrity; CNS: None; CL: Analyze; DIFFICULTY: Challenge

24. 1. A client who engages in high-risk behaviors such as polysubstance use should undergo HIV testing. This client would benefit from an entire chemistry profile as part of a complete medical examination, rather than a single test for electrolytes. An anxiety screen isn't needed for a client with antisocial personality disorder. Information from psychological testing is valuable when developing a treatment plan but isn't an immediate concern.
CN: Safe, effective care environment; CNS: Coordinated care; CL: Apply; DIFFICULTY: Difficult

25. 4. By working on appropriate expression of feelings, the client learns how to talk about what's stressful, rather than hurt himself or others. The most pressing need is to learn to cope and talk about problems rather than act out. Developing goals for personal improvement is a long-term goal, not a short-term one. Although it's important to differentiate what is and isn't under the client's control, the most important goal for handling distress is to talk about feelings appropriately. The identification of traumatic life events will occur only after the client begins to express feelings appropriately.
CN: Psychosocial integrity; CNS: None; CL: Apply; DIFFICULTY: Moderate

26. 1. Clients with antisocial personality disorder tend to engage in acts of dishonesty, shown by lying. Clients with schizotypal personality disorder tend to be superstitious. Clients with histrionic personality disorder tend to overreact to frustrations and disappointments, have temper tantrums, and seek attention.
CN: Psychosocial integrity; CNS: None; CL: Apply; DIFFICULTY: Difficult

27. When reviewing a client's chart, the nurse sees the progress note below. Which statement about the client's condition is **most** accurate?

Progress notes	
9/4/2017	Client, age 28, admitted to unit with
1130	diagnosis of antisocial personality
	disorder and suicide attempt after
	cutting his right wrist. Right wrist
	dressing appears dry and intact. Client
	states, "I don't want to be here and I'm
	not following your treatment plan or any
	of your rules. I'm going to tell everyone
	here not to follow your rules."
	— Barbara Jones, LPN

1. The client requires psychotropic drugs to treat his condition, but he is refusing.
2. The client manipulates other clients but not his family.
3. The client may not be motivated to change his behavior or his lifestyle.
4. The client could quickly make behavior changes if motivated.

27. 3. Clients with antisocial personality disorder feel nothing is wrong with their behavior and have no desire to change. These clients don't benefit from psychotropic drug therapy. They attempt to manipulate all people with whom they come in contact. A quick behavior change isn't a realistic expectation for clients with this disorder.

CN: Psychosocial integrity; CNS: None; CL: Apply; DIFFICULTY: Moderate

28. During a family meeting for a client with an antisocial personality disorder, which statement is expected from an exasperated family member?
1. "Today I'm the enemy, but tomorrow I'll be a saint."
2. "There is never an apology when my spouse is wrong."
3. "Sometimes I can't believe how my spouse exaggerates about everything."
4. "There are times when the compulsive behavior is too much to handle."

A client's personality disorder affects everyone in the family.

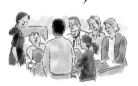

28. 2. The client with antisocial personality disorder has no remorse. The client with a borderline personality disorder shows splitting. The client with an antisocial personality disorder doesn't tend to exaggerate about life events or to be compulsive.

CN: Psychosocial integrity; CNS: None; CL: Analyze; DIFFICULTY: Moderate

29. Which goal is appropriate for a client with antisocial personality disorder who possesses a high risk of violence directed at others?
1. The client will discuss the desire to hurt others rather than act.
2. The client will be given something to destroy to displace the anger.
3. The client will develop a list of resources to use when anger escalates.
4. The client will understand the difference between anger and physical symptoms.

29. 1. By discussing the desire to be violent toward others, the nurse can help the client get in touch with the pain associated with the angry feelings. It isn't helpful to give the client something to destroy. The client needs to talk about strong feelings in a nonviolent manner, not refer to a list of crisis resources. Helping the client understand the relationship between feelings and physical symptoms can be done after discussing the desire to hurt others.

CN: Psychosocial integrity; CNS: None; CL: Analyze; DIFFICULTY: Challenge

30. A client with antisocial personality disorder says, "I always want to blow things off." Which response is **most** appropriate?
  1. "Try to focus on what needs to be done and just do it."
  2. "Let's work on considering some options and strategies."
  3. "Procrastinating is a part of your illness that we'll work on."
  4. "The best thing to do is decide on some useful goals to accomplish."

31. Which goal for the family of a client with antisocial disorder should the nurse stress in the education?
  1. The family must assist the client to decrease ritualistic behavior.
  2. The family must learn to live with the client's impulsive behavior.
  3. The family must stop reinforcing inappropriate negative behavior.
  4. The family must start to use negative reinforcement of the client's behavior.

32. Which nursing intervention is appropriate for inclusion in the plan of care for a client with antisocial personality disorder who shows defensive behaviors?
  1. Help the client accept responsibility for his own decisions and behaviors.
  2. Work with the client to feel better about himself by taking care of basic needs.
  3. Educate the client on identifying the defense mechanisms used to cope with distress.
  4. Confront the client about the disregard of social rules and the feelings of others.

33. A client with antisocial personality disorder is trying to manipulate the health care team. Which strategy is important for the staff to use?
  1. Focus on how to educate the client more effectively on behaviors for meeting basic needs.
  2. Help the client verbalize underlying feelings of hopelessness and learn coping skills.
  3. Remain calm and don't respond emotionally to the client's manipulative actions.
  4. Help the client eliminate the intense desire to have everything in life turn out perfectly.

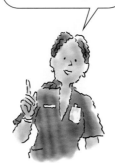

It's easy for family members to contribute to a client's negative behaviors without even realizing it.

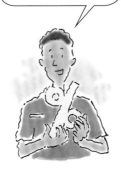

Looks like you're giving 150% on this test. Way to go!

30. 2. By considering options or strategies, the client gains skills to overcome ineffective behaviors. The client tends to be irresponsible and needs guidance on what specifically to focus on to change behavior. Clients with an antisocial personality disorder don't tend to struggle with procrastination; instead, they act recklessly and irresponsibly. It's premature to decide on goals when the client needs to address the mental mindset and work to change the irresponsible behavior.
CN: Psychosocial integrity; CNS: None; CL: Analyze; DIFFICULTY: Easy

31. 3. The family needs help learning how to stop reinforcing inappropriate client behavior. Clients with antisocial personality disorder don't show ritualistic behaviors. The family can set limits and reinforce consequences when the client shows shortsightedness and poor planning. Negative reinforcement is an inappropriate strategy for the family to use to support this client.
CN: Psychosocial integrity; CNS: None; CL: Analyze; DIFFICULTY: Moderate

32. 1. Clients with antisocial personality disorder tend to blame other people for their behaviors and must learn how to take responsibility for their actions. Clients with antisocial personality disorder don't tend to have problems with self-care habits or meeting basic needs. Clients with antisocial personality disorder will deny they're defensive or distressed. Most commonly, these clients feel justified in their retaliatory behavior. To confront the client would only cause him to become even more defensive.
CN: Psychosocial integrity; CNS: None; CL: Analyze; DIFFICULTY: Challenge

33. 3. The best strategy to use with a client trying to manipulate staff is to stay calm and refrain from responding emotionally. Negative reinforcement of inappropriate behavior increases the chance it will be repeated. Later, it may be possible to address how to meet the client's basic needs. Clients with antisocial personality disorder don't tend to experience feelings of hopelessness or the desire for life events to turn out perfectly. In most cases, these clients negate responsibility for their behavior.
CN: Psychosocial integrity; CNS: None; CL: Analyze; DIFFICULTY: Moderate

34. A client with dependent personality disorder is working to increase self-esteem. Which statement by the client shows that the education was successful?
1. "I'm not just going to look at the negative things about myself."
2. "I'm most concerned about my level of competence and progress."
3. "I'm not as envious of the things other people have as I used to be."
4. "I find I can't stop myself from taking over things others should be doing."

Clients with dependent personality disorder often can only see their flaws and weaknesses.

35. A client is suspected of having antisocial personality disorder. Which finding by the nurse would support this diagnosis?
1. The client has delusional thinking.
2. The client has feelings of inferiority.
3. The client has disorganized thinking.
4. The client has multiple criminal charges.

36. A nurse on the psychiatric unit is caring for a client with antisocial personality disorder. Which behavior is the nurse **most** likely to observe?
1. Manipulation, shallowness, and the need for immediate gratification
2. Tendency to profit from mistakes or learn from past experiences
3. Expression of guilt and anxiety regarding behavior
4. Acceptance of authority and discipline

Too ... many ... questions. I need a break.

37. When gathering data from a client with antisocial personality disorder, which finding is consistent with this diagnosis?
1. Problematic work history
2. Struggle with severe anxiety
3. Severe physical health conditions
4. Criticism of positive feedback

38. A nurse determines that a client with antisocial personality disorder is beginning to practice several socially acceptable behaviors in the group setting. Which behavior if observed by the nurse would indicate this is taking place?
1. Fewer panic attacks
2. Acceptance of reality
3. Improved self-esteem
4. Decreased physical symptoms

34. 1. As the client makes progress on improving self-esteem, feelings of self-blame and negative self-evaluations will decrease. Clients with dependent personality disorder tend to feel fragile and inadequate and would be extremely unlikely to discuss their level of competence and progress. These clients focus on self and aren't envious or jealous. Individuals with dependent personality disorders don't take over situations because they see themselves as inept and inadequate.
CN: Psychosocial integrity; CNS: None; CL: Apply; DIFFICULTY: Moderate

35. 4. Clients with antisocial personality disorder are commonly sent for treatment by the court after multiple crimes or for the use of illegal substances. Clients with antisocial personality disorder don't tend to have delusional thinking, feelings of inferiority, or disorganized thinking.
CN: Psychosocial integrity; CNS: None; CL: Apply; DIFFICULTY: Difficult

36. 1. Because of the lack of scruples and underlying powerlessness of the client with antisocial personality disorder, the nurse expects to see manipulation, shallowness, impulsivity, and self-centered behavior. This client doesn't profit from mistakes and learn from past experiences, lacks anxiety and guilt, and is unable to accept authority and discipline.
CN: Psychosocial integrity; CNS: None; CL: Apply; DIFFICULTY: Easy

37. 1. Clients with a diagnosis of antisocial personality disorder tend to have problems in their job roles and poor work histories. They don't have severe anxiety disorders or severe physical health problems and are able to accept positive feedback from others.
CN: Psychosocial integrity; CNS: None; CL: Understand; DIFFICULTY: Moderate

38. 3. When clients with antisocial personality disorder begin to practice socially acceptable behaviors, they also commonly experience a more positive sense of self. Clients with antisocial personality disorder don't tend to have panic attacks, alteration in their perception of reality, or somatic manifestations of their illness.
CN: Psychosocial integrity; CNS: None; CL: Apply; DIFFICULTY: Moderate

39. A client with a diagnosis of borderline personality disorder is admitted to the unit after slashing their wrist. When assisting with the planning of care, which goal is **most** appropriate for this client?
1. Establish a therapeutic relationship with the client.
2. Identify if splitting is present in the client's thoughts.
3. Talk about his acting out and self-destructive tendencies.
4. Encourage the client to understand why they blame others.

40. Which nursing intervention would be of assistance in helping a client with a borderline personality disorder identify appropriate behaviors?
1. Schedule a family meeting.
2. Place the client in seclusion.
3. Formulate a behavioral contract.
4. Perform a mental status assessment.

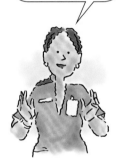

Nursing interventions can help outline what's appropriate and what's not.

41. Which statement is typical of a client with borderline personality disorder who has recurrent suicidal thoughts?
1. "I can't believe how everyone has suddenly stopped believing in me."
2. "I don't care what other people say, I know how bad I looked to them."
3. "I might as well check out because my boyfriend doesn't want me anymore."
4. "I won't stop until I've gotten revenge on all those people who blamed me."

42. The nurse is taking a health history on a client with borderline personality disorder. Which finding would the nurse expect to observe?
1. A negative sense of self
2. A tendency to be compulsive
3. A problem with communication
4. An inclination to be philosophical

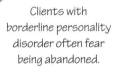

Clients with borderline personality disorder often fear being abandoned.

43. Which characteristic or situation is indicated when a client with borderline personality disorder has a crisis?
1. Antisocial behavior
2. Suspicious behavior
3. Relationship problems
4. Auditory hallucinations

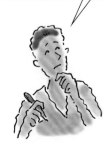

39. 1. After promoting client safety, the nurse establishes a rapport with the client to facilitate appropriate expression of feelings. At this time, the client isn't ready to address unhealthy behavior. A therapeutic relationship must be established before the nurse can effectively work with the client on splitting, self-destructive tendencies, and blaming others.
CN: Safe, effective care environment; CNS: Coordinated care; CL: Apply; DIFFICULTY: Moderate

40. 3. The use of a behavioral contract establishes a framework for healthier functioning and places responsibility for actions back on the client. Seclusion will reinforce the fear of abandonment found in clients with borderline personality. Performing a mental status assessment or scheduling a family meeting won't help the client identify appropriate behaviors.
CN: Psychosocial integrity; CNS: None; CL: Apply; DIFFICULTY: Challenge

41. 3. The client with borderline personality disorder who's suicidal typically exhibits a tendency toward all-or-nothing thinking. The first statement indicates the client has experienced a credibility problem; the second statement indicates the client is extremely embarrassed; and the last statement indicates the client has an antisocial personality disorder.
CN: Safe, effective care environment; CNS: Safety and infection control; CL: Apply; DIFFICULTY: Moderate

42. 1. Clients with a borderline personality disorder have low self-esteem and a negative sense of self. They have little or no problem expressing themselves and communicating with others. Although they have a tendency to be impulsive, they usually aren't compulsive or philosophical.
CN: Psychosocial integrity; CNS: None; CL: Apply; DIFFICULTY: Difficult

43. 3. Relationship problems can precipitate a crisis because they bring up issues of abandonment. Clients with borderline personality disorder aren't usually suspicious; they're more likely to be depressed or highly anxious. They don't have symptoms of antisocial behavior or auditory hallucinations.
CN: Psychosocial integrity; CNS: None; CL: Analyze; DIFFICULTY: Difficult

44. The nurse is gathering data from a client with borderline personality disorder. Which finding does the nurse determine is relevant to this diagnosis?
1. Abrasions in various healing stages
2. Intermittent episodes of hypertension
3. Alternating tachycardia and bradycardia
4. Mild state of euphoria with disorientation

45. Which short-term goal is appropriate for a client with borderline personality disorder who displays low self-esteem?
1. Write in a journal daily.
2. Express fears and feelings.
3. Stop obsessive-compulsive behaviors.
4. Decrease dysfunctional family conflicts.

46. Which intervention is important to include in an education plan for the family of a client diagnosed with borderline personality disorder? Select all that apply.
1. Educate the family about methods for handling the client's anxiety.
2. Explore behaviors the family employs which can reinforce the client's undesirable behaviors.
3. Encourage the family to have the client express intense emotions.
4. Help the family to pressure the client to improve current behavior.
5. Educate the family about the borderline personalities.

47. Which statement to the nurse is expected from a client with borderline personality disorder who also has a history of dysfunctional relationships?
1. "I won't get involved in another relationship."
2. "I'm determined to look for the perfect partner."
3. "I've decided to learn better communication skills."
4. "I'm going to be an equal partner in a relationship."

48. In assisting with the planning of care for a client with borderline personality disorder, a nurse must be aware that this client is prone to developing which condition?
1. Binge eating
2. Memory loss
3. Cult membership
4. Delusional thinking

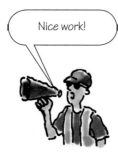
Nice work!

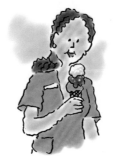
Just one more triple-scoop ice cream cone—then I'll stop eating, I promise.

44. 1. Clients with borderline personality disorder tend to self-mutilate and have abrasions in various stages of healing. Intermittent episodes of hypertension, alternating tachycardia and bradycardia, or a mild state of euphoria with disorientation don't tend to occur with this disorder.
CN: Psychosocial integrity; CNS: None; CL: Apply; DIFFICULTY: Challenge

45. 2. Acknowledging fears and feelings can help the client identify areas of self that cause discomfort to be able to develop a positive sense of self. Writing in a daily journal isn't a short-term goal to enhance self-esteem. A client with borderline personality disorder doesn't struggle with obsessive-compulsive behaviors. Decreasing dysfunctional family conflicts is a long-term goal.
CN: Psychosocial integrity; CNS: None; CL: Analyze; DIFFICULTY: Easy

46. 1, 2, 5. The family needs to learn how to handle the client's intense stress and low tolerance for frustration. Family members need to understand how they can impact behaviors of the client. Education about the disorder is paramount to the success of their involvement in the plan of care. Clients with borderline personality disorder already maintain intense emotions and it's not safe to encourage further expression of them. The family doesn't need to pressure the client to change behavior; this approach will only cause inappropriate behavior to escalate.
CN: Psychosocial integrity; CNS: None; CL: Apply; DIFFICULTY: Challenge

47. 2. Clients with borderline personality disorder would decide to look for a perfect partner. This characteristic is a result of the dichotomous manner in which these clients view the world. They go from relationship to relationship without taking responsibility for their behavior. It's unlikely an unsuccessful relationship will cause these clients to change. Because they tend to blame others for problems, it's unlikely they would express a desire to learn communication skills. They tend to be demanding and impulsive in relationships. There's no thought given to what one wants or needs from a relationship.
CN: Psychosocial integrity; CNS: None; CL: Analyze; DIFFICULTY: Moderate

48. 1. Clients with borderline personality disorder are likely to develop dysfunctional coping and act out in self-destructive ways, such as binge eating. They aren't prone to develop memory loss or delusional thinking. Joining a cult may be seen in some clients with antisocial personality disorder.
CN: Psychosocial integrity; CNS: None; CL: Analyze; DIFFICULTY: Challenge

49. The nurse is caring for a client with borderline personality disorder. When working with the client on developing healthy, lasting relationships which intervention would be encouraged **first**?
1. Encourage the client to assess current behaviors.
2. Work with the client to develop outgoing behavior.
3. Limit the client's interactions to family members only.
4. Encourage the client to approach others for interactions.

50. Which defense mechanism is the nurse **most** likely to hear when having a conversation with a client who has borderline personality disorder?
1. Compensation
2. Displacement
3. Identification
4. Projection

51. Which nursing intervention has **priority** for a client with borderline personality disorder?
1. Maintain consistent, realistic limits.
2. Give instructions for meeting basic self-care needs.
3. Arrange for participation in daytime activities to stimulate wakefulness.
4. Schedule the client to attend group therapy on a daily basis.

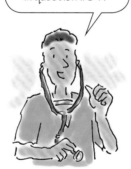

What's the priority intervention in question #51?

52. Which action by a client with borderline personality disorder indicates adequate learning about personal behavior?
1. The client talks about intense anger.
2. The client smiles while making demands.
3. The client decides never to engage in conflict.
4. The client stops the family from controlling finances.

53. Which behavior observed by the nurse is **most** likely to coexist in clients with a diagnosis of borderline personality disorder?
1. Avoidance
2. Delirium
3. Depression
4. Disorientation

49. 1. Self-assessment of behavior enables the client to look at himself and identify social behaviors that need to be changed. Clients with borderline personality disorder don't tend to have difficulty approaching and interacting with other people. It's unrealistic to limit clients with borderline personality disorder to interactions with family members only. Clients with borderline personality disorder tend to be demanding and enjoy being the center of attention. It isn't useful for these clients to develop outgoing behavior.
CN: Psychosocial integrity; CNS: None; CL: Analyze; DIFFICULTY: Moderate

50. 4. Clients with borderline personality disorder tend to blame others and project their feelings and inadequacies onto others. They don't identify with other people or use compensation to handle distress. Clients with borderline personality disorder are impulsive and tend to react immediately. It's unlikely they would displace their feelings onto others.
CN: Psychosocial integrity; CNS: None; CL: Analyze; DIFFICULTY: Difficult

51. 1. Clients with borderline personality disorder who are needy, dependent, and manipulative will benefit greatly from maintaining consistent, realistic limits. They don't tend to have difficulty meeting their self-care needs and don't tend to have sleeping difficulties. They enjoy attending group therapy because they typically attempt to use the opportunity to become the center of attention.
CN: Safe, effective care environment; CNS: Coordinated care; CL: Apply; DIFFICULTY: Easy

52. 1. Learning has occurred when anger is discussed rather than acted out in unhealthy ways by the client with borderline personality disorder. The behavior to change would be the demands placed on others. Smiling while making these demands shows manipulative behavior. Not engaging in conflict is unrealistic. It's important to help this client slowly develop financial responsibility rather than just stopping the family from monitoring the client's tendency to overspend.
CN: Psychosocial integrity; CNS: None; CL: Apply; DIFFICULTY: Moderate

53. 3. Chronic feelings of emptiness and sadness predispose this client to depression. About 40% of the clients with borderline personality disorder struggle with depression. They tend to disregard boundaries and limits. Avoidance isn't an issue with these clients. They don't tend to develop delirium or become disoriented. These conditions are only a possibility if the client becomes intoxicated.
CN: Safe, effective care environment; CNS: Coordinated care; CL: Understand; DIFFICULTY: Moderate

54. In planning care for a client with borderline personality disorder, the nurse must account for which behavioral trait?
1. An inability to make decisions independently
2. A propensity to act out when feeling afraid, alone, or devalued
3. A belief she deserves special privileges not accorded to others
4. A display of inappropriately seductive appearance and behavior

54. 2. Clients with borderline personality disorder have an intense fear of abandonment, so they act out when feeling afraid, alone, or devalued. These clients are able to make decisions independently. A person who feels deserving of special privileges is characteristic of narcissistic personality disorder. Inappropriate seductive appearance and behavior are characteristics of someone with histrionic personality disorder.
CN: Psychosocial integrity; CNS: None; CL: Apply; DIFFICULTY: Moderate

55. A client is admitted to a medical–surgical unit for treatment of an orthopedic injury. In addition to this admitting diagnosis, the nurse notes that the client has a history of borderline personality disorder with episodes of cutting/self-mutilation. Which type of behavior would the nurse expect to be present due to this self-mutilation history? Select all that apply.
1. No presence of cuts or burns found during assessment
2. No unexplained frequent injuries
3. Knife or razor in purse or bag
4. Insistence on wearing long-sleeved shirt even in warm temperatures
5. Overly hesitant behavior when the nurse attempts to assist with bathing or dressing

55. 3, 4, 5. The client who self-mutilates can be expected to have numerous small cuts over the body, unexplained frequent injuries, and may have a knife or razor in possession. The client will wear long-sleeved shirts even in warm weather to prevent anyone from seeing self-inflicted cuts or burns. The client may be overly hesitant for medical personnel to assist with bathing or dressing due to the presence of cuts or burns over the body.
CN: Psychosocial integrity; CNS: None; CL: Apply; DIFFICULTY: Easy

56. The nurse is caring for a client with dependent personality disorder. Which action by the nurse would be appropriate?
1. Orient the client to current surroundings.
2. Reassure the client about personal safety.
3. Ask questions to help the client recall problems.
4. Differentiate between positive and negative feedback.

Expect clients with dependent personality disorder to be hypersensitive to your comments.

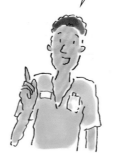

56. 4. Clients with dependent personality disorder tend to view all feedback as criticism; they commonly misinterpret another's remarks. Clients with dependent personality disorder don't need orientation to their surroundings. Personal safety isn't an issue because these clients typically aren't self-destructive. Memory problems aren't associated with this disorder, so asking questions to stimulate memory isn't necessary.
CN: Psychosocial integrity; CNS: None; CL: Apply; DIFFICULTY: Difficult

57. Which short-term goal is appropriate for a client with dependent personality disorder experiencing excessive dependency needs?
1. Verbalize self-confidence in own abilities.
2. Decide relationships don't take energy to sustain.
3. Discuss feelings related to frequent mood swings.
4. Stop obsessive thinking that impedes daily social functioning.

57. 1. Individuals with dependent personalities believe they must depend on others to be competent for them. They need to gain more self-confidence in their own abilities. The client must realize relationships take energy to develop and sustain. Clients with dependent personality disorder usually don't have mood swings or obsessive thinking that interferes with their socialization.
CN: Psychosocial integrity; CNS: None; CL: Apply; DIFFICULTY: Easy

58. A client with dependent personality disorder is thinking about getting a part-time job. Which nursing intervention will help this client when employment is obtained?

1. Help the client develop strategies to control impulses.
2. Explain there are consequences for inappropriate behaviors.
3. Encourage the client to work to sustain healthy interpersonal relationships.
4. Help the client decrease the use of regression as a defense mechanism.

59. A client with dependent personality disorder has difficulty expressing personal concerns. Which communication technique is **best** to teach the client?

1. Questioning
2. Reflection
3. Silence
4. Touch

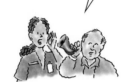

If your client seems confused about instructions you are giving, try rephrasing them.

60. A nurse is evaluating the effectiveness of an assertiveness group attended by a client with dependent personality disorder. Which client statement indicates the group had therapeutic value?

1. "I can't seem to do the things other people do."
2. "I wish I could be more organized like other people."
3. "I want to talk about something that's bothering me."
4. "I just don't want people in my family to fight anymore."

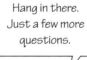

Hang in there. Just a few more questions.

61. After a family visit, a client with dependent personality disorder becomes anxious. Which situation is a possible cause of the anxiety?

1. Sensitivity to criticism
2. Discussion of family rules
3. Being asked personal questions
4. Identification of eccentric behavior

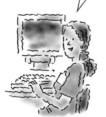

As beneficial as medications can be, never force a client to take them.

62. A client undergoing treatment for paranoia refuses to take his risperidone, stating, "I think it's poisoned." Which action by the nurse is appropriate?

1. Omit the dose and notify the health care provider.
2. Tell the client he will receive an injection if the medication is refused.
3. Put the medication in juice without informing the client.
4. Allow the client to examine the medication to see that it isn't poisoned.

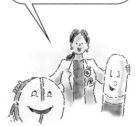

58. 3. Sustaining healthy relationships will help the client be comfortable with peers in the job setting. Clients with dependent personality disorder don't usually have trouble with impulse control or offensive behavior that would lead to negative consequences. They don't usually use regression as a defense mechanism. It's common to see denial and introjection used.
CN: Psychosocial integrity; CNS: None; CL: Analyze; DIFFICULTY: Challenge

59. 1. Questioning is a way to learn to identify feelings and express self. The use of reflection isn't a communication technique that will help the client with dependent personality disorder to express personal feelings and concerns. Using silence won't help the client identify and discuss personal concerns. The use of touch to express feelings and personal concerns must be used very judiciously.
CN: Psychosocial integrity; CNS: None; CL: Apply; DIFFICULTY: Challenge

60. 3. By asking to talk about a bothersome situation, the client with dependent personality disorder has taken the first step toward assertive behavior. Noting an inability to do things other people do reflects a lack of self-confidence; it isn't assertive. Expressing wishes isn't assertive. To smooth over or minimize troubling events such as family fights isn't an assertive action.
CN: Psychosocial integrity; CNS: None; CL: Apply; DIFFICULTY: Easy

61. 1. Clients with dependent personality disorder are extremely sensitive to criticism and can become very anxious when they feel interpersonal conflict or tension. When they have discussions about family rules, they try to become submissive and please others rather than become anxious. When they're asked personal questions, they don't necessarily become anxious. Clients with dependent personality disorder don't tend to behave eccentrically.
CN: Psychosocial integrity; CNS: None; CL: Apply; DIFFICULTY: Difficult

62. 1. The nurse's best response is to omit the dose and notify the health care provider; insisting that the client take the medication will only increase paranoia and agitation. Forcing injections and tricking a client into taking medication by putting it in juice without informing him is illegal. A rational approach (such as allowing the client to examine the medication) to irrational ideas seldom works.
CN: Safe, effective care environment; CNS: Coordinated care; CL: Apply; DIFFICULTY: Challenge

63. A client has a dependent personality disorder. Which emotional health problem should the nurse monitor the client for that may coexist with dependent personality disorder?
1. Psychotic disorder
2. Acute stress disorder
3. Alcohol-related disorder
4. Posttraumatic stress disorder (PTSD)

64. While obtaining data from a client diagnosed with impulse control disorder who is displaying violent, aggressive, and assaultive behavior, what can the nurse can expect to discover about the client? Select all that apply:
1. The client functions well in other areas of life.
2. The degree of aggressiveness is out of proportion to the stressor.
3. The client typically uses a stressor to justify the violent behavior.
4. The client has a history of parental alcoholism and a chaotic, abusive family life.
5. The client shows no remorse about the inability to control behavior.

65. A nurse is monitoring a client who is hallucinating and notes paranoid content in the client's speech, along with agitation. The client is gesturing at a figure on the television. Which nursing interventions are appropriate? Select all that apply.
1. In a firm voice, instruct the client to stop the behavior.
2. Reinforce that the client is not in any danger.
3. Acknowledge the presence of the hallucinations.
4. Instruct other team members to ignore the client's behavior.
5. Immediately implement physical restraint procedures.
6. Use a calm voice and simple commands.

66. A client has borderline personality disorder. Which behaviors would substantiate this diagnosis? Select all that apply.
1. Recurrent suicidal behaviors, gestures, or threats
2. Chronically depressed affect, slowed thinking, and slurred speech
3. Frantic attempts to avoid real or imagined abandonment
4. Chronic feelings of emptiness
5. Binging and purging

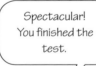
Spectacular! You finished the test.

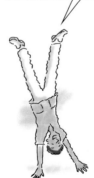

63. 2. Because they have placed their own needs in the hands of others, clients with dependent personalities are extremely vulnerable to acute stress disorder. They don't tend to have coexisting problems of psychotic disorder, alcohol-related disorder, or PTSD.
CN: Psychosocial integrity; CNS: None; CL: Analyze; DIFFICULTY: Difficult

64. 1, 2, 4. A client with an impulse control disorder who displays violent, aggressive, and assaultive behavior generally functions well in other areas of life. The degree of the client's aggressiveness is disproportionate to the stressor, and the client commonly has a history of parental alcoholism as well as a chaotic family life. The client usually verbalizes sincere guilt and remorse for the aggressive behavior.
CN: Psychosocial integrity; CNS: None; CL: Apply; DIFFICULTY: Difficult

65. 2, 3, 6. Using a calm voice, the nurse should reassure the client that he's safe. The nurse shouldn't challenge the client; rather, acknowledge hallucinatory experience. It's not appropriate to request that the client stop the behavior. Implementing restraints isn't warranted at this time. Although the client is agitated, no evidence exists that the client is at risk for harming self or others.
CN: Psychosocial integrity; CNS: None; CL: Apply; DIFFICULTY: Moderate

66. 1, 3, 4. Recurrent suicidal behaviors, gestures, or threats; frantic attempts to avoid real or imagined abandonment; and chronic feelings of emptiness are typical behaviors seen in borderline personality disorder. Though the etiology of this disorder is unknown, it's believed to result from a severely disrupted or disconnected attachment with the primary caregiver at an early developmental age. This disruption of normal emotional development causes a sense of "core emptiness" that persists for life and is generally resistant to treatment. Chronically depressed affect, slowed thinking, and slurred speech are more indicative of a mood disorder. Binging and purging are consistent with an eating disorder.
CN: Psychosocial integrity; CNS: None; CL: Analyze; DIFFICULTY: Difficult

Chapter 16

Schizophrenia Spectrum & Other Psychotic Disorders

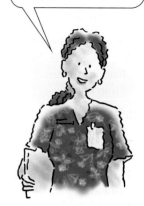

It's no delusion. You'll do great on this chapter if you use your nursing skills—knowledge, experience, compassion, insight …

Schizophrenia spectrum & other psychotic disorders refresher

Schizophrenia

Disturbances in thought content and form, perception, emotions and affect, movements and behavior; this results in difficulty thinking clearly, managing emotions, making decisions and relating to others

Key signs and symptoms

Positive or hard symptoms
- Hallucinations (auditory, visual, tactile)
- Delusions
- Bizarre behavior
- Thought disorders (disorganized thinking)
- Agitated movements (psychomotor agitation)
- Echopraxia (involuntary imitation of another person's movements and gestures)
- Loose associations

Negative or soft symptoms
- Catatonia (psychomotor slowing)
- Flat or blunted affect
- Alogia (speak very little)
- Anhedonia (lack of pleasure in things that used to bring pleasure)
- Lack of focus

Key test results
- Magnetic resonance imaging (MRI) shows possible enlargement of lateral ventricles, enlarged third ventricle, and enlarged sulci
- Impaired performance on neuropsychological and cognitive tests

Key treatments
- Milieu therapy
- Supportive psychotherapy
- Social skills training
- Antipsychotic medication therapy: haloperidol, aripiprazole, olanzapine, risperidone, quetiapine, thioridazine, mesoridazine, fluphenazine, clozapine

Key interventions
- Monitor client for adverse effects of antipsychotic drugs, such as dystonic reactions, tardive dyskinesia, and akathisia

- Be aware of client's personal space, use gestures, and touch judiciously
- Provide appropriate measures to ensure client's safety
- Collaborate with client to identify anxious behaviors as well as probable causes
- Help client meet basic needs for food, comfort, and a sense of safety
- During an acute psychotic episode, remove any potentially hazardous items from client's environment
- If client experiences hallucinations, ensure safety and provide comfort and support
- Encourage client to participate in one-on-one interactions and then help progress to small groups
- Provide positive reinforcement for socially acceptable behavior, such as an effort to improve hygiene and table manners
- Encourage client to express feelings about the hallucinations experienced
- Set limits on aggressive behavior
- Maintain a low level of stimuli
- Provide reality-based diversional activities
- Provide a safe environment
- Reorient the client to time and place when appropriate

Schizoaffective disorder

Psychosis occurring with a mood disturbance at the same time

Key signs and symptoms
- Client is extremely ill, with symptoms of psychotic behavior as well as mood symptoms
- Symptoms may alternate between the psychotic behavior and the mood symptoms

Key treatments
- Milieu therapy
- Atypical antipsychotics, mood stabilizers, and antidepressants are first-line medications for treatment

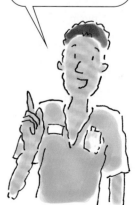

No, you're not hallucinating … this really is the psychotic disorders chapter.

Key interventions
- Supportive psychotherapy
- Milieu therapy

Delusional disorder

Psychotic disorder characterized by delusions (false, fixed beliefs); these delusions can be plausible or bizarre and impossible

Key signs and symptoms
- Delusions (false, fixed beliefs)
- Inability to trust
- Projection

Key test results
- Blood and urine tests eliminate an organic or chemical cause
- Endocrine function tests rule out hyperadrenalism, pernicious anemia, and thyroid disorders

- Neurologic evaluations rule out an organic cause

Key treatments
- Milieu therapy
- Supportive psychotherapy
- Antipsychotics: chlorpromazine, clozapine, fluphenazine, haloperidol, olanzapine, risperidone, thioridazine, aripiprazole, mesoridazine

Key interventions
- Explore events that trigger delusions
- Don't directly attack the delusion
- After the dynamics of the delusions are understood, discourage repetitious talk about delusions and refocus the conversation on the client's underlying feelings
- Recognize the delusion as the client's perception of the environment

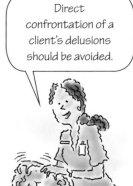

Direct confrontation of a client's delusions should be avoided.

thePoint® You can download tables of drug information to help you prepare for the NCLEX®! View Generic Drug Names, Drug Classifications, Drug Actions, and Nursing Implications for the drugs discussed in this refresher at **http://thePoint.lww.com**.

Schizophrenia spectrum & other psychotic disorders questions, answers, and rationales

1. A client with schizophrenia tells the nurse, "I am scheduled to meet the King of Samoa at a special time," making it impossible for the client to leave the room for dinner. Which response by the nurse is the **most** appropriate?
1. "It's meal time. Let's go so you can eat."
2. "The King of Samoa told me to take you to dinner."
3. "Your health care provider expects you to follow the unit's schedule."
4. "People who don't eat on this unit aren't being cooperative."

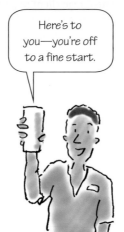

Here's to you—you're off to a fine start.

2. While looking out the window, a client with schizophrenia remarks, "That school across the street has creatures in it that are waiting for me." Which nursing action is the **most** appropriate for this client?
1. Ask the client what the creatures look like.
2. Acknowledge the client's fears and insecurities.
3. Explain to the client that there are no creatures in the school.
4. Ignore the remark and redirect the client to group activities.

1. 1. A delusional client is so wrapped up in the false beliefs that there tends to be a disregard for activities of daily living, such as nutrition and hydration. The client needs clear, concise, firm directions from a caring nurse to meet needs. Telling the client a false story belittles and tricks the client, possibly evoking mistrust on the part of the client. Talking about the health care provider's expectations evades the issue of meeting the client's basic needs. Telling the client that not eating equates to being uncooperative is demeaning and doesn't address the delusion.
CN: Psychosocial integrity; CNS: None; CL: Apply;
DIFFICULTY: Moderate

2. 2. Acknowledging the client's fears and insecurities helps to establish a trusting relationship and increase feelings of safety. Asking the client what the creatures look like only serves to reinforce the delusional thoughts. Challenging the client's delusion may lead to agitation. Ignoring the remark doesn't reassure the client. A delusional client isn't able to participate in group activities.
CN: Psychosocial integrity; CNS: None; CL: Apply;
DIFFICULTY: Difficult

3. The nurse is reviewing the plan of care for a client diagnosed with schizophrenia who has just been admitted to the psychiatric unit. Which intervention would the nurse identify as the **priority** for this client?

1. Teaching the client about the illness
2. Initiating a behavioral contract with the client
3. Requiring the client to attend all unit functions
4. Providing a consistent, predictable environment

4. A client with schizophrenia was admitted to the psychiatric unit during the night. The next morning, the client begins to call the nurse by a sibling's name. Which intervention is **best**?

1. Assessing the client for potential violence
2. Taking the client to the room, where the client will feel safer
3. Assuming the misidentification makes the client feel more comfortable
4. Correcting the misidentification and orienting the client to the unit and staff

5. A client is diagnosed with schizoaffective disorder. When working with the interdisciplinary team on developing a treatment plan for the client, the nurse would anticipate addressing the signs and symptoms of which condition? Select all that apply.

1. Schizophrenia
2. Mood disorder
3. Personality disorder
4. Eating disorder
5. Anxiety disorder

6. A client diagnosed with schizophrenia several years ago tells the nurse about feeling "very sad." The nurse observes that the client is smiling when saying it. When documenting this observation, the nurse would describe it using which term?

1. Inappropriate affect
2. Extrapyramidal
3. Insight
4. Inappropriate mood

7. A client on the psychiatric unit is imitating the movements of the nurse during recovery, saying, "I thought the nurse was my mirror. I felt connected only when I saw my nurse." What does the nurse document this behavior as?

1. Modeling
2. Echopraxia
3. Ego-syntonicity
4. Ritualism

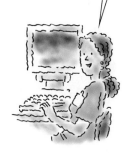

Check out that word "priority" in question #3—it looks important.

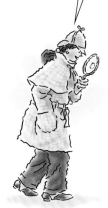

Look over question #7 carefully, and the answer is sure to come to you ... come to you ... come to you.

3. **4.** A consistent, predictable environment helps the client remain as functional as possible and prevents sensory overload. Teaching the client about his illness is important but not a priority. A behavioral contract and required attendance at all functions aren't particularly effective for clients with schizophrenia.
CN: Safe, effective care environment; CNS: Coordinated care; CL: Apply; DIFFICULTY: Easy

4. **4.** Misidentification can contribute to anxiety, fear, aggression, and hostility. Orienting a new client to the hospital unit, staff, and other clients, along with establishing a nurse–client relationship, can decrease these feelings and help the client feel in control. Assessing for potential violence is an important nursing function for any psychiatric client, but a perceived supportive environment reduces the risk of violence. Withdrawing to the room, unless interpersonal relationships have become nontherapeutic, encourages the client to remain in the fantasy world.
CN: Psychosocial integrity; CNS: None; CL: Apply; DIFFICULTY: Easy

5. **1, 2.** A client with schizoaffective disorder experiences signs and symptoms of a mood disorder (major depression, mania, or mixed episode) along with signs and symptoms of schizophrenia. Therefore, the treatment plan would need to address these signs and symptoms. Personality disorder, eating disorder, or anxiety disorder are not involved with schizoaffective disorder.
CN: Safe, effective care environment; CNS: Coordinated care; CL: Apply; DIFFICULTY: Challenge

6. **1.** Affect refers to behaviors, such as facial expression, that can be observed when a person is expressing and experiencing feelings. If the client's affect doesn't reflect the emotional content of the statement, the affect is considered inappropriate. Extrapyramidal symptoms are adverse effects of some categories of medication. Insight is a component of the mental status examination and is the ability to perceive oneself realistically and understand if a problem exists. Mood is an extensive and sustained feeling.
CN: Psychosocial integrity; CNS: None; CL: Apply; DIFFICULTY: Easy

7. **2.** Echopraxia is the involuntary copying of another's behaviors and is the result of the loss of ego boundaries. Modeling is the conscious copying of someone's behaviors. Ego-syntonicity refers to behaviors that correspond with the individual's sense of self. Ritualistic behaviors are repetitive and compulsive.
CN: Psychosocial integrity; CNS: None; CL: Apply; DIFFICULTY: Challenge

8. A nurse is providing care to a client with delusional disorder who has been admitted to the inpatient psychiatric unit. The client states, "I can't stand this itching and burning any more. All these bugs are crawling all over my skin. See, it's like they're swarming all around me and drilling holes in my skin." On inspection, the skin is clean, dry and intact without any evidence of redness or irritation. The nurse suspects that the client is experiencing which type of delusion?

1. Somatic
2. Grandiose
3. Jealous
4. Erotomanic

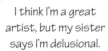

I think I'm a great artist, but my sister says I'm delusional.

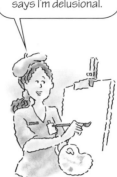

8. **1.** Somatic delusions involve bodily functions or sensations such as insects invading the skin. This type of delusion is often accompanied by tactile hallucinations, such as the intense itching or burning voiced by the client. Grandiose delusions reflect the belief that the person has some great, unrecognized talent; made some important discovery; or has a special relationship with a prominent person. Jealous delusions involve unfaithfulness or infidelity of a spouse or significant other and are based on incorrect inferences on the part of the client. Erotomanic delusions involve the belief that the client is loved intensely by another who is, under normal circumstances, out of the client's usual environment.

CN: Psychosocial integrity; CNS: None; CL: Apply; DIFFICULTY: Easy

9. An adolescent child of a parent with schizophrenia is worried about having schizophrenia as well. Based on the nurse's understanding of the disorder, which behavior would be an indication that should be evaluated for signs of the disorder?

1. Moodiness
2. Preoccupation with his body
3. Spending more time away from home
4. Changes in sleep patterns

9. **4.** In conjunction with other signs, changes in sleep patterns are distinctive initial signs of schizophrenia. Other signs include changes in personal care habits and social isolation. Moodiness, preoccupation with the body, and spending more time away from home are normal adolescent behaviors.

CN: Physiological integrity; CNS: Reduction of risk potential; CL: Apply; DIFFICULTY: Challenge

10. The nurse is reviewing the teaching provided to the family of a client with a psychiatric disorder about traditional antipsychotic drugs and their effect on symptoms. The nurse understands that which symptom would be **most** responsive to these types of drugs?

1. Apathy
2. Delusions
3. Social withdrawal
4. Attention impairment

10. **2.** Positive symptoms, such as delusions, hallucinations, thought disorder, and disorganized speech, respond to traditional antipsychotic drugs. Apathy, social withdrawal, and attention impairment are part of the category of negative symptoms, which also includes affective flattening, restricted thought and speech, and anhedonia. These symptoms are more responsive to the atypical antipsychotics, such as clozapine, risperidone, and olanzapine.

CN: Physiological integrity; CNS: Pharmacological therapies; CL: Apply; DIFFICULTY: Moderate

11. A client was hospitalized after his son filed a petition for involuntary hospitalization for safety reasons. The son seeks out the nurse because his father is angry and refuses to talk with him. The son is frustrated and states, "I feel so guilty about my decision." Which response to this client's son is the **most** empathic?

1. "Your father is here because he needs help."
2. "Your father will feel differently about you as he gets better."
3. "It's common for family members to feel this way. Can you tell me more?"
4. "This is a stressful time for you, but you'll feel better as your father gets well."

11. **3.** This response is most empathic because it focuses on the son and helps him understand that he is not alone. In addition, by asking the son to tell the nurse more about it helps him to discuss and deal with his feelings. Unresolved feelings of guilt, shame, isolation, and loss of hope impact the family's ability to manage the crisis and be supportive of the client. The other responses offer premature reassurance and cut off the opportunity for the son to discuss his feelings.

CN: Psychosocial integrity; CNS: None; CL: Apply; DIFFICULTY: Moderate

12. A client has followed an antipsychotic medication regimen for a number of years. The health care provider treats a urinary tract infection with antibiotic therapy. Which action would be **most** appropriate?
1. Arrange for possible hospitalization so that the client adheres to the new therapy.
2. Let a visiting nurse give the medication to reduce the risk for nonadherence.
3. Give instruction on the medication, possible adverse effects, and a return demonstration for teaching effectiveness.
4. Develop a psychoeducational program to address the client's emotional and physical problems arising from physiologic problems.

13. While providing care to a client receiving antipsychotic therapy, the nurse suspects that the client is experiencing tardive dyskinesia based on which finding?
1. Involuntary movements
2. Blurred vision
3. Restlessness
4. Sudden fever

14. A client with schizophrenia approaches a nurse and states, "I hear voices telling me that you are evil and deserve to die." The nurse interprets the client's statement as indicating which sign or symptom?
1. Delusion
2. Disorganized speech
3. Hallucination
4. Idea of reference

15. A client is admitted to the emergency department frightened and reports hearing voices with instructions to do bad things. Which intervention should be the nurse's **priority**?
1. Tell the client that he or she is safe and the voices aren't real.
2. Tell the client that he or she is safe now and promise the staff will protect them.
3. Assess the nature of the commands by asking the client what the voices are saying.
4. Administer a neuroleptic medication.

16. A nurse working on an inpatient psychiatric unit is caring for a client diagnosed with schizophrenia. The client is scheduled to attend an inpatient therapy group. The nurse understands that the group would be **most** successful if the group consisted of how many members?
1. One to four
2. Four to seven
3. 7 to 10
4. 10 to 15

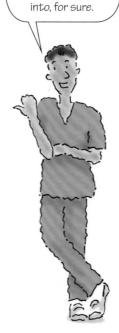

I wonder what the client means by "bad things?" Something to look into, for sure.

12. 3. The client has been successful and reliable in carrying out current medication regimen. The nurse should assume the competency includes self-administration of antibiotics if the instructions are understood. No evidence exists that the client is having a relapse as a result of the infection, so the client wouldn't need a psychoeducational program or hospitalization. Arranging for a community nurse to give the medication encourages dependency as opposed to self-care.
CN: Safe, effective care environment; CNS: Coordinated care; CL: Apply; DIFFICULTY: Easy

13. 1. Symptoms of tardive dyskinesia include tongue protrusion, lip smacking, chewing, blinking, grimacing, choreiform movements of limbs and trunk, and foot tapping. Blurred vision is a common adverse reaction of antipsychotic drugs and usually disappears after a few weeks of therapy. Restlessness is associated with akathisia. Sudden fever may be a symptom of a malignant neurologic disorder.
CN: Physiological integrity; CNS: Reduction of risk potential; CL: Apply; DIFFICULTY: Easy

14. 3. Hallucinations are sensory experiences that are misrepresentations of reality or have no basis in reality. Delusions are beliefs not based in reality. Disorganized speech is characterized by jumping from one topic to the next or using unrelated words. An idea of reference is a belief that an unrelated situation holds special meaning for the client.
CN: Psychosocial integrity; CNS: None; CL: Apply; DIFFICULTY: Challenge

15. 3. Safety is the priority. The nurse should directly ask the client about the nature of the auditory commands to adequately assess the safety of the client and the staff. The nurse should never make promises to the client that may not be fulfilled. The health care provider may order a neuroleptic medication, but the nurse's priority is to address safety.
CN: Psychosocial integrity; CNS: None; CL: Apply; DIFFICULTY: Moderate

16. 3. The ideal number of members to have in an inpatient group is 7 to 10. Fewer than seven members provides inadequate interaction and material for successful group process. More than 10 group members doesn't allow adequate time for individual participation.
CN: Psychosocial integrity; CNS: None; CL: Apply; DIFFICULTY: Challenge

17. A client admitted to an inpatient unit approaches the assigned nursing student. The client tells the student, "I am descended from a long line of people of a 'super-race.'" Which action by the student is correct?
1. Smile and walk into the nurse's station.
2. Challenge the client's false belief.
3. Listen for hidden messages in themes of delusion, indicating unmet needs.
4. Provide an introduction, shake hands and sit down with the client in the dayroom.

17. 4. The first goal is to establish a relationship with the client, which includes creating psychological space for the creation of trust. The student should sit and be available, reflecting concern and interest. Walking into the nurse's station would indicate disinterest and lack of concern about the client's feelings. Delusions are firmly maintained false beliefs, and attempts to dismiss or challenge them don't work. After establishing a relationship and lessening the client's anxiety, the student can orient the client to reality, clarify the meaning of the delusion, listen to concerns and fears, and try to understand the feelings reflected in the delusions.
CN: Safe, effective care environment; CNS: Coordinated care; CL: Apply; DIFFICULTY: Challenge

18. The nurse obtains data related to auditory hallucinations from a client with schizophrenia. Which behavior is **most** suggestive of this symptom?
1. Speaking loudly when engaged in conversation
2. Ignoring comments by the nurse
3. Limiting any responses made to the same person
4. Tilting the head to one side

18. 4. A client who's having auditory hallucinations may tilt the head to one side, as if listening to someone or something. Speaking loudly, ignoring comments, and responding only to one person are indicative of hearing deficit, anxiety, and paranoid behavior, respectively.
CN: Psychosocial integrity; CNS: None; CL: Analyze; DIFFICULTY: Moderate

19. A nurse is assisting with morning care when a client suddenly throws off the covers and starts shouting, "My body is changing and disintegrating because I'm not of this world!" The nurse interprets this statement as indicating which behavior?
1. Depersonalization
2. Ideas of reference
3. Looseness of association
4. Paranoid ideation

19. 1. Depersonalization is a state in which the client feels unreal or believes parts of the body are being distorted. Ideas of reference are beliefs unrelated to situations and hold special meaning for the individual. The term looseness of association refers to sentences that have a vague connection to one another. Paranoid ideations are beliefs that others intend to harm the client in some way.
CN: Psychosocial integrity; CNS: None; CL: Analyze; DIFFICULTY: Challenge

20. When collecting data from a client with schizophrenia, the nurse notes that the client is exhibiting opposing emotions simultaneously. How will the nurse document this finding?
1. Double bind
2. Ambivalence
3. Loose associations
4. Inappropriate affect

20. 2. Ambivalence, one of the symptoms associated with schizophrenia, immobilizes the person from acting. A double bind presents two conflicting messages—for example, saying that you trust someone but not allowing the person in your room. Loose association involves rapid shifts of ideas from one subject to another in an unrelated manner. Inappropriate affect refers to an observable expression of emotion incongruent with the emotion felt.
CN: Psychosocial integrity; CNS: None; CL: Apply; DIFFICULTY: Difficult

21. An adolescent client with a diagnosis of schizophrenia has become very clingy and begins sucking the thumb while interacting with the nurse. The nurse understands that these behaviors indicate which defense mechanism?
1. Repression
2. Regression
3. Rationalization
4. Projection

21. 2. Regression, a return to earlier behavior in order to reduce anxiety, is the basic defense mechanism in schizophrenia. Repression is the blocking of unacceptable thoughts or impulses from the consciousness. Rationalization is a defense mechanism used to justify one's behavior. Projection is a defense mechanism in which one blames others and attempts to justify actions.
CN: Psychosocial integrity; CNS: None; CL: Apply; DIFFICULTY: Easy

22. A nurse on a psychiatric unit observes a client in the corner of the room moving the lips as if talking to himself. Which action is the **most** appropriate?
1. Ask the client why he is talking to himself.
2. Leave the client alone until he stops talking.
3. Tell the client it isn't good to talk to himself.
4. Inviting the client to join in a card game.

23. A client makes vague statements with no logical connections and asks whether the nurse understands. Which response is **best**?
1. "Why don't we wait until later to talk about it?"
2. "You're not making sense, so I won't talk about this topic."
3. "Yes, I understand the overall sense of the logical connections from the idea."
4. "I want to understand what you're saying, but I'm having difficulty following you."

24. A client asks a nurse, "Do you hear the voices speaking to me?" Which response by the nurse is **best**?
1. "Stop asking about voices. No one is in your room except you."
2. "Yes, I hear, but I won't listen."
3. "What has the voice told you? Is it helpful advice?"
4. "No, I don't hear anything, but I know you do. What are they saying?"

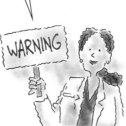

Remember to "keep it real" when discussing a client's hallucination. Lying is a violation of the therapeutic relationship.

WARNING

25. A client is taking chlorpromazine as part of a treatment plan. Which response by the client indicates an understanding of the education about the drug?
1. "I can reduce the dosage if I feel better."
2. "It's okay if I have an occasional drink once in a while."
3. "I should stop taking the drug immediately if adverse reactions develop."
4. "I need to schedule appointments for routine medication checks."

26. A client is referred to a mental health clinic by the court for harassing a couple next door and claiming that the husband was in love with her. She wrote love notes and called him on the telephone throughout the night. The client is employed and has had no problems with her job. The nurse interprets these findings as suggesting which condition?
1. Major depression
2. Paranoid schizophrenia
3. Delusional disorder
4. Bipolar disorder

22. 4. Joining the nurse and playing a game provide stimulation that competes with the hallucinations. Asking the client why he is talking to himself reinforces and challenges the hallucination. Remaining alone keeps the client in the fantasy world. Telling the client it isn't good to talk to himself fails to recognize how real the fantasy world and hallucinations are.
CN: Psychosocial integrity; CNS: None; CL: Apply; DIFFICULTY: Easy

23. 4. The nurse must communicate the desire to understand without blaming the client for the lack of understanding. Asking the client to wait because he's too confused to communicate is asking too much of the client in the current state. Telling the client that he isn't making sense is judgmental and could impair the therapeutic relationship. Pretending to understand is a violation of trust that can damage the therapeutic relationship.
CN: Psychosocial integrity; CNS: None; CL: Apply; DIFFICULTY: Easy

24. 4. The nurse who admits to not hearing the voice but is interested in what has been said points out reality and shows concern and support for the client. Attempting to argue the client out of the belief might entrench the client more firmly in the belief, making him feel more out of control because of the negative and fearful nature of hallucinations. The other two responses violate the trust of the therapeutic relationship because they don't maintain reality orientation.
CN: Psychosocial integrity; CNS: None; CL: Apply; DIFFICULTY: Easy

25. 4. Ongoing assessment by a practitioner is important to assess for adverse reactions to chlorpromazine and continued therapeutic effectiveness. The dosage should be cut only after checking with the practitioner. Alcoholic beverages are contraindicated while taking an antipsychotic drug. Adverse reactions should be reported immediately to determine if the drug should be discontinued.
CN: Physiological integrity; CNS: Pharmacological therapies; CL: Analyze; DIFFICULTY: Challenge

26. 3. The client's signs and symptoms suggest delusional disorder with erotomanic delusions as her primary symptom. She believes she's loved intensely by a married person showing no interest in her. No symptoms of major depression exist. The client doesn't believe someone is trying to harm her (the hallmark characteristic of paranoia). Bipolar disorder is characterized by cycles of extreme emotional highs (mania) and lows (depression).
CN: Psychosocial integrity; CNS: None; CL: Apply; DIFFICULTY: Easy

27. A homebound client taking clozapine tells the nurse he has been feeling tired for 5 days. Temperature is 99.6° F (37.6° C); pulse 110 beats/minute; and respirations 20 breaths/minute. Based on the client's report, which instruction would be **most** appropriate?

1. Take the medication with milk.
2. Stop the medication at once and see the health care provider immediately.
3. Understand that the symptoms will disappear as soon as the client gets more rest.
4. Stop the medication gradually and see the health care provider next week.

27. 2. The client should stop the medication and see the health care provider immediately because fever can be a sign of agranulocytosis, which is a medical emergency. Taking an antipsychotic medication with milk, nicotine, or caffeine decreases its effectiveness. Rest won't relieve the client's symptoms. Fatigue associated with clozapine use usually disappears with continued therapy.
CN: Physiological integrity; CNS: Pharmacological therapies; CL: Analyze; DIFFICULTY: Moderate

28. A client is admitted to the inpatient facility with a diagnosis of schizophrenia. During the initial assessment, the client points to the nurse's stethoscope and says it's a snake. The nurse understands that the client is exhibiting which phenomenon?

1. Abstraction
2. Delusion
3. Hallucination
4. Illusion

28. 4. An illusion is a misinterpretation of an actual sensory stimulation. An abstraction is an idea or concept, such as love, or a belief that can't be represented by a concrete object. A delusion is a fixed belief. A hallucination is a false sensory perception without a stimulus.
CN: Psychosocial integrity; CNS: None; CL: Apply; DIFFICULTY: Difficult

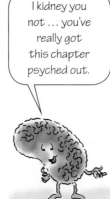

I kidney you not ... you've really got this chapter psyched out.

29. A client with schizophrenia was admitted to the hospital 2 days ago and began medication treatment with haloperidol. When reviewing the progress record, the nurse notes the entry below. Which laboratory results would the nurse need to report **immediately**?

Progress notes	
9/4/16	Client is pale and diaphoretic, with warm
1345	skin. She has tremors and difficulty speaking.
	Vital signs: Temp, 102.6° F (39.2° C); BP,
	160/98 mm Hg;
	heart rate, 94 beats/minute;
	respiratory rate, 20 breaths/minute.
	Laboratory results received: CK, 500 units/L
	(500 U/L); WBC,
	15,000/μmm³ (15.0 × 109/L); HCT, 38%
	(0.38); Hb, 14 g/dL
	— Barbara Smith, L.P.N

1. CK and HCT
2. WBC and HCT
3. CK and WBC
4. WBC and Hb

29. 3. The client's symptoms and elevated CK level and WBC count indicate possible neuroleptic malignant syndrome (NMS), a potentially fatal reaction to antipsychotic medications. Signs and symptoms of NMS include elevated blood pressure, hyperthermia, muscle rigidity, diaphoresis, and pale skin. HCT and Hb are within normal range.
CN: Physiological integrity; CNS: Pharmacological therapies; CL: Analyze; DIFFICULTY: Moderate

30. A nurse is reviewing the interdisciplinary plan of care for a client experiencing hallucinations. Which intervention would the nurse **most** likely identify as being included in the plan?
1. Confining the client to the room until feeling better
2. Providing a competing stimulus that distracts from the hallucinations
3. Discouraging attempts to understand what precipitates the hallucinations
4. Supporting perceptual distortions until the client gives them up on own accord

30. **2.** Providing a competing stimulus acknowledges the presence of the hallucinations and teaches the client ways to decrease their frequency. The other nursing actions support and maintain hallucination occurrence or deny its existence.
CN: Safe, effective care environment; CNS: Coordinated care; CL: Apply; DIFFICULTY: Easy

31. A client with schizophrenia reports that hallucinations have decreased in frequency. Which intervention would be appropriate to begin addressing the client's problem with social isolation?
1. Encourage the client to join in a group game.
2. Name the client the leader of the client support group.
3. Suggest that the client play solitaire.
4. Ask the client to participate in a group sing-along.

31. **4.** Inviting the client to participate in a noncompetitive group activity such as a sing-along doesn't require individual participation and won't present a threat to the client with schizophrenia. Games can become competitive and can lead to anxiety or hostility. The client probably lacks sufficient social skills to lead a group at this time. Playing solitaire doesn't encourage socialization.
CN: Psychosocial integrity; CNS: None; CL: Apply; DIFFICULTY: Challenge

32. A client is admitted with acute exacerbation of schizophrenia. The nurse anticipates that which therapy will **most** likely be initiated?
1. Counseling to produce insight into behavior
2. Biofeedback to reduce agitation associated with schizophrenia
3. Drug therapy to reduce symptoms associated with acute schizophrenia
4. Electroconvulsive therapy to treat the mood component of schizophrenia

32. **3.** Drug therapy is usually successful in normalizing behavior and reducing or eliminating hallucinations, delusions, thought disorder, affect flattening, apathy, avolition, and asociality. Counseling to produce insight into the client's behavior usually isn't effective in an acute schizophrenic reaction. Biofeedback reduces anxiety and modifies behavioral responses but isn't the major component in the treatment of schizophrenia. Electroconvulsive therapy might be considered for schizoaffective disorder (which has a mood component) and is a treatment of choice for clinical depression.
CN: Psychosocial integrity; CNS: None; CL: Apply; DIFFICULTY: Moderate

33. A client states to the nurse, "The voices are telling me to do terrible things." As part of the client's initial therapy, which action would be **most** likely included?
1. Find out what the voices are saying.
2. Let the client go to his room to decrease anxiety.
3. Begin to talk to the client about an unrelated topic.
4. Tell the client the voices aren't real.

33. **1.** For safety purposes, the nurse must find out whether the voices are directing the client to harm himself or others. Further assessment can help identify appropriate therapeutic interventions. Isolating a person during this intense sensory confusion commonly reinforces the psychosis. Changing the topic indicates that the nurse isn't concerned about the client's fears. Dismissing the voices shuts down communication between the client and the nurse.
CN: Safe, effective care environment; CNS: Safety and infection Control; CL: Apply; DIFFICULTY: Easy

34. A newly admitted client diagnosed with schizophrenia tells the nurse, "The police are looking for me and will kill me if I am found." The nurse recognizes that the client is exhibiting which type of delusion?
1. Paranoid
2. Religious
3. Grandiose
4. Somatic

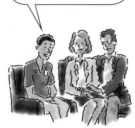

No, Mrs. Johnston, I'm not an operative with the CIA. I'm just your nurse.

35. A client is prescribed haloperidol. When reinforcing the teaching plan about the drug, which instruction would the nurse emphasize?
1. "You should report feelings of restlessness or agitation at once."
2. "You can take your herbal supplements safely with this drug."
3. "Be aware that you'll feel increased energy taking this drug."
4. "This drug will indirectly control essential hypertension."

36. The nurse is interacting with a client experiencing delusions. Which action would be **most** appropriate for the nurse to do?
1. Tell the client the delusions aren't real.
2. Explain the delusion to the client.
3. Encourage the client to remain delusional.
4. Identify the meaning of the delusion.

37. A nurse is collecting data from a client diagnosed with schizophrenia. Which symptoms would the nurse identify as supporting the client's diagnosis?
1. Persistent, intrusive thoughts leading to repetitive, ritualistic behaviors
2. Feelings of helplessness and hopelessness
3. Unstable moods and delusions of grandeur
4. Hallucinations or delusions and decreased ability to function in society

38. The nurse is caring for a client diagnosed with schizophrenia. The client says, "The earth and the roof of the house rule the political structure with particles of rain." The nurse interprets this statement as which type of expression?
1. Tangentiality
2. Perseveration
3. Loose association
4. Thought blocking

34. 1. This client is exhibiting paranoid delusions, which are excessive or irrational suspicions or distrust of others. A religious delusion is the belief that one is favored by a higher being or is an instrument of a higher being. A grandiose delusion is the belief that one possesses greatness or special powers. A somatic delusion is the belief that one's body or body parts are distorted or diseased.
CN: Psychosocial integrity; CNS: None; CL: Apply; DIFFICULTY: Easy

35. 1. Agitation and restlessness are adverse effects of haloperidol that can be treated with anticholinergic drugs. Using herbal supplements while taking haloperidol may interfere with the drug's effectiveness. Although the client may experience increased concentration and activity, these effects are due to a decrease in symptoms, not to the drug itself. Haloperidol isn't likely to cause essential hypertension.
CN: Physiological integrity; CNS: Pharmacological therapies; CL: Apply; DIFFICULTY: Easy

36. 4. Identifying the meaning of the delusion helps the client understand and begin to develop strategies for dealing with these thought processes. Never argue with or try to talk the client out of a delusion. The delusions are very real to the client. Explaining the delusions helps the nurse, not the client. Encouraging the client to remain delusional isn't therapeutic.
CN: Psychosocial integrity; CNS: None; CL: Apply; DIFFICULTY: Moderate

37. 4. Schizophrenia is a brain disease characterized by a variety of symptoms, including hallucinations, delusions, and asociality. Clients with obsessive-compulsive disorder experience intrusive thoughts and ritualistic behaviors. Feelings of helplessness and hopelessness are pivotal symptoms of clinical depression. Unstable moods and delusions of grandeur are characteristics of bipolar affective disorder.
CN: Psychosocial integrity; CNS: None; CL: Apply; DIFFICULTY: Easy

38. 3. Loose association refers to changing ideas from one unrelated theme to another, as exhibited by this client. Tangentiality is wandering from topic to topic. Perseveration is involuntary repetition of the answer to a question in response to a new question. Thought blocking is difficulty articulating a response or stopping in midsentence.
CN: Psychosocial integrity; CNS: None; CL: Apply; DIFFICULTY: Moderate

39. During the initial interview, a client with schizophrenia tells the nurse, "I don't enjoy things anymore. I used to love to read mystery books, but even that isn't enjoyable now." The nurse correctly identifies that the client is experiencing which condition?

1. Avolition
2. Anhedonia
3. Alogia
4. Flat affect

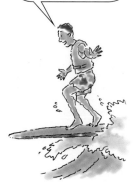

I don't know what my therapist is talking about … I feel perfectly balanced.

39. 2. Anhedonia is the loss of pleasure in things that are usually pleasurable. Avolition is the lack of motivation. Alogia, also called poverty of speech, is a decrease in the amount of richness of speech. A flat affect is absence of emotional expression.
CN: Psychosocial integrity; CNS: None; CL: Apply;
DIFFICULTY: Moderate

40. A client is admitted after being found on a highway, throwing rocks and debris and yelling at motorists. When approached by the nurse, the client shouts, "You're the one who stole my husband from me." The nurse interprets the client's statement as indicating which condition?

1. Hallucinatory experience
2. Delusional experience
3. Disorientation to the environment
4. Need for limit-setting from the staff

40. 2. A delusion is a false belief manufactured without appropriate or sufficient evidence to support it. The client's statement isn't a hallucination because it isn't a perceptual disorder. The question doesn't provide information about orientation. Although limit-setting is integral to a safe environment, the client's statement reflects self-esteem issues.
CN: Psychosocial integrity; CNS: None; CL: Apply;
DIFFICULTY: Easy

41. A nurse is working with the interdisciplinary team on a teaching plan for educating the family of a client with schizophrenia. Which information would be **most** important to include?

1. Relapse can be prevented if the client takes medication.
2. Support is available to help family members meet their own needs.
3. Improvement should occur if the client has a stimulating environment.
4. Stressful situations in the family can precipitate a relapse in the client.

41. 2. Because family members of a client with schizophrenia face difficult situations and great stress, the nurse should inform them of support services that can help them cope. The nurse should also teach them that medication can't prevent relapses and that environmental stimuli may precipitate symptoms. Although stress can trigger symptoms, the nurse shouldn't make the family feel responsible for the client's relapses.
CN: Health promotion and maintenance; CNS: None; CL: Apply;
DIFFICULTY: Challenge

42. A nurse on an inpatient unit is having a discussion with a client with schizophrenia about the schedule for the day. The client comments being highly active at home, then explains the volunteer job held. The nurse interprets this discussion as reflecting which aspect about the client's thinking?

1. Circumstantiality
2. Loose associations
3. Referential
4. Tangentiality

42. 4. Tangentiality describes thought patterns loosely connected, but not directly related, to the topic. In circumstantiality, the person digresses with unnecessary details. Loose associations are rapid shifts in the expression of ideas from one subject to another in an unrelated manner. An individual who demonstrates referential thinking incorrectly interprets neutral incidents and external events as having a particular or special meaning for him.
CN: Psychosocial integrity; CNS: None; CL: Apply;
DIFFICULTY: Difficult

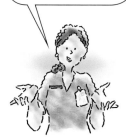

I come up with neo worgs all the time … do you think it's anything to be consterned about?

43. While talking to a client with schizophrenia, a nurse notes that the client frequently uses unrecognizable words that have not been accepted into mainstream language. How does the nurse document this finding?

1. Echolalia
2. Clang association
3. Neologism
4. Word salad

43. 3. Neologisms are newly coined words with personal meaning to the client with schizophrenia. Word salads are words strung in sequence that have no connection to one another. Echolalia is parrotlike echoing of spoken words or sounds. Clanging is the association of words by sound rather than meaning.
CN: Psychosocial integrity; CNS: None; CL: Apply; DIFFICULTY: Moderate

44. While caring for a hospitalized client diagnosed with schizophrenia, a nurse observes the client watching television. The client states, "The television is speaking directly to me." The nurse interprets the client's statement as indicating which type of thinking?
1. Autistic
2. Concrete
3. Paranoid
4. Referential

44. 4. Referential, or primary process, thinking is a belief that incidents and events in the environment have special meaning for the client. Autistic thinking is a disturbance in thought due to the intrusion of a private, internally stimulated fantasy world, resulting in abnormal responses to people. Concrete thinking is the literal interpretation of words and symbols. A client with paranoid thinking believes that others are trying to harm him.
CN: Psychosocial integrity; CNS: None; CL: Understand; DIFFICULTY: Challenge

45. A client diagnosed with schizophrenia has been taking haloperidol for 1 week when a nurse observes that the client's gaze is fixed on the ceiling. The nurse reports this finding as which condition?
1. Akathisia
2. Neuroleptic malignant syndrome
3. Oculogyric crisis
4. Tardive dyskinesia

45. 3. An oculogyric crisis involves a fixed positioning of the eyes, typically in an upward gaze. The condition is uncomfortable but not life-threatening. Akathisia is a restlessness that can cause pacing and tapping of the fingers or feet. High fever, sweating, unstable blood pressure, stupor, and muscular rigidity are signs of neuroleptic malignant syndrome. Stereotyped involuntary movements (tongue protrusion, lip smacking, chewing, blinking, and grimacing) characterize tardive dyskinesia.
CN: Physiological integrity; CNS: Pharmacological therapies; CL: Apply; DIFFICULTY: Moderate

46. A client with schizophrenia becomes agitated and confronts the nurse with clenched fists. Which action would be the **priority** for the nurse to do?
1. Take the client by the hand and lead him to the activity room for a game of cards.
2. Step up to the client and state that this behavior is inappropriate.
3. Call for security to take the client to a seclusion room.
4. Speak to the client in a quiet voice and offer medication to help calm down.

> Understanding medication side effects can help keep a client healthy.

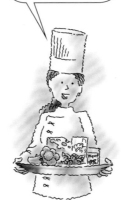

46. 4. Always use the least restrictive means to calm a client. Never touch an agitated client; touch can be misinterpreted as a threat and further escalate the situation. Stepping up to an agitated client can be seen as an aggressive act. Seclusion is a last resort.
CN: Safe, effective care environment; CNS: Safety and infection control; CL: Apply; DIFFICULTY: Moderate

47. A client is prescribed fluphenazine and is given discharge instructions. Which statement by a client indicates that the discharge education was successful?
1. "I need to stay out of the sun."
2. "I need to drink plenty of fluids."
3. "I can't eat any aged cheese."
4. "I need to plan rest periods throughout the day."

47. 1. Fluphenazine is an antipsychotic drug that can cause photosensitivity and sunburn. Clients taking this drug don't need to increase fluid intake, avoid cheeses, or plan rest periods.
CN: Physiological integrity; CNS: Pharmacological therapies; CL: Analyze; DIFFICULTY: Difficult

48. A client approaches the nurse and points at the sky, showing the nurse where the scary people would be coming from to get them. Which response is **most** therapeutic?
1. "Why do you think the people are coming here?"
2. "You're safe here; we won't let them harm you."
3. "It seems like the world is pretty scary for you, but you're safe here."
4. "There are no bad people in the sky because no one lives that close to Earth."

48. 3. Explaining that the world is scary but that the client is safe acknowledges the client's fears and feelings and offers a sense of security as the nurse tries to understand the symbolism. The nurse reflects these concerns to the client, along with reassurance of safety. The first response validates the delusion, not the feelings and fears, and doesn't orient the client to reality. The second response gives false reassurance; since the nurse isn't sure of the symbolism, and can't make this promise. The last response rejects the client's feelings and doesn't address the fears.
CN: Psychosocial integrity; CNS: None; CL: Apply; DIFFICULTY: Moderate

49. The nurse monitoring a client who appears to be hallucinating notes paranoid content in the client's speech. The client appears agitated, gesturing at a figure on the television. Which nursing intervention is appropriate? Select all that apply.
1. Instruct the client to stop the behavior.
2. Reassure the client that there is no danger.
3. Acknowledge the presence of the hallucinations.
4. Instruct other team members to ignore the client's behavior.
5. Immediately apply physical restraints.
6. Use a calm voice and simple commands.

50. A client with schizophrenia is taking clozapine, an atypical antipsychotic medication. On a follow-up visit, while collecting data, which signs and symptoms would be **most** concerning to the nurse? Select all that apply.
1. Sore throat
2. Pill-rolling movements
3. Polyuria
4. Fever
5. Polydipsia
6. Orthostatic hypotension

51. A health care provider starts a client on haloperidol. Based on the nurse's understanding of possible extrapyramidal adverse effects with this medication, which measure should the nurse take when administering this drug? Select all that apply.
1. Review subcutaneous injection technique.
2. Closely monitor vital signs, especially temperature.
3. Provide the client with the opportunity to pace.
4. Monitor blood glucose levels.
5. Provide the client with sugarless hard candy.
6. Monitor for signs and symptoms of urticaria.

49. 2, 3, 6. Using a calm voice, the nurse should reassure the client that he is safe. Do not challenge the client; rather, acknowledge the hallucinatory experience. It isn't appropriate to request that the client stop the behavior or instruct other team members to ignore the client's behavior. Implementing restraints isn't warranted at this time. Although the client is agitated, no evidence exists that there is a risk for harming self or others.
CN: Psychosocial integrity; CNS: None; CL: Apply; DIFFICULTY: Moderate

50. 1, 4. Sore throat, fever, and sudden onset of other flulike symptoms are signs of agranulocytosis, an adverse effect of clozapine caused by an insufficient number of granulocytes. This causes the client to be susceptible to infection. The client's white blood cell count should be monitored at least weekly throughout the course of treatment. Pill-rolling movements can occur in those experiencing extrapyramidal adverse effects associated with antipsychotic medication that is prescribed for much longer than a medication such as clozapine. Polydipsia (excessive thirst) and polyuria (increased urine) are common adverse effects of lithium. Orthostatic hypotension is an adverse effect of tricyclic antidepressants.
CN: Physiological integrity; CNS: Pharmacological therapies; CL: Apply; DIFFICULTY: Difficult

51. 2, 3, 5. Neuroleptic malignant syndrome is a life-threatening extrapyramidal adverse effect of antipsychotic medications such as haloperidol. It's associated with a rapid increase in temperature. The most common extrapyramidal adverse effect, akathisia, is a form of psychomotor restlessness that can commonly be relieved by pacing. The anticholinergic medications provided to alleviate the extrapyramidal effects of haloperidol can result in dry mouth. Providing the client with sugarless hard candy to suck on can help alleviate this problem. Haloperidol isn't given subcutaneously and doesn't affect blood glucose levels. Urticaria isn't usually associated with this drug's administration.
CN: Physiological integrity; CNS: Pharmacological therapies; CL: Analyze; DIFFICULTY: Challenge

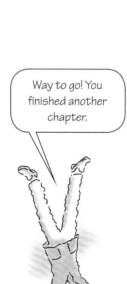

Way to go! You finished another chapter.

Chapter 17

Substance Use Disorders

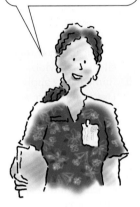

Substance use is serious business—as is answering these questions carefully and thoughtfully.

Substance use disorders refresher

Alcohol disorder

Problem drinking that becomes severe whether it be use or dependency

Key signs and symptoms
- History of alcohol intake
- History of blackouts
- Pathologic intoxication
- Symptoms of withdrawal

Key test results
- CAGE questionnaire responses indicate alcoholism
- Michigan Alcoholism Screening Test results indicate alcoholism

Key treatments
- Alcoholics Anonymous
- Individual therapy
- Rehabilitation
- Antidepressants: bupropion
- Anxiolytics: chlordiazepoxide, diazepam, lorazepam
- Disulfiram to prevent relapse into alcohol use
  - client must be alcohol-free for 12 hours before administering this drug
- Naltrexone to prevent relapse into alcohol use
- Selective serotonin reuptake inhibitors (SSRIs): fluoxetine, paroxetine

Key interventions
- Evaluate the client's use of alcohol as a coping mechanism
- Set limits on denial and rationalization
- Ask client to formulate goals for actions that will help maintain a lifestyle free from substance use

Cocaine use disorder

When use of cocaine harms a person's health or social functioning, or when a person has physical withdrawal symptoms when attempting to discontinue use of the drug

Key signs and symptoms
- Elevated energy and mood

- Grandiose thinking
- Impaired judgment

Key test results
- A drug screening is positive for cocaine

Key treatments
- Detoxification
- Rehabilitation (inpatient or outpatient)
- Narcotics Anonymous
- Individual therapy
- Anxiolytics: lorazepam, alprazolam
- Dopamine agent: bromocriptine
- Selective serotonin reuptake inhibitors (SSRIs): fluoxetine, paroxetine

Key interventions
- Establish a trusting relationship with client
- Provide client with well-balanced meals
- Set limits on client's attempts to rationalize behavior

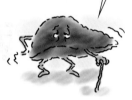

I've definitely been working too hard!

Other substance use disorders

Use or dependence on a drug leading to consequences that are negative to the individual's physical and/or mental health, and/or the well-being of others

Key signs and symptoms
- Blaming others for problems
- Development of physiologic or psychological need for a substance
- Dysfunctional anger
- Feelings of grandiosity
- Impulsiveness
- Use of denial and rationalization to explain consequences of behavior

Key test results
- A drug screening is positive for the used substance

Key treatments
- Individual therapy
- Clonidine for opiate withdrawal symptoms
- Methadone maintenance for opiate addiction detoxification

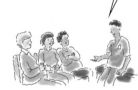

Discussing substance abuse is especially important during pregnancy, as many drugs can harm the fetus.

Key interventions

- Ensure a safe, quiet environment free from stimuli
- Monitor for withdrawal symptoms, such as tremors, seizures, and anxiety
- Help the client understand the consequences of substance use
- Encourage the client to vent fear and anger

the Point® You can download tables of drug information to help you prepare for the NCLEX®! View Generic Drug Names, Drug Classifications, Drug Actions, and Nursing Implications for the drugs discussed in this refresher at **http://thePoint.lww.com**.

Substance use disorders questions, answers, and rationales

1. Family members of a client who uses alcohol ask a nurse to help them intervene. Which action is essential for a successful intervention?
   1. All family members must tell the client they're powerless.
   2. All family members must describe how the addiction affects them.
   3. All family members must come up with their share of financial support.
   4. All family members must become caregivers during the detoxification period.

2. A client who uses alcohol tells a nurse, "I'm sure I can become a social drinker." Which response is **most** appropriate?
   1. "When do you think you can become a social drinker?"
   2. "What makes you think you'll learn to drink normally?"
   3. "What examples of major problems in your life are related to your alcohol use?"
   4. "How many alcoholic beverages does a social drinker consume?"

3. A nurse is observing a client for signs of alcohol withdrawal. During the period of early withdrawal, what would the nurse expect to find?
   1. Depression
   2. Hypotension
   3. Insomnia
   4. Nausea

4. A client asks a nurse not to tell the parents about an alcohol problem. Which response is **most** appropriate?
   1. "How can you not tell them? Is that being honest?"
   2. "Don't you think you'll need to tell them someday?"
   3. "Do alcohol problems run in either side of your family?"
   4. "What do you think will happen if you tell your parents?"

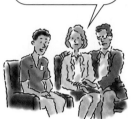

With substance abuse, the whole family needs to be involved in treatment.

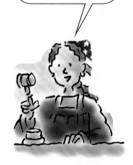

Avoid being judgmental with clients struggling with addiction problems.

1. 2. After the family is taught about addiction, they must write down examples of how the addiction has affected each of them and use this information during the intervention. The client shouldn't be told the family is powerless. The family is empowered through this intervention experience. In many cases, a third-party payer will help with treatment costs. Participating in an intervention doesn't make family members responsible for financial support or for providing care and support during the detoxification period.
CN: Psychosocial integrity; CNS: None; CL: Analyze; DIFFICULTY: Easy

2. 3. Asking the client to name the problems in the life related to alcohol use may help the client recall the troublesome results of using alcohol, as well as the reasons why treatment began. Asking when the client believes he can begin social drinking only encourages the addicted client to deny the problem and develop an unrealistic, self-defeating goal. Asking how many alcoholic beverages a social drinker can consume and why the client thinks he can drink normally encourages the addicted client to defend himself and deny alcohol use problem.
CN: Psychosocial integrity; CNS: None; CL: Apply;
DIFFICULTY: Challenge

3. 4. Nausea and subsequent vomiting are early signs of alcohol withdrawal. Depression, hypotension, and insomnia aren't associated with early alcohol withdrawal.
CN: Psychosocial integrity; CNS: None; CL: Apply;
DIFFICULTY: Moderate

4. 4. Clients who struggle with addiction problems commonly believe people will be judgmental, rejecting, and uncaring if they're told that the client is recovering from alcohol use. The first response challenges the client and will put him on the defensive. The second response will make the client defensive and apt to construct rationalizations about why the parents don't need to know. The third response is a good assessment question, but it isn't appropriate to ask a client who's afraid to tell others about the addiction.
CN: Psychosocial integrity; CNS: None; CL: Analyze DIFFICULTY: Easy

CN: Client needs category   CNS: Client needs subcategory   CL: Cognitive level

5. The nurse is assessing a client with prolonged, chronic alcohol intake. Which finding would the nurse expect?
   1. Enlarged liver
   2. Nasal irritation
   3. Muscle wasting
   4. Limb paresthesia

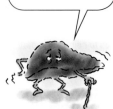

When you abuse alcohol, you abuse me.

6. Within 8 hours of the last drink, an alcoholic client experiences tremors, loss of appetite, and disordered thinking. The nurse believes this client is exhibiting signs of alcohol withdrawal. What is the **priority** action by the nurse?
   1. Give disulfiram as prescribed.
   2. Obtain a health care provider's order for lorazepam.
   3. Help the client engage in progressive muscle-relaxation techniques.
   4. Provide the client with constant one-on-one monitoring.

7. A client who uses alcohol tells a nurse, "Alcohol helps me sleep." Which information about alcohol use affecting sleep is **most** accurate?
   1. Alcohol doesn't help promote sleep.
   2. Continued alcohol use causes insomnia.
   3. One glass of alcohol at dinnertime can induce sleep.
   4. Sometimes, alcohol can make one drowsy enough to fall asleep.

8. A client withdrawing from alcohol is given lorazepam. The nurse reinforces education for the client and family about the drug. Which response by a family member indicates that the nurse's education has been successful?
   1. "Short-term use of lorazepam can lead to dependency."
   2. "The lorazepam will reduce the symptoms of withdrawal."
   3. "The lorazepam will make the client forget about the symptoms of withdrawal."
   4. "The lorazepam will also help with heart disease."

9. A client with chronic alcoholism may be predisposed to develop which condition?
   1. Arteriosclerosis
   2. Heart failure
   3. Heart valve damage
   4. Pericarditis

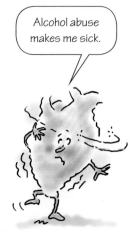

Alcohol abuse makes me sick.

5. 1. A major effect of alcohol on the body is liver impairment, and an enlarged liver is a common physical finding. Nasal irritation is commonly seen in clients who snort cocaine. Muscle wasting and limb paresthesia don't tend to occur in clients who use alcohol.
CN: Physiological integrity; CNS: Physiological adaptation; CL: Apply; DIFFICULTY: Easy

6. 2. A client in alcohol withdrawal should be medicated with a benzodiazepine, such as lorazepam, to prevent progression of symptoms to delirium tremens, a life-threatening withdrawal syndrome. Disulfiram is used during early recovery, not during detoxification. Progressive muscle relaxation isn't particularly effective during withdrawal. Close monitoring during withdrawal is appropriate after the client has been medicated for withdrawal symptoms.
CN: Psychosocial integrity; CNS: None; CL: Apply; DIFFICULTY: Moderate

7. 2. Alcohol use may initially promote sleep but, with continued use, it causes insomnia. Evidence shows that alcohol doesn't facilitate sleep. One glass of alcohol at dinnertime won't induce sleep. Stating that alcohol can make one drowsy enough to fall asleep doesn't give information about how alcohol adversely affects sleep. It encourages the client to think alcohol use to induce sleep is an appropriate strategy.
CN: Psychosocial integrity; CNS: None; CL: Analyze; DIFFICULTY: Moderate

8. 2. Lorazepam is a short-acting benzodiazepine that may be given for approximately 4 days to help the client in alcohol withdrawal. However, there's some debate over its use due to a potential risk for cross-addiction. The medication isn't given to help forget the experience. Benzodiazepines counteract the central nervous system stimulation of the withdrawal syndrome to lessen the symptoms of withdrawal. Lorazepam isn't used to treat coexisting cardiovascular problems or promote a sense of well-being.
CN: Physiological integrity; CNS: Pharmacological therapies; CL: Apply; DIFFICULTY: Easy

9. 2. Heart failure is a severe cardiac consequence associated with long-term alcohol use. Arteriosclerosis, heart valve damage, and pericarditis aren't medical consequences of alcoholism.
CN: Physiological integrity; CNS: Reduction of risk potential; CL: Understand; DIFFICULTY: Moderate

10. A client who uses alcohol tells a nurse that everyone in the family has an alcohol problem, and nothing can be done about it. Which response is **most** appropriate?
1. "You're right; it's much harder to become a recovering person."
2. "This is just an excuse for you so you don't have to work on becoming sober."
3. "Sometimes nothing can be done, but you may be the exception in your family."
4. "Alcohol problems can occur in families, but you can decide to take the steps to become and stay sober."

11. Which finding does the nurse recognize is commonly associated with use of alcohol in a young, depressed adult woman?
1. Defiant responses
2. Infertility
3. Memory loss
4. Sexual abuse

12. A nurse determines that a client who used alcohol has nutritional problems. Which strategy is **best** for addressing the client's nutritional needs?
1. Encourage the client to eat a diet high in calories.
2. Help the client to recognize and follow a balanced diet.
3. Provide the client with liquid protein supplements daily.
4. Ask the client to monitor the calories consumed each day.

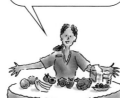

Just look at all these nutritious choices.

13. A client with a history of alcohol use refuses to take vitamins. Which statement is **most** appropriate for explaining why vitamins are important?
1. "It's important to take vitamins to stop your craving."
2. "Prolonged use of alcohol can cause vitamin depletion."
3. "For every vitamin you take, you'll help your liver heal."
4. "By taking vitamins, you won't need to worry about your diet."

14. A client arrives in the emergency department via rescue squad with a suspected opiate overdose. Which medication prescribed by the health care provider does the nurse prepare to administer?
1. Bupropion
2. Fluoxetine
3. Diazepam
4. Naloxone

10. 4. Stating that alcohol problems can run in families, but that a decision can be made to become sober, challenges the client to become proactive and take the steps necessary to maintain a sober lifestyle. Telling the client he is right and that recovery is hard agrees with the client's denial and isn't a useful response. Telling the client that his statement is just an excuse confronts the client and may make the client more adamant to continue alcohol use. Telling the client that he may be the exception to a typically hard-to-combat problem agrees with the client's denial and isn't a useful response.
CN: Psychosocial integrity; CNS: None; CL: Apply; DIFFICULTY: Easy

11. 4. Many women diagnosed with substance use problems also have a history of physical or sexual abuse. Alcohol use isn't a common finding in a young woman showing defiant behavior or experiencing infertility. Memory loss isn't expected in a young woman dealing with alcohol use.
CN: Psychosocial integrity; CNS: None; CL: Understand; DIFFICULTY: Easy

12. 2. Clients who use alcohol are commonly malnourished and need help to follow a balanced diet; this is especially important because episodes of hypoglycemia and hyperglycemia may occur due to the high sugar content of alcohol. Increasing calories may cause the client to eat empty calories. The client must be involved in the decision to supplement daily dietary intake; the nurse can't force the client to drink liquid protein supplements. Asking the client to monitor calorie intake could be done only after the client recognizes the need to maintain a balanced diet. Calorie counts aren't needed in most recovering clients who begin to eat from basic food groups.
CN: Physiological integrity; CNS: Basic care and comfort; CL: Understand; DIFFICULTY: Easy

13. 2. Chronic alcoholism interferes with the metabolism of many vitamins. Vitamin supplements can prevent deficiencies. Taking vitamins won't stop the craving for alcohol or help a damaged liver heal. A balanced diet is essential in addition to taking multivitamins.
CN: Physiological integrity; CNS: Basic care and comfort; CL: Apply; DIFFICULTY: Easy

14. 4. The antidote for opiate overdose is naloxone.
CN: Physiological integrity; CNS: Pharmacological therapies; CL: Apply; DIFFICULTY: Easy

15. A nurse is caring for a client who typically consumes 15 to 20 beers per week and is extremely defensive about alcohol intake. The client admits to experiencing blackouts and has had three alcohol-related motor vehicle crashes. What's the **best** action for this client?
1. Monitor alcohol intake.
2. Switch to low-alcohol beer or wine coolers.
3. Limit intake to no more than three beers per drinking occasion.
4. Abstain from alcohol altogether.

16. A nurse is caring for a client who's undergoing treatment for acute alcohol dependence. The client tells the nurse, "I don't have a problem. My spouse made me come here." Which defense mechanism does the nurse determine the client is using?
1. Projection and suppression
2. Denial and rationalization
3. Rationalization and repression
4. Suppression and denial

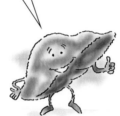

Encourage clients with alcohol disorder to seek treatment. Their livers will thank you.

17. Which short-term goal should be a **priority** for a client with a knowledge deficit about the effects of alcohol on the body?
1. Test blood chemistries daily.
2. Verbalize the results of substance use.
3. Talk to a pharmacist about the substance.
4. Attend a weekly aerobic exercise program.

18. A nurse is assigned to care for a recently admitted client who has attempted suicide. What is a **priority** nursing action?
1. Search the client's belongings and room carefully for items that could be used to attempt suicide.
2. Express trust that the client won't cause self-harm while in the facility.
3. Respect the client's privacy and don't search any belongings.
4. Remind all staff members to check on the client frequently.

15. 4. This client demonstrates behaviors consistent with addiction. Once addicted, the only way to control intake is to abstain altogether—monitoring or limiting intake or switching to low-alcoholic drinks won't work for this client.
CN: Psychosocial integrity; CNS: None; CL: Apply; DIFFICULTY: Moderate

16. 2. The client is using denial and rationalization. Denial is the unconscious disclaimer of unacceptable thoughts, feelings, needs, or certain external factors. Rationalization is the unconscious effort to justify intolerable feelings, behaviors, and motives. The client isn't using projection, suppression, or repression. Emotions, behavior, and motives, which are consciously intolerable, are denied and then attributed to others in projection. Suppression is a conscious effort to control and conceal unacceptable ideas and impulses into the unconscious. Repression is the unconscious placement of unacceptable feelings into the unconscious mind.
CN: Physiological integrity; CNS: Physiological adaptation; CL: Apply; DIFFICULTY: Easy

17. 2. It's important for the client to talk about the health consequences of the continued use of alcohol. Testing blood chemistries daily gives the client minimal knowledge about the effects of alcohol on the body and isn't the most useful information in an education plan. A pharmacist isn't the appropriate health care professional to educate the client about the effects of alcohol use on the body. Although exercise is an important goal of self-care, it doesn't address the client's knowledge deficit about the effects of alcohol on the body.
CN: Safe, effective care environment; CNS: Coordinated care; CL: Apply; DIFFICULTY: Easy

18. 1. Because a client who has attempted suicide could try again, the nurse should search the client's belongings and room to remove any items that could be used in another suicide attempt; the need to maintain a safe environment supersedes the client's right to privacy. Expressing trust that the client won't cause self-harm may increase the client's guilt and pain if he can't live up to that trust. Frequent checks by staff members aren't enough because the client may attempt suicide between checks.
CN: Safe, effective care environment; CNS: Safety and infection control; CL: Apply; DIFFICULTY: Easy

19. A client experiencing alcohol withdrawal says he is worried about periodic hallucinations. Which intervention is **best** for this client's problem?
1. Pointing out that the sensation doesn't exist
2. Allowing the client to talk about the experience
3. Encouraging the client to wash body areas well
4. Determining if the client has a cognitive impairment

20. A client who has been drinking alcohol for 30 years asks a nurse if the immune system has suffered permanent damage. Which response is **best**?
1. "There's usually less resistance to infections."
2. "Sometimes, the body's metabolism will increase."
3. "Put your energies into maintaining sobriety for now."
4. "Drinking puts you at high risk for disease later in life."

21. A client experiencing alcohol withdrawal is upset about going through detoxification. Which goal is the **priority**?
1. The client will commit to a drug-free lifestyle.
2. The client will work with the nurse to remain safe.
3. The client will drink plenty of fluids on a daily basis.
4. The client will make a personal inventory of strengths.

22. A client recovering from alcohol use needs to develop effective coping skills to handle daily stressors. Which intervention is **most** useful to the client?
1. Determining the client's verbal skills
2. Helping the client avoid conflict
3. Discussing examples of successful coping behavior
4. Educating the client about accepting uncomfortable situations

23. A client is struggling with alcohol dependence. Which communication strategy would be **most** effective for the nurse?
1. Speak briefly and directly.
2. Avoid blaming or preaching to the client.
3. Confront feelings and examples of perfectionism.
4. Determine if nonverbal communication will be more effective.

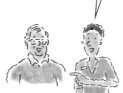

When your client expresses concern about his symptoms, listen up!

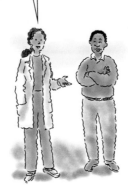

Alcohol dependence is a disease. Listen empathetically to your client.

19. 2. The client needs to talk about the periodic hallucinations to prevent them from becoming triggers to aggressive behaviors and possible self-injury. The client's experience of sensory-perceptual alterations must be acknowledged. Determining if the client has a cognitive impairment and encouraging the client to wash body areas well don't address the problem of periodic hallucinations.
CN: Psychosocial integrity; CNS: None; CL: Apply; DIFFICULTY: Easy

20. 1. Chronic alcohol use depresses the immune system and causes increased susceptibility to infections. A nutritionally well-balanced diet that includes foods high in protein and B vitamins will help develop a strong immune system. The potential damage to the immune system doesn't increase the body's metabolism. Encouraging sobriety negates the client's concern and isn't an appropriate or caring response by the nurse. Drinking alcohol may put the client at risk for immune system problems at any time in life.
CN: Physiological integrity; CNS: Physiological adaptation; CL: Analyze; DIFFICULTY: Challenge

21. 2. The most important goal is client safety. Although drinking enough fluids, identifying personal strengths, and committing to a drug-free lifestyle are important goals, promoting client safety must be the nurse's priority.
CN: Psychosocial integrity; CNS: None; CL: Analyze; DIFFICULTY: Moderate

22. 3. The client needs help identifying a successful coping behavior and developing ways to incorporate that behavior into daily functioning. There are many skills for coping with stress; determining the client's level of verbal skills may be unrelated. Encouraging the client to avoid conflict or to accept uncomfortable situations prevents him from learning skills to handle daily stressors.
CN: Psychosocial integrity; CNS: None; CL: Analyze; DIFFICULTY: Easy

23. 2. Blaming or preaching to the client should be avoided because the negativity created prevents the client from hearing what the nurse has to say. Speaking briefly to the client may not allow time for adequate communication. Perfectionism doesn't tend to be an issue. Determining if nonverbal communication will be more effective is better suited to a client with a cognitive impairment.
CN: Psychosocial integrity; CNS: None; CL: Analyze; DIFFICULTY: Easy

24. A client signed herself into an alcohol treatment program. During the first visit with the nurse, the client vehemently maintains there is no problem with alcohol and states that she is in the program only because the spouse issued an ultimatum. What is the **best** response by the nurse?
1. "I wonder why your spouse would issue such an ultimatum."
2. "Because you came voluntarily, you're free to leave anytime you wish."
3. "From your point of view, what is most important for me to know about you?"
4. "You sound pretty definite about not having a problem with alcohol."

25. A client recovering from alcohol addiction has limited coping skills. Which characteristic would indicate relationship problems?
1. The client is prone to panic attacks.
2. The client doesn't pay attention to details.
3. The client has poor problem-solving skills.
4. The client ignores the need to relax and rest.

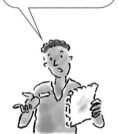

In question #26, you are looking for the best rationale for the suggested intervention.

26. A nurse suggests to a client struggling with alcohol addiction that keeping a journal may be helpful. Which reason **best** explains this?
1. The client can identify stressors and responses to them.
2. The client will be better able to understand the diagnosis.
3. The client can help others by reading the journal to them.
4. The client will develop an emergency plan for use in a crisis.

27. Which information is **most** important to use in an education plan for a client who has used alcohol?
1. Personal needs
2. Illness exacerbation
3. Cognitive distortions
4. Communication skills

28. A nurse is preparing for an education session with a client who uses alcohol. Which client assessment would be **most** important for the nurse to obtain?
1. Sleep patterns
2. Decision making
3. Willingness to learn
4. Communication skills

24. 3. Asking the client what is most important for the nurse to know about her allows the nurse to collect more information. Wondering why the spouse would issue an ultimatum focuses on the spouse, not the client. Telling the client she is free to leave is abrasive and blocks communication. Telling the client that she sounds definite about not having an alcohol problem doesn't allow for further exploration of the problem.
CN: Psychosocial integrity; CNS: None; CL: Apply;
DIFFICULTY: Moderate

25. 3. To have satisfying relationships, a person must be able to communicate and problem-solve. Relationship problems don't predispose people to panic attacks more than other psychosocial stressors. Paying attention to details isn't a major concern when addressing the client's relationship difficulties. Although ignoring the need for rest and relaxation is unhealthy, it shouldn't pose a major relationship problem.
CN: Psychosocial integrity; CNS: None; CL: Analyze;
DIFFICULTY: Moderate

26. 1. Keeping a journal enables the client to identify problems and patterns of coping. From this information, the difficulties the client faces can be addressed. A journal may help to promote better understanding of the client's illness. However, its primary purpose is to help the client gain insight. Journals aren't read to other people unless the client wants to share a particular part. Journals aren't typically used for identifying an emergency plan for use in a crisis.
CN: Psychosocial integrity; CNS: None; CL: Apply; DIFFICULTY: Easy

27. 4. Addicted clients commonly have difficulty communicating their needs in an appropriate way. Learning appropriate communication skills is a major goal of treatment. Next, behavior that focuses on the self and on meeting personal needs will be addressed. Educating clients about illness exacerbation isn't a skill, but it is essential for relaying information about relapse. Identifying cognitive distortions would be difficult if the client has poor communication skills.
CN: Psychosocial integrity; CNS: None; CL: Analyze;
DIFFICULTY: Difficult

28. 3. It's important to know if the client's current situation helps or hinders the potential to learn. Sleep patterns, decision making, and communication skills aren't factors that must be assessed before educating clients about addiction.
CN: Psychosocial integrity; CNS: None; CL: Analyze;
DIFFICULTY: Moderate

CN: Client needs category   CNS: Client needs subcategory   CL: Cognitive level

29. A nurse is developing strategies to prevent relapse with a client who uses alcohol. Which client intervention is important?
  1. Avoiding taking over-the-counter (OTC) medications
  2. Limiting monthly contact with the family
  3. Refraining from becoming involved in group activities
  4. Avoiding people, places, and activities from the former lifestyle

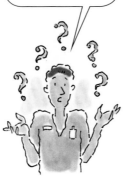

Is fielding clients' questions a key communication skill for nurses?

30. A client asks a nurse, "Why is it important to talk to my peers in group therapy?" Which response is **most** appropriate?
  1. "Group therapy lets you see what you're doing wrong in your life."
  2. "Group therapy acts as a defense against your disorganized behavior."
  3. "Group therapy provides a way to ask for support as well as to support others."
  4. "In group therapy, you can express your frustrations, and others will listen."

31. A family meeting is held with a client who uses alcohol. While listening to the family, which unhealthy communication pattern might be identified?
  1. Use of descriptive jargon
  2. Disapproval of behaviors
  3. Avoidance of issues that cause conflict
  4. Unlimited expression of nonverbal communication

32. A client addicted to alcohol begins individual therapy with a nurse. Which goal should be a **priority** for the client?
  1. Learning to express feelings
  2. Establishing new roles in the family
  3. Determining new strategies for socializing
  4. Decreasing preoccupation with physical health

33. When gathering data from a client with a history of polysubstance use, which information is a **priority** to obtain after the names of the drugs used?
  1. Oral administration of any drug
  2. Time of last use of each drug
  3. How the drugs were obtained
  4. The place the drugs were used

29. 4. Changing the client's old habits is essential for sustaining a sober lifestyle. Certain OTC medications that don't contain alcohol will probably need to be used by the client at certain times. It's unrealistic to have the client abstain from all such medications. Contact with the client's family may not be a trigger to relapse, so limiting contact wouldn't be useful. Refraining from group activities isn't a good strategy to prevent relapse. Attending Alcoholics Anonymous meetings and other support groups will help prevent relapse.
CN: Psychosocial integrity; CNS: None; CL: Analyze; DIFFICULTY: Easy

30. 3. The best response about attending group therapy is that it provides opportunities to communicate, learn, and give and get support. Group members will give a client feedback, not simply point out what a client is doing wrong. Group therapy isn't a defense against disorganized behavior. People can express all kinds of feelings and discuss a variety of topics in group therapy. Interactions are goal oriented and not just vehicles to express one's frustrations.
CN: Psychosocial integrity; CNS: None; CL: Apply; DIFFICULTY: Easy

31. 3. The interaction pattern of a family with a member who uses alcohol commonly revolves around denying the problem, avoiding conflict, or rationalizing the addiction. Health care providers are more likely to use jargon. The family might have problems setting limits and expressing disapproval of the client's behavior. Nonverbal communication usually gives the nurse insight into family dynamics.
CN: Psychosocial integrity; CNS: None; CL: Analyze; DIFFICULTY: Moderate

32. 1. The client must address issues, learn ways to cope effectively with life stressors, and express needs appropriately. Only after the client establishes sobriety can the possibility of taking on new roles become a reality. Determining new strategies for socializing isn't the priority goal for an addicted client. Usually, these clients need to change unhealthy socializing habits. Clients addicted to alcohol don't tend to be preoccupied with physical health problems.
CN: Safe, effective care environment; CNS: Coordinated care; CL: Analyze; DIFFICULTY: Easy

33. 2. The time of last use of each drug gives information about expected withdrawal symptoms of the drugs and what immediate treatment is necessary. How the drugs were obtained and places they were used aren't essential information for treatment, nor is the fact that they were consumed orally.
CN: Psychosocial integrity; CNS: None; CL: Apply; DIFFICULTY: Easy

34. A client recovering from alcohol addiction asks a nurse how to talk to the children about the impact of addiction on them. Which response by the nurse is **most** appropriate?
  1. "Try to limit references to the addiction and focus on the present."
  2. "Talk about all the hardships you've had in working to remain sober."
  3. "Tell them you're sorry and emphasize that you're doing so much better now."
  4. "Talk to them by acknowledging the difficulties and pain your drinking caused."

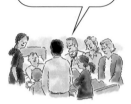

Families that suffer together also need to heal together.

34. 4. Part of the healing process for the family is to acknowledge the pain, embarrassment, and overall difficulties the client's drinking problem caused family members. Limiting references to the addiction facilitates the client's ability to deny the problem. Talking about the hardships of remaining sober prevents the client from acknowledging the difficulties his children endured. Just telling the children "I'm sorry" leads the client to believe only a simple apology is needed. The addiction must be addressed, and the children's pain acknowledged.
CN: Psychosocial integrity; CNS: None; CL: Apply; DIFFICULTY: Easy

35. A client with alcoholism has just completed a residential treatment program. What can this client reasonably expect?
  1. The family will no longer be dysfunctional.
  2. The client will need ongoing support to remain abstinent.
  3. The client doesn't need to be concerned about abusing alcohol in the future.
  4. The client can learn to consume alcohol without problems.

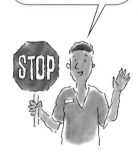

Remember to look for multiple right answers in "select all that apply" questions.

35. 2. Addiction is a relapsing illness. Support is helpful to most people in maintaining an abstinent lifestyle. The family dynamics probably will change as a result of the client's abstinence; however, there's no way to predict whether these changes will be healthy. A client with alcoholism will always remain at risk for abusing alcohol. Addicted people can't consume alcohol in moderation.
CN: Psychosocial integrity; CNS: None; CL: Apply; DIFFICULTY: Easy

36. A client says amphetamines are used to be productive at work. Which symptoms should the nurse monitor when the drug is discontinued? Select all that apply.
  1. Severe anxiety
  2. Increased agitation
  3. Altered perceptions
  4. Amotivational syndrome
  5. Nausea and vomiting

36. 1, 2. When amphetamines are abruptly discontinued, the client may experience severe anxiety or agitation. Altered perceptions occur when a client is withdrawing from hallucinogens. Amotivational syndrome is seen in clients using marijuana. Nausea and vomiting is often seen in heroin use when the drug is withheld.
CN: Psychosocial integrity; CNS: None; CL: Apply; DIFFICULTY: Difficult

37. A client is admitted with bone marrow depression and tells the nurse he has been abusing drugs for 7 years. Which drug should the nurse expect to find in the history?
  1. Amphetamines
  2. Cocaine
  3. Inhalants
  4. Marijuana

37. 3. Inhalants cause severe bone marrow depression. Amphetamines, cocaine, and marijuana don't cause bone marrow depression.
CN: Physiological integrity; CNS: Pharmacological therapies; CL: Apply; DIFFICULTY: Difficult

38. Which statement **best** explains why it's important to monitor behavior in a client who has stopped using phencyclidine (PCP)?
  1. Fatigue can cause feelings of being overwhelmed.
  2. Agitation and mood swings can occur during withdrawal.
  3. Bizarre behavior can be a precursor to a psychotic episode.
  4. Memory loss and forgetfulness can cause unsafe conditions.

38. 3. Bizarre behavior and speech are associated with PCP withdrawal and can indicate psychosis. Fatigue isn't necessarily a problem when a client stops using PCP. Agitation, mood swings, memory loss, and forgetfulness don't tend to occur when a client has stopped using PCP.
CN: Psychosocial integrity; CNS: None; CL: Analyze; DIFFICULTY: Challenge

39. Which information is **most** important for the nurse to teach a client who uses prescription drugs?
1. Herbal substitutes are safer to use.
2. Medication should be used only for the reason prescribed.
3. The client should consult a health care provider before using a drug.
4. Consider if family members influence the client to use drugs.

40. The family of an adolescent who smokes marijuana asks a nurse if the use of marijuana can be addicting. Which response is **best**?
1. "Use of marijuana is a stage your child will go through."
2. "Many people use marijuana and don't use other street drugs."
3. "Use of marijuana can lead to psychological dependence."
4. "It's difficult to answer that question, as I don't know your child."

41. Which test might be ordered for a client with a history of cocaine use who exhibits behavior changes following a return to an inpatient treatment facility?
1. Antibody screen
2. Glucose screen
3. Hepatic screen
4. Urine screen

42. A nurse is obtaining data from a client admitted to the emergency department with suspected overdose of an antianxiety agent. Which clinical manifestations does the nurse recognize correlate with this diagnosis?
1. Combativeness, sweating, and confusion
2. Agitation, hyperactivity, and grandiose ideation
3. Diminished reflexes, sedation, and impaired memory
4. Suspiciousness, dilated pupils, and increased blood pressure

43. Which clinical condition is commonly seen in substance use clients who repeatedly use cocaine?
1. Panic attacks
2. Bipolar cycling
3. Attention deficits
4. Expressive aphasia

44. A client who formerly used lysergic acid diethylamide (LSD) is seeking counseling. Which condition would be seen in this client's mental health history?
1. Lack of trust
2. Panic attacks
3. Recurrent depression
4. Loss of ego boundaries

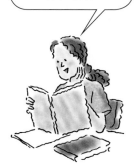

Do you remember which body system cocaine is most likely to affect?

39. 2. Drug users usually take prescribed drugs for reasons other than those intended, primarily to self-medicate or experience a sense of euphoria. The safety and efficacy of most herbal remedies hasn't been established. Sometimes, over-the-counter medications are necessary for minor problems that don't require consulting with a health care provider. There may be a family history of substance use, but it isn't the most important information to teach a client who uses prescription drugs.
CN: Psychosocial integrity; CNS: None; CL: Apply; DIFFICULTY: Easy

40. 3. Marijuana can cause psychological dependence. There is controversy over whether physiologic dependency can occur and whether it is a "gateway" drug leading to the use of more potent drugs. Marijuana use isn't part of a developmental stage that adolescents go through. It isn't important that the nurse know the child to address this question.
CN: Psychosocial integrity; CNS: None; CL: Apply; DIFFICULTY: Easy

41. 4. A urine toxicology screen would show the presence of cocaine in the body. Antibody, glucose, or hepatic screening wouldn't show the presence of cocaine in the body.
CN: Psychosocial integrity; CNS: None; CL: Apply; DIFFICULTY: Easy

42. 3. Signs of antianxiety agent overdose include diminished reflexes, sedation, and impaired memory. Phencyclidine overdose can cause combativeness, sweating, and confusion. Amphetamine overdose can result in agitation, hyperactivity, and grandiose ideation. Hallucinogen overdose can produce suspiciousness, dilated pupils, and increased blood pressure.
CN: Physiological integrity; CNS: Reduction of risk potential; CL: Apply; DIFFICULTY: Easy

43. 2. Clients who frequently use cocaine will experience the rapid cycling effect of excitement and then severe depression. They don't tend to experience panic attacks, attention deficits, or expressive aphasia.
CN: Psychosocial integrity; CNS: None; CL: Understand; DIFFICULTY: Difficult

44. 2. Clients who used LSD typically have a history of panic attacks or psychotic behavior, often referred to as a "bad trip." Loss of ego boundaries, recurrent depression, and lack of trust don't tend to be problems for former LSD users.
CN: Psychosocial integrity; CNS: None; CL: Analyze; DIFFICULTY: Difficult

CN: Client needs category   CNS: Client needs subcategory   CL: Cognitive level

45. Which statements by a client indicate that education about cocaine use has been effective? Select all that apply.
1. "I wasn't using cocaine to feel better about myself."
2. "I started using cocaine more and more until I couldn't stop."
3. "I'm addicted to cocaine even if I go days or weeks between use."
4. "I'm not going to be a chronic user. I only use it on holidays."
5. "I can still hang out with all my friends even though they use."

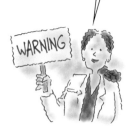

Clients recovering from cocaine use are at risk for experiencing depression.

WARNING

45. 2, 3. Using cocaine more and more until one can't stop reflects the trajectory, or common pattern, of cocaine use and indicates successful education. Cocaine users tend to be binge users and can be drug-free for days or weeks between use, but they still have a drug problem. The client who says he wasn't using cocaine to feel better about himself is in denial. People gravitate to the drug and continue its use because it gives them a sense of well-being, competency, and power. The client who decides to use cocaine on "holidays only" is in denial about the drug's potential to become habit forming; effective education hasn't occurred. "Hanging out" with old friends may create an environment that makes it difficult to avoid cocaine use.
CN: Psychosocial integrity; CNS: None; CL: Analyze; DIFFICULTY: Moderate

46. A nurse is assisting with the development of a care plan for a client recovering from cocaine use. Which intervention should be the nurse's **priority** for this client?
1. Providing meticulous skin care
2. Initiating suicide precautions
3. Establishing frequent orientation
4. Obtaining nutritional consultation

46. 2. Clients recovering from cocaine use are prone to "postcoke depression" and are likely to become suicidal if they can't take the drug. Skin care and frequent orientation are routine nursing interventions but aren't the most immediate considerations for this client. Nutrition consultation isn't the most pressing intervention for this client.
CN: Safe, effective care environment; CNS: Coordinated care; CL: Analyze; DIFFICULTY: Moderate

47. What should the nurse monitor the client for when the client is using phencyclidine (PCP)?
1. Cardiac arrest
2. Seizure disorder
3. Violent behavior
4. Delirium reaction

47. 3. When a client is using PCP, an acute psychotic reaction can occur. The client is capable of sudden, explosive, violent behavior. PCP doesn't tend to cause cardiac arrest or a seizure disorder. Delirium is associated with inhalant intoxication.
CN: Physiological integrity; CNS: Reduction of risk potential; CL: Apply; DIFFICULTY: Difficult

48. A client who smoked marijuana daily for 10 years tells a nurse, "I don't have any goals, and I just don't know what to do." Which communication technique is the **most** useful when talking to this client?
1. Focusing the interaction
2. Using nonverbal methods
3. Using reflection techniques
4. Using open-ended questions

Looks like all your studying has paid off. Well done!

48. 1. A client with amotivational syndrome from chronic use of marijuana tends to talk in tangents and needs the nurse to focus the conversation. Nonverbal communication or reflection techniques wouldn't be useful, as this client must focus and learn to identify and accomplish goals. Using only open-ended questions won't allow the client to focus and establish specific goals.
CN: Psychosocial integrity; CNS: None; CL: Apply; DIFFICULTY: Challenge

49. A nurse is obtaining data for physical health problems in a client who uses heroin. Which medical consequence of heroin does the nurse recognize commonly occurs?
1. Hepatitis
2. Peptic ulcers
3. Hypertension
4. Chronic pharyngitis

49. 1. Hepatitis is the most common medical complication of heroin use. Peptic ulcers are more likely to be a complication of caffeine use, hypertension is a complication of amphetamine use, and chronic pharyngitis is a complication of marijuana use.
CN: Physiological integrity; CNS: Reduction of risk potential; CL: Apply; DIFFICULTY: Easy

50. The family of a client who is a recovering heroin addict asks a nurse why the client is receiving naltrexone. Which response is correct?
1. "It's used to block the effects or 'high' produced by heroin."
2. "It's used to keep the client sedated during withdrawal."
3. "It takes the place of detoxification with methadone."
4. "It's given to decrease the client's memory of the withdrawal experience."

51. Which nursing intervention comprises the major component of a cocaine addiction treatment program?
1. Helping the client find ways to be happy and competent
2. Fostering the creative use of self in community activities
3. Educating the client about handling stresses in the work setting
4. Helping the client acknowledge the current level of dependency

52. A client tells a nurse, "I've been clean from drugs for the past 5 years, but my life really hasn't changed." Which concept should be explored with this client?
1. Further education
2. Conflict resolution
3. Career development
4. Personal development

53. A client discusses how drug addiction has made life unmanageable. Which information does the client need in the **later** part of the treatment process? Select all that apply.
1. How peers have committed to sobriety
2. How to accomplish family of origin work
3. The addiction process and tools for recovery
4. How environmental stimuli serve as drug triggers
5. Identification of addiction as a problem

54. A nurse is collecting data from a client with a history of cocaine use. Which condition might typically be found with this client?
1. Glossitis
2. Pharyngitis
3. Bilateral ear infections
4. Perforated nasal septum

50. 1. Naltrexone is an opioid antagonist that is used to help maintain sobriety by blocking and reversing the effects of opioids. Keeping the client sedated during withdrawal isn't the reason for giving this drug. The drug isn't used in place of detoxification with methadone and doesn't decrease the client's memory of the withdrawal experience.
CN: Physiological integrity; CNS: Reduction of risk potential; CL: Apply; DIFFICULTY: Challenge

51. 1. The major component of a treatment program for a client addicted to cocaine is to help the client discover ways to feel happy and competent without using the drug. Because clients typically credit cocaine for their achievements, helping them discover ways of achieving happiness and success without the drug are paramount. Fostering the creative use of self in community activities may encourage cocaine use because the client hasn't yet discovered drug-free ways of engaging in challenging activities. Educating the client about handling stress at work is appropriate but isn't the major component of treatment. Helping the client acknowledge the current level of dependency isn't a major treatment component because the client must first work on remaining drug-free.
CN: Psychosocial integrity; CNS: None; CL: Apply; DIFFICULTY: Challenge

52. 4. True recovery involves changing the client's distorted thinking and working on personal and emotional development. Before the client pursues further education, conflict resolution skills, or career development, it's imperative to devote energy to emotional and personal development.
CN: Psychosocial integrity; CNS: None; CL: Analyze; DIFFICULTY: Easy

53. 2, 4. Information about how peers have committed themselves to sobriety would be shared with the client as the treatment process *begins*. Family of origin work dealing with past family issues would be a *later* part of the treatment process. *Initially*, the client must commit to sobriety and learn skills for recovery. Identifying how environmental stimuli serve as drug triggers would be a *later* part of the treatment process. Identification of addiction as a problem is the *first* step in the recovery process.
CN: Psychosocial integrity; CNS: None; CL: Analyze; DIFFICULTY: Challenge

54. 4. The client who snorts cocaine frequently commonly develops a perforated nasal septum. Glossitis, bilateral ear infections, and pharyngitis aren't common physical findings for a client with a history of cocaine use.
CN: Physiological integrity; CNS: Physiological adaptation; CL: Apply; DIFFICULTY: Easy

55. A client recovering from cocaine use is participating in group therapy. Which statements by the client indicate that group participation has been beneficial? Select all that apply.
1. "I think the laws about drug possession are too strict in this country."
2. "I'll be more careful about mentioning my drug use to my children."
3. "I finally realize the short high from cocaine isn't worth the depression."
4. "I understand how I could get all these problems that we talked about in group."
5. "I was not responsible for using drugs since all my friends do it."

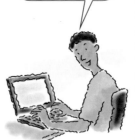

Stuck on a question? Try to eliminate as many wrong options as you can before answering.

55. 3, 4. Realizing that the short high created by cocaine isn't worth the depression is a realistic appraisal of a client's experience with cocaine and indicative of how harmful the experience is. Understanding of the problems resulting from drug use indicates the client is no longer in denial about the consequences of cocaine use. A comment about drug possession laws indicates the client is distracting from personal issues and isn't working on goals in the group setting. Talking about drugs to children must be reinforced with nonverbal behavior, while not mentioning drug use may give children the wrong message about drug use. Not accepting responsibility for the use of drugs demonstrates behaviors that determine the client has not benefitted from the group.
CN: Psychosocial integrity; CNS: None; CL: Analyze; DIFFICULTY: Moderate

56. A family expresses concern that a relative who stopped using amphetamines 3 months ago is acting paranoid. Which explanation by the nurse is **best**?
1. A person gets symptoms of paranoia with polysubstance use.
2. When a person uses amphetamines, paranoid tendencies may continue for months.
3. Sometimes, family dynamics and a high suspicion of continued drug use make a person paranoid.
4. Amphetamine users may have severe anxiety and paranoid thinking.

56. 2. After a client uses amphetamines, there may be long-term effects that exist for months after use. Two common effects are paranoia and ideas of reference. Even with polysubstance use, the paranoia stems from the chronic use of amphetamines. Holding the family responsible for the paranoia because they suspect continued drug use incorrectly places blame on the family; the paranoia actually comes from the drug use. Severe anxiety isn't typically manifested in paranoid thinking.
CN: Psychosocial integrity; CNS: None; CL: Analyze; DIFFICULTY: Easy

57. A nurse is trying to determine if a client who uses heroin has any drug-related legal problems. Which assessment question is the **best** to ask the client?
1. "When did your spouse become aware of your use of heroin?"
2. "Do you have a probation officer you report to periodically?"
3. "Have you received any legal violations related to your drug use?"
4. "Do you have a history of frequent visits with the employee assistance program manager?"

57. 3. Asking about legal violations related to drug use provides direct information about drug-related legal problems. When a spouse becomes aware of a partner's substance use, the first action isn't necessarily to institute legal action. Even if the client reports to a probation officer, the offense isn't necessarily a drug-related problem. Asking if the client has a history of frequent visits with the employee assistance program manager isn't useful; it assumes any such visit is related to drug issues.
CN: Psychosocial integrity; CNS: None; CL: Analyze; DIFFICULTY: Easy

58. A nurse has developed a therapeutic relationship with a client who has an addiction problem. Which information would indicate that their interaction is in the working stage? Select all that apply.
1. The client addresses how the addiction has contributed to family distress.
2. The client reluctantly shares a family history of addiction.
3. The client verbalizes difficulty identifying personal strengths.
4. The client discusses the financial problems related to the addiction.
5. The client expresses uncertainty about meeting with the nurse.
6. The client acknowledges the addiction's effects on the children.

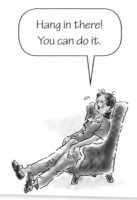

Hang in there! You can do it.

58. 1, 4, 6. Addressing how the addiction has contributed to family distress, discussing financial problems related to addiction, and acknowledging the addiction's effects on the children are examples of the nurse–client working phase of an interaction. In the working phase, the client explores, evaluates, and determines solutions to identified problems. Reluctant sharing of family addiction history, difficulty identifying personal strengths, and expressing uncertainty about meeting with the nurse are examples of what happens during the *introductory* phase of the nurse–client interaction.
CN: Psychosocial integrity; CNS: None; CL: Analyze; DIFFICULTY: Challenge

59. A client returns to the psychiatric unit after returning from a 6-hour pass. The nurse observes that the client is agitated, and is ataxic with nystagmus and general muscle hypertonicity. The nurse suspects that the client was using drugs while away from the unit. These symptoms are most indicative of intoxication with which drug?
1. Phencyclidine (PCP)
2. Crack cocaine
3. Heroin
4. Marijuana

60. A client who's recovering from an appendectomy is alert and ambulatory and reports pain. The team leader asks the nurse to give the client PRN-ordered oral analgesic. The nurse is aware that this client has had a long history of substance use. List in ascending chronologic order the steps the nurse would take to administer this particular medication. Use all the options.

1. Check the client's two identifiers with the medication administration record.

2. Stay with the client while taking the medication to ensure the medication hasn't been pocketed in cheeks or under the tongue.

3. Document on the medication sheet that the medication has been given.

4. Administer the medication.

5. Check the health care provider's orders with the medication administration record to see if it's time for the medication.

6. Place the correct medication and dose in a medication cup.

61. The health care provider has prescribed oral diazepam 50 mg once daily. The drug is available as oral suspension with a strength of 25 mg/5 mL. How many milliliters should the nurse administer? Record your answer using a whole number.

_____ mL

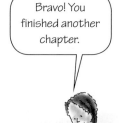

Bravo! You finished another chapter.

59. 1. The client's behavior suggests the use of PCP. Crack cocaine intoxication is characterized by euphoria, grandiosity, aggressiveness, paranoia, and depression. Heroin intoxication is characterized by euphoria, followed by sleepiness. Marijuana intoxication is characterized by a panic state and visual hallucinations.
CN: Psychosocial integrity; CNS: None; CL: Analyze;
DIFFICULTY: Difficult

60. Ordered Response:

5. Check the health care provider's orders with the medication administration record to see if it's time for the medication.

6. Place the correct medication and dose in a medication cup.

1. Check the client's two identifiers with the medication administration record.

4. Administer the medication.

2. Stay with the client as the medication is taken to ensure the medication hasn't been pocketed in the cheeks or under the tongue.

3. Document on the medication sheet that the medication has been given.

The first step is to check the health care provider's orders to ensure accuracy. The nurse should check for the appropriate time because this is a PRN order. Once the correct medication and dose are obtained and placed in a medication cup, the nurse would go to the client with the medication orders and check the client's two identifiers. Medication is always administered after establishing the correct identity of the client. Because this client has a history of substance use, the nurse should remain with the client as the medication is taken; check the mouth to be sure it has been swallowed, and then document the medication administration on the medication sheet.
CN: Safe, effective care environment; CNS: Coordinated care;
CL: Apply; DIFFICULTY: Challenge

61. 10.
The correct formula to calculate a drug dose is:

$$\frac{\text{Dose on hand}}{\text{Quantity on hand}} = \frac{\text{Dose desired}}{\text{X}}$$

The health care provider prescribes 50 mg, which is the dose desired. The drug available is 25 mg/5 mL, which is the dose on hand.

$$\frac{25\,\text{mg}}{5\,\text{mL}} = \frac{50\,\text{mg}}{\text{X}}$$

$$\text{X} = 10\,\text{mL}$$

CN: Physiological integrity; CNS: Pharmacological therapies;
CL: Apply; DIFFICULTY: Easy

CN: Client needs category CNS: Client needs subcategory CL: Cognitive level

Chapter 18

Dissociative Disorders

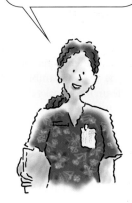

Caring for clients with dissociative disorders can be challenging and rewarding. Get ready … this chapter is a real out-of-body experience.

Dissociative disorders refresher

Depersonalization/derealization disorder

Feelings of being detached or disconnected from one's own thoughts or body, often described as feeling as if a person is "outside of one's own body" or living in a dream; the person does not lose touch with reality

Key signs and symptoms
- Fear of going "insane"
- Impaired occupational functioning
- Impaired social functioning
- Persistent or recurring feelings of detachment from mind and body

Key test results
- Standard dissociative disorder tests demonstrate a high degree of dissociation. These tests include:
  - diagnostic drawing series
  - dissociative experience scale
  - dissociative interview schedule
  - structured clinical interview for dissociative disorders

Key treatments
- Benzodiazepines: alprazolam, lorazepam, clonazepam

Key interventions
- Encourage the client to recognize that depersonalization is a defense mechanism used to deal with anxiety and trauma
- Assist the client in establishing supportive relationships

Dissociative amnesia

An inability to remember important personal information, often as a result of a stressful or traumatic event

Key signs and symptoms
- Altered identity
- Low self-esteem
- No conscious recollection of a traumatic event, yet colors, sounds, sites, or odors of the event may trigger distress or depression
- Sudden onset of amnesia and inability to recall personal information

Key test results
- Standard dissociative disorder tests demonstrate a degree of dissociation. These tests include:
  - diagnostic drawing series
  - dissociative experience scale
  - dissociative interview schedule
  - structured clinical interview for dissociative disorders

Key treatments
- Individual therapy
- Benzodiazepines: alprazolam, lorazepam
- Selective serotonin reuptake inhibitors (SSRIs): paroxetine

Key interventions
- Encourage the client to verbalize feelings of distress
- Encourage the client to recognize that memory loss is a defense mechanism used to deal with anxiety and trauma

Dissociative identity disorder

Disturbance in a person's identity, with the development of two or more distinct personalities or identities, called "alters," that control the person's behavior at different times; formerly called multiple personality disorder

Key signs and symptoms
- Guilt and shame
- Lack of recall (beyond ordinary forgetfulness)
- Presence of two or more distinct identities or personality states

Key test results
- Standard dissociative disorder tests demonstrate a degree of dissociation. These tests include:
  - diagnostic drawing series
  - dissociative experience scale
  - dissociative interview schedule
  - structured clinical interview for dissociative disorders
- EEG readings may vary markedly among the different identities

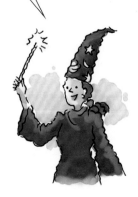

There are no magic cures for dissociative identity disorder, but benzodiazepines and psychotherapy can help.

Key treatments
- Long-term reconstructive psychotherapy
- Benzodiazepines: alprazolam, lorazepam, clonazepam
- SSRIs: paroxetine
- Tricyclic antidepressants: imipramine, desipramine

Key interventions
- Assist the client in identifying each personality
- Encourage the client to identify emotions that occur under duress

thePoint® You can download tables of drug information to help you prepare for the NCLEX®! View Generic Drug Names, Drug Classifications, Drug Actions, and Nursing Implications for the drugs discussed in this refresher at **http://thePoint.lww.com**.

Dissociative disorders questions, answers, and rationales

1. The nurse is gathering data from a client with dissociative identity disorder (DID). Which statement would the nurse **most** likely hear from the client?
1. "My father wasn't around much."
2. "I feel good about myself."
3. "I can recall many traumatic events from my childhood."
4. "My father loved me one day and hit me the next."

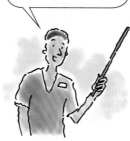

Several answers to question #1 could be true, but you are looking for the one that is *most likely.*

2. A nurse is working with the interdisciplinary team to develop an appropriate plan of care for a client with depersonalization/derealization disorder. Which factor would be a **priority** for the team to address?
1. Ritualistic behavior
2. Out-of-body experiences
3. History of sexual abuse
4. Inability to give a thorough personal history

3. A nurse is providing care to a client with dissociative identity disorder who was recently admitted to the inpatient psychiatric facility. Based on the nurse's understanding of this disorder (DID), the nurse would expect the plan of care to focus on which situation as the reason for the client's hospitalization?
1. Delusional ideations
2. Risk for self-harm
3. Lack of diversional activities
4. Hallucinations

4. A nurse is carrying out the plan of care developed for a client diagnosed with dissociative identity disorder (DID). Which intervention would be the **priority** for this client?
1. Giving antipsychotic medications as prescribed
2. Maintaining consistency when interacting with the client
3. Confronting the client about the use of alter personalities
4. Preventing client interaction with others when one of the alter personalities is in control

1. 4. Repeated exposure to a childhood environment that alternates between highly stressful and then loving and supportive can be a factor in the development of DID. Many children grow up in a household without a father but don't develop DID. Because of dissociation from the trauma, a client with DID usually can't recall traumatic childhood events. Clients with DID commonly have low self-esteem.
CN: Psychosocial integrity; CNS: None; CL: Apply; DIFFICULTY: Moderate

2. 2. Out-of-body experiences are commonly associated with depersonalization/derealization disorder and must be addressed as the priority for this client. Ritualistic behavior is seen with obsessive-compulsive disorders. DID is theorized to develop as a protective response to traumatic experiences such as sexual abuse. An inability to give a personal history would be more often associated with DID or dissociative amnesia.
CN: Safe, effective care environment; CNS: Coordinated care; CL: Apply; DIFFICULTY: Difficult

3. 2. A common reason clients with DID are admitted to a psychiatric facility is because one of the alternate personalities is trying to kill another personality, thus the risk for self-harm. Delusions and hallucinations are commonly associated with schizophrenia. Because of the assortment of alter personalities controlling the client with DID, lack of diversional activities is rarely a problem.
CN: Safe, effective care environment; CNS: Coordinated care; CL: Apply; DIFFICULTY: Challenge

4. 2. Using consistency to establish trust and support is important when interacting with a client with DID. Many of these clients have had few healthy relationships. Medication hasn't proven effective in the treatment of DID. Confronting the client about the alter personalities would be ineffective because the client has little, if any, knowledge of the presence of these other personalities. Isolating the client wouldn't be therapeutic.
CN: Safe, effective care environment; CNS: Coordinated care; CL: Analyze; DIFFICULTY: Easy

CN: Client needs category   CNS: Client needs subcategory   CL: Cognitive level

5. A nurse is caring for a client with dissociative amnesia who is exhibiting signs of low self-esteem. The nurse determines that the interventions have been successful when the client demonstrates which behavior?

1. Participation in new activities.
2. Sleeping without interruption at night.
3. Inability to confront fear of failure.
4. Greater time spent with the nurse.

6. A nurse is caring for a client diagnosed with dissociative identity disorder (DID). The nurse reviews the plan of care for the client and implements interventions to achieve which outcome?

1. The client is able to confront the abuser.
2. The client attends the unit's milieu meetings.
3. The client prevents alter personalities from emerging.
4. The client reports reduced feelings of anger about childhood traumas.

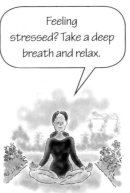

Feeling stressed? Take a deep breath and relax.

7. A nurse is caring for a client with a diagnosis of dissociative identity disorder (DID). Which client behavior should the nurse identify as a safety risk?

1. The client experiences periods of lost time.
2. The client expresses a desire to do self harm.
3. The client expresses gladness to be in the unit.
4. The client is hearing loud voices.

8. The nurse is gathering data from a client with dissociative identity disorder (DID). What statement by the client would the nurse expect to hear?

1. "I have a close relationship with my mother."
2. "I never did well in school."
3. "I can't recall certain events or experiences."
4. "I can perform a skill or task consistently."

9. A hospitalized client with dissociative identity disorder (DID) tells the nurse about hearing voices. Which nursing intervention is **most** appropriate?

1. Telling the client to lie down and rest
2. Giving an as-needed dose of haloperidol
3. Encouraging the client to continue with daily activities
4. Notifying the health care provider that the client is having a psychotic episode

5. 1. Interventions for persons with dissociative amnesia and low self-esteem would be demonstrated by participation in new activities and the ability to confront the fear of failure. There isn't an issue related to sleeping. Spending more time with the nurse would be inappropriate. The client needs to participate in new activities with others.

CN: Psychosocial integrity; CNS: None; CL: Apply; DIFFICULTY: Moderate

6. 2. The desired outcome would be that the client attends milieu meetings. Doing so decreases feelings of isolation and shows that the client has begun to trust the nurse. Typically, the abuser was a part of the client's childhood, and confrontation in adulthood may not be possible or therapeutic. The client with DID is commonly unaware of alter personalities and thus can't prevent them from emerging. Clients with DID have dissociated from painful experiences, so the host personality usually doesn't have negative feelings about such experiences.

CN: Psychosocial integrity; CNS: None; CL: Apply; DIFFICULTY: Difficult

7. 2. The nurse needs to initiate safety precautions to prevent self-harm. The sensation of lost periods of time isn't a safety issue. Being glad to be in the unit indicates a feeling of security. The client with DID hearing voices doesn't indicate a psychotic episode.

CNS: Safe, effective care environment;

CN: Safety and infection control; CL: Apply; DIFFICULTY: Easy

8. 3. Clients with DID commonly experience bouts of amnesia when alter personalities are in control. Clients with DID have learned in childhood how to live in two separate worlds: one in the daytime, in which they're able to perform well in school and have friendships, and one at nighttime, when the abuse occurs. The alter personalities may vary in the ability and type of skills and tasks performed. A close relationship with a parent is unlikely because of probable abuse in childhood.

CN: Psychosocial integrity; CNS: None; CL: Understand; DIFFICULTY: Easy

9. 3. Because many clients with DID hear voices, it's appropriate to have the client continue with daily activities. The voices are probably alter personalities communicating, which doesn't indicate a psychotic episode. Telling the client to lie down and rest wouldn't be therapeutic. The health care provider wouldn't be notified to prescribe antipsychotic medication such as haloperidol for the client with DID.

CN: Safe, effective care environment; CNS: Coordinated care; CL: Apply; DIFFICULTY: Difficult

---

CN: Client needs category   CNS: Client needs subcategory   CL: Cognitive level

10. A client has just been diagnosed with dissociative identity disorder (DID). When implementing the plan of care for the client, the nurse would initially assist the client in achieving which goal?
1. Learning how to control periods of mania
2. Learning how to integrate all the alternate personalities
3. Developing coping strategies to deal with a traumatic childhood
4. Determining what's causing the client to feel periods time are lost

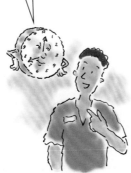

Oh—there you are! I thought I had lost you.

10. **4.** The initial symptom many clients with DID experience is the sensation of "lost time." These are times the alter personalities are in control. Therefore, the nurse would assist the client in determining the underlying cause of "lost time." Depression, not mania, may be another early symptom of clients with DID. Initially, the client with DID isn't aware of the presence of alternate personalities. Before therapeutic interventions, clients with DID may not even be aware of childhood trauma because of dissociation from the event.
CN: Psychosocial integrity; CNS: None; CL: Apply; DIFFICULTY: Difficult

11. A client with dissociative identity disorder (DID) reports hearing voices and asks the nurse if that means the client is "crazy." Which response would be **most** therapeutic?
1. "What do the voices tell you?"
2. "Why would you think you're crazy?"
3. "People with your condition sometimes report hearing voices."
4. "Hearing voices is typically a symptom of schizophrenia."

11. **3.** The most therapeutic answer is to give the client the correct information: people with DID sometimes hear voices. Asking what the voices tell the client would be changing the topic without answering the question. Asking "why" questions can put the client on the defensive. Schizophrenia isn't the only cause of hearing voices, and this response suggests the client may have schizophrenia.
CN: Psychosocial integrity; CNS: None; CL: Analyze; DIFFICULTY: Moderate

12. A client with dissociative identity disorder (DID) requires hospitalization. Which intervention would **most** likely appear in the client's plan of care plan?
1. Arrange to have staff check on the client every 15 to 30 minutes.
2. Prevent all family from visiting until the third day of hospitalization.
3. Make sure the staff understands the client will be on seizure precautions.
4. Place the client in a quiet room away from the noise of the nurses' station.

12. **1.** A common reason for hospitalization in clients with DID is suicidal ideations or gestures. For the client's safety, frequent checks should be done. Family interactions might be therapeutic for the client, and the family may be able to provide a more thorough history because of the client's dissociation from traumatic events. Seizure activity isn't an expected symptom of DID. Because of the possibility of suicide, the client's room should be close to the nurses' station.
CN: Safe, effective care environment; CNS: Safety and infection control; CL: Apply; DIFFICULTY: Moderate

13. A client is diagnosed with depersonalization/derealization disorder. Which statements would the nurse likely hear when collecting data from the client? Select all that apply.
1. "I feel like I'm going crazy."
2. "It's like I'm outside my body looking down on it."
3. "Everything around me seems so real."
4. "I know what's real but I feel disconnected."
5. "I don't remember ever being in a fire."

I just feel disconnected...am I going insane?

13. **1, 2, 4.** Clients with depersonalization/derealization disorder exhibit feelings of being detached or disconnected from their body or thoughts. They often report feeling like they are going crazy, or looking down on their body from the outside. Clients with this disorder often report feeling like everything around them is unreal and experience a disconnectedness, but they are in touch with reality. The inability to remember a traumatic event would most likely occur with dissociative amnesia.
CN: Psychosocial integrity; CNS: None; CL: Apply; DIFFICULTY: Difficult

14. A client is being treated at a community mental health clinic. A nurse has been instructed to observe for any behaviors indicating dissociative identity disorder (DID). Which behavior would be included?
1. Delusions of grandeur
2. Reports of fatigue
3. Changes in dress, mannerisms, and voice
4. Refusal to make a follow-up appointment

14. **3.** When alter personalities are in control, the person will have complete personality changes. Delusions of grandeur are more commonly associated with such disorders as manic states and schizophrenia. Reports of fatigue aren't a main symptom of DID. The refusal to make a follow-up appointment could indicate many problems, including noncompliance.
CN: Psychosocial integrity; CNS: None; CL: Apply; DIFFICULTY: Easy

CN: Client needs category   CNS: Client needs subcategory   CL: Cognitive level

15. A nurse is interacting with a client with a dissociative identity disorder. During the interaction, the nurse observes that one of the alter personalities is in control. Which intervention is **most** appropriate?
1. Recognize the alter personality.
2. Notify the health care provider.
3. Immediately stop interaction with the client.
4. Ignore the alter personality and ask to speak to the host personality.

16. The nurse reinforces the education provided to a client diagnosed with dissociative identity disorder (DID). The nurse determines that the client understands the need to continue therapy when what statement is made?
1. "Therapy will help eliminate my family problems."
2. "I must continue going to outpatient treatment for the next 2 months."
3. "I understand that I need to integrate all my alter personalities into one."
4. "Once therapy is complete, I won't have the traits of my alter personalities."

17. A family member of a client with depersonalization/derealization disorder asks a nurse if hypnotic therapy might help the client. Which response would be **most** appropriate?
1. "What would make you think that?"
2. "Unfortunately, hypnosis is usually not used to treat this condition."
3. "Yes, but this treatment is used only after other types of therapy have failed."
4. "Yes, it will help make him more conscious of his alters."

18. When caring for a client with dissociative identity disorder (DID), the nurse would most likely implement which intervention **first**?
1. Reminding the alter personalities that they're part of the host personality
2. Limiting interaction with the client to those when the host personality is in control
3. Establishing an empathic relationship with each emerging personality
4. Providing positive reinforcement to the client when calm, not angry, alter personalities are present

15. 1. By recognizing the alter personality, the nurse conveys to the client that she believes the alter personality exists. Asking to speak to the host personality or immediately stopping interaction with the client won't stop the client from being controlled by alter personalities. The health care provider doesn't need to be notified because this is an expected occurrence.
CN: Psychosocial integrity; CNS: None; CL: Analyze; DIFFICULTY: Easy

16. 3. The main goal of therapy of clients with DID is to integrate the alter personalities. Complete elimination of personalities may not be possible. Therapy is often long term. Through therapy, the client can learn how to cope with family problems.
CN: Psychosocial integrity; CNS: None; CL: Analyze; DIFFICULTY: Moderate

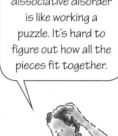

Working with a client with dissociative disorder is like working a puzzle. It's hard to figure out how all the pieces fit together.

17. 2. Depersonalization/derealization disorder is typically not treated with hypnosis. The mainstay of treatment usually includes cognitive behavioral therapy or psychodynamic therapy. The first response could place the family member on the defensive. Hypnosis is used in a variety of psychiatric conditions; however, it is not used with depersonalization/derealization disorder. Dissociative identity disorder is associated with "alters," not depersonalization/derealization disorder.
CN: Psychosocial integrity; CNS: None; CL: Apply; DIFFICULTY: Moderate

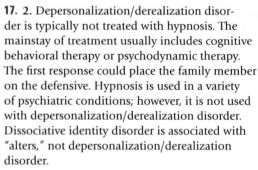

Working with clients alter personalities can go a long way toward soothing their symptoms.

18. 3. Establishing an empathic relationship with each emerging personality (including those that may seem unpleasant) provides a therapeutic environment in which to care for the client. This is a priority intervention. As time goes on, it may be appropriate to remind the alter personalities that they are part of the host. Interacting with the client only when the host personality is in control would be useless because the client has limited, if any, control or awareness when alter personalities are in control.
CN: Psychosocial integrity; CNS: None; CL: Apply; DIFFICULTY: Challenge

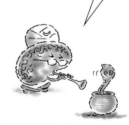

19. While interacting with a client with dissociative identity disorder (DID), a nurse observes characteristics of an alter personality. The client goes from being calm to being angry and shouting. Which response would be **most** appropriate?
  1. "Is one of you upset?"
  2. "Why have you become angry?"
  3. "Tell me how you're feeling right now."
  4. "Let me speak to someone who isn't angry."

20. A client with dissociative amnesia has been receiving therapy for the past several years to uncover memories that have been buried as a result of sexual abuse by the father during childhood. The client has just learned the father passed away. Which intervention would be **most** appropriate?
  1. Urge the client to seek inpatient therapy immediately.
  2. Encourage the client to verbalize any feelings that she may have.
  3. Encourage the client to repress her feelings about the father for the time being.
  4. Impress upon the client that the father's death should be helpful in the healing process.

21. A nurse finds a client with dissociative identity disorder trying to commit suicide. To preserve the client's self-esteem and safety, which action would be the **priority**?
  1. Place the client in seclusion with checks every 15 minutes.
  2. Assign a nursing staff member to remain with the client at all times.
  3. Make the client stay with the group at all times.
  4. Refuse to let the client in a private room.

22. A nurse observes that an alternate personality (a child) of an adult client with dissociative identity disorder (DID) is in control. The client is sitting in the dayroom, interacting with others. Which action would be **most** appropriate?
  1. Allow the client to continue interacting with clients in the dayroom.
  2. Ask to speak to one of the adult alter personalities of the host personality.
  3. Remove the client from the dayroom and allow the client to play with toys.
  4. Remove the client from the dayroom and reorient in a safe place.

19. 3. Asking the client how she's feeling now encourages integration and discourages dissociation. When interacting with clients with DID, the nurse always wants to remind the client that the alter personalities are a component of one person. Responses reinforcing interaction with only one alter personality instead of trying to interact with the individual as a single person aren't appropriate. Asking "why" questions can put the client on the defensive and impede further communication.
CN: Psychosocial integrity; CNS: None; CL: Apply;
DIFFICULTY: Easy

20. 2. The death of the abuser may cause the client to experience a wide range of feelings, such as anger and guilt. The nurse should encourage the client to verbalize feelings. Unless the client becomes suicidal or rapidly deteriorates, inpatient treatment wouldn't be necessary. Encouraging the client to repress feelings would be inappropriate and unhealthy. The death of the abuser can be a stressful event and can leave the client with unresolved feelings.
CN: Physiological integrity; CNS: Reduction of risk potential;
CL: Analyze; DIFFICULTY: Easy

21. 2. Implementing a one-to-one, staff-to-client ratio is the nurse's highest priority. Doing so allows the client to maintain self-esteem and keep them safe. Seclusion would damage the client's self-esteem. Forcing the client to stay with the group and refusing to let the client in a private room will not guarantee safety.
CN: Safe, effective care environment; CNS: Safety and infection control; CL: Apply; DIFFICULTY: Easy

22. 4. Removing the client at this time may protect from future embarrassment. Reorienting the client discourages dissociation and encourages integration. Asking to speak to an alter personality encourages dissociation. Allowing the client to play with toys would reinforce this behavior and encourage dissociation.
CN: Safe, effective care environment; CNS: Safety and infection control; CL: Analyze; DIFFICULTY: Challenge

23. The nurse is working as part of the interdisciplinary team in caring for a client with dissociative identity disorder. Which behavior reported by a family member would indicate that the client's therapy is effective?
1. The client is forgetful.
2. The client sleeps through the night.
3. The client has had several unsuccessful relationships.
4. The client hears voices.

24. The nurse reinforces the discharge education for a client diagnosed with dissociative identity disorder (DID). Which statement by the client indicates successful teaching?
1. "I need to confront my abuser before I can get well."
2. "I will need to stick with my psychotherapy for a long time."
3. "I'm going to name my alters Joe and Sam."
4. "It is important for me to take my prescribed antipsychotic drugs."

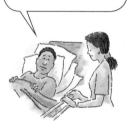

Before discharging a client, make sure he has an accurate understanding of the course of treatment he faces.

25. A client diagnosed with dissociative amnesia is prescribed alprazolam as part of the treatment plan. After reviewing the medication with the client, the nurse determines that the teaching was successful when the client identifies the need to avoid which substance to reduce the risk for an interaction? Select all that apply.
1. Alcohol
2. Nicotine
3. Grapefruit juice
4. St. John's wort
5. Green, leafy vegetables
6. Dairy products

26. A client with dissociative identity disorder (DID) is admitted to an inpatient psychiatric unit. A nurse manager asks all staff to attend a meeting. Which is the **most** likely reason for the meeting?
1. To review the restraint protocol with the staff
2. To inform the staff that no one should refuse to work with the client
3. To warn the staff that this client may be difficult to work with
4. To allow staff members to discuss concerns about working with a client with DID

27. The nurse is providing care to a client. The history reveals that the client was reported missing after being the victim of a violent crime. Two months later, a family member found the client working in a city 100 miles from home. The client wasn't able to recognize the family member or recall being the victim of a crime. The nurse would suspect which condition?
1. Depersonalization disorder
2. Dissociative amnesia
3. Dissociative fugue
4. Dissociative identity disorder (DID)

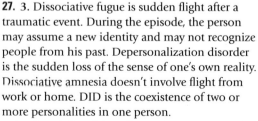

Sometimes I just don't know who I am.

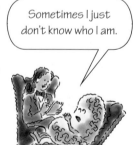

23. 2. Because clients with DID often have sleep disorders, sleeping through the night is a sign of effective therapy. Forgetfulness, difficulty forming relationships, and hallucinations are signs of unsuccessful treatment.
CN: Psychosocial integrity; CNS: None; CL: Analyze;
DIFFICULTY: Easy

24. 2. Clients with DID need long-term psychotherapy in order to improve and maintain their mental health. The client with DID has repressed the abuse and would be unable to confront the abuser. Suggesting the client name subpersonalities is nontherapeutic. Antipsychotic drugs aren't prescribed for DID.
CN: Psychosocial integrity; CNS: None; CL: Analyze;
DIFFICULTY: Challenge

25. 1, 2, 3, 4. Alprazolam can interact with alcohol, causing additive effects on the central nervous system. Cigarette smoking (nicotine) may decrease the effectiveness of alprazolam and should be discouraged. Grapefruit juice may increase alprazolam levels; St. John's wort may decrease drug levels. Alprazolam does not interact with green, leafy vegetables or dairy products.
CN: Physiological integrity; CNS: Pharmacological therapies;
CL: Analyze; DIFFICULTY: Difficult

26. 4. Allowing all staff members to meet together may prevent them from splitting into groups of those who believe the diagnosis is valid and those who don't. Unless this client shows behaviors harmful to self or others, restraints aren't needed. Telling the staff that no one should refuse to work with the client or that this client will probably be difficult sets a negative tone for the staff as they develop a plan of care for the client and implement it.
CN: Safe, effective care environment; CNS: Coordinated care;
CL: Apply; DIFFICULTY: Easy

27. 3. Dissociative fugue is sudden flight after a traumatic event. During the episode, the person may assume a new identity and may not recognize people from his past. Depersonalization disorder is the sudden loss of the sense of one's own reality. Dissociative amnesia doesn't involve flight from work or home. DID is the coexistence of two or more personalities in one person.
CN: Psychosocial integrity; CNS: None; CL: Apply;
DIFFICULTY: Challenge

28. The nurse is providing care to a client who has just had an episode of dissociative fugue. Which nursing intervention would be **most** appropriate for this client?
1. Let the client verbalize the fear and anxiety that is felt.
2. Encourage the client to share experiences during the episode.
3. Ask the client to sign a contract committing to not leaving the premises.
4. Tell the client there will be no resolving of problems by running away from them.

29. While reading a journal article, a nurse comes across a discussion of the causes of dissociative disorders. Which information would the nurse **most** likely find in the discussion?
1. They occur as a result of incest.
2. They occur as a result of substance abuse.
3. They occur in more than 40% of all people.
4. They occur as a result of the brain trying to protect the person from severe stress.

30. A client is experiencing recurrent episodes of dissociative fugue. Which nursing intervention would be **most** helpful to reduce these recurrent episodes?
1. Placing the client on elopement precautions
2. Helping the client identify resources to deal with stressful situations
3. Allowing the client to share experiences about the dissociative fugue episodes
4. Confronting the client about running away from problems instead of dealing with them

31. A client lost his home in a flood last month. When questioned about feelings about the loss, there is no memory of being in a flood or owning a home. Based on the client's report, the nurse suspects that the client is most likely experiencing which condition?
1. Depersonalization disorder
2. Dissociative amnesia
3. Dissociative fugue
4. Dissociative identity disorder (DID)

32. The nurse is gathering data from a client with dissociative amnesia. A report of which event would the nurse interpret as the **most** likely contributing factor?
1. Binge drinking
2. A hostage situation
3. A closed-head injury
4. A fight with a family member

Word on the street is that you are dominating this test. Care to comment?

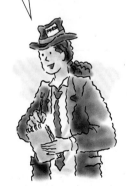

28. 1. An episode of dissociative fugue can be a frightening experience; encouraging the client to discuss fears will help establish a plan for coping with them. The client rarely remembers the events during the fugue episode, and asking to recall them can increase anxiety. Signing a contract would have little effect because a dissociative fugue episode isn't something the client consciously wants. Because the client isn't conscious of "running away," telling the client there will be no resolving of problems by fleeing isn't helpful.
CN: Psychosocial integrity; CNS: None; CL: Apply; DIFFICULTY: Challenge

29. 4. The best description of the cause of a dissociative disorder is that the brain tries to protect the person from severe stress. Incest is only one of many reasons dissociative disorders occur. Typically, substance abuse isn't a cause (but may be an effect) of a dissociative disorder. Dissociative disorders are actually rare.
CN: Psychosocial integrity; CNS: None; CL: Apply; DIFFICULTY: Easy

30. 2. Dissociative fugue is precipitated by stressful situations. Helping the client identify resources could prevent recurrences. When the dissociative fugue episode is over, the client returns to normal functioning; he wouldn't be an elopement risk. Clients commonly have amnesia about the events during the dissociative fugue episode; therefore, asking them to share or remember their experiences or confronting them about running away from their problems can increase their anxiety.
CN: Psychosocial integrity; CNS: None; CL: Apply; DIFFICULTY: Challenge

31. 2. Dissociative amnesia commonly occurs after a person has experienced a traumatic event. Depersonalization disorder is characterized by recurrent sensations of loss of one's own reality. Dissociative fugue is the sudden departure from one's home or work. DID is the coexistence of two or more personalities within the same individual.
CN: Psychosocial integrity; CNS: None; CL: Analyze; DIFFICULTY: Moderate

32. 2. Dissociative amnesia typically occurs after the person has experienced a significantly stressful, traumatic situation, such as a hostage situation. Binge drinking doesn't cause dissociative amnesia. A closed-head injury could result in physiologic, but not dissociative, amnesia. A fight with a family member typically wouldn't be stressful enough to cause dissociative amnesia.
CN: Psychosocial integrity; CNS: None; CL: Apply; DIFFICULTY: Moderate

33. A client was the driver in an automobile accident in which a 3-year-old child was killed; the client is now experiencing dissociative amnesia. After reviewing the treatment plan with the client, the nurse determines that the client demonstrates understanding by which statement?
1. "I won't drive a car again for at least 1 year."
2. "I'll take my lorazepam any time I feel upset about this situation."
3. "I'll visit the child's grave as soon as I'm released from the hospital."
4. "I'll attend my hypnotic therapy sessions prescribed by my psychiatrist."

34. A nurse is reinforcing the teaching plan with a client diagnosed with dissociative identity disorder (DID). Which statement by the client indicates that the education has been effective?
1. "I'll probably never be able to regain my memories of the fire."
2. "I have problems with my memory due to my abuse of tranquilizers."
3. "If I concentrate hard enough, I'll be able to bring up memories of the car accident."
4. "My brain has temporarily hidden my memories of the rape to protect me."

35. Which nursing intervention would be the **priority** when caring for a client with a dissociative disorder?
1. Encouraging the client to participate in unit activities and meetings
2. Questioning the client about the events triggering the dissociative disorder
3. Allowing the client to remain in the client's room anytime the client is experiencing feelings of dissociation
4. Encouraging the client to form friendships with other clients in therapy groups to decrease feelings of isolation

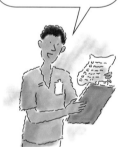

Decreasing a sense of isolation is a key goal for clients with dissociative disorders.

36. A client with depersonalization/derealization disorder is prescribed drug therapy as part of the treatment plan. Which medication would the nurse **most** likely administer if prescribed? Select all that apply.
1. Alprazolam
2. Lorazepam
3. Clonazepam
4. Paroxetine
5. Imipramine

33. 4. Hypnosis can be beneficial to this client because it allows repressed feelings and memories to surface. Visiting the child's grave upon release from the hospital may be too traumatic and could encourage continuation of the amnesia. The client needs to learn coping mechanisms other than taking a highly addictive drug such as lorazepam. The client may be ready to drive again, and circumstances may dictate driving again before 1 year has passed.
CN: Psychosocial integrity; CNS: None; CL: Analyze; DIFFICULTY: Moderate

34. 4. One of the cardinal features of DID is that the person has loss of memory of a traumatic event. With this disorder, the loss of memory is a protective function performed by the brain and isn't within the person's conscious control. With therapy and time, the person will probably be able to recall the traumatic event. This type of amnesia isn't related to substance abuse.
CN: Psychosocial integrity; CNS: None; CL: Analyze; DIFFICULTY: Easy

35. 1. Individuals with certain dissociative disorders feel detached from their environment and can experience impaired social functioning. Attending unit activities and meetings helps decrease the client's sense of isolation. Often, the client can't recall the events that triggered the dissociative disorder, so the client would need to be isolated from others only if the client couldn't interact appropriately. A client with a dissociative disorder has typically had few healthy relationships. Forming friendships with others in therapy could result in the client establishing unhealthy relationships.
CN: Safe, effective care environment; CNS: Coordinated care; CL: Apply; DIFFICULTY: Moderate

36. 1, 2, 3. Depersonalization/derealization disorder may be treated with benzodiazepines such as alprazolam, lorazepam, or clonazepam. Paroxetine may be prescribed for dissociative amnesia or dissociative identity disorder. Imipramine may be prescribed to treat dissociative identity disorder.
CN: Physiological integrity; CNS: Pharmacological therapies; CL: Analyze; DIFFICULTY: Moderate

37. A client with dissociative amnesia says, "You must think I'm really stupid because I have no recollection of the accident." Which response would be **most** appropriate?
1. "Why would I think you're stupid?"
2. "Have I acted like I think you're stupid?'
3. "You'll be fine soon. Don't worry about it."
4. "The brain sometimes protects us by not letting us remember traumatic events."

38. A client with dissociative disorder is hospitalized. The client has threatened to commit suicide. When gathering data from the client, which set of circumstances would the nurse identify as indicating the **highest** risk of suicide?
1. Suicide plan, handy means of carrying out plan, and history of previous attempt
2. Preoccupation with morbid thoughts and limited support system
3. Suicidal ideation, active suicide planning, and family history of suicide
4. Threats of suicide, recent job loss, and intact support system

39. A nurse is reviewing a client's history. Which characteristic would lead the nurse to suspect that a client is experiencing a depersonalization/derealization disorder?
1. Disorientation to time, place, and person
2. Sensation of detachment from body or mind
3. Unexpected and sudden travel to another location
4. A feeling that one's environment will never change

40. A nurse is working with a client diagnosed with a depersonalization/derealization disorder on ways to decrease symptoms. The nurse determines that the client understands what to do when which statement is made?
1. "I'll avoid any stressful situation."
2. "Meditation will help control my symptoms."
3. "I'll need to practice meditation regularly."
4. "I may need to remain on antipsychotic medication for the rest of my life."

41. A client with depersonalization/derealization disorder spends much of the day in a dreamlike state, during which they ignore personal care needs. The nurse understands that this is most likely related to which situation?
1. Organic brain damage
2. Impaired memory
3. Perceptual impairment
4. Lack of information

37. 4. The nurse's response that the brain sometimes doesn't let humans remember traumatic events as a means of protection provides a simple explanation for the client. The use of "why" questions can put the client on the defensive. The nurse asking "Have I acted like I think you're stupid" takes the focus off the client. Telling the client he'll be fine soon gives false reassurance.
CN: Psychosocial integrity; CNS: None; CL: Apply; DIFFICULTY: Easy

38. 1. A lethal plan with a handy means of carrying it out along with a previous attempt poses the highest risk and requires immediate intervention. Although all the remaining risk factors can lead to suicide, they aren't considered as high a risk as a formulated, lethal plan and the means at hand. However, a client exhibiting any of these risk factors should be taken seriously and considered at risk for suicide.
CN: Safe, effective care environment; CNS: Coordinated care; CL: Apply; DIFFICULTY: Easy

39. 2. In depersonalization/derealization disorder, the client feels detached from his body and mental processes. The client is usually oriented to time, place, and person. Unexpected and sudden travel to another location is one of the characteristics of dissociative fugue. Clients with depersonalization/derealization disorder commonly feel the outside world has changed.
CN: Psychosocial integrity; CNS: None; CL: Apply; DIFFICULTY: Moderate

40. 3. Relaxation can lead to a decrease in maladaptive responses. Although stress can be a predisposing factor in depersonalization disorder, it's impossible to avoid all stressful situations. Meditation is the voluntary induction of the sensation of depersonalization. Depersonalization disorder isn't a psychotic disorder, so antipsychotic medication wouldn't be therapeutic.
CN: Psychosocial integrity; CNS: None; CL: Analyze; DIFFICULTY: Moderate

41. 3. Because of time spent in a dreamlike state, the client's perception is impaired. Thus, many clients with depersonalization/derealization disorder ignore self-care needs. There's no known organic brain damage with this disorder. Memory impairment is more of a problem with other dissociative disorders, such as dissociative identity disorder and dissociative amnesia. The dreamlike state does not indicate a lack of information.
CN: Safe, effective care environment; CNS: Safety and infection control; CL: Apply; DIFFICULTY: Easy

42. A severely depressed client who has made multiple suicide attempts matter-of-factly tells the nurse that family life was normal and uneventful. Which behaviors would lead the nurse to suspect the diagnosis of a dissociative identity disorder (DID) in this client? Select all that apply.

1. Inability to recall important personal information too severe to be explained by ordinary forgetfulness
2. Absence of any physiologic effects of a substance such as alcohol or drugs
3. Ability to selectively and consciously choose to avoid certain painful topics
4. A sense of grandiosity, feelings of being special, and having a particular mission for mankind
5. Posttraumatic symptoms, such as flashbacks, nightmares, and an exaggerated startle response

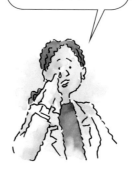

Being depressed without any memory of traumatic events could be a sign of dissociative identity disorder.

42. 1, 2, 5. A dissociative disorder is a persistent state of being disconnected from the totality of one's personhood, particularly painful emotions. With dissociative disorder, the inability to recall personal information is far more extensive than ordinary forgetfulness. Posttraumatic symptoms, such as flashbacks, nightmares, and an exaggerated startle response, are also signs and symptoms of DID. The symptoms occur apart from any chemical inducement, and the individual doesn't have the ability to consciously make a decision to separate from painful emotions or topics. A sense of grandiosity isn't a characteristic of this disorder.
CN: Psychosocial integrity; CNS: None; CL: Analyze; DIFFICULTY: Difficult

43. The wife of a client reports that her husband often disappears for days at a time, not showing up for work and then returning with no memory of anything unusual occurring. Which scenarios might the nurse suspect? Select all that apply.

1. The client is experiencing sleep terror disorder interfering with his activities of daily life.
2. The client is taking drugs, possibly of a hallucinogenic nature.
3. The client is experiencing dissociative fugue.
4. The client has a form of a severe dissociative identity disorder.
5. The client may have a neurologic disorder requiring examination by a competent neurologist.

43. 3, 4. Dissociative fugue is a type of dissociative identity disorder (DID) characterized by sudden, unexpected travel away from home, with the inability to recall what took place during this time frame. DIDs are considered severe, chronic identity disorders. Sleep terror disorder involves recurrent episodes in which the client awakens abruptly from sleep and experiences feelings of panic. Use of hallucinogenic drugs is unlikely because drugs wouldn't explain the inability to recover lengthy periods of lost time such as this client experiences. A serious neurologic disorder is possible, but not likely, because there are no other physiologic symptoms and the predominant report from the wife is more characteristic of a severe dissociative disorder.
CN: Psychosocial integrity; CNS: None; CL: Analyze; DIFFICULTY: Challenge

44. A client is awake and sitting quietly in a chair but doesn't respond to verbal or tactile stimuli. There are repeated episodes of staring into the distance, seemingly oblivious to events or persons in the immediate vicinity. When the client emerges from these episodes, life continues as usual. Which statements are accurate based on these assessment findings? Select all that apply.

1. The client has entered a state of self-induced hypnosis.
2. The client may be involved in ritual activity that leads into a trancelike state.
3. The client is demonstrating signs of a dissociative trance disorder.
4. The client is in a state of factitious disease to obtain a secondary, emotional gain.
5. The client is demonstrating psychotic behavior and decompensation.
6. The client has no control over his behavior.

Impressive! Another chapter down.

44. 3, 6. The client is demonstrating typical signs of a dissociative trance that isn't consciously induced. There's no basis to make the assumption that the client is in a state of self-induced hypnosis or has any involvement in ritual activities that would account for this behavioral state. There's no evidence to suggest that factitious disease is a reasonable explanation. The client, though not responsive, does come out of the trances and demonstrates normal behavior, so psychosis with decompensation can be ruled out.
CN: Psychosocial integrity; CNS: None; CL: Analyze; DIFFICULTY: Difficult

Chapter 19

Sexual Dysfunctions & Gender Dysphoria

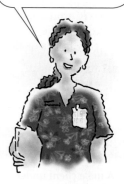

This chapter will test your knowledge of disorders of a highly sensitive nature. You'll do great. Good luck!

Sexual dysfunctions & gender dysphoria refresher

Gender dysphoria

Conflict between a person's physical gender and the gender he or she identifies with

Key signs and symptoms
- Dreams of cross-gender identification
- Finding one's own genitals "disgusting"
- Persistent distress about sexual orientation
- Preoccupation with appearance
- Self-hatred

Key test results
- Psychological testing may reveal cross-gender identification or behavior patterns

Key treatments
- Group and individual psychotherapy
- Hormonal therapy
- Sex-reassignment surgery

Key interventions
- Demonstrate a nonjudgmental attitude
- Help the client to identify positive aspects of himself

Paraphilic disorders

Sexual arousal and satisfaction that depend on engaging in, and fantasizing about, sexual behaviors that are uncharacteristic and risky

Key signs and symptoms
- Development of a hobby or change in occupation that makes the paraphilia more accessible
- Recurrent paraphilic fantasies
- Social isolation
- Troubled social or sexual relationships

Key treatments
- Individual therapy

Key interventions
- Demonstrate a nonjudgmental attitude
- Institute safety precautions as needed according to facility protocol

- Initiate a discussion about how emotional needs for self-esteem, respect, love, and intimacy influence sexual expression
- Encourage the client to identify feelings (such as pleasure, reduced anxiety, increased control, and shame) associated with sexual behavior and fantasies

Sexual dysfunction

Any physical or psychological problem that prevents the client or partner from getting sexual satisfaction

Key signs and symptoms
Female sexual interest/arousal disorder and genito-pelvic pain/penetration disorder
- Anxiety
- Decreased sexual desire
- Delayed or absent orgasm
- Depression
- Pain with sexual intercourse

Male sexual dysfunction
- Anxiety
- Inability to maintain an erection
- Premature ejaculation

Key test results
Female sexual interest/arousal disorder and genito-pelvic pain/penetration disorder
- Diagnostic tests are used to rule out a physiologic cause for the dysfunction

Male sexual dysfunction
- Diagnostic tests are used to rule out a physiologic cause for the dysfunction

Key treatments
Female sexual interest/arousal disorder and genito-pelvic pain/penetration disorder
- Individual therapy

Male sexual dysfunction
- Individual therapy
- Hormone replacement therapy; testosterone
- Sildenafil, tadalafil, vardenafil for impotence

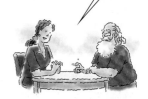

A nonjudgmental attitude is essential when discussing sensitive issues with clients.

Key interventions

Female sexual interest/arousal disorder and genito-pelvic pain/penetration disorder
- Encourage client to discuss feelings and perceptions about sexual function
- Offer client suggestions about alternative ways of expressing her affection
- Encourage client to seek evaluation and therapy from a qualified professional

Male sexual dysfunction
- Encourage client to discuss feelings and perceptions about his sexual dysfunction
- Teach client and his partner alternative ways of expressing their affection
- Encourage client to seek evaluation and therapy from a qualified professional

thePoint® You can download tables of drug information to help you prepare for the NCLEX®! View Generic Drug Names, Drug Classifications, Drug Actions, and Nursing Implications for the drugs discussed in this refresher at **http://thePoint.lww.com**.

Sexual dysfunctions & gender dysphoria questions, answers, and rationales

1. A male client underwent surgery for repair of an abdominal aortic aneurysm, and asks the nurse if he will be impotent. Which response is **most** appropriate?
1. "Don't worry; you'll be okay."
2. "You have other problems to worry about."
3. "We'll cross that bridge when we come to it."
4. "There may be a chance of erectile dysfunction following this type of surgery."

2. Which discharge instruction would be **most** accurate for a female client who has suffered a spinal cord injury at the C4 level?
1. "After a spinal cord injury, women usually remain fertile; therefore, you may consider contraception if you don't want to become pregnant."
2. "After a spinal cord injury, women are usually unable to conceive a child."
3. "Sexual intercourse shouldn't be different for you."
4. "After a spinal cord injury, menstruation usually stops."

3. While obtaining data from a client, the nurse observes that the client has been prescribed tadalafil. What should the nurse carefully monitor for this client?
1. Urine output
2. Temperature
3. Blood pressure
4. Urine specific gravity

4. A client with chronic obstructive pulmonary disease (COPD) tells the nurse, "I no longer have enough energy to make love to my husband." Which nursing intervention would be **most** appropriate?
1. Refer the couple to a sex therapist.
2. Refer the woman to a gynecologist.
3. Suggest methods and measures that conserve energy.
4. Tell the client to discuss it with her husband.

Don't forget to cover sexual function considerations during discharge, when needed.

1. 4. Erectile dysfunction and retrograde ejaculation are sexual dysfunctions commonly experienced after abdominal aortic aneurysm repair. Telling the client that he will be all right offers false assurance. Stating that the client has other problems isn't therapeutic and doesn't address the concern. Telling the client that "we'll cross that bridge when we come to it" ignores the client's concerns and isn't therapeutic. CN: Psychosocial integrity; CNS: None; CL: Apply; DIFFICULTY: Easy

2. 1. After a spinal cord injury, women remain fertile and can conceive and deliver a child. If a woman doesn't want to become pregnant, she *must* use contraception. Menstruation isn't affected by a spinal cord injury, but sexual functioning may be different. CN: Physiological integrity; CNS: Physiological adaptation; CL: Apply; DIFFICULTY: Easy

3. 3. When a client is receiving tadalafil, the nurse should monitor the client's blood pressure carefully because this drug causes hypotension. CN: Physiological integrity; CNS: Pharmacological therapies; CL: Apply; DIFFICULTY: Moderate

4. 3. Sexual dysfunction in clients with COPD is the direct result of dyspnea and reduced energy levels. Measures to reduce physical exertion, enhance oxygenation, and accommodate decreased energy levels may aid sexual activity. If the problem persists, a consult with a sex therapist might be necessary. A gynecologic consult isn't necessary. Discussing this with her husband may not resolve the problem. CN: Physiological integrity; CNS: Reduction of risk potential; CL: Apply; DIFFICULTY: Easy

CN: Client needs category   CNS: Client needs subcategory   CL: Cognitive level

5. A client with an ileostomy tells the nurse he can't have an erection. Which pertinent information should the nurse know?
1. The client will never regain function.
2. The client needs an abdominal x-ray.
3. The client has no problem with self-control.
4. Impotence is uncommon after an ileostomy.

6. A nurse is reinforcing education for a client regarding the medication vardenafil. What statement made by the client demonstrates that education has been successful?
1. "I will take the medication 3 hours before sexual intercourse"
2. "I will take the medication 2 hours before sexual intercourse"
3. "I will take the medication 1 hour before sexual intercourse"
4. "I will take the medication immediately before sexual intercourse"

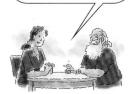

Be open and honest when discussing sexual dysfunction with your client—just as you would with any other condition.

7. Which action should the nurse be sure is included in the education plan of a newly married female client with a cervical spinal cord injury who doesn't wish to become pregnant at this time?
1. Provide the client with brochures on sexual practice.
2. Provide the client's husband with information on vasectomy.
3. Instruct the client on the rhythm method of contraception.
4. Instruct the client's husband on proper insertion of a diaphragm with contraceptive jelly.

8. A client tells the nurse she's having her menstrual period every 2 weeks, and it lasts for 1 week. How will the nurse **best** document this finding?
1. Amenorrhea
2. Dyspareunia
3. Menorrhagia
4. Metrorrhagia

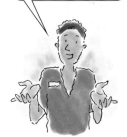

Caring for a client's psychological health following surgery can be just as important as caring for physical health.

9. A nurse is caring for a client who recently had surgery and is having difficulty accepting changes in body image. Which nursing intervention is appropriate?
1. Actively listen to the client when the client expresses positive and negative feelings about body image.
2. Restrict the client's opportunity to view the incision and dressing because it's upsetting.
3. Assist the client to focus on future plans for recovery.
4. Assist the client to repress anger while discussing the body image alteration.

5. 4. Sexual dysfunction is uncommon after an ileostomy; psychological causes of impotence should be explored. An abdominal x-ray isn't indicated for sexual dysfunction. An ileostomy can change a person's perception of self-control, making sexual functioning difficult.
CN: Psychosocial integrity; CNS: None; CL: Analyze; DIFFICULTY: Easy

6. 3. Vardenafil is given for the treatment of impotence and should be taken one hour before sexual activity.
CN: Physiological integrity; CNS: Pharmacological therapies; CL: Apply; DIFFICULTY: Moderate

7. 4. Because the client experienced a cervical spinal cord injury, she can't insert any form of contraception protection; therefore, it's vital to provide her husband with instructions on inserting a diaphragm in order to prevent pregnancy. Providing the couple with literature on sexual practice doesn't address the client's concerns. During this time of crisis, the couple doesn't wish to have children, but they may reconsider, so providing information on vasectomy isn't appropriate. The rhythm method isn't the most effective way to prevent pregnancy.
CN: Psychosocial integrity; CNS: None; CL: Apply; DIFFICULTY: Difficult

8. 3. Menorrhagia is excessive menstrual period. Amenorrhea is lack of menstruation. Dyspareunia is painful intercourse. Metrorrhagia is uterine bleeding from a cause other than menstruation.
CN: Physiological integrity; CNS: Reduction of risk potential; CL: Apply; DIFFICULTY: Moderate

9. 1. The nurse must observe for any indication that the client is ready to address body image change. The client should be allowed to look at the incision and dressing if so inclined. It's too soon to focus on the future with this client. The nurse should allow the client to express feelings and not repress them, because repression prolongs recovery.
CN: Psychosocial integrity; CNS: None; CL: Apply; DIFFICULTY: Easy

10. A client must undergo a hysterectomy for uterine cancer. Which nursing action would **best** meet the woman's body image changes?
1. Ask her if she's having pain.
2. Refer her to a psychotherapist.
3. Don't discuss the subject with her.
4. Encourage her to verbalize her feelings.

11. A client who had a myocardial infarction 8 weeks ago tells a nurse, "My wife wants to make love, but I don't think I can. I'm worried that it might kill me." Which response from the nurse would be **most** appropriate?
1. "Tell me about your feelings."
2. "Let's have you do more rehabilitation."
3. "Let me call the health care provider for you."
4. "Tell your wife that, when you're able, you'll make love."

12. A client who's in cardiac rehabilitation tells a nurse that she can't make love to her husband because she often feels excessively fatigued and has a sense of doom. Which nursing intervention is **most** appropriate?
1. Instruct her not to have intercourse until she's ready.
2. Instruct her to take a nitroglycerin tablet prior to intercourse.
3. Encourage her to learn additional methods to use for sexual intercourse.
4. Encourage her to verbalize her feelings while a physical examination is performed.

13. A client tells the nurse she has never had an orgasm and her partner is upset that he can't meet her needs. Which nursing intervention is **most** appropriate?
1. Ask the client if she desires intercourse.
2. Assess the couple's perception of the problem.
3. Tell the client that most women don't reach orgasm.
4. Refer the client to a therapist because she has sexual aversion disorder.

There is that word "priority" again. Think about which action is important to take right away.

14. A client is in the emergency department after being sexually assaulted by a stranger. Which nursing intervention has **priority**?
1. Assisting in identifying which behaviors placed the client at risk for the attack
2. Making an appointment in 6 weeks at a local sexual assault crisis center
3. Encouraging discussion of early childhood experiences
4. Assisting in identifying family or friends who could provide immediate support

EMERGENCY

10. 4. Encourage the client to verbalize her feelings because loss of reproductive organs may bring on feelings of loss related to body image and sexuality. Pain is a concern after surgery, but it has no bearing on body image. Referring her to a psychotherapist may be premature; the client should be given time to work through her feelings. Avoiding the subject isn't a therapeutic nursing intervention.
CN: Psychosocial integrity; CNS: None; CL: Apply; DIFFICULTY: Easy

11. 1. The nurse should address the client's concerns. Asking the client to verbalize his feelings will permit the nurse to gain insight into the problem. Rehabilitation shouldn't be increased until the nurse assesses the situation and is sure no harm will come to the client. Calling the health care provider before a complete assessment is made is inappropriate. Telling the wife that eventually the client will be able to make love may place strain on the marriage.
CN: Psychosocial integrity; CNS: None; CL: Apply; DIFFICULTY: Easy

12. 4. Because the client reports fatigue, she should be examined, and her feelings should be explored. Instructing her not to have intercourse doesn't address her concerns. She shouldn't take nitroglycerin before intercourse until her fatigue is evaluated. Before recommending alternative methods for intercourse, the client should be assessed physically and psychologically.
CN: Psychosocial integrity; CNS: None; CL: Apply; DIFFICULTY: Moderate

13. 2. Assessing the couple's perception of the problem will define it and assist the couple and the nurse in understanding it. A nurse can't make a medical diagnosis such as sexual aversion disorder. Most women can be taught to reach orgasm if there's no underlying medical condition. When assessing the client, the nurse should be professional and matter-of-fact; she shouldn't make the client feel inadequate or defensive.
CN: Psychosocial integrity; CNS: None; CL: Apply; DIFFICULTY: Moderate

14. 4. The client who has been sexually assaulted by a stranger needs tremendous support to help through this ordeal. Assisting the client in identifying behaviors that were risk factors for the attack places the blame on the client. Waiting 6 weeks to make an appointment at a local crisis center is incorrect—the center must be called immediately. Some psychiatric disorders are related to early childhood experiences, but rape isn't one of them.
CN: Psychosocial integrity; CNS: None; CL: Apply; DIFFICULTY: Easy

15. A client is taking antihypertensive medication and tells the nurse who's monitoring the blood pressure that he can't have sexual intercourse with his wife anymore. What likely cause should the nurse discuss with the client?
1. His advancing age
2. His blood pressure
3. His stressful lifestyle
4. His blood pressure medication

16. The nurse is caring for an adult victim of childhood sexual abuse. For which behaviors should the nurse monitor the client?
1. Depression and substance abuse disorders
2. Bipolar and somatic symptom disorder
3. Narcissistic disorders and bulimia nervosa
4. Obsessive-compulsive and posttraumatic stress disorders

17. The nurse is gathering data from a female client that states she has had difficulty conceiving. Which statement made by the client would the nurse find **most** significant related to the difficulty getting pregnant?
1. "I have used oral contraceptives for 2 years."
2. "I had gonorrhea that went untreated for about 3 months."
3. "I had iron deficiency anemia"
4. "I was told I had the beginning of osteoporosis."

18. A client reports to the nurse that he has a strong desire to live and be treated as a woman. He confesses that he's uncomfortable with his assigned sex. Which term **best** describes the client's feelings?
1. Delusions
2. Gender dysphoria
3. Homosexuality
4. Hormone imbalances

19. Sildenafil has been prescribed for a client. While reviewing his medical records, the nurse would question which order?
1. Use of nitroglycerin
2. Insomnia
3. Use of multivitamins
4. Neuralgia

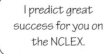

I predict great success for you on the NCLEX.

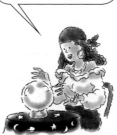

20. Which statement by a client with paraphilia indicates a potential for relapse?
1. "I'll go to outpatient therapy."
2. "I'm going to try to attend all therapy sessions."
3. "I can't imagine why the judge sent me here."
4. "The health care provider wants me to take leuprolide acetate. I think that will help."

15. 4. Antihypertensive medication may cause impotence in men. Blood pressure itself doesn't cause impotence, but its treatment does. Stress may cause erectile dysfunction, but there's no evidence that the client is under stress. Men are usually able to have an erection throughout their lives.
CN: Physiological integrity; CNS: Pharmacological therapies; CL: Apply; DIFFICULTY: Easy

16. 1. Childhood sexual abuse is closely linked to the development of depression and substance abuse disorders. It's also linked to the development of somatic symptoms and posttraumatic stress disorders and bulimia nervosa. Victims of childhood sexual abuse aren't predisposed to developing bipolar, narcissistic, or obsessive-compulsive disorders.
CN: Psychosocial integrity; CNS: None; CL: Analyze; DIFFICULTY: Easy

17. 2. If left untreated, some STIs can interfere with fertility. A history of taking oral contraceptives doesn't lead to infertility. Anemia doesn't lead to infertility; however, correcting this condition can increase fertility and help maintain a pregnancy. Osteoporosis is a condition in which bone loss occurs; the risk of developing osteoporosis increases after menopause.
CN: Health promotion and maintenance; CNS: None; CL: Apply; DIFFICULTY: Easy

18. 2. A persistent, cross-gender identification and dissatisfaction with one's assigned gender are major characteristics of gender dysphoria. Delusions are firmly held beliefs not substantiated in reality. Homosexuality is an attraction to members of the same sex. Hormone imbalances aren't relevant to the diagnosis of gender dysphoria.
CN: Psychosocial integrity; CNS: None; CL: Apply; DIFFICULTY: Easy

19. 1. Use of nitroglycerin; when sildenafil and nitroglycerin are used concurrently it may cause hypotension, therefore it is contraindicated to use nitrates. Insomnia and neuralgia are side effects of the medication and sildenafil is not contraindicated with the use of vitamins.
CN: Physiological integrity; CNS: Pharmacological therapies; CL: Apply; DIFFICULTY: Easy

20. 3. A lack of insight into his problem may indicate a potential for relapse for this client. Attending all therapy sessions and outpatient therapy demonstrates compliance with the treatment. Leuprolide acetate is an antiandrogenic that lowers testosterone levels and decreases the libido.
CN: Psychosocial integrity; CNS: None; CL: Analyze; DIFFICULTY: Easy

CN: Client needs category   CNS: Client needs subcategory   CL: Cognitive level

21. A client returning home from the store late one evening was sexually assaulted. When brought to the emergency department, she's crying. Which intervention for this client should be the nurse's **priority**?
1. Filing a police report
2. Calling the client's family
3. Encouraging the client to enroll in a self-defense class
4. Remaining with the client and assisting her through the crisis

22. A client in college who has recently been diagnosed with human papillomavirus (HPV) infection comes to the health clinic and is anxious and tearful. Which nursing intervention would be **most** appropriate?
1. Ask the client to discuss concerns.
2. Provide the client with reliable information about this condition.
3. Refer the client to a gynecologist.
4. Discuss the dangers of multiple sex partners.

23. A client is admitted to the hospital for treatment of pedophilia and tells the nurse that he doesn't want to talk about sexual behaviors. Which response from the nurse is **most** appropriate?
1. "I need to ask you the questions on the database."
2. "It's your right not to answer my questions."
3. "OK, I'll just write 'no comment.'"
4. "I know this must be difficult for you."

24. A client with ulcerative colitis has recently had a colostomy and is anxious. The client states to the nurse, "I don't think I can ever have a sexual relationship now that I have this." Which response by the nurse would be **most** appropriate?
1. Offer to refer to a support group.
2. Allow the client to express concerns.
3. Offer to research statistics on this topic.
4. Explore the positive aspects of her treatment regimen.

25. Which outcome developed by the health care team is appropriate for a client diagnosed with pedophilia?
1. Attending all meetings on the unit
2. Using triggers to initiate sexual behaviors
3. Informing the client's employer of the reason for hospitalization
4. Verbalizing appropriate methods to meet sexual needs upon discharge

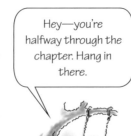

Hey—you're halfway through the chapter. Hang in there.

21. 4. Sexual assault is treated as a medical emergency, and the client requires constant attention and assistance during the crisis. Filing a police report doesn't take precedence over a medical emergency. Comforting the client by contacting her family should be carried out after her injuries are treated. Encouraging the client to enroll in a self-defense class isn't appropriate during crisis.
CN: Psychosocial integrity; CNS: None; CL: Apply; DIFFICULTY: Easy

22. 1. Encouraging the client to discuss concerns establishes a nonjudgmental, therapeutic relationship and would be the best initial response. Other interventions might be appropriate at some point. After a therapeutic relationship is established, the nurse should discuss the dangers of multiple sex partners in a nonjudgmental manner.
CN: Psychosocial integrity; CNS: None; CL: Apply; DIFFICULTY: Easy

23. 4. Telling the client that his condition must be difficult for him acknowledges the client's feelings and opens communication. Insisting that the form must be completed doesn't open up communication or acknowledge the client's feelings. Clients have rights, but data collection is necessary so that help with the problem can be offered. Writing "no comment" alone would be inappropriate and not therapeutic.
CN: Psychosocial integrity; CNS: None; CL: Apply; DIFFICULTY: Challenge

24. 2. Allowing the client to express her concerns is a therapeutic first step. Referring to a support group is premature. Offering to research statistics or to explore positive aspects of treatment negates the emotional aspect of this problem, and the client might conclude that it isn't acceptable to discuss her feelings.
CN: Physiological integrity; CNS: Reduction of risk potential; CL: Apply; DIFFICULTY: Easy

25. 4. Upon discharge, the client should be able to verbalize an alternative, appropriate method to meet sexual needs, as well as effective strategies to prevent relapse. It isn't imperative that the client attend all meetings on the unit, but it's important that the client attend the required group sessions. A client with pedophilia should recognize triggers that initiate inappropriate sexual behavior and learn ways to direct impulses. The client may wish to discuss the disorder with his spouse but not necessarily with his employer.
CN: Psychosocial integrity; CNS: None; CL: Analyze; DIFFICULTY: Easy

26. A client is brought to the emergency department after being sexually assaulted by a rival gang member. The nurse observes that the client appears relaxed and is calmly talking to a relative. The nurse determines that the client may be using which defense mechanism?
1. Rationalization
2. Denial
3. Displacement
4. Projection

27. A client admitted to the behavioral health unit with a diagnosis of pedophilia tells his roommate about the problems he is having. The roommate runs down the hall yelling to the nurse, "I don't want to be in here with a child molester." Which response from the nurse is **most** appropriate?
1. "Stop acting out."
2. "Calm down and go back to your room."
3. "Your roommate isn't a child molester."
4. "I can see you're upset. Let's sit down and we'll talk."

28. A client has been diagnosed with voyeurism. The nurse knows that which action is characteristic of a voyeur?
1. Observing others while they disrobe
2. Wearing clothing of the opposite sex
3. Rubbing against a nonconsenting person
4. Using rubber sheeting for sexual arousal

29. A client being treated for infertility confides to the nurse that he hasn't told his partner about being treated for a sexually transmitted infection in the past. What would be the **most** therapeutic response for the nurse to give?
1. "Do you think withholding this information is the basis for a trusting relationship?"
2. "Don't you think your partner deserves to know?"
3. "What concerns do you have about sharing this information?"
4. "I can understand why you would want to keep this information private."

30. After learning that his gay roommate has tested positive for human immunodeficiency virus (HIV), a client asks the nurse about moving to another room on the psychiatric unit because he doesn't feel "safe" now. What should the nurse do **first**?
1. Move the client to another room.
2. Ask the client to describe any fears.
3. Move the client's roommate to a private room.
4. Explain that such a move wouldn't be therapeutic for the client or his roommate.

26. 2. The client is demonstrating the defense mechanism of denial, in which a client retreats into himself to reduce the threat of what has happened to his self-concept. Rationalization prevents admitting an inadequacy. Displacement transfers feelings about one person to another. Projection places blame on someone else or on circumstances.
CN: Psychosocial integrity; CNS: None; CL: Analyze; DIFFICULTY: Moderate

27. 4. Acknowledging that the client is upset and sitting down and talking with him allows the client to verbalize feelings. Telling the client to stop acting out isn't a therapeutic response. It wouldn't be therapeutic or safe to keep these clients together without intervention if one is agitated or anxious over the other. Stating that the client with pedophilia isn't a child molester doesn't acknowledge the roommate's feelings.
CN: Psychosocial integrity; CNS: None; CL: Apply; DIFFICULTY: Easy

28. 1. Voyeurism is sexual arousal from secretly observing someone who's disrobing. Transvestic fetishism describes the enjoyment of cross-dressing. Rubbing against someone who is nonconsenting is frottage. Using objects for sexual arousal is fetishism.
CN: Psychosocial integrity; CNS: None; CL: Understand; DIFFICULTY: Easy

29. 3. Asking about the client's concerns on sharing the information encourages the client to verbalize the concerns in a safe environment and begin to choose a course of action for dealing with this issue now. Telling the client that withholding information may cause distrust in a relationship (and that the partner deserves to know) conveys negative judgments. The nurse who supports withholding of information doesn't encourage discussion or problem solving.
CN: Psychosocial integrity; CNS: None; CL: Apply; DIFFICULTY: Easy

30. 2. To intervene effectively, the nurse must first understand the client's fears. After exploring the client's fears, the nurse may move the client or his roommate or explain why such a move wouldn't be therapeutic.
CN: Psychosocial integrity; CNS: None; CL: Apply; DIFFICULTY: Easy

31. A client with a sexual arousal disorder asks the nurse if taking sildenafil is the only method to treat erectile dysfunction. What is the **best** response by the nurse?
1. "It is the best treatment for sexual arousal."
2. "Taking sildenafil is the only method that works."
3. "Group therapy reduces the anxiety connected with erectile difficulties."
4. "Reducing the pressure to perform only helps the woman."

32. A nurse is obtaining data for a client admitted to the clinic with a paraphilic disorder. Which interventions **best** demonstrate the appropriate care of this client? Select all that apply.
1. Demonstrate a nonjudgmental attitude.
2. Institute safety precautions as needed according to facility protocol.
3. Inform the client that behaviors like "that" will not be tolerated in the facility.
4. Encourage the client to identify feelings.
5. Have the client sign a contract stating the client will not have inappropriate sexual feelings.

33. A client and spouse are seeking treatment for infertility after having difficulty becoming pregnant. Which statement made by the client does the nurse determine is causing the **most** "stressful aspect of treatment"?
1. "I am having an examination today to determine if I have an infection."
2. "My husband is giving a specimen today to determine his sperm count."
3. "We have to schedule sexual intercourse with our busy lives."
4. "We are not sure who has the problem."

34. A nurse is conducting a sexual awareness group of known pedophiles. What will the nurse highlight as the primary focus of this group?
1. Socialization
2. Cognitive restructuring
3. Insight
4. Punishment

35. A nurse knows that gender is part of one's identity. Which event signifies when gender is first ascribed?
1. A neonate is born.
2. A child attends school.
3. A child receives sex-specific toys.
4. A child receives sex-specific clothing.

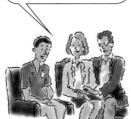

Remember to present all treatment options to a client, pharmacological and nonpharmacological.

31. 3. Group therapy is a successful treatment to reduce the anxiety connected with erectile dysfunction.
CN: Psychosocial integrity; CNS: None; CL: Apply; DIFFICULTY: Challenge

32. 1, 2, 4. The nurse should always maintain a nonjudgmental attitude when caring for any client. Safety precautions should be taken for the client as well as other clients. Informing a client that his behaviors will not be tolerated is threatening behavior and the nurse should abstain from making this type of statement. Encouraging the client to identify feelings is a key factor in attempting a behavior change. It is unrealistic to expect a client to suppress feelings without therapeutic interventions.
CN: Psychosocial integrity; CNS: None; CL: Apply; DIFFICULTY: Easy

33. 3. The major cause of stress in infertile couples is planning sexual intercourse to correlate with fertility cycles. The inconvenience and discomfort of receiving examinations and producing specimens aren't major stressors. Most couples undergoing fertility treatment understand that one partner is usually infertile.
CN: Health promotion and maintenance; CNS: None; CL: Analyze; DIFFICULTY: Challenge

34. 2. The nurse's focus is on education. The priority is to obtain an awareness of the sexual behaviors and the consequences. Cognitive restructuring is used in an attempt to change the individual's maladaptive behaviors.
CN: Psychosocial integrity; CNS: None; CL: Apply; DIFFICULTY: Easy

35. 1. As soon as a neonate is born, gender is ascribed. In the hospital, a neonate is given either a pink or blue name band, card, or blanket. Sexual identity is reaffirmed throughout the school years. Gender identification is perpetuated throughout life with sex-specific clothing and toys.
CN: Psychosocial integrity; CNS: None; CL: Understand; DIFFICULTY: Moderate

36. A parent brings a 14-year-old son to the psychiatric crisis room and states, "He's always dressing in female clothing. There must be something wrong with him." Which response from the nurse would be **most** appropriate?
1. "Your son will be evaluated shortly."
2. "I'll tell your son that this isn't appropriate."
3. "You seem to be upset. Would you like to talk?"
4. "I wouldn't want my son to dress in girls' clothing."

37. A client taking antidepressant medication reports a decreased desire for sex, which is causing significant marital stress. Which response by the nurse would be **most** appropriate?
1. "Don't stop taking the medication."
2. "What are your thoughts on how you should handle this?"
3. "Doesn't your spouse understand the importance of your medication?"
4. "Have you discussed this with your health care provider?"

38. A male client is undergoing estrogen therapy for future sexual reassignment surgery. Which outcome should the nurse assist in evaluating?
1. The client will develop breasts.
2. The client will begin menstruating.
3. The client will be able to cross-dress.
4. The client will develop body hair.

39. A nurse is assisting in developing an education plan on rape prevention. Which guideline would have **priority** in this plan?
1. Avoid drinking heavily at a party.
2. Avoid walking alone at night.
3. Learn ways to defend yourself.
4. Always take the shortest driving route home.

40. A nurse is obtaining data from a client with the potential diagnosis of gender dysphoria. The nurse knows that the diagnostic criteria for this disorder in a male must include a persistent identification with femaleness and which other sign or symptom?
1. Significant impairment in social, occupational, or other important areas of functioning
2. Coexisting physical intersex condition
3. Simple rejection of sex-role stereotypes without distress
4. Delusional ideas of belonging to the female sex with a secondary diagnosis of schizophrenia

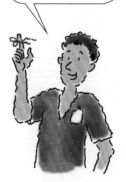

Remember—you're looking for the most appropriate response in question #36.

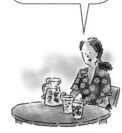

Sweet. You've already finished 40 questions.

36. 3. Acknowledging the parent's feelings and offering her an opportunity to verbalize concerns provides a forum for open communication. Telling the client's parent that he'll be evaluated shortly doesn't address her concerns. Telling the client that this behavior isn't appropriate doesn't assess his feelings nor does it analyze the behavior. The nurse shouldn't offer an opinion by stating she wouldn't want her son dressing in female clothing.
CN: Psychosocial integrity; CNS: None; CL: Apply; DIFFICULTY: Easy

37. 2. Encouraging the client to verbalize her thoughts will help to problem-solve. Telling the client not to stop taking the medication is too direct and doesn't encourage exploration on the part of the client. Asking the client if the spouse understands the importance of taking the medication conveys negative judgment. Asking if the client has discussed the issue with her health care provider might be appropriate, but it may also give the impression that the nurse doesn't want to discuss the problem with the client.
CN: Psychosocial integrity; CNS: None; CL: Apply; DIFFICULTY: Challenge

38. 1. A male who receives long-term estrogen therapy will develop female secondary sexual characteristics such as breasts. A male on estrogen won't menstruate, as he doesn't have a uterus. Estrogen has no bearing on cross-dressing. Androgens would be taken by a female to develop body hair and stop menstruation.
CN: Psychosocial integrity; CNS: None; CL: Analyze; DIFFICULTY: Easy

39. 3. Learning a self-defense method helps protect an individual in various situations. Drinking heavily at a party, especially if unescorted, and walking alone at night would tend to compromise safety. The shortest driving route might take an individual through a high-crime neighborhood; one should learn alternative routes in order to have options if safety seems compromised.
CN: Health promotion and maintenance; CNS: None; CL: Apply; DIFFICULTY: Moderate

40. 1. Diagnostic criteria for male gender dysphoria include a pervasive identification with femaleness and feelings of discomfort or inappropriateness with maleness. These feelings cause significant distress and disturbances in functioning and aren't simply a rejection of sex-role stereotypes. Gender dysphoria doesn't usually occur as a result of an intersex condition and rarely occurs along with a diagnosis of schizophrenia.
CN: Psychosocial integrity; CNS: None; CL: Analyze; DIFFICULTY: Moderate

CN: Client needs category   CNS: Client needs subcategory   CL: Cognitive level

41. A group of college students were walking back to their dorm at night when someone suddenly jumped out and exposed themselves. One of the students was extremely upset and went to the clinic. Which response by the nurse would be **most** helpful psychologically to this student?
1. "Can you imagine a flasher on campus?"
2. "I'll call security right away."
3. "I can see you're upset. Tell me more about this."
4. "Please describe this person to me."

42. A client who has been married for 10 years arrives at the psychiatric clinic stating, "I can't live this lie anymore. I wish I were a woman. I don't want my wife. I need a man." Which nursing intervention would be **most** appropriate?
1. Call the primary health care provider.
2. Encourage the client to speak to his wife.
3. Admit the client.
4. Sit down with the client and talk about his feelings

43. A client states he has little or no sexual desire and says this is causing great distress in his marriage. What further information would be **most** useful in assessing the situation? Select all that apply.
1. The client's age when he had his first girlfriend
2. When the problem first appeared and potential contributing factors
3. Medications and dosages
4. Report of recent bladder or prostate problems
5. Age of the client's wife

44. A male client is seeking treatment by court order after being released from jail for actions indicating pedophilia. Which behavior demonstrated by the client would correlate with this diagnosis? Select all that apply.
1. A strong sexual attraction to prepubescent children exists.
2. Male children are more commonly the focus of attention than female children.
3. The pedophile is usually very attentive to a child's needs to gain their attention.
4. The disorder generally begins in early adulthood.
5. The pedophile must be age 16 or older or at least 5 years older than the child.

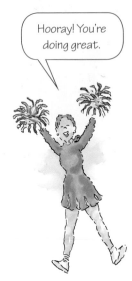

Hooray! You're doing great.

41. 3. Acknowledging the client's emotions is the best initial step in helping her talk about her concerns. Making a comment about a flasher on campus isn't therapeutic. Calling security and asking for the man's description are appropriate interventions but don't help the student deal with her emotional reaction.
CN: Psychosocial integrity; CNS: None; CL: Analyze; DIFFICULTY: Easy

42. 4. Sitting down with the client and exploring his feelings allows the nurse to assess him. The primary health care provider shouldn't be notified until an assessment is made. The client shouldn't speak to his wife until he has processed his feelings. An assessment of the client should be made *before* admitting him to the unit.
CN: Psychosocial integrity; CNS: None; CL: Apply; DIFFICULTY: Easy

43. 2, 3. In assessing this situation, it would be most useful to know when the problem first appeared and what contributed to it. These questions provide opportunity to gather a great deal of useful information to better understand the client's current condition. Knowing the client's medications and dosages is very important because certain medications profoundly affect sexual desire. The client's age when he started dating has no bearing on the current problem. Reporting previous problems is useful but wouldn't provide a sufficient explanation for the lack of sexual desire. The age of the client's wife is irrelevant and doesn't provide assessment data.
CN: Psychosocial integrity; CNS: None; CL: Analyze; DIFFICULTY: Challenge

44. 1, 3, 5. Pedophilia is a disorder characterized by a strong sexual attraction to prepubescent children that generally begins to manifest itself in adolescence, not early adulthood. By definition, the pedophile must be age 16 or older or at least 5 years older than the child. The pedophile generally is attentive to the needs of children in order to gain their trust, loyalty, and attention. Female, not male, children are more commonly the focus of attention.
CN: Psychosocial integrity; CNS: None; CL: Understand; DIFFICULTY: Difficult

45. The nurse uses the PLISSIT model to help clients with gender issues or sexual problems. Place the levels in progressive order.

1. Specific suggestions

2. Limited information

3. Permission giving

4. Intensive therapy

46. A client tells the nurse that he is only interested in sex when his partner wears cowboy boots and a scanty nightgown. Which term will the nurse use to describe this behavior?
1. Pedophile
2. Homosexual
3. Voyeurism
4. Fetishism

47. A client in the behavioral health unit with a history of noncoercive paraphilia is experiencing an auditory hallucination. What is the **priority** nursing action?
1. Stay with the client
2. Call the health care provider
3. Give the client medication
4. Alert the staff on the unit

48. A homosexual client tells the nurse that "my family is not supportive." What is the **best** response by the nurse?
1. "What do you mean by not supportive?"
2. "They will understand later."
3. "How do they treat you?"
4. "Would you like to arrange for counseling?"

49. A client confides to a nurse, "I have urges and desires to have sex with children." What should the nurse's **most** appropriate response be?
1. Ask the client, "Have you ever acted on these desires?"
2. Question the client, "Are you able to control your thoughts about sexual relations with children?"
3. Explain that these thoughts are unacceptable and intensive therapy is need.
4. Inform child protective services about the client and the thoughts the client reported.

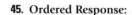

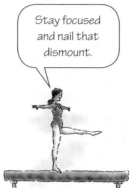
Stay focused and nail that dismount.

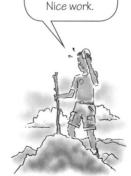
You made it! Nice work.

45. Ordered Response:

3. Permission giving

2. Limited information

1. Specific suggestions

4. Intensive therapy

CN: Psychosocial integrity; CNS: None; CL: Apply; DIFFICULTY: Difficult

46. 4. A client with fetishism uses sexually arousing objects as part of sexual activity. Pedophile refers to sexual arousal and preference for a prepubescent child. Homosexual is sexual attraction or preference for persons of the same sex. Voyeurism refers to viewing others, who are unaware they are being observed, in intimate situations.
CN: Psychosocial integrity; CNS: None; CL: Apply; DIFFICULTY: Easy

47. 1. Staying with the client, listening, and offering methods of controlling the hallucinations will calm the client. This will be an effective action to keep the client and others safe. Calling the health care provider is not necessary at this time. The nurse can initiate interventions to assist the client to cope with the hallucinations. Giving the client medication may be useful but the nurse will begin with the least restrictive interventions. Alerting the staff is not a priority at this time.
CN: Psychosocial integrity; CNS: None; CL: Apply; DIFFICULTY: Easy

48. 1. "What do you mean by not supportive?" The nurse is encouraging the client to talk about the difficulty and the feelings connected to the client's perception. "They will understand later" is a false promise. "How do they treat you?" This question focuses on the family and does not give the client the opportunity to explore the meaning of not feeling supported by family. "Would you like to arrange for counseling?" This is a closed-ended question. The nurse would focus on the client's perceptions before initiating a solution to the problem.
CN: Psychosocial integrity; CNS: None; CL: Apply; DIFFICULTY: Moderate

49. 1. If a client reports a desire for pedophilia, then it is important to assess if the client ever acted upon these thoughts; the best predictor of future behaviors is past behaviors. Humans may have sexual fantasies but it is their behavior by which they are judged. No human thoughts are unacceptable, but therapy is required if the client is dystonic. Informing child protective services is premature; the nurse has not obtained information whether the client has acted on these thoughts.
CN: Psychosocial integrity; CNS: None; CL: Apply; DIFFICULTY: Moderate

Chapter 20

Eating Disorders

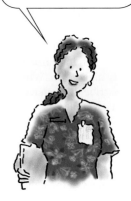

New information about eating disorders is released continuously. Start educating yourself by considering these questions carefully!

Eating disorders refresher

Anorexia nervosa

Obsession for thinness achieved by self-starvation

Key signs and symptoms

- Decreased blood volume, evidenced by lowered blood pressure and orthostatic hypotension
- Electrolyte imbalance, evidenced by muscle weakness, seizures, or dysrhythmias
- Low body weight for developmental stage
- Need to achieve and please others
- Obsessive rituals concerning food
- Refusal to eat
- Persistent behavior that interferes with weight gain

Key test results

- Eating Attitude Test suggests eating disorder
- Electrocardiogram reveals nonspecific ST-segment changes and a prolonged PR interval
- Laboratory tests show elevated blood urea nitrogen (BUN) level and electrolyte imbalances
- Female clients exhibit low estrogen levels
- Male clients exhibit low serum testosterone levels

Key treatments

- Psychotherapy: individual, family-based, group
- Nutritional counseling
- Antianxiety agents: lorazepam, alprazolam
- Antidepressants: amitriptyline, imipramine
- Selective serotonin reuptake inhibitors (SSRIs): paroxetine, fluoxetine

Key interventions

- Contract for specific amount of food to be eaten at each meal
- Provide one-on-one support before, during, and after meals
- Prevent client from using the bathroom for 2 hours after eating
- Help client identify coping mechanisms for dealing with anxiety

- Weigh client once or twice a week at the same time of day using the same scale
- Help client understand the cycle of anorexia

Bulimia nervosa

Uncontrolled consumption of large amounts of food followed by compensatory behaviors to prevent weight gain

Key signs and symptoms

- Alternating episodes of binge eating and purging
- Constant preoccupation with food
- Disruptions in interpersonal relationships
- Eroded tooth enamel
- Extreme need for acceptance and approval
- Irregular menses
- Russell sign (bruised knuckles due to induced vomiting)
- Sporadic, excessive exercise

Key test results

- Beck Depression Inventory may reveal depression
- Eating Attitude Test suggests eating disorder
- Metabolic acidosis may occur from diarrhea caused by enemas and excessive laxative use
- Metabolic alkalosis may occur from frequent vomiting

Key treatments

- Cognitive therapy to identify triggers for binge eating and purging
- SSRIs: paroxetine, fluoxetine

Key interventions

- Explain the purpose of a nutritional contract
- Avoid power struggles about food
- Prevent client from using the bathroom for 2 hours after eating
- Provide one-on-one support before, during, and after meals
- Weigh client once or twice per week at the same time of day using the same scale
- Help client identify cause of the disorder
- Point out cognitive distortions

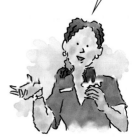

My relationship with food is complicated.

thePoint® You can download tables of drug information to help you prepare for the NCLEX®! View Generic Drug Names, Drug Classifications, Drug Actions, and Nursing Implications for the drugs discussed in this refresher at **http://thePoint.lww.com**.

Eating disorders questions, answers, and rationales

1. A parent whose adolescent child is diagnosed with bulimia nervosa asks a nurse, "How can my child have an eating disorder without being underweight?" Which response is **best**?
1. "A person with bulimia nervosa may be normal weight, overweight, or underweight."
2. "It's hard to face this problem in a person you love."
3. "At first there's no weight loss; it comes later in the disease."
4. "This is a serious problem even though there's no weight loss."

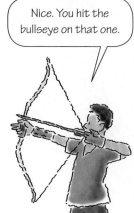

Nice. You hit the bullseye on that one.

1. 1. A person with bulimia nervosa may be of normal weight, overweight, or underweight. Weight loss isn't a clinical criterion for bulimia nervosa. The responses about facing the problem in a loved one, and the severity of the problem despite lack of weight loss, don't address the need for information about the relationship between weight change and bulimia nervosa. The statement about weight loss coming later in the disease is incorrect because the client may experience little or no weight loss.
CN: Psychosocial integrity; CNS: None; CL: Apply; DIFFICULTY: Easy

2. A nurse is reviewing the chart of an adolescent client who has been admitted to the unit. When reading the progress notes below, the nurse sees a laboratory result that indicates a condition consistent with a diagnosis of bulimia nervosa. Which condition does the nurse suspect?

Progress notes	
4/25/17	Received 15-year-old female admitted with
1015	diagnosis of bulimia nervosa. Vital signs:
	blood pressure, 100/70 mm Hg; heart
	rate, 82 beats/minute; respiratory rate, 20
	breaths/minute; temperature, 98° F (36.7°
	C). Laboratory results: Na, 136 mEg/L; K, 3.0
	mEg/L; Cl, 104 mEg/L; Ca, 9.5 mg/dL; fasting
	blood glucose, 90 g/dL. Results called to
	Dr. L. Smith, M.D.
	— Barbara Smith, L. P. N

1. Hypocalcemia
2. Hypoglycemia
3. Hypokalemia
4. Hyponatremia

2. 3. Clients who are bulimic have hypokalemia (decreased potassium levels) due to purging behaviors. Hyponatremia, hypoglycemia, and hypocalcemia don't tend to occur in clients with bulimia nervosa; all the lab results are at normal levels for this client.
CN: Physiological integrity; CNS: Physiological adaptation;
CL: Analyze; DIFFICULTY: Moderate

3. A client with bulimia and a history of purging by vomiting is hospitalized for further observation because of the risk for which conditions? Select all that apply.
1. Diabetes
2. Electrolyte imbalances
3. Cardiac dysrhythmias
4. GI obstruction
5. Esophageal erosion
6. Septicemia from a low white blood cell count

3. 2, 3, 5. People who purge by vomiting are at increased risk for electrolyte imbalance and resulting cardiac dysrhythmias. Purging leads to possible electrolyte imbalance and esophageal erosion; it is not disease producing.
CN: Physiological integrity; CNS: Reduction of risk potential;
CL: Apply; DIFFICULTY: Challenge

4. Which statement about the binge-purge cycle that occurs with bulimia nervosa is correct?
1. There are emotional triggers connected to bingeing.
2. Over time, people usually grow out of bingeing behaviors.
3. Bingeing isn't the problem; purging is the issue to address.
4. When a person gets too hungry, there's a tendency to binge.

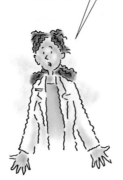

Ack! I'm so stressed. I need a doughnut ... or six.

5. A client with a diagnosis of bulimia nervosa is working on relationship issues. Which nursing intervention is **most** important?
1. Assist the client to work on developing social skills.
2. Help the client identify how relationships cause bulimic behavior.
3. Facilitate the client's ability to identify feelings about relationships.
4. Discuss ways to prevent getting overinvolved in relationships.

6. A young client with bulimia nervosa wants to lessen feelings of powerlessness. Which short-term goal is initially **most** important?
1. Learning problem-solving skills
2. Decreasing symptoms of anxiety
3. Performing self-care activities daily
4. Verbalizing how to set limits with others

7. A client with bulimia nervosa tells a nurse that their parents don't know about the eating disorder. Which goal is appropriate for this client and family?
1. Decreasing the chaos in the family unit
2. Learning effective communication skills
3. Spending time together in social situations
4. Discussing the client's need to be responsible

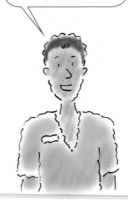

Changing the way the client thinks is half the battle with eating disorders.

8. When the nurse is discussing self-esteem with a client with bulimia nervosa, which area is **most** important?
1. Assess personal fears.
2. Identify family strengths.
3. Discuss negative thinking patterns.
4. Reduce environmental stimuli.

4. 1. It's important for the client to understand the emotional triggers for bingeing, such as disappointment, depression, and anxiety. People don't outgrow eating disorders. This response leads a person to believe binge eating is a normal part of growth and development when it definitely isn't. Addressing purging negates the seriousness of bingeing and leads the client to believe only vomiting is a problem. Physiologic hunger doesn't predispose a client to bingeing behaviors.
CN: Physiological integrity; CNS: Reduction of risk potential; CL: Apply; DIFFICULTY: Easy

5. 3. The client must address personal feelings about relationships, especially uncomfortable ones because they may trigger bingeing behavior. Social skills are important to a client's well-being, but they aren't typically a major problem for the client with bulimia nervosa. Relationships *don't cause* bulimic behaviors. It's the inability to handle stress or conflict that arises from interactions that causes the client to be distressed. The client isn't necessarily overinvolved in relationships; the issue may be the lack of satisfying relationships in their life.
CN: Psychosocial integrity; CNS: None; CL: Apply; DIFFICULTY: Moderate

6. 1. When the client can learn effective problem-solving skills, they will gain a sense of control and power over life. Development of these skills is essential to recovery. Anxiety is commonly caused by feelings of powerlessness. Performing daily self-care activities won't reduce one's sense of powerlessness. Verbalizing how to set limits to protect themself from the intrusive behavior of others is a necessary life skill, but problem-solving skills take priority in this case.
CN: Psychosocial integrity; CNS: None; CL: Analyze; DIFFICULTY: Difficult

7. 2. A major goal for the client with bulimia nervosa and family is to learn to communicate directly and honestly in a peaceful environment. To change the chaotic environment, the family must first learn to communicate effectively. Families with a member who has an eating disorder are commonly enmeshed and don't need to spend more time together. Before discussing the client's level of responsibility, the family needs to establish effective ways of communicating with one another.
CN: Psychosocial integrity; CNS: None; CL: Apply; DIFFICULTY: Easy

8. 3. Clients with bulimia nervosa need to work on identifying and changing their negative thinking and distortion of reality. Personal fears are related to negative thinking. Exploring family strengths isn't a priority; it's more appropriate to explore the client's strengths. Environmental stimuli don't cause bulimic behaviors.
CN: Psychosocial integrity; CNS: None; CL: Apply; DIFFICULTY: Challenge

9. The nurse is caring for a client with bulimia nervosa. Which observation by the nurse is life-threatening and should be reported to the health care provider immediately?
1. Serum calcium 10.1 mg/dL
2. Heart rate 56 beats/minute
3. Serum potassium 2.9 mEq/L *3.0–5*
4. Respiratory rate 16 breaths/minute

10. A nurse is talking to a client with bulimia nervosa about the complications of laxative abuse. Which statement by the client indicates an initial understanding of the risks associated with laxative abuse?
1. "I don't really have much taste for food, so there's no loss in getting it out of my system more quickly."
2. "Laxatives help me get rid of extra calories before they're added to my body. I know I just shouldn't eat the extra calories to begin with."
3. "Laxatives are over-the-counter medications that have no harmful effect."
4. "Using laxatives prevents my body from absorbing essential nutrients, such as protein, fat, and calcium."

11. The nurse is caring for an adolescent client receiving a selective serotonin reuptake inhibitor (SSRI) as part of the treatment plan for anorexia nervosa. Which action is a priority intervention related to the SSRI therapy?
1. Monitor for suicidal thoughts.
2. Weigh the client regularly.
3. Document the food intake without comment.
4. Explore the client's strengths and positive coping mechanisms.

12. A client is talking with a nurse about the binge-purge cycle. Which question should the nurse ask about the cycle?
1. "Do you know how to stop the binge-purge cycle?"
2. "Does the binge-purge cycle help you lose weight?"
3. "Can the binge-purge cycle take away your anxiety?"
4. "How often do you go through the binge-purge cycle?"

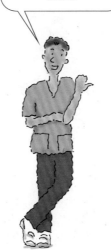

Only one of these questions in question #12 will yield valuable information from the client.

9. 3. Electrolyte imbalance such as hypokalemia (low serum potassium) can be a life-threatening complication of bulimia nervosa due to purging behaviors. Normal serum potassium is 3.5 to 4.5 mEq/L. A serum calcium level of 10.1 mg/dL is within normal range. A heart rate of 56 beats/minute indicates bradycardia, but it isn't life-threatening. A respiratory rate of 16 breaths/minute is within the normal range (16 to 20 breaths/minute), therefore not life-threatening.
CN: Physiological integrity; CNS: Reduction of risk potential; CL: Apply; DIFFICULTY: Easy

10. 4. A serious complication of laxative abuse is malabsorption of nutrients, such as proteins, fats, and calcium. Laxative abuse doesn't tend to affect the client's sense of taste. Overuse of over-the-counter laxatives can be harmful, either when taken alone or in combination with other over-the-counter or prescription medications. Clients with bulimia nervosa need to change their negative thinking in regard to calories and the use of laxatives.
CN: Physiological integrity; CNS: Pharmacological therapies; CL: Apply; DIFFICULTY: Easy

11. 1. The FDA has issued a black box warning that alerts health providers to the increased risk of suicidal ideation and behavior in children, adolescents and young adults (18-24 years of age) when taking antidepressants. Weighing the client, documenting food intake, and exploring the client's strengths are important interventions, but do not relate to the SSRI administration.
CN: Physiological integrity; CNS: Pharmacological therapies; CL: Analyze; DIFFICULTY: Moderate

12. 4. This question is important because there's usually a range of frequencies, such as from a once-a-week pattern to multiple times each day. Asking about ability to stop the binge-purge cycle isn't appropriate because it generates feelings of self-blame and shame. It's common for clients with bulimia nervosa to experience daily fluctuations in their weight. Some clients report weight variations of up to 10 pounds (4.5 kg). The binge-purge cycle may initially relieve mood symptoms, but it tends to generate overall negative feelings about self.
CN: Psychosocial integrity; CNS: None; CL: Apply; DIFFICULTY: Easy

13. A nurse is assessing a client with bulimia nervosa for possible substance abuse. Which question is **best** for obtaining information about this possible problem?
1. "Have you ever used diet pills?"
2. "Where would you go to buy drugs?"
3. "At what age did you start drinking?"
4. "Do your peers ever offer you drugs?"

14. A client with bulimia nervosa is discussing abnormal eating behaviors. Which statement indicates the client is beginning to understand this eating disorder?
1. "When I am feeling lonely, I start to binge."
2. "I know that when my life gets better, I'll eat right."
3. "I know I waste food and waste my money on food."
4. "After my parents' divorce is final, I'll talk about bingeing and purging."

15. The nurse is caring for a client with a diagnosis of bulimia nervosa. After reviewing the client's lab results, the primary health care provider has written a prescription for 20 mEq of potassium chloride oral solution to be administered today. The label on the oral solution states potassium chloride oral solution 40 mEq/15 mL. How many mL should the nurse administer? Record your answer using one decimal place.

_____ mL

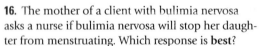

16. The mother of a client with bulimia nervosa asks a nurse if bulimia nervosa will stop her daughter from menstruating. Which response is **best**?
1. "All women with anorexia nervosa or bulimia nervosa will have amenorrhea."
2. "When your daughter is bingeing and purging, she won't have normal periods."
3. "The eating disorder must be ongoing for your daughter's menstrual cycle to change."
4. "Your daughter may have a normal or abnormal menstrual cycle, depending on the severity of her problem."

17. The nurse is working with a client with bulimia nervosa. What would the nurse expect to observe in the client's family dynamic?
1. Mental illness
2. Multiple losses
3. Chronic anxiety
4. Substance abuse

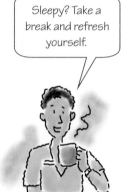

Sleepy? Take a break and refresh yourself.

Now you're cooking.

13. 1. Some clients with bulimia nervosa have a history of, or actively use, amphetamines to control weight. The use of alcohol and street drugs is also common. The questions "Where would you go to buy drugs?" or "Do your peers ever offer you drugs?" could be answered by the client without revealing drug use. The age a client starts drinking may not reveal current substance use.
CN: Psychosocial integrity; CNS: None; CL: Apply; DIFFICULTY: Moderate

14. 1. Binge eating is a way to handle the uncomfortable feelings of frustration, loneliness, anger, and fear. The statement about eating better when life improves indicates the client is experiencing denial of the eating disorder. The statement about wasting food and money addresses the client's guilt feelings; it doesn't demonstrate knowledge of the eating disorder. The statement about the parents' divorce shows the client isn't ready to discuss the eating disorder.
CN: Psychosocial integrity; CNS: None; CL: Analyze; DIFFICULTY: Easy

15. 7.5.
The correct formula to calculate a drug dose is:

$$\frac{\text{Dose on hand}}{\text{Quantity on hand}} = \frac{\text{Dose desired}}{X}$$

The health care provider prescribes 20 mEq, which is the dose desired. The available solution states 40 mEq/15 mL, which is the dose on hand.

$$\frac{40\,\text{mEq}}{15\,\text{mL}} = \frac{20\,\text{mEq}}{X}$$
$$40x = 300$$
$$X = 7.5\,\text{mL}$$

CN: Physiological integrity; CNS: Pharmacological therapies; CL: Apply; DIFFICULTY: Difficult

16. 4. Women with bulimia nervosa may have a normal or abnormal menstrual cycle, depending on the severity of the eating disorder. Not all women with eating disorders have amenorrhea. The eating disorder can disrupt the menstrual cycle at any point in the illness.
CN: Physiological integrity; CNS: Physiological adaptation; CL: Analyze; DIFFICULTY: Easy

17. 2. Families with a member who has bulimia nervosa usually struggle with multiple losses. Mental illness, chronic anxiety, and substance abuse don't tend to be themes in the family background of the client with bulimia nervosa.
CN: Psychosocial integrity; CNS: None; CL: Analyze; DIFFICULTY: Difficult

18. A client with bulimia nervosa tells a nurse that the major problem is eating too much food in a short period of time and then vomiting. Which short-term goal is **most** important?
1. Helping the client understand every person has a satiety level
2. Encouraging the client to verbalize fears and concerns about food
3. Determining the amount of food the client will eat without purging
4. Obtaining a therapy appointment to look at the emotional causes of bulimia nervosa

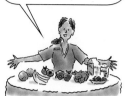

Encourage clients with bulimia to eat small portions of healthy food.

18. 3. The client must meet nutritional needs to prevent further complications and identify the amount of food that can be eaten without purging as a first short-term goal. Determining satiety level or verbalizing fears and feelings about food are *not* priority goals for this client. All clients must first take steps to meet their nutritional needs. Therapy is an important part of dealing with this disorder, but it isn't the first step.
CN: Physiological integrity; CNS: Reduction of risk potential; CL: Apply; DIFFICULTY: Challenge

19. Which statement indicates a client with bulimia nervosa is making progress in interrupting the binge-purge cycle?
1. "I called my friend the last two times I got upset."
2. "I know I'll have this problem with eating forever."
3. "I started asking my family to watch me eat each meal."
4. "I will have my friend bring me home from parties if I want to purge."

19. 1. The client who verbalizes feelings and interacts with people instead of turning to food for comfort shows signs of progress. Feeling that the eating problem will last forever indicates the client needs more information on how to handle the disorder. Having another person watch the client eat isn't a helpful strategy, as the client will depend on others to help control food intake. Asking a friend to take the client home from parties to purge indicates they are in denial about the severity of the problem.
CN: Psychosocial integrity; CNS: None; CL: Apply; DIFFICULTY: Challenge

20. A client with bulimia nervosa asks a nurse, "How can I ask for help from my family?" Which response is **most** appropriate?
1. "When you ask for help, make sure you really need it."
2. "Have you ever asked your family for help in the past?"
3. "Ask family members to spend time with you at mealtime."
4. "Think about how you can handle this situation without help."

20. 2. The nurse should determine whether the client has ever been successful in asking for help because previous experiences affect the client's ability to ask for help now. The client needs to be able to ask for help anytime without analyzing the level of need. Asking other people to be present at mealtime isn't the only way to ask for help. Developing a support system is imperative for this client, not trying to handle the situation independently.
CN: Psychosocial integrity; CNS: None; CL: Analyze; DIFFICULTY: Challenge

21. A client with bulimia nervosa tells a nurse he or she does not eat during the day, but after 5 p.m. begins to binge and vomit. Which intervention would be **most** useful to this client?
1. Help the client to stop eating the foods on which they binge on.
2. Discuss the effects of fasting on the client's pattern of eating.
3. Encourage the client to become involved in food preparation.
4. Educate the client to eat earlier in the day and decrease intake at night.

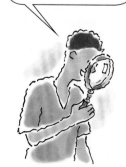

Look carefully for the *most useful* intervention in question #21.

21. 2. It's common for a person who fasts for most of the day to become extremely hungry, overeat by bingeing, and then feel the need to purge. Restricting food intake can actually trigger the binge-purge cycle. In treatment, the client is taught to identify foods that trigger eating, discuss the feelings associated with these foods, and work to eat them in normal amounts. Involvement in food preparation won't promote changes in the client's behaviors. Eating earlier or decreasing nighttime intake doesn't address how fasting can trigger the binge-purge cycle.
CN: Psychosocial integrity; CNS: None; CL: Apply; DIFFICULTY: Difficult

22. A client with bulimia nervosa tells a nurse the client was doing well until last week, after having a fight with a parent. Which nursing intervention would be **most** helpful?
1. Examine the relationship between feelings and eating.
2. Discuss the importance of therapy for the entire family.
3. Encourage the client to avoid certain family members.
4. Identify daily stressors and learn stress management skills.

22. 1. The client must understand their feelings and develop healthy coping skills to handle unpleasant situations. Family therapy may be indicated but shouldn't be an immediate intervention. Avoidance isn't a useful coping strategy; eventually, the underlying issues must be explored. All clients can benefit from stress management skills but, for this client, care must focus on the relationship between feelings and eating behaviors.
CN: Psychosocial integrity; CNS: None; CL: Apply;
DIFFICULTY: Challenge

23. Which statement from a client with bulimia shows that the client understands the concept of relapse?
1. "If I can't maintain control over things, I'll have problems."
2. "If I have problems, then I haven't learned much."
3. "If this illness becomes chronic, I won't be able to handle it."
4. "If I have problems, I can start over again and not feel hopeless."

23. 4. The client with bulimia who knows they can try again and not feel hopeless following a relapse realizes that a relapse is just a slip, and positive gains made from treatment haven't been lost. Control issues relate to powerlessness, which contributes to relapse. Negative self-statements can lead to relapse.
CN: Psychosocial integrity; CNS: None; CL: Understand; DIFFICULTY: Challenge

24. A client with bulimia nervosa has a history of severe gastrointestinal (GI) problems caused by excessive purging. Based on this finding, this nurse must stay alert for which physiologic problem(s)? Select all that apply.
1. Renal calculi - stones
2. Esophageal tears
3. Focal seizures
4. Rectal bleeding
5. Muscle atrophy

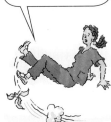
Don't let this question trip you up. Slow down and read it again.

24. 1, 2. A client with bulimia who has severe GI problems from excessive purging is at increased risk for esophageal tears and irritation, or esophagitis. In addition, clients with eating disorders may develop renal calculi. Purging by excessive laxative use can result in rectal bleeding. Focal seizures and muscle atrophy aren't related to severe GI problems.
CN: Physiological integrity; CNS: Reduction of risk potential;
CL: Analyze; DIFFICULTY: Difficult

25. Which intervention is the treatment team's **priority** in planning the care of a client with an eating disorder?
1. Prevent the client from performing any muscle-building exercises.
2. Keep the client on bed rest until they attain a specified weight.
3. Meet daily to discuss manipulation and countertransference.
4. Monitor the client's weight and vital signs daily.

25. 3. Clients with eating disorders commonly use manipulative ploys and countertransference to resist weight gain (if they restrict food intake) or maintain purging practices (if they have bulimia). They commonly play staff members against one another and hone in on their caretaker's vulnerabilities. Muscle building is acceptable because, compared with aerobic exercise, it burns relatively few calories. Keeping the client on bed rest until they reach a specified weight can result in unnecessary power struggles and prevent staff from focusing on more pertinent problems. Monitoring the client's weight and vital signs on a daily basis is important, but not vital, unless the client's physiologic condition warrants such close scrutiny.
CN: Safe, effective care environment; CNS: Coordinated care;
CL: Apply; DIFFICULTY: Challenge

26. The nurse caring for a client with anorexia nervosa determines what goal will take **priority**?

1. The client will establish adequate daily nutritional intake.
2. The client will make a contract with the nurse that sets a target weight.
3. The client will identify unrealistic self-perceptions about body size.
4. The client will verbalize the possible physiologic consequences of self-starvation.

26. **1.** According to Maslow hierarchy of needs, all humans need to meet basic physiologic needs first. Because a client with anorexia nervosa eats little or nothing, the nurse must plan to help the client meet this basic, immediate physiologic need first. The nurse may give lower priority to goals that address long-term plans, self-perception, and potential complications.
CN: Safe, effective care environment; CNS: Coordinated care;
CL: Apply; DIFFICULTY: Easy

27. A nurse is caring for a client with anorexia nervosa who is receiving lorazepam for anxiety. The nurse concludes the teaching has been effective when the client makes which statements? Select all that apply.

1. "I can still drive after I have taken this medication."
2. "I should not discontinue this medication without notifying my health care provider."
3. "I will only be taking this medication until I learn to manage my anxiety."
4. "I should avoid drinking alcohol while taking this medication."
5. "I can take this medication without worrying about becoming addicted."

27. **2, 3, 4.** Lorazepam is a benzodiazepine and is known to cause drowsiness and sedation. Activities that require alertness, like driving a car, should be avoided while taking this drug. The drug should be tapered, not stopped abruptly. These drugs are only recommended for short-term use. Long-term use can result in dependency. Alcohol use with the benzodiazepines will cause an additive CNS depression, so alcohol should be avoided.
CN: Physiological integrity; CNS: Pharmacological therapies;
CL: Analyze; DIFFICULTY: Challenge

28. A client with anorexia nervosa tells a nurse, "I'll never have the slender body I want." Which intervention is **best** to handle this problem?

1. Call a family meeting to get help from the parents.
2. Help the client work on developing a realistic body image.
3. Make an appointment for the client to see the dietitian on a weekly basis.
4. Develop an exercise program the client can participate in twice per week.

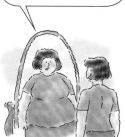

Clients with anorexia nervosa have a distorted view of their bodies.

28. **2.** The client with anorexia nervosa pursues thinness and has a distorted view of self. A family meeting may not help the client develop a more realistic view of the client's body. Although meeting with a dietitian might be helpful, it isn't a priority. Clients with anorexia nervosa typically exercise excessively.
CN: Psychosocial integrity; CNS: None; CL: Apply; DIFFICULTY: Easy

29. A client with anorexia nervosa attended psychoeducational sessions on principles of adequate nutrition. Which statement by the client indicates the education was effective?

1. "I should eat while I'm doing things to distract myself."
2. "I should eat all my food at night just before I go to bed."
3. "I should eat small amounts of food slowly at every meal."
4. "I should eat only when I'm with my family and trying to be social."

29. **3.** Slowly eating small amounts of food facilitates adequate digestion and prevents distention. Healthy eating is best accomplished when a person isn't doing other things while eating. Eating just before bedtime isn't a healthy eating habit. A client, who eats only when the family is present, or when trying to be social, ties eating to social or emotional cues rather than nutritional needs.
CN: Health promotion and maintenance; CNS: None; CL: Apply;
DIFFICULTY: Easy

30. Which communication strategy is **best** to use with a client with anorexia nervosa who is having problems with peer relationships?
1. Use concrete language and maintain a focus on reality.
2. Direct the client to talk about what's causing the anxiety.
3. Teach the client to communicate feelings and express self appropriately.
4. Confront the client about being depressed and self-absorbed.

31. A nurse plans to include the parents of a client with anorexia nervosa in therapy sessions along with the client. Which fact should the nurse remember about the parents of clients with anorexia?
1. They tend to overprotect their children.
2. They usually have a history of substance abuse.
3. They maintain emotional distance from their children.
4. They alternate between loving and rejecting their children.

32. A nurse is talking to the family of a client with anorexia nervosa. Which family behavior is **most**-likely to be seen during the family's interaction?
1. Sibling rivalry
2. Rage reactions
3. Parental disagreement
4. Excessive independence

33. A nurse is working with a client with anorexia nervosa who has acrocyanosis in the extremities. Which short-term goal is **most** important for the client?
1. Do daily range-of-motion exercises.
2. Eat some fatty foods daily.
3. Check neurologic reflexes.
4. Promote adequate circulation.

34. A client with anorexia nervosa tells a nurse about always feeling fat. Which intervention is **best** for this client?
1. Identify positive characteristics to boost self-esteem.
2. Encourage the client to honestly evaluate him or herself in a mirror.
3. Educate about the dynamics of the disorder.
4. Talk about how they are different from peers.

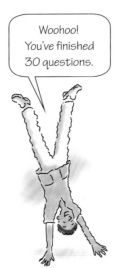

Woohoo! You've finished 30 questions.

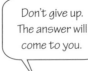

Don't give up. The answer will come to you.

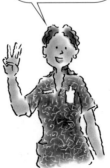

30. 3. Clients with anorexia nervosa commonly communicate on a superficial level and avoid expressing feelings. Identifying feelings and learning to express them are initial steps in decreasing isolation. Clients with anorexia nervosa are usually able to discuss abstract and concrete issues. Confrontation or directing the client to talk about what's causing the anxiety usually isn't effective communication strategy, because it may cause the client to withdraw and become more depressed.
CN: Psychosocial integrity; CNS: None; CL: Apply; DIFFICULTY: Easy

31. 1. Clients with anorexia nervosa typically come from a family with parents who are controlling and overprotective. These clients use eating to gain control of an aspect of their lives. Having a history of substance abuse, maintaining an emotional distance, and alternating between love and rejection aren't characteristic of parents of children with anorexia nervosa.
CN: Psychosocial integrity; CNS: None; CL: Apply;
DIFFICULTY: Moderate

32. 3. In many families with a member suffering from anorexia nervosa, there's marital conflict and parental disagreement. Sibling rivalry is common and not specific to a family with a member who suffers from anorexia nervosa. In these families, the members tend to be enmeshed and dependent on each other. The family with an anorexic member is usually one that looks good to the outside observer. Emotions are over-controlled, and there's difficulty appropriately expressing negative feelings.
CN: Psychosocial integrity; CNS: None; CL: Apply;
DIFFICULTY: Moderate

32. 4. Circulation decrease causes extremities to be cold, numb, and have dry and flaky skin. Exercise may help prevent contractures and muscle atrophy, but it may have only a limited secondary effect in promoting circulation. Intake of fatty foods won't impact the client's circulation problems. Checking neurologic reflexes won't necessarily assist with improving circulation problems.
CN: Physiological integrity; CNS: Reduction of risk potential;
CL: Apply; DIFFICULTY: Easy

34. 3. The client can benefit from understanding the underlying dynamics of the eating disorder. The client with anorexia nervosa has low self-esteem and won't believe the positive statements. Although the client may look at his or herself in the mirror, in their mind, they'll still see themself as fat. Pointing out differences will only diminish already low self-esteem.
CN: Psychosocial integrity; CNS: None; CL: Apply;
DIFFICULTY: Challenge

35. A client with anorexia nervosa is discharged from the hospital after gaining 12 lb. What client statement best indicates that the nurse's reinforcement of discharge education has been effective? Select all that apply.
1. "I plan to eat two small meals a day."
2. "I will need to work on this for a prolonged period of time."
3. "I feel this is scary, but I'm not going to write about it in my journal."
4. "I have to cut back on my calorie intake because I've gained 12 lb."
5. "I'll need to attend therapy for support to stay healthy."

36. The grandparents of a client with anorexia nervosa want to support the clients but aren't sure what they should do. Which intervention is **best**?
1. Encourage positive expressions of affection.
2. Encourage behaviors that promote socialization.
3. Discuss how eating disorders create powerlessness.
4. Discuss the meaning of hunger and body sensations.

37. A nurse is analyzing the need for health education in a female client with anorexia nervosa who lives in a chaotic family situation. Which question is **most** important for the nurse to ask the client?
1. "For how many months have your menstrual periods been irregular?"
2. "How often do you think about food in a 24-hour period?"
3. "What were the circumstances before your eating disorder?"
4. "How much and what kinds of exercise do you engage in every day?"

38. An adolescent client with anorexia nervosa tells a nurse about his or her outstanding academic achievements and thoughts about suicide. Which factor must the nurse consider when contributing to the care plan for this client?
1. Self-esteem
2. Physical illnesses
3. Paranoid delusions
4. Relationship avoidance

39. How can the nurse **best** help a client with anorexia nervosa recognize self-distortions?
1. Identify the client's misperceptions of self.
2. Acknowledge immature and childlike behaviors.
3. Determine the consequences of a faulty support system.
4. Recognize the age-appropriate tasks to be accomplished.

35. 2, 5. The client is planning to attend therapy after discharge, and this shows an understanding of the need for continued counseling. Recovery from eating disorders may take years and clients may relapse. Eating only two small meals a day is an unrealistic plan for meeting nutritional needs. Feeling insecure when leaving a controlled environment is a common response to discharge; however, writing about feelings in a journal would be therapeutic. Gaining 12 pounds indicates that the client's nutritional needs are being met at the present caloric intake levels.
CN: Psychosocial integrity; CNS: None; CL: Analyze;
DIFFICULTY: Moderate

36. 1. Clients with eating disorders need emotional support and expressions of affection from family members. It wouldn't be appropriate for the grandparents to promote socialization. Clients with eating disorders feel powerless, but it's better to have the grandparents focus on something positive. Talking about hunger and other body sensations isn't a useful strategy.
CN: Psychosocial integrity; CNS: None; CL: Apply;
DIFFICULTY: Moderate

37. 3. The circumstances before the onset of the eating disorder provide the nurse information about the family and background situations that influenced the client's needs and distorted eating. Menstrual history, exercise pattern, and food obsessions are relevant, but they don't provide information related to the family situation.
CN: Psychosocial integrity; CNS: None; CL: Analyze; DIFFICULTY:
Moderate

38. 1. The client lacks self-esteem, which contributes to her level of depression and feelings of personal ineffectiveness, which, in turn, may lead to suicidal thoughts. Physical illnesses are common with clients with anorexia nervosa, but they don't relate to this situation. Paranoid delusions refer to an individual's false idea that others want to cause harm. No evidence exists that this client is socially isolated.
CN: Psychosocial integrity; CNS: None; CL: Analyze; DIFFICULTY: Easy

39. 1. Questioning the client's misperceptions and distortions will create doubt about how the client views herself. Acknowledging immature behaviors or determining the consequences of a faulty support system won't promote recognition of self-distortions. Recognizing the age appropriate tasks to be accomplished won't help the client recognize distortions.
CN: Psychosocial integrity; CNS: None; CL: Analyze; DIFFICULTY: Easy

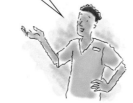

When developing a care plan, don't forget to include measures that have worked well for the client previously.

40. The nurse is assisting with the development of a care plan for a client with anorexia nervosa. Which information should the nurse ensure is included?
   1. Coping mechanisms used in the past
   2. Concerns about changes in lifestyle and daily activities
   3. Rejection of feedback from family and significant others
   4. Appropriate eating habits and social behaviors centering on eating

41. The parents of a client with anorexia nervosa ask the nurse about the risk factors for this disorder. After reinforcement of the education plan by the nurse, which statement by the parents **best** indicates that it has been effective?
   1. "Risk factors include the inability to be still and emotional lability."
   2. "Risk factors include a high level of anxiety and disorganized behavior."
   3. "Risk factors include low self-esteem and problems with family relationships."
   4. "Risk factors include a lack of life experiences and opportunities to learn life skills."

42. A client with anorexia nervosa has started taking fluoxetine. The nurse should closely monitor the client for which adverse reaction?
   1. Drowsiness
   2. Dry mouth
   3. Light-headedness
   4. Nausea

43. A client with anorexia nervosa is worried about rectal bleeding. Which question by the nurse will help obtain more information about the problem?
   1. "How often do you use laxatives?"
   2. "How many days ago did you stop vomiting?"
   3. "Are you eating anything that causes irritation?"
   4. "Do you bleed before or after exercise?"

44. Which characteristics are typical findings in a client with anorexia nervosa? Select all that apply.
   1. Intense fear of gaining weight
   2. Weight 70% or less than her ideal body weight
   3. Awareness that she has a problem but refusal to admit it
   4. Self-esteem that's dependent on how she looks
   5. Weight loss accomplished through the use of diet pills

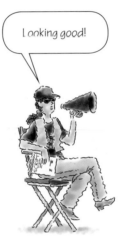

Looking good!

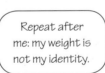

Repeat after me: my weight is not my identity.

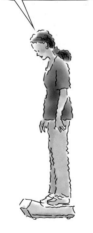

40. **1.** Examination of positive and negative coping mechanisms used by the family allows the nurse to build a care plan specific to the family's strengths and weaknesses. The way the family copes with concerns is more important than the concerns themselves. Feedback from the family and significant others is vital when building a care plan. Providing information on appropriate eating habits and social behaviors centered on eating won't assist the family in coping with the illness.
CN: Psychosocial integrity; CNS: None; CL: Apply; DIFFICULTY: Challenge

41. **3.** There are several risk factors for eating disorders, including low self-esteem, history of depression, substance abuse, and dysfunctional family relationships. Restlessness and emotional lability are symptoms of manic-depressive illness. Anxiety and disorganized behavior could be signs of a psychotic disorder. A lack of life experiences and an absence of opportunities to learn life skills may be a *result* of anorexia.
CN: Psychosocial integrity; CNS: None; CL: Analyze; DIFFICULTY: Easy

42. **4.** Nausea is an adverse reaction to the drug that compounds the eating disorder problem, and the client must be closely monitored. Although the adverse reactions of drowsiness, dry mouth, and light-headedness may occur, they aren't likely to interfere with treatment.
CN: Physiological integrity; CNS: Pharmacological therapies; CL: Apply; DIFFICULTY: Difficult

43. **1.** Excessive use of laxatives will cause GI irritation and rectal bleeding. If the client stopped vomiting but is still using laxatives, rectal bleeding can occur. Clients with anorexia eat very little, and what they eat wouldn't cause rectal bleeding. Exercise doesn't cause rectal bleeding.
CN: Health promotion and maintenance; CNS: None; CL: Apply; DIFFICULTY: Easy

44. **1, 4.** Individuals with anorexia are intensely afraid of gaining weight. Self-esteem depends on how she looks. The diagnostic criteria state that a person has anorexia when weight is 85% below the expected weight for height. Individuals with the disorder typically don't believe they have a problem and don't consider their behavior abnormal. They don't accomplish weight loss through the use of diet pills but rather through avoidance of food and with excessive exercise.
CN: Psychosocial integrity; CNS: None; CL: Apply; DIFFICULTY: Difficult

45. The nurse is participating in a care planning conference for a client with anorexia nervosa. Which interventions should be included in the plan of care? Select all that apply.
  1. Provide small, frequent feedings.
  2. Monitor weight frequently, but randomly.
  3. Allow the client to skip meals until the antidepressant levels are therapeutic.
  4. Encourage journaling to promote the expression of feelings.
  5. Encourage the client to eat three substantial meals per day.

45. 1, 2, 4. Smaller, more frequent meals may be better tolerated by the client and will gradually increase her daily caloric intake. Weight should be monitored randomly to prevent the client from water loading (drinking excessive water and not urinating prior to being weighed). Clients with anorexia are emotionally restrained and afraid of their feelings, so journaling can be a powerful tool that assists in recovery. Clients with anorexia are obsessed with gaining weight and will skip all meals if given the opportunity, so encouraging the client to skip meals isn't therapeutic. Because of self-starvation, clients with anorexia seldom tolerate large meals three times per day.
CN: Safe, effective care environment; CNS: Coordinated care;
CL: Analyze; DIFFICULTY: Challenge

46. A nurse should be alert for which findings in a client with bulimia nervosa? Select all that apply.
  1. Severe electrolyte imbalances
  2. Damaged teeth due to the eroding effects of gastric acids on tooth enamel
  3. Pneumonia from aspirated stomach contents
  4. Cessation of menses
  5. Esophageal tears and gastric rupture
  6. Intestinal inflammation

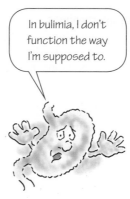
In bulimia, I don't function the way I'm supposed to.

46. 1, 2, 4, 5. Constant bingeing and purging behaviors can result in severe electrolyte imbalances, erosion of tooth enamel from constant exposure to gastric acids, menstrual irregularities, esophageal tears and, in severe cases, gastric rupture. Aspiration pneumonia is unlikely because the vomiting is voluntary and controlled. Intestinal inflammation isn't typically associated with bulimia nervosa.
CN: Physiological integrity; CNS: Physiological adaptation;
CL: Apply; DIFFICULTY: Challenge

47. The nurse is caring for a client with bulimia nervosa requiring IV fluids for dehydration and electrolyte imbalances. The primary health care provider has prescribed 1,000 mL of 0.9% sodium chloride with 40 mEq of potassium chloride to infuse over 6 hours. The drop factor of the IV tubing is 10 drops per mL. How many drops per minute should the nurse infuse the fluids? Record your answer as a whole number.

_____ drops/min

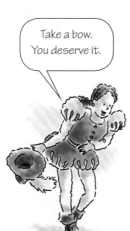
Take a bow. You deserve it.

47. 28.
The correct formula to calculate a drug dose is:

$$\frac{\text{drops}}{\text{min}} = \frac{\text{drops}}{\text{mL}} \times \frac{\text{Dose desired}}{\text{Time desired}} \times \frac{1\,\text{hr}}{60\,\text{min}}$$

$$\frac{10\,\text{drops}}{\text{mL}} \times \frac{1,000\ \cancel{\text{mL}}}{6\ \cancel{\text{hrs}}} \times \frac{1\ \cancel{\text{hr}}}{60\,\text{min}}$$

$$= \frac{10,000}{360} = 27.7 = 28\,\text{drops}\,/\,\text{min}$$

CN: Physiological integrity; CNS: Pharmacological therapies;
CL: Apply, DIFFICULTY: Moderate

Chapter 21

Antepartum Care

Antepartum care refresher

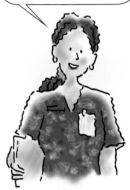

Looking for information about antepartum care before tackling this chapter? Visit www.obgyn.net/, an independent Web site dedicated to obstetric and gynecologic health problems.

Acquired immunodeficiency syndrome (AIDS)

Condition caused by the human immunodeficiency virus (HIV); infection places the client at high risk for opportunistic infections, unusual cancers, and other abnormalities

Key signs and symptoms
- Diarrhea
- Fatigue
- Kaposi sarcoma
- Mild flulike symptoms
- Opportunistic infections, such as toxoplasmosis, oral and vaginal candidiasis, herpes simplex, *Pneumocystis jiroveci,* and *Candida esophagitis*
- Weight loss

Key test results
- CD4+ T-cell level is less than 200 cells/µL
- Enzyme-linked immunosorbent assay shows positive HIV antibody titer
- Western blot test is positive

Key treatments
- Treatment depends upon clinical situation
- Anti-HIV medications should be combination of at least three medications: two NRTI class (one should be AZT) and either one NNRTI class or one protease inhibitor

Key interventions
- Determine whether client will be able to care for her infant after delivery

Adolescent pregnancy

Pregnancy that occurs in females between the ages of 11 to 19 years; the pregnant adolescent is considered high-risk due to the physical and psychological demands associated with her own growth and development along with the demands of pregnancy

Key signs and symptoms
- Denial of pregnancy, which may deter the client from seeking medical attention early in pregnancy

Key test results
- Pregnancy test is positive

Key treatments
- Diet with caloric intake that supports the growing adolescent and developing fetus

Key interventions
- Monitor client's weight gain
- Advise client of her options, including:
  ○ terminating the pregnancy
  ○ continuing the pregnancy and giving up the infant for adoption
  ○ continuing the pregnancy and keeping the infant

Gestational diabetes

Endocrine disorder that involves problems of glucose metabolism; women who enter pregnancy and develop diabetes during pregnancy are said to have gestational diabetes

Key signs and symptoms
- Glycosuria
- Ketonuria
- Polyuria

Key test results
- Diagnosed if the client has two or more of the following results:
  ○ fasting blood sugar level equals or exceeds 105 mg/dL
  ○ three-hour glucose tolerance test reveals 1-hour level at or above 180 mg/dL
  ○ three-hour glucose tolerance test reveals 2-hour level at or above 155 mg/dL
  ○ three-hour glucose tolerance test reveals 3-hour level at or above 140 mg/dL

Key treatments
- 1,800- to 2,200-calorie diet divided into three meals and three snacks
- Diet should also include low fat and cholesterol and high fiber
- Administration of insulin or glyburide after the first trimester

Key interventions
- Encourage adherence to dietary regulations

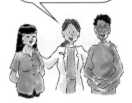

I have great expectations for this chapter … it's pregnant with possibilities.

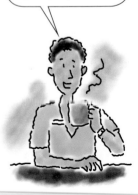

I don't know about you, but drinking lots of coffee always gives me polyuria.

- Encourage client to exercise moderately
- Prepare the client for antepartum fetal surveillance testing, including:
  - oxytocin challenge testing
  - nipple stimulation stress testing
  - amniotic fluid index
  - biophysical profile
  - nonstress test

Ectopic pregnancy

Pregnancy in which the fertilized ovum implants outside the uterine cavity; although implantation can occur on the ovarian surface or in the cervix, the most common site of implantation is the fallopian tube

Key signs and symptoms

- Irregular vaginal bleeding and dull abdominal pain on the affected side early in pregnancy
- Positive Cullen sign (bluish discoloration around the umbilicus)
- Rupture of tubes, causing sudden and severe abdominal pain, syncope, and referred shoulder pain as the abdomen fills with blood

Key test results

- Human chorionic gonadotropin (HCG) titers are abnormally low when compared to a normal pregnancy
- Transvaginal ultrasound confirms pregnancy placement

Key treatments

- Laparotomy to ligate the bleeding vessels and remove or repair damaged fallopian tube
- If tube hasn't ruptured, methotrexate followed by leucovorin to stop the trophoblastic cells from growing (therapy continues until negative HCG levels are achieved)

Key interventions

- Monitor for signs of rupturing ectopic pregnancy, such as:
  - severe abdominal pain
  - orthostatic hypotension
  - tachycardia
  - dizziness
- Maintain IV fluid replacement
- Monitor blood product administration

Heart disease

Pregnant woman with heart disease is at high risk for complications due to the physiologic changes that occur during pregnancy, primarily the increase in circulating blood volume

Key signs and symptoms

- Crackles at the base of the lungs
- Diastolic murmur at the heart's apex

- Dyspnea
- Fatigue
- Tachycardia

Key test results

- Echocardiography, electrocardiography, and chest x-ray may reveal cardiac abnormalities, dysrhythmias, impaired cardiac function, increased workload on the heart, and cardiovascular decompensation

Key treatments

Class III and class IV disease

- Anticoagulants: heparin
- Antiarrhythmics: digoxin, procainamide, beta-blockers
- Thiazide diuretics and furosemide to control heart failure if activity restriction and reduced sodium intake don't prevent it

Key interventions

- Monitor cardiovascular and respiratory status
- Administer oxygen by nasal cannula or face mask during labor
- Position client on her left side with her head and shoulders elevated during labor

Hydatidiform mole

Abnormal growth and degeneration of the trophoblastic villi cells; cells become fluid-filled vesicles and the embryo fails to develop (also known as gestational trophoblastic disease)

Key signs and symptoms

- Intermittent or continuous bright red or brownish vaginal bleeding by the 12th week of gestation
- Absence of fetal heart tones

Key test results

- HCG levels much higher than normal
- Ultrasound fails to reveal a fetal skeleton

Key treatments

- Therapeutic abortion (suction and curettage) if spontaneous abortion doesn't occur
- Weekly monitoring of HCG levels until they remain normal for 3 consecutive weeks
- Periodic follow-up for 1 to 2 years because of increased risk of neoplasm

Key interventions

- Monitor vaginal bleeding
- Send contents of uterine evacuation to laboratory for analysis

Hyperemesis gravidarum

Nausea and vomiting that persist past the 12th week of pregnancy or that is so severe that it interferes with the pregnant woman's nutrition

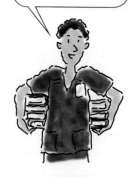

Do you remember where the fertilized egg implants in an ectopic pregnancy?

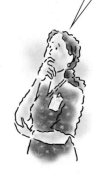

A client has continuous bright red bleeding in her 12th week of gestation, no fetal heart tones are heard, and HCG levels are sky-high. What condition would you suspect?

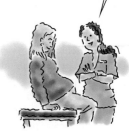

"Hyperemesis gravidarum" is just a fancy way of saying "lots of vomiting when you're pregnant."

Key signs and symptoms
- Continuous, severe nausea and vomiting
- Dehydration
- Oliguria
- Significant weight loss (≥5% prepregnancy weight)

Key test results
- Arterial blood gas analysis reveals metabolic alkalosis
- Hemoglobin level and hematocrit are elevated
- Serum potassium level reveals hypokalemia

Key treatments
- Restoration of fluid and electrolyte balance

Key interventions
- Monitor fundal height and client's weight
- Provide small, frequent meals
- Maintain IV fluid replacement and total parenteral nutrition

Hypertension in pregnancy
High blood pressure during pregnancy (termed gestational hypertension if condition develops during pregnancy)

Key signs and symptoms
Gestational hypertension
- Systolic blood pressure ≥140 mm Hg or diastolic blood pressure ≥90 mm Hg at 20 weeks' gestation and was previously normotensive
- No proteinuria

Preeclampsia
- Systolic blood pressure ≥140 mm Hg or diastolic blood pressure ≥90 mm Hg
- Proteinuria (0.3 g protein in 24-hour specimen)
- Headaches, blurred vision, hyperreflexia, nausea, vomiting, irritability, cerebral disturbances, and epigastric pain
- Presence of HELLP syndrome (hemolysis, elevated liver enzymes, and low platelet count)

Key test results
- Blood chemistry reveals:
  - increased blood urea nitrogen, creatinine, and uric acid levels
  - elevated liver function studies

Key treatments
- Bed rest in a left lateral position
- Delivery:
  - with mild preeclampsia: when fetus is mature and safe induction is possible
  - with severe preeclampsia: regardless of gestational age

- High-protein diet with restriction of excessively salty foods
- With chronic hypertension: methyldopa or labetalol
- With preeclampsia:
  - hydralazine or labetalol to control blood pressure
  - betamethasone to accelerate fetal lung maturation
  - magnesium sulfate to reduce the amount of acetylcholine produced by motor nerves, thereby preventing seizures

Key interventions
All clients
- Evaluate client for edema and proteinuria
- Maintain seizure precautions in hospitalized clients
- Encourage bed rest in a left lateral recumbent position
- Monitor blood pressure

Severe preeclampsia
- Monitor maternal blood pressure every 4 hours or more frequently if unstable
- Be prepared to obtain a blood sample for typing and cross-matching
- Keep calcium gluconate (antidote to magnesium sulfate) nearby for administration at first sign of magnesium sulfate toxicity (elevated serum levels, decreased deep tendon reflexes, muscle flaccidity, central nervous system depression, and decreased respiratory rate and renal function)

Multifetal pregnancy
Pregnancy with more than one fetus present in the uterus

Key signs and symptoms
- More than one set of fetal heart sounds
- Uterine size greater than expected for dates

Key test results
- Alpha-fetoprotein levels are elevated
- Ultrasonography is positive for multifetal pregnancy

Key treatments
- Bed rest if early dilation occurs before or at 24 to 28 weeks' gestation
- Biweekly nonstress test to document fetal growth, beginning with the 28th week of gestation
- Increased intake of calories, iron, folate, and vitamins
- Ultrasound examinations monthly to document fetal growth

Key interventions
- Monitor fetal heart sounds

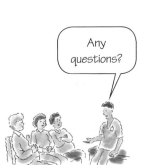

If your client has high blood pressure, protein in the urine, and severe headaches, suspect preeclampsia.

Any questions?

- Monitor maternal vital signs and weight
- Monitor cardiovascular and pulmonary status

Placenta previa

Abnormal implantation of the placenta in the uterus; a common cause of painless bleeding during the second half of pregnancy

Key signs and symptoms

- Painless, bright red vaginal bleeding, especially during third trimester

Key test results

- Early ultrasound evaluation reveals placenta implanted in the lower uterine segment

Key treatments

- Depends on gestational age, when first episode occurs, and amount of bleeding
- If gestational age less than 34 weeks, hospitalize client and restrict her to bed rest to avoid preterm labor.
- Surgical intervention by cesarean delivery depending on placental placement and maternal and fetal stability

Key interventions

- Avoid rectal or vaginal examinations unless equipment is available for vaginal and cesarean delivery

thePoint® You can download tables of drug information to help you prepare for the NCLEX®! View Generic Drug Names, Drug Classifications, Drug Actions, and Nursing Implications for the drugs discussed in this refresher at **http://thePoint.lww.com.**

Antepartum care questions, answers, and rationales

1. During an examination, a client who's 32 weeks' pregnant becomes dizzy, light-headed, and pale while supine. What should the nurse do **first**?
 1. Listen to fetal heart tones.
 2. Take the client's blood pressure.
 3. Ask the client to breathe deeply.
 4. Turn the client on her left side.

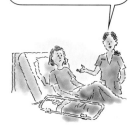

Watch out for that vena cava. If your client starts feeling light-headed while supine, it might be time to roll over.

1. 4. As the enlarging uterus increases pressure on the inferior vena cava, it compromises venous return, which can cause dizziness, light-headedness, and pallor when the client is supine. The nurse can relieve these symptoms by turning the client on her left side, which relieves pressure on the vena cava and restores venous return. Although they're valuable assessments, fetal heart tone and maternal blood pressure measurements don't correct the problem. Because deep breathing has no effect on venous return, it can't relieve the client's symptoms. CN: Physiological integrity; CNS: Reduction of risk potential; CL: Apply; DIFFICULTY: Easy

2. A nurse is reinforcing the instructions given to a client in her education plan about the signs of labor. The nurse determines that the client has an accurate understanding of the instructions when which statement is made by the client?
 1. "False contractions are regular."
 2. "False contractions intensify with walking."
 3. "False contractions usually occur in the abdomen."
 4. "False contractions move from the back to the front of the abdomen."

2. 3. False labor contractions are usually felt in the abdomen, are irregular, and are typically relieved by walking. True labor contractions move from the back to the front of the abdomen, are regular, and aren't relieved by walking. CN: Health promotion and maintenance; CNS: None; CL: Analyze; DIFFICULTY: Moderate

3. Antepartum testing from a client pregnant with twins reveals a twin-to-twin transfusion syndrome. The nurse is assisting with development of a plan of care. Which condition will the nurse likely provide interventions for?
 1. Anemia
 2. Oligohydramnios
 3. Polycythemia
 4. Small size

3. 3. The recipient twin in twin-to-twin transfusion syndrome (also known as twin-twin transfusion syndrome) is transfused by the other twin. The recipient twin then becomes polycythemic and commonly has heart failure due to circulatory overload. The donor twin becomes anemic. The recipient twin has polyhydramnios, not oligohydramnios. The recipient twin is usually large, whereas the donor twin is usually small in size. CN: Physiological integrity; CNS: Physiological adaptation; CL: Analyze; DIFFICULTY: Difficult

CN: Client needs category   CNS: Client needs subcategory   CL: Cognitive level

4. A pregnant client who reports painless vaginal bleeding at 28 weeks' gestation is diagnosed with placenta previa, in which the placental edge reaches the internal os. The nurse would suspect the client has which type of placenta previa?
1. Low-lying placenta previa
2. Marginal placenta previa
3. Partial placenta previa
4. Total placenta previa

5. A client is diagnosed with placenta previa at 28 weeks' gestation. Which procedure should the nurse prepare the client for?
1. Stat culture and sensitivity
2. Antenatal steroids after 34 weeks' gestation
3. Ultrasound examination every 2 to 3 weeks
4. Scheduled birth of the fetus before fetal maturity

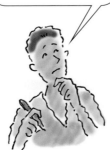

What would be the best way to find out whether the placenta is implanted in the wrong spot?

6. A client with painless vaginal bleeding is suspected of having placenta previa. The nurse will assist in preparing the client for which procedure?
1. Amniocentesis
2. Speculum examination
3. External fetal monitoring
4. Ultrasound

7. A client is diagnosed with hyperemesis gravidarum after coming to the antepartum unit with persistent vomiting, weight loss, and hypovolemia. While gathering data from the client, which information is most significant?
1. Trophoblastic disease
2. Maternal age older than 35 years
3. Malnutrition
4. Low levels of human chorionic gonadotropin (HCG)

8. A client has just been diagnosed with having a hydatidiform mole. When reviewing the client's medical record, what is the **most** significant risk factor?
1. Age in 20s or 30s
2. High socioeconomic status
3. Primigravida
4. Prior molar gestation

4. 2. A marginal placenta previa is characterized by implantation of the placenta in the margin of the cervical os, not covering the os. A low-lying placenta is implanted in the lower uterine segment but doesn't reach the cervical os. A partial placenta previa is the partial occlusion of the cervical os by the placenta. The internal cervical os is completely covered by the placenta in a total placenta previa.
CN: Physiological integrity; CNS: Physiological adaptation; CL: Apply; DIFFICULTY: Difficult

5. 3. Fetal surveillance through ultrasound examination every 2 to 3 weeks is indicated to evaluate fetal growth, amniotic fluid, and placental location in clients with placenta previa being expectantly managed. A stat culture and sensitivity would be done for severe bleeding, or maternal or fetal distress, and isn't part of expectant management. Antenatal steroids may be given to clients between 26 and 32 weeks' gestation to enhance fetal lung maturity. In a hemodynamically stable mother, birth of the fetus should be delayed until fetal lung maturity is attained.
CN: Physiological integrity; CNS: Reduction of risk potential; CL: Apply; DIFFICULTY: Moderate

6. 4. When the mother and fetus are stabilized, ultrasound evaluation of the placenta should be done to determine the cause of the bleeding. Amniocentesis is contraindicated in placenta previa. A digital or speculum examination shouldn't be done, as this may lead to severe bleeding or hemorrhage. External fetal monitoring won't detect a placenta previa, although it will detect fetal distress, which may result from blood loss or placental separation.
CN: Physiological integrity; CNS: Reduction of risk potential; CL: Apply; DIFFICULTY: Easy

7. 1. Trophoblastic disease is associated with hyperemesis gravidarum. Obesity and maternal age younger than 20 years are risk factors for developing hyperemesis gravidarum. High levels of estrogen and HCG have been associated with hyperemesis.
CN: Physiological integrity; CNS: Reduction of risk potential; CL: Apply; DIFFICULTY: Difficult

8. 4. A previous molar gestation increases a woman's risk for developing a subsequent molar gestation by four to five times. Adolescents and women age 40 years and older are at increased risk for molar pregnancies. Multigravidas, especially women with a prior pregnancy loss, and those with lower socioeconomic status are at an increased risk for this problem.
CN: Physiological integrity; CNS: Physiological adaptation; CL: Apply; DIFFICULTY: Easy

CN: Client needs category   CNS: Client needs subcategory   CL: Cognitive level

9. A nurse is reinforcing education for a client entering the third trimester of pregnancy. The nurse determines that the client understands the education when stating she will immediately report which symptom?
1. Hemorrhoids
2. Blurred vision
3. Dyspnea on exertion
4. Increased vaginal mucus

9. 2. During pregnancy, blurred vision may be a danger sign of preeclampsia or eclampsia, complications that require immediate attention because they can cause severe maternal and fetal consequences. Although hemorrhoids may occur during pregnancy, they don't require immediate attention. Dyspnea on exertion and increased vaginal mucus are common discomforts caused by the physiologic changes of pregnancy.
CN: Physiological integrity; CNS: Reduction of risk potential;
CL: Analyze; DIFFICULTY: Easy

10. The nurse is caring for a client suspected of having a hydatidiform mole. Which signs and symptoms would confirm this diagnosis?
1. Heavy, bright red bleeding every 21 days
2. Fetal cardiac motion after 6 weeks' gestation
3. Benign tumors found in the smooth muscle of the uterus
4. "Snowstorm" pattern on ultrasound with no fetus or gestational sac

10. 4. Ultrasound is the technique of choice in diagnosing a hydatidiform mole. The chorionic villi of a molar pregnancy resemble a "snowstorm" pattern on ultrasound. Bleeding with a hydatidiform mole is usually dark brown and may occur erratically for weeks or months. There's no cardiac activity because there's no fetus. Benign tumors found in the smooth muscle of the uterus are leiomyomas or fibroids.
CN: Physiological integrity; CNS: Reduction of risk potential;
CL: Understand; DIFFICULTY: Challenge

11. A client arrives at the emergency department reporting cramping, abdominal pain, and mild vaginal bleeding. Pelvic examination shows a left adnexal mass that's tender when palpated. Culdocentesis shows blood in the cul-de-sac. The nurse would suspect which condition?
1. Abruptio placentae
2. Ectopic pregnancy
3. Hydatidiform mole
4. Pelvic inflammatory disease

Looking good! You're putting on quite a performance.

11. 2. Most ectopic pregnancies don't appear as obvious life-threatening medical emergencies. Ectopic pregnancies must be considered in any woman of childbearing age who reports menstrual irregularity, cramping abdominal pain, and mild vaginal bleeding. Blood in the cul-de-sac is typically not seen with pelvic inflammatory disease, abruptio placentae, and hydatidiform mole.
CN: Physiological integrity; CNS: Reduction of risk potential;
CL: Apply; DIFFICULTY: Moderate

12. A client who is 34 weeks' pregnant arrives at the emergency department with severe abdominal pain, uterine tenderness, and increased uterine tone between contractions, but no vaginal bleeding. The external fetal monitor shows fetal distress with severe, variable decelerations. Which condition does the nurse anticipate this client will be treated for?
1. Abruptio placentae
2. Ectopic pregnancy
3. Molar pregnancy
4. Placenta previa

12. 1. A client with severe abruptio placentae will commonly have severe abdominal pain. The uterus will have increased tone with little to no return to resting tone between contractions. The fetus will start to show signs of distress, with decelerations in the heart rate or even fetal death with a large placental separation. An ectopic pregnancy, which usually occurs in the fallopian tubes, would rupture well before 34 weeks. A molar pregnancy generally would be detected before 34 weeks' gestation. Placenta previa usually involves painless vaginal bleeding without uterine contractions.
CN: Physiological integrity; CNS: Reduction of risk potential;
CL: Apply ; DIFFICULTY: Moderate

13. During a routine visit to the clinic, a client tells the nurse that she thinks she may be pregnant. Which pregnancy test result would the nurse identify as **most** accurate in confirming pregnancy?
1. Increase in human chorionic gonadotropin (HCG)
2. Decrease in HCG
3. Increase in luteinizing hormone (LH)
4. Decrease in LH

13. 1. HCG increases in a woman's blood and urine to fairly large concentrations until the 15th week of pregnancy. The other hormone values aren't indicative of pregnancy.
CN: Health promotion and maintenance; CNS: None;
CL: Apply; DIFFICULTY: Easy

14. A client arrives at the clinic for a scheduled amniocentesis. Which question should the nurse ask?
1. "Have you had at least 1 L of water to drink?"
2. "Have you emptied your bladder?"
3. "Did you fast for the last 12 hours?"
4. "Do you have any problems lying on your left side?"

15. A client who is 27 weeks' pregnant arrives at her health care provider's office reporting fever, nausea, vomiting, malaise, unilateral flank pain, and costovertebral angle tenderness. About which condition does the nurse anticipate reinforcing education?
1. Asymptomatic bacteriuria
2. Bacterial vaginosis
3. Pyelonephritis
4. Urinary tract infection (UTI)

16. A pregnant client is visiting the clinic and reports tiny, blanched, slightly raised-end arterioles on her face, neck, arms, and chest. The nurse documents this finding on the medical record as which condition?
1. Epulis
2. Linea nigra
3. Striae gravidarum
4. Telangiectasias

17. A nurse is collecting data as part of an initial history on a pregnant client. The client asks about the chances of having dizygotic twins. Which statement by the nurse would be **most** accurate?
1. They occur most frequently in Asian women.
2. There's a decreased risk with increased parity.
3. There's an increased risk with increased maternal age.
4. Use of fertility drugs poses no additional risk.

18. A client in her fifth month of pregnancy is having a routine clinic visit. When gathering data from the client, the nurse would be alert for which common second trimester condition?
1. Mastitis
2. Metabolic alkalosis
3. Physiologic anemia
4. Respiratory acidosis

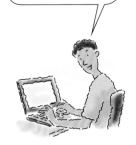

Remember—amniocentesis involves inserting a needle into the client's uterus to remove amniotic fluid, very near the bladder.

14. 2. Before amniocentesis, the client should void to empty the bladder, reducing the risk of bladder perforation. The client doesn't need to drink fluids before amniocentesis nor does she need to fast. The client should be placed in a supine position for the procedure.
CN: Health promotion and maintenance; CNS: None; CL: Analyze; DIFFICULTY: Moderate

15. 3. The symptoms indicate acute pyelonephritis, a serious condition in a pregnant client. Asymptomatic bacteriuria doesn't cause symptoms. Bacterial vaginosis causes milky-white vaginal discharge but no systemic symptoms. UTI symptoms include dysuria, urgency, frequency, and suprapubic tenderness.
CN: Physiological integrity; CNS: Reduction of risk potential; CL: Apply; DIFFICULTY: Moderate

16. 4. The dilated arterioles that occur during pregnancy are due to the elevated level of circulating estrogen and are called telangiectasias. An epulis is a red raised nodule on the gums that may develop at the end of the first trimester and continue to grow as the pregnancy progresses. The linea nigra is a pigmented line extending from the symphysis pubis to the top of the fundus during pregnancy. Striae gravidarum, or stretch marks, are slightly depressed streaks that commonly occur over the abdomen, breasts, and thighs during the second half of pregnancy.
CN: Health promotion and maintenance; CNS: None; CL: Apply; DIFFICULTY: Difficult

17. 3. Dizygotic twinning is influenced by race (most frequent in black women and least frequent in Asian women), age (increased risk with increased maternal age), parity (increased risk with increased parity), and fertility drugs (increased risk with the use of fertility drugs, especially ovulation-inducing drugs). The incidence of monozygotic twins isn't affected by race, age, parity, heredity, or fertility medications.
CN: Health promotion and maintenance; CNS: None; CL: Apply; DIFFICULTY: Moderate

18. 3. Hemoglobin level and hematocrit decrease during pregnancy as the increase in plasma volume exceeds the increase in red blood cell production. The result is physiologic anemia. Mastitis is an infection in the breast characterized by a swollen, tender breast and flulike symptoms. This condition is most commonly seen in breast-feeding clients. Alterations in acid-base balance during pregnancy result in a state of respiratory alkalosis, compensated by mild metabolic acidosis.
CN: Health promotion and maintenance; CNS: None; CL: Apply; DIFFICULTY: Moderate

19. A client, 6 weeks' pregnant, is diagnosed with hyperemesis gravidarum. The nurse should monitor the client for the development of which condition?
1. Bowel perforation
2. Electrolyte imbalance
3. Miscarriage
4. Gestational hypertension

20. A client has gestational diabetes. When assisting with developing the plan of care for this client, which therapy would the nurse **most** likely identify as important for this client to manage her glucose levels?
1. Diet
2. Long-acting insulin
3. Oral hypoglycemic drugs
4. Glucagon

21. The nurse is providing care to a pregnant client with preeclampsia. Magnesium sulfate has been ordered. The nurse understands that this drug is being given to prevent which condition?
1. Hemorrhage
2. Hypertension
3. Hypomagnesemia
4. Seizures

22. A pregnant client has a contraction stress test (CST). Which findings would the nurse interpret as indicative of a negative CST result?
1. Persistent late decelerations in fetal heartbeat occurred, with at least three contractions in a 10-minute window.
2. Accelerations of fetal heartbeat occurred, with at least 15 beats/minute, lasting 15 to 30 seconds in a 20-minute period.
3. Accelerations of fetal heartbeat were absent or didn't increase by 15 beats/minute for 15 to 30 seconds in a 20-minute period.
4. There was moderate fetal heart rate variability, and no decelerations from contraction, in a 10-minute period in which there were three contractions.

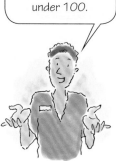

Glucose level is like a golf score ... try to keep it under 100.

19. 2. Excessive vomiting in clients with hyperemesis gravidarum commonly causes weight loss and fluid, electrolyte, and acid-base imbalances. Gestational hypertension and bowel perforation aren't related to hyperemesis. The effects of hyperemesis on the fetus depend on the severity of the disorder. Clients with severe hyperemesis may have a low-birth-weight infant, but the disorder isn't generally life-threatening.
CN: Physiological integrity; CNS: Reduction of risk potential; CL: Apply; DIFFICULTY: Easy

20. 1. Clients with gestational diabetes are usually managed by diet alone to control their glucose intolerance. Long-acting insulin usually isn't needed for blood glucose control in the client with gestational diabetes. Oral hypoglycemic drugs are contraindicated in pregnancy. Glucagon raises blood glucose and is used to treat hypoglycemic reactions.
CN: Safe, effective care environment; CNS: Coordinated care; CL: Apply; DIFFICULTY: Easy

21. 4. For clients with preeclampsia, magnesium sulfate is believed to depress seizure foci in the brain and peripheral neuromuscular blockade, thus preventing eclampsia. Magnesium doesn't help prevent hemorrhage in clients with preeclampsia. Antihypertensive drugs other than magnesium are preferred for sustained hypertension. Hypomagnesemia isn't a complication of preeclampsia.
CN: Physiological integrity; CNS: Pharmacological therapies; CL: Analyze; DIFFICULTY: Easy

22. 4. A CST measures the fetal response to uterine contractions. A client must have three contractions in a 10-minute period. A negative CST shows moderate fetal heart rate variability with no decelerations from uterine contractions. Persistent late decelerations with contractions is a positive CST. Reactive nonstress tests (NSTs) show accelerations in the fetal heartbeat of at least 15 beats/minute, lasting 15 to 30 seconds in a 20-minute period. No accelerations in the heartbeat of at least 15 beats/minute, for 15 to 30 seconds in a 20-minute period, indicate a non-reactive NST.
CN: Health promotion and maintenance; CNS: None; CL: Analyze; DIFFICULTY: Moderate

23. A pregnant client at 12 weeks' gestation comes to the clinic for a follow up visit and tells the nurse that she is "feeling really constipated." Which suggestion would be appropriate for the nurse to give the client? Select all that apply.
1. "Make sure that you attempt to move your bowels regularly."
2. "Try increasing the amount of fruits and vegetables in your diet."
3. "Be sure to increase the amount of fluids that you drink each drink each day."
4. "Use mineral oil as a gentle laxative to get things moving."
5. "An enema once a week should give you adequate relief."

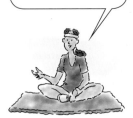

What do pregnant women and nurses have in common? A need to relax and destress.

23. 1, 2, 3. For constipation during pregnancy, appropriate suggestions would include making sure to attempt to move one's bowels regularly (i.e., making time to have a bowel movement), ingesting an increase in foods high in fiber (such as fruits and vegetables), and increasing the amount of fluid ingested each day. Mineral oil interferes with the absorption of fat-soluble vitamins and should be avoided. Enemas also should be avoided because they can stimulate labor.
CN: Physiological integrity; CNS: Basic care and comfort; CL: Apply; DIFFICULTY: Challenge

24. The nurse is gathering information from the chart of a pregnant client. Which finding would the nurse determine does **not** require intervention?
1. Cardiac tamponade
2. Heart failure
3. Endocarditis
4. Systolic murmur

24. 4. Systolic murmur is heard in up to 90% of pregnant clients, and the murmur disappears soon after the birth. Cardiac tamponade, which causes effusion of fluid into the pericardial sac, isn't normal during pregnancy. Despite the increases in intravascular volume and workload of the heart associated with pregnancy, heart failure isn't normal in pregnancy. Endocarditis is most commonly associated with IV drug use and isn't a normal finding in pregnancy.
CN: Health promotion and maintenance; CNS: None; CL: Apply; DIFFICULTY: Moderate

25. A client in her 24th week of pregnancy is exhibiting signs and symptoms of preeclampsia. The nurse would be alert for which finding indicating that the client has developed eclampsia?
1. Seizures
2. Headaches
3. Blurred vision
4. Weight gain

25. 1. The primary difference between preeclampsia and eclampsia is the occurrence of seizures, which occur when the client develops eclampsia. Headaches, blurred vision, weight gain, increased blood pressure, and edema of the hands and feet are all indicative of preeclampsia.
CN: Physiological integrity; CNS: Physiological adaptation; CL: Apply; DIFFICULTY: Moderate

26. A client with preeclampsia is prescribed magnesium sulfate to prevent seizure activity. The nurse is reviewing the results of the client's serum magnesium level and determines that the client's level is therapeutic based on which result?
1. 6.8 mEq/L (3.4 mmol/L)
2. 9.2 mEq/L (4.6 mmol/L)
3. 11.5 mEq/L (5.75 mmol/L)
4. 16 mEq/L (8 mmol/L)

26. 1. The therapeutic level of magnesium for clients with preeclampsia ranges 4 to 8 mEq/L (2 to 4 mmol/L). A serum magnesium level of 8 to 10 mEq/L (4 to 5 mmol/L) may cause the absence of reflexes in the client. Serum levels of 10 to 12 mEq/L (5 to 6 mmol/L) may cause respiratory depression, and a serum level of magnesium greater than 15 mEq/L (7.5 mmol/L) may result in respiratory paralysis.
CN: Physiological integrity; CNS: Pharmacological therapies; CL: Apply; DIFFICULTY: Moderate

27. A client with severe preeclampsia is receiving an intravenous infusion of magnesium sulfate. The client is exhibiting signs and symptoms of magnesium toxicity. Which medication would the nurse expect to be given?
1. Calcium gluconate
2. Hydralazine
3. Naloxone
4. Rho(D) immune globulin

27. 1. Calcium gluconate is the antidote for magnesium toxicity. Ten milliliters of 10% calcium gluconate is given by IV push over 3 to 5 minutes. Hydralazine is given for sustained elevated blood pressures in clients with preeclampsia. Naloxone is used to correct narcotic toxicity. Rho(D) immune globulin is given to women with Rh-negative blood to prevent antibody formation from Rh-positive conceptions.
CN: Physiological integrity; CNS: Pharmacological therapies; CL: Apply; DIFFICULTY: Easy

CN: Client needs category   CNS: Client needs subcategory   CL: Cognitive level

28. A client is receiving IV magnesium sulfate for severe preeclampsia. While monitoring the client, the nurse would immediately report which finding?
1. Anemia
2. Decreased urine output
3. Hyperreflexia
4. Increased respiratory rate

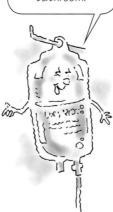

When you're administering me, get ready for a lot of trips to the bathroom.

28. **2.** Magnesium is excreted through the kidneys, so a decreased urine output may result in retention of magnesium, which can accumulate to toxic levels. Urine output should be monitored closely and be greater than 30 mL/hour. Anemia isn't associated with magnesium therapy. Magnesium infusions may cause depression of deep tendon reflexes. The client should be monitored for respiratory depression and paralysis when serum magnesium levels reach approximately 15 mEq/L (7.5 mmol/L).
CN: Physiological integrity; CNS: Pharmacological therapies; CL: Apply; DIFFICULTY: Difficult

29. A pregnant client is screened for tuberculosis during her first prenatal visit. An intradermal injection of purified protein derivative (PPD) of the tuberculin bacilli is given. The nurse determines that the result is positive based on which finding?
1. An indurated wheal under 10 mm in diameter appearing in 6 to 12 hours.
2. An indurated wheal over 10 mm in diameter appearing in 48 to 72 hours.
3. A flat, circumscribed area under 10 mm in diameter appearing in 6 to 12 hours.
4. A flat, circumscribed area over 10 mm in diameter appearing in 48 to 72 hours.

29. **2.** A positive PPD result would be indicated by an indurated wheal over 10 mm in diameter that appears in 48 to 72 hours. The area must be a raised wheal, not a flat, circumscribed area, to be considered positive. The test is read in 48 to 72 hours, not 6 to 12 hours.
CN: Health promotion and maintenance; CNS: None; CL: Apply; DIFFICULTY: Easy

30. A nurse is discussing nutrition with a primigravida. The client states that she knows that calcium is important during pregnancy but that she and her family don't consume many milk or dairy products. What advice should the nurse give?
1. "The prenatal vitamins that are recommended will satisfy all dietary requirements."
2. "You could supplement your diet with 1,800 mg of over-the-counter calcium tablets."
3. "You should consume other nondairy foods that are high in calcium."
4. "After the first trimester, calcium isn't as important since all fetal organ structures are formed."

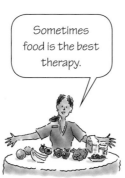

Sometimes food is the best therapy.

30. **3.** Food is considered the ideal source of nutrients. However, milk and dairy aren't the only food sources of calcium. The client should consume other nondairy foods that are high in calcium, such as dark green leafy vegetables. While prenatal vitamins are generally recommended, they don't satisfy all requirements. The calcium requirement for pregnancy is 1,300 mg/day. Over-the-counter supplements aren't always safe and should be specifically recommended by the health care provider. While it's true that all fetal organs are formed by the end of the first trimester, development continues throughout pregnancy. Calcium requirements remain at 1,300 mg/day throughout pregnancy.
CN: Heath promotion and maintenance; CNS: None; CL: Apply; DIFFICULTY: Easy

31. A nurse is assisting with the education of a client who receives a dose of human Rho(D) immune globulin at 28 weeks' gestation to prevent Rh isoimmunization. What should the nurse inform the client regarding the reason for administering the medication?
1. Rh-positive maternal blood crosses into fetal blood, stimulating fetal antibodies.
2. Rh-positive fetal blood crosses into maternal blood, stimulating maternal antibodies.
3. Rh-negative fetal blood crosses into maternal blood, stimulating maternal antibodies.
4. Rh-negative maternal blood crosses into fetal blood, stimulating fetal antibodies.

31. **2.** Rh isoimmunization occurs when Rh-positive fetal blood cells cross into the maternal circulation and stimulate maternal antibody production. In subsequent pregnancies with Rh-positive fetuses, maternal antibodies may cross back into the fetal circulation and destroy the fetal blood cells.
CN: Physiological integrity; CNS: Reduction of risk potential; CL: Apply; DIFFICULTY: Moderate

32. A pregnant client develops iron-deficiency anemia and is prescribed supplemental iron along with prenatal vitamins. After reviewing possible adverse effects of iron supplementation with the client, the nurse determines that the education was successful when the client identifies which adverse effect? Select all that apply.

1. Gastric upset
2. Bright red blood in stools
3. Constipation
4. Anorexia
5. Metallic taste

33. A client hospitalized for premature labor tells the nurse she's having occasional contractions. Which nursing intervention would be **most** appropriate?

1. Inform the client about the possible complications of premature birth.
2. Tell the client to walk around to see if she can get rid of the contractions.
3. Give IV and oral fluids, encouraging her to empty her bladder.
4. Notify the anesthesia department for immediate epidural placement for pain relief.

34. A client's prenatal history shows her to be a 23-year-old gravida 4, para 2. The nurse has correctly interpreted this information when she makes this statement?

1. The client has been pregnant four times and had two miscarriages.
2. The client has been pregnant four times and delivered two live-born children.
3. The client has been pregnant four times and had two cesarean deliveries.
4. The client has been pregnant four times and had two spontaneous abortions.

35. A client is diagnosed with an unruptured ectopic pregnancy. Which medication does the nurse expect to administer to the client?

1. Methotrexate
2. Labetalol
3. Magnesium sulfate
4. Indomethacin

36. A nurse is assisting with the development of a plan of care for a pregnant client. The interdisciplinary team determines that the client will require more frequent prenatal visits based on which data gathered?

1. Blood type O-positive
2. First pregnancy at age 33
3. History of allergy to honey bee pollen
4. Type 1 diabetes

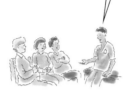

Supplemental iron helps treat anemia but can cause adverse effects. That's what I call iron-y.

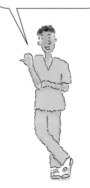

One of these conditions in question #36 is notorious for increasing risk for complications; can you remember which one?

32. 1, 3, 4, 5. Adverse effects of iron supplementation include gastric upset, nausea, vomiting, anorexia, diarrhea, metallic taste, and constipation. Typically, iron makes stools appear black and tarry. Bright red blood in the stools is not associated with iron therapy.
CN: Physiological integrity; CNS: Pharmacological therapies; CL: Analyze; DIFFICULTY: Difficult

33. 3. An empty bladder and adequate hydration may help decrease or stop labor contractions. Educating the client on potential complications is likely to increase her anxiety rather than help her relax. Walking may encourage contractions to become stronger. It would be inappropriate to call the anesthesia department to have an epidural placed because further assessment of the contractions is necessary.
CN: Physiological integrity; CNS: Reduction of risk potential; CL: Apply; DIFFICULTY: Difficult

34. 2. Gravida refers to the number of times a client has been pregnant; para refers to the number of viable children born. Therefore, the client who's gravida 4, para 2 has been pregnant four times and delivered two live-born children.
CN: Health promotion and maintenance; CNS: None; CL: Analyze; DIFFICULTY: Easy

35. 1, 2. Unruptured ectopic pregnancies can be treated with medication therapy, most commonly methotrexate. Labetalol is used to treat hypertension. Magnesium sulfate is used to treat preeclampsia and eclampsia. Indomethacin would be used to slow contractions of preterm labor.
CN: Physiological integrity; CNS: Pharmacological therapies; CL: Apply; DIFFICULTY: Moderate

36. 4. A woman with a history of diabetes has an increased risk for perinatal complications, including hypertension, preeclampsia, and neonatal hypoglycemia; therefore, she needs to be more closely monitored. The age of 33 without other risk factors doesn't necessarily increase the client's risk, nor does having type O-positive blood or environmental allergens.
CN: Safe, effective care environment; CNS: Coordinated care; CL: Apply; DIFFICULTY: Easy

37. A pregnant client at term is in early labor. Over the past 12 hours, she has been experiencing contractions every 10 to 12 minutes and has not progressed. The nurse would anticipate which medication as being prescribed to help stimulate uterine contractions?
1. Estrogen
2. Fetal cortisol
3. Oxytocin
4. Progesterone

37. 3. Oxytocin is the hormone responsible for stimulating uterine contractions and may be given to clients to induce or augment uterine contractions. Although estrogen has a role in uterine contractions, it isn't given to help uterine contractility. Fetal cortisol is believed to slow the production of progesterone by the placenta. Progesterone has a relaxing effect on the uterus.
CN: Physiological integrity; CNS: Pharmacological therapies; CL: Apply; DIFFICULTY: Easy

38. A client, 8 weeks' pregnant, comes to the emergency department with reports of severe, stabbing, lower abdominal pain. A ruptured ectopic pregnancy is suspected based on which signs and symptoms? Select all that apply.
1. Thready, rapid pulse
2. Increased blood pressure
3. Scant vaginal bleeding
4. Abdominal tenderness with distention
5. Referred shoulder pain

38. 1, 3, 4, 5. Signs and symptoms associated with an ectopic pregnancy include a rapid, thready pulse and decreased blood pressure due to internal bleeding, scant vaginal bleeding, abdominal tenderness with distention, and referred shoulder pain due to irritation of the phrenic nerve.
CN: Physiological integrity; CNS: Physiological adaptation; CL: Apply; DIFFICULTY: Difficult

39. A client in her third trimester has come to the clinic for a routine check-up. The nurse reinforces the importance of lying on the left side when resting or sleeping. Which rationale should the nurse give to the client for this position?
1. It will relieve heartburn.
2. It will facilitate bladder emptying.
3. It will prevent compression of the vena cava.
4. It will prevent the development of fetal anomalies.

39. 3. The weight of the pregnant uterus is sufficiently heavy to compress the vena cava, which could impair blood flow to the uterus, and subsequently interfere with supplying sufficient oxygen to the fetus. The side-lying position, especially the left side-lying position, helps to prevent compression, thereby ensuring adequate blood flow and oxygenation to the fetus. The side-lying position hasn't been shown to prevent fetal anomalies, nor does it facilitate bladder emptying or heartburn.
CN: Health Promotion and Maintenance; CNS: None; CL: Apply; DIFFICULTY: Easy

40. A pregnant client is concerned about lack of fetal movement. Which response by the nurse would be most therapeutic?
1. "You need to start taking additional prenatal vitamins."
2. "Try taking a warm bath to facilitate fetal movement."
3. "Eat foods that contain a high sugar content to stimulate the fetus."
4. "Lie down once a day and count the number of fetal movements for 15 to 30 minutes."

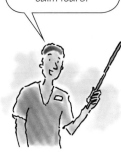

Helping your client become more attuned to fetal movement can help calm fears.

40. 4. Instructing the client to lie down once during the day will allow her to concentrate on detecting fetal movement, making it easier to accomplish. The ability to feel fetal movement is reassuring and comforting to the mother. The mother who is up and actively walking around tends to soothe the fetus, resulting in sleep promotion. Instructing her to take an additional prenatal vitamin is beyond the nurse's scope of practice and isn't recommended because vitamins can be toxic. Taking a warm bath is likely to soothe and relax the fetus. There's also a risk for hyperthermia if the water is too warm or the client is immersed too long. Eating additional sugary foods isn't recommended because some pregnant clients are more susceptible to cavities. The additional sugar intake is not associated with stimulating fetal activity.
CN: Psychosocial integrity; CNS: None; CL: Apply; DIFFICULTY: Easy

41. A pregnant client comes to the clinic for a follow-up visit and reports swelling in her feet and ankles. Which recommendation would be **most** appropriate for the nurse to suggest?
1. Limit oral fluid intake.
2. Buy a good pair of walking shoes.
3. Sit and elevate the feet at least twice daily.
4. Start taking a diuretic as needed daily.

42. A client in her early second trimester tells the nurse that she is experiencing a significant amount of heartburn. Which suggestion would be **most** appropriate for the nurse to make? Select all that apply.
1. Eat small, frequent meals throughout the day.
2. Eat crackers on waking every morning.
3. Drink a preparation of salt and vinegar.
4. Drink orange juice frequently during the day.
5. Keep the head of the bed elevated.

43. A pregnant client is obese. The nurse is working as part of the interdisciplinary team developing the client's plan of care. Based on the understanding of potential complications, the nurse would expect to monitor the client closely for which condition on follow-up visits?
1. Mastitis
2. Placenta previa
3. Preeclampsia
4. Rh isoimmunization

44. A client with preeclampsia is scheduled to undergo a nonstress test (NST) and asks the nurse why this test is being performed. When responding to the client, which condition would the nurse **most** likely include as the reason?
1. Anemia
2. Fetal well-being
3. Intrauterine growth restriction (IUGR)
4. Oligohydramnios

45. A client is 33 weeks' pregnant and has had diabetes since age 21. When checking her fasting blood glucose level, which value would indicate the client's disease is controlled?
1. 45 mg/dL (2.5 mmol/L)
2. 85 mg/dL (4.7 mmol/L)
3. 120 mg/dL (6.67 mmol/L)
4. 136 mg/dL (7.56 mmol/L)

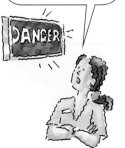

Obesity is a critical risk factor for a serious blood pressure-related condition.

DANGER

41. 3. Sitting down and putting the feet up at least twice daily helps to promote venous return in the pregnant client and, therefore, decrease edema. Limiting fluid intake isn't recommended unless there are additional medical complications such as heart failure. Walking shoes won't necessarily decrease edema. Diuretics aren't recommended during pregnancy because it's important to maintain an adequate circulatory volume.
CN: Physiological integrity; CNS: Basic care and comfort; CL: Apply; DIFFICULTY: Easy

42. 1, 5. Eating small, frequent meals and keeping the head of the bed elevated place less pressure on the esophageal sphincter, reducing the likelihood of the regurgitation of stomach contents into the lower esophagus. Eating crackers, drinking a salt and vinegar solution, or drinking orange juice have not been shown to decrease heartburn.
CN: Physiological integrity; CNS: Basic care and comfort; CL: Apply; DIFFICULTY: Challenge

43. 3. The incidence of preeclampsia in obese clients is significantly greater than in a pregnant client who is not obese. Placenta previa, mastitis, and Rh isoimmunization aren't associated with increased incidence in pregnant clients who are obese.
CN: Safe, effective care environment; CNS: Coordinated care; CL: Apply; DIFFICULTY: Easy

44. 2. An NST is based on the theory that a healthy fetus has transient fetal heart rate accelerations with fetal movement. Because uteroplacental circulation is compromised in clients with preeclampsia, an NST would usually show a lack of these accelerations, which indicate a nonreactive NST. An NST can't detect anemia in a fetus. Serial ultrasounds will detect IUGR and oligohydramnios in a fetus.
CN: Physiological Integrity; CNS: Reduction of risk potential; CL: Apply; DIFFICULTY: Easy

45. 2. The recommended fasting blood glucose level in the pregnant client with diabetes is 60 to 95 mg/dL (3.33 to 5.28 mmol/L). A fasting blood glucose level of 45 mg/dL (2.5 mmol/L) is low and may result in symptoms of hypoglycemia. A blood glucose level below 120 mg/dL (6.67 mmol/L) is recommended for 2-hour postprandial values. A blood glucose level above 136 mg/dL (7.56 mmol/L) in a pregnant client indicates hyperglycemia.
CN: Health promotion and maintenance; CNS: None; CL: Apply; DIFFICULTY: Easy

46. A client with diabetes in the late third trimester has a nonstress test (NST) twice weekly. The 20-minute test showed three fetal heart rate accelerations that exceeded the baseline by 15 beats/minute and lasted longer than 15 seconds. The nurse knows these results are consistent with which interpretation of a nonstress test?
1. Reactive test
2. Nonreactive test
3. Positive test
4. Negative test

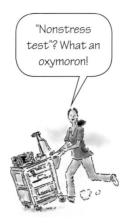

"Nonstress test"? What an oxymoron!

47. A client is pregnant with triplets and is at greater risk for complications. The nurse reinforces education about the signs and symptoms of which conditions? Select all that apply.
1. Placenta previa
2. Preterm labor
3. Anemia
4. Hypertension of pregnancy
5. Hydatidiform mole

48. A pregnant client at 26 weeks' gestation undergoes a glucose tolerance test. The nurse identifies the need for further action based on which results?
1. A glucose level of 120 mg/dL (6.67 mmol/L) during a 1-hour glucose tolerance test
2. A 1-hour glucose level of 160 mg/dL (8.88 mmol/L) during a 3-hour glucose tolerance test
3. A 2-hour glucose level of 150 mg/dL (8.32 mmol/L) during a 3-hour glucose tolerance test
4. A 3-hour glucose level of 130 mg/dL (7.22 mmol/L) during a 3-hour glucose tolerance test

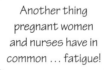

Another thing pregnant women and nurses have in common ... fatigue!

49. A client with a history of hypertension is 15 weeks' pregnant. For which condition should the nurse closely monitor this client?
1. Abruptio placentae
2. Preterm labor
3. Spontaneous abortion
4. Anemia

50. The nurse is providing care to a pregnant adolescent client in her first trimester. Which intervention would the nurse identify as the **highest priority**?
1. Schedule the client for a screening glucose tolerance test.
2. Make sure the client receives nutritional counseling and reinforce the education.
3. Teach the client that she's at increased risk for having a macrosomic neonate.
4. Monitor the client for signs and symptoms of placenta previa.

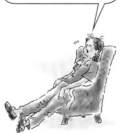

46. 1. The nonstress test is the preferred antepartum heart rate screening test for pregnant clients with diabetes. A reactive nonstress test is two or more fetal heart rate accelerations that exceed baseline by at least 15 beats/minute and last longer than 15 seconds within a 20-minute period. A nonreactive nonstress test lacks accelerations in the fetal heart rate with fetal movement. The terms positive and negative aren't used to describe the interpretation of nonstress tests.
CN: Physiological integrity; CNS: Reduction of risk potential
CL: Analyze; DIFFICULTY: Moderate

47. 1, 2, 3, 4. Women with multifetal pregnancies are at greater risk for complications such as hypertension of pregnancy, placenta previa, preterm labor, and anemia. They are not considered to be a greater risk for the development of a hydatidiform mole.
CN: Physiological integrity; CNS: Reduction of risk potential ;
CL: Apply; DIFFICULTY: Moderate

48. 2. Gestational diabetes is diagnosed when a 3-hour glucose tolerance test has a 1-hour glucose level of 140 mg/dL (7.78 mmol/L) or greater. Other diagnostic test indications of gestational diabetes include a 2-hour glucose level 165 mg/dL (9.16 mmol/L) during a 3-hour glucose tolerance test; a 1-hour glucose test greater than 140 mg/dL (7.78 mmol/L) ; a 3-hour glucose tolerance test with a 2-hour glucose level of 165 mg/dL (9.16 mmol/L) or greater; or a 3-hour glucose tolerance test with a 3-hour glucose level of 145 mg/dL (8.06 mmol/L) or greater.
CN: Physiological integrity; CNS: Reduction of risk potential;
CL: Analyze; DIFFICULTY: Moderate

49. 1. A history of hypertension predisposes the client to developing abruptio placentae. She isn't at risk for developing preterm labor, spontaneous abortion, or anemia.
CN: Safe, effective care environment; CNS: Coordinated care;
CL: Apply; DIFFICULTY: Difficult

50. 2. Nutritional counseling must be emphasized as part of the prenatal care for adolescent clients. Adolescents need to meet nutritional needs for this rapid period of growth and development. The needs are further increased due to the pregnancy. Adolescents aren't at increased risk for developing gestational diabetes or placenta previa. Adolescent clients are at risk for delivering low-birth-weight neonates, not macrosomic neonates.
CN: Safe, effective care environment; CNS: Coordinated care;
CL: Apply; DIFFICULTY: Easy

51. A nurse is teaching a group of pregnant adolescents about the anatomy and physiology of reproduction. The nurse determines that the teaching was effective when the adolescents identify the area where fertilization occurs. Mark that area on the illustration.

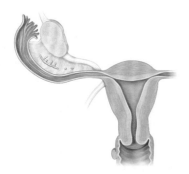

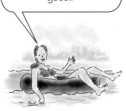

Floating around in a warm, comfortable environment with not a care in the world … life as a fetus sounds pretty good!

51. After ejaculation, the sperm travel by flagellar movement through the fluids of the cervical mucus into the fallopian tube to meet the descending ovum in the ampulla, where fertilization occurs.

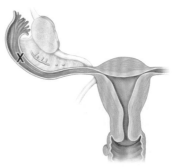

CN: Health promotion and maintenance; CNS: None; CL: Analyze; DIFFICULTY: Difficult

52. When assisting with the education of an antepartum client on the passage of the fetus through the birth canal during labor, the nurse describes the cardinal mechanisms of labor. Place these events in the proper ascending chronological order.

| 1. Flexion |
| 2. External rotation |
| 3. Descent |
| 4. Expulsion |
| 5. Internal rotation |
| 6. Extension |

52.

| 3. Descent |
| 1. Flexion |
| 5. Internal rotation |
| 6. Extension |
| 2. External rotation |
| 4. Expulsion |

The fetus moving through the birth canal changes position to ensure that the smallest diameter of the fetal head always presents to the smallest diameter of the birth canal. Termed the cardinal mechanisms of labor, these position changes occur in this sequence: descent, flexion, internal rotation, extension, external rotation, and expulsion.

CN: Health Promotion and Maintenance; CNS: None; CL: Apply; DIFFICULTY: Moderate

53. A pregnant client in the second trimester is scheduled for amniocentesis. What should the nurse do to prepare the client for the procedure? Select all that apply.
1. Ask the client to void.
2. Have the client drink 1 L of fluid.
3. Ask the client to lie on her left side.
4. Assess fetal heart rate.
5. Insert an IV catheter.
6. Monitor maternal vital signs.

Congratulations! You've delivered another healthy test performance.

53. 1, 4, 6. To prepare a client for amniocentesis, the nurse should ask her to empty her bladder to reduce the risk of bladder perforation. Before the procedure, the nurse should also assess fetal heart rate and maternal vital signs to establish baselines. The client should be asked to drink 1 L of fluid before transabdominal ultrasound, not amniocentesis. The client should be supine during amniocentesis; afterward, she should be placed on her left side to avoid supine hypotension, promote venous return, and ensure adequate cardiac output. IV access isn't necessary for this procedure.

CN: Physiological integrity; CNS: Reduction of risk potential; CL: Apply; DIFFICULTY: Difficult

Chapter 22

Intrapartum Care

Intrapartum care refresher

Abruptio placentae

Premature separation of the placenta from the uterus; a common cause of third trimester bleeding

Key signs and symptoms
- Acute abdominal pain and rigid abdomen
- Hemorrhage with dark red vaginal bleeding

Key test result
- Ultrasonography locates the placenta and may reveal a clot or hematoma

Key treatments
- Transfusion: packed red blood cells (RBCs), platelets, and fresh frozen plasma if necessary
- Cesarean delivery

Key interventions
- Avoid pelvic or vaginal examinations and enemas
- Monitor administration of packed RBCs, platelets, or fresh frozen plasma
- Position client in a left lateral recumbent position

Amniotic fluid embolism

Amniotic fluid entering the maternal circulation through some break in the normal barrier mechanism; the fluid contains debris such as hair, skin and vernix, subsequently causing obstruction of the pulmonary vessels and resulting in severe respiratory distress

Key signs and symptoms
- Cyanosis and chest pain
- Tachypnea and sudden dyspnea

Key test result
- Electronic fetal monitor reveals fetal distress (during the intrapartum period)
- Arterial blood gas results (ABG) reveal hypoxemia

Key treatments
- Oxygen therapy: face mask, cannula, or endotracheal (ET) intubation and mechanical ventilation if respiratory arrest occurs

- Cardiopulmonary resuscitation (CPR) if client is apneic and pulseless
- Emergency delivery using forceps or by cesarean birth

Key interventions
- Monitor respiratory and cardiovascular status
- Monitor fetal heart rate (FHR)
- Perform CPR if necessary
- Assist with immediate delivery of neonate

Disseminated intravascular coagulation (DIC)

Clotting system is abnormally activated and leads to increased coagulation along with a bleeding defect

Key signs and symptoms
- Abnormal bleeding (petechiae, hematomas, ecchymosis, cutaneous oozing)
- Oliguria

Key test result
- Coagulation studies reveal:
  - decreased fibrinogen level
  - positive D-dimer test specific for disseminated intravascular coagulation (DIC)
  - prolonged prothrombin time (PT)
  - prolonged partial thromboplastin time (PTT)
- Hematology studies reveal decreased platelet count

Key treatments
- Transfusion therapy: packed RBCs, fresh frozen plasma, platelets, and cryoprecipitate
- Treatment of the underlying condition
- Immediate delivery of the fetus

Key interventions
- Monitor cardiovascular, respiratory, neurologic, GI, and renal status
- Monitor vital signs frequently
- Closely monitor intake and output
- Monitor client closely for signs and symptoms of a transfusion reaction
- Monitor the results of serial blood studies

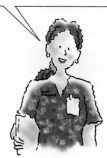
The antepartum and postpartum periods are important to know about. However, the intrapartum period—that's where the action is! This chapter covers the intrapartum period, perhaps the most critical of the three.

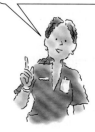
Take a deep breath and bear down ... this chapter will be a labor of love.

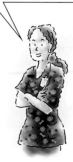
Abnormal bleeding and bruising, decreased urine output, and prolonged clotting time—what condition does this sound like?

Dystocia

Difficult or abnormal labor that results from a myriad of factors; typically associated with a slow and abnormal progression of labor

Key signs and symptoms

- Arrested descent
- Hypotonic contractions

Key test result

- Ultrasonography shows fetal position or malformation

Key treatments

- Delivery of fetus by cesarean birth if labor fails to progress and mother or fetus shows signs of compromise
- Oxytocic agent: oxytocin if contractions are ineffective

Key interventions

- Monitor vital signs
- Assist the client to a left side-lying position
- Monitor the effectiveness of oxytocin therapy and watch for complications

Emergency birth

Situation in which immediate birth of the fetus is necessary to reduce the risk of injury and death to the mother or fetus or both

Key signs and symptoms

Prolapsed umbilical cord
- Cord visible at vaginal opening
- Cord palpable during vaginal examination
- Variable decelerations or bradycardia noted on fetal monitor strip

Uterine rupture
- Abdominal pain and tenderness, especially at the peak of a contraction, or the feeling that "something ripped"
- Excessive external bleeding
- Late decelerations, reduced fetal heart rate (FHR) variability, tachycardia and bradycardia, cessation of FHR
- Palpation of the fetus outside the uterus

Amniotic fluid embolism
- Chest pain
- Coughing with pink, frothy sputum
- Increasing restlessness and anxiety
- Sudden dyspnea
- Tachypnea

Key test result

Prolapsed umbilical cord
- Ultrasonography confirms that the cord is prolapsed

Uterine rupture
- Ultrasonography may reveal absence of the amniotic cavity within the uterus

Amniotic fluid embolism
- ABG analysis reveals hypoxemia

Key treatments

- Administration of oxygen by nasal cannula or mask (endotracheal intubation and mechanical ventilation may be necessary in the case of amniotic fluid embolism)
- Emergency cesarean delivery

Key interventions

- Monitor maternal vital signs, pulse oximetry, and intake and output as well as FHR
- Administer maternal oxygen by cannula or mask at 8 to 10 L/minute
- Maintain IV fluid replacement
- Place client in left lateral recumbent position
- Obtain blood samples to determine hematocrit (HCT), hemoglobin (Hgb) level, PT and PTT, fibrinogen level, and platelet count, and to type and crossmatch blood
- Monitor administration of blood products as necessary
- Prepare client and her family for possibility of cesarean delivery

Fetal distress

Signs exhibited by fetus that indicate an inability to cope with the demands of labor, as evidenced by changes in fetal heart rate and rhythm

Key signs and symptoms

- Change in FHR

Key test result

- Fetal scalp blood sampling reveals acidosis

Key treatments

- Supplemental oxygen by face mask, typically at 6 to 8 L/minute
- IV fluid administration
- Emergent fetal delivery by cesarean birth

Key interventions

- Monitor FHR, fetal activity, and fetal heart variability
- Assist client to a left side-lying position

Inverted uterus

Uterine fundus prolapses to (or through) the cervix, causing uterus to turn inside out after birth

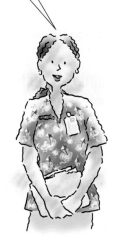

Your client is exhibiting signs of dystocia. What should you do?

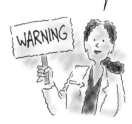

The umbilical cord being visible at the vaginal opening is a critical sign of a prolapsed cord, and an indication for an emergency birth.

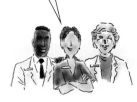

If you suspect uterine rupture, call the doctor STAT—a cesarean delivery may be in order.

Key signs and symptoms

- Large, sudden gush of blood from vagina
- Severe uterine pain

Key test result

- Hematology tests reveal decreased Hgb levels and HCT

Key treatments

- Fluid resuscitation with IV fluids and blood products
- Supplemental oxygen administration
- Immediate manual replacement of uterus
- Possible emergency hysterectomy

Key interventions

- Administer supplemental oxygen
- Monitor vital signs frequently
- Closely monitor intake and output

Laceration

Injury to the vaginal tissue during labor; can range from a tear involving only the lining or the tissue of the vagina to a tear involving the vaginal lining, submucosal tissues, anal sphincter, and rectal lining

Key signs and symptoms

- Increased vaginal bleeding after delivery of placenta

Key test result

- Hematology studies may reveal decreased levels of Hgb and HCT

Key treatments

- Laceration repair
- Analgesics: ibuprofen, acetaminophen and oxycodone, acetaminophen

Key interventions

- Monitor vital signs, including temperature
- Monitor laceration site for signs of infection

Precipitate labor

Abrupt onset of strong contractions that occur in a short period of time (instead of the typical gradually increasing contractions associated with labor)

Key signs and symptoms

- Cervical dilation greater than 5 cm/hour in a nulliparous woman; more than 10 cm/hour in a multiparous woman

Key test result

- No key test result specific to this complication

Key treatments

- Controlled delivery to prevent maternal and fetal injury

Key interventions

- Monitor FHR and variability

Premature rupture of membranes

Membrane breaks before client goes into labor

Key signs and symptoms

- Blood-tinged amniotic fluid gushing or leaking from vagina
- Uterine tenderness

Key test result

- Nitrazine or ferning test is positive, indicating possible ruptured membranes
- Vaginal probe ultrasonography allows detection of amniotic sac tear or rupture

Key treatments

- Hospitalization to monitor for maternal fever, leukocytosis, and fetal tachycardia if pregnancy is between 28 and 34 weeks; if infection is confirmed, labor must be induced
- Oxytocic agent: oxytocin for labor induction if term pregnancy and if labor doesn't result within 24 hours after membrane rupture
- Betamethasone administered IM to increase fetal lung maturity if gestational age is 24 to 34 weeks

Key interventions

- Monitor for signs of infection or fetal distress
- Administer antibiotics as prescribed
- Encourage client to express her feelings and concerns

Preterm labor

Labor that occurs before the end of the 37th week of gestation; involves regular uterine contractions in conjunction with cervical effacement and dilation

Key signs and symptoms

- Feeling of pelvic pressure or abdominal tightening
- Increased vaginal discharge
- Intestinal cramping
- Uterine contractions that result in cervical dilation and effacement

Key test result

- Electronic fetal monitoring confirms uterine contractions
- Vaginal examination confirms cervical effacement and dilation

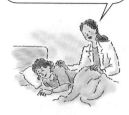

Side-lying is often preferred during early labor for optimal circulation and maternal comfort.

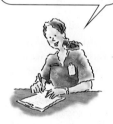

Immediately after birth, there is a large, sudden gush of blood from your client's vagina and she reports severe uterine pain. What's going on?

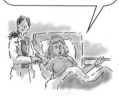

Wow—you're progressing rapidly. This must be a case of precipitate labor.

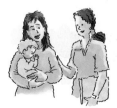

Proper care helps to ensure delivery of a healthy baby.

Key treatments

- Betamethasone administered IM at regular intervals over 48 hours to increase fetal lung maturity in a fetus expected to be delivered preterm
- Magnesium sulfate to maintain uterine relaxation
- Tocolytic agents, such as terbutaline, to inhibit uterine contractions

Key interventions

- Monitor maternal vital signs, contractions, and FHR every 15 minutes during tocolytic therapy (otherwise, provide continuous fetal monitoring)
- Monitor for magnesium sulfate toxicity and make sure calcium gluconate is available

Prolapsed umbilical cord

Umbilical cord protrusion alongside (or ahead of) the fetal presenting part; occlusion of the cord can lead to impaired fetal perfusion

Key signs and symptoms

- Cord visible at the vaginal opening
- Variable decelerations or bradycardia noted on fetal monitor strip

Key test result

- Ultrasonography may reveal the cord as the presenting part

Key treatments

- Immediate delivery of the fetus

Key interventions

- Place client in Trendelenburg position (client's hips higher than head in a knee-to-chest position)
- Monitor FHR and variability

Uterine rupture

Uterus tears and opens into the abdominal cavity; site of the rupture is usually a previous scar

Key signs and symptoms

- Abdominal pain and tenderness, especially at the peak of a contraction, or the feeling that "something ripped"
- Late decelerations, reduced FHR variability, tachycardia and bradycardia, cessation of FHR

Key test result

- Hematology tests reveal decreased levels of Hgb and HCT

Key treatments

- Fluid resuscitation: IV fluids and blood products via rapid infusion
- Surgery to remove the fetus and repair the tear or hysterectomy if necessary
- Oxytocic agent: oxytocin to help contract the uterus

Key interventions

- Monitor vital signs frequently
- Prepare client for immediate surgery

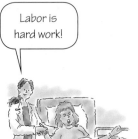

Labor is hard work!

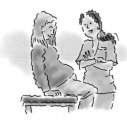

Expectant mothers should discuss any concerns with their health care provider.

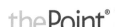

thePoint® You can download tables of drug information to help you prepare for the NCLEX®! View Generic Drug Names, Drug Classifications, Drug Actions, and Nursing Implications for the drugs discussed in this refresher at **http://thePoint.lww.com**.

Intrapartum care questions, answers, and rationales

1. A client with a full-term, uncomplicated pregnancy comes into the labor and delivery unit in early labor states, "I think my water has broken." Which action by the nurse would be the **priority**?
1. Prepare the client for birth.
2. Note the color, amount, and odor of the fluid.
3. Immediately contact the health care provider.
4. Collect a sample of the fluid for microbial analysis.

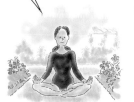

Staying calm will help your client stay calm. Remember to manage your own breathing while helping manage hers.

1. 2. Noting the color, amount, and odor of the fluid will help guide the nurse in her next action. There's no need to call the client's health care provider immediately or prepare the client for birth if the fluid is clear and birth isn't imminent. Rupture of membranes isn't unusual in the early stages of labor. Fluid collection for microbial analysis isn't routine if there's no concern of infection (maternal fever).

CN: Safe, effective care environment; CNS: Coordinated care; CL: Apply; DIFFICULTY: Moderate

CN: Client needs category   CNS: Client needs subcategory   CL: Cognitive level

2. A client who is 36 weeks' pregnant comes into the labor and delivery unit with mild contractions. While collecting data from the client, which signs would alert the nurse that the client is experiencing abruptio placentae? Select all that apply.
  1. Sudden rupture of membranes
  2. Profuse amounts of dark red vaginal bleeding
  3. Emesis
  4. Fever
  5. Rigid abdomen

3. A client's labor doesn't progress. The health care provider orders IV administration of 1,000 mL normal saline solution with oxytocin 10 units to run at 2 milliunits/minute. At which rate will the nurse administer the infusion? Record your answer using one decimal place.

_____ mL/minute

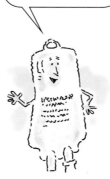

Careful with your calculation—it helps me know how fast to flow.

4. Cervical effacement and dilation aren't progressing for a client in labor. The health care provider orders IV administration of oxytocin. Which rationale does the nurse give the client for the close monitoring of her fluid intake and urine output?
  1. Oxytocin causes water intoxication.
  2. Oxytocin causes excessive thirst.
  3. Oxytocin is toxic to the kidneys.
  4. Oxytocin has a diuretic effect.

5. A client in labor has been receiving oxytocin to aid her progress. The nurse caring for her notes that a contraction has remained strong for 60 seconds. Which action should the nurse take **first**?
  1. Stop the oxytocin infusion.
  2. Notify the health care provider.
  3. Monitor fetal heart tones as usual.
  4. Turn the client on her left side.

6. A pregnant client in labor has an amniotomy. Which outcome would the nurse identify as the **highest priority**?
  1. The client will express increased knowledge about amniotomy.
  2. The fetus will maintain adequate tissue perfusion.
  3. The fetus will display no signs of infection.
  4. The client will report relief of pain.

2. 2, 5. In a client with abruptio placentae, the client would most likely exhibit a rigid abdomen and hemorrhage with dark red vaginal bleeding. Sudden rupture of membranes, emesis, or fever are not associated with abruptio placentae.
cn: Physiological integrity; cns: Reduction of risk potential;
cl: Apply; difficulty: Difficult

3. 0.2.
The answer is found by setting up a ratio and following through with the calculations shown below. Each unit of oxytocin contains 1,000 milliunits. Therefore, 10 units of oxytocin is equivalent to 10,000 milliunits. Thus 1,000 mL of IV fluid contains 10,000 milliunits (10 units) of oxytocin. Use the following equation:

$$10,000 / 1,000 = 2/X;$$
$$10,000 \, X = 2,000;$$
$$X = 0.2 \text{ mL}.$$

cn: Physiological integrity; cns: Pharmacological therapies;
cl: Analyze; difficulty: Moderate

4. 1. The nurse should monitor fluid intake and output because prolonged oxytocin infusion may cause severe water intoxication, leading to seizure, coma, and death. Excessive thirst results from the work of labor and limited oral fluid intake, not oxytocin. Oxytocin has no nephrotoxic or diuretic effects; in fact, it produces an antidiuretic effect.
cn: Physiological integrity; cns: Pharmacological therapies;
cl: Apply; difficulty: Difficult

5. 1. A contraction that remains strong for 60 seconds with no sign of letting up signals impending tetany and could cause rupture of the uterus. Oxytocin stimulates contractions and should be stopped. The nurse should monitor the fetal heart tones and notify the health care provider but only after stopping the oxytocin. The client should already be on her left side, but the tonic contraction is more than likely due to the oxytocin.
cn: Safe, effective care environment; cns: Coordinated care;
cl: Apply; difficulty: Difficult

6. 2. Amniotomy increases the risk of umbilical cord prolapse, which would impair the fetal blood supply and tissue perfusion. Because the fetus's life depends on the oxygen carried by that blood, maintaining fetal tissue perfusion takes priority over goals related to increased knowledge, infection prevention, and pain relief.
cn: Safe, effective care environment; cns: Coordinated care;
cl: Analyze; difficulty: Challenge

7. A client at term arrives in the labor unit experiencing contractions every 4 minutes. When reviewing the client's medical record, the nurse would monitor the client closely for fetal distress based on which finding?
1. Total weight gain of 30 lb (13.6 kg)
2. Maternal age of 32 years
3. Blood pressure of 146/90 mm Hg
4. Treatment for syphilis at 15 weeks' gestation

7. 3. A blood pressure of 146/90 mm Hg may indicate gestational hypertension. Over time, gestational hypertension reduces blood flow to the placenta and can cause intrauterine growth retardation and other problems that make the fetus less able to tolerate the stress of labor. A weight gain of 30 lb is within expected parameters for a healthy pregnancy. A woman at age 32 doesn't have a greater risk of complications if her general condition is healthy before pregnancy. Increased risk of complications begins around age 35. Syphilis that has been treated doesn't pose an additional risk.
CN: Physiological integrity; CNS: Reduction of risk potential; CL: Apply; DIFFICULTY: Easy

8. A client at 42 weeks' gestation is 3 cm dilated and 30% effaced with membranes intact and the fetus at +2 station. Fetal heart rate (FHR) is 140 to 150 beats/minute. After 2 hours, the nurse notes on the external fetal monitor that for the past 10 minutes, the FHR ranged from 160 to 190 beats/minute. The client states that her baby has been extremely active. Uterine contractions are strong, occurring every 3 to 4 minutes and lasting 40 to 60 seconds. The nurse suspects fetal hypoxia based on which finding?
1. Abnormally long uterine contractions
2. Abnormally strong uterine intensity
3. Excessively frequent contractions, with rapid fetal movement
4. Excessive fetal activity and fetal tachycardia

8. 4. Fetal tachycardia and excessive fetal activity are the first signs of fetal hypoxia. The duration of uterine contractions is within normal limits. Uterine intensity can be mild to strong and still be within normal limits. The frequency of contractions is within the normal limits for the active phase of labor.
CN: Physiological integrity; CNS: Reduction of risk potential; CL: Apply; DIFFICULTY: Moderate

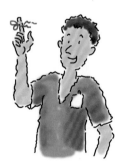

Don't forget to inform your client of any side effects associated with prescribed medications.

9. A client at 32 weeks' gestation and leaking amniotic fluid is placed on an external fetal monitor. The monitor indicates uterine irritability, and contractions are occurring every 4 to 6 minutes. The health care provider orders nifedipine. Which educational statement is appropriate for this client?
1. "This medicine will make you breathe better."
2. "You may feel flushed and feel your heart beating faster."
3. "This will dry your mouth and make you feel thirsty."
4. "You'll need to replace the potassium lost by this drug."

9. 2. Maternal tachycardia and flushing are common adverse reactions to nifedipine. The drug is being given to reduce the client's uterine irritability, not relieve bronchospasm. Dry mouth, feelings of thirst, and potassium loss are not common with this drug.
CN: Physiological integrity; CNS: Pharmacological therapies; CL: Apply; DIFFICULTY: Difficult

10. A primigravida client with severe gestational hypertension is admitted to the labor unit. She has been receiving magnesium sulfate IV for 3 hours. The latest data reveals deep tendon reflexes (DTRs) of +1, blood pressure of 150/100 mm Hg, a pulse of 92 beats/minute, a respiratory rate of 10 breaths/minute, and urine output of 20 mL/ hour. Which action would be most appropriate?
1. Continue monitoring per standards of care.
2. Stop the magnesium sulfate infusion.
3. Increase the infusion rate by 5 gtt/minute.
4. Decrease the infusion rate by 5 gtt/minute.

10. 2. Magnesium sulfate should be withheld if the client's respiratory rate or urine output falls, or if reflexes are diminished or absent, all of which are true for this client. The client may also show other signs of impending toxicity, such as flushing and feeling warm. Continuing to monitor the client won't resolve suppressed DTRs and low respiratory rate and urine output. The client is already showing central nervous system depression because of excessive magnesium sulfate, so increasing the infusion rate is inappropriate. Impending toxicity indicates that the infusion should be stopped rather than just slowed.
CN: Physiological integrity; CNS: Pharmacological therapies; CL: Apply; DIFFICULTY: Easy

11. Vaginal examination of a client in labor reveals the fetus's larger, diamond-shaped fontanel is toward the anterior portion of the client's pelvis. The nurse interprets this finding as indicative of what situation?
1. The client can expect a brief and intense labor, with potential for lacerations.
2. The client is at risk for uterine rupture and needs constant monitoring.
3. The client may need interventions to ease her back labor and change the fetal position.
4. The client must be told that birth of the fetus will require forceps or a vacuum extractor.

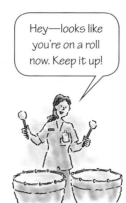

Hey—looks like you're on a roll now. Keep it up!

12. A primigravida is in labor. Her cervix is 5 cm dilated and 75% effaced, and the fetus is at 0 station. The health care provider prescribes an epidural regional block. When assisting with the procedure, the nurse would expect to place the client in which position when the epidural is administered?
1. Lithotomy
2. Supine
3. Prone
4. Lateral

13. While gathering data on a client in labor, the nurse reviews the client's medical record and observes that client's cervix is 70% effaced. The nurse interprets this to indicate which change is occurring in the cervix? Select all that apply.
1. Thinning
2. Shortening
3. Widening
4. Lowering
5. Engaging

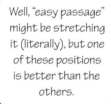

Well, "easy passage" might be stretching it (literally), but one of these positions is better than the others.

14. The nurse is providing care to a pregnant woman in early labor. Which position is the fetus in that will provide an easy passage through the birth canal?
1. Vertex position
2. Transverse lie position
3. Frank breech position
4. Posterior position of the fetal head

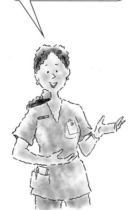

15. A nurse is providing care to a client in labor and reviewing the plan of care. The nurse determines that the client understands the information when identifying birth as occurring during which stage?
1. First stage of labor
2. Second stage of labor
3. Third stage of labor
4. Fourth stage of labor

11. 3. The fetal position is occiput posterior, a position that commonly produces intense back pain during labor. Most of the time, the fetus rotates during labor to occiput anterior position. Positioning the client on her side can facilitate this rotation. An occiput posterior position would most likely result in prolonged labor. Occiput posterior position alone doesn't create a risk of uterine rupture. Forceps or vacuum extractor would be necessary only if the fetus didn't rotate spontaneously.
CN: Safe, effective care environment; CNS: Safety and infection control; CL: Analyze; DIFFICULTY: Moderate

12. 4. The client should be placed on her left side (lateral position) or sitting upright, with her shoulders parallel and legs slightly flexed. Her back shouldn't be flexed because this position increases the possibility that the dura may be punctured and the anesthetic will inadvertently be given as spinal, not epidural, anesthesia. None of the other positions allows proper access to the epidural space.
CN: Physiological integrity; CNS: Reduction of risk potential; CL: Understand; DIFFICULTY: Easy

13. 1, 2. Cervical effacement refers to a thinning and shortening of the cervix. Dilation refers to the widening of the cervix. Both facilitate opening the cervix in preparation for birth. Lowered is not a term used to describe a pregnant woman's cervix. Engagement refers to the movement of the fetal head into the mother's pelvis and is unrelated to changes in the woman's cervix.
CN: Health promotion and maintenance; CNS: None; CL: Apply; DIFFICULTY: Difficult

14. 1. Vertex position (flexion of the fetal head) is the optimal position for passage through the birth canal. Transverse lie positioning generally results in poor labor contractions and an unacceptable fetal position for birth. Frank breech positioning, in which the buttocks present first, is a difficult birth. Posterior positioning of the fetal head makes it difficult for the fetal head to pass under the maternal symphysis pubis bone.
CN: Health promotion and maintenance; CNS: None; CL: Apply; DIFFICULTY: Challenge

15. 2. The second stage of labor begins with complete dilation (10 cm) and ends with the expulsion of the fetus. The first stage of labor is the stage of dilation, which is divided into three distinct phases: latent, active, and transition. The third stage of labor begins immediately following the birth of the neonate and ends with the expulsion of the placenta. The fourth stage of labor is the first 1 to 4 hours after placental expulsion, in which the client's body begins the recovery process.
CN: Health promotion and maintenance; CNS: None; CL: Analyze; DIFFICULTY: Challenge

16. A nurse is assigned to assist with the admission of a client in labor. Which action would be **most** appropriate? Select all that apply.
1. Asking about the estimated date of delivery (EDD)
2. Estimating fetal size
3. Taking maternal and fetal vital signs
4. Asking about the woman's last menses
5. Administering an analgesic
6. Asking about the amount of time between contractions

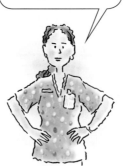

Remember—health care is a team sport, and you don't play all the positions. Know when to call in a team mate.

16. 1, 3, 6. The nurse should ask about the EDD and then compare the response to the information in the prenatal record. If the fetus is preterm, special precautions and equipment are necessary. Maternal and fetal vital signs should be obtained to evaluate the well-being of the client and fetus. Determining how far apart the contractions are provides the health care team with valuable baseline information. The health care provider estimates the size of the fetus. It wouldn't be appropriate at this time for the nurse to ask about the client's last menses; this information would be collected at the first prenatal visit. It would be premature to administer an analgesic, which could slow or stop labor contractions.
CN: Health promotion and maintenance; CNS: None; CL: Apply; DIFFICULTY: Difficult

17. A pregnant client is admitted to the labor unit in early labor. When reviewing the plan of care for the client, which laboratory test would the nurse identify as being critical to obtain?
1. Blood type
2. Calcium level
3. Iron level
4. Oxygen saturation

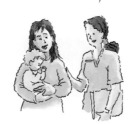

The labor in the hospital is nothing compared to the labor over the next 18 years or so.

17. 1. Blood type is a critical laboratory test to be done because the risk of blood loss is always a potential complication during the labor and birth process. Approximately 40% of a woman's cardiac output is delivered to the uterus; therefore, blood loss can occur quite rapidly in the event of uncontrolled bleeding. Calcium, iron, and oxygen saturation are not critical tests.
CN: Safe, effective care environment; CNS: Coordinated Care; CL: Analyze; DIFFICULTY: Moderate

18. A pregnant client is at term and in labor. The nurse is checking the fetal heart rate. Which finding would the nurse interpret as indicating appropriate fetal perfusion?
1. 88 beats/minute
2. 100 beats/minute
3. 135 beats/minute
4. 180 beats/minute

18. 3. A rate of 120 to 160 beats/minute in the fetal heart is appropriate for filling the heart with blood and pumping it out to the system. A fetal heart rate of 135 beats per minute falls within this range. Faster or slower rates don't accomplish perfusion adequately.
CN: Health promotion and maintenance; CNS: None; CL: Analyze; DIFFICULTY: Easy

19. The nurse is gathering data on a client in the early stages of labor with an external monitor applied. The nurse interprets the monitor data as indicative of which of the following?
1. Gender of the fetus
2. Fetal position
3. Labor progress
4. Oxygenation

19. 4. Oxygenation of the fetus may be indirectly determined through fetal monitoring by closely examining the fetal heart rate strip. Accelerations in the fetal heart rate indicate normal oxygenation, while decelerations in the fetal heart rate sometimes indicate abnormal fetal oxygenation. The fetal heart rate strip can't determine the gender of the fetus or fetal position. Labor progress can be directly monitored only through cervical examination.
CN: Physiological integrity; CNS: Reduction of risk potential; CL: Apply; DIFFICULTY: Challenge

20. A client in labor is scheduled to receive epidural analgesia. In preparation for this procedure, which action would be **most** important for the nurse to do?
1. Giving a fluid bolus of 500 mL
2. Checking for maternal pupil dilation
3. Testing maternal reflexes
4. Observing maternal gait

20. 1. One of the major adverse effects of epidural administration is hypotension. Therefore, a 500-mL fluid bolus is usually administered to help prevent hypotension in the client who wishes to receive an epidural for pain relief. Checking maternal reflexes, pupil response, and gait aren't necessary.
CN: Physiological integrity; CNS: Reduction of risk potential; CL: Apply; DIFFICULTY: Moderate

21. A client in labor requires an episiotomy. Which complication should the nurse have the client report to the health care provider after the procedure?
1. Blood loss
2. Uterine disfigurement
3. Prolonged dyspareunia
4. Postpartum hormonal fluctuation

22. A client in labor tells the nurse, "I'm noticing that I have a clear, milky discharge from both of my breasts." Based on the client's statement, which action by the nurse would be **most** appropriate?
1. Tell the client that her milk is starting to come in because she's in labor.
2. Complete a thorough breast examination, and document the results in the chart.
3. Perform a culture on the discharge, and inform the client that she might have mastitis.
4. Inform her that the discharge is colostrum, normally present after the fourth month of pregnancy.

23. A nurse is participating in developing the plan of care for a client in labor. When reviewing the collected data, which finding would the nurse identify as requiring additional action?
1. Urine output of 100 mL every 2 hours after epidural placement
2. Increase in blood pressure to 154/96 mm Hg during contractions
3. Decrease in respirations to 12 breaths/minute at the acme of contractions
4. Increase in temperature from 98° F to 99.6° F (36.7° C to 37.6° C)

24. A client concerned about the pinkish "stretch marks" on her abdomen asks the nurse about them. Which response by the nurse would be **most** appropriate?
1. "They will go away completely once the uterus goes back to its prepregnant state."
2. "Although they will fade, they won't disappear."
3. "You need to use an emollient cream to remove them."
4. "They are a sign of that your muscle has separated."

21. 3. Prolonged dyspareunia (painful intercourse) may result when complications such as infection interfere with wound healing. Minimal blood loss occurs when an episiotomy is performed. The uterus isn't affected by episiotomy; the perineum is cut to accommodate the fetus. Hormonal fluctuations that occur during the postpartum period aren't the result of an episiotomy.
CN: Physiological integrity; CNS: Basic care and comfort; CL: Understand; DIFFICULTY: Challenge

22. 4. After the fourth month of pregnancy, colostrum may be noticed. The breasts normally produce colostrum for the first few days after birth. Milk production begins 1 to 3 days postpartum. A clinical breast examination isn't usually indicated in the intrapartum setting. Although a culture may be indicated, it requires advanced assessment as well as a medical order.
CN: Health promotion and maintenance; CNS: None; CL: Apply; DIFFICULTY: Easy

23. 2. During contractions, blood pressure increases and blood flow to the intervillous spaces changes, compromising the fetal blood supply. Therefore, the nurse should assess the client's blood pressure frequently to determine if it returns to precontraction level and allows adequate fetal blood flow again. A urine output of 100 mL every 2 hours, respirations of 12 breaths/minute, and temperature changes are normal.
CN: Physiological integrity; CNS: Reduction of risk potential; CL: Analyze; DIFFICULTY: Moderate

24. 2. Striae are wavy, depressed streaks that may occur over the abdomen, breasts, or thighs as pregnancy progresses. They fade with time to a silvery color but won't disappear. Creams may soften the skin and reduce the appearance of striae, but they won't remove the striae completely. Separation of the rectus muscle, or diastasis recti, is a condition of pregnancy whereby the abdominal wall has difficulty stretching enough to accommodate the growing fetus, causing the muscle to separate. Striae are not an indication of this separation.
CN: Health promotion and maintenance; CNS: None; CL: Apply; DIFFICULTY: Easy

25. A client is admitted to the labor unit in early labor. The nurse would encourage the client to assume which position to promote tissue perfusion?
1. Supine
2. Sitting
3. Side-lying
4. Semi-Fowler's

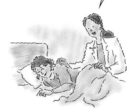

Like my nursing instructor used to say, "perfused tissue is happy tissue."

26. A client has given birth vaginally several minutes ago. The nurse notes blood gushing from the vagina, the umbilical cord lengthening, and a globe-shaped uterus. The nurse should monitor the client closely for which condition?
1. Uterine involution
2. Cervical laceration
3. Placental separation
4. Postpartum hemorrhage

27. While cervical dilation and effacement are being evaluated in a client in labor, a prolapsed cord is discovered. Which intervention would be **most** important? Select all that apply.
1. Give medication to hasten a vaginal birth.
2. Keep the client in the supine position.
3. Position the client in Trendelenburg position.
4. Prepare the client for an emergency cesarean section.
5. Move the cord back to its original location.
6. Monitor fetal heart rate.

28. A client comes to the labor unit reporting contractions. After gathering data, it is determined the client is having Braxton Hicks contractions and education regarding the difference between true and false labor is given. Which statement by the client indicates the teaching has been effective?
1. "Braxton Hicks contractions begin irregularly and become regular."
2. "Braxton Hicks contractions cause cervical dilation and effacement."
3. "Braxton Hicks contractions begin in the lower back and radiate to the abdomen."
4. "Braxton Hicks contractions begin in the abdomen and remain irregular."

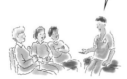

Don't be fooled by Braxton Hicks contractions.

25. 3. In the side-lying position, cardiac output increases, stroke volume increases, and the pulse rate decreases, thereby promoting tissue perfusion. In the supine position, the blood pressure can drop severely due to the pressure of the fetus on the vena cava, resulting in supine hypotensive syndrome or vena cava syndrome. Neither the sitting nor semi-Fowler's position increases cardiac output or stroke volume.
CN: Health promotion and maintenance; CNS: None; CL: Apply; DIFFICULTY: Moderate

26. 3. Placental separation causes a sudden gush or trickle of blood from the vagina, rise of the fundus in the abdomen, increased umbilical cord length at the introitus, and a globe-shaped uterus. Uterine involution causes a firmly contracted uterus, which can't occur until the placenta is delivered. Cervical lacerations produce a steady flow of bright red blood in a client with a firmly contracted uterus. Postpartum hemorrhage results in excessive vaginal bleeding and signs of shock, such as pallor and a rapid, thready pulse.
CN: Health promotion and maintenance; CNS: None; CL: Apply; DIFFICULTY: Moderate

27. 3, 4, 6. A prolapsed cord is an emergency situation and necessitates an emergency cesarean section. Placing the client in the Trendelenburg position relieves pressure of the fetal head on the umbilical cord. Keeping the client supine is inappropriate. It is important to not attempt to move the cord. Monitoring fetal heart rate will reveal any compromise in fetal oxygenation.
CN: Physiological integrity; CNS: Physiological adaptation; CL: Analyze; DIFFICULTY: Difficult

28. 4. Braxton Hicks contractions begin and remain irregular. They're felt in the abdomen and remain confined to the abdomen and groin. They commonly disappear with ambulation and don't dilate the cervix. True contractions begin irregularly but become regular and predictable, causing cervical effacement and dilation. True contractions are felt initially in the lower back and radiate to the abdomen in a wavelike motion.
CN: Health promotion and maintenance; CNS: None; CL: Analyze; DIFFICULTY: Easy

29. A client in active labor requests a holistic approach to labor and birth. Which intervention provided would meet this client's needs during the labor and birth process?
1. A warm bath
2. A foot massage
3. Use of Reiki
4. Use of heated stones

29. 3. The use of Reiki—a gentle technique focusing on the body's energy centers by loosening blocked energy, promoting total relaxation, and establishing spiritual equilibrium and mental well-being—is the most realistic holistic approach. A warm bath or foot massage might help any client, not just those who approach their health holistically. The use of heated stones might be difficult to arrange in a labor and birth unit.
CN: Physiological integrity; CNS: Basic care and comfort; CL: Apply; DIFFICULTY: Difficult

30. A client in labor is prescribed oxytocin and asks the nurse, "What's this medication for?" The nurse would incorporate knowledge of which action in the response?
1. Stimulates labor and prevents hemorrhage
2. Decreases maternal heart rate and stimulates labor
3. Slows labor progression and increases diuresis
4. Prevents hemorrhage and increases diuresis

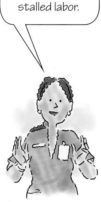

Oxytocin is like a pair of jumper cables for a stalled labor.

30. 1. Oxytocin is the synthetic form of the pituitary hormone used to stimulate uterine contractions, stimulate labor, and prevent hemorrhage. It may increase maternal heart rate and has an antidiuretic effect.
CN: Physiological integrity; CNS: Pharmacological therapies; CL: Apply; DIFFICULTY: Easy

31. A client is in the first stage of labor. Her cervical dilation has progressed from 4 to 7 cm. The nurse understands that the client is **most** likely in which phase?
1. Preparatory phase
2. Latent phase
3. Active phase
4. Transition phase

31. 3. Cervical dilation occurs more rapidly during the active phase than any of the previous phases. The active phase is characterized by cervical dilation that progresses from 4 to 7 cm. The preparatory, or latent, phase begins with the onset of regular uterine contractions and ends when rapid, cervical dilation begins. Transition is defined as cervical dilation beginning at 8 cm and lasting until 10 cm or complete dilation.
CN: Health promotion and maintenance; CNS: None; CL: Apply; DIFFICULTY: Moderate

32. The nurse is reviewing information about the stages of labor with a pregnant client. The nurse determines that the client has understood the information when stating that crowning occurs during which stage of labor?
1. First
2. Second
3. Third
4. Fourth

32. 2. The second stage of labor begins at full cervical dilation (10 cm) and ends when the infant is born. Crowning is present during this stage as the fetal head, pushed against the perineum, causes the vaginal introitus to open, allowing the fetal scalp to be visible. The first stage of labor begins with true labor contractions and ends with complete cervical dilation. The third stage is from the time the infant is born until the delivery of the placenta. The fourth stage is the first 1 to 4 hours following delivery of the placenta.
CN: Health promotion and maintenance; CNS: None; CL: Analyze; DIFFICULTY: Moderate

33. For a client in active labor, the health care provider plans to use an internal electronic fetal monitoring (EFM) device. Which finding from the client's medical record would the nurse interpret as supporting the use of internal EFM? Select all that apply.
1. The membranes have ruptured.
2. Fetus is at -3 station.
3. The cervix is 10 cm dilated
4. The client has received anesthesia.
5. Fetal head is engaged

33. 1, 3, 5. Internal EFM can be applied only after the client's membranes have ruptured, when the fetus is at least at the -1 station and when the cervix is dilated at least 2 cm. A fetus whose head is engaged is at 0 station. Although the client may receive anesthesia, it isn't required before application of an internal EFM device. A fetus at -3 station is above the ischial spines and the head has not yet engaged (0 station).
CN: Physiological integrity; CNS: Reduction of risk potential; CL: Analyze; DIFFICULTY: Difficult

34. A nurse is collecting data from a client in labor and suspects that the client may have been physically abused by her male partner. Which intervention by the nurse would be **most** appropriate?
1. Confront the male partner.
2. Question the woman in front of her partner.
3. Contact hospital security.
4. Collaborate with the health care provider to make a referral to social services.

34. 4. Collaborating with the health care provider to make a referral to social services aids the client by creating a plan and providing support. Additionally, by law in most states, the nurse or nursing supervisor is legally mandated to report the suspected abuse to law enforcement. Although confrontation can be used therapeutically, this action will most likely provoke anger in the suspected abuser. Questioning the woman in front of her partner doesn't allow her the privacy required to address this issue and may place her in greater danger. If the woman isn't in imminent danger, there's no need to call hospital security.
CN: Psychosocial Integrity; CNS: None; CL: Apply;
DIFFICULTY: Easy

35. A pregnant client with diabetes is admitted to the labor unit. Which action by the nurse would be **most** appropriate for this situation?
1. Ask the client about her most recent blood glucose levels.
2. Prepare oral hypoglycemic medications for administration during labor.
3. Notify the neonatal intensive care unit that the newborn of a woman with diabetes will be coming.
4. Prepare the client for cesarean birth.

35. 1. It would be most important to find out about the client's most recent blood glucose levels because this would provide information about how well her diabetes has been controlled. Oral hypoglycemic drugs are never used during labor because they cross the placental barrier, stimulate fetal insulin production, and are potentially teratogenic. Plans to admit the neonate to the neonatal intensive care unit are premature. Cesarean birth is no longer the preferred birth for clients with diabetes. Vaginal birth is preferred and presents a lower risk to the mother and fetus.
CN: Physiological integrity; CNS: Reduction of risk potential;
CL: Apply; DIFFICULTY: Moderate

36. Vaginal examination of a client in labor reveals that the biparietal diameter of the fetal head has reached the level of the ischial spines. The nurse would interpret this as indicating which fetal station?
1. −1
2. 0
3. +1
4. +2

The critical thing here is to estimate the delivery date. What information do you need to do that?

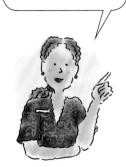

36. 2. When the largest diameter of the presenting part (typically the biparietal diameter of the fetal head) is level with the ischial spines, the fetus is at station 0. A station of −1 indicates that the fetal head is 1 cm above the ischial spines. At +1, it's 1 cm below the ischial spines. At +2, it's 2 cm below the ischial spines.
CN: Health promotion and maintenance; CNS: None; CL: Apply;
DIFFICULTY: Moderate

37. A multiparous client admitted to the labor unit hasn't received prenatal care for this pregnancy. When collecting information from this client, which data would be **most** important to obtain?
1. Date of last menstrual period (LMP)
2. Family history of sexually transmitted infections (STIs)
3. Name of insurance provider
4. Number of siblings

37. 1. The date of the LMP is essential to estimate the date of birth. The nursing history would also include subjective information, such as personal (but not necessarily family) history of STIs, gravidity, and parity. Although beneficial to the hospital for financial reimbursement, the insurance provider has no bearing on the nursing history. Likewise, the number of siblings isn't pertinent to the assessment.
CN: Health promotion and maintenance; CNS: None; CL: Apply;
DIFFICULTY: Easy

38. A pregnant client has received dinoprostone for cervical ripening. The nurse would monitor the client for which **most** common adverse effect of this drug?
1. Vomiting
2. Euphoria
3. Uterine inversion
4. Constipation

38. 1. Headache, nausea, vomiting, chills, fever, and hypertension are adverse effects of dinoprostone. Euphoria and uterine inversion are rare adverse effects of this drug. Diarrhea, not constipation, is a possible adverse effect.
CN: Physiological integrity; CNS: Pharmacological therapies;
CL: Apply; DIFFICULTY: Challenge

CN: Client needs category   CNS: Client needs subcategory   CL: Cognitive level

39. The nurse is providing care to a client with gestational hypertension who is in labor. Which finding would the nurse **immediately** report?
1. Decreasing blood pressure
2. Increasing oliguria
3. Decreasing edema
4. Trace levels of protein in the urine

40. The nurse is assisting with the birth of a fetus in a frank breech presentation. Which image illustrates this position?

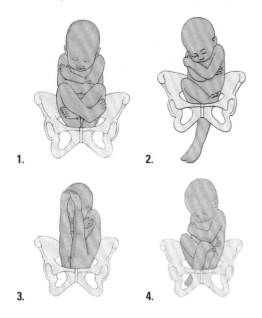

1.　　　2.

3.　　　4.

41. A client in labor has been given an epidural anesthetic. When collecting data on the client immediately following the epidural administration, which finding would be **most** important for the nurse to report?
1. Maternal respirations decrease from 20 to 14 breaths/minute.
2. Maternal blood pressure decreases from 130/70 to 98/50 mm Hg.
3. Maternal pulse increases from 78 to 96 beats/minute.
4. Maternal temperature increases from 99° F (37.2° C) to 100° F (37.8° C).

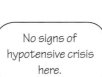

No signs of hypotensive crisis here.

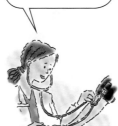

42. A pregnant client has a total hemoglobin level of 9 g/dL. The nurse understands that the client is at **greatest** risk for which condition during the intrapartum period?
1. Small-for-gestational-age neonate
2. Fetal distress
3. Excessive postpartum bleeding
4. Shortness of breath

39. 2. Renal plasma flow and glomerular filtration are decreased in gestational hypertension, so increasing oliguria indicates a worsening condition. Blood pressure increases as a result of increased peripheral resistance. Increasing (not decreasing) edema would suggest a worsening condition. Trace levels to +1 proteinuria are acceptable; higher levels would indicate a worsening condition.

CN: Safe, effective care environment; CNS: Coordinated care; CL: Apply; DIFFICULTY: Challenge

40. 3. In a frank breech presentation, the buttocks are the presenting part, with the hips flexed and the knees remaining straight. In a complete breech (option 1), the knees and hips are flexed. In a footling breech (option 2), neither the hips nor the lower legs are flexed, and one or both feet may present. In an incomplete breech (option 4), one or both hips remain extended, and one or both feet or knees lie below the breech.

CN: Physiological integrity; CNS: Physiological adaptation; CL: Apply; DIFFICULTY: Easy

41. 2. As the epidural anesthetic agent spreads through the spinal canal, it may produce hypotensive crisis, which is characterized by maternal hypotension, decreased beat-to-beat variability, and fetal bradycardia. Maternal blood pressure that decreases from 130/70 to 98/50 mm Hg is the most important finding following administration of epidural anesthesia. The respiratory rate, pulse rate, and temperature listed are within normal limits for a laboring client.

CN: Safe, effective care environment; CNS: Coordinated care; CL: Analyze; DIFFICULTY: Moderate

42. 2. Fetal distress is more common in women with anemia (hemoglobin level <11 g/dL) than in the general nonanemic population. A small-for-gestational-age neonate and excessive postpartum bleeding are diagnosed after the intrapartum period. Shortness of breath occurs more commonly during the antepartum period; the risk for developing shortness of breath doesn't increase during the intrapartum period.

CN: Physiological integrity; CNS: Reduction of risk potential; CL: Apply; DIFFICULTY: Difficult

43. A client in labor is receiving magnesium sulfate as an intravenous infusion. Which medication should the nurse ensure is at the bedside while the magnesium sulfate is being infused?
1. Oxytocin
2. Terbutaline
3. Calcium gluconate
4. Naloxone

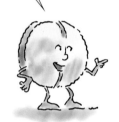

A lot of clients say that I make them sick to their stomach, but I try not to take it personally.

44. A client in labor is prescribed an IV of 5% dextrose in lactated Ringer's solution to run at 125 mL/hour. The IV tubing delivers 10 drops per mL. At which infusion rate should the nurse set the IV? Record your answer using a whole number.

_____ gtt/minute

45. A nurse is assisting in monitoring a client in labor. Which data obtained by the nurse is indicative of fetal well-being?
1. Fetal heart rate of 145 to 155 beats/minute with 15-second accelerations to 160
2. Fetal heart rate of 130 to 140 beats/minute with late decelerations to 110
3. Fetal heart rate of 110 to 120 beats/minute with variable decelerations to 90
4. Fetal heart rate of 165 to 175 beats/minute with late decelerations to 140

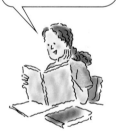

Normal fetal heart rates are way higher than those for adults, and short bursts of acceleration are nothing to be concerned about.

46. A nurse is assisting in monitoring a client who's receiving oxytocin to induce labor. The nurse would be alert for which maternal adverse reactions? Select all that apply.
1. Hypertension
2. Jaundice
3. Dehydration
4. Fluid overload
5. Uterine tetany
6. Bradycardia

43. 3. Calcium gluconate should be kept at the bedside while a client is receiving a magnesium infusion. If magnesium toxicity occurs, administering calcium gluconate is an antidote. Oxytocin is the synthetic form of the naturally occurring pituitary hormone used to initiate or augment uterine contractions. Terbutaline is a smooth muscle relaxant sometimes used to relax the uterus, especially for preterm labor and uterine hyperstimulation. Naloxone is an opiate antagonist administered to reverse the respiratory depression that sometimes follows doses of opiates.
CN: Physiological integrity; CNS: Pharmacological therapies; CL: Understand; DIFFICULTY: Easy

44. 21.
Multiply the number of milliliters to be infused (125) by the drop factor (10).

$$125 \times 10 = 1,250.$$

Then divide the answer by the number of minutes to run the infusion (60). Use the following equation:

$$1,250 \div 60 = 20.83 \,(\text{or 20 to 21 gtt/minute}).$$

CN: Physiological integrity; CNS: Pharmacological therapies; CL: Analyze; DIFFICULTY: Moderate

45. 1. Accelerations of up to 15 beats/minute above baseline for a duration of 15 seconds are signs of fetal well-being. Decelerations initiated 30 to 40 seconds after the onset of the contraction are termed late decelerations, and are due to uteroplacental insufficiency from decreased blood flow during uterine contractions. Variable decelerations are an indication of cord compression. Variable decelerations can occur with or without contractions.
CN: Physiological integrity; CNS: Physiological adaptation; CL: Apply; DIFFICULTY: Moderate

46. 1, 4, 5. Maternal adverse effects of oxytocin include hypertension, fluid overload, and uterine tetany. Oxytocin's antidiuretic effect increases renal reabsorption of water, leading to fluid overload, not dehydration. Jaundice and bradycardia are adverse effects that may occur in the neonate. Tachycardia, not bradycardia, is reported as a maternal adverse effect.
CN: Physiological integrity; CNS: Pharmacological therapies; CL: Apply; DIFFICULTY: Challenge

47. Obtaining data for a client progressing through labor reveals the findings below. Order them in the most likely sequence in which they would have occurred.

1.	Uncontrollable urge to push

2.	Cervical dilation of 4 cm

3.	100% cervical effacement

4.	Strong Braxton Hicks contractions

5.	Mild contractions lasting 20 to 40 seconds

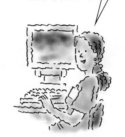

Sweet! I love these ordering questions. Now, which is most likely to occur first?

47.

4.	Strong Braxton Hicks contractions

5.	Mild contractions lasting 20 to 40 seconds

2.	Cervical dilation of 4 cm

3.	100% cervical effacement

1.	Uncontrollable urge to push

Strong Braxton Hicks contractions typically occur before the onset of true labor and are considered a preliminary sign of labor. During the latent phase of the first stage of labor, contractions are mild, lasting about 20 to 40 seconds. As the client progresses through labor, contractions increase in intensity and duration, and cervical dilation occurs. Cervical dilation of 4 cm indicates that the client has entered the active phase of the first stage of labor. Cervical effacement also occurs; effacement of 100% characterizes the transition phase of the first stage of labor. Progression into the second stage of labor is noted by the client's uncontrollable urge to push.
CN: Health promotion and maintenance; CNS: None: CL: Analyze; DIFFICULTY: Moderate

48. A client is receiving a tocolytic agent to help stop preterm labor contractions. The nurse would be alert for signs and symptoms of which potentially life-threatening complication?
1. Diabetic ketoacidosis
2. Hyperemesis gravidarum
3. Pulmonary edema
4. Sickle cell anemia

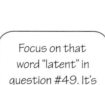

Focus on that word "latent" in question #49. It's important.

48. 3. Tocolytics are used to stop labor contractions. The most common adverse effect associated with the use of these drugs is pulmonary edema. Clients who don't have diabetes don't need to be observed for diabetic ketoacidosis. Hyperemesis gravidarum doesn't result from tocolytic use. Sickle cell anemia is an inherited genetic condition that doesn't develop spontaneously.
CN: Physiological integrity; CNS: Pharmacological therapies; CL: Apply; DIFFICULTY: Moderate

49. A pregnant client is admitted to the labor unit. When gathering data, which finding would the nurse identify as an indication that the client is in the latent phase of the first stage of labor? Select all that apply.
1. Cervical dilation of 5 cm
2. Contractions occurring every 6 to 7 minutes
3. Contractions lasting about 30 to 45 seconds
4. Cervical effacement of 50%
5. Moderate contraction intensity

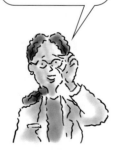

49. 2, 3. Signs indicating the latent phase of the first stage of labor include contractions occurring every 5 to 10 minutes and lasting about 30 to 45 seconds. Signs indicating the active phase of the first stage of labor include cervical dilation from 4 to 7 cm, cervical effacement from 40% to 80%, and moderate contraction intensity.
CN: Health promotion and maintenance; CNS: None; CL: Analyze; DIFFICULTY: Difficult

50. A woman is in the third stage of labor after having just given birth to a healthy newborn. Which actions would be **most** important during this stage? Select all that apply.
1. Assisting with skin-to-skin contact of the mother with the newborn.
2. Providing the woman with cool compresses to prevent overheating.
3. Encouraging the woman to breast-feed if appropriate.
4. Assisting the woman into a comfortable position.
5. Applying a heating pad to the episiotomy site.

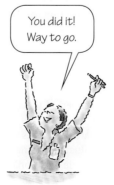

You did it! Way to go.

50. 1, 3, 4. During the third stage of labor, the nurse should assist with skin-to-skin contact between the mother and the newborn, provide warm blankets to prevent shivering, encourage the woman to breast-feed if appropriate, assist the woman to a comfortable position, and apply ice to the episiotomy site.
CN: Safe, effective care environment; CNS: Coordinated care; CL: Apply; DIFFICULTY: Moderate

Chapter 23

Postpartum Care

Postpartum care refresher

Mastitis

Inflammation and infection of the breast that results from the stasis of milk; the most common infecting organism is *Staphylococcus aureus*

Key signs and symptoms
- Chills
- Localized area of redness, inflammation, and tenderness
- Temperature of 101.1° F (38.4° C) or higher

Key test results
- Culture of purulent discharge may test positive for *Staphylococcus aureus*

Key treatments
- Incision and drainage if abscess occurs
- Moist heat application
- Feed or pump breasts every 2 to 4 hours to preserve breast-feeding ability if abscess occurs
- Analgesics: acetaminophen, ibuprofen
- Antibiotics: cephalexin, cefaclor, clindamycin

Key interventions
- Administer antibiotic therapy
- Apply moist heat

Postpartum hemorrhage

Blood loss of 500 mL or more after a vaginal birth or 1,000 mL or more after cesarean birth; can occur within the first 24 hours (early postpartum hemorrhage) or from 24 hours to 6 weeks after birth (late postpartum hemorrhage)

Key signs and symptoms
- Blood loss greater than 500 mL within a 24-hour period; may occur up to 6 weeks after delivery
- Signs of shock (tachycardia, hypotension, oliguria)
- Uterine atony

Key test results
- Hematology studies show decreased hemoglobin and hematocrit levels, low fibrinogen level, and decreased partial thromboplastin time

Key treatments
- Bimanual compression of the uterus and dilation and curettage (D & C) to remove clots
- IV replacement of fluids and blood
- Parenteral administration of methylergonovine maleate
- Rapid IV infusion of dilute oxytocin

Key interventions
- Massage the fundus and express clots from the uterus
- Perform a pad count
- Monitor the fundus for location
- Monitor IV infusion of dilute oxytocin

Psychological maladaptation

Changes in the mother's mood, which can range from postpartum blues (or baby blues) to postpartum depression to postpartum psychosis

Key signs and symptoms
- Inability to stop crying
- Increased anxiety about self and infant's health
- Overall feeling of sadness
- Unwillingness to be left alone

Key treatments
- Counseling for the client and family at risk
- Psychotherapy for the client
- Antidepressants: imipramine, nortriptyline

Key interventions
- Obtain a health history during the antepartum period to determine risk of postpartum depression
- Evaluate client's support systems
- Evaluate maternal-infant bonding
- Provide emotional support and encouragement

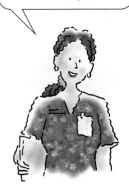

Before taking off through the chapter, why not spend a few minutes browsing the birthing stories at www.birthstories.com/? It will get you in just the right mood to tackle care of the postpartum client. Enjoy!

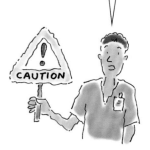

Postpartum blood loss greater than 500 mL within a 24-hour period is considered hemorrhage and should be addressed immediately.

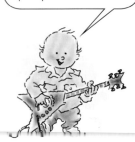

I'd like to dedicate this next song to my mom. "Don't you go singing those low-down, postpartum blues ..."

Puerperal infection

Fever occurring after the first 24 hours after birth, and occurring on at least two of the first 10 days after birth; can occur in the reproductive tract, the urinary tract, or wound

Key signs and symptoms
- Abdominal pain and tenderness
- Purulent, foul-smelling lochia
- Tachycardia
- Temperature of 101.5° F (38.6° C) or higher

Key test results
- Complete blood count may show an elevated white blood cell count in the upper ranges of normal (more than 30,000/μL) for the postpartum period
- Cultures of the blood or the endocervical and uterine cavities may reveal the causative organism

Key treatments
- Broad-spectrum IV antibiotic therapy unless a causative organism is identified

Key interventions
- Monitor vital signs every 4 hours
- Place client in Fowler's position
- Maintain IV fluid administration as ordered
- Administer antibiotics as prescribed

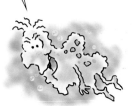

We bacteria love the postpartum period. So many opportunities to invade and multiply.

thePoint® You can download tables of drug information to help you prepare for the NCLEX®! View Generic Drug Names, Drug Classifications, Drug Actions, and Nursing Implications for the drugs discussed in this refresher at **http://thePoint.lww.com**.

Postpartum care questions, answers, and rationales

1. A nurse enters a postpartum client's room to collect data and observes the perineal pad is completely saturated with lochia rubra. Which action by the nurse is the **priority**?
1. Vigorously massage the fundus.
2. Immediately call the health care provider.
3. Have the charge nurse review the finding.
4. Ask the client when she last changed her perineal pad.

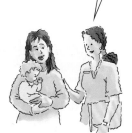

Other than being chronically sleep-deprived and having sore breasts and hemorrhoids—I'm doing fantastic.

1.   4. If the morning assessment is done relatively early, it's possible that the client hasn't yet been to the bathroom, in which case her perineal pad may have been in place all night. Secondly, her lochia may have pooled during the night, resulting in a heavy flow in the morning. Vigorous massage of the fundus isn't recommended for heavy bleeding or hemorrhage. It would be inappropriate at this time to call the health care provider. More information is needed to determine the status of the situation. If the nurse was uncertain, she should ask a more experienced nurse to check the client but only after a complete assessment of the client's status.

CN: Safe, effective care environment; CNS: Coordinated care; CL: Analyze; DIFFICULTY: Easy

2. A nurse is assisting a postpartum client to breastfeed her newborn. The client is having difficulty in establishing an adequate supply of breast milk. The nurse understands that which factor might play a role?
1. Supplemental formula feedings
2. Maternal diet high in vitamin C
3. An alcoholic drink
4. Frequent feedings

2.   1. Routine formula supplementation may interfere with establishing an adequate milk volume because decreased stimulation to the client's nipples affects hormonal levels and milk production. Vitamin C levels haven't been shown to influence milk volume. One drink containing alcohol generally tends to relax the client, facilitating letdown. Excessive consumption of alcohol may block letdown of milk to the infant, though supply isn't necessarily affected. Frequent feedings are likely to increase milk production.

CN: Health promotion and maintenance; CNS: None; CL: Apply; DIFFICULTY: Moderate

3. A postpartum client is experiencing breast engorgement. When providing care to the client, which action would the nurse anticipate as being **most** helpful?
1. Applying ice
2. Applying a breast binder
3. Informing the client how to express her breasts in a warm shower
4. Restricting oral intake of fluids

4. A postpartum client has given birth to a healthy newborn by cesarean. Which information would the nurse most likely reinforce?
1. Frequent douching after she's discharged
2. Coughing and deep-breathing exercises
3. Sit-ups for 2 weeks postoperatively
4. Side-rolling exercises

5. A postpartum client who had a cesarean birth reports right calf pain to the nurse. The nurse observes that the client has nonpitting edema from her right knee to her foot. Based on this finding, the nurse would anticipate which test as the **priority**?
1. Venous duplex ultrasound of the right leg
2. Transthoracic echocardiogram
3. Venogram of the right leg
4. Noninvasive arterial studies of the right leg

6. A nurse is providing care to a postpartum client. As part of the client's plan of care, the nurse reinforces the need to perform Kegel exercises based on which reason?
1. To assist with lochia removal.
2. To promote the return of normal bowel function.
3. To promote blood flow, enabling healing and muscle strengthening.
4. To assist the client in burning calories for rapid, postpartum weight loss.

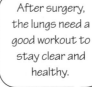

After surgery, the lungs need a good workout to stay clear and healthy.

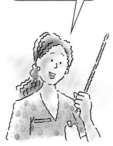

3. 3. Informing the client on how to express her breasts in a warm shower aids with letdown and will give temporary relief. Ice promotes comfort by decreasing blood flow (vasoconstriction), numbing the area, and discouraging further letdown of milk; however, this is followed by a rebound reaction of more letting down once the ice is removed. Restricting fluids doesn't reduce engorgement and shouldn't be encouraged. Breast binders aren't effective in relieving the discomforts of engorgement.
CN: Physiological integrity; CNS: Basic care and comfort; CL: Apply; DIFFICULTY: Easy

4. 2. As for any postoperative client, coughing and deep-breathing exercises should be reinforced to keep the alveoli open and prevent infection. Frequent douching isn't recommended and is contraindicated in clients who have just given birth. Sit-ups at 2 weeks postpartum could potentially damage the healing of the incision. Side-rolling exercises aren't an accepted medical practice.
CN: Physiological integrity; CNS: Reduction of risk potential; CL: Apply; DIFFICULTY: Easy

5. 1. Right calf pain and nonpitting edema may indicate deep vein thrombosis (DVT). Postpartum clients and clients who have had abdominal surgery are at increased risk for DVT. Venous duplex ultrasound is a noninvasive test that visualizes the veins and assesses blood flow patterns. A venogram is an invasive test that utilizes dye and radiation to create images of the veins; it wouldn't be the first test to perform. Transthoracic echocardiography looks at cardiac structures and isn't indicated at this time. Right calf pain and edema are symptoms of venous outflow obstruction, not arterial insufficiency.
CN: Safe, effective care environment; CNS: Coordinated care; CL: Apply; DIFFICULTY: Moderate

6. 3. Exercising the pubococcygeal muscle increases blood flow to the area. The increased blood flow brings oxygen and other nutrients to the perineal area to aid in healing. Additionally, these exercises help strengthen the musculature, thereby decreasing the risk of future complications, such as incontinence and uterine prolapse. Kegel exercises may assist with lochia removal but that isn't their main purpose. Bowel function isn't influenced by Kegel exercises. Kegel exercises don't generate sufficient energy expenditure to burn many calories.
CN: Health promotion and maintenance; CNS: None; CL: Analyze; DIFFICULTY: Easy

7. A nurse is providing care to a postpartum client in the immediate postpartum period. The nurse suspects that the client may be experiencing a pulmonary embolus based on which finding? Select all that apply.
1. Sudden dyspnea
2. Chest pain
3. Chills
4. Bradycardia
5. Hypertension

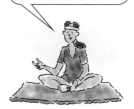

Being a nurse requires a lot of flexibility; you never know what's coming next.

8. A client had an emergency cesarean birth. Afterward, the client expresses disappointment about not being able to give birth vaginally. The nurse understands that this feeling may be based on which concept?
1. Cesarean births cost more.
2. Depression is more common after a cesarean birth.
3. The client is usually more fatigued after cesarean birth.
4. The client may feel a loss for not having experienced a "normal" birth.

9. The nurse is reinforcing discharge instructions to a postpartum client after a vaginal birth. The nurse determines that the client has understood the information when the client states what finding as expected? Select all that apply.
1. Redness or swelling in the calves
2. A nonpalpable uterine fundus after 6 weeks
3. Vaginal dryness after the lochial flow has ended
4. Dark red lochia for approximately 6 weeks after the birth
5. Strong smelling lochia by end of the first week

Remember to look for the priority action in question #10.

10. A nurse checks the fundus of a postpartum client and notes that the fundus is situated in the client's left abdomen. What is the **priority** action by the nurse?
1. Ask the client to empty her bladder.
2. Straight catheterize the client immediately.
3. Call the client's primary health care provider for direction.
4. Straight catheterize the client for half of her urine volume.

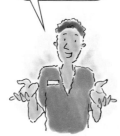

11. A nurse is reinforcing the teaching plan for a postpartum client diagnosed with mastitis. The nurse determines that the client has understood the information when she states which organism as most likely responsible?
1. Escherichia coli
2. Group beta-hemolytic streptococci (GBS)
3. Staphylococcus aureus
4. Streptococcus pyogenes

7. **1, 2.** Signs of pulmonary embolus include sudden dyspnea and chest pain. Chills would most likely signal an infection. The client with a pulmonary embolus would have tachycardia and hypotension.
CN: Physiological integrity; CNS: Reduction of risk potential; CL: Analyze; DIFFICULTY: Moderate

8. **4.** Clients occasionally feel a loss after a cesarean birth. They may feel they're inadequate because they couldn't give birth to their newborn vaginally. The cost of cesarean birth doesn't generally apply because the client usually isn't directly responsible for payment. No conclusive studies support the theory that depression is more common after cesarean birth than after vaginal birth. Although clients are usually more fatigued after a cesarean birth, fatigue hasn't been shown to cause feelings of disappointment over the method of birth.
CN: Psychosocial integrity; CNS: None; CL: Analyze; DIFFICULTY: Easy

9. **2, 3.** Vaginal dryness is a normal finding during the postpartum period due to hormonal changes. The fundus shouldn't be palpable beyond 6 weeks. Redness or swelling in the calves is not normal and may indicate thrombophlebitis. Dark red lochia (indicating fresh bleeding) should last only 2 to 3 days postpartum. Lochia at any stage should have a fleshy odor. Any other strong odor suggests an infection.
CN: Physiological integrity; CNS: Physiological adaptation; CL: Apply; DIFFICULTY: Moderate

10. **1.** A full bladder may displace the uterine fundus to the left or right side of the abdomen. Therefore, the nurse should have the client empty her bladder and then check the fundus again. A straight catheterization is unnecessarily invasive if the client can urinate on her own. Nursing interventions should be completed before notifying the primary health care provider in a nonemergency situation.
CN: Physiological integrity; CNS: Physiological adaptation; CL: Apply; DIFFICULTY: Easy

11. **3.** The most common cause of mastitis is S. aureus, which can be transmitted from the lining of the infant's nostrils when an opportunity such as a crack in the nipple presents itself. Mastitis isn't harmful to the neonate. E. coli, GBS, and S. pyogenes aren't associated with mastitis. GBS infection is associated with neonatal sepsis and death.
CN: Safe and Effective Care Environment; CNS: Safety and Infection Control; CL: Analyze; DIFFICULTY: Moderate

12. The nurse is monitoring a client who gave birth vaginally yesterday. The nurse determines that the client is progressing as expected when the nurse finds the top of the client's fundus at which location?
1. One fingerbreadth above the umbilicus
2. One fingerbreadth below the umbilicus
3. At the level of the umbilicus
4. Below the symphysis pubis

13. The nurse is providing care to a postpartum client with type 1 diabetes who developed polyhydramnios. The client's newborn was macrosomic. The nurse would monitor the client closely for which complication?
1. Postpartum mastitis
2. Increased insulin needs
3. Postpartum hemorrhage
4. Gestational hypertension

14. The nurse is caring for a postpartum client with diabetes who has developed an infection. The nurse would monitor this client for which complication?
1. Anemia
2. Ketoacidosis
3. Respiratory acidosis
4. Respiratory alkalosis

15. The nurse is providing care to a postpartum client with mastitis. As part of the client's teaching plan, the nurse is reinforcing information about the condition. Which information should the nurse emphasize?
1. The most common pathogen is group A beta-hemolytic streptococci.
2. A breast abscess is a common complication of mastitis.
3. Mastitis usually develops in both breasts of a breast-feeding client.
4. Symptoms include fever, chills, malaise, and localized breast tenderness.

16. A 7-day postpartum client comes to the emergency department with vaginal bleeding. A diagnosis of delayed postpartum hemorrhage is made. When reviewing the client's medical record, which condition would the nurse expect to find as a likely cause? Select all that apply.
1. Retained placental fragments
2. Uterine atony
3. Intrauterine infection
4. Uterine fibroids
5. Uterine rupture

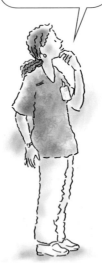

Let's see … mastitis is an infection of the breast. What symptoms should we expect to see?

12. 2. After a client gives birth vaginally, the height of her fundus should decrease by about one fingerbreadth (about 1 cm) each day. So by the end of the first postpartum day, the fundus should be one fingerbreadth below the umbilicus. Immediately after birth, the fundus may be above the umbilicus; 6 to 12 hours after birth, it should be at the level of the umbilicus; and 10 days after birth, it should be below the symphysis pubis.
CN: Health Promotion and Maintenance; CNS: None; CL: Apply; DIFFICULTY: Moderate

13. 3. The client with diabetes is at risk for a postpartum hemorrhage from the overdistention of the uterus because of the extra amniotic fluid (polyhydramnios) and the large neonate (macrosomia). The uterus may not be able to contract as well as it would normally. The client with diabetes usually has decreased insulin needs for the first few days postpartum. Neither polyhydramnios nor macrosomia increases the client's risk of hypertension in pregnancy or mastitis.
CN: Physiological integrity; CNS: Reduction of risk potential; CL: Apply; DIFFICULTY: Moderate

14. 2. Clients with diabetes who become pregnant tend to become sicker and develop illnesses more quickly than pregnant clients without diabetes. Severe infections in diabetes can lead to diabetic ketoacidosis. Anemia, respiratory acidosis, and respiratory alkalosis aren't generally associated with infections in clients with diabetes.
CN: Physiological integrity; CNS: Reduction of risk potential; CL: Analyze; DIFFICULTY: Easy

15. 4. Mastitis is an infection of the breast characterized by flulike symptoms, along with redness and tenderness in the breast. The most common causative agent is Staphylococcus aureus. Breast abscess is rarely a complication of mastitis if the client continues to empty the affected breast. Mastitis usually occurs in one breast, not bilaterally.
CN: Physiological integrity; CNS: Physiological adaptation; CL: Apply; DIFFICULTY: Easy

16. 1, 3, 4. The most common causes of a delayed postpartum hemorrhage include retained placental fragments, intrauterine infection, and fibroids. Uterine atony and uterine rupture are common causes of early postpartum hemorrhage.
CN: Physiological integrity; CNS: Reduction of risk potential; CL: Apply; DIFFICULTY: Difficult

17. The nurse receives a report on a client who delivered a healthy neonate 1 hour ago. What is the priority for the nurse to monitor during the immediate postpartum period ? Select all that apply.
1. Blood glucose level
2. Heart rhythm via electrocardiogram (ECG)
3. Height of fundus
4. Stool test for occult blood
5. Urine output

17. 3. A focused physical examination should be performed every 15 minutes for the first 1 to 2 hours postpartum, including assessment of the fundus, lochia, perineum, blood pressure, pulse, and bladder function (urine output). A blood glucose level would be obtained if the client has risk factors for an unstable blood glucose level or if she has symptoms of an altered blood glucose level. An ECG would be necessary only if the client is at risk for cardiac difficulty. A stool test for occult blood generally wouldn't be valid during the immediate postpartum period because it's difficult to sort out lochial bleeding from rectal bleeding.
CN: Health maintenance and promotion; CNS: None; CL: Apply; DIFFICULTY: Difficult

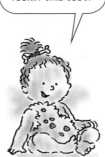

Yabba dabba doo! You're really rockin' this test.

18. When monitoring a postpartum client 2 hours after birth of her newborn, the nurse notices heavy bleeding with large clots. Which action would the nurse perform first?
1. Massaging the fundus firmly
2. Performing bimanual compression
3. Administering ergonovine
4. Notifying the primary health care provider

18. 1. Initial management of excessive postpartum bleeding is firm massage of the fundus and administration of oxytocin. Bimanual compression is performed by a primary health care provider. Ergonovine should be used only if the bleeding doesn't respond to massage and oxytocin. The primary health care provider should be notified if the client doesn't respond to fundal massage, but other measures can be taken in the meantime.
CN: Physiological integrity; CNS: Reduction of Risk Potential; CL: Analyze; DIFFICULTY: Easy

19. A postpartum client reports that her afterpains have increased in severity. When reviewing the client's history, which condition would the nurse most likely find to support the client's statement?
1. Bottle-feeding
2. Diabetes
3. Multiple gestation
4. Primiparity

19. 3. Multiple gestation, breast-feeding, multiparity, and conditions that cause overdistention of the uterus increase the intensity of afterpains. Bottle-feeding and diabetes aren't directly associated with increasing severity of afterpains, unless the client has delivered a macrosomic neonate.
CN: Health promotion and maintenance; CNS: None; CL: Apply; DIFFICULTY: Moderate

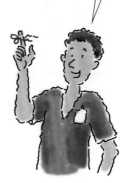

Remember to keep your priorities in order when answering question #20.

20. A multiparous postpartum client is being discharged 48 hours after a successful 16-hour vaginal birth of an 8-lb, 14-oz (4,036-g) neonate. The nurse notes that the mother is rubella-immune with Rh-positive blood type. When assisting with the discharge plan, which outcome would be the priority?
1. The client will receive Rho(D) immune globulin IM before discharge.
2. The client will understand the need for planned rest periods and identify a support system.
3. The client will understand and consent to a rubella vaccine before discharge.
4. The client will verbalize the importance of reporting any change in character of lochia.

20. 4. A multiparous client who has a history of prolonged labor and birth of a large infant is at a higher risk for developing late postpartum hemorrhage. The nurse should ensure that the client understands the importance of reporting a change in lochia pattern, including increased amount, resumption of a brighter color, passage of clots, or foul odor. The client with Rh-positive blood doesn't require a Rho(D) immune globulin injection. Postpartum hemorrhage instruction takes precedence over planning adequate rest. A client who is rubella-immune doesn't require immunization.
CN: Safe, effective care environment; CNS: Coordinated care; CL: Analyze; DIFFICULTY: Challenge

21. The nurse is caring for a postpartum client after giving birth to a healthy neonate. When checking the client's fundus, which finding would the nurse most likely note?
1. Fundus 1 cm above the umbilicus 1 hour postpartum
2. Fundus 1 cm above the umbilicus on postpartum day 3
3. Fundus palpable in the abdomen at 2 weeks postpartum
4. Fundus slightly to right; 2 cm above umbilicus on postpartum day 2

22. When reviewing self-care instructions with a postpartum client, the nurse emphasizes the need for the client to report heavy or excessive bleeding. The nurse would describe "heavy bleeding saturating one sanitary pad within which time span?"
1. 15 minutes
2. 1 hour
3. 4 hours
4. 8 hours

23. A nurse is about to give a client with type 1 diabetes insulin before breakfast on her first day postpartum. Which statement by the client indicates an understanding of insulin requirements immediately postpartum?
1. "I will need less insulin now than during my pregnancy."
2. "I will need more insulin now than during my pregnancy."
3. "I will need less insulin now than before I was pregnant."
4. "I will need more insulin now than before I was pregnant."

24. A client and her neonate have a blood incompatibility. The neonate has had a positive direct Coombs test. Which nursing intervention is appropriate?
1. Because the client has been sensitized, give Rho(D) immune globulin.
2. Because the client hasn't been sensitized, give Rho(D) immune globulin.
3. Because the client has been sensitized, don't give Rho(D) immune globulin.
4. Because the client hasn't been sensitized, don't give Rho(D) immune globulin.

25. A postpartum client experiences postpartum hemorrhage. Fundal massage has failed to maintain uterine contraction and the client continues to experience hemorrhage. The nurse would anticipate which medication to be prescribed? Select all that apply.
1. Oxytocin
2. Carboprost
3. Methylergonovine
4. Heparin
5. Amoxicillin

No thanks. I think I'll just hang out in here a while longer.

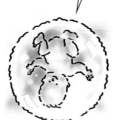

21. 1. Within the first 12 hours postpartum, the fundus is usually approximately 1 cm above the umbilicus. The fundus should be below the umbilicus by postpartum day 3. The fundus shouldn't be palpated in the abdomen after day 10. A uterus that isn't midline or is above the umbilicus on postpartum day 3 might be caused by a full, distended bladder or a uterine infection.
CN: Health promotion and maintenance; CNS: None; CL: Apply; DIFFICULTY: Easy

22. 2. Bleeding is considered heavy when a woman saturates one sanitary pad in 1 hour. Excessive bleeding occurs when a postpartum client saturates one pad in 15 minutes. Moderate bleeding occurs when the bleeding saturates less than 6 in (15 cm) of one pad in 1 hour. Light bleeding occurs when bleeding saturates one pad in 4 hours or more.
CN: Health promotion and maintenance; CNS: None; CL: Apply; DIFFICULTY: Challenge

23. 3. Postpartum insulin requirements are usually significantly lower than prepregnancy requirements. Occasionally, clients may require little to no insulin during the first 24 to 48 hours postpartum.
CN: Physiological integrity; CNS: Reduction of risk potential; CL: Analyze; DIFFICULTY: Challenge

24. 3. A positive Coombs test means that the Rh-negative client is now producing antibodies to the Rh-positive blood of the neonate. Rho(D) immune globulin shouldn't be given to a sensitized client because it won't be able to prevent antibody formation.
CN: Physiological integrity; CNS: Reduction of risk potential; CL: Apply; DIFFICULTY: Challenge

25. 1, 2, 3. If fundal massage fails to maintain uterine contraction, oxytocin, carboprost or methylergonovine may be ordered to maintain uterine tone and control hemorrhage. Heparin would be appropriate as treatment for deep vein thrombosis. Amoxicillin may be ordered to treat an infection.
CN: Physiological integrity; CNS: Pharmacological Therapies; CL: Apply; DIFFICULTY: Moderate

26. A nurse reads the progress note entry below and knows she must report the client's data because the client may be developing which condition?

Progress notes	
09/04/17	Client is 5 hours postvaginal birth with
1030	vacuum extraction. Fundus is firm;
	moderate lochia. VS: Temperature, 100.8° F
	(38.2° C) orally; heart rate, 110 beats/minute;
	respiratory rate, 22 breaths/minute; blood
	pressure, 110/78 mm Hg
	— Barbara Smith L. V. N

1. Urine retention
2. Pulmonary embolus
3. Shock from blood loss
4. Puerperal infection or endometritis

27. A nurse is providing care to a postpartum client who gave birth vaginally to a healthy newborn 48 hours ago. When talking with the client, which information would cause the nurse concern?
1. The client is nervous about taking the baby home.
2. The client feels empty since she delivered the neonate.
3. The client would like to watch the nurse give the baby her first bath.
4. The client would like the nurse to take her baby to the nursery so she can sleep.

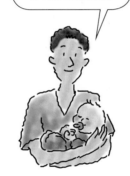

The "baby blues" might sound harmless, but it can develop into depression; monitor any client with signs of this condition.

28. A postpartum client has continuous seepage of blood from the vagina. Her fundus is firm and 1 cm below the umbilicus. A nurse would monitor this client closely for which condition?
1. Retained placental fragments
2. Urinary tract infection
3. Cervical laceration
4. Uterine atony

29. A postpartum client is receiving anticoagulant therapy for deep venous thrombophlebitis, After assisting with the discharge teaching plan the nurse determines that the client has understood the information when what statement is made?
1. "I need to avoid taking any iron supplements."
2. "I should not take any over-the-counter (OTC) salicylates."
3. "It's important for me to wear knee-high stockings when possible."
4. "Shortness of breath is a common adverse effect."

26. 4. The client's elevated temperature along with her prolonged labor and the instrumentation associated with the birth place her at risk for postpartum infection. Her temperature should be reported to the health care provider. At 5 hours post vaginal birth, , the nurse wouldn't expect the client to have voided yet and wouldn't become concerned until after 8 hours had passed. Urine retention without infection wouldn't cause an elevation in temperature. The client's respiratory rate is normal and there's no evidence to support pulmonary embolus. Shock from blood loss can be ruled out because the pulse rate is within normal limits and the firm fundus and moderate lochia are also normal.
CN: Physiological integrity; CNS: Reduction of risk potential; CL: Analyze; DIFFICULTY: Moderate

27. 2. A client experiencing postpartum blues may say she feels empty now that the infant is no longer in her uterus. She may also verbalize that she feels unprotected now. The other situations are considered normal and wouldn't be cause for concern. Many first-time mothers are nervous about caring for their neonates by themselves after discharge. New mothers may want a demonstration before doing a task themselves. A client may want to get some uninterrupted sleep, so she may ask that the neonate be taken to the nursery.
CN: Psychosocial integrity; CNS: None; CL: Analyze; DIFFICULTY: Moderate

28. 3. Continuous seepage of blood may be due to cervical or vaginal lacerations if the uterus is firm and contracting. Retained placental fragments and uterine atony may cause subinvolution of the uterus, making it soft, boggy, and larger than expected. Urinary tract infection won't cause vaginal bleeding, although hematuria may be present.
CN: Physiological integrity; CNS: Reduction of risk potential; CL: Apply; DIFFICULTY: Difficult

29. 2. Discharge education should include informing the client to avoid OTC salicylates, which may potentiate the effects of anticoagulant therapy. Iron won't affect anticoagulation therapy. Restrictive clothing such as knee-high stockings should be avoided to prevent the recurrence of thrombophlebitis. Shortness of breath should be reported immediately because it may be a symptom of pulmonary embolism.
CN: Physiological integrity; CNS: Reduction of risk potential; CL: Apply; DIFFICULTY: Moderate

30. A client is 2 days postpartum and is experiencing bleeding. She asks the nurse, "Will it always be like this?" Which statement by the nurse would be the most accurate?
1. "This is lochia alba and will last 4 weeks."
2. "This is lochia serosa and will last 2 days."
3. "This is lochia rubra and will last 3 to 4 days."
4. "This is your menstrual cycle and will last 6 weeks."

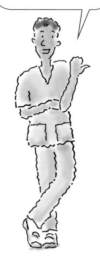

Inform your client that if heavy bleeding lasts longer than a few days, she should contact her health care provider immediately.

31. A client experienced a perinatal loss 3 days ago. The nurse is concerned that the client may be experiencing dysfunctional grieving based on which finding?
1. Lack of appetite
2. Denial of the death
3. Blaming herself
4. Frequent crying spells

32. A nurse obtains the vital signs of a client who is 2 days postpartum and finds the temperature is 100.8° F (38.2° C). Additional data indicates that infection is not present. The nurse interprets the findings suspecting that the fever may be the result of which condition?
1. Breast engorgement
2. Endometritis
3. Mastitis
4. Uterine involution

33. An Rh-positive client gives birth vaginally to a 6-lb, 10-oz (3,007-g) neonate after 17 hours of labor. The nurse monitors the client for possible infection based on the understanding that the client is at risk due to which factor?
1. Length of labor
2. Maternal Rh status
3. Method of birth
4. Size of the neonate

34. A client who gave birth by cesarean 3 days ago is bottle-feeding her neonate. While collecting data, the nurse notes that vital signs are stable, the fundus is four fingerbreadths below the umbilicus, small amount of lochia rubra, and the client reports discomfort in her breasts, which are hard and warm to touch. Which action would be most appropriate?
1. Encouraging the client to wear a supportive bra.
2. Having the client stand in a warm shower.
3. Informing the health care provider that the client is showing early signs of breast infection.
4. Recommending use of a breast pump to facilitate removal of stagnant breast milk.

30. 3. Lochia rubra, which is made up of blood, mucus, and tissue debris, lasts 3 to 4 days. Lochia serosa, which consists of blood, mucus, and leukocytes, lasts from day 3 to day 10 postpartum. Lochia alba, which consists largely of mucus, lasts from day 10 to day 14 postpartum. Lochia alba may last up to 6 weeks postpartum. Postpartum bleeding is not the menstrual cycle.
CN: Physiological integrity; CNS: Physiological adaptation; CL: Apply; DIFFICULTY: Easy

31. 2. Denial of the perinatal loss reflects dysfunctional grieving in the client. Lack of appetite, blaming oneself, and frequent crying spells are part of a normal grieving process.
CN: Psychosocial integrity; CNS: None; CL: Analyze; DIFFICULTY: Moderate

32. 1. Breast engorgement and dehydration are noninfectious causes of postpartum fevers. Mastitis and endometritis are postpartum infections. Involution of the uterus doesn't cause temperature elevations.
CN: Health promotion and maintenance; CNS: None; CL: Apply; DIFFICULTY: Moderate

33. 1. A prolonged length of labor, such as 17 hours, places the mother at increased risk for developing an infection. The average size of the neonate, vaginal birth, and Rh status of the client don't place the mother at increased risk.
CN: Safe and Effective Care Environment; CNS: Safety and Infection Control; CL: Analyze; DIFFICULTY: Moderate

34. 1. These assessment findings are normal for the third postpartum day. Hard, warm breasts indicate engorgement, which occurs at about three days after birth. The client should be encouraged to wear a supportive bra to help minimize engorgement and decrease nipple stimulation. The client's vital signs are stable and don't indicate signs of infection. Ice packs can reduce vasocongestion and relieve discomfort. Warm water and a breast pump will stimulate milk production.
CN: Physiological integrity; CNS: Basic care and comfort; CL: Apply; DIFFICULTY: Moderate

35. The nurse is assisting in developing a plan of care for a client who had an episiotomy. Which interventions would most likely be included? Select all that apply:

1. Apply an ice pack intermittently to the perineal area for 3 days.
2. Avoid the use of topical pain gels.
3. Administer sitz baths three to four times per day.
4. Encourage the client to do Kegel exercises.
5. Limit the number of times the perineal pad is changed.

36. A client needs to void 3 hours after a vaginal birth. The nurse implements safety precautions when getting the client out of bed based on an understanding that the client is at risk for which condition?

1. Chest pain
2. Breast engorgement
3. Orthostatic hypotension
4. Separation of episiotomy incision

37. A client who had an emergency cesarean birth for fetal distress 3 days ago is preparing for discharge. When reviewing the home care instructions with the nurse, the client reveals she is saddened about her cesarean and feels let down that she wasn't able to have a vaginal birth. When questioned further, the client states she feels "weepy about everything" and can't stop crying. Which action would be the priority?

1. Contact the health care provider to report the client's deteriorating mental status.
2. Discuss the client's potential depression with her family members.
3. Ask the client to elaborate on her feelings.
4. Document the conversation.

38. A postpartum client who has developed mastitis is being discharged. What recommendation would be most appropriate when the client voices concern about breast-feeding her neonate with this condition?

1. Stop breast-feeding until completing the antibiotic.
2. Supplement feeding with formula until the infection resolves.
3. Don't use analgesics because they aren't compatible with breast-feeding.
4. Continue to breast-feed; mastitis won't infect the neonate.

35. 3, 4. Sitz baths help decrease inflammation and tension in the perineal area. Kegel exercises improve circulation to the area and help reduce edema. Ice packs should be applied to the perineum for the first 24 hours only; after that time, heat should be used. Topical pain gels should be applied to the suture area to reduce discomfort, as ordered. The perineal pad should be changed frequently to prevent irritation caused by the discharge.

CN: Physiological integrity; CNS: Basic care and comfort; CL: Apply; DIFFICULTY: Challenge

36. 3. The rapid decrease in intra-abdominal pressure occurring after birth causes splanchnic engorgement. The client is at risk for orthostatic hypotension when standing due to the blood pooling in this area. Breast engorgement is caused by vascular congestion in the breast through lactation. The client shouldn't experience separation of the episiotomy incision or chest pain when standing. None of these conditions are risks related to the need to assist the client out of bed.

CN: Safe and Effective Care Environment; CNS: Safety and Infection Control ; CL: Apply; DIFFICULTY: Easy

37. 3. The client's affect is consistent with postpartum blues, a transient source of sadness experienced during the first week after birth. The nurse should offer support to the client and encourage her to elaborate on her concerns and feelings. The client's emotional state is normal and contacting the health care provider isn't indicated at this point. Discussing the client's feelings with family members is a violation of confidentiality and isn't an appropriate action. Documenting the interaction is indicated but should take place after the encounter is completed and additional information is gathered.

CN: Psychosocial integrity; CNS: None; CL: Analyze; DIFFICULTY: Easy

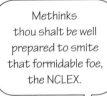

Methinks thou shalt be well prepared to smite that formidable foe, the NCLEX.

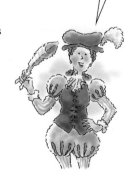

38. 4. The client with mastitis should be encouraged to continue breast-feeding while taking antibiotics for the infection. Mastitis won't infect the neonate. No supplemental feedings are necessary because breast-feeding doesn't need to be altered and actually encourages resolution of the infection. Analgesics are safe and should be administered as needed.

CN: Safe and Effective Care Environment; CNS: Safety and Infection Control ; CL: Apply; DIFFICULTY: Moderate

---

CN: Client needs category   CNS: Client needs subcategory   CL: Cognitive level

39. A postpartum client is brought to the emergency department by her husband after he noticed she was acting strangely. The client gave birth to a healthy newborn about 3 ½ weeks ago. The husband reports that the client has been having trouble sleeping, experiencing extreme fatigue and crying all the time. The healthcare team suspects that the client may be experiencing postpartum psychosis based on which additional finding? Select all that apply.

1. Euphoria
2. Preoccupation with guilt
3. Statements about being worthless
4. Thoughts of hurting herself
5. Hallucinations

39. 2, 3, 4, 5. Signs and symptoms associated with postpartum psychosis include: sleep disturbances, fatigue, depression, tearfulness, confusion, and preoccupation with feelings of guilt and worthlessness that may escalate to delirium, hallucinations, anger toward herself or her infant, bizarre behavior, mania, and thoughts of hurting herself or her infant. There may be a loss of touch with reality and a high risk for suicide or infanticide.
CN: Psychosocial Integrity; CNS: None; CL: Apply; DIFFICULTY: Difficult

40. The nurse is reviewing the medical record of a client who is 6 weeks postpartum and came for a follow up appointment with her health care provider. The client's uterus is enlarged and soft, and is experiencing vaginal bleeding. Based on the findings, which condition would the nurse most likely suspect?

1. Cervical laceration
2. Clotting deficiency
3. Perineal laceration
4. Uterine subinvolution

40. 4. Late postpartum bleeding is usually the result of subinvolution of the uterus. Retained products of conception or infection commonly cause subinvolution. Cervical or perineal lacerations can cause an immediate postpartum hemorrhage. A client with a clotting deficiency may have an immediate postpartum hemorrhage if the deficiency isn't corrected at the time of birth.
CN: Physiological integrity; CNS: Physiological adaptation; CL: Apply; DIFFICULTY: Easy

41. A client who gave birth vaginally 16 hours ago states she doesn't need to void at this time. The nurse reviews the documentation and finds that the client hasn't voided for 7 hours. Which response by the nurse is indicated?

1. "If you don't attempt to void, I'll need to catheterize you."
2. "It's common for you to have a full bladder even though you can't sense it."
3. "I'll need to contact your health care provider right away for instructions."
4. "I'll come back and check on you in a few hours to see if you can go."

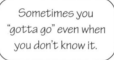

Sometimes you "gotta go" even when you don't know it.

41. 2. After a vaginal birth, the client should be encouraged to void every 4 to 6 hours. As a result of anesthesia and trauma, the client may be unable to sense the filling bladder. It's premature to catheterize the client without allowing her to attempt to void first. Additionally the statement is threatening to the client. There's no need to contact the health care provider at this time, as the client is demonstrating common adaptations in the early postpartum period. Allowing the client's bladder to fill for another 2 to 3 hours might cause overdistention.
CN: Physiological integrity; CNS: Physiological adaptation; CL: Analyze; DIFFICULTY: Moderate

42. A nurse is reinforcing discharge education with a postpartum client who isn't immune to rubella. Which statement by the client indicates the need for further education?

1. "I can continue to breast-feed my baby after taking the rubella vaccine."
2. "There may be some soreness or tenderness at the injection site for a few days."
3. "The immunization will be given at my 6-week postpartum examination."
4. "Although I've had a tubal ligation, the rubella vaccine will still be needed."

42. 3. The rubella vaccine is administered at the time of discharge, not at the 6-week postpartum examination. It's safe for both bottle- and breast-feeding mothers. The medication is given as an intramuscular injection; there may be some localized tenderness, which will subside. To promote community health and wellness, the vaccine is administered to women who've had a tubal ligation.
CN: Health promotion and maintenance; CNS: None; CL: Analyze; DIFFICULTY: Moderate

43. A nurse received a client from the surgical suite following a cesarean birth. The report given reveals the client has received magnesium sulfate for management of gestational hypertension just before the emergency surgery. The nurse should monitor the client for adverse effects from the magnesium sulfate by checking which parameter?
  1. Consistency of the fundus
  2. Heart rate
  3. Homans sign
  4. Gag reflex

44. A health care provider has prescribed magnesium sulfate for a client with premature labor. Data collection reveals the client's respiratory rate is 12 breaths/minute, and urine output is 30 mL/hour. The magnesium sulfate serum levels are 7 mg/dL. The client reports feeling warm and flushed. Which action by the nurse is most appropriate?
  1. The client is demonstrating early signs of toxicity and the dosage should be reduced.
  2. The client is demonstrating an allergic reaction and the medication should be discontinued immediately.
  3. The client's response is appropriate and within normal limits; therefore, no action is necessary.
  4. The client is demonstrating potential complications and the health care provider should be notified.

45. Which change **best** describes the insulin needs of a client with type 1 diabetes who has just given birth vaginally to a newborn without complications?
  1. Increased
  2. Decreased
  3. The same as before pregnancy
  4. The same as during pregnancy

46. A postpartum client with diabetes wants to breast feed but is concerned about the effects of breast-feeding on her health? Which response would be most appropriate?
  1. Mothers with diabetes who breast-feed have a hard time controlling their insulin needs.
  2. Mothers with diabetes shouldn't breast-feed because of potential complications.
  3. Mothers with diabetes shouldn't breast-feed; insulin requirements usually are doubled.
  4. Mothers with diabetes may breast-feed; insulin requirements may decrease from breast-feeding.

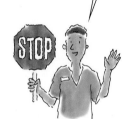

Birth significantly changes the insulin needs of clients with type 1 diabetes. Note any dosage changes and monitor blood glucose levels closely.

43. 1. Magnesium sulfate has properties that act as a smooth-muscle relaxant; therefore, the uterus may fail to adequately contract after administration. The nurse should monitor the consistency of the fundus. Failure of the uterus to contract may result in excessive blood loss. The heart rate, Homans sign, and gag reflex aren't affected by the administration of magnesium sulfate.
CN: Physiological integrity; CNS: Pharmacological therapies; CL: Apply; DIFFICULTY: Challenge

44. 3. Magnesium sulfate is associated with feelings of warmth and flushing; these symptoms do not indicate toxicity or allergic reaction. Respirations of 12 breaths/minute are considered normal. Urine output should be at least 30 mL/hour. Serum levels of magnesium sulfate should be between 4 and 8 mg/dL (2 to 4 mmol/L) to promote a therapeutic response.
CN: Physiological integrity; CNS: Pharmacological therapies; CL: Analyze; DIFFICULTY: Difficult

45. 2. The placenta produces the hormone human placental lactogen, an insulin antagonist. After birth, the placenta, the major source of insulin resistance, is gone. Insulin needs decrease, and women with type 1 diabetes may need only one-half to two-thirds of the prenatal insulin dose during the first few postpartum days. Blood glucose levels should be monitored and insulin dosages adjusted as needed. The client should be encouraged to maintain appropriate dietary schedules, even if her infant is feeding on demand.
CN: Physiological integrity; CNS: Physiological adaptation; CL: Apply; DIFFICULTY: Moderate

46. 4. Breast-feeding has an antidiabetic effect. Insulin needs are decreased because carbohydrates are used in milk production. Breast-feeding clients are at a higher risk for hypoglycemia in the first postpartum days after birth because glucose levels are lower. Diabetic clients should be encouraged to breast-feed.
CN: Physiological integrity; CNS: Pharmacological therapies; CL: Apply; DIFFICULTY: Easy

47. A multiparous client has given birth vaginally to a healthy neonate. It is now her first postpartum day. Which factor would the nurse identify as putting this client at risk for developing hemorrhage?
1. Hemoglobin level of 12 g/dL
2. Uterine atony
3. Thrombophlebitis
4. Moderate amount of lochia rubra

47. 2. Multiparous women typically experience a loss of uterine tone due to frequent distentions of the uterus from previous pregnancies. As a result, this client is at higher risk for hemorrhage. Thrombophlebitis doesn't increase the risk of hemorrhage during the postpartum period. The client's hemoglobin level and lochia flow are within acceptable limits.
CN: Physiological Integrity; CNS: Reduction of Risk Potential; CL: Applys; DIFFICULTY: Easy

48. The nurse is assisting with the development of a care plan for a postpartum client who had an uncomplicated vaginal birth of an 8-lb, 2-oz (3,693-g) neonate over an intact perineum 24 hours ago. While planning care for this client, the registered nurse collaborates with the licensed practical nurse to achieve which priority outcome in the next 8 hours?
1. Encouraging high-fiber foods to achieve a soft bowel movement.
2. Encouraging the client to demonstrate an ability to breast-feed the neonate.
3. Administering a rubella vaccination if the client isn't immune.
4. Completing an initial sitz bath.

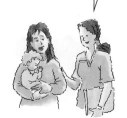

> Emotional support and encouragement can be invaluable to a new mother.

48. 2. With an uncomplicated vaginal birth, the average client will be hospitalized for 48 hours or less. By 24 hours postpartum, it's important for the client to start demonstrating the ability to care for her neonate. The first bowel movement occurs on average 2 to 3 days postpartum. The rubella vaccine is given, when indicated, on the day of discharge. This client delivered over an intact perineum, so a sitz bath isn't a priority.
CN: Safe, effective care environment; CNS: Coordinated care; CL: Analyze; DIFFICULTY: Moderate

49. On the first postpartum night, a client requests that her neonate be sent back to the nursery so she can get some sleep. The nurse identifies that the client is most likely in which phase?
1. Depression phase
2. Letting-go phase
3. Taking-hold phase
4. Taking-in phase

49. 4. The taking-in phase occurs in the first 24 hours after birth. The client is concerned with her own needs and requires support from staff and relatives. The taking-hold phase occurs when the client is ready to take responsibility for her care as well as her neonate's care. The letting-go phase begins several weeks later, when the client incorporates the new infant into the family unit. The depression phase isn't a postpartum phase.
CN: Health promotion and maintenance; CNS: None; CL: Apply; DIFFICULTY: Moderate

50. The nurse observes several interactions between a mother and her new son. Which behaviors by the mother would the nurse identify as evidence of mother-infant attachment? Select all that apply.
1. Talks and coos to her son
2. Cuddles her son close to her
3. Doesn't make eye contact with her son
4. Requests the nurse to take the baby to the nursery for feedings
5. Encourages the father to hold the baby
6. Takes a nap when the baby is sleeping

50. 1, 2. Talking to, cooing to, and cuddling with her son are positive signs that the mother is adapting to her new role. Avoiding eye contact is a sign that the mother isn't bonding with her baby. Eye contact, touching, and speaking are important to establish attachment with an infant. Feeding a neonate is an important role of a new mother and facilitates attachment. Encouraging the dad to hold the baby facilitates attachment between the neonate and the father. Resting while the infant is sleeping conserves needed energy and allows the mother to be alert and awake when her infant is awake, however, it isn't evidence of bonding.
CN: Psychosocial integrity; CNS: None; CL: Apply; DIFFICULTY: Difficult

51. The nurse is performing a postpartum check on a client. Which nursing measure is appropriate?

1. Place the client supine position with arms overhead to examine her breasts and fundus.
2. Instruct the client to empty her bladder before the examination.
3. Wear sterile gloves when assessing the pad and perineum.
4. Perform the examination as quickly as possible.

52. The nurse finds that a client who gave birth 3 hours ago has completely saturated a perineal pad within 15 minutes. Which action should the nurse take? Select all that apply:

1. Begin an IV infusion of lactated Ringer solution.
2. Assess the client's vital signs.
3. Palpate the client's fundus.
4. Place the client in high Fowler position.
5. Administer a pain medication.

53. A nurse is assisting a postpartum woman with breast feeding her newborn. Which action would the nurse recommend to help the new mother breast feed? Select all that apply.

1. Suggesting the mother cuddle and caress the infant while feeding him.
2. Reminding her that breast feeding is a natural skill.
3. Encouraging her to breast feed when the infant is alert and hungry.
4. Showing her the different positions for holding the infant for feeding.
5. Reminding her to limit feedings to about 5 to 10 minutes each time.

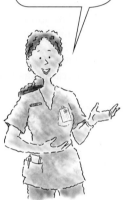

Watch out for boggy uteruses. They are a common cause of postpartum hemorrhage.

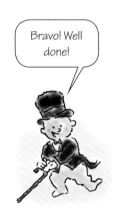

Bravo! Well done!

51. 2. An empty bladder facilitates the examination of the fundus. The client should be in a supine position with her arms at her sides and her knees bent. Clean gloves should be used when assessing the perineum; sterile gloves aren't necessary. The postpartum examination shouldn't be done quickly. The nurse can take this time to review information with the client about the changes in her body after birth.
CN: Health promotion and maintenance; CNS: None; CL: Apply; DIFFICULTY: Easy

52. 2, 3. Assessing vital signs provides information about the client's circulatory status and identifies significant changes to report to the health care provider. By palpating the client's fundus, the nurse also gains valuable data. A boggy uterus may lead to excessive bleeding. Starting an IV infusion requires a health care provider's order. Placing the client in high Fowler's position may lower blood pressure and harm the client. Administration of a pain medication doesn't address the client's perineal pad saturated in 15 minutes.
CN: Physiological integrity; CNS: Reduction of risk potential; CL: Apply; DIFFICULTY: Moderate

53. 1, 3, 4. Breast feeding is a learned skill and some newborns are able to adapt immediately while others take more time. The nurse should suggest that the mother cuddle and caress the infant during feedings, making sure that the infant is alert and awake and showing signs of hunger. In addition, the nurse should show the mother different positions that can be used for feeding and encourage her to allow sufficient time to enjoy each other in an unhurried atmosphere.
CN: Health Promotion and Maintenance; CNS: None; CL: Apply; DIFFICULTY: Moderate

Chapter 24

Neonatal Care

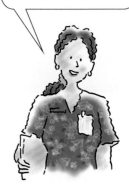

Neonates depend on you for everything. Let's show 'em you've got what it takes for neonatal care!

Neonatal care refresher

Fetal alcohol spectrum disorder

Spectrum of birth defects and behavioral and neurocognitive disabilities resulting from maternal use of alcohol during pregnancy

Key signs and symptoms
- Difficulty establishing respirations
- Lethargy
- Opisthotonos
- Seizures
- Slow pre- and postnatal growth
- Distinctive facial features
- Microcephaly

Key test results
- Chest x-ray may reveal congenital heart defect

Key treatments
- Swaddling
- IV phenobarbital

Key interventions
- Provide a stimulus-free environment for the neonate; darken the room, if necessary
- Provide gavage feedings, if necessary
- Early diagnosis improves outcome of birth defects and cognitive development

Human immunodeficiency virus (HIV)

Infection with the HIV virus can be transmitted to the fetus in utero or during the birth process or through breast milk; incidence can be reduced if the HIV-positive pregnant woman receives treatment with antiretroviral therapy

Key signs and symptoms
- Produces no symptoms at birth

Key test results
- Test interpretation is problematic because most neonates with an HIV-positive mother test positive at birth
- Uninfected neonates lose this maternal antibody between 8 and 15 months, and infected neonates remain seropositive
- Testing should be repeated at age 15 months

Key treatments
- Antimicrobial therapy to treat opportunistic infections
- Zidovudine administration based on neonate's lymphocyte count

Key interventions
- Monitor cardiovascular and respiratory status
- Keep umbilical stump meticulously clean
- Maintain standard precautions

Hypothermia

Neonates are at risk for hypothermia due to their immature temperature regulating system

Key signs and symptoms
- Kicking and crying (a mechanism used to increase the metabolic rate to produce body heat)
- Core body temperature lower than 97.7° F (36.5° C)

Key test results
- Arterial blood gas (ABG) analysis shows hypoxemia
- Blood glucose level reveals hypoglycemia

Key treatments
- Radiant warmer

Key interventions
- Dry the neonate immediately after delivery
- Allow mother to hold the neonate skin to skin
- Monitor vital signs every 15 to 30 minutes
- Provide a knitted cap for the neonate
- Place the neonate in a radiant warmer

Neonatal drug dependency

Dependency caused by exposure to an addictive drug while in the womb

Key signs and symptoms
- Neonatal abstinence syndrome (including seizures, hyperactive reflexes, poor feeding, respiratory disturbances)
- High-pitched cry

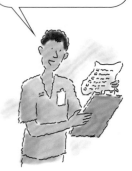

Why are neonates especially at risk for hypothermia?

416

- Irritability
- Jitteriness
- Poor sleeping pattern
- Tremors

Key test results
- Urine toxicology screen determines drug exposure
- Meconium screening reveals drug exposure

Key treatments
- Gavage feedings, if necessary

Opioid withdrawal
- Methadone, morphine

Nonopioid withdrawal
- Phenobarbital, chlorpromazine, diazepam

Key interventions
- Monitor cardiovascular status
- Use tight swaddling for comfort
- Place the neonate in a dark, quiet environment
- Encourage use of a pacifier
- Be prepared to administer gavage feedings (in cases of methadone withdrawal)
- Maintain fluid and electrolyte balance

Neonatal infections
Neonates are at risk for infections due to their need to rely on maternal antibodies for protection; with birth, the neonate is no longer protected by the intrauterine environment and must develop own defenses against the environment

Key signs and symptoms
- Feeding pattern changes, such as poor sucking or decreased intake
- Sternal retractions
- Subtle, nonspecific behavioral changes, such as lethargy or hypotonia
- Temperature instability

Key test results
- Blood and urine cultures positive for the causative organism, most commonly gram-positive beta-hemolytic streptococci and the gram-negative Escherichia coli, Aerobacter, Proteus, and Klebsiella
- Complete blood count shows an increased white blood cell count

Key treatments
- IV therapy to provide adequate hydration
- Antibiotic therapy: broad-spectrum until causative organism is identified and then specific antibiotic

Key interventions
- Monitor cardiovascular and respiratory status

- Administer broad-spectrum antibiotics before culture results are received
- Administer specific antibiotic therapy after culture results are received

Neonatal jaundice
Yellowing of the skin caused by the accumulation of bilirubin in the blood and deposited in the skin and mucous membranes; in the newborn, the rate of bilirubin production must balance the rate of excretion; if production exceeds excretion, hyperbilirubinemia and jaundice result

Key signs and symptoms
- Jaundice
- Lethargy

Key test results
- Bilirubin levels exceed 12 mg/dL in premature or term neonates

Key treatments
- Increased fluid intake
- Phototherapy

Key interventions
- Monitor neurologic status
- Monitor serum bilirubin levels
- Initiate and maintain phototherapy
  - provide eye protection while under phototherapy lights
  - remove eye shields promptly when removed from the phototherapy lights

Respiratory distress syndrome
Respiratory disorder commonly seen in premature neonates that results from lung immaturity and a lack of surfactant in the alveoli

Key signs and symptoms
- Cyanosis and pallor
- Expiratory grunting
- Fine crackles and diminished breath sounds
- Seesaw respirations
- Sternal, substernal, and intracostal retractions
- Tachypnea (more than 60 breaths/minute)

Key test results
- ABG analysis reveals respiratory acidosis
- Chest x-ray reveals bilateral diffuse reticulogranular density

Key treatments
- Oxygenation and continuous positive airway pressure (CPAP)
- Endotracheal (ET) intubation and mechanical ventilation

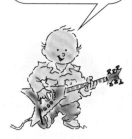

A healthy baby is the goal; any other accomplishment is a bonus!

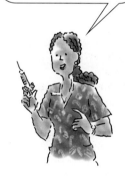

What type of antibiotic therapy is called for initially to treat a neonatal infection?

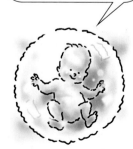

With all that's waiting for me out there—cold, infections, diseases—I think I'll just stay put.

- Nutrition supplements (total parenteral nutrition [TPN] or enteral feedings if possible)
- Surfactant replacement by way of ET tube
- Temperature regulation with a radiant warmer

Key interventions
- Monitor cardiovascular, respiratory, and neurologic status
- Monitor vital signs
- Maintain ventilatory support status
- Administer medications, including ET surfactant as prescribed
- Provide adequate nutrition through enteral feedings, if possible, or TPN

Tracheoesophageal fistula
Abnormal opening between the trachea and the esophagus; during embryonic development, the esophagus and trachea do not separate as they normally should

Key signs and symptoms
- Difficulty feeding, such as choking or aspiration; cyanosis during feeding
- Signs of respiratory distress

Key test results
- Abdominal x-ray shows the fistula and a gas-free abdomen

Key treatments
- Emergency surgical intervention to prevent pneumonia, dehydration, and fluid and electrolyte imbalances
- Maintenance of patent airway

Key interventions
- Monitor cardiovascular, respiratory, and GI status
- Place neonate in high Fowler position
- Keep a laryngoscope and ET tube at bedside
- Provide neonate with a pacifier
- Provide gastrostomy tube feedings postoperatively

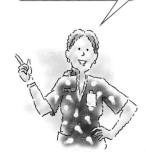

A neonate you are caring for chokes, aspirates, and turns blue during feeding. What condition should you suspect?

thePoint® You can download tables of drug information to help you prepare for the NCLEX®! View Generic Drug Names, Drug Classifications, Drug Actions, and Nursing Implications for the drugs discussed in this refresher at **http://thePoint.lww.com.**

Neonatal care questions, answers, and rationales

1. The nurse is working as part of multidisciplinary team in developing the plan of care for a premature neonate. Breast milk is being encouraged as part of the plan. The nurse understands that the use of breast milk for this neonate would help prevent which condition?
  1. Down syndrome
  2. Hyaline membrane disease
- 3. Necrotizing enterocolitis
  4. Turner syndrome

2. The parents of a neonate receiving surfactant therapy ask the nurse about why their baby is receiving this therapy. What is the **best** response by the nurse?
  1. "Surfactant helps regulate the baby's breathing pattern."
  2. "Surfactant helps clear mucus and fluid from the respiratory system to make breathing easier."
  3. "Surfactant helps mature the upper airways to make breathing easier."
- 4. "Surfactant helps in keeping the lungs expanded after the baby starts breathing on its own."

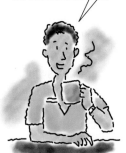

No worries. This chapter is child's play.

1. **3.** Components specific to breast milk have been shown to lower the incidence of necrotizing enterocolitis in premature neonates. Hyaline membrane disease isn't directly influenced by breast milk or breast-feeding. Down syndrome and Turner syndrome are genetic defects that aren't influenced by breast milk.
CN: Safe, effective care environment; CNS: Coordinated care;
CL: Apply; DIFFICULTY: Easy

2. **4.** Surfactant works by reducing surface tension in the lung, which allows the lung to remain slightly expanded, decreasing the amount of work required for inspiration. Surfactant hasn't been shown to influence upper airway maturation, clear the respiratory tract, or regulate the neonate's breathing pattern.
CN: Physiological integrity; CNS: Pharmacological therapies;
CL: Apply; DIFFICULTY: Moderate

3.   The nurse observes that a 2-hour-old neonate has acrocyanosis. Which nursing action is a **priority**?
1. Activate the code blue or emergency system.
2. Do nothing because acrocyanosis is normal in a neonate.
3. Immediately take the neonate's temperature according to facility policy.
4. Notify the health care provider of the need for genetic counseling.

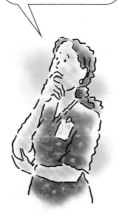

A bluish discoloration of the hands and feet— what should I do?

3.   **2.** Acrocyanosis, or bluish discoloration of the hands and feet in the neonate (also called peripheral cyanosis), is a normal finding and shouldn't last more than 24 hours after birth. Activating the emergency system, taking the neonate's temperature, or notifying the health care provider is inappropriate because the finding is a normal finding.
CN: Physiological integrity; CNS: Physiological adaptation;
CL: Apply; DIFFICULTY: Easy

4.   The nurse is teaching a group of parents about infant cardiopulmonary resuscitation prior to discharge of their newborns. Where should the nurse teach the parents to place their fingers to correctly perform chest compressions?

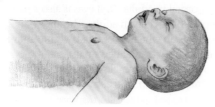

4.   The correct position for the fingers is one fingerbreadth below the nipple line.

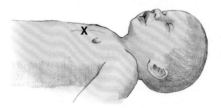

CN: Health promotion and maintenance; CNS: None;
CL: Comprehension; DIFFICULTY: Easy

5.   The nurse is caring for a neonate. Which action would be the **priority** for the nurse to prevent and control infection?
1. Check frequently for signs of infection.
2. Use sterile technique for all caregiving.
3. Practice meticulous hand washing.
4. Wear gloves at all times.

This next song goes out to Nurse Joy: "Keep on a rockin' me baby. Keep on a rockin' me baby ..."

5.   **3.** To prevent and control infection, the nurse should practice meticulous hand washing, scrubbing for 3 minutes before entering the nursery, washing frequently during caregiving activities, and scrubbing for 1 minute after providing care. Checking for signs of infection can detect, not prevent, infection. The nurse should use sterile technique for invasive procedures, not all caregiving. The nurse should wear gloves whenever contact with blood or body fluids is possible.
CN: Safe, effective care environment; CNS: Safety and infection control; CL: Apply; DIFFICULTY: Easy

6.   The nurse is gathering data from a neonate. The nurse determines that the neonate is adequately hydrated based on which finding?
1. Soft, smooth skin
2. A sunken fontanel
3. Excessive spitting up
4. No urine output in the first 24 hours of life

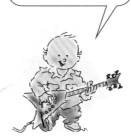

6.   **1.** Soft, smooth skin is a sign of adequate hydration. A sunken fontanel and no urine output in the first 24 hours of life are signs of poor hydration. In the case of no urine output, kidney dysfunction would also be a concern. Frequent spitting up is normal in neonates. Excessive spitting up, however, may result in poor hydration.
CN: Physiological integrity; CNS: Basic care and comfort;
CL: Analyze; DIFFICULTY: Easy

7.   A nurse is providing care to a neonate who has received prolonged mechanical ventilation following birth. For which condition should the nurse carefully monitor this neonate?
1. Bronchopulmonary dysplasia
2. Esophageal atresia
3. Hydrocephalus
4. Renal failure

7.   **1.** Bronchopulmonary dysplasia commonly results from the high pressures that must sometimes be used to maintain adequate oxygenation. Esophageal atresia, a structural defect in which the esophagus and trachea do not communicate with each other, doesn't relate to mechanical ventilation. Hydrocephalus and renal failure don't typically occur in neonates who received prolonged mechanical ventilation following birth.
CN: Physiological integrity; CNS: Reduction of risk potential;
CL: Analyze; DIFFICULTY: Easy

8. The nurse is providing care to a neonate whose mother has diabetes. The nurse would monitor the neonate for which complication?
1. Anemia
2. Hypoglycemia
3. Nitrogen loss
4. Thrombosis

8. 2. Neonates of mothers with diabetes are at risk for hypoglycemia due to increased insulin levels. During gestation, an increased amount of glucose is transferred to the fetus through the placenta. The neonate's liver can't initially adjust to the changing glucose levels after birth. This inability may result in an overabundance of insulin in the neonate, causing hypoglycemia. Neonates of mothers with diabetes aren't at increased risk for anemia, nitrogen loss, or thrombosis.
CN: Physiological integrity; CNS: Physiological adaptation; CL: Analyze; DIFFICULTY: Easy

9. When collecting data on a neonate, which finding would the nurse identify as expected?
1. Doll eyes
2. "Sunset" eyes
3. Positive Babinski sign
4. Pupils that don't react to light

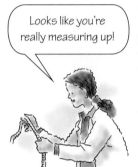

Looks like you're really measuring up!

9. 3. A positive Babinski sign is present in infants until approximately age 1 and is normal in neonates, though abnormal in adults. Doll eyes is also a neurologic response but occurs in adults. The appearance of "sunset" eyes, in which the sclera is visible above the iris, results from cranial nerve palsies and may indicate increased intracranial pressure. A neonate's pupils normally react to light as an adult's would.
CN: Health promotion and maintenance; CNS: None; CL: Analyze; DIFFICULTY: Easy

10. When bathing a neonate who is 1-hour old, which nursing action is **most** important?
1. Place on a table covered with blankets, and give a sponge bath.
2. Bathe in a tub of warm water.
3. Keep under a radiant warmer, and give a sponge bath.
4. Wash only hands and head because the condition isn't stable enough to have a complete bath.

10. 3. During the first several hours after birth, a neonate's thermal regulatory system is adapting to extrauterine life. When bathing a neonate under a radiant warmer, the external heat decreases the chances for cold stress by decreasing the number of internal mechanisms the neonate must use to stay warm. Bathing a neonate on a table, where she's exposed to air drafts and cooler air currents, can set her up for cold stress. Bathing the neonate in a tub and then removing her increases her heat loss and metabolism. Washing only the hands and head would chill the neonate and reduce thermoregulation because most heat is lost through the head.
CN: Health promotion and maintenance; CNS: None; CL: Analyze; DIFFICULTY: Easy

11. A mother asks the nurse why her neonate is getting an injection of vitamin K. Which response by the nurse would be **most** appropriate?
1. "It helps with coagulation."
2. "The vitamin assists the gut to mature."
3. "It gets the immune system functioning."
4. "The vitamin prevents excess fluid production in the brain."

Read the answers to question #12 carefully—it's all about the timing.

11. 1. Vitamin K, deficient in the neonate, is needed to activate clotting factors II, VII, IX, and X. In the event of trauma, the neonate would be at risk for excessive bleeding. Vitamin K doesn't assist the gut to mature, but the gut produces vitamin K after maturity is achieved. Vitamin K doesn't affect fluid production in the brain or the immune system function.
CN: Physiological integrity; CNS: Pharmacological therapies; CL: Apply; DIFFICULTY: Easy

12. A client with group AB blood whose husband has group O blood has just given birth. Which sign would indicate ABO blood incompatibility in the neonate?
1. Negative Coombs test
2. Bleeding from the nose or ear
3. Jaundice after the first 24 hours of life
4. Jaundice within the first 24 hours of life

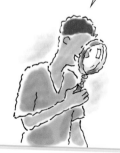

12. 4. The neonate with an ABO blood incompatibility with its mother will have jaundice within the first 24 hours of life. The neonate would have a positive Coombs test result. Jaundice after the first 24 hours of life is physiologic jaundice. Bleeding from the nose and ear should be investigated for possible causes, but it probably isn't related to ABO incompatibility.
CN: Physiological integrity; CNS: Reduction of risk potential; CL: Analyze; DIFFICULTY: Moderate

13. The nurse is caring for a neonate whose mother is infected with hepatitis B. The nurse would inform the mother that her child will receive which treatment?
1. Hepatitis B vaccine at birth and age 1 month
2. Hepatitis B immune globulin at birth; no hepatitis B vaccine
3. Hepatitis B immune globulin within 48 hours of birth and hepatitis B vaccine at age 1 month
4. Hepatitis B immune globulin within 12 hours of birth and hepatitis B vaccine at birth, age 1 month, and age 6 months

13. 4. Hepatitis B immune globulin should be given as soon as possible after birth but within 12 hours. Neonates should also receive hepatitis B vaccine at regularly scheduled intervals. This sequence of care is considered superior to the other treatment options.
CN: Health promotion and maintenance; CNS: None; CL: Analyze; DIFFICULTY: Moderate

14. The nurse is preparing to give a neonate the initial hepatitis B vaccine. Where should the nurse give this injection?

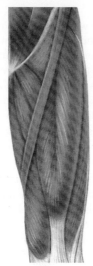

14. The vastus lateralis should be used for infant IM injections.

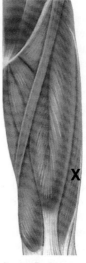

CN: Physiological integrity; CNS: Basic care and comfort; CL: Apply; DIFFICULTY: Moderate

15. The amniotic fluid of a neonate who is about to be born is stained with meconium. During the birth process, the nurse understands that which sequence of actions will most effectively decrease the risk of meconium aspiration?
1. Deliver the thorax, then suction the neonate's mouth.
2. Clamp the umbilical cord, then suction the mouth.
3. Deliver the head, then suction the mouth and then the nose.
4. Deliver the thorax, then suction the nose and then the mouth.

15. 3. To minimize the risk of meconium aspiration after birth, the neonate's mouth, then nose, should be suctioned after the head is born. This suctioning shouldn't be delayed until after the thorax is born because the neonate will take its first breath with meconium in its mouth.
CN: Physiological integrity; CNS: Reduction of risk potential; CL: Analyze; DIFFICULTY: Easy

16. The nurse is reviewing the medical records of several neonates. The nurse determines that one of the neonates is at risk for respiratory distress syndrome (RDS) based on which information?
1. Premature birth
2. Vaginal birth
3. First born of twins
4. Postdate pregnancy

16. 1. Prematurity is the single most important risk factor for developing RDS. The second born of twins and neonates born by cesarean birth are also at increased risk for RDS. Surfactant deficiency, which commonly results in RDS, isn't a problem for postdate neonates.
CN: Physiological integrity; CNS: Reduction of risk potential; CL: Analyze; DIFFICULTY: Easy

17. A nurse is assisting with the care of a neonate and is preparing to administer erythromycin ointment to the neonate's eyes shortly after birth. Which condition is the nurse preventing by administering this medication to the neonate?
1. Cataracts
2. Diabetic retinopathy
3. Ophthalmia neonatorum
4. Strabismus

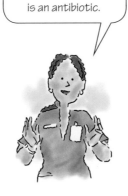

Hint: erythromycin is an antibiotic.

17. 3. Eye prophylaxis is administered to the neonate immediately, or soon after birth, to prevent ophthalmia neonatorum (conjunctivitis contracted during birth from passage through the birth canal). Erythromycin ointment is not given to prevent cataracts, diabetic retinopathy, or strabismus. Cataracts are opacities of the lens of the eye in children with congenital rubella, galactosemia, or cortisone therapy. Diabetic retinopathy occurs in clients with diabetes when the retina bleeds into the vitreous humor causing scarring, after which neovascularization occurs. Strabismus is neuromuscular incoordination of the eye alignment.

CN: Health promotion and maintenance; CNS: None; CL: Apply; DIFFICULTY: Easy

18. Two days after circumcision, while providing care to a male neonate, the nurse notes yellow-white exudate around the site of the circumcision. Which action by the nurse would be **most** appropriate?
1. Leave the area alone.
2. Report the findings to the health care provider.
3. Take the neonate's temperature.
4. Remove the exudate with a warm wash cloth.

18. 1. The yellow-white exudate is part of the granulating process and a normal finding for a healing penis after circumcision. There is no need to act. Therefore, notifying the health care provider isn't necessary. There's no indication of an infection that would necessitate taking the neonate's temperature. The exudate shouldn't be removed.

CN: Health promotion and maintenance; CNS: None; CL: Analyze; DIFFICULTY: Difficult

19. A client has just given birth at 42 weeks' gestation. When collecting data about the neonate, which finding would the nurse expect?
1. A sleepy, lethargic neonate
2. Lanugo covering the neonate's body
3. Desquamation of the neonate's epidermis
4. Vernix caseosa covering the neonate's body

19. 3. Postdate neonates lose the vernix caseosa, and the epidermis may become desquamated. A neonate at 42 weeks' gestation is usually very alert and missing lanugo.

CN: Health promotion and maintenance; CNS: None; CL: Analyze; DIFFICULTY: Moderate

20. After collecting data from a neonate, the nurse suspects that the neonate may have an infection based on which finding?
1. Flushed cheeks
2. Temperature of 98° F (36.7° C)
3. Temperature of 96.8° F (36.0° C)
4. Increased activity level

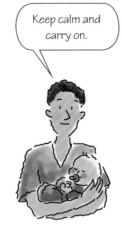

Keep calm and carry on.

20. 3. A decreased temperature in the neonate, such as 96.8° F (36.0° C) may be a sign of infection. The neonate's color commonly changes with an infectious process but generally becomes ashen or mottled, not flushed. The neonate with an infection will usually show a decrease in activity level or lethargy. Temperature of 98° F (36.7° C) would be considered normal.

CN: Physiological integrity; CNS: Reduction of risk potential; CL: Analyze; DIFFICULTY: Challenge

21. A nurse is providing care to a small-for-gestation neonate who is in the transitional period. For which complication should the nurse monitor the neonate?
1. Anemia probably due to chronic fetal hypoxia
2. Hyperthermia due to decreased glycogen stores
3. Hyperglycemia due to decreased glycogen stores
4. Polycythemia probably due to chronic fetal hypoxia

21. 4. The small-for-gestation neonate is at risk for developing polycythemia, not anemia, during the transitional period in an attempt to decrease hypoxia. This neonate is also at increased risk for developing hypoglycemia and hypothermia due to decreased glycogen stores.

CN: Physiological integrity; CNS: Reduction of risk potential; CL: Apply; DIFFICULTY: Difficult

22. Which finding would indicate the neonate was adapting normally to extrauterine life without difficulty? Select all that apply.
1. Nasal flaring
2. Light, audible grunting
3. Respiratory rate of 40 to 60 breaths/minute
4. Respiratory rate of 60 to 80 breaths/minute
5. Heart rate of 130 to 140 beats/minute

23. The nurse is caring for a neonate whose mother received magnesium sulfate during labor. The nurse would closely monitor the neonate for which potential problem? Select all that apply.
1. Hypoglycemia
2. Twitching
3. Respiratory depression
4. Tachycardia
5. Bradycardia

24. The nurse is caring for a neonate of a diabetic mother. For which condition should the nurse monitor the neonate?
1. Atelectasis
2. Microcephaly
3. Pneumothorax
4. Macrosomia

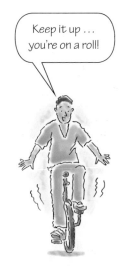

Keep it up ... you're on a roll!

25. A nurse is caring for a neonate whose mother was using drugs during the pregnancy. The nurse anticipates that the neonate may experience drug withdrawal. Which intervention would be the **priority**?
1. Placing the Isolette in a quiet area of the nursery.
2. Withholding all medication to help the liver metabolize drugs.
3. Dressing the neonate in loose clothing so he won't feel restricted.
4. Placing the Isolette near the nurses' station for frequent contact with health care workers.

26. A nurse is assisting with the administration of erythromycin ointment to a neonate. Place the actions in the sequence in which the nurse would complete them.

| **1.** Obtain a single-dose application tube. |
| **2.** Close the eye for several seconds. |
| **3.** Pull down on the lower eyelid. |
| **4.** Place a line of ointment into the conjunctival sac of the lower lid. |
| **5.** Wipe away any excess ointment after about 1 minute. |

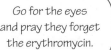

Go for the eyes and pray they forget the erythromycin.

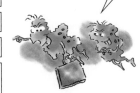

22. 3, 5. A respiratory rate of 40 to 60 breaths/minute and a heart rate between 120 to 160 beats per minute are normal for a neonate during the transitional period. Nasal flaring, respiratory rate of more than 60 breaths/minute, and audible grunting are signs of respiratory distress.
CN: Health promotion and maintenance; CNS: None; CL: Analyze;
DIFFICULTY: Moderate

23. 3, 5. Magnesium sulfate crosses the placenta, and adverse neonatal effects include respiratory depression, hypotonia, and bradycardia. The serum blood glucose level isn't affected by magnesium sulfate. The neonate would experience hypotonia, not twitching.
CN: Physiological integrity; CNS: Pharmacological therapies;
CL: Analyze; DIFFICULTY: Moderate

24. 4. Neonates of diabetic mothers are at increased risk for macrosomia (excessive fetal growth) due to the increased supply of maternal glucose combined with an increase in fetal insulin. Along with macrosomia, neonates of diabetic mothers are at risk for respiratory distress syndrome, hypoglycemia, hypocalcemia, hyperbilirubinemia, and congenital anomalies. They aren't at greater risk for atelectasis or pneumothorax. Microcephaly is usually the result of cytomegalovirus or rubella virus infection.
CN: Health promotion and maintenance; CNS: None; CL: Apply;
DIFFICULTY: Easy

25. 1. Neonates experiencing drug withdrawal commonly have sleep disturbance. The neonate should be moved to a quiet area of the nursery to minimize environmental stimuli. Medications such as phenobarbital, methadone, and diazepam should be given as needed. The neonate should be swaddled to prevent him from flailing and stimulating himself.
CN: Physiological integritiy; CNS: Reduction of risk potential;
CL: Analyze; DIFFICULTY: Moderate

26. Ordered Response:

| **1.** Obtain a single-dose application tube. |
| **3.** Pull down on the lower eyelid. |
| **4.** Place a line of ointment into the conjunctival sac of the lower lid. |
| **2.** Close the eye for several seconds. |
| **5.** Wipe away any excess ointment after about 1 minute. |

CN: Physiological integrity; CNS: Pharmacological therapies;
CL: Analyze; DIFFICULTY: Easy

27. A neonate is 3-hours old. When collecting data on the neonate, the nurse would suspect that the neonate is experiencing newborn distress based on which finding? Select all that apply.
1. Respiratory rate of 45 breaths/minute
2. Sternal retractions
3. Acrocyanosis
4. Grunting
5. Nasal flaring

28. A nurse is maintaining a neutral thermal environment for a neonate by keeping the nursery temperature warm and wrapping the neonate in blankets. The nurse's actions reflect prevention of heat loss by which mechanism?
1. Conduction
2. Convection
3. Evaporation
4. Radiation

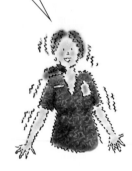

Ugh. I can't stand hypothermia. I wish someone would wrap me in warm blankets.

29. A nurse is caring for a 36-hour-old neonate and observes jaundice from physiologic hyperbilirubinemia. When describing this condition to the parents, which information would the nurse incorporate into the discussion?
1. The neonate usually also has a medical problem.
2. In full-term neonates, it usually appears after 24 hours.
3. It results in unusually elevated conjugated bilirubin levels.
4. It's usually progressive from the neonate's feet to his head.

30. A nurse who is part of the multidisciplinary team is assigned to care for four neonates and is reviewing each neonate's plan of care. The nurse would closely monitor which neonate considered to be at **highest** risk for developing hyperbilirubinemia?
1. Neonate of a black mother
2. Neonate of an Rh-positive mother
3. Neonate with ABO incompatibility
4. Neonate with Apgar scores 9 and 10 at 1 and 5 minutes

27. 2, 4, 5. Sternal retractions, or the use of accessory chest muscles, indicate distress. Grunting and nasal flaring indicate the infant is working very hard to breathe. A respiratory rate greater than 60 breaths/minute indicates distress. Acrocyanosis is normal cyanosis as indicated by discoloring of the hands and feet.
CN: Physiological integrity; CNS: Physiological adaptation;
CL: Apply; DIFFICULTY: Moderate

28. 2. Convection heat loss is the flow of heat from the body surface to cooler air. Keeping the nursery temperature warm and wrapping in blankets helps to prevent this type of heat loss. Conduction is the loss of heat from the body surface to cooler surfaces in direct contact. Covering surfaces with warmed blankets helps to prevent this type of heat loss. Evaporation is the loss of heat that occurs when a liquid is converted to a vapor. Drying neonates quickly and applying caps to the dried hair help to reduce this type of heat loss. Radiation is the loss of heat from the body surface to cooler, solid surfaces that are not in direct contact but are in relative proximity. Keeping neonates away from cooler surfaces helps to prevent this type of heat loss.
CN: Health promotion and maintenance; CNS: None; CL: Apply;
DIFFICULTY: Difficult

29. 2. Physiologic hyperbilirubinemia, or jaundice, in full-term neonates first appears after 24 hours. Neonates with this condition are otherwise healthy and have no medical problems. Hyperbilirubinemia is caused almost exclusively by unconjugated bilirubin. Jaundice usually appears in a cephalocaudal progression from head to feet.
CN: Physiological integrity; CNS: Reduction of risk potential;
CL: Apply; DIFFICULTY: Challenge

30. 3. The mother's blood type, which is different from the neonate's, impacts the neonate's bilirubin level due to the antigen-antibody reaction. Therefore, a neonate with ABO incompatibility would be at highest risk for developing hyperbilirubinemia. Black neonates tend to have lower mean levels of bilirubin. Chinese, Japanese, Korean, and Greek neonates tend to have higher incidences of hyperbilirubinemia. Neonates of Rh-negative, not Rh-positive, mothers tend to have hyperbilirubinemia. Low Apgar scores, not high ones such as 9 or 10, may indicate a risk for hyperbilirubinemia.
CN: Safe, effective care environment; CNS: Coordinated care;
CL: Analyze; DIFFICULTY: Moderate

31. A 3-day-old neonate needs phototherapy for hyperbilirubinemia. The nurse is reviewing the plan of care for this neonate. Which interventions would the nurse **most** likely find?
1. Administration of tube feedings
2. Feeding the neonate while under phototherapy lights
3. Use of eye patches to prevent retinal damage
4. Temperature monitoring every 6 hours during phototherapy

32. The nurse is reviewing information with a new parent about her neonate's stools. After describing meconium as the first stool, which description of the stool by the parent would demonstrate understanding?
1. Soft, pale yellow
2. Hard, pale brown
3. Sticky, greenish black
4. Loose, golden yellow

33. A neonate has been diagnosed with caput succedaneum. Which information would the nurse reinforce with the parent about this condition?
1. It usually resolves in 3 to 6 weeks.
2. It doesn't cross the cranial suture line.
3. It's a collection of blood between the skull and the periosteum.
4. It is tissue swelling over the presenting part of the fetal scalp.

34. A nurse is caring for a neonate and suspects the development of early-onset sepsis. Which finding would indicate to the nurse that this is occurring? Select all that apply.
1. Tachypnea
2. Hypoglycemia
3. Lethargy
4. Constipation
5. Exaggerated sucking reflex

35. A neonate develops significant respiratory distress about 14 hours after birth. After reviewing the neonate's medical record, the nurse finds that the neonate's mother experienced prolonged rupture of membranes. The nurse suspects that which organism **most** likely contributed to this problem?
1. *Candida albicans*
2. *Chlamydia trachomatis*
3. *Escherichia coli*
4. Group B beta-hemolytic streptococci

31. 3. The neonate's eyes must be covered with eye patches to prevent damage. The neonate can be removed from the lights and held for feeding. Tube feedings are not necessary. The neonate's temperature should be monitored at least every 2 to 4 hours because of the risk of hyperthermia with phototherapy.
CN: Physiological integrity; CNS: Reduction of Risk Potential; CL: Apply; DIFFICULTY: Easy

32. 3. Meconium collects in the GI tract during gestation and is initially sterile. Meconium is viscous and greenish black because of occult blood. The stools of formula-fed babies are typically soft and pale-yellow after feeding is well established. The stools of breast-fed neonates are loose and golden-yellow after the transition to extrauterine life. Neonate stools typically are not hard or pale brown.
CN: Health promotion and maintenance; CNS: None; CL: Analyze; DIFFICULTY: Easy

33. 4. Caput succedaneum is the swelling of tissue over the presenting part of the fetal scalp due to sustained pressure. This boggy, edematous swelling is present at birth, crosses the suture line, and most commonly occurs in the occipital area. A cephalohematoma is a collection of blood between the skull and periosteum that doesn't cross cranial suture lines and resolves in 3 to 6 weeks. Caput succedaneum resolves within 3 to 4 days.
CN: Health promotion and maintenance; CNS: None; CL: Apply; DIFFICULTY: Moderate

34. 1, 2, 3. Signs and symptoms of early-onset neonatal sepsis include respiratory distress such as tachypnea, hypoglycemia, lethargy, and diarrhea, not constipation. The sucking reflex is usually diminished.
CN: Physiological integrity; CNS: Physiological adaptation; CL: Apply; DIFFICULTY: Moderate

Some infections can be transmitted to the fetus in utero.

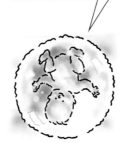

35. 4. Transmission of group B beta-hemolytic streptococci to the fetus results in respiratory distress that can rapidly lead to septic shock. This organism is a major cause of infection in the neonate. *E. coli* is the second most common cause. *Candida albicans* may be acquired from the birth canal. *C. trachomatis* infection causes neonatal conjunctivitis and pneumonia.
CN: Physiological integrity; CNS: Physiological adaptation; CL: Apply; DIFFICULTY: Easy

36. The nurse observes a neonate who was born at 28 weeks' gestation. Which finding would the nurse expect to see? Select all that apply.
1. The skin is pale, and no vessels show through it.
2. Creases appear on the interior two-thirds of the sole.
3. The pinna of the ear is soft, flat, and stays folded.
4. The neonate has 5 to 6 mm of breast tissue.
5. The neonate shows little extremity recoil.

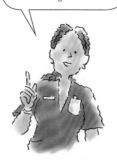

Twenty-eight weeks' gestation is significantly premature. What findings are consistent with this age?

37. A nurse is attempting to interact with a neonate experiencing drug withdrawal. The nurse determines that the neonate is willing to interact based on which behavior?
1. Gaze aversion
2. Hiccups
3. Quiet, alert state
4. Yawning

38. A nurse is caring for a neonate at risk for the development of ophthalmia neonatorum. Which medication will the nurse administer within 1 hour of birth to eliminate this risk?
1. Erythromycin ophthalmic ointment
2. Gentamicin
3. Nystatin
4. Vitamin A

39. When caring for a neonate of a mother with diabetes, the nurse suspects the neonate is experiencing hypoglycemia based on which finding? Select all that apply.
1. Hyperalert state
2. Jitteriness
3. Excessive crying
4. Serum glucose level of 60 mg/dL
5. Diaphoresis

40. A nurse is reviewing a neonate's discharge instructions about umbilical cord care with new parents. The nurse determines that the parents understand the information when they state that the cord will most likely fall off how many days after birth?
1. 1 to 2 days
2. 3 to 4 days
3. 7 to 10 days
4. 15 to 30 days

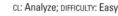

White, cheesy coating? I'm guessing mozzarella is out.

41. A neonate is born at 38 weeks' gestation. The parent asks what the thick, white, cheesy coating is on his skin. What does the nurse document related to this finding?
1. Lanugo
2. Milia
3. Nevus flammeus
4. Vernix

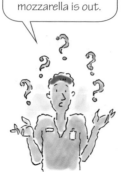

36. 3, 5. In a preterm neonate, the ear has a soft pinna that's flat and stays folded, and the infant exhibits minimal to no extremity recoil. Pale skin with no vessels showing through, and 5 to 6 mm of breast tissue, are characteristic of a neonate at 40 weeks' gestation. Creases on the anterior two-thirds of the sole are characteristic of a neonate at 36 weeks' gestation.
CN: Physiological integrity; CNS: Physiological adaptation; CL: Analyze; DIFFICULTY: Difficult

37. 3. When caring for neonates experiencing drug withdrawal, the nurse must be alert for distress signals from the infant. Stimuli should be introduced one at a time when the neonate is in a quiet, alert state. Gaze aversion, yawning, sneezing, hiccups, and body arching are distress signals that indicate the neonate can't handle stimuli at that time.
CN: Psychosocial integrity; CNS: None; CL: Analyze; DIFFICULTY: Easy

38. 1. Erythromycin ophthalmic ointment is given for prophylactic treatment of ophthalmia neonatorum, usually within 1 hour of birth. Gentamicin is an antibiotic used to treat an infection in the neonate. Nystatin is used for treatment of thrush. Vitamin K, not vitamin A, is given to help the neonate's blood to clot.
CN: Physiological integrity; CNS: Pharmacological therapies; CL: Analyze; DIFFICULTY: Easy

39. 2, 5. Hypoglycemia in a neonate is expressed as jitteriness, lethargy, diaphoresis, and a serum glucose level below 40 mg/dL. A hyperalert state in a neonate is more suggestive of neuralgic irritability and has no correlation to blood glucose levels. Excessive crying isn't found in hypoglycemia. A serum glucose level of 60 mg/dL is a normal level.
CN: Physiological integrity; CNS: Reduction of risk potential; CL: Analyze; DIFFICULTY: Moderate

40. 3. The umbilical stump deteriorates over the first 7 to 10 days postpartum due to dry gangrene and usually falls off by day 10.
CN: Health promotion and maintenance; CNS: None; CL: Analyze; DIFFICULTY: Easy

41. 4. Vernix is a white, cheesy material present on the neonate's skin at birth. Lanugo is the fine body hair on a neonate at birth. Milia are small, white papules on the skin. Nevus flammeus is a reddish discoloration of an area of skin.
CN: Health promotion and maintenance; CNS: None; CL: Understand; DIFFICULTY: Easy

25

42. A nurse is assisting with the care of neonate immediately after birth. The neonate is to receive vitamin K intramuscularly. The new parents asks the nurse, "Where are you going to give it to him?" Which site would the nurse include in the response to the parents?
1. Deltoid
2. Ventrogluteal
3. Abdomen
4. Vastus lateralis

42. 4. Vitamin K is given IM into the middle third of the vastus lateralis muscle in a neonate. It is not given in the deltoid or ventrogluteal site. Subcutaneous injections are given in the abdomen.
CN: Physiological integrity; CNS: Pharmacologic therapies; CL: Apply; DIFFICULTY: Easy

43. The nurse is collecting data on a healthy neonate. Which finding would the nurse most likely document? Select all that apply.
1. Simian crease
2. Oral moniliasis
3. Cystic hygroma
4. Bulging fontanel
5. Head circumference 14 inches (35.5 cm)

43. 2, 5. Also known as thrush, oral moniliasis is a common finding in neonates, usually acquired from the mother during birth. Another normal finding is the head circumference, which normally ranges from 13 to 15 inches (32 to 38 cm). A Simian crease is present in 40% of neonates with trisomy 21 (Down syndrome). Cystic hygroma is a neck mass that can destruct the airway. Bulging fontanels are a sign of intracranial pressure.
CN: Health promotion and maintenance; CNS: None; CL: Analyze; DIFFICULTY: Difficult

44. A nurse is working as part of the team providing nursing care for a neonate immediately after birth. Which intervention has the highest nursing **priority**?
1. Obtain a glucose reading.
2. Give the initial bath.
3. Give the vitamin K injection.
4. Cover the neonate's head with a cap.

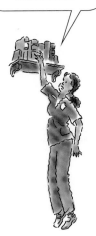

Erythematous dermatitis—hmm … I remember reading about that somewhere.

44. 3. The American Academy of Pediatrics recommends that vitamin K be given within 1 hour of birth. Glucose reading, appropriate for neonates with risk factors for hyperglycemia, are obtained at 30 minutes to 1 hour of age. Initial baths aren't given until the neonate's temperature is stable. The neonate's head shouldn't be covered until the hair is dried under a radiant warmer.
CN: Safe, effective care environment; CNS: Coordinated care; CL: Analyze; DIFFICULTY: Challenge

45. The nurse observes small, white papules surrounded by erythematous dermatitis on a neonate's skin. How will the nurse document this finding?
1. Cutis marmorata
2. Epstein pearls
3. Erythema toxicum
4. Mongolian spots

45. 3. Erythema toxicum has lesions that appear and disappear on the face, trunk, and limbs. They're small, white, or yellow papules or vesicles with erythematous dermatitis. Cutis marmorata is bluish mottling of the skin. Epstein pearls, found in the mouth, are similar to facial milia. Mongolian spots are large macules or patches that are gray or blue-green.
CN: Health promotion and maintenance; CNS: None; CL: Apply; DIFFICULTY: Difficult

46. A nurse is reviewing the medical record of a neonate. Which data from the record would the nurse identify as the **best** indicator of fetal lung maturity?
1. Meconium in the amniotic fluid
2. Glucocorticoid treatment just before birth
3. Lecithin to sphingomyelin ratio of more than 2:1
4. Absence of phosphatidylglycerol in amniotic fluid

46. 3. Lecithin and sphingomyelin are phospholipids that help compose surfactant in the lungs; lecithin peaks at 36 weeks, and sphingomyelin concentrations remain stable. Meconium is released due to fetal stress before birth, but it's chronic fetal stress that matures lungs. Glucocorticoids must be given at least 48 hours before birth. The presence of phosphatidylglycerol indicates lung maturity.
CN: Physiological integrity; CNS: Physiological adaptation; CL: Analyze; DIFFICULTY: Moderate

47. A nurse is preparing to give a neonate his first bath. Which action would be the **priority**?
1. Giving a tub bath
2. Using water and mild soap
3. Giving the bath right after birth
4. Using hexachlorophene soap

47. 2. Use only water and mild soap on a neonate to prevent drying out the skin. Tub baths are delayed until the umbilical cord falls off. The initial bath is given when the neonate's temperature is stable. Hexachlorophene soaps should be avoided; they're neurotoxic and may be absorbed through a neonate's skin.
CN: Health promotion and maintenance; CNS: None; CL: Analyze; DIFFICULTY: Easy

48. A nurse is caring for a neonate and is using measures to help maintain the neonate's temperature. Which intervention would be **most** effective in helping to prevent evaporative heat loss?
1. Administering warm oxygen
2. Controlling the drafts in the room
3. Immediately drying the neonate
4. Placing the neonate on a warm, dry towel

48. 3. Immediately drying the neonate decreases evaporative heat loss from his moist body from birth. Placing the neonate on a warm, dry towel decreases heat loss through conduction. Controlling the drafts in the room and administering warm oxygen help reduce heat loss through convection.
CN: Health promotion and maintenance; CNS: None; CL: Analyze; DIFFICULTY: Easy

49. A male neonate has just been circumcised. When reviewing the neonate's plan of care after this procedure, which intervention would the nurse most likely perform **first**?
1. Apply alcohol to the site.
2. Change the diaper every 10 minutes.
3. Keep the neonate in the prone position.
4. Apply petroleum gauze to the site for 24 hours.

49. 4. Petroleum gauze is applied to the site for the first 24 hours to prevent the skin edges from sticking to the diaper. Alcohol is contraindicated for circumcision care. Diapers are changed more frequently to inspect the site, but not every 10 minutes. Neonates are initially kept in the supine position.
CN: Health promotion and maintenance; CNS: None; CL: Apply; DIFFICULTY: Easy

50. A nurse is caring for several neonates in a busy nursery. When weighing a neonate, which action should the nurse take?
1. Leave the diaper on for comfort.
2. Place a sterile paper on the scale for infection control.
3. Keep a hand on the neonate's abdomen for safety.
4. Weigh the neonate at the same time each day for accuracy.

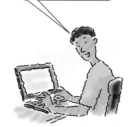

When it comes to measurement, there's a lot to be said for consistency.

50. 4. A neonate of any age should be weighed at the same time each day, using the same technique. A neonate should be weighed while undressed. Clean scale paper should be used when weighing the neonate; sterile scale paper is unnecessary. The nurse should keep a hand above, not on, the abdomen when weighing the neonate.
CN: Health promotion and maintenance; CNS: None; CL: Apply; DIFFICULTY: Moderate

51. The nurse is administering the initial bath to a neonate who's 4 hours old and weighs 7 lb, 2 oz (3,235 g). Vital signs before the bath were pulse, 126 beats/minute; respiratory rate, 42 breaths/minute; and rectal temperature, 98.4° F (36.9° C). Crying has occurred lustily throughout the bath. When drying the child, color becomes slightly dusky, the child cries weakly, and stops moving vigorously. Which action would the nurse do **first**?
1. Obtain a pulse oximetry reading and administer oxygen.
2. Immediately place the neonate under the warmer.
3. Use a bulb syringe to suction the neonate's nose and oropharynx.
4. Apply an oxygen mask over the neonate's nose and mouth and give two rescue breaths.

51. 2. Because this neonate is receiving a bath, he's at risk for becoming cold and metabolizing brown fat. Immediately placing him under the warmer helps restore his body temperature and stops the acidosis that occurs with the metabolism of brown fat. After placing the neonate under the warmer, data collection will continue. If the neonate continues to deteriorate, the other actions may be necessary and should be performed under the warmer. There's no initial evidence that the neonate's respirations are compromised; he continues to cry, although weakly. His dusky color is not respiratory in origin but is due to metabolic acidosis. Based on the findings, there's no need to suction or give rescue breaths.
CN: Physiological integrity; CNS: Reduction of risk potential; CL: Analyze; DIFFICULTY: Difficult

52. A nurse is gathering data about a neonate. The nurse suspects that the neonate is experiencing a metabolic response to cold stress based on which finding?
1. Dysrhythmia
2. Hypoglycemia
3. Elevated liver function tests
4. Increased blood pressure

53. A nurse is caring for a full-term neonate who is receiving phototherapy for hyperbilirubinemia. Which finding should the nurse report **immediately**?
1. Maculopapular rash
2. Absent Moro reflex
3. Greenish stool
4. Bronze-colored skin

54. A neonate is receiving phototherapy treatment. The nurse would monitor the neonate closely for which condition?
1. Hyperglycemia
2. Increased insensible water loss
3. Severe decrease in platelet count
4. Increased GI transit time

55. A nurse is working with the team to develop a neonate's plan of care. Which action would be the **highest priority** in regulating the neonate's temperature?
1. Supply extra heat sources to the neonate.
2. Keep the ambient room temperature less than 100° F (37.8° C).
3. Minimize the energy needed for the neonate to produce heat.
4. Block sources of radiant, convective, conductive, and evaporative losses.

56. A nurse is reviewing data on a neonate. Which finding would lead the nurse to suspect physiologic hyperbilirubinemia?
1. Clinical jaundice before age 36 hours
2. Clinical jaundice lasting beyond 14 days
3. Bilirubin levels of 12 mg/dL (205.2 µmol/L) by the third day of life
4. Serum bilirubin level increasing by more than 5 mg/dL (85.5 µmol/L)/day

57. A 2-day-old boy is scheduled for circumcision without anesthesia. When reviewing the neonate's plan of care, which measure would the nurse likely find as **most** important after the procedure?
1. Charting the time of the neonate's voiding
2. Keeping the neonate's penis exposed to air
3. Feeding the neonate only clear fluids for the first 12 hours
4. Placing a small ice cap on the neonate's penis

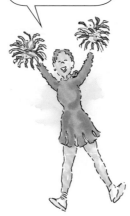

Hooray! You're doing awesome! Keep it up.

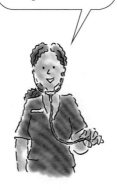

Check out the words "highest priority"—they'll point you to the right answer.

52. 2. Hypoglycemia occurs as the consumption of glucose increases with the increase in metabolic rate. Dysrhythmia and increases in blood pressure occur due to cardiorespiratory manifestations. Liver function declines in cold stress.
CN: Health promotion and maintenance; CNS: None; CL: Analyze; DIFFICULTY: Moderate

53. 2. An absent Moro reflex, lethargy, and seizures are symptoms of bilirubin encephalopathy, which can be life threatening. A maculopapular rash, greenish stools, and bronze-colored skin are minor adverse effects of phototherapy that should be monitored but don't require immediate intervention.
CN: Physiological integrity; CNS: Physiological adaptation; CL: Apply; DIFFICULTY: Moderate

54. 2. Increased insensible water loss is due to absorbed photon energy from the lights. Hyperglycemia isn't a characteristic effect of phototherapy treatment. Phototherapy may cause a mild decrease in platelet count. GI transit time may decrease with the use of phototherapy.
CN: Physiological integrity; CNS: Reduction of risk potential; CL: Apply; DIFFICULTY: Moderate

55. 4. Prevention of heat loss is always the first goal in thermoregulation to avoid hypothermia in the neonate by blocking the sources of loss. The second goal is to minimize the energy necessary for the neonate to produce heat. Adding extra heat sources is a means of correcting hypothermia. The ambient room temperature should be kept at approximately 100° F (37.8° C).
CN: Safe, effective care environment; CNS: Coordinated care; CL: Apply; DIFFICULTY: Moderate

56. 3. Increased bilirubin levels in the liver usually cause bilirubin levels of 12 mg/dL (205.2 µmol/L) by the third day of life. This rise results from the impaired conjugation and excretion of bilirubin and difficulty clearing bilirubin from plasma. The other findings suggest nonphysiologic jaundice.
CN: Physiological integrity; CNS: Reduction of risk potential; CL: Analyze; DIFFICULTY: Difficult

57. 1. After a circumcision, urine retention may occur. Therefore the nurse should monitor and document the time of the neonate's voiding. Although the penis should be inspected for swelling and bleeding, further care is unnecessary. A petroleum dressing is commonly applied to the penis; then the neonate is diapered. Because no anesthetic was given, feeding restrictions are unnecessary. Ice should not be used on a neonate.
CN: Safe, effective care environment; CNS: Safety and infection control; CL: Apply; DIFFICULTY: Moderate

58. A nurse is reviewing the plan of care for a neo-nate receiving phototherapy. Which action would be **most** important for the nurse to do?
1. Decrease the amount of formula given.
2. Dress the neonate warmly.
3. Massage the neonate's skin with lotion.
4. Reposition the neonate frequently.

58. 4. Phototherapy works by the chemical inter-action between a light source and the bilirubin in the neonate's skin. Therefore, the larger the skin area exposed to light, the more effective the treatment. Changing the neonate's position fre-quently ensures maximum exposure. Because the neonate loses water through the skin as a result of evaporation, the amount of formula or water may need to be increased. The neonate is typically undressed to ensure maximum skin exposure. The eyes are covered to protect them from light, and an abbreviated diaper is used to prevent soiling. The skin should be clean and patted dry. Use of lotions would interfere with phototherapy.

CN: Physiological integrity; CNS: Reduction of risk potential; CL: Apply; DIFFICULTY: Easy

59. A nurse suspects that a neonate may be expe-riencing breast-milk jaundice based on which finding?
1. History of poor breast-feeding
2. Decreased bilirubin level around day 3 of life
3. Clinical jaundice evident after 96 hours
4. Increased bilirubin levels between 24 to 72 hours due to interrupted breast-feeding

59. 3. Breast-milk jaundice is an elevation of indi-rect bilirubin in a breast-fed neonate that develops 7 days after birth and peaks during weeks 2 and 3 of life. History of being a poor breast-feeder and interruption of breast-feeding are indicative of breast-feeding jaundice, which occurs in the first week of life and is caused by insufficient pro-duction or intake of breast milk. Jaundice is an elevation, not a decrease, in bilirubin.

CN: Health promotion and maintenance; CNS: None; CL: Analyze; DIFFICULTY: Challenge

60. While caring for a neonate, which finding early on would lead the nurse to suspect that the neo-nate is developing respiratory distress syndrome (RDS)?
1. Bilateral crackles
2. Pale-gray skin color
3. Tachypnea more than 60 breaths/minute
4. Poor capillary filling time (3 to 4 seconds)

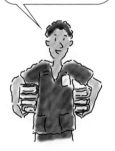

I get tachypnea every time I run up a flight of stairs.

60. 3. Tachypnea and expiratory grunting occur early in respiratory distress syndrome to help improve oxygenation. Poor capillary filling time, a later manifestation, occurs if signs and symptoms of RDS aren't treated. Crackles occur as the res-piratory distress progressively worsens. A pale-gray skin color obscures earlier cyanosis as respiratory distress symptoms persist and worsen.

CN: Physiological integrity; CNS: Physiological adaptation; CL: Apply; DIFFICULTY: Moderate

61. A neonate was born 2 days ago. The mother is being prepared for discharge and voices concern because her neonate's birth weight has declined by 2 oz. She states that she'll continue to breast-feed but will supplement after each breast-feeding with 4 oz of formula. Which response by the nurse would be **best**?
1. "That's a good idea. It's difficult to determine if your breast-fed baby is getting enough to eat."
2. "To determine if the baby is getting enough, you should weigh the baby before and after each feeding."
3. "It's normal for a neonate to lose 6% to 10% of its birth weight. While supplementing is acceptable, remember your baby's stomach can hold only about 3 oz."
4. "Supplementing with formula is never recom-mended for breast-feeding infants."

61. 3. Normal neonatal weight loss can range from 6% to 10% of birth weight. A decrease in weight of 2 oz would be considered within normal range. The normal neonate's stomach holds about 3 oz (90 mL). A breast-fed neonate's continued weight gain is an indication that he is eating a sufficient amount. While the premature or low-birth-weight neonate is weighed before and after eating in the clinical setting, this isn't an action that's ordi-narily taken for the normal neonate at home. Supplementation of breast-fed neonates, especially with large amounts (such as 4 oz), should be dis-couraged because it would reduce milk supply and volume. Additionally, it would distend the neo-nate's stomach and lead to possible regurgitation.

CN: Health promotion and maintenance; CNS: None; CL: Apply; DIFFICULTY: Easy

62. A neonate develops a mild respiratory disorder. After evaluation, the condition is determined to be self-limiting. The nurse understands that this disorder is most likely which condition?
1. Pneumonia
2. Meconium aspiration syndrome
3. Transient tachypnea
4. Persistent pulmonary hypertension

62. **3.** Transient tachypnea is a mild respiratory disorder that is self-limiting. It has an invariably favorable outcome after several hours to several days. The outcome of pneumonia depends on the causative agent involved and may lead to complications. Meconium aspiration, depending on severity, may have long-term adverse effects. In persistent pulmonary hypertension, mortality is more than 50%.
CN: Physiological integrity; CNS: Physiological adaptation; CL: Analyze; DIFFICULTY: Moderate

One of these immunoglobulins crosses the placenta and provides passive immunity. Which one is it?

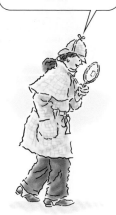

63. A nurse is providing care to a 1-day-old neonate, ensuring the safety of the neonate and using appropriate infection control measures. The new mother asks the nurse, "I thought that my baby had all the protection he needed from me." When responding to the mother, the nurse would integrate information about which immunoglobulin (Ig) that provides the neonate with passive immunity against bacterial and viral pathogens?
1. IgA
2. IgE
3. IgG
4. IgM

63. **3.** IgG is a major Ig of serum and interstitial fluid that crosses the placenta and provides passive immunity to the neonate. IgE plays a major role in allergic reactions. IgM and IgA don't cross the placenta.
CN: Health promotion and maintenance; CNS: None; CL: Apply; DIFFICULTY: Moderate

64. A 10-hour-old neonate appears exceptionally irritable, crying easily and startles when touched. A drug screen test indicates that the neonate is positive for cocaine. When assisting with developing the plan of care for this neonate, which action would be **most** helpful in soothing the neonate?
1. Leaving the light on beside the bassinet at night
2. Wrapping the neonate snugly in a blanket
3. Providing multisensory stimulation while the neonate is awake
4. Giving the neonate a warm bath

It's a wrap! Swaddling can help soothe both healthy and struggling neonates.

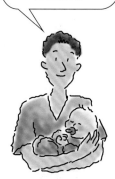

64. **2.** The practice of tightly wrapping, or swaddling, a cocaine-addicted neonate provides a safe, secure environment and maintains body warmth, both of which are soothing. A cocaine-addicted neonate typically experiences withdrawal 8 to 10 hours after birth; signs and symptoms include constant crying, jitteriness, poor feeding, emesis, respiratory distress, and seizures. To minimize or prevent these signs and symptoms, sensory stimulation is kept to a minimum and the neonate is typically kept in a quiet, dimly lit environment. A bath would necessitate the removal of clothing and exposure to changes in temperature, both of which are too stimulating for the cocaine-addicted neonate.
CN: Physiological integrity; CNS: Basic care and comfort; CL: Apply; DIFFICULTY: Easy

65. A nurse is caring for a neonate diagnosed with fetal alcohol syndrome (FAS). When gathering data on this neonate, which craniofacial change would the nurse **most** likely find?
1. Macrocephaly
2. Microcephaly
3. Wide, palpebral fissures
4. Well-developed philtrum

65. **2.** Distinctive facial dysmorphology of children with FAS most commonly involves the eyes (microphthalmia). Microcephaly is generally seen with FAS, as are short palpebral fissures and a poorly developed philtrum.
CN: Physiological integrity; CNS: Physiological adaptation; CL: Analyze; DIFFICULTY: Moderate

66. A neonate was diagnosed as having cystic fibrosis. When reviewing a neonate's medical record, the nurse would **most** likely find which condition?
1. Duodenal obstruction
2. Jejunal atresia
3. Malrotation
4. Meconium ileus

66. **4.** Meconium ileus is a luminal obstruction of the distal small intestine by abnormal meconium, seen in neonates with cystic fibrosis. Duodenal obstruction, jejunal atresia, and malrotation aren't characteristic findings in neonates with cystic fibrosis.
CN: Physiological integrity; CNS: Physiological adaptation; CL: Understand; DIFFICULTY: Moderate

67. A neonate was born at 36-weeks' gestation weighing 4 pounds (1,800 g). The neonate also has microcephaly and microphthalmia. The nurse is reviewing the maternal history in preparation for care. Which risk factor would the nurse **most** likely expect to find?

1. Use of alcohol
2. Use of marijuana
3. Gestational diabetes
4. Positive group B streptococci

68. A nurse is caring for a 4-hour-old male neonate. The heel stick hematocrit test result is 55% (0.55). How does the nurse interpret this finding?

1. Indicating serious anemia
2. Being within normal limits
3. Suggesting the sample has been hemolyzed
4. Requiring repeat testing with a venous blood sample

69. A neonate of a diabetic mother was born full-term and weighing 10 lb, 1 oz (4.6 kg). While caring for this large-for-gestational age (LGA) neonate, the nurse checks the clavicles for which reason?

1. Neonates of diabetic mothers have brittle bones.
2. Clavicles are commonly absent in neonates of diabetic mothers.
3. One of the neonate's clavicles may have been broken during birth.
4. LGA neonates have glucose deposits on their clavicles.

70. A nurse is working with the parents of a neonate who will be discharged soon. The neonate has just been circumcised. Which information would the nurse emphasize with the parents? Select all that apply.

1. The infant must void before being discharged to home.
2. Apply petroleum jelly to the glans of the penis with each diaper change.
3. Tub baths for the infant are acceptable while the circumcision heals.
4. Report spots of blood on the front of the diaper.
5. The circumcision requires care for 2 to 4 days after discharge.

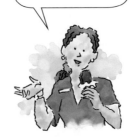

Hang in there—you're almost done. Then you can have a treat.

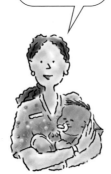

Remember to "select all that apply" in question 70.

67. 1. The most common sign of the effects of alcohol on fetal development is retarded growth in weight, length, and head circumference (microcephaly). Intrauterine growth retardation isn't characteristic of marijuana use. Gestational diabetes usually produces large-for-gestational-age neonates. Positive group B streptococci isn't a relevant risk factor.

CN: Physiological integrity; CNS: Reduction of risk potential; CL: Apply; DIFFICULTY: Easy

68. 2. Hematocrit of 52% (0.52) to 58% (0.58) is normal in a neonate because of increased blood supply during intrauterine life. Hematocrit of 55% (0.55) doesn't indicate serious anemia because the value is within the normal range for a neonate. If the heel-stick blood test shows hematocrit greater than 58% (0.58), a venous blood sample is obtained for testing because hemolysis of the heel-stick sample can show a false reading. Hematocrit greater than 58% (0.58) requires treatment after the health care provider has been notified.

CN: Health promotion and maintenance; CNS: None; CL: Analyze; DIFFICULTY: Easy

69. 3. Because of the neonate's large size, clavicular fractures are common during birth. The nurse should gather data on all LGA neonates for this occurrence. Neonates of diabetic mothers do not have brittle bones or glucose deposits, nor are the clavicles absent.

CN: Physiological integrity; CNS: Reduction of risk potential; CL: Apply; DIFFICULTY: Easy

70. 2, 5. Petroleum jelly should be applied to the glans with each diaper change. Typically, the circumcised penis heals within 2 to 4 days. Although voiding after circumcision is important, discharge need not be delayed. Parents are encouraged to monitor the neonate's voiding and to call if there is no voiding in 24 hours. Tub baths should be avoided until the circumcision heals to prevent infection. A small amount of blood is expected after circumcision; parents should report any large amount of bleeding.

CN: Health promotion and maintenance; CNS: None; CL: Apply; DIFFICULTY: Moderate

71. The nurse is eliciting reflexes in a neonate during a physical examination. Identify the area the nurse would touch to elicit a plantar grasp reflex.

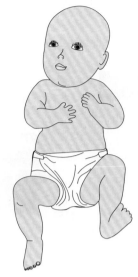

71. Touching the sole near the base of the digits elicits a plantar grasp reflex and causes flexion or grasping. This reflex disappears around age 9 months.

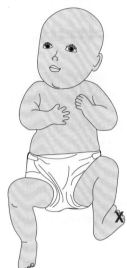

CN: Health promotion and maintenance; CNS: None; CL: Apply; DIFFICULTY: Easy

72. The nurse notes that a neonate is pink with acrocyanosis at 5 minutes after birth; his knees are flexed, his fists are clinched, he has a whimpering cry, and his heart rate is 128 beats/minute. He withdraws his foot to a slap on the sole. What 5-minute Apgar score should the nurse record for this neonate?

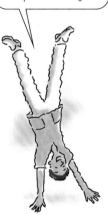

Yeah, baby! You finished another chapter. Great job.

Apgar Scoring Chart			
	Score		
Sign	0	1	2
Heart rate	Absent	Slow (<100)	>100
Breathing	Absent	Slow, irregular; weak cry	Good; strong cry
Muscle tone	Flaccid	Some flexion of extremities	Well flexed
Reflex response			
Response to catheter in nostril	No response	Grimace	Cough or sneeze
or			
Slap of sole of foot	No response	Grimace	Cry and withdrawal of foot
Color	Blue, pale	Body pink, extremities blue	Completely pink

72. 8. The Apgar score quantifies neonatal heart rate, respiratory effort, muscle tone, reflexes, and color. Each category is assessed 1 minute after birth and again 5 minutes later. Scores in each category range from 0 to 2. This neonate has a heart rate above 100 beats/minute, which equals 2; is pink in color with acrocyanosis, which equals 1; is well-flexed, which equals 2; has a weak cry, which equals 1; and has a good response to slapping the soles, which equals 2. Therefore, the nurse should record a total Apgar score of 8 for this neonate.

CN: Physiological integrity; CNS: Physiological adaptation; CL: Analyze; DIFFICULTY: Difficult

Growth & Development

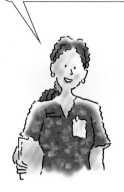

Growth & development refresher

Infant (birth to age 1)

Neonatal period

- All behavior is under reflex control; extremities are flexed
- Normal pulse rate ranges from 110 to 160 beats/minute
- Normal blood pressure is 65/40 to 78/52 mm Hg
- Normal respiratory rate is 32 to 60 breaths/ minute. Respirations are irregular and from the abdomen; the neonate is an obligate nose breather
- Temperature regulation is poor

1 to 4 months

- Posterior fontanel closes
- Begins to hold up his head
- Cries to express needs

5 to 6 months

- Rolls over from stomach to back
- Cries when parent leaves

7 to 9 months

- Fear of strangers appears to peak during the 8th month
- Sits alone with assistance
- Creeps on hands and knees with belly off floor
- Verbalizes all vowels and most consonants but speaks no intelligible words

10 to 12 months

- Holds onto furniture while walking (cruising) at age 10 months, walks with support at age 11 months, and stands alone and takes first steps at age 12 months
- Says "mama" and "dada" and responds to own name at age 10 months; can say about five words but understands many more

Toddler (ages 1 to 3)

- Normal pulse rate is 70 to 110 beats/minute
- Normal blood pressure is 90/55 to 105/70 mm Hg

- Normal respiratory rate is 20 to 30 breaths/ minute
- Separation anxiety arises
- Toilet-trained; day dryness is achieved between ages 18 months and 3 years and night dryness between ages 2 and 5

Preschool child (ages 3 to 5)

- Normal pulse rate ranges from 90 to 100 beats/minute
- Normal blood pressure ranges from 85/60 to 90/70 mm Hg
- Normal respiratory rate is 20 to 25 breaths/ minute
- May express fear of animal noises, new experiences, and the dark

School-age child (ages 5 to 12)

- Normal pulse rate ranges from 75 to 115 beats/minute
- Normal blood pressure ranges from 106/69 to 117/76 mm Hg
- Normal respiratory rate ranges from 20 to 25 breaths/minute
- Accidents are a major cause of death and disability during this period
- Plays with peers, develops a first true friendship, and develops a sense of belonging, cooperation, and compromise
- Learns to read and spell

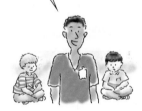

Adolescent (ages 12 to 18)

- Experiences puberty-related changes in body structure and psychosocial adjustment
- Vital signs approach adult values
- Peers influence behavior and values

Infants and nutrition

Primary nutrition guidelines for first year of life

- Begin with formula or breast milk; give no more than 30 oz (887 mL) of formula each day

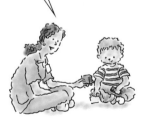

- Iron supplements may be necessary after 4 months
- No solid foods should be given for the first 4 to 6 months
- Provide rice cereal as the first solid food, followed by any other cereal except wheat
- Yellow and green vegetables may be given at 8 to 9 months
- Provide noncitrus fruits at 6 1/2 to 8 months, followed by citrus fruits late in the first year
- Give junior foods or soft table foods after 9 months

Growth & development questions, answers, and rationales

1. A 2-year-old child's parent informs the nurse of a concern that the child may have attention deficit hyperactivity disorder (ADHD) because "my child has so much energy, doesn't pay attention for long, and is always getting into things." Which response by the nurse would be **best**?
1. "This behavior is normal. The child is exploring and learning about the world."
2. "You should talk to your pediatrician. You have definite concerns."
3. "Keep intake of sugar and sugary treats to a minimum.
4. "I'd suggest going to a child psychologist for evaluation."

2. The parent of a 12-month-old infant expresses concern about the effect of frequent thumb sucking on the child's teeth. After the nurse reinforces education, which response by the parent indicates that teaching has been effective?
1. "Thumb sucking should be discouraged at 12 months."
2. "I'll give the baby a pacifier instead."
3. "Sucking is important to the baby."
4. "I'll wrap the thumb in a bandage."

3. Which developmental milestones would the nurse expect a 10-month-old infant to display during a routine health maintenance visit? Select all that apply.
1. Holding the head erect
2. Self-feeding
3. Demonstrating good bowel and bladder control
4. Sitting on a firm surface without support
5. Bearing the majority of his weight on the legs
6. Walking alone

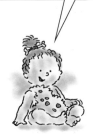

"All by myself!" Infants and toddlers are constantly learning new skills.

1. 1. It's normal for a 2-year-old child to eagerly explore the environment for new sensory experiences. Talking to the pediatrician is inappropriate because the nurse is assuming a corrective, parental role toward the parent without addressing concerns. Restricting the child's intake of sugar and sugary treats is incorrect because the nurse is making assumptions and recommendations that don't relate to the parent's concerns. Suggesting evaluation by a psychologist reinforces the parent's fear that something is wrong with the child.
CN: Health promotion and maintenance; CNS: None; CL: Analyze;
DIFFICULTY: Easy

2. 3. Sucking is the infant's chief pleasure. However, thumb sucking can cause malocclusion if it persists after age 4. Many fetuses begin sucking their fingers in utero and, as infants, refuse a pacifier as a substitute. A young child is likely to chew on a bandage, which could lead to airway obstruction.
CN: Health promotion and maintenance; CNS: None; CL: Apply;
DIFFICULTY: Moderate

3. 1, 4, 5. By age 10 months, an infant should be able to hold the head erect—a developmental milestone achieved by age 3 months. The child should also be able to sit on a firm surface without support and bear the majority of weight on the legs (for example, walking while holding on to furniture). Self-feeding and bowel and bladder control are developmental milestones of toddlers. By age 12 months, the infant should be able to stand alone and may take first steps.
CN: Health promotion and maintenance; CNS: None; CL: Apply;
DIFFICULTY: Challenge

CN: Client needs category   CNS: Client needs subcategory   CL: Cognitive level

4. A parent brings a child to the clinic for a routine wellness check. The nurse gathers data that reveals a BP 90/65 mm Hg, pulse 94 beats/minute, and respirations 20 breaths/minute. Which age group could this child represent based on these vital signs? Select all that apply.

1. Infant
2. Toddler
3. Preschool child
4. School-age child
5. Adolescent

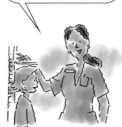

Looks like you really measure up. Keep up the good work.

4. 2, 3. Normal vital signs for preschoolers (ages 3 to 5) are blood pressure 85/60 to 90/70 mm Hg, pulse 90 to 100 beats per minute and respirations 20 to 25 breaths per minute. For toddlers (ages 1 to 3), normal pulse rate is 70 to 110 beats per minute, blood pressure is 90/55 to 105/70 mm Hg, and respiratory rate is 20 to 30 breaths per minute. For the school aged child (ages 5-12), normal pulse rate ranges from 75 to 115 beats per minute, blood pressure ranges from 106/69 to 117/76 mm Hg, and respiratory rate ranges from 20 to 25 breaths per minute. For infants (birth to 1 year), normal pulse rate ranges from 110 to 160 beats per minute, blood pressure is 65/40 to 78/52 mm Hg, and respiratory rate is 32 to 60 breaths per minute. Respirations are irregular and from the abdomen; the neonate is an obligate nose breather. Adolescent heart rate is close to the adult range: 55 to 95 beats per minute, respiratory rate is 12 to 18 breaths per minute, and blood pressure is the same range as an adult.

CN: Health promotion and maintenance: CNS: None; CL: Analyze; DIFFICULTY: Difficult

5. A 14-month-old is admitted to the pediatric floor with a diagnosis of croup. After gathering data, which characteristics exhibited by the toddler does the nurse determine represent expected developmental milestones? Select all that apply.

1. Strong hand grasp
2. Tendency to hold one object while looking for another
3. Recognition of familiar voices (smiles in recognition)
4. Presence of Moro reflex
5. Weight that's triple his birth weight
6. Closed anterior fontanel

5. 1, 2, 3, 5. A strong hand grasp is demonstrated within the first month of life. Holding one object while looking for another is accomplished by the 20th week. Within the first year of life, the toddler masters smiling at familiar faces and voices, his birth weight triples, and the Moro reflex disappears. The anterior fontanel closes at approximately age 18 months.

CN: Health promotion and maintenance; CNS: None; CL: Apply; DIFFICULTY: Challenge

6. When discussing death and dying with 10- and 11-year-old children which guides would be **best** for the nurse to incorporate? Select all that apply.

1. Logical explanations aren't appropriate.
2. The children will be curious about the physical aspects of death.
3. The children will know that death is inevitable and irreversible.
4. The children will be influenced by the attitudes of the adults in their lives.
5. Educating children about death and dying shouldn't start before age 11.
6. Telling children that death is the same as going to sleep, as a way of alleviating fear, is appropriate.

6. 2, 3, 4. School-age children are curious about the physical aspects of death and may wonder what happens to the body. By age 9 or 10, most children know that death is universal, inevitable, and irreversible. Their cognitive abilities are advanced and they respond well to logical explanations. They should be encouraged to ask questions. Because adults influence children's attitudes toward death, they should be encouraged to include children in the family rituals and be prepared to answer questions that may seem shocking. Educating children about death should begin early in childhood. Comparing death to sleep can be frightening for children and cause them to fear falling asleep.

CN: Psychosocial integrity; CNS: None; CL: Apply; DIFFICULTY: Moderate

7. The nurse obtaining data from an adolescent boy classifies his sexual maturity as Tanner stage 3. Which image depicts this stage?

1.
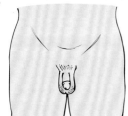

2.
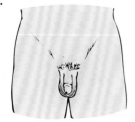

3.
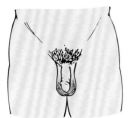

4.
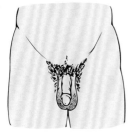

7. 2. In Tanner stage 3, pubic hair extends across the pubis. Testes and scrotum begin to enlarge, and the penis increases in length. Option 1 depicts Tanner stage 2, option 3 shows Tanner stage 4, and option 4 depicts Tanner stage 5.

CN: Physiological integrity; CNS: Physiological adaptation; CL: Apply; DIFFICULTY: Moderate

Chapter 26

Cardiovascular Disorders

Pediatric cardiovascular refresher

Increased pulmonary blood flow defects and obstructions to blood flow from the ventricles

Key signs and symptoms
- Congested cough
- Diaphoresis
- Fatigue
- Machinelike heart murmur (in patent ductus arteriosus)
- Mild cyanosis (if the condition leads to right-sided heart failure)
- Respiratory distress
- Tachycardia
- Tachypnea

Key test results
- Chest x-ray, echocardiography, and cardiac catheterization confirm type of heart defect

Key treatments
- Surgical repair
- Digoxin
- Diuretic (e.g., furosemide)

Key interventions
- Monitor vital signs, pulse oximetry, and intake and output
- Monitor cardiovascular and respiratory status
- Take apical pulse for 1 minute before giving digoxin (bradycardia is considered to be a pulse below 100 beats/minute in infants)
- Monitor fluid status

Decreased pulmonary blood flow and mixed blood flow defects

Key signs and symptoms
- Clubbing
- Crouching position assumed frequently

- Cyanosis
- History of inadequate feeding
- Irritability
- Tachycardia
- Tachypnea

Key test results
- Arterial blood gas analysis shows diminished arterial oxygen saturation
- Complete blood count shows polycythemia

Key treatments
- For transposition of the great vessels or arteries: corrective surgery to redirect blood flow
- For tetralogy of Fallot: complete repair or palliative treatment
- For hypoplastic left-heart syndrome: surgery to restructure the heart or heart transplantation
- For truncus arteriosus: surgery to recreate the pulmonary trunk and repair the ventricular septal defect

Key interventions
- Monitor cardiovascular and respiratory status
- Monitor vital signs, pulse oximetry, and intake and output
- Administer prophylactic antibiotics

Rheumatic fever

Inflammatory condition that may result as a complication after experiencing a Group A streptococcus infection; may cause chronic cardiac complications

Key signs and symptoms
- Carditis
- Chorea
- Erythema marginatum (temporary, disk-shaped, nonpruritic, reddened macules that fade in the center, leaving raised margins)

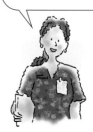

Ah, there you are. You've reached our test on cardiovascular disorders in children. Before starting these practice questions, why not bolster yourself with a heart-healthy snack of celery and low-fat cream cheese? Yum!

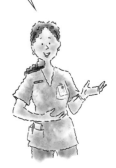

Now this chapter has a lot of heart.

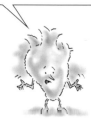

When I'm defective, not enough oxygen gets to the rest of the body, which is bad news.

- Polyarthritis
- Subcutaneous nodules

Key test results
- Erythrocyte sedimentation rate is increased
- Electrocardiogram shows prolonged PR interval
- Echocardiography shows damage to heart structures

Key treatments
- Bed rest until the sedimentation rate normalizes
- Penicillin to prevent additional damage from future attacks
- Anti-inflammatory drug to reduce pain and inflammation

Key interventions
- Monitor vital signs and intake and output

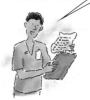

Why is rheumatic fever in a cardiovascular chapter? What's the connection?

thePoint® You can download tables of drug information to help you prepare for the NCLEX®! View Generic Drug Names, Drug Classifications, Drug Actions, and Nursing Implications for the drugs discussed in this refresher at **http://thePoint.lww.com.**

Cardiovascular disorders questions, answers, and rationales

1. When auscultating heart sounds on a 2-year-old child, where would the nurse place the stethoscope to hear the first heart sound **best**?
1. Third or fourth intercostal space
2. The apex with the stethoscope bell
3. Second intercostal space, midclavicular line
4. Fifth intercostal space, left midclavicular line

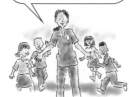

Kids love me ... until I pull out my syringe. Then they can't run away fast enough.

2. The nurse has auscultated the first heart sound. When does the nurse determine this sound is occurring?
1. Late in diastole
2. Early in diastole
3. With closure of the mitral and tricuspid valves
4. With closure of the aortic and pulmonic valves

Hmm. I think the first heart sound occurs in systole.

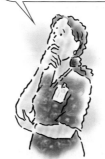

3. A child is seen at the health care provider's office. During the interview period the child's parent reports the child has a grade 1 heart murmur. The nurse is aware that this murmur has which characteristic?
1. A sound equal to the heart sounds
2. A sound softer than the heart sounds
3. A sound that can be heard with the naked ear
4. A sound associated with a precordial thrill

4. A patent ductus arteriosus (PDA) is suspected in a newborn. When reviewing the assessment data, which findings are supportive of this potential diagnosis? Select all that apply.
1. Heart rate weak, thready at 110 beats per minute
2. Heart rate pounding at 150 beats per minute
3. Acrocyanosis
4. Jaundice
5. Tachypnea

1. 4. The first heart sound can best be heard at the fifth intercostal space, left midclavicular line. The second heart sound is heard at the second intercostal space. The third heart sound is heard with the stethoscope bell at the apex of the heart. The fourth heart sound can be heard at the third or fourth intercostal space.
CN: Health promotion and maintenance; CNS: None; CL: Apply; DIFFICULTY: Moderate

2. 3. The first heart sound occurs during systole with closure of the mitral and tricuspid valves. The second heart sound occurs during diastole with closure of the aortic and pulmonic valves. The third heart sound is heard early in diastole. The fourth heart sound is heard late in diastole and may be a normal finding in children.
CN: Health promotion and maintenance; CNS: None; CL: Analyze; DIFFICULTY: Moderate

3. 2. A grade 1 heart murmur is usually difficult to hear and softer than the heart sounds. A grade 2 murmur is usually equal to the heart sounds. A grade 4 murmur can be associated with a precordial thrill. A thrill is a palpable manifestation associated with a loud murmur. A grade 6 murmur can be heard with the naked ear or with the stethoscope off the chest.
CN: Health promotion and maintenance; CNS: None; CL: Apply; DIFFICULTY: Moderate

4. 2, 5. A PDA results when the ductus arteriosus does not close at birth. This usually results within 15 hours of life. Symptoms that are consistent with the condition include a full, bounding pulse; dyspnea; and tachypnea. A weak pulse is not associated with PDA. Acrocyanosis refers to a blue discoloration in the extremities. This is commonly seen in the first hours after birth. Jaundice is not associated with PDA.
CN: Physiological integrity; CNS: Physiological adaptation; CL: Apply; DIFFICULTY: Difficult

5. A child is diagnosed with cardiogenic shock. Which statement by the child's parents indicates an understanding of the condition? Select all that apply.

1. "My child has a reduction in cardiac output."
2. "There is less blood circulating in my child's body."
3. "My child's body tissues and organs are not getting enough oxygen."
4. "My child's condition has resulted from an inflow or outflow obstruction of the main bloodstream."
5. "My child has a bacterial infection that is causing him to become septic."

6. The nurse is caring for a child in a shock state. Which clinical manifestation does the nurse determine indicates a late sign of shock in this child?

1. Tachycardia
2. Hypotension
3. Delayed capillary refill
4. Pale, cool, mottled skin

7. The nurse is gathering data from a 1-month-old infant. Which data obtained by the parents indicate the infant may have a cardiac defect?

1. The infant is gaining weight
2. The infant has been hyperactive
3. The infant is not taking formula well
4. The infant has pink, mucous membranes

8. A 2-year-old child is showing signs of shock. A 10 mL/kg bolus of normal saline solution is ordered. The child weighs 20 kg. How many milliliters should be administered? Record your answer using a whole number.

_____ mL

9. The nurse is attending an educational program about dysrhythmias in children. In which populations are premature atrial contractions common? Select all that apply.

1. Fetuses
2. Neonates
3. Infants
4. School age children
5. Adolescents

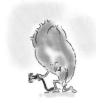

Speaking of "cardiogenic shock," check this out ...

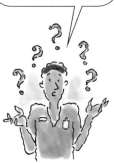

That word "late" in question #6 looks important. Which sign would be the last to appear?

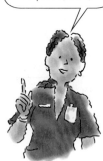

Try not to overthink question #8. As math problems go, it's pretty easy.

5. 1, 3. Cardiogenic shock occurs when cardiac output is decreased, and tissue oxygen needs aren't adequately met. Hypovolemic shock describes a reduction in circulating blood volume. Septic shock occurs with overwhelming sepsis and circulating bacterial toxins. Obstructive shock is seen with an inflow or outflow obstruction of the main bloodstream.

CN: Physiological integrity; CNS: Physiological adaptation; CL: Understand; DIFFICULTY: Difficult

6. 2. Hypotension is considered a late sign of shock in children. This represents a decompensated state and impending cardiopulmonary arrest. Tachycardia, delayed capillary refill, and pale, cool, mottled skin are earlier indicators of shock that may show compensation.

CN: Physiological integrity; CNS: Physiological adaptation; CL: Analyze; DIFFICULTY: Difficult

7. 3. Infants and children with heart defects tend to have poor nutritional intake and weight loss, indicating poor cardiac output, heart failure, or hypoxemia. The child appears lethargic or tired because of the heart failure or hypoxia. Gray, pale, or mottled skin may indicate hypoxia or poor cardiac output. Pink, moist mucous membranes are normal.

CN: Health promotion and maintenance; CNS: None; CL: Analyze; DIFFICULTY: Moderate

8. 200.
Use the following equation:

$$10 \text{ mL} / \text{kg} \times 20 \text{ kg} = 200 \text{ mL}$$

CN: Physiological integrity; CNS: Pharmacological therapies; CL: Analyze; DIFFICULTY: Moderate

9. 1, 2, 3. Premature atrial contractions are common in fetuses, neonates, and infants. They occur from increased automaticity of an atrial cell anywhere except the sinoatrial node. Atrial fibrillation is an uncommon dysrhythmia in children occurring from a disorganized state of electrical activity in the atria. Bradyarrhythmias are usually congenital, surgically acquired, or caused by infection. Premature ventricular contractions are more common in adolescents.

CN: Physiological integrity; CNS: Physiological adaptation; CL: Understand; DIFFICULTY: Moderate

10. The nurse is caring for a child who has recently been diagnosed with a cardiovascular disorder. The child's parents do not seem to be accepting of the diagnosis and the changes the diagnosis will make in their lives. What initial action by the nurse will be **most** therapeutic?
 1. Encourage the parents to consider genetic counseling to consider the risk for future children born to them.
 2. Review the planned treatments with the parents and assess understanding of them.
 3. Encourage the parents to discuss their feelings about the loss of their child's health.
 4. Refer the parents to a counselor.

11. The nurse is talking with the parent of a 3-year-old child who has congenital heart disease. The parent reports feeling concerns that the child does not seem to be maturing emotionally in a manner that is at the same rate as the two older children in the family. Which response by the nurse is **most** appropriate?
 1. "All children mature at different rates so comparisons are not really fair."
 2. "Children who have chronic health issues may experience developmental delays."
 3. "The emotional immaturity you are seeing may just be your child's manner of acting out in response to being sick so much."
 4. "You will need to lower your expectations for your child's level of maturity."

12. A neonate with a patent ductus arteriosus was delivered 6 hours earlier and is being held by the mother. As the nurse enters the room to assess the neonate's vital signs, the mother says, "The health care provider says that my baby has a heart murmur. Does that mean the baby has a bad heart?" Which responses by the nurse would be appropriate? Select all that apply.
 1. "The baby will need more tests to determine the heart condition."
 2. "The baby will require oxygen therapy at home for a while."
 3. "The baby will be fine. Don't worry."
 4. "The murmur is caused by the natural opening, which can take a day or two to close."
 5. "Many newborns experience murmurs in their transition after being born."

13. A 3-year-old child is experiencing distress after having cardiac surgery. Which findings are characteristic of cardiac tamponade? Select all that apply.
 1. Hypertension
 2. Muffled heart sounds
 3. Widened pulse pressures
 4. Increased chest tube drainage
 5. Tachypnea

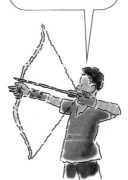

When providing information, don't just aim to please. Be honest and direct.

10. 3. Grief and feelings of loss by the parents are expected phenomena when a child receives a diagnosis of a chronic health concern. Parents will need to work through the feelings that the anticipated future of their child may be modified. Genetic counseling may be needed if the disorder is hereditary, but in this case it is premature and the focus needs to be on assisting the family to navigate through their feelings and focus on the care of their child. Education about the treatment plan is needed but it does not meet the needs discussed in this scenario. Counseling may be of benefit but the nurse must first promote communication with the parents.
CN: Psychosocial integrity; CNS: None; CL: Apply; DIFFICULTY: Easy

11. 2. Chronic illnesses can impact a child's growth and development both emotionally and cognitively. The child with a cardiac disorder may experiences delays as a result of hypoxic episodes or because of repeated hospitalizations. Educating parents about these possibilities will be helpful in initiating the discussion about the child's level of maturity. Although children mature at different rates this is not the best response. Children may act out in response to illness or other factors but there is no information that supports this reason for the child's behavior. Encouraging parents to lower their expectations is not therapeutic.
CN: Psychosocial integrity; CNS: None; CL: Evaluation; DIFFICULTY: Moderate

12. 4, 5. Although the nurse may want to tell the mother not to worry, the most appropriate response would be to explain the neonate's present condition, to relieve her, and to acknowledge an awareness of the condition. A neonate's vascular system changes with birth; certain factors help to reverse the flow of blood through the ductus and ultimately favor its closure. This closure typically begins within the first 24 hours after birth and ends within a few days after birth. The other responses aren't appropriate.
CN: Health promotion and maintenance; CNS: None; CL: Analyze; DIFFICULTY: Challenge

13. 2, 5. Symptoms of cardiac tamponade include muffled heart sounds, hypotension, sudden cessation of chest tube drainage, rapid respirations and a narrowing pulse pressure. Cardiac tamponade occurs when a large volume of fluid interferes with ventricular filling and pumping, and collects in the pericardial sac, decreasing cardiac output.
CN: Physiological integrity; CNS: Physiological adaptation; CL: Analyze; DIFFICULTY: Difficult

14. A child is scheduled to have a cardiac catheterization. Both the child and parents report increasing anxiety as day of the scheduled procedure approaches. Which activity would be beneficial for the child and his parents prior to the procedure? Select all that apply.
1. Supply a map of the hospital.
2. Limit visitors to parents only.
3. Offer a guided tour of the hospital and catheterization laboratory.
4. Explain that the child can't eat or drink for 1 to 2 days postoperatively.
5. Allow the child and parents to meet with a nurse from the department where the procedure will be performed.

14. 3, 5. A guided tour will help minimize fears and allay anxieties for the child and parents. It gives the opportunity for questions and education. Having familiarity with a staff member of the department will be of assistance. It will also allow a time for questions to be asked. A map of the hospital will not reduce concerns about the procedure. A tour provides the family with information about what they will hear and see in the unit. The child will be able to start clear liquids and advance as tolerated after the procedure is completed and the child is fully awake. The preoperative education should indicate that siblings and all significant others are appropriate visitors for the child.
CN: Physiological integrity; CNS: Physiological adaptation; CL: Analyze; DIFFICULTY: Challenge

15. A 15-year-old child has been scheduled to have a cardiac catheterization. Which statements by the teen or parent indicate the need for further instruction? Select all that apply.
1. "A consent will need to be signed by my parents for this procedure."
2. "My health care provider will put me to sleep for the catheterization."
3. "The sound waves will let the health care providers see how my heart moves."
4. "It provides visualization of the heart and great vessels with radiopaque dye."
5. "They will pass a small catheter through one of my veins to look at the inside of my heart."

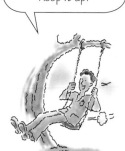

Now you've got the swing of things. Keep it up!

15. 2, 3. Cardiac catheterization provides visualization of the heart and great vessels. It's an invasive procedure in which a thin catheter is passed into the chambers of the heart through a peripheral vein or artery. A consent will be required. Conscious sedation is usually given before cardiac catheterization. General anesthesia is not generally done. High-frequency sound waves are used during ultrasound and echocardiography.
CN: Health promotion and maintenance; CNS: None; CL: Apply; DIFFICULTY: Difficult

16. The nurse is caring for a child who underwent a cardiac catheterization 1 hour ago. Which interventions are appropriate for inclusion in the care delivered? Select all that apply.
1. Elevate the head of the bed to 90 degrees.
2. Encourage the child to remain flat in bed.
3. Assess vital signs every half hour.
4. Replace the dressing if it becomes soiled.
5. Maintain NPO status until the child is 24 hours post procedure.

16. 2, 3. During recovery, the child should remain flat in bed, keeping the punctured leg straight for the prescribed time. The child should avoid raising the head, sitting, straining the abdomen, or coughing. Vital signs are taken every 15 minutes until the child is awake and stable, then every half hour, and then hourly as ordered. If bleeding occurs at the insertion site, the nurse should reinforce the dressing and monitor for changes. There is no reason for the child to be NPO after the procedure.
CN: Physiological integrity; CNS: Physiological adaptation; CL: Analyze; DIFFICULTY: Difficult

17. A child is preparing for discharge to home after undergoing a cardiac catheterization. Which statements by the child indicates the need for further instruction? Select all that apply.
1. "Once I go home I will be able to go back to my normal diet."
2. "Drinking extra water is recommended."
3. "I will be able to go to school tomorrow."
4. "It will be at least 2 to 4 weeks before I can participate in gym class."
5. "By next week I will be able to take a bath or shower."

17. 3, 4. After a cardiac catheterization a regular diet may be resumed. Increased fluid intake is recommended as it will help to flush the dye from the system. A return to school will normally wait for about 3 to 5 days. Most regular activities including exercise will be permissible after 3 to 5 days. Taking a bath or shower is permissible after a few days.
CN: Physiological integrity; CNS: Physiological adaptation; CL: Analyze; DIFFICULTY: Challenge

---

CN: Client needs category   CNS: Client needs subcategory   CL: Cognitive level

18. A 2-year-old child is being monitored after cardiac surgery. Which findings signal a potential decrease in cardiac output? Select all that apply.
1. Blood pressure 80/45
2. Urinary output of 45 mL in the past 2 hours
3. Weak peripheral pulses
4. Capillary refill less than 2 seconds
5. Heart rate 100 BMP

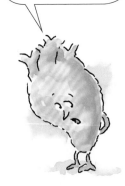

When my blood pressure is down, I just can't pump out the red stuff like usual.

19. A nurse is reviewing the laboratory testing for a 17-year-old teenager in the postoperative period. Which findings indicate the need for follow up? Select all that apply.
1. Potassium 3.1 mEq/L
2. Sodium 151 mEq/L
3. Calcium 9 mg/dL
4. Chloride 2.5 mg/dL
5. Magnesium 2.0 mg/dL

20. A nurse is discussing wound and skin care after cardiac surgery. Which information should be included in the discussion? Select all that apply.
1. "Using powders near the incision location will need to be avoided."
2. "Your child can take a bath tomorrow."
3. "Tingling, itching, and numbness are normal sensations at the wound site."
4. "The surgical incision will remain covered by a dressing for several days."
5. "If the sterile adhesive strips over the incision fall off, call the health care provider."

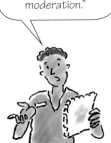

As my grandpa always says, "everything in moderation."

21. Parents ask a nurse about a child's activity level after cardiac surgery. Which response would be **best**?
1. There are no exercise limitations.
2. The child may resume school in 3 days.
3. Encourage a balance of rest and exercise.
4. Climbing and contact sports are restricted for 1 week.

22. Which home care instruction is **most** appropriate for a child after cardiac surgery?
1. Maintain the prescribed medication regimen until the health care provider makes a change.
2. Maintain a sodium-restricted diet.
3. Routine dental care can be resumed.
4. Immunizations are delayed indefinitely.

18. 1, 2, 3. Signs of decreased cardiac output include weak peripheral pulses, low urine output, delayed capillary refill, hypotension, and cool extremities. The normal blood pressure for a child of this age may range from 95-110/60-75. This blood pressure represented is well below this value. Urinary output less than 30 mL per hour signals reduced cardiac output. A heart rate of 100 beats per minute is within normal limits for a 2-year-old child.
CN: Physiological integrity; CNS: Physiological adaptation; CL: Analyze; DIFFICULTY: Moderate

19. 1, 2. The normal range for serum potassium is 3.5 to 5.5 mEq/ L. Serum sodium levels should range from 135 to 147 mEq/L. Those values found for both sodium and potassium are not within normal limits and require follow up. The calcium, chloride and magnesium levels are within normal limits.
CN: Health promotion and maintenance; CNS: None; CL: Analyze; DIFFICULTY: Difficult

20. 1, 3. As the area heals, tingling, itching, and numbness are normal sensations that will eventually go away. Lotions and powders should be avoided during the first 2 weeks after surgery. A complete bath should be delayed for the first week. The initial surgical dressing will be removed by the surgeon and the incision assessed the day after surgery. Adhesive strips may loosen or fall off on their own. This is a common and normal occurrence.
CN: Physiological integrity; CNS: Physiological adaptation; CL: Analyze; DIFFICULTY: Difficult

21. 3. Activity should be increased gradually each day, allowing for a sensible balance of rest and exercise. School and large crowds should be avoided for at least 2 weeks to prevent exposure to people with active infections. Sports and contact activities should be restricted for about 6 weeks, giving the sternum enough time to heal.
CN: Physiological integrity; CNS: Physiological adaptation; CL: Analyze; DIFFICULTY: Easy

22. 1. Drugs such as digoxin and furosemide shouldn't be stopped abruptly. There are no diet restrictions, so the child may resume his regular diet. Routine dental care is usually delayed 4 to 5 months after surgery. Immunizations may be delayed 6 to 8 weeks after surgery.
CN: Physiological integrity; CNS: Physiological adaptation; CL: Analyze; DIFFICULTY: Challenge

23. A 4-year-old client with a chest tube is placed on water seal. Which statement is correct?
1. The water level rises with inhalation.
2. Bubbling is seen in the suction chamber.
3. Bubbling is seen in the water seal chamber.
4. Water seal is obtained by clamping the tube.

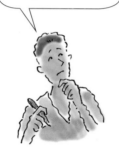

Make sure your priorities are in order in question #24.

24. The nurse is caring for a client when the chest tube becomes dislodged. Which action by the nurse should be performed **first**?
1. Place a dry gauze dressing over the insertion site.
2. Place a petroleum gauze dressing over the insertion site.
3. Wipe the tube with alcohol and reinsert it.
4. Call the health care provider immediately.

25. The nurse is assigned to care for a child who has been diagnosed with heart failure. Which data gathered is consistent with this condition? Select all that apply.
1. Bradycardia
2. Bradypnea
3. Gallop murmur
4. Strong, bounding pulses
5. Tachycardia

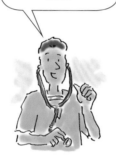

All the sounds I'm hearing from your heart are good ones.

26. A nurse is obtaining data from a child with left-sided heart failure. Which symptoms does the nurse correlate with the diagnosis? Select all that apply.
1. Weight gain
2. Peripheral edema
3. Neck vein distention
4. Tachypnea
5. Dyspnea

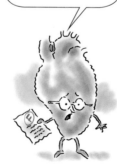

What do you mean I'm a failure? I'm pumping as hard as I can!

27. The nurse is caring for a child with heart failure. What should the nurse recognize when monitoring administration of oxygen to avoid complications?
1. Oxygen is contraindicated in this situation.
2. Oxygen is given at high levels only.
3. Oxygen is a pulmonary bed constrictor.
4. Oxygen decreases the work of breathing.

23. 1. The water seal chamber is functioning appropriately when the water level rises in the chamber with inhalation and falls with expiration. This shows that negative pressure required in the lung is being maintained. Bubbling in the suction chamber should only be seen when suction is being used. Bubbling in the water seal chamber generally indicates the presence of an air leak. The chest tube should never be clamped; a tension pneumothorax may occur. Water seal is activated when the suction is disconnected.
CN: Physiological integrity; CNS: Physiological adaptation; CL: Apply; DIFFICULTY: Challenge

24. 2. Petroleum gauze should be placed over the insertion site immediately to prevent a pneumothorax. The health care provider should be notified after this step. A dry gauze dressing will allow air to escape, leading to a pneumothorax. The tube is only reinserted by a health care provider using a sterile thoracotomy tray.
CN: Physiological integrity; CNS: Physiological adaptation; CL: Apply; DIFFICULTY: Moderate

25. 3, 5. When the heart stretches beyond efficiency, an extra heart sound or S3 gallop murmur may be audible. This is related to excessive preload and ventricular dilation. Tachycardia occurs as a compensatory mechanism to the decrease in cardiac output. It also attempts to increase the force and rate of myocardial contraction and increase oxygen consumption of the heart. The respiratory rate increases, not decreases, in an attempt to increase oxygenation. Pulses are usually weak and thready.
CN: Physiological integrity; CNS: Physiological adaptation; CL: Analyze; DIFFICULTY: Difficult

26. 4, 5. Respiratory symptoms, such as tachypnea and dyspnea, are seen due to pulmonary congestion. Weight gain, peripheral edema, and neck vein distention are seen with systemic venous congestion or right-sided failure. Fluid accumulates in the interstitial spaces due to blood pooling in the venous circulation.
CN: Physiological integrity; CNS: Physiological adaptation; CL: Apply; DIFFICULTY: Difficult

27. 4. Oxygen decreases the work of breathing and increases arterial oxygen levels, so it's indicated in this situation. Oxygen usually is administered at low levels with humidification. Oxygen is a pulmonary bed dilator, not constrictor, and can exacerbate any condition in which the lungs are overloaded.
CN: Physiological integrity; CNS: Physiological adaptation; CL: Analyze; DIFFICULTY: Moderate

28. Which nursing intervention is **most** appropriate when caring for an infant with heart failure?
1. Limit fluid intake.
2. Avoid using infant seats.
3. Cluster nursing activities.
4. Place the infant prone or supine.

29. The nurse is reinforcing education for parents of an infant with heart failure. Which diet plan will the nurse discuss with the parents?
1. Restrict fluids.
2. Weigh once per week.
3. Use low-sodium formula.
4. Increase caloric content per ounce.

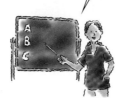

Teach parents the ABCs of nutrition for kids with heart failure.

30. The nurse is preparing to administer digoxin to a child. Which symptoms related to the digoxin require the nurse to withhold administration and notify the health care provider? Select all that apply.
1. Weight gain
2. Tachycardia
3. Nausea and vomiting
4. Seizures
5. Bradycardia

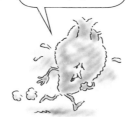

Phew! I sure could use a hit of digoxin. I'm feeling beat after all this running.

31. A teenager with heart failure prescribed digoxin asks the nurse, "What will this drug do for my heart?" What is the best response by the nurse?
1. It will cause vasodilation and help with chest pain.
2. It will decrease the workload of the heart.
3. It will cause sodium excretion.
4. It will increase your heart rate.

32. An 11-month-old infant with heart failure weighs 10 kg. Digoxin is prescribed as 0.01 mg/kg in divided doses every 12 hours. How much is given per dose? Record your answer using two decimal places.

_____ mg/dose

28. 3. Energy expenditures need to be limited to reduce metabolic and oxygen needs. Nursing care should be clustered, followed by long periods of undisturbed rest. Fluid may be restricted in older children, but infants' nutritional requirements depend on fluid needs. Infants should be placed in the semi-Fowler or upright position. Infant seats help maintain an upright position. This facilitates lung expansion, provides less restrictive movement of the diaphragm, relieves pressure from abdominal organs, and decreases pulmonary congestion.

CN: Physiological integrity; CNS: Physiological adaptation; CL: Analyze; DIFFICULTY: Challenge

29. 4. Formulas with increased caloric content are given to meet the greater caloric requirements from the overworked heart and labored breathing. Fluid restriction and low-sodium formulas aren't recommended. An infant's nutritional needs depend on fluid. Daily weights at the same time of day on the same scale before feedings are recommended to follow trends in nutritional stability and diuresis. Low-sodium formulas may cause hyponatremia.

CN: Physiological integrity; CNS: Basic care and comfort; CL: Apply; DIFFICULTY: Challenge

30. 3, 5. Digoxin toxicity in infants and children may present with nausea, vomiting, anorexia, or a slow, irregular apical heart rate. Weight gain, tachycardia, or seizures aren't seen in digoxin toxicity.

CN: Physiological integrity; CNS: Pharmacological therapies; CL: Analyze; DIFFICULTY: Challenge

31. 2. Digoxin is a cardiac glycoside. It decreases the workload of the heart and improves myocardial function. It will not cause vasodilation and increase sodium excretion. Diuretics help remove excess fluid. Digoxin is not a vasodilator and it will slow the heart rate, not increase it.

CN: Physiological integrity; CNS: Pharmacological therapies; CL: Apply; DIFFICULTY: Easy

32. 0.05.
Use the following equations:
$$10 \text{ kg} \times 0.01 \text{ mg/kg} = 0.1 \text{ mg}$$
$$24 \text{ hours}/12 \text{ hours/dose} = 2 \text{ doses}$$
$$0.1 \text{ mg}/2 \text{ doses} = 0.05 \text{ mg/dose}$$

CN: Physiological integrity; CNS: Pharmacological therapies; CL: Analyze; DIFFICULTY: Difficult

33. A child with heart failure is given captopril. The nurse should reinforce education of the child's parents on which action of captopril?
1. It increases vasoconstriction.
2. It increases sodium excretion.
3. It decreases sodium excretion.
4. It increases vascular resistance.

33. 2. ACE inhibitors block the conversion of angiotensin I to angiotensin II in the kidney. This causes decreased aldosterone, vasodilation, and increased sodium excretion. As a vasodilator, it also acts to reduce vascular resistance by the manipulation of afterload.
CN: Physiological integrity; CNS: Pharmacological therapies; CL: Apply; DIFFICULTY: Moderate

34. Which statement would the nurse need to keep in mind when assisting with the education plan for the parents of a child with patent ductus arteriosus?
1. Heart failure is uncommon.
2. The ductus normally closes completely by age 6 weeks.
3. An open ductus arteriosus causes decreased blood flow to the lungs.
4. It represents a cyanotic defect with decreased pulmonary blood flow.

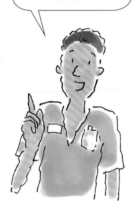

Sounds like the client would like a little more control. What's the best way to accomplish that?

34. 2. At birth, oxygenated blood normally causes the ductus to constrict, and the vessel closes completely by age 6 weeks. This defect is considered an acyanotic defect with increased pulmonary blood flow. Heart failure is common in premature infants with patent ductus arteriosus. The open ductus arteriosus can cause excessive blood flow to the lungs because of the high pressure in the aorta.
CN: Physiological integrity; CNS: Physiological adaptation; CL: Understand; DIFFICULTY: Difficult

35. A hospitalized teen diagnosed with a cardiac disorder reports feeling "trapped in a diseased body." Which action the by the nurse will be **most** therapeutic?
1. Provide the teen with information on the medical diagnosis.
2. Encourage the teen to participate in planning the day.
3. Ask the teen to invite friends to visit in the hospital.
4. Encourage the teen's parents to bring familiar items from home.

35. 2. All of the interventions listed should be considered in the plan of care. The most important would be allowing the teen to become more involved in the plan of treatment to promote feelings of control. Although not all of the teen's requests may be incorporated in the plan of care, some may — and this will increase feelings of value and worth.
CN: Psychosoical integrity; CNS: None; CL: Analyze; DIFFICULTY: Difficult

36. Which nursing action would be appropriate for an infant after cardiac catheterization?
1. Keep the leg on the operative site flexed to reduce bleeding.
2. Change the catheterization dressing immediately to reduce the risk of infection.
3. Apply pressure if oozing or bleeding is noted.
4. Keep the infant's temperature below normal to promote vasoconstriction and decrease bleeding.

36. 3. Applying pressure to the site is appropriate if bleeding is noted. The leg should be kept straight and immobile to prevent trauma and bleeding. The pressure dressing shouldn't be changed, but it may be reinforced if bleeding occurs. Hypothermia causes stress in infants and should be avoided.
CN: Physiological integrity; CNS: Reduction of risk potential; CL: Apply; DIFFICULTY: Moderate

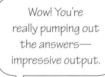

Wow! You're really pumping out the answers— impressive output.

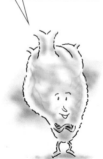

37. The nurse has observed that the mother of a 6-month-old child diagnosed with a cardiac disorder seems to be disinterested in her child's daily routine. Which action by the nurse will be **most** appropriate?
1. Make a referral to the hospital's social services department.
2. Refer the parent to a local support group.
3. Invite the child's parent to assist with care delivery.
4. Set up a care conference with the parent and the discipline involved in the child's care.

37. 3. Caring for a child with a cardiac disorder may be overwhelming for the parent. She may fear harming the child and may have a sense of powerlessness. The focus should be to bring the parent an increase in involvement in the child's care. This may be a gradual process. There is no indication that a social services referral is needed. A support group may be of benefit but it is not the initial intervention needed. A care conference may be of benefit to allow the parent to have a better understanding of the care being provided and plans for future care but it is not the initial action to be taken.
CN: Psychosocial integrity; CNS: None; CL: Apply; DIFFICULTY: Difficult

38. Which finding is expected when obtaining data from a child with an acyanotic heart defect?
1. Excess weight gain
2. Bradycardia
3. Hepatomegaly
4. Decreased respiratory rate

38. 3. Hepatomegaly may result from blood backing up into the liver due to increased resistance in the right side of the heart. Poor growth and development, not excess weight gain, may be seen because of the increased energy required for breathing. The increase in blood flow to the lungs may cause tachycardia (not bradycardia) and an increased respiratory rate to compensate.
CN: Physiological integrity; CNS: Physiological adaptation; CL: Apply; DIFFICULTY: Difficult

39. A child hospitalized with right-sided heart failure is tearful and states "My parents do not want me to have any activity and I always needs to rest." Which action by the nurse is **most** appropriate?
1. Explain to the child that becoming tired is a concern with this condition.
2. Explain to the child that the parents are just showing love and care.
3. Ask the child if assistance is needed to share concerns with the parents.
4. Ask the child if he would like to visit the unit's playroom.

39. 3. Fatigue is a concern in a child with heart failure. Efforts should be made to ensure adequate periods of rest. Activity and play are normal needs for a child. Parents of chronically ill children may at times be over protective. Encouraging a meeting with the parents and child may be of benefit to highlight the child's concerns. Explaining that fatigue is a concern and that there is parental love, while true, does not address the child's concerns. Visiting the play room does not address the concerns.
CN: Safe, effective care environment; CNS: Management of care; CL: apply; DIFFICULTY: Difficult

40. The nurse is caring for a child with a ventricular septal defect. Which signs may be seen when the nurse gathers data from this child? Select all that apply.
1. Cyanosis of the nail beds
2. Anorexia
3. Unexplained weight gain
4. Pink nail beds with capillary refill less than 2 seconds
5. Fatigue

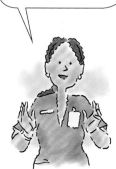

A ventricular septal defect causes decreased perfusion. What does this look like?

40. 1, 2, 3, 5. A ventricular septal defect refers to an abnormal opening in the wall of the heart. The clinical manifestations will vary depending upon the size and location. Symptoms that are characteristic include cyanotic nail beds can be seen when pulmonary resistance increases and causes the left-to-right shunt to reverse and shunt right to left. This shift leads to signs of heart failure and cyanosis. Children with the defect usually present with symptoms of heart failure, poor growth and development, and failure to thrive. A loss of appetite is also seen. Weight gain may result from edema.
CN: Physiological integrity; CNS: Physiological adaptation; CL: Analyze; DIFFICULTY: Difficult

41. When caring for a child diagnosed with a ventricular septal defect, which description would the nurse incorporate when talking with the parents about this condition?
1. Narrowing of the aortic arch
2. Failure of a septum to develop completely between the atria
3. Narrowing of the valves at the entrance of the pulmonary artery
4. Failure of a septum to develop completely between the ventricles

41. 4. Failure of a septum to develop between the ventricles results in a left-to-right shunt, which is noted as a ventricular septal defect. When the septum fails to develop between the atria, it's considered an atrial septal defect. The narrowing of the aortic arch describes coarctation of the aorta. Narrowing of the valves at the pulmonary artery describes pulmonary stenosis.
CN: Physiological integrity; CNS: Physiological adaptation; CL: Apply; DIFFICULTY: Easy

42. A child with a ventricular septal repair is receiving dopamine postoperatively. The nurse should reinforce education to the child's parents that this medication is **most** likely to be given for which action?
1. To decrease the heart rate
2. To decrease urine output
3. To increase cardiac output
4. To decrease cardiac contractility

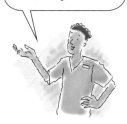

If you're having trouble finding the right answer, try eliminating a few wrong ones; it will increase your odds.

42. 3. Dopamine stimulates beta-1 and beta-2 receptors. It's a selective cardiac stimulant that increases cardiac output, heart rate, and cardiac contractility. Urine output increases in response to dilation of the blood vessels to the mesentery and kidneys.
CN: Physiological integrity; CNS: Pharmacological therapies; CL: Apply; DIFFICULTY: Moderate

CN: Client needs category CNS: Client needs subcategory CL: Cognitive level

43. A 6-month-old infant with uncorrected tetralogy of Fallot suddenly becomes increasingly cyanotic and diaphoretic, with weak peripheral pulses and an increased respiratory rate. What is the **priority** action by the nurse?
1. Administer oxygen.
2. Administer morphine sulfate.
3. Place the infant in a knee-chest position
4. Place the infant in Fowler position.

44. A child returns to the unit after a cardiac catheterization. The nurse should reinforce education for the child and parents on which point regarding mobility?
1. The child may sit in a chair with the affected extremity immobilized.
2. The child will be maintained on bed rest with no further activity restrictions.
3. The child will be maintained on bed rest with the affected extremity immobilized.
4. The child may get out of bed to go to the bathroom, if necessary.

45. A parent is taught to administer digoxin to a 6-month-old infant at home. Which statement by the parent indicates the need for additional education?
1. "I'll count the baby's pulse before every dose."
2. "I'll make sure the pulse is regular before every dose."
3. "I'll measure the dose carefully."
4. "I'll withhold the medication if the pulse is below 60."

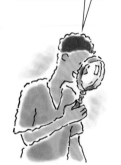

Remember—"need for additional education" is code for "wrong."

46. Which finding would concern the nurse who's caring for an infant after a right femoral cardiac catheterization?
1. Weak right dorsalis pedis pulse
2. Elevated temperature
3. Decreased urine output
4. Slight bloody drainage around catheterization site dressing

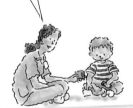

Remember: kids with heart conditions are still kids. Encourage them to play, as appropriate.

47. A child with an atrial septal repair is entering postoperative day 2. Which intervention would be appropriate for inclusion in the plan of care? Select all that apply.
1. Give the child nothing by mouth.
2. Maintain strict bed rest.
3. Take vital signs every 2 to 4 hours.
4. Administer an analgesic as needed.
5. Monitor intake and output.

43. 3. The knee-chest position reduces the workload of the heart by increasing the blood return to the heart and keeping the blood flow more centralized. Oxygen should be administered quickly but only after placing the infant in the knee-chest position. Morphine should be administered after positioning and oxygen administration are completed. Fowler position wouldn't improve tetralogy of Fallot.
CN: Physiological integrity; CNS: Physiological adaptation; CL: Apply; DIFFICULTY: Challenge

44. 3. Following cardiac catheterization, the child should be maintained on bed rest with the affected extremity immobilized to prevent hemorrhage. Allowing the child to sit in a chair with the affected extremity immobilized, to move the affected extremity while on bed rest, or to have bathroom privileges places him at risk for hemorrhage.
CN: Physiological integrity; CNS: Reduction of risk potential; CL: Apply; DIFFICULTY: Moderate

45. 4. A pulse rate under 60 beats/minute is an indication for withholding digoxin from an *adult*. Withholding digoxin from an infant is appropriate if the infant's pulse is under 90 beats/minute. The pulse rate must be counted before each dose of digoxin is given to an infant. An irregular pulse may be a sign of digoxin toxicity; if this occurs, the health care provider should be consulted before the drug is given. The dose must be measured carefully to decrease the risk of toxicity.
CN: Physiological integrity; CNS: Pharmacological therapies; CL: Apply; DIFFICULTY: Challenge

46. 1. The pulse below the catheterization site should be strong and equal to the unaffected extremity. A weakened pulse may indicate vessel obstruction or perfusion problems. Elevated temperature and decreased urine output are relatively normal findings after catheterization and may be the result of decreased oral fluids. A small amount of bloody drainage is normal; however, the site must be assessed frequently for increased bleeding.
CN: Physiological integrity; CNS: Reduction of risk potential; CL: Apply; DIFFICULTY: Moderate

47. 3, 4, 5. Vital signs should be monitored every 2 to 4 hours. Pain management is always a priority and should be given on an as-needed basis. By day 3, the child should be advancing to a regular diet. Monitoring intake and output to ensure there is no fluid overload or deficits should be included into the plan of care. Activity should be allowed as able in the step-down unit, with coughing and deep-breathing exercises.
CN: Physiological integrity; CNS: Physiological adaptation; CL: Apply; DIFFICULTY: Challenge

48. Propranolol has been prescribed for a teen who has been diagnosed with hypertension. When discussing the medication with the teen which statement indicates the need for further instruction?
1. "I should take this medication daily on an empty stomach."
2. "It is best to take this medication at the same time each day."
3. "I may experience dizziness with this medication."
4. "If I experience weight gain I need to contact my health care provider."

48. 1. Propranolol is used in the management of hypertension. The medication is taken daily. It is recommended that it should be taken at the same time each day. The drug is administered with food. Side effects include changes in sleep pattern, dizziness, and light headedness. Side effects such as skin afflictions, weight gain, and difficulty breathing should be reported promptly to the health care provider.
CN: Physiological integrity; CNS: Pharmacological therapies; CL: Apply; DIFFICULTY: Moderate

49. The parents of a 14-year-old child who underwent an atrial septal repair 5 days ago have asked if a few family members can visit. Which response by the nurse is appropriate?
1. "Your child is extremely fragile and visitations are not recommended."
2. "Let's have your child communicate with phone calls with friends and family members instead."
3. "We should not have visitors for another few days to best protect your child from infection."
4. "While controlling infection and promoting rest are important, a few visitors would not be a problem at this stage of recovery."

49. 4. Prevention of infection after any surgical procedure is important. After a week the child's risk for infection while still present is lessened. If all visitors are free of infection a visit would be fine.
CN: Safe, effective care environment; CNS: Safety and infection control; CL: Apply; DIFFICULTY: Moderate

50. When reinforcing family education regarding coarctation of the aorta, which statement describing the condition should be included?
1. Absent tricuspid valve
2. Narrowing in the area of the aortic valve
3. Localized constriction or narrowing of the aortic wall
4. Narrowing at some location along the right ventricular outflow tract

50. 3. Coarctation of the aorta consists of a localized constriction or narrowing of the aortic wall. Tricuspid atresia is characterized by an absent tricuspid valve. Aortic stenosis is a narrowing in the area of the aortic valve. Pulmonary stenosis consists of a narrowing along the right ventricular outflow tract.
CN: Health promotion and maintenance; CNS: None; CL: Apply; DIFFICULTY: Challenge

51. A child is diagnosed with coarctation of the aorta. Which finding would the nurse expect when observing this child?
1. Normal blood pressure
2. Increased blood pressure in the upper extremities
3. Decreased blood pressure in the upper extremities
4. Decreased or absent pulses in the upper extremities

51. 2. As blood is pumped from the left ventricle to the aorta, some blood flows to the head and upper extremities while the rest meets obstruction and jets through the constricted area. Pressures and pulses are greater in the upper extremities. Decreased or absent pulses are found in the lower extremities.
CN: Physiological integrity; CNS: Physiological adaptation; CL: Analyze; DIFFICULTY: Moderate

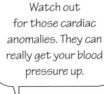
Watch out for those cardiac anomalies. They can really get your blood pressure up.

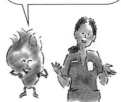

52. Which factor is an important part of observing a child with a possible cardiac anomaly?
1. Skin turgor
2. Temperature
3. Pupil size and reaction to light
4. Blood pressure in four extremities

52. 4. Measuring blood pressure in all four extremities in a child with a possible cardiac anomaly is necessary to document hypertension and the blood pressure gradient between the upper and lower extremities. Temperature, skin turgor, and pupillary assessment are also important, but they are not as specific for cardiac assessment as blood pressure.
CN: Physiological integrity; CNS: Physiological adaptation; CL: Apply; DIFFICULTY: Easy

53. A child with coarctation of the aorta experiences a postsurgical recoarctation. Which treatment should the nurse expect the health care provider to recommend?
1. Bypass graft repair
2. Patch aortoplasty
3. Balloon angioplasty
4. Left subclavian flap angioplasty

54. Which intervention is recommended postoperatively for a child with repair of a coarctation of the aorta?
1. Give a vasoconstrictor.
2. Maintain hypothermia.
3. Maintain a low blood pressure.
4. Give a bolus of IV fluids.

55. Which observation is expected in a child with tetralogy of Fallot?
1. Machinelike murmur
2. Eisenmenger complex
3. Increasing cyanosis with crying or activity
4. Higher pressure in the upper extremities than in the lower extremities

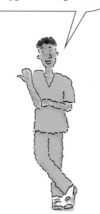

No, not that kind of clubbing. We're talking about fingers and toes swelling due to a lack of oxygen, not nightlife.

56. A child with tetralogy of Fallot has clubbing of the fingers and toes. The nurse understands that this finding is related to which condition?
1. Polycythemia
2. Chronic hypoxia
3. Pansystolic murmur
4. Abnormal growth and development

57. The parents of a 3-year-old with a congenital heart disease are being seen for a check-up. They report that they are concerned about giving a flu vaccine to their child. Which statement is appropriate for inclusion in the nurse's response?
1. "Since there are troubling side effects in the vaccine for your child I would instead recommend the other members of the household be immunized instead."
2. "The flu vaccine is both safe and recommended to children who have chronic illness such as heart disease."
3. "You are right to be concerned since this vaccine should be provided to children who are older than 3 years of age."
4. "As long as you are careful who your child is exposed to you should be fine to avoid giving this vaccine."

53. 3. Balloon angioplasty is the treatment of choice for postsurgical recoarctation. Bypass graft repair, patch aortoplasty, and left subclavian flap angioplasty are surgical options to treat the original coarctation.
CN: Physiological integrity; CNS: Physiological adaptation; CL: Analyze; DIFFICULTY: Moderate

54. 3. Blood pressure is tightly managed and kept low, so there's no excessive pressure on the fresh suture lines. Vasoconstrictors would be contraindicated. Normal body temperature is maintained, and diuretics may be given to decrease fluid volume.
CN: Physiological integrity; CNS: Physiological adaptation; CL: Analyze; DIFFICULTY: Moderate

55. 3. A child with tetralogy of Fallot will be mildly cyanotic at rest and have increasing cyanosis with crying, activity, or straining, as with a bowel movement. A machinelike murmur is a characteristic of patent ductus arteriosus. Eisenmenger complex is a complication of ventricular resistance exceeding systemic pressure. Higher pressures in the upper extremities are characteristic of coarctation of the aorta.
CN: Physiological integrity; CNS: Physiological adaptation; CL: Apply; DIFFICULTY: Moderate

56. 2. Chronic hypoxia causes clubbing of the fingers and toes when untreated. Hypoxia varies with the degree of pulmonary stenosis. Polycythemia is an increased number of red blood cells as a result of chronic hypoxemia. A pansystolic murmur is heard at the middle to lower left sternal border but has no impact on clubbing. Growth and development may appear normal.
CN: Physiological integrity; CNS: Physiological adaptation; CL: Understand; DIFFICULTY: Moderate

57. 2. Children who have heart disease and other chronic illnesses are vulnerable to the flu. Immunization is recommended for the child. Any possible side effects are of lesser concern than contracting the flu. Children ages 2 or older may receive the flu vaccine. It is important to avoid exposing a vulnerable child to at-risk populations but this is not as large a safeguard as providing the immunization.
CN: Safe, effective care environment; CNS: Safety and infection control; CL: Apply; DIFFICULTY: Moderate

58. A child with tetralogy of Fallot may assume which position of comfort during exercise?
1. Prone
2. Semi-Fowler's
3. Side-lying
4. Squat

59. A child diagnosed with tetralogy of Fallot has been ordered to undergo testing. Which test would the nurse prepare the child for that will indicate the direction and amount of shunting in this child?
1. Chest radiography
2. Echocardiography
3. Electrocardiography
4. Cardiac catheterization

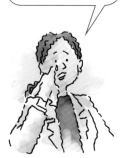

Don't get upset if you can't figure out a question— just move on to the next one.

60. The nurse is talking with the parents of a child who has been diagnosed with tricuspid atresia. Which statements indicate the need for further instruction? Select all that apply.
1. "There's a narrowing at the aortic outflow tract."
2. "The pulmonary veins don't return to the left atrium."
3. "There's a narrowing at the entrance of the pulmonary artery."
4. "The child's tricuspid valve did not fully develop."
5. "There is no communication between the right atrium and the right ventricle."

61. Which characteristic can the nurse document when gathering data from a child with tricuspid atresia?
1. Cyanosis
2. Machinelike murmur
3. Decreased respiratory rate
4. Capillary refill more than 2 seconds

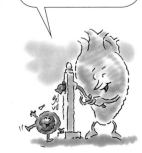

Hearts are the most important pumps in the world. They keep us healthy so we can do our job.

62. When reviewing the laboratory studies from a child with tricuspid atresia, which finding would the nurse expect to observe?
1. Acidosis
2. Alkalosis
3. Normal red blood cell (RBC) count
4. Normal arterial oxygen saturation

58. 4. A child may squat or assume a knee-chest position to reduce venous blood flow from the lower extremities and to increase systemic vascular resistance, which diverts more blood flow into the pulmonary artery. Prone, semi-Fowler, and side-lying positions won't produce this effect.
CN: Physiological integrity; CNS: Physiological adaptation; CL: Analyze; DIFFICULTY: Moderate

59. 4. Cardiac catheterization provides specific information about the direction and amount of shunting, coronary anatomy, and each portion of the heart defect. Chest radiographs show right ventricular hypertrophy pushing the heart apex upward, resulting in a boot-shaped silhouette. Echocardiogram scans define such defects as large ventricular septal defects, pulmonary stenosis, and malposition of the aorta. Electrocardiograms show right ventricular hypertrophy with tall R waves.
CN: Physiological integrity; CNS: Physiological adaptation; CL: Apply; DIFFICULTY: Moderate

60. 4, 5. Tricuspid atresia is failure of the tricuspid valve to develop, leaving no communication between the right atrium and the right ventricle. Narrowing at the aortic outflow tract is aortic stenosis. Total anomalous pulmonary venous return is a defect in which the pulmonary veins don't return to the left atrium but abnormally return to the right side of the heart. Narrowing at the entrance of the pulmonary artery represents pulmonic stenosis.
CN: Physiological integrity; CNS: Physiological adaptation; CL: Analyze; DIFFICULTY: Difficult

61. 1. Cyanosis is the most consistent clinical sign of tricuspid atresia. A machinelike murmur is characteristic of a patent ductus arteriosus. Tricuspid atresia doesn't have a characteristic murmur. Tachypnea and dyspnea are typically present because of the pulmonary blood flow and right-to-left shunting. Decreased oxygenation increases capillary refill time.
CN: Physiological integrity; CNS: Physiological adaptation; CL: Analyze; DIFFICULTY: Difficult

62. 1. In tricuspid atresia, the tricuspid valve is completely closed so that no blood flows from the right atrium to the right ventricle. Therefore, no oxygenation of blood occurs. The child has chronic hypoxemia and acidosis, not alkalosis, due to decreased atrial oxygenation. This chronic hypoxemia leads to polycythemia, so a normal RBC wouldn't result. Arterial oxygenation isn't normal, as the blood bypasses the lungs and the step of oxygenation.
CN: Physiological integrity; CNS: Physiological adaptation; CL: Analyze; DIFFICULTY: Difficult

63. Which action is appropriate for the nurse to perform when administering digoxin to an infant?
1. Mix the digoxin with the infant's food.
2. Double the subsequent dose if a dose is missed.
3. Give the digoxin with antacids when possible.
4. Withhold the dose if the apical pulse rate is less than 90 beats/minute.

63. 4. Digoxin is used to decrease heart rate; however, the apical pulse must be carefully monitored to detect a severe reduction. Administering digoxin to an infant with a heart rate of less than 90 beats/minute could further reduce the rate and compromise cardiac output. Mixing digoxin with other food may interfere with accurate dosing. Double-dosing should never be done. Antacids may decrease absorption of digoxin.

CN: Physiological integrity; CNS: Pharmacological therapies; CL: Apply; DIFFICULTY: Easy

64. The nurse is reviewing a listing of assigned clients. Which client should be seen **first**?
1. A 13-year-old child who is hospitalized with suspected cardiomyopathy and is scheduled for a cardiac catheterization the following day.
2. An 8 year old child who had a cardiac catheterization 3 hours prior who reportedly has a 2 cm spot of drainage on the dressing.
3. A 9 year old child who had cardiac surgery 2 days ago and is reporting pain rated a level of 5 on a 10 point scale.
4. A 14 year old child who had cardiac surgery 2 days ago and who had urinary output of 200 mL over the past 8 hours.

64. 4. A urinary output of 200 mL/hr is less than an average of 30 mL each hour. This signals potential complications. This child should be seen first. The other children are considered stable in relation.

CN: Safe, effective care environment; CNS: Coordinated care; CL: Analyze; DIFFICULTY: Moderate

65. The nurse is caring for a child who is experiencing a hypercyanotic episode. Which actions by the nurse will be of benefit to the child? Select all that apply.
1. Encourage the child to take deep breaths.
2. Assist the child to a semi-Fowler position.
3. Provide supplemental oxygen.
4. Assist the child into a knee-chest position.
5. Use a soothing tone of voice when interacting with the child during the episode.

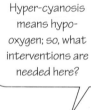

Hyper-cyanosis means hypo-oxygen; so, what interventions are needed here?

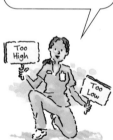

65. 1, 3, 4, 5. Cyanosis has resulted from a lack of oxygenation. Activities should focus on relieving anxiety and promoting oxygenation and perfusion to the body's tissues. Deep breaths and supplemental oxygen will provide increased oxygen intake. Knee-chest positioning improves pulmonary oxygenation. A soothing tone of voice will enhance relaxation and calm the child. The use of a semi-Fowler position will not improve oxygenation.

CN: Physiological integrity; CNS: Basic care and comfort; CL: Apply, DIFFICULTY: Difficult

66. Which finding is common when gathering data from a child with a total anomalous pulmonary venous return defect?
1. Hypertension
2. Frequent respiratory infections
3. Normal growth and development
4. Above average weight gain on the growth chart

66. 2. Children with total anomalous pulmonary venous return defects are prone to repeated respiratory infections due to increased pulmonary blood flow. Hypertension usually occurs with coarctation of the aorta, an acyanotic defect with obstructive flow. Poor feeding and failure to thrive are also signs of a total anomalous pulmonary venous return defect, as are infants that look thin and malnourished.

CN: Physiological integrity; CNS: Physiological adaptation; CL: Apply; DIFFICULTY: Moderate

67. A child has undergone a repair of total anomalous pulmonary venous return and develops pulmonary hypertension postoperatively. Which finding would the nurse be **most** likely to observe in a child with this condition?
1. Hypotension
2. Hypertension
3. Bradycardia
4. Tachypnea

67. 4. Pulmonary hypertension may result as a postoperative complication of this procedure, which can cause hypoxia. Symptoms of hypoxia include tachypnea, cyanosis, chest retractions, and fatigue.

CN: Physiological integrity; CNS: Physiological adaptation; CL: Apply; DIFFICULTY: Moderate

68. The nurse is reviewing orders from the primary health care provider for a child scheduled for cardiac surgery the following day. Which orders will likely be included? Select all that apply.
1. Complete blood count
2. Electrolyte levels
3. Urinalysis
4. 2 step TB test
5. Partial prothrombin time (PTT)

68. 1, 2, 3, 5. During the preoperative period diagnostic testing is anticipated. The information obtained provides a baseline for comparison after the test and, additionally, it can alert the health care provider to any problems prior to the procedure. Tests that are commonly ordered during the preoperative period include a complete blood count, electrolyte levels, urinalysis, and bleeding time studies such as a partial prothrombin time (PTT). A 2 step TB test is not needed for the client scheduled for a cardiac procedure. The partial prothrombin time does provide information about clotting times but is not a part of routine preoperative testing.
CN: Health promotion and maintenance; CNS: None; CL: Apply; DIFFICULTY: Difficult

69. Which finding would a nurse expect to observe in a child with truncus arteriosus?
1. Weak, thready pulses
2. Narrowed pulse pressure
3. Pink, moist mucous membranes
4. Harsh systolic ejection murmur

69. 4. As a result of the ventricular septal defect of truncus arteriosus, a harsh systolic ejection murmur is heard along the left sternal border and is usually accompanied by a thrill. Increasing pulmonary blood flow causes bounding pulses and a widened pulse pressure. Pulmonary stenosis leads to mild or moderate cyanosis, so mucous membranes may appear dull or gray.
CN: Physiological integrity; CNS: Physiological adaptation; CL: Apply; DIFFICULTY: Challenge

70. The health care provider has prescribed digoxin and a diuretic for a child. How should the nurse administer the drug to the child?
1. Use a measuring spoon.
2. Use a graduated dropper.
3. Mix the drug with baby food.
4. Mix the drug in a bottle with juice or milk.

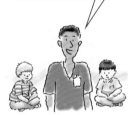
When administering digoxin, it's important for the dosage to be exact.

70. 2. Using a graduated dropper allows the exact dosage to be given. A measuring spoon isn't as exact as a graduated dropper. Mixing drugs with juice, milk, or food is problematic because, if the child doesn't completely finish the meal, the nurse can't determine the exact amount ingested. In addition, this may prevent the child from drinking or eating for fear of tasting the drug.
CN: Physiological integrity; CNS: Pharmacological therapies; CL: Apply; DIFFICULTY: Easy

71. The nurse is caring for a newborn who has transposition of the great arteries. When reviewing the neonate's medical record which findings are consistent with this disorder? Select all that apply.
1. The newborn's mother has diabetes.
2. The newborn's mother was treated with bacterial pneumonia during the pregnancy.
3. The newborn's mother reported excessive alcohol use during the pregnancy.
4. The newborn's mother has a history of chronic hypertension.
5. The newborn's mother became pregnant while taking combination oral contraceptives.

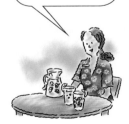
Feeling weary? Take a short break and refresh yourself.

71. 1, 3. The exact cause of transposition of the great arteries is unknown. There are a series of factors which are associated with the condition. Maternal diabetes and excessive alcohol intake in pregnancy are associated with the occurrence of the condition. Viral infections, not bacterial infections, during pregnancy are tied to the condition. Hypertension in the mother is not tied to the condition. Oral contraceptive use in the mother prior to or during pregnancy is not tied to the condition.
CN: Physiological integrity; CNS: Reduction of risk potential; CL: apply; DIFFICULTY: Challenge

72. Which change would the nurse expect after administering oxygen to an infant with uncorrected tetralogy of Fallot?
1. Disappearance of the murmur
2. No evidence of cyanosis
3. Improvement of finger clubbing
4. Less agitation

72. 4. Supplemental oxygen will help the infant breathe more easily and feel less anxious or agitated. None of the other findings occurs as the result of supplemental oxygen administration.
CN: Physiological integrity; CNS: Basic care and comfort; CL: Apply; DIFFICULTY: Challenge

CN: Client needs category   CNS: Client needs subcategory   CL: Cognitive level

73. The nurse is caring for a gravid woman whose health care provider is concerned that the fetus may have transposition of the great arteries. Which procedure will provide the **most** definitive information about this condition?
1. Amniocentesis
2. Echocardiography
3. Percutaneous umbilical cord sampling
4. Nuchal translucency measurement

74. A nurse is caring for a child with transposition of the great arteries. Which associated defect should the nurse expect to see in this client?
1. Mitral atresia
2. Atrial septal defect
3. Patent foramen ovale
4. Hypoplasia of the left ventricle

75. A 9-year-old child had cardiac surgery 2 days ago. The child reports being sore and doesn't want to move much today. Which action by the nurse is **most** appropriate?
1. Agree to allow the child to rest today after promising to get up tomorrow.
2. Medicate the child for discomfort and then begin activities related to ambulation.
3. Inform the child that soreness will get worse without moving from the bed.
4. Ask the parents to encourage the child to get up.

76. Balloon dilation valvuloplasty treatment is planned for an adolescent with valvular pulmonic stenosis. When reviewing information with the teen which statement indicates the need for further instruction? Select all that apply.
1. "I will be prescribed diuretic therapy for an indefinite period after my procedure."
2. "The outcomes for this procedure are positive for the majority of clients."
3. "This procedure may need to be repeated in 10 years or so."
4. "I will likely need to have open heart surgery within 6 to 12 months of this procedure to achieve the best outcome for my health."
5. "Unfortunately, I will not be able to participate in sporting activities after my recovery."

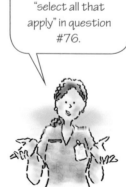

Remember to "select all that apply" in question #76.

73. 2. An echocardiogram can be used to diagnose transposition of the great arteries. It can be done to assess the fetus in utero. An ultrasound may be performed to assess gross cardiac anatomy. Percutaneous umbilical cord sampling is used to collect a fetal blood sample. This can be used to determine genetic information. Nuchal translucency is used to assess for the presence of Down syndrome.
CN: Health promotion and maintenance; CNS: None; CL: Apply; DIFFICULTY: Moderate

74. 3. A patent foramen ovale, patent ductus arteriosus, and ventricular septal defect are associated defects related to transposition of the great arteries. A patent foramen ovale is the most common atrial septal defect and is necessary to provide adequate mixing of blood between the two circulations. An atrial septal defect is common in association with total anomalous pulmonary venous return. Hypoplasia of the left ventricle and mitral atresia are two defects associated with hypoplastic left heart syndrome.
CN: Physiological integrity; CNS: Physiological adaptation; CL: Analyze; DIFFICULTY: Challenge

75. 2. Postoperative pain is an anticipated occurrence. Despite the discomfort the client must ambulate. Prolonging ambulation for a day may promote complications. Medicating the child will allow achievement of an increased level of comfort prior to the activity. The child should know that ambulation does aid in preventing complications but it does not manage the root problem, which is pain. The parents should be involved in the care being delivered but they should not be used to threaten the child; this again does not alleviate the issue, which is pain.
CN: Health promotion and maintenance; CNS: None; CL: Apply; DIFFICULTY: Moderate

76. 1, 4, 5. The narrowing in the vessels for the client with valvular pulmonic stenosis is often successfully managed with balloon dilation valvuloplasty. This procedure has a positive outcome rating for adolescents. This procedure is usually all that is needed, and if successful open heart surgery will not be necessary. Diuretic therapy is not indicated in the management of this condition. Participation in sports is not prohibited for those with condition.
CN: Health promotion and maintenance; CNS: None; CL: Apply; DIFFICULTY: Difficult

77. The parents of a 3-week-old infant diagnosed with tricuspid atresia are discussing the planned courses of therapy with the nurse. Which statements indicate an understanding of the condition and traditional courses of treatment? Select all that apply.

1. "My child will likely need a series of corrective procedures."
2. "It will be difficult but the surgical repairs will be completed by my child's first birthday.
3. "The initial procedures will be performed to increase blood flow."
4. "Children with this disorder often have a significantly reduced life expectancy."
5. "The final procedures to manage this condition should be completed once she is in her later teen years and has stopped growing."

78. Which finding is seen during cardiac catheterization of a child with pulmonic stenosis?

1. Right-to-left shunting
2. Left-to-right shunting
3. Decreased pressure in the right side of the heart
4. Increased oxygenation in the left side of the heart

79. A nurse is caring for a 16-year-old adolescent with aortic stenosis. Which finding is associated with aortic stenosis when the teen is active?

1. Chest pain
2. Right ventricular failure
3. Increased cardiac output
4. Loud systolic murmur with a thrill

80. A nurse is reinforcing education for the parents of a child with congenital aortic stenosis. Which statement should the nurse include in the education about this disorder?

1. "It can result from rheumatic fever (infection with group A streptococci)."
2. "It accounts for 25% of all congenital defects."
3. "It causes an increase in cardiac output."
4. "It's classified as an acyanotic defect with increased pulmonary blood flow."

81. Which instruction by the nurse would be **most** appropriate for a child with symptomatic aortic stenosis?

1. Restrict exercise.
2. Avoid prostaglandin E1.
3. Avoid digoxin and diuretics.
4. Allow the child to exercise freely.

Yo. The name's strep. Let's just say I'm a real heartbreaker.

77. 1, 3. In tricuspid atresia one of the tricuspid valves has not developed and is instead a solid band of tissue. Management of the condition traditionally includes a series of surgical corrections. The first procedure can be done between 3 and 6 months of age. The final procedure can usually be completed once the child reaches 2 years of age. Procedures performed initially are to increase flood flow. The children who have this condition usually have corrective procedures and then are able to live a relatively normal life into adulthood.
CN: Physiological integrity; CNS: Reduction of risk potential; CL: Apply; DIFFICULTY: Challenge

78. 1. In pulmonic stenosis, right-to-left shunting develops through a patent foramen ovale due to right ventricular failure and an increase in pressure in the right side of the heart. Decreased oxygenation in the left side of the heart is noted due to the right-to-left shunt.
CN: Physiological integrity; CNS: Physiological adaptation; CL: Analyze; DIFFICULTY: Difficult

79. 1. Children with aortic stenosis may develop chest pain similar to angina when they're active. They're also at risk for hypotension, tachycardia, angina, syncope, left ventricular failure, dyspnea, fatigue, and palpitations. Poor left ventricular ejection leads to decreased cardiac output. Loud systolic murmurs are heard with ventricular septal defects.
CN: Physiological integrity; CNS: Physiological adaptation; CL: Apply; DIFFICULTY: Moderate

80. 1. Aortic stenosis can result from rheumatic fever, which can damage the aortic valve in the first 8 weeks of pregnancy. It accounts for about 5% of all congenital heart defects. It causes a decrease in cardiac output. It's classified as an acyanotic defect with obstructed flow from the ventricles.
CN: Physiological integrity; CNS: Physiological adaptation; CL: Analyze; DIFFICULTY: Difficult

81. 1. In a child with symptomatic aortic stenosis, exercise should be restricted due to low cardiac output and left ventricular failure. Prostaglandin E1 is recommended to maintain the patency of the ductus arteriosus in neonates. This allows for improved systemic blood flow. Digoxin and diuretics may be required for critically ill children experiencing heart failure as a result of severe aortic stenosis. Strenuous activity has been reported to result in sudden death from the development of myocardial ischemia.
CN: Physiological integrity; CNS: Physiological adaptation; CL: Apply; DIFFICULTY: Moderate

82. The nurse is discussing nutritional needs with the mother of a newborn diagnosed with hypoplastic left heart syndrome. What information should be included in the discussion? Select all that apply.
1. Feeding should be limited to 15 minute sessions to avoid overtiring the baby.
2. High-calorie formulas may be added to the baby's diet.
3. Frequent weighing is of the baby is needed.
4. Tube feedings may be instituted to ensure adequate nutritional intake.
5. Bottle feeding is recommended for the child with hypoplastic left heart syndrome.

83. The nurse is talking with the parent of a 5-year-old child. The parent reports having recently read an article about rheumatic fever and heart disease and questions how to prevent this from happening to the child. What is the **best** response by the nurse?
1. "Making sure your child has the annual influenza vaccine is the most important thing you can do."
2. "Your child is not susceptible since there is no history of cardiac problems."
3. "Prompt treatment of strep infections is a key to preventing this condition."
4. "The pneumococcal vaccine is needed to reduce your child's risk."

84. A 3-year-old child has a high red blood cell count and polycythemia. When assisting with the planning of care which action will be of **greatest** impact in preventing complications?
1. Promote adequate fluid intake.
2. Encourage the appropriate number of calories daily.
3. Administer iron supplements as prescribed.
4. Encourage daily period of exercise.

85. A child receives prednisone after a heart transplant. For which adverse reaction to prednisone would a nurse monitor in this child?
1. Weight loss
2. Hyperpyrexia
3. Anorexia
4. Poor wound healing

86. A child is given 0.5 mg/kg/day of prednisone divided into two doses. The child weighs 10 kg. How much is given in each dose? Record your answer using one decimal place.

_____ mg

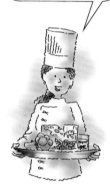

Make sure your neonatal clients are plumping up—especially after surgery.

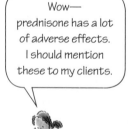

Wow—prednisone has a lot of adverse effects. I should mention these to my clients.

82. 2, 3, 4. The infant with hypoplastic left heart syndrome may experience difficulty with feeding. Feeding may be tiring. This may result in inadequate weight gain or weight loss. High-caloric formulas maybe prescribed. Frequent weighing will be needed to assess weight gain. Tube feedings may be instituted if weight loss becomes a concern. Limiting feedings may be done but 15 minutes is not excessive. Bottle feeding is not encouraged over breast-feeding.
CN: Physiological integrity; CNS: Basic care and comfort; CL: Analyze; DIFFICULTY: Difficult

83. 3. Rheumatic fever is often caused by a strep infection in children. Seeking prompt care and following treatment recommendations is key in prevention of complications. Although the influenza vaccine and pneumococcal vaccine are recommended for a 5-year-old child, they will not reduce the risk of rheumatic fever or rheumatic heart disease.
CN: Safe, effective care environment; CNS: Safety and infection control; CL: Apply; DIFFICULTY: Easy

84. 1. Dehydration is a concern with polycythemia. Adequate fluid intake will be assistive in preventing complications. The other items may be included in the plan of care but are not of the highest priority.
CN: Health promotion and maintenance; CNS: None; CL: Apply; DIFFICULTY: Moderate

85. 4. Common adverse reactions to prednisone include poor wound healing, weight gain, delayed temperature response, increased appetite, delayed sexual maturation, growth impairment, and a Cushingoid appearance. The school-aged child who has received prednisone is usually overweight and has a moon-shaped face.
CN: Physiological integrity; CNS: Pharmacological therapies; CL: Apply; DIFFICULTY: Moderate

86. 2.5.
Use the following equations:

$$0.5 \text{ mg} / \text{kg} \times 10 \text{ kg} = 5 \text{ mg}$$
$$5 \text{ mg} / 2 \text{ doses} = 2.5 \text{ mg} / \text{dose}$$

CN: Physiological integrity; CNS: Pharmacological therapies; CL: Analyze; DIFFICULTY: Moderate

87. The nurse is discussing bacterial/infective endocarditis with the parent of a teen who has been diagnosed with the disorder. Which statement about bacterial/infective endocarditis indicates an understanding of the condition?
1. It is caused by bacteria invading only tissues of the heart.
2. It is an infection of the valves and inner lining of the heart.
3. It is an inappropriate fusion of the endocardial cushions in fetal life.
4. It is caused by alterations in cardiac preload, afterload, contractility, or heart rate.

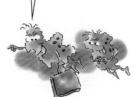

Ooh, look! It's the heart—my favorite organ to infect. We can do some real damage there.

87. 2. Bacterial/infective endocarditis is an infection of the valves and inner lining of the heart. It's usually caused by the bacteria *Streptococcus viridans* and frequently affects children with acquired or congenital anomalies of the heart or great vessels. Bacteria may grow into adjacent tissues and may break off and embolize elsewhere, such as the spleen, kidney, lung, skin, and central nervous system. Endocardial cushion defects result from inappropriate fusion of the endocardial cushions in fetal life. Alterations in preload, afterload, contractility, or heart rate occur in heart failure.
CN: Physiological integrity; CNS: Physiological adaptation; CL: Analyze; DIFFICULTY: Easy

88. A child receives prednisone after undergoing a heart transplant. What is the desired outcome of this medication?
1. Stimulate appetite
2. Suppress immune response
3. Improve wound healing
4. Prevent fluid retention

88. 2. The goal of prednisone for this client is to suppress the immune system, thereby preventing organ rejection. Prednisone is often used in combination with other immunosuppressant medications in order to prevent rejection. While corticosteroids do stimulate appetites, that is not the desired effect for this child. Prednisone and other corticosteroids decrease wound healing; fluid retention is one of their side effects.
CN: Physiological integrity; CNS: Physiological adaptation; CL: Apply; DIFFICULTY: Moderate

89. A child with suspected bacterial endocarditis arrives at the emergency department. Which finding is expected during data collection?
1. Weight gain
2. Bradycardia
3. Low-grade fever
4. Increased hemoglobin level

89. 3. Symptoms may include a low-grade intermittent fever, tachycardia, anorexia, weight loss, decreased activity level, and a decrease in hemoglobin level.
CN: Physiological integrity; CNS: Physiological adaptation; CL: Apply; DIFFICULTY: Moderate

90. The nurse is gathering data from a parent of a child with possible bacterial endocarditis who also has an underlying heart condition. What data indicates the child has a risk factor for this disease?
1. History of a cold for 3 days
2. Dental work pretreated with antibiotics
3. Peripheral IV catheter in place for 1 day
4. Indwelling urinary catheter for 2 days leading to a urinary tract infection

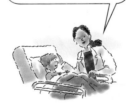

Routes for infection abound in the hospital. Become an expert at identifying them and taking preventive measures.

90. 4. Bacterial organisms can enter the bloodstream from any site of infection, such as a urinary tract infection. Gram-negative bacilli are common causative agents. A peripheral IV catheter is an entry site but only if signs and symptoms of infection are present. Colds are usually viral, not bacterial. Dental work is a common portal of entry if not pretreated with antibiotics. Long-term indwelling catheters pose a higher risk of infection. Heart surgery is also a common cause of endocarditis, especially if synthetic material is used.
CN: Physiological integrity; CNS: Physiological adaptation; CL: Analyze; DIFFICULTY: Moderate

91. Erythromycin is given to a 6-year-old child before dental work to prevent endocarditis. The child weighs 44 lb (20 kg). The order is for 20 mg/kg by mouth 2 hours before the procedure. How many milligrams should be given to this child? Record your answer using a whole number.

_____ mg

91. 400.
Use the child's weight in kilograms. Then, use the following equation:

$$20 \text{ mg}/\text{kg} \times 20 \text{ kg} = 400 \text{ mg}$$

CN: Physiological integrity; CNS: Pharmacological therapies; CL: Analyze; DIFFICULTY: Moderate

92. What would be the **most** common adverse reaction a nurse might observe after administering enteric-coated erythromycin?
1. Weight gain
2. Constipation
3. Increased appetite
4. Nausea and vomiting

93. Which characteristic indicates a child with Kawasaki disease has entered the subacute phase?
1. Polymorphous rash
2. Normal blood values
3. Cervical lymphadenopathy
4. Desquamation of the hands and feet

94. An adolescent with endocarditis is preparing for discharge from the hospital. The parents and child have had instruction about symptoms that may signal further cardiac complications. Which symptoms indicate potential cardiac complications? Select all that apply.
1. Skin rash
2. Diarrhea
3. Increasing fatigue
4. Swelling in the lower extremities
5. Temperature elevations

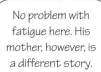

No problem with fatigue here. His mother, however, is a different story.

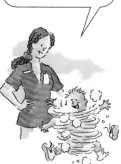

95. When obtaining data from a child with suspected Kawasaki disease, which symptom is common?
1. Low-grade fever
2. "Strawberry" tongue
3. Pink, moist mucous membranes
4. Abdominal pain

96. A nurse is reinforcing education for the parents of a child with Kawasaki disease. Which statement should the nurse include in the education about this disorder?
1. "It mostly occurs in the summer and fall."
2. "Diagnosis can be determined by laboratory testing."
3. "It's an acute systemic vasculitis of unknown cause."
4. "It manifests in two different stages: acute and subacute."

97. A child is prescribed aspirin as part of the therapy for Kawasaki disease. The order is for 80 mg/kg/day orally in four divided doses until the child is afebrile. The child weighs 15 kg. How much is given in one dose? Record your answer using a whole number.

_____ mg

92. 4. Erythromycin is an antibacterial antibiotic. Common adverse effects include nausea, vomiting, anorexia, diarrhea, and abdominal pain. It should be given with a full glass (8 oz) of water after meals or with food to lessen GI symptoms.
CN: Physiological integrity; CNS: Pharmacological therapies;
CL: Apply; DIFFICULTY: Easy

93. 4. The subacute phase shows characteristic desquamation of the hands and feet. Blood values return to normal at the end of the convalescent phase. Polymorphous rash and cervical lymphadenopathy can be seen in the acute phase because of the onset of inflammation and fever.
CN: Physiological integrity; CNS: Physiological adaptation;
CL: Analyze; DIFFICULTY: Moderate

94. 3, 4. The adolescent with endocarditis is at risk for the development of further cardiac complications. Increasing fatigue may signal cardiac insufficiency. Swelling and edema are associated with heart failure. The client with endocarditis will be discharged to home with continued antibiotic therapy. A skin rash and diarrhea signal possible reactions to the antibiotic therapy and are not likely cardiac in nature.
CN: Heath promotion and maintenance; CNS: none; CL: Apply;
DIFFICULTY: Challenge

95. 2. Inflammation of the pharynx and oral mucosa develops in Kawasaki disease, causing red, cracked lips and a "strawberry" tongue, in which the normal coating of the tongue sloughs off. A high fever of 5 or more days unresponsive to antibiotics and antipyretics is also part of the diagnostic criteria. Abdominal pain would suggest a possible GI problem. Pink, moist mucous membranes are a normal finding.
CN: Physiological integrity; CNS: Physiological adaptation;
CL: Apply; DIFFICULTY: Easy

96. 3. Kawasaki disease can best be described as an acute systemic vasculitis of unknown cause. Most cases are geographic and seasonal, occurring in the late winter and early spring. Diagnosis is based on clinical findings of five of the six diagnostic criteria and associated laboratory results. There's no specific laboratory test for diagnosis. There are three stages: acute, subacute, and convalescent.
CN: Physiological integrity; CNS: Physiological adaptation;
CL: Apply; DIFFICULTY: Moderate

97. 300.
Use the following equations:

$$80 \text{ mg} / \text{kg} \times 15 \text{ kg} = 1{,}200 \text{ mg}$$
$$1{,}200 \text{ mg} / 4 \text{ doses} = 300 \text{ mg} / \text{dose}$$

CN: Physiological integrity; CNS: Pharmacological therapies;
CL: Analyze; DIFFICULTY: Moderate

CN: Client needs category   CNS: Client needs subcategory   CL: Cognitive level

98. The nurse is caring for a child who is in the second phase of Kawasaki disease. Which findings are consistent with this stage of the illness? Select all that apply.
1. Diarrhea
2. Abdominal pain
3. Joint pain
4. Swollen, reddened palms
5. Peeling skin

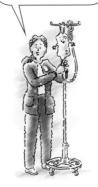

My little friend here is not that great at math. Can you calculate his dose in question #99?

99. Therapy for Kawasaki disease includes IV gamma globulin, prescribed at 400 mg/kg/day for 4 days. The child weighs 10 kg. What's the daily dose for this child? Record your answer using a whole number.

_____ mg

100. A 2-month-old infant arrives in the emergency department with a heart rate of 180 beats/minute and a temperature of 103.1° F (39.5° C) rectally. Which intervention is **most** appropriate?
1. Administer acetaminophen.
2. Encourage fluid intake.
3. Apply carotid massage.
4. Place the infant's hands in cold water.

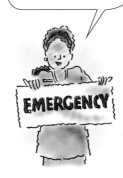

Gotta get that temperature down, STAT!

EMERGENCY

101. A nurse is caring for a child with Kawasaki disease. Which symptom concerns the nurse the **most**?
1. Mild diarrhea
2. Pain in the joints
3. Abdominal pain with vomiting
4. Increased erythrocyte sedimentation rate

102. A nurse is reinforcing discharge instructions to the parents of a child with Kawasaki disease. Which statement shows an understanding of the treatment plan?
1. "A regular diet can be resumed at home."
2. "Black, tarry stools are considered normal."
3. "My child should use a soft-bristled toothbrush."
4. "My child can return to playing football next week."

98. 1, 2, 3, 5. Kawasaki disease is characterized by inflammation of the walls of the body's arteries, including those of the heart. The condition has three phases. In the second phase symptoms include gastrointestinal problems such as abdominal pain and diarrhea. Joint pain is also seen in the second phase. Skin peeling on the hands and feet is also seen in the second phase. Red, swollen palms are seen in the initial phase of the disease.
CN: Physiological integrity; CNS: Physiological adaptation; CL: Apply; DIFFICULTY: Difficult

99. 4,000.
Use the following equation:

$$400 \text{ mg / kg} \times 10 \text{ kg} = 4,000 \text{ mg (or 4 g)}$$

CN: Physiological integrity; CNS: Pharmacological therapies; CL: Analyze; DIFFICULTY: Moderate

100. 1. Acetaminophen should be given first to decrease the infant's temperature. A heart rate of 180 beats/minute is normal in an infant with a fever. Fluid intake is encouraged after the acetaminophen is given to help replace insensible fluid losses. Carotid massage is an attempt to decrease the heart rate as a vagal maneuver; it won't work in this infant because the source of the increased heart rate is fever. A tepid sponge bath may be given to help decrease the temperature and calm the infant.
CN: Physiological integrity; CNS: Physiological adaptation; CL: Apply; DIFFICULTY: Easy

101. 3. The most serious complication of Kawasaki disease is cardiac involvement. Abdominal pain, vomiting, and restlessness are the main symptoms of an acute myocardial infarction in children. Mild diarrhea can be treated with oral fluids. Pain in the joints is an expected sign of arthritis that usually occurs in the subacute phase. An increased erythrocyte sedimentation rate is a reflection of the inflammatory process and may be seen for 2 to 4 weeks after the onset of symptoms.
CN: Physiological integrity; CNS: Physiological adaptation; CL: Analyze; DIFFICULTY: Challenge

102. 3. Because of the anticoagulant effects of aspirin therapy, a soft-bristled toothbrush will prevent bleeding of the gums. A low-cholesterol diet should be followed until coronary artery involvement resolves, usually within 6 to 8 weeks. Black, tarry stools are abnormal and are signs of bleeding that should be reported to the health care provider immediately. Contact sports should be avoided because of the cardiac involvement and excessive bruising that may occur due to aspirin therapy.
CN: Physiological integrity; CNS: Physiological adaptation; CL: Analyze; DIFFICULTY: Easy

103. The parent of a 10-year-old who has been diagnosed with an upper respiratory infection questions the nurse about the potential development of rheumatic heart disease. What information is appropriate for the nurse to include in the response? Select all that apply.
1. The condition is genetically more likely to occur in some individuals.
2. The condition will be more likely to occur if there is a family history of heart disease.
3. Not all strains of streptococcus bacteria will result in the development of rheumatic heart disease.
4. Antiviral therapy administered at the onset of the infection will aid in reducing the likelihood of developing complications.
5. The condition will begin manifestation within 3 to 5 days of the initial infection.

104. The nurse is caring for a child with acute rheumatic fever. Which finding does the nurse anticipate observing in this child?
1. Leukocytosis
2. Normal electrocardiogram
3. High fever for 5 or more days
4. Normal erythrocyte sedimentation rate

105. A 17-year-old client is preparing for discharge from the hospital after receiving care for rheumatic fever with cardiac inflammation. Which statement indicates the need for further instruction?
1. "I will be able to go back to school in a few days."
2. "By taking all of medications prescribed I have a greater chance of avoiding further complications."
3. "I may have an extended need for bed rest."
4. "We may not know the extent of damage to my heart for quite some time."

106. Which criteria is required to establish a diagnosis of acute rheumatic fever?
1. Laboratory tests
2. Fever and four Jones criteria
3. Positive blood cultures for *Staphylococcus organisms*
4. Use of Jones criteria and presence of a streptococcal infection

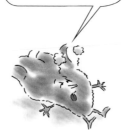

Ugh. I feel a little warm. Maybe I should have my white blood cells checked out.

103. 1, 3, 5. Rheumatic heart disease may result in individuals who have been experiencing Group A streptococcus infections. The condition will manifest a few weeks after the initial infection. The condition is more likely to result in individuals with certain genetic makeups. Not all strains of the bacteria will cause the infection. A family history of heart disease does not increase the occurrence of this complication. Antiviral therapy is not used in the prevention of the complication.
CN: Health promotion and maintenance; CNS: none; CL: apply; DIFFICULTY: Difficult

104. 1. Leukocytosis can be seen as an immune response triggered by colonization of the pharynx with group A streptococci. The electrocardiogram will show a prolonged PR interval as a result of carditis. A low-grade fever is a minor manifestation. A high fever for 5 or more days may indicate Kawasaki disease. The inflammatory response will cause an elevated erythrocyte sedimentation rate.
CN: Physiological integrity; CNS: Physiological adaptation; CL: Apply; DIFFICULTY: Challenge

105. 1. After rheumatic fever rest will be needed. The cardiac involvement will require an extended period of rest and relaxation. The remaining statements indicate understanding.
CN: Health promotion and maintenance; CNS: None; CL: Apply; DIFFICULTY: Moderate

106. 4. Two major (or one major and two minor) manifestations from Jones criteria, and the presence of a streptococcal infection, indicate the diagnosis of rheumatic fever. There's no single laboratory test for diagnosis. Fever and four diagnostic criteria are required to diagnose Kawasaki disease. Blood cultures would be positive for streptococcus, not staphylococcus, organisms.

Jones criteria for diagnosing rheumatic fever

Major criteria	Minor criteria
• Carditis	• Fever
• Migratory polyarthritis	• Arthralgia
• Sydenham chorea	• Elevated acute phase
• Subcutaneous nodules	reactants
• Erythema marginatum	• Prolonged PR interval

CN: Physiological integrity; CNS: Physiological adaptation; CL: Analyze; DIFFICULTY: Moderate

107. Criteria for rheumatic fever are being discussed with parents. The nurse realizes that the parents understand chorea when they make which statement?
1. "My child may not be able to walk."
2. "Long movies may help for relaxation."
3. "My child might have difficulty in school."
4. "Many activities and visitors are recommended."

108. A 3-year-old child has a positive culture for streptococcus organisms. Which intervention is **most** appropriate?
1. Give aspirin.
2. Give antibiotics.
3. Give corticosteroids.
4. Encourage fluid intake.

109. A nurse is preparing to discharge a child with rheumatic fever without carditis. Which instructions should the nurse give the parents?
1. "Give aspirin for signs of chorea."
2. "Give penicillin for 1 month."
3. "Only give penicillin for dental procedures."
4. "It isn't necessary to give penicillin before dental procedures."

110. When planning care for a child with rheumatic fever which is the **greatest** area of concern?
1. Nutrition
2. Anxiety management
3. Cognitive delays
4. Prevention of falls

111. Treatment for a child with sinus bradycardia includes atropine 0.02 mg/kg. If the child weighs 20 kg, how much is given per dose? Record your answer using one decimal place.

_____ mg

112. The nurse is reviewing the telemetry for a group of assigned clients. In which client would sinus bradycardia be considered a normal finding?
1. Preterm neonate
2. Term neonate
3. Growth-delayed adolescent
4. Physically conditioned adolescent

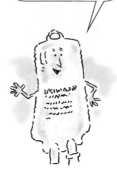

Strep infection? No worries. I've got a nice dose of penicillin heading your way.

107. 3. Chorea may last 1 to 6 months. Central nervous system involvement contributes to a shortened attention span, so children might have difficulty learning in school. Muscle incoordination may cause the child to be more clumsy than usual when walking. A quiet environment is required for treatment.
CN: Physiological integrity; CNS: Physiological adaptation; CL: Analyze; DIFFICULTY: Difficult

108. 2. Infection caused by streptococcus organisms is treated with antibiotics, mainly penicillin. Antipyretics, such as acetaminophen, may be given for fever. Aspirin isn't recommended. Corticosteroids are not indicated. Fluid intake is encouraged to prevent dehydration from decreased oral intake due to a sore throat, or to replace fluids lost due to possible diarrhea from the antibiotics.
CN: Physiological integrity; CNS: Physiological adaptation; CL: Analyze; DIFFICULTY: Easy

109. 4. Children who might benefit from prophylactic penicillin include those with unrepaired congenital heart defects, those with heart defects repaired with synthetic material, those with prior infective endocarditis, and some children with heart transplants. Prophylactic antibiotic therapy isn't otherwise recommended.
CN: Physiological integrity; CNS: Pharmacological therapies; CL: Apply; DIFFICULTY: Difficult

110. 4. The child with rheumatic fever has a risk for chorea. This can lead to falls. In addition, the child may experience weakness, thus increasing the risk for falls. The remaining items are not typical concerns for rheumatic fever.
CN: Safe, effective care environment; CNS: Safety and infection control; CL: Apply; DIFFICULTY: Challenge

111. 0.4.
Use the following equation:

$$0.02 \text{ mg} / \text{kg} \times 20 \text{ kg} = 0.4 \text{ mg}$$

CN: Physiological integrity; CNS: Pharmacological therapies; CL: Analyze; DIFFICULTY: Moderate

112. 4. A physically conditioned adolescent might have a lower-than-normal heart rate, which is of no significance. Growth-delayed adolescents don't have bradycardia as a normal finding. Neonates have characteristic elevated heart rates.
CN: Physiological integrity; CNS: Physiological adaptation; CL: Analyze; DIFFICULTY: Moderate

113. Atropine is being administered to a child with sinus bradycardia. Which statement is most accurate about the administration of this medication?
   1. It increases heart rate.
   2. It raises blood pressure.
   3. It dilates bronchial tubes.
   4. It decreases heart rate.

114. A nurse has given atropine to an 11-month-old infant to treat sinus bradycardia. Which adverse reaction does the nurse anticipate observing?
   1. Lethargy
   2. Diarrhea
   3. No tears when crying
   4. Increased urine output

115. When performing the assessment on a child the nurse notes sinus tachycardia. Which findings in the child's health history would be associated with this?
   1. Febrile illness
   2. Hypothermia
   3. Hypothyroidism
   4. Hypoxia

116. The nurse is talking with the parents of a child who has had surgery to manage tetralogy of Fallot. Which statements demonstrate an understanding of the condition? Select all that apply.
   1. "My son will not be able to play any sports when he gets older."
   2. "My son's life expectancy has been diminished by this diagnosis."
   3. "My son will need to be seen throughout his life by a cardiologist."
   4. "My son's heart may at times have irregular rhythm patterns."
   5. "Repeated surgical procedures will likely be needed to manage my son's condition."

117. The health care provider orders digoxin 0.1 mg orally every morning for a 6-month-old infant with heart failure. Digoxin is available in a 400 mcg/mL concentration. How many milliliters of digoxin should the nurse give? Record your answer using two decimal places.

_____ mL

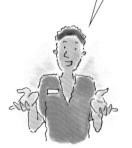

If the whole point of atropine is to treat bradycardia, then what effect should it have?

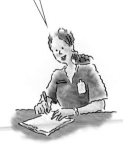

Oh look, another math problem—my favorite. Don't forget to convert.

113. **1.** Atropine blocks vagal impulses to the myocardium and stimulates the cardio-inhibitory center in the medulla, thereby increasing heart rate and cardiac output. Atropine is not given to directly increase blood pressure or dilate the bronchial tubes.
CN: Physiological integrity; CNS: Pharmacological therapies; CL: Apply; DIFFICULTY: Moderate

114. **3.** Atropine dries up secretions and also lessens the response of ciliary and iris sphincter muscles in the eye, causing mydriasis. It usually causes paradoxical excitement in children. Constipation and urinary retention can be seen because of a decrease in smooth-muscle contractions of the GI and genitourinary tracts.
CN: Physiological integrity; CNS: Pharmacological therapies; CL: Apply; DIFFICULTY: Difficult

115. **1.** Sinus tachycardia is commonly seen in children with a fever. It's usually a result of a noncardiac cause. Hypothermia, hypothyroidism, and hypoxia all result in sinus bradycardia.
CN: Physiological integrity; CNS: Physiological adaptation; CL: Analyze; DIFFICULTY: Challenge

116. **3, 4.** Tetralogy of Fallot is a congenital cardiac condition in which there are four primary defects of the heart's structure and function. These include a large ventricular septal defect, pulmonary stenosis, right ventricular hypertrophy, and an overriding aorta. The condition is typically managed with surgical intervention in infancy. This procedure is usually all that is needed to manage the condition. The ability to live a full life with few restrictions is possible for these clients. There is not a significant loss of life years with the condition. The child with this condition will need lifelong monitoring by a cardiologist. Individuals with this condition have an increased risk for the development of cardiac dysrhythmias.
CN: Physiological integrity; CNS: Physiological adaptation; CL: Analyze; DIFFICULTY: Challenge

117. **0.25.**
First, convert milligrams to micrograms:
$$1{,}000 \text{ mcg} / 1 \text{ mg} = X \text{ mcg} / 0.1 \text{ mg}$$
$$X = 100 \text{ mcg}$$
Then, calculate drug dose:
Dose on hand / Quantity on hand = Dose desired / X.
$$400 \text{ mcg} / \text{mL} = 100 \text{ mcg} / X$$
$$X = 0.25 \text{ mL}$$
CN: Physiological integrity; CNS: Pharmacological therapies; CL: Apply; DIFFICULTY: Moderate

118. The nurse is providing preoperative education to the parents of a 9-month-old infant who's having surgery to repair a ventricular septal defect. Identify the area of the heart where the defect is located.

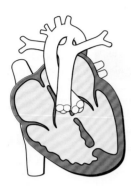

119. An infant who weighs 8 kg is to receive ampicillin 25 mg/kg IV every 6 hours. How many milligrams should the nurse administer per dose? Record your answer using a whole number.

_____ mg

120. A 6-year-old arrives in the emergency department reporting dizziness and collapses before taken into an examination room. Prioritize in ascending chronologic order the steps to take during initial intervention. Use all the options.

1.	Begin chest compressions.
2.	Tilt the child's head back to open up the airway.
3.	Check the carotid pulse.
4.	Give two rescue breaths.
5.	Establish unresponsiveness and call for help.

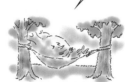

All done? Super! Time for a nap.

118.
A ventricular septal defect is a hole in the septum between the ventricles. The defect can be anywhere along the septum but is most commonly located in the middle of the septum.

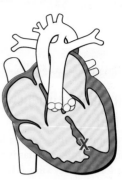

CN: Physiological integrity; CNS: Physiological adaptation; CL: Understand; DIFFICULTY: Moderate

119. 200.
Use the following equation:

$$25\,mg\,/\,kg \times 8\,kg = 200\,mg$$

CN: Physiological integrity; CNS: Pharmacological therapies; CL: Analyze; DIFFICULTY: Moderate

120. Ordered Response:

5.	Establish unresponsiveness and call for help.
3.	Check the carotid pulse.
1.	Begin chest compressions (30).
2.	Tilt the child's head back to open up the airway.
4.	Give two rescue breaths.

According to the 2010 American Heart Association guidelines, the first step is to establish unresponsiveness and call for help. Then check the carotid pulse for no more than 10 seconds. If there's no pulse, begin chest compressions (30 compressions for a single rescuer). Then tilt the child's head back to open the airway and give two breaths.

CN: Safe, effective care environment; CNS: Coordinated care; CL: Apply; DIFFICULTY: Difficult

Chapter 27

Hematologic & Immune Disorders

Pediatric hematologic & immune refresher

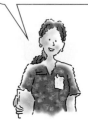

This chapter covers sickle cell disease, varicella, Rocky Mountain spotted fever, leukemia, and many other blood and immune system disorders in kids. It's a whopper of a chapter on a critical area. If you're ready, let's begin!

Acquired immunodeficiency syndrome (AIDS)

Grouping of symptoms that signal a loss of immune response in one who has is positive for human immunodeficiency virus (HIV)

Key signs and symptoms
- Failure to thrive
- Mononucleosis-like prodromal symptoms
- Night sweats
- Recurring diarrhea
- Weight loss

Key test results
- CD4+ T-cell count measures the severity of immunosuppression
- Enzyme-linked immunosorbent assay and Western blot are positive for HIV antibody
- Viral culture or p24 antigen test reveals presence of HIV in children younger than age 18 months

Key treatments
- Antibiotic therapy according to sensitivity of infecting organisms
- Antiviral agents such as zidovudine
- Monthly gamma globulin administration

Key interventions
- Monitor vital signs, intake and output, and growth and development
- Monitor respiratory and neurologic status
- Maintain standard precautions

Hemophilia

Deficiency of clotting factors, in which the absence of these clotting factors results in abnormal bleeding times

Key signs and symptoms
- Multiple bruises without petechiae
- Prolonged bleeding after circumcision, immunizations, or minor injuries

Key test results
- Prolonged partial thromboplastin time (PTT)

Key treatments
- Cryoprecipitate (frozen factor VIII) administration to maintain an acceptable serum level of the clotting factor; usually done by the family at home
- Fresh frozen plasma

Key interventions
- Monitor vital signs and intake and output
- When bleeding occurs:
  - elevate the affected extremity above the heart
  - immobilize the site
  - apply pressure to the site for 10 to 15 minutes
  - decrease the child's anxiety

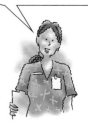

Careful—this refresher will really get in your blood.

Iron deficiency anemia

Deficiency of red blood cells, which are responsible for carrying oxygen in the body

Key signs and symptoms
- Fatigue, listlessness
- Increased susceptibility to infection
- Pallor
- Tachycardia
- Numbness and tingling of the extremities
- Vasomotor disturbances

Key test results
- Hemoglobin (Hb), hematocrit, and serum ferritin levels are low
- Serum iron levels are low, with high binding capacity

Key treatments
- Oral preparation of iron or a combination of iron and ascorbic acid (which enhances iron absorption)

Key interventions
- Administer iron before meals with citrus juice
- Give liquid iron through a straw; for infants, administer by oral syringe toward the back of the mouth
- Do not give iron with milk products

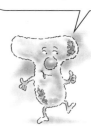

No immunosuppression here. I'm feeling T-rrific.

Iron and milk products don't mix. Serve iron with a citrus juice and have your client sip it through a straw.

WARNING

Leukemia
Cancer of the blood-forming cell of the body

Key signs and symptoms
- Fatigue
- History of infections
- Low-grade fever
- Lymphadenopathy
- Pallor
- Petechiae and ecchymosis
- Poor wound healing and oral lesions

Key test results
- Blast cells appear in the peripheral blood
- Blast cells may be as high as 95% in the bone marrow
- Initial white blood cell count may be 10,000/$\propto$L at time of diagnosis in a child ages 3 to 7 with acute lymphocytic leukemia (ALL)

Key treatments
- Bone marrow transplantation
- Radiation therapy
- Chemotherapy

Key interventions
- Provide pain relief
- Monitor vital signs and intake and output
- Inspect the skin frequently
- Provide nursing measures to ease adverse effects of radiation and chemotherapy

Reye syndrome
Serious condition impacting all organs and tissues of the body, but acts most severely on the brain and liver, where it is associated with swelling; many affected will experience a viral infection prior to syndrome development

Key signs and symptoms
- Stage V: seizures, loss of deep tendon reflexes, flaccidity, respiratory arrest (death is usually a result of cerebral edema or cardiac arrest)

Key test results
- Blood test results show elevated serum ammonia levels; serum fatty acid and lactate levels are also elevated
- Coagulation studies reveal prolonged prothrombin time (PT) and partial thromboplastin time (PTT).
- Liver biopsy shows fatty droplets distributed through cells
- Liver function studies show aspartate aminotransferase and alanine aminotransferase elevated to twice normal levels

Key treatments
- Endotracheal intubation and mechanical ventilation
- Exchange transfusion
- Induced hypothermia

Key interventions
- Monitor vital signs and pulse oximetry
- Monitor cardiac, respiratory, and neurologic status
- Monitor fluid intake and output
- Monitor blood glucose levels
- Maintain seizure precautions
- Keep head of bed at 30-degree angle
- Maintain oxygen therapy, which may include intubation and mechanical ventilation
- Administer blood products as necessary
- Administer medications, as ordered, and monitor for adverse effects
- Maintain hypothermia blanket as needed and monitor temperature every 15 to 30 minutes while in use
- Check for loss of reflexes and signs of flaccidity

Sickle cell anemia
Condition in which the red blood cells are sickle shaped, resulting in ineffective ability to carry oxygen to the body's tissues; the cells become lodged in the body's organs and vessels

Key signs and symptoms
- In infants: colic and splenomegaly
- In toddlers and preschoolers: hypovolemia, shock, and pain at site of crisis
- In school-age children and adolescents: enuresis, extreme pain at site of crisis, and priapism

Key test results
- More than 50% Hb S indicates sickle cell disease; a lower level of Hb S indicates sickle cell trait

Key treatments
- Hydration with IV fluid administration
- Transfusion therapy as necessary
- Treatment for acidosis
- Analgesics: morphine or hydromorphone
- Oral penicillin prophylactically until age 5 to 6 years
- Daily folic acid supplementation

Key interventions
- Monitor vital signs and intake and output
- Administer pain medications and note effectiveness

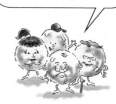

Leukemia mutates white blood cells, turning them from heroes to villains.

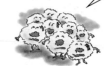

Time for a head count! Elevated white blood cell count can be an indicator of a problematic immune response.

Hematologic & immune questions, answers, and rationales

1. What should the nurse anticipate is most important for successful management of the child with Reye syndrome?
1. Early diagnosis
2. Initiation of antibiotics
3. Isolation of the child
4. Staging of the illness

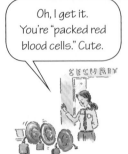

Oh, I get it. You're "packed red blood cells." Cute.

1. 1. Early diagnosis and therapy are essential because of the rapid, clinical course of the disease and its high mortality. Reye syndrome is associated with a viral illness, and antibiotic therapy isn't effective to prevent the initial progression of the illness. Isolation isn't necessary because the disease isn't communicable. Staging, although important to therapy, occurs after a differential diagnosis is made.
CN: Physiological integrity; CNS: Reduction of risk potential; CL: Analyze; DIFFICULTY: Easy

2. A child with Reye syndrome is in stage I of the illness. Which measure would help prevent further progression of the illness?
1. Invasive monitoring
2. Endotracheal intubation
3. Hypertonic glucose solution
4. Pancuronium

2. 3. For children in stage I of Reye syndrome, treatment is primarily supportive and directed toward restoring blood glucose levels and correcting acid-base imbalances. IV administration of dextrose solutions with added insulin helps to replace glycogen stores and may help prevent progression of the syndrome. Noninvasive monitoring is adequate to assess status at this stage. Endotracheal intubation may be necessary later. Pancuronium is used as an adjunct to endotracheal intubation and wouldn't be used in stage I of Reye syndrome.
CN: Physiological integrity; CNS: Reduction of risk potential; CL: Apply; DIFFICULTY: Difficult

3. The nurse is caring for a 9-month-old with Reye syndrome. Which nursing interventions should be included when assisting with the plan of care?
1. Check the skin for signs of breakdown every shift.
2. Perform range-of-motion (ROM) exercises every 4 hours.
3. Monitor the child's intake and output.
4. Place the child in protective isolation.

Heads up! Finding the right position is critical in question #4.

3. 3. Monitoring intake and output alerts the nurse to the development of dehydration and cerebral edema, complications of Reye syndrome. Although checking the skin for signs of breakdown is important because the child may not be as active as normal, it isn't as critical as monitoring the infant's intake and output. Active ROM exercises may not be needed and aren't as important as monitoring the child's intake and output. Placing the child in protective isolation isn't necessary.
CN: Physiological integrity; CNS: Reduction of risk potential; CL: Apply; DIFFICULTY: Easy

4. A child with Reye syndrome is exhibiting signs of increased intracranial pressure (ICP). Which nursing intervention would be most appropriate for this child?
1. Position the child with the head elevated and the neck in a neutral position.
2. Maintain the child in the prone position.
3. Cluster together interventions that may be perceived as noxious.
4. Position the child in the supine position, with head turned to the side.

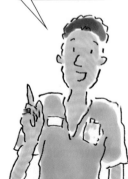

4. 1. Positioning the child with Reye syndrome with the head elevated and the neck in neutral position helps decrease ICP. The prone and supine positions cause increased ICP. Interventions that may be perceived as noxious should be spaced over time because if clustered together, they may have a cumulative effect in increasing ICP. Turning the head to the side may impede venous return from the head and increase ICP.
CN: Physiological integrity; CNS: Physiological adaptation; CL: Apply; DIFFICULTY: Easy

5. The nurse is comforting a child upset at the loss of hair related to the administration of chemotherapy. Which statements should be included in the information provided by the nurse? Select all that apply.
1. "Options to cover your hair loss include a cap, scarf or wig."
2. The hair loss is temporary and will begin to regrow in about 1 to 2 months."
3. "You should begin to interact with your friends as soon as possible."
4. "Please share your feelings about this change with your parents."
5. "There is no requirement to wear head covering unless it is for protection from the sun or cold."

5. 1, 3, 4, 5. The loss of hair is a common reaction to chemotherapy. This loss is temporary. New hair growth begins in 3 to 6 months. The new hair may be a different color or texture than the hair that was lost. Children may choose to cover their scalps with wigs, hats or scarves. Covering should be done to protect from elements such as cold and sun when present. Sharing feelings is important so that support may be received from those closest to the child. Remaining in contact with peers is helpful. It is important to avoid social isolation.
CN: Psychosocial integrity; CNS: None; CL: Apply;
DIFFICULTY: Difficult

6. A child with pauciarticular juvenile rheumatoid arthritis (JRA) is being seen for an annual physical examination. The child's parent reports not understanding why the child will need to have an annual eye examination if there are no visual problems. Which statement by the nurse is **most** appropriate?
1. "Detached retinas are commonly associated with the disease."
2. "Painless iritis (inflammation of the iris) is commonly seen with the disease."
3. "Glaucoma is commonly seen with the disease."
4. "Strabismus is commonly seen with the disease."

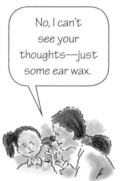

No, I can't see your thoughts—just some ear wax.

6. 2. Painless iritis may be found in up to 75% of children with pauciarticular JRA. If it's not detected and is left untreated, permanent scarring in the anterior chamber of the eye may occur, with loss of vision. Children should have annual slit-lamp examinations by an ophthalmologist. Detached retinas, glaucoma, and strabismus aren't commonly associated with pauciarticular JRA.
CN: Health promotion and maintenance; CNS: None; CL: Apply;
DIFFICULTY: Moderate

7. An 8-year-old child is brought to the clinic with watery eyes, clear nasal drainage that has lasted more than 10 days, without fever. The nurse observes that the child has dark circles under the eyes and a crease above the tip of the nose. Which intervention should be the nurse's **priority**?
1. Collect data about potential environmental allergy triggers.
2. Prepare to administer amoxicillin 25 mg/kg PO every 12 hours.
3. Prepare to administer trivalent inactivated influenza vaccine 0.5 mL PO.
4. Prepare the child for sinus x-rays.

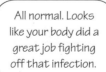

All normal. Looks like your body did a great job fighting off that infection.

7. 1. Cold symptoms that last longer than 10 days without fever, dark circles under the eyes (from increased blood flow near the sinuses), and a crease near the tip of the nose (from upward nose wiping) are all signs and symptoms of perennial allergic rhinitis. The nurse's priority is to collect data about potential indoor and outdoor environmental allergen triggers. Amoxicillin is used to treat bacterial infections, not allergies. Additionally the nurse will not prepare medication for administration without the appropriate orders from the health care provider. Influenza vaccination is indicated annually. Sinus x-rays may be necessary to check for structural abnormalities, but they are not the priority at this time.
CN: Safe and effective care environment; CNS: Safety and infection control; CL: Analyze; DIFFICULTY: Easy

8. A nurse is caring for a child with juvenile arthritis (JA) prescribed oral prednisone. The nurse knows that the drug will be given at the lowest possible dosage and for a short time in order to avoid which adverse effects?
1. Growth retardation and increased risk of infection
2. Deafness and severe weight loss
3. Hypoglycemia and hypovolemia
4. Fibrotic skin changes and increased muscle mass

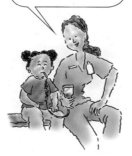

8. 1. Long-term prednisone use is associated with poor growth and immunosuppression; it may aggravate or mask serious infections. Prednisone is associated with weight gain and cataract formation but not deafness. It may cause hyperglycemia, significant sodium and fluid retention, edema, and heart failure. Long-term use of prednisone may cause muscle wasting, weakness, and thin, fragile skin.
CN: Physiological integrity; CNS: Pharmacological therapies;
CL: Analyze; DIFFICULTY: Moderate

9. A nurse is reinforcing the education plan with the parent of a 12-year-old child recently diagnosed with systemic juvenile arthritis (JA). Which statements by the parent best indicate that education has been effective? Select all that apply.
  1. "Maintaining an appropriate, regular exercise program is very important."
  2. "Systemic JA typically appears at or before the age of 12."
  3. "High fevers that spike in the morning may be the first sign of the disease."
  4. "It's important that my child's diet includes 1,300 mg of calcium daily."
  5. "Warm showers in the morning may be very beneficial to easing my child's morning discomforts."

10. The parents of a healthy 4-month old child are seen for a well-child check-up. Which statement indicates an understanding of the recommended immunization schedule?
  1. "My child should have the DTaP on this visit."
  2. "My child will need to have the measles, mumps, and rubella (MMR) during this appointment."
  3. "It is time for my child to receive the Hep B booster."
  4. "I can request the influenza vaccine at any time for my child."

11. The nurse is caring for a child with leukemia. Which nursing intervention would be helpful in reducing stress and alleviating the parent's fear for their child?
  1. Not accepting aggressive behavior from parents
  2. Minimizing the expression of feelings and concerns
  3. Letting parents interpret the child's behaviors and responses
  4. Encouraging parents to talk about their feelings

12. The nurse is preparing to administer an immunization to a 2-month old child. The child's parent states, "I am going to put off the immunizations because I hate to see my child hurt." Which response by the nurse is **most** appropriate?
  1. "I understand that it is hard to see your child feel any type of discomfort."
  2. "Your child will not even remember this little shot."
  3. "Although your baby will feel discomfort now, it will be short lived."
  4. "Deciding to forgo the planned immunizations is actually not in the baby's best interests."

> Leukemia is a scary diagnosis. Help parents to verbalize their emotions about it.

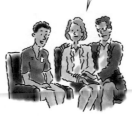

9. **1, 4, 5.** Maintaining a regular, appropriate exercise program is important to maintain muscle strength and joint flexibility. All types of JA occur at or before the age of 16. High fevers that spike at night and then suddenly disappear typically may be the first sign of systemic JA. It's important for a 12-year-old child to consume 1,300 mg of calcium daily to maintain bone health. Morning pain and stiffness are concerns of the child with juvenile arthritis. The longer a joint has been inactive the more discomfort that may be experienced. Heat related treatments are often effective in managing these concerns.
CN: Health promotion and maintenance; CNS: None; CL: Analyze; DIFFICULTY: Moderate

10. **1.** The child at the age of 4 months should be given the DTaP. The measles, mumps, and rubella, Hep B booster and influence vaccine will be administered at 6 months of age if the child is on target with the recommended immunizations.
CN: Health promotion and maintenance; CNS: None; CL: Apply; DIFFICULTY: Challenge

11. **4.** As the parents are encouraged to talk about their feelings, stress is reduced. Aggressive behavior shouldn't be tolerated, but instead recognized as a symptom of poor coping skills, indicating their need for greater emotional support. It's critical to not minimize the feelings and concerns of the parents because this may increase their stress. It's important for the nurse to explain the child's behavior to the parents so they don't misinterpret the meaning.
CN: Psychosocial integrity; CNS: None; CL: Apply; DIFFICULTY: Easy

12. **3.** Parents often experience anxiety when care that causes discomfort or stress is administered to a child. The nurse is most correct when the stress or anxiety is acknowledged. Telling the parent that there is understanding of the discomfort is not therapeutic. While the child will not recall the shot in the future this does not address the parent's current concerns. Immunizations are recommended but telling the parent that the decision is not in the baby's best interest is inappropriate.
CN: Psychological integrity; CNS: None; CL: Apply; DIFFICULTY: Challenge

13. A parent asks the nurse when it is **most** appropriate for her infant to begin receiving the measles vaccine? What is the **best** response by the nurse?
1. At age 6 months
2. At age 12 months
3. At age 18 months
4. At age 24 months

14. Parents of a child with Kawasaki disease should be taught the importance of keeping follow-up appointments to monitor and prevent which complication?
1. Encephalitis
2. Glomerulonephritis
3. Myocardial infarction
4. Idiopathic thrombocytopenic purpura (ITP)

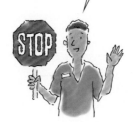

Kawasaki disease can damage blood vessels and lead to life-threatening heart complications.

15. A child is considered immunocompromised. What education should the nurse reinforce to the parents concerning immunizations? Select all that apply.
1. The immunization schedule should be followed as usual.
2. Immunizations may be delayed.
3. The child should be put on an accelerated immunization schedule.
4. The child should receive no further immunizations.
5. The child may be prescribed a modified schedule, changing the number of immunizations administered in a single visit.

16. The parents of an infant report they are concerned about giving their child immunizations due to their association with autism. Which response by the nurse is appropriate?
1. "Studies do not support a link between autism and immunizations."
2. "There are limited risks of autism with the use of 'live' vaccines."
3. "The administration of more than one immunization at a time has shown a slight relationship with the development of autism."
4. "The use of inactivated vaccines has been linked to a slight increase in the development of autism in populations at risk."

17. A child is admitted to the hospital for an asthma exacerbation. The nursing history reveals this client was exposed to chickenpox 1 week ago. When would this client require isolation if he were to remain hospitalized?
1. Isolation isn't required.
2. Immediate isolation is required.
3. 10 days after exposure
4. 12 days after exposure

13. 2. According to the American Academy of Pediatrics, the first dose of the measles vaccine should be administered at age 12 to 15 months. CN: Health promotion and maintenance; CNS: None; CL: Apply; DIFFICULTY: Challenge

14. 3. In Kawasaki disease, inflammation of small and medium blood vessels can result in weakening of the vessels and aneurysm formation, especially in the heart. Blood flow through damaged vessels can cause thrombosis formation and myocardial infarction. Encephalitis, glomerulonephritis, and ITP aren't associated with Kawasaki disease. CN: Health promotion and maintenance; CNS: None; CL: Apply; DIFFICULTY: Difficult

15. 2, 5. Immunizations should be delayed until the health care provider has determined that the child is ready. The particular type and number of immunizations given at one time may vary for this child. The child may be put on a schedule to catch up eventually, but that would not be the first response. The child would not typically be excluded from immunizations in the future. CN: Health promotion and maintenance; CNS: None; CL: Apply; DIFFICULTY: Difficult

16. 1. There has been a great deal of discussion about the risk of autism being increased with the administration of immunizations. Studies do not presently show a correlation regardless of whether they are live or inactivated vaccines. CN: Health promotion and maintenance; CNS: None; CL: Apply; DIFFICULTY: Moderate

17. 2. The incubation period for chickenpox is 2 to 3 weeks, commonly 13 to 17 days. A client is commonly isolated 1 week after exposure to avoid the risk of an earlier breakout. A person is infectious from 1 day before eruption of lesions until after the vesicles have formed crusts. CN: Safe, effective care environment; CNS: Safety and infection control; CL: Apply; DIFFICULTY: Moderate

18. The nurse is caring for a child who is receiving steroid therapy as a part of a cancer treatment plan. The child tearfully asks the nurse," Why does my face looks so "fat?" What information should be included in the nurse's response?
  1. The facial tissues are retaining fluid as a result of the cancer.
  2. An activity plan to promote calorie use will be helpful in reducing this facial appearance.
  3. Drinking more fluids will help ensure toxins are flushed from the system and will reduce this appearance.
  4. This change is temporary and will subside once the steroid medication has been discontinued.

18. 4. Steroid therapy is associated with an increased roundness of the face. This may be a source of distress to the child and parents. It is important to explain that this is the result of the medication therapy and will subside.
CN: Physiologic integrity; CNS: Pharmacological therapies; CL: Apply; DIFFICULTY: Easy

19. The nurse is observing a student nurse preparing to administer the measles, mumps, and rubella (MMR) vaccine to a 6 year-old child. Which action would prompt the nurse to provide additional instruction?
  1. The student nurse obtains a 5/8-inch needle.
  2. The student nurse selects the deltoid muscle of the arm for the site of administration.
  3. The nurse discusses plans to administer the immunization intramuscularly.
  4. The nurse reports the correct dose is 0.5 mL.

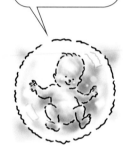

Vaccinations are like a protective bubble. Remind my parents to get them for me.

19. 3. The measles, mumps, and rubella (MMR) vaccine is administered subcutaneously. It is appropriate to utilize a 5/8-inch needle for the administration. The use of the deltoid muscle is appropriate. The correct dosage is 0.5 mL
CN: Health promotion and maintenance; CNS: none; CL: Apply; DIFFICULTY: Difficult

20. While gathering data about a child's skin integrity, the nurse observes a papular pruritic rash with some vesicles. The rash is profuse on the trunk and sparse on the distal limbs. What does the nurse correlate this finding with?
  1. Measles
  2. Mumps
  3. Roseola
  4. Chickenpox

20. 4. Chickenpox begins with a macule, rapidly progresses to a highly pruritic papule, then becomes a vesicle. All three stages are present in varying degrees at one time. Measles begin as an erythematous maculopapular eruption on the face and gradually spread downward. Mumps doesn't manifest a skin rash. Roseola rash is nonpruritic and appears as discrete rose-pink macules, first on the trunk and then spreading to the neck, face, and extremities.
CN: Health promotion and maintenance; CNS: None; CL: Analyze; DIFFICULTY: Moderate

21. Which response would be appropriate to a parent inquiring, "When can my child with chickenpox return to school"?
  1. "When the child is afebrile"
  2. "When all vesicles have dried"
  3. "When vesicles begin to crust over"
  4. "When lesions and vesicles are gone"

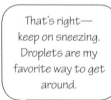

That's right— keep on sneezing. Droplets are my favorite way to get around.

21. 2. Chickenpox is contagious. It's transmitted through direct contact, droplet spread, and contact with contaminated objects. Vesicles break open; therefore, the child is considered contagious until all vesicles have dried. A child may be fever-free but continue to have vesicles and remain contagious. Some vesicles may be crusted over, but new ones may have formed so the child remains contagious. It isn't necessary to wait until dried lesions have disappeared. Isolation is usually necessary only for about 1 week after the onset of the disease.
CN: Health promotion and maintenance; CNS: None; CL: Apply; DIFFICULTY: Difficult

22. Parents report their child has roseola. Which clinical manifestations would the nurse expect to find?
1. Apparent sickness, fever, and rash
2. Fever for 3 to 4 days, followed by rash
3. Rash, without history of fever or illness
4. Rash for 3 to 4 days, followed by high fever

23. The nurse would advise a child with chickenpox and the parents to avoid scratching and irritating open vesicles to prevent which condition?
1. Myocarditis
2. Neuritis
3. Obstructive laryngitis
4. Secondary bacterial infection

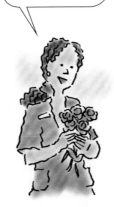

I'd much rather have roses than roseola.

24. The nurse is caring for a child suspected of having roseola. Which finding is consistent with a roseola rash?
1. Maculopapular red spots on the torso
2. Pruritic papules and vesicles on the extremities
3. Rose-pink macules that blanch on pressure
4. Red maculopapular eruptions on the face

25. The nurse is reviewing the plan of treatment for a 4 month old infant born to an HIV positive woman. The child has also recently tested positive for the infection. What can the nurse anticipate will be in the plan of care for the child's first year of life? Select all that apply.
1. Prophylactic administration of sulfamethoxazole-trimethoprim for the first year of life.
2. The administration of sulfamethoxazole-trimethoprim for the first 6 months after the diagnosis of HIV in the child.
3. Immunization with varicella vaccine at age 12 months if there is no evidence of severe immunosuppression.
4. Immunization with varicella vaccine at age 6 months if there is no evidence of severe immunosuppression.
5. Initiation of antirectoviral medications at age 6 months.

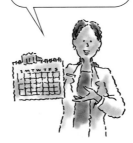

Remember that certain conditions will affect children's vaccination schedules.

26. Which communicable disease requires isolating infected children from pregnant women?
1. Pertussis
2. Roseola
3. Rubella
4. Varicella

22. 2. Roseola is manifested by persistent high fever for 3 to 4 days followed by a rash. When the rash appears, a precipitous drop in fever occurs and the temperature returns to normal.
CN: Health promotion and maintenance; CNS: None; CL: Understand; DIFFICULTY: Moderate

23. 4. Secondary bacterial infections can occur as a complication of chickenpox. Further irritation of skin lesions can lead to cellulitis or even an abscess. Myocarditis isn't considered a complication of chickenpox but has been noted as a complication of mumps. Neuritis has been associated with diphtheria. Obstructive laryngitis occurs as a complication of measles.
CN: Physiological integrity; CNS: Reduction of risk potential; CL: Apply; DIFFICULTY: Easy

24. 3. Roseola rashes are discrete, rose-pink macules or maculopapules that blanch on pressure and usually last 1 to 2 days. Chickenpox rash is macular, with papules and vesicles. Roseola isn't pruritic. Maculopapular red spots may be indicative of fifth disease. Measles begin as a maculopapular eruption on the face.
CN: Health promotion and maintenance; CNS: None; CL: Apply; DIFFICULTY: Moderate

25. 1, 3. The HIV positive infant will begin antiretroviral medications at the time of diagnosis. These medications are used to delay the onset of illness and to strengthen the body's response in the event of infection. Pneumocystis carinii pneumonia is a common infection encountered by HIV positive children. Health care providers will initiate prophylactic sulfamethoxazole-trimethoprim for the first year of life. Children will be scheduled to receive immunizations in the first year per the recommended schedule as long as there is no evidence of severe immunosuppression. The varicella vaccine is scheduled to be administered at 12 months of age.
CN: Physiological integrity; CNS: Pharmacologic therapies; CL: Apply; DIFFICULTY: Difficult

26. 3. Rubella (German measles) has a teratogenic effect on the fetus. An infected child must be isolated from pregnant women. Pertussis, roseola, and varicella don't have any teratogenic effects on a fetus.
CN: Safe, effective care environment; CNS: Safety and infection control; CL: Understand; DIFFICULTY: Moderate

27. The nurse would expect the health care provider to prescribe which medication as the treatment of choice for scarlet fever?
1. Acyclovir
2. Amphotericin B
3. Ibuprofen
4. Penicillin

27. 4. The causative agent of scarlet fever is group A beta-hemolytic streptococci, which is susceptible to penicillin. Erythromycin is used for penicillin-sensitive children. Acyclovir is used in the treatment of herpes infections. Amphotericin B is used to treat fungal infections. Anti-inflammatory drugs, such as ibuprofen, aren't indicated for children with scarlet fever.

CN: Physiological integrity; CNS: Pharmacological therapies; CL: Apply; DIFFICULTY: Moderate

28. A 2-year-old hospitalized child is HIV positive with severe thrush. The child's anxious grandparents are at the bedside, continually calling the nurses with various concerns. The staff speaks disparagingly about them because they're tired of responding to the frequent call lights. When working with the unit's staff, which response by the nurse manager would be appropriate in creating a more optimal care environment for the child?
1. "This situation will improve as you respond to the call light more promptly."
2. "This couple is demanding, but we need to handle things in a professional manner."
3. "It might be best to have the child transferred to a facility that's better staffed."
4. "If we stop by the room before the light goes on, they may be less anxious."

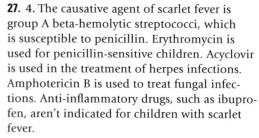

This is the part of the job I love.

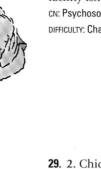

28. 4. Although the situation may improve with more prompt responses to the call light, stopping by the room before the light goes on addresses the needs of the family. This response encourages the staff to be proactive and compassionate and provide prompt nursing intervention. The staff should handle the situation more professionally, providing individualized care based on the needs of the family. Transferring the child to a better-staffed facility isn't a therapeutic solution.

CN: Psychosocial integrity; CNS: None; CL: Analyze; DIFFICULTY: Challenge

29. Which instructions would the nurse include when reinforcing education to the parents about caring for a child with chickenpox?
1. Administer antibiotics as ordered.
2. Administer antipruritics as ordered.
3. Provide peer interaction as a distraction.
4. Avoid varicella-zoster immunizations if the child has been taking aspirin.

29. 2. Chickenpox is highly pruritic. Preventing the child from scratching is necessary to prevent scarring and secondary infection caused by irritation of lesions. Antibiotics aren't usually used to treat chickenpox. Interaction with other children would be contraindicated due to the risk of disease transmission, unless the other children have previously had chickenpox or have been immunized. Varicella-zoster immune globulin should be given to exposed children who are taking aspirin because of the possible risk of Reye syndrome.

CN: Physiological integrity; CNS: Pharmacological therapies; CL: Apply; DIFFICULTY: Moderate

30. The nurse is caring for a child diagnosed with scarlet fever. Which period of isolation is indicated?
1. Until the associated diaper rash disappears
2. Until completion of antibiotic therapy
3. Until the child is free from fever for 24 hours
4. Until 24 hours after initiation of treatment

30. 4. A child requires respiratory isolation until 24 hours after initiation of treatment. Rash may persist for 3 weeks. It isn't necessary to wait until the end of treatment. The child usually becomes afebrile 24 hours after therapy has begun. It isn't necessary to maintain isolation for an additional 24 hours.

CN: Safe, effective environment; CNS: Safety and infection control; CL: Apply; DIFFICULTY: Challenge

31. A mother infected with human immunodeficiency virus (HIV) asks about breast-feeding her infant. Which response would be **best**?
1. "It is not advisable to breast-feed if you have HIV."
2. "Breast-feeding is safe if you have HIV."
3. "You can breast-feed your infant only if you are taking zidovudine."
4. "It's best to supplement breast-feeding with formula to reduce exposure to HIV."

32. The nurse is caring for a teen who was recently sexually assaulted and has concerns about becoming infected with HIV as a result. Which symptoms associated with early infection should the nurse inform the client to report? Select all that apply.
1. Night sweats
2. Diarrhea
3. Enlarged lymph nodes in the groin region
4. Fatigue
5. Weight loss

33. A nurse working in a public health clinic is talking with a teen about having HIV testing. The teen is concerned about people finding out the results. What information can be provided to the individual?
1. "When you have HIV testing the only people who will be told are your parents."
2. "HIV test results must be released to the local health department to allow them to begin looking for sexual contacts."
3. "You may choose to have confidential testing which will allow only you to know your results."
4. "Anonymous testing will allow you to use a private ID number to retrieve your test results."

34. A pregnant woman has recently found out she is HIV positive. When discussing the impact of the condition and care of the infant what information should be provided? Select all that apply.
1. Definitively diagnosing a newborn with HIV is challenging in the first year of life.
2. HIV symptoms will not develop in an infant before 6 months of age.
3. Taking the prescribed antiviral medications during the pregnancy will significantly lower the risk of HIV transmission to the baby.
4. Vaginal birth will be permissible if the woman has been compliant with prescribed antiviral therapies.
5. Breast-feeding is permissible in the first few weeks life if the mother is compliant with prescribed antiviral therapies.

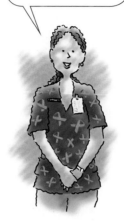

Keep an eye on that word "early" in question #32. It will point you to the right answers.

31. 1. Mothers infected with HIV shouldn't breast-feed because the virus has been isolated in breast milk and can be transmitted to the infant. Taking zidovudine doesn't prevent transmission of the virus in breast milk, and supplementing breast-feeding with formula wouldn't reduce exposure of the infant to the HIV virus in breast milk.
CN: Health promotion and maintenance; CNS: None;
CL: Apply; DIFFICULTY: Challenge

32. 3, 4. Early HIV infection has few clinical symptoms. These symptoms may be attributed to other factors or overlooked. Symptoms seen in the first weeks after infection include fever, headache, fatigue, swollen lymph nodes in the neck or groin regions. *Later* symptoms seen in HIV infection include weight loss, night sweats and diarrhea.
CN: Physiological integrity; CNS: Physiological adaptation;
CL: Analyze; DIFFICULTY: Challenge

33. 4. HIV testing is recommended for every individual ages 13 to 64 years at least once as a part of routine care. HIV testing may be performed either confidentially or anonymously. The confidential test allows the results to be tied to the individual. These results then become a part of the individual's permanent medical record. This makes the results available to insurance companies and health care providers who are involved with the individual. Anonymous testing assigns a personal identification number to the individual to retrieve the results and no other individuals or agencies will be privy to the results.
CN: Safe, effective care environment; CNS: Coordinated care;
CL: Analyze; DIFFICULTY: Challenge

34. 1, 3. A confirmed diagnosis is difficult during the first 15 months because of the presence of maternal antibody. Symptoms may present prior to 1 year of age in an infected newborn. The use of antiviral therapies in an HIV pregnant woman can reduce transmission to the newborn to less than 1%. The recommended method of birth is cesarean section. Breast-feeding is not recommended for women who are HIV positive.
CN: Health promotion and maintenance; CNS: None;
CL: Apply; DIFFICULTY: Difficult

35. The nurse is gathering data from a child with sickle cell anemia. Which bone-related complications would the nurse be alert for during the data collection?
1. Arthritis
2. Osteoporosis
3. Osteogenic sarcoma
4. Spontaneous fractures

36. A child with sickle cell anemia is being treated for a vasoocclusive crisis and reports significant discomfort. Which actions can promote increased levels of comfort for the child? Select all that apply.
1. Cluster care interventions.
2. Encourage fluid intake.
3. Perform passive range of motion.
4. Oxygen therapy as prescribed
5. Assist to knee-chest position.

Remember to "select all that apply" in question #36.

37. The nurse educator is providing an inservice about the care and clinical manifestations of children with sickle cell anemia experiencing vasoocclusive crisis. Which statement by a staff member indicates an understanding?
1. "I should avoid palpating the abdomen of this child to prevent causing a splenic rupture."
2. "I should avoid palpating the abdomen of this child to avoid causing him to vomit."
3. "I should avoid palpating the abdomen to avoid increasing the child's abdominal pain."
4. "I should avoid palpating the abdomen to avoid promoting blood cell destruction."

38. A child tests positive for the sickle cell trait, and the parents ask the nurse what this means. Which response by the nurse would be **most** appropriate?
1. "Your child has sickle cell anemia."
2. "Your child is a carrier but doesn't have the disease."
3. "Your child is a carrier and will pass the disease to any offspring."
4. "Your child doesn't have the disease now but may develop the disease as he gets older."

Great job! You really know how to stick to it.

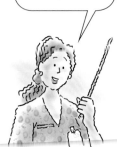

35. 2. Sickle cell anemia causes hyperplasia and congestion of the bone marrow, resulting in osteoporosis. Arthritis doesn't occur secondary to sickle cell anemia; however, a crisis can cause localized swelling over joints, resulting in arthralgia. Bones do weaken, but spontaneous fractures don't occur as a result. Osteogenic sarcoma is bone cancer; sickle cell anemia doesn't cause bone cancer.
CN: Physiological integrity; CNS: Physiological adaptation; CL: Apply; DIFFICULTY: Difficult

36. 1, 2, 4. Sickle cell anemia is a condition that is characterized by red blood cells that are crescent or "sickle" in shape. At times these cells may become clumped in the blood vessels, resulting in what is referred to as a vasoocclusive crisis. Interventions that will promote increased comfort for this client include clustering of care activities. Clustering of care will allow the child to have periods of rest and periods of organized activity. This will reduce fatigue and discomfort for the child. Hydration is important in managing and prevention further facilitation of the crisis. Oxygen is often prescribed for the child in crisis. Range of motion, although beneficial to promote joint mobility, does not improve comfort to the individual who is experiencing pain related to a vasoocclusive crisis. Knee-chest positioning will not be of benefit to this client.
CN: Physiological integrity; CNS: Basic care and comfort; CL: Apply; DIFFICULTY: Difficult

37. 1. Palpating a child's abdomen in vasoocclusive crisis should be avoided because sequestered red blood cells may precipitate splenic rupture. Abdominal pain alone isn't a reason to avoid palpation. Vomiting or blood cell destruction doesn't occur from palpation of the abdomen.
CN: Physiological integrity; CNS: Reduction of risk potential; CL: Analyze; DIFFICULTY: Moderate

38. 2. A child with sickle cell trait is only a carrier and may never show any symptoms, except under special hypoxic conditions. A child with sickle cell trait doesn't have the disease and will never test positive for sickle cell anemia. Sickle cell anemia would be transmitted to offspring only as the result of a union between two individuals who are positive for the trait.
CN: Health promotion and maintenance; CNS: None; CL: Apply; DIFFICULTY: Moderate

39. When caring for a child with sickle cell anemia in vasoocclusive crisis, what does the nurse identify as the **priority** nursing intervention?

1. Manage pain.
2. Provide a cool environment.
3. Immobilize the affected part.
4. Restrict fluids.

40. Which nursing intervention is most effective in maximizing tissue perfusion for a child in vasoocclusive crisis?

1. Administer analgesics.
2. Monitor fluid restrictions.
3. Encourage activity as tolerated.
4. Administer oxygen as prescribed.

Tissue perfusion is all about getting oxygen to the cells of the body.

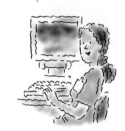

41. Which nursing action is **most** important to decrease the risk of postoperative complications in a child with sickle cell anemia?

1. Increasing fluids
2. Preparing the child psychologically
3. Discouraging coughing
4. Limiting the use of analgesics

42. Which instruction should the nurse include as a **priority** in reinforcing the education of parents about prevention of infection in their child with sickle cell anemia?

1. Provide adequate nutrition.
2. Avoid emotional stress.
3. Visit the health care provider when sick.
4. Avoid strenuous physical exertion.

39. 1. Pain management is an important aspect in the care of a child with sickle cell anemia in vasoocclusive crisis. The goal is to prevent sickling. This can be accomplished by promoting tissue oxygenation, adequate hydration, and rest, which minimize energy expenditure and oxygen utilization. A cool environment can cause vaso-constriction and thus more sickling and pain. Immobilization can promote stasis and increase sickling.

CN: Physiological integrity; CNS: Basic care and comfort; CL: Analyze; DIFFICULTY: Easy

40. 4. Administering oxygen is the most effective way to maximize tissue perfusion. Short-term oxygen therapy helps to prevent hypoxia, which leads to metabolic acidosis, causing sickling. Long-term oxygen therapy depresses erythropoiesis. Analgesics are used to control pain. Hydration is essential to promote hemodilution and maintain electrolyte balance. Bed rest should be promoted to reduce oxygen utilization.

CN: Physiological integrity; CNS: Reduction of risk potential; CL: Apply; DIFFICULTY: Moderate

41. 1. The main surgical risk from anesthesia is hypoxia; however, emotional stress, demands of wound healing, and the potential for infection can each increase the sickling phenomenon. Increased fluids are encouraged because keeping the child well-hydrated is most important for hemodilution to prevent sickling. Preparing the child psychologically to decrease fear minimizes undue emotional stress. Deep coughing is encouraged to promote pulmonary hygiene and prevent respiratory tract infection. Analgesics are used to control wound pain and to prevent abdominal splinting and decreased ventilation.

CN: Health promotion and maintenance; CNS: None; CL: Apply; DIFFICULTY: Easy

42. 1. The nurse must emphasize adequate nutrition as the priority to prevent infection in children with sickle cell anemia. Frequent medical supervision can prevent infection, often a predisposing factor toward development of a crisis. Avoiding stress and strenuous physical exertion helps prevent sickling, but adequate nutrition remains a priority.

CN: Health promotion and maintenance; CNS: None; CL: Apply; DIFFICULTY: Moderate

43. The health care provider has ordered diagnostic testing for a client suspected of having thalassemia. When gathering data from this client, which findings does the nurse determine are consistent with the disorder? Select all that apply.
1. Hgb: 8.8 g/dL
2. Hgb: 13.4 g/dL
3. HCT 36%
4. RBC 2.9
5. RBC 5.2

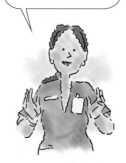

The two biggest problems in a sickle cell crisis are dehydration and pain. What interventions are best at addressing these?

44. The nurse is working in the emergency department when a child is admitted in sickle cell crisis. Which interventions should the nurse expect to perform? Select all that apply.
1. Give blood transfusions.
2. Give antibiotics.
3. Increase fluid intake.
4. Administered prescribed analgesics.
5. Prepare the child for a splenectomy.

45. When collecting data on a child with sickle cell anemia, which finding would indicate the child is experiencing vasoocclusive crisis?
1. Pain upon urination
2. Pain with ambulation
3. Reports of throat pain
4. Fever with associated rash

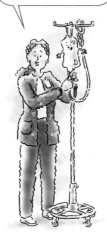

Remember to keep clients who are having a vasoocclusive crisis properly hydrated.

46. The nurse is caring for a child who has just been diagnosed with sickle anemia. Which initial action will be **most** therapeutic?
1. Discuss plans for contraception to prevent pregnancies at this time.
2. Referral for genetic counseling.
3. Offer emotional support.
4. Reinforce the idea that transmission is unlikely in subsequent pregnancies.

47. A 14-year-old is admitted for sickle cell crisis. Which nursing intervention would be **most** important?
1. Gather information about the child's ability to cope with this condition.
2. Monitor the child's temperature every 2 hours.
3. Provide adequate oxygenation, hydration, and pain management.
4. Make sure the family is involved in every step of the child's care.

43. 1, 4. A complete blood cell count can be anticipated in the client suspected of having thalassemia. In thalassemia the number of red blood cells and hemoglobin levels are reduced. A normal hemoglobin level for the client in this age group would be 12.5 to 16.1 g/dL. The normal range for red blood cell count for a client in this age range would be 4.1 to 5.3. The hematocrit level of 36% is within normal limits.
CN: Physiological integrity; CNS: Physiological adaptation; CL: Analyze; DIFFICULTY: Difficult

44. 3, 4. The primary therapy for sickle cell crisis is to increase fluid intake (according to age) and to give analgesics. Blood transfusions are only given conservatively to avoid iron overload. Antibiotics are given to children with fever. Routine splenectomy isn't recommended. Splenectomy in a child with sickle cell anemia is controversial.
CN: Physiological integrity; CNS: Physiological adaptation; CL: Apply; DIFFICULTY: Difficult

45. 2. Bone pain is one of the major symptoms of vasoocclusive crisis. Hand-foot syndrome, characterized by edematous painful extremities, is usually exhibited in the refusal of the child to bear weight and ambulate. Painful urination doesn't occur, but sickle cell anemia can cause kidney abnormalities. Throat pain isn't a symptom of vasoocclusive crisis. Fever is one of the major symptoms of vasoocclusive crisis but isn't associated with rash.
CN: Physiological integrity; CNS: Physiological adaptation; CL: Analyze; DIFFICULTY: Moderate

46. 3. The nurse can be instrumental in providing support, encouragement, and correct information to the parents of a child newly diagnosed with sickle cell anemia. Selective birth methods, such as in vitro fertilization of an embryo without markers for sickle cell disease, are discussed, but parents make their own decisions. All heterozygous, or trait-positive, parents should be referred for genetic counseling. The risk of transmission of sickle cell anemia in subsequent pregnancies remains the same.
CN: Psychological integrity; CNS: None; CL: Apply; DIFFICULTY: Easy

47. 3. The most critical need of a child in sickle cell crisis is to provide adequate oxygenation, hydration, and pain management until the crisis passes. Obtaining a temperature every 2 hours is not the priority intervention. While assessing the child's ability to cope and involving the family in the child's care are important, they aren't the priority interventions during a sickle cell crisis.
CN: Safe, effective care environment; CNS: Coordinated care; CL: Analyze; DIFFICULTY: Easy

48. The nurse is administering a blood transfusion to a child with sickle cell anemia. Which finding would indicate development of a transfusion reaction?
1. Diaphoresis and hot flashes
2. Urticaria, flushing, and wheezing
3. Fever, urticaria, and red, raised rash
4. Fever, disorientation, and abdominal pain

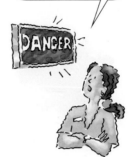

Be on the lookout for these symptoms of a transfusion reaction—it's serious business.

48. 2. Allergic reactions may occur when the recipient reacts to allergens in the donor's blood; this reaction causes urticaria, flushing, and wheezing. A febrile reaction can occur, causing fever and urticaria, but it wouldn't be accompanied by rash. Diaphoresis, hot flashes, disorientation, and abdominal pain aren't symptoms of a transfusion reaction.
CN: Physiological integrity; CNS: Reduction of risk potential; CL: Analyze; DIFFICULTY: Moderate

49. A parent asks the clinic nurse how often the influenza virus vaccine should be given to a child. Which response would be **most** accurate?
1. "The vaccine is usually given annually to children with certain risk factors."
2. "I wouldn't worry; your child doesn't need the vaccine."
3. "The vaccine is given monthly."
4. "The vaccine is given every 6 months."

49. 1. The influenza virus vaccine is usually administered annually to children at risk, not at monthly or 6-month intervals. The vaccine isn't contraindicated in children but is targeted at clients with chronic cardiac, pulmonary, hematologic, and neurologic problems.
CN: Health promotion and maintenance; CNS: None; CL: Apply; DIFFICULTY: Easy

50. A 3-year-old sibling of a neonate is diagnosed with pertussis. The parent gives a history of having been immunized as a child. What should be included in reinforcing education of the parent about possible infection of the neonate?
1. The neonate will inevitably contract pertussis.
2. Immune globulin is effective in protecting the neonate.
3. The risk to the neonate depends on the parent's immune status.
4. Erythromycin should be administered prophylactically to the neonate.

50. 4. In exposed, high-risk clients, such as neonates, erythromycin may be effective in preventing or lessening the severity of pertussis if administered during the preparoxysmal stage. Immune globulin isn't indicated; it's used as an immunization against hepatitis A. Neonates exposed to pertussis are at considerable risk for infections, regardless of the parent's immune status; however, infection isn't inevitable.
CN: Health promotion and maintenance; CNS: None; CL: Apply; DIFFICULTY: Difficult

51. A child has recently been admitted to the pediatric unit with laboratory values indicating an increase in hemoglobin A2. Based on this finding, the nurse should expect to follow a care plan based on which condition?
1. Beta-thalassemia trait
2. Iron deficiency
3. Lead poisoning
4. Sickle cell anemia

Confused by all the data in question #52? Try focusing on the words "petechial rash."

51. 1. The concentration of hemoglobin A2 is increased with beta-thalassemia trait. In severe iron deficiency, hemoglobin A2 may be decreased. The hemoglobin A2 level is normal in lead poisoning and sickle cell anemia.
CN: Physiological integrity; CNS: Reduction of risk potential; CL: Apply; DIFFICULTY: Difficult

52. A 4-year-old is asymptomatic but has a petechial rash. The platelet count is 20,000/∝L, and the hemoglobin level and white blood cell (WBC) count are normal. Which diagnosis would the nurse **most** likely suspect?
1. Acute lymphocytic leukemia (ALL)
2. Disseminated intravascular coagulation (DIC)
3. Idiopathic thrombocytopenic purpura (ITP)
4. Systemic lupus erythematosus (SLE)

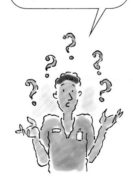

52. 3. The onset of ITP typically occurs between ages 1 and 6. Children with ITP are asymptomatic, except for petechial rash. ALL is associated with a low platelet count but an abnormal hemoglobin level and WBC count. DIC is secondary to a severe underlying disease. SLE is rare in a 4-year-old child.
CN: Physiological integrity; CNS: Physiological adaptation; CL: Analyze; DIFFICULTY: Moderate

53. A child has been diagnosed with leukemia. Which finding yields a poor prognosis for this child?
1. Presence of a mediastinal mass
2. Late central nervous system leukemia
3. Normal white blood cell (WBC) count at diagnosis
4. Disease presents between ages 2 and 10.

53. 1. The presence of a mediastinal mass indicates a poor prognosis for children with leukemia. Early central nervous system leukemia and a WBC count of 100,000/∝L or higher indicate a poor prognosis for a child with leukemia. The prognosis is poorer if age at onset is less than 2 years or greater than 10 years.
CN: Physiological integrity; CNS: Physiological adaptation; CL: Analyze; DIFFICULTY: Challenge

54. Which action would the nurse incorporate when reinforcing education for the parents of a neonate diagnosed with sickle cell anemia?
1. Stress the importance of iron supplementation.
2. Stress the importance of monthly vitamin B_{12} injections.
3. Demonstrate how to take an accurate temperature.
4. Explain that immunizations are contraindicated.

54. 3. Parents should be able to take an accurate temperature. A temperature of 101.3° to 102.2° F (38.5° to 39° C) calls for emergency evaluation, even if the neonate appears well. Folic acid requirement is increased in sickle cell anemia; therefore, supplementation is prudent. Vitamin B_{12} supplementation and iron supplementation aren't necessary. Parents should be encouraged to keep the immunizations up to date.
CN: Health promotion and maintenance; CNS: None; CL: Apply; DIFFICULTY: Difficult

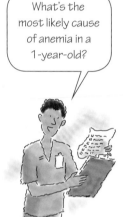

What's the most likely cause of anemia in a 1-year-old?

55. A 1-year-old infant is pale, but the physical examination is normal. Blood studies reveal a hematocrit of 24%. Which question by the nurse to the parents would be **most** useful in helping to establish a diagnosis of anemia?
1. "Is the infant on any medications?"
2. "What's the infant's usual daily diet?"
3. "Did the infant receive phototherapy for jaundice?"
4. "What's the pattern and appearance of bowel movements?"

55. 2. Iron deficiency anemia is the most common nutritional deficiency in infants between ages 9 months and 15 months. Anemia in a 1-year-old is mostly nutritional in origin, and its cause will be suggested by a detailed nutritional history. The other questions would not be helpful in diagnosing anemia.
CN: Health promotion and maintenance; CNS: None; CL: Apply; DIFFICULTY: Moderate

56. A nurse is reinforcing education for the parents of a child newly diagnosed with Hodgkin lymphoma. Which statement should the nurse include when reinforcing the education?
1. "Staging laparotomy is mandatory for every client."
2. "Excessive weight gain can be a symptom."
3. "Hodgkin lymphoma is rare before age 5."
4. "The incidence of Hodgkin lymphoma peaks between ages 11 and 15."

56. 3. Hodgkin lymphoma is rare before age 5. Staging laparotomy isn't recommended for children who have obvious intra-abdominal disease easily diagnosed by noninvasive studies. Systemic symptoms of Hodgkin lymphoma include fever, night sweats, malaise, weight loss, and pruritus. The peak incidence of Hodgkin lymphoma occurs in late adolescence and young adulthood (ages 15 to 34).
CN: Physiological integrity; CNS: Physiological adaptation; CL: Analyze; DIFFICULTY: Difficult

57. The nurse is caring for a child with perinatally acquired human immunodeficiency virus (HIV). At which age do children usually demonstrate symptoms of acquired immunodeficiency syndrome (AIDS)?
1. Within the first month of life
2. At 1 to 3 months of age
3. At 18 to 24 months of age
4. At 3 to 5 years of age

57. 3. The majority of children with perinatally transmitted AIDS appear normal in early infancy. Symptoms usually develop at 18 to 24 months of age.
CN: Physiological integrity; CNS: Physiological adaptation; CL: Understand; DIFFICULTY: Difficult

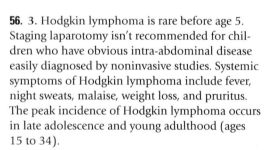

58. A 14-year-old is seen in the pediatrician's office with a history of mild sore throat, low-grade fever, a diffuse maculopapular rash, and reports swelling of the wrists and redness in the eyes. The nurse interprets these findings as indications of which condition?
1. Rubella
2. Rubeola
3. Roseola
4. Varicella

58. 1. Rubella presents with a diffuse maculopapular rash, mild sore throat, low-grade fever and, occasionally, conjunctivitis, arthralgia, or arthritis. Rubeola is associated with high fever, which reaches its peak at the height of a generalized macular rash and typically lasts for 5 days. Roseola involves high fever and is abruptly followed by a rash. Varicella presents with fever; small erythematous macules on the trunk or scalp, which progress to papules; and clear vesicles on an erythematous base.
CN: Physiological integrity; CNS: Physiological adaptation; CL: Analyze; DIFFICULTY: Moderate

59. The nurse is caring for a child diagnosed with iron deficiency anemia. Which treatment option deemed necessary by the health care provider does the nurse reinforce education?
1. Blood transfusion
2. Oral ferrous sulfate
3. An iron-fortified cereal
4. Intramuscular iron dextran

59. 2. A prompt rise in hemoglobin level and hematocrit follows the administration of oral ferrous sulfate. Blood transfusion is rarely indicated unless a child becomes symptomatic or is further compromised by a superimposed infection. Dietary modifications are appropriate long-term measures, but these modifications won't make enough iron quickly available to replenish iron stores. Intramuscular iron dextran is reserved for use when compliance can't be achieved; it's expensive, painful, and no more effective than oral iron.
CN: Physiological integrity; CNS: Pharmacological therapies; CL: Apply; DIFFICULTY: Challenge

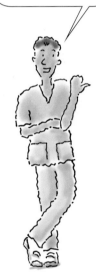

Drinking too much milk means not eating enough solid food. Those little tummies can only hold so much, after all.

60. Which statement by a caregiver indicates that a 10-month-old is at high risk for iron deficiency anemia?
1. "The baby is sleeping through the night without a bottle."
2. "The baby drinks about five 8-oz bottles of milk per day."
3. "The baby likes egg yolk in his cereal."
4. "The baby likes all vegetables except carrots."

60. 2. The recommended intake of milk, which doesn't contain iron, is 24 oz per day; 40 oz per day exceeds the recommended allotment and may reduce iron intake from solid food sources, risking iron deficiency anemia. Sleeping through the night without a bottle is an anticipated behavior at this age. Egg yolk is a good source of iron and would minimize any risk factor related to nutritional anemia. Because only dark-green vegetables are good sources of iron, a dislike of carrots wouldn't be significant for this client.
CN: Physiological integrity; CNS: Basic care and comfort; CL: Analyze; DIFFICULTY: Moderate

61. An iron dextran injection has been ordered for an 8-month-old baby with iron deficiency anemia. When reinforcing information about the medication to the parents, which statement indicates the need for further instruction?
1. "Most side effects of this medication will be noted within 12 hours of administration."
2. "If there are any side effects experienced by my child they will likely subside within 3 to 4 days."
3. "This medication will work to increase my baby's blood count."
4. "To check to see how effective this medication is the health care provider will order blood testing in the future."

61. 1. When iron dextran injection is administered to clients with anemia, the majority of side effects will manifest within about 24 hours of administration. The remaining statements are correct.
CN: Physiological integrity; CNS: Pharmacological therapies; CL: Analyze; DIFFICULTY: Difficult

62. When reinforcing education to parents about preventing nutritional iron deficiency, the nurse should emphasize which foods are significant sources of dietary iron? Select all that apply.
1. Peas
2. Fish
3. Spinach
4. Milk products
5. Dried fruits

62. **1, 3, 5.** Good dietary sources of iron include red meat, peas, beans, leafy green vegetables and dried fruits such as apricots and raisins. Fish isn't a good source of dietary iron. Milk is deficient in iron and should be limited in cases of nutritional anemia.

CN: Physiological integrity; CNS: Basic care and comfort;
CL: Apply; DIFFICULTY: Difficult

63. Which instructions would the nurse incorporate into the education plan for parents about the proper administration of oral iron supplements? Select all that apply.
1. Give the supplements with food.
2. Stop medication if vomiting occurs.
3. Follow the medication's administration with a glass of milk.
4. Give the medicine via a dropper or through a straw.
5. Increase dietary intake of fruits, vegetables and fiber to prevent constipation.

63. **4, 5.** Liquid iron preparations may temporarily stain the teeth; therefore, the drug should be given by dropper or through a straw. Constipation can be decreased by increasing intake of fruits and vegetables. Supplements should be given between meals, when the presence of free hydrochloric acid is greatest. If vomiting occurs, supplementation shouldn't be stopped; instead, it should be administered with food.

CN: Physiological integrity; CNS: Pharmacological therapies;
CL: Apply; DIFFICULTY: Difficult

64. While collecting data, a nurse should recognize which symptom as the primary clinical manifestation of hemophilia?
1. Petechiae on the face
2. Prolonged bleeding time
3. Decreased clotting time
4. Decreased white blood cell (WBC) count

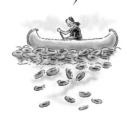

Looks like there's no absence of clotting factors here.

64. **2.** The effect of hemophilia is prolonged bleeding, anywhere from or within the body. With severe deficiencies, hemorrhage can occur as a result of minor trauma. Petechiae are uncommon in persons with hemophilia because repair of small hemorrhages depends on platelet function, not on blood clotting mechanisms. Clotting time is increased in a client with hemophilia. A decrease in WBCs is not indicative of hemophilia.

CN: Physiological integrity; CNS: Physiological adaptation;
CL: Apply; DIFFICULTY: Moderate

65. The nurse would be alert for signs and symptoms of internal bleeding **most** commonly at which site for a child with hemophilia?
1. Brain tissue
2. GI tract
3. Joint cavities
4. Spinal cord

65. **3.** The joint cavities, especially the knees, ankles, and elbows, are the most common site of internal bleeding. This bleeding typically results in bone changes and crippling, disabling deformities. Intracranial hemorrhage occurs less commonly than expected because the brain tissue has a high concentration of thromboplastin. Hemorrhage along the GI tract and spinal cord can occur but less commonly.

CN: Physiological integrity; CNS: Physiological adaptation;
CL: Apply; DIFFICULTY: Challenge

66. The nurse is reinforcing education for the parents of a child with hemophilia. The nurse should prepare them to initiate which immediate treatments to prevent excessive blood loss? Select all that apply.
1. Apply heat to the affected area.
2. Withhold factor replacement.
3. Apply pressure for at least 5 minutes.
4. Immobilize the affected area.
5. Elevate the affected area.

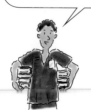

Your client with hemophilia begins to bleed profusely from a cut. What should you do?

66. **4, 5.** Immobilizing and elevating the area above the level of the heart will decrease blood flow. Cold, not heat, should be applied to promote vasoconstriction. Factor replacement should not be delayed. Pressure should be applied to the area for at least 10 to 15 minutes to allow clot formation.

CN: Physiological integrity; CNS: Physiological adaptation;
CL: Apply; DIFFICULTY: Challenge

CN: Client needs category   CNS: Client needs subcategory   CL: Cognitive level

67. A child with hemophilia is hospitalized with bleeding into the knee. Which action should the nurse take **first**?
   1. Prepare to administer a whole blood transfusion.
   2. Prepare to administer a plasma transfusion.
   3. Perform active range-of-motion (ROM) exercise on the affected part.
   4. Elevate the affected part.

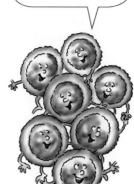

Look, guys—there's the laceration. Now clump together and chant, "Hemostasis."

67. 4. Bleeding into the joints is the most common type of bleeding episode in the more severe hemophilia forms. Elevating the affected part and applying pressure and cold are indicated. The nurse should anticipate transfusing the missing clotting factor—not whole blood or plasma, which won't stop the bleeding promptly and may pose a risk of fluid overload. Active ROM exercises are contraindicated because they may cause more bleeding, injury, and pain.
CN: Safe, effective care environment; CNS: Coordinated care; CL: Apply; DIFFICULTY: Easy

68. What should the nurse be sure to discuss with the parents of a child with hemophilia to prevent the crippling effects of joint degeneration?
   1. Avoiding the use of analgesics
   2. Using aspirin for pain relief
   3. Administering replacement factor
   4. Using active range-of-motion (ROM) exercises

68. 3. Prevention of bleeding is the ideal goal and is achieved by factor replacement therapy. Analgesics should be administered before physical therapy to control pain and provide the maximum benefit. Acetaminophen should be used for pain relief because aspirin has anticoagulant effects and has been linked to Reye syndrome. Passive ROM exercises are usually instituted after the acute phase.
CN: Physiological integrity; CNS: Physiological adaptation; CL: Apply; DIFFICULTY: Challenge

69. A client is diagnosed with von Willebrand disease. Where should the nurse most closely monitor bleeding?
   1. Brain tissue
   2. GI tract
   3. Mucous membranes
   4. Spinal cord

69. 3. The most characteristic clinical feature of von Willebrand disease is an increased tendency to bleed from mucous membranes, which may be seen as frequent nosebleeds or menorrhagia. In hemophilia, the joint cavities are the most common site of internal bleeding. Bleeding into the GI tract, spinal cord, and brain tissue can occur, but these are not the most common sites for bleeding.
CN: Physiological integrity; CNS: Physiological adaptation; CL: Analyze; DIFFICULTY: Difficult

70. Which nursing actions may be employed for the child with von Willebrand disease (VWD) who's having epistaxis? Select all that apply.
   1. Lay the client in a supine position.
   2. Pack the nostrils.
   3. Avoid pressure to the nose.
   4. Apply pressure to the nose.
   5. Sit leaning forward.

70. 2, 4, 5. Applying pressure to the nose may stop bleeding because most bleeds occur in the anterior part of the nasal septum. The child should be instructed to sit up and lean forward to avoid aspiration of blood. Pressure should then be maintained for at least 10 minutes to allow clotting to occur. Packing with tissue or cotton may be used to help stop bleeding, although care must be taken in removing packing to avoid dislodging the clot.
CN: Physiological integrity; CNS: Physiological adaptation; CL: Apply; DIFFICULTY: Difficult

71. A nurse is reinforcing education for the parents of a child with acute lymphocytic leukemia (ALL). The parents ask for information about what helps determine long-term survival. On what should the nurse base the response?
   1. Histologic type of the disease, initial platelet count, and type of treatment.
   2. Type of treatment, stage at diagnosis, and age at diagnosis.
   3. Histologic type of the disease, initial white blood cell (WBC) count, and age at diagnosis.
   4. Progression of illness, initial WBC count, and age at diagnosis.

71. 3. The histologic type of the disease has the greatest prognostic value in determining long-term outcome. Children with normal or low WBC counts at diagnosis tend to have much better prognoses than those with high WBC counts. Children diagnosed between the ages of 2 and 10 years consistently demonstrate better prognoses than those who are younger than 2 years or older than 10 years when diagnosed.
CN: Physiological integrity; CNS: Physiological adaptation; CL: Analyze; DIFFICULTY: Difficult

CN: Client needs category   CNS: Client needs subcategory   CL: Cognitive level

72. The nurse is reinforcing education to the parents of a child with leukemia about the three main consequences. What should the nurse inform the parents they should monitor for?
1. Bone deformities, spherocytosis, and infection
2. Anemia, infection, and bleeding tendencies
3. Lymphocytopoiesis, growth delays, and hirsutism
4. Polycythemia, decreased clotting time, and infection

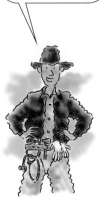

Ready for some adventures in assessment? Make sure you're equipped with all the right gear.

73. A child is seeing the health care provider for reports of bone and joint pain. Which other signs and symptoms may suggest leukemia?
1. Abdominal pain
2. Increased activity level
3. Increased appetite
4. Petechiae

74. Which findings in a child with leukemia would the nurse determine are indicators that the cancer has metastasized to the brain?
1. Headache and vomiting
2. Restlessness and tachycardia
3. Hypervigilant and anxious behavior
4. Increased heart rate and decreased blood pressure

75. The nurse is caring for a teen diagnosed with acute lymphocytic leukemia (ALL). A review of the laboratory report indicates a platelet count of 125,500/$\propto$L. When gathering data, which finding is **most** consistent with this laboratory result?
1. Abdominal swelling
2. Joint swelling
3. Bruising
4. Swollen axillary lymph nodes

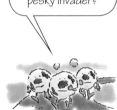

Never fear! The white blood cells are here. Now where's that pesky invader?

72. 2. The three main consequences of leukemia are anemia, caused by decreased erythrocyte production; infection secondary to neutropenia; and bleeding tendencies from decreased platelet production. Bone deformities don't occur with leukemia, although bones may become painful because of the proliferation of cells in the bone marrow. Spherocytosis refers to erythrocytes taking on a spheroid shape and isn't a feature of leukemia. Mature cells aren't produced in adequate numbers. Hirsutism and growth delay can be a result of large doses of steroids but aren't common in leukemia. Anemia, not polycythemia, occurs. Clotting times would be prolonged.
CN: Physiological integrity; CNS: Physiological adaptation; CL: Apply; DIFFICULTY: Moderate

73. 4. The most common signs and symptoms of leukemia result from infiltration of the bone marrow. These include petechiae, fever, pallor, and joint pain with decreased activity level. Abdominal pain is caused by areas of inflammation from normal flora in the GI tract. Increased appetite can occur, but it usually isn't a presenting symptom.
CN: Physiological integrity; CNS: Physiological adaptation; CL: Apply; DIFFICULTY: Challenge

74. 1. The usual effect of leukemic infiltration of the brain is increased intracranial pressure. The proliferation of cells interferes with the flow of cerebrospinal fluid in the subarachnoid space and at the base of the brain. The increased fluid pressure causes dilation of the ventricles, which creates symptoms of severe headache, vomiting, irritability, lethargy, increased blood pressure, decreased heart rate, and, eventually, coma. Children with a variety of illnesses are typically hypervigilant and anxious when hospitalized.
CN: Physiological integrity; CNS: Physiological adaptation; CL: Analyze; DIFFICULTY: Moderate

75. 3. Platelet production may be impaired in the client with leukemia. A platelet count of 125,000/$\propto$L is less than normal. This may be accompanied with bruising or reports of nosebleeds. The child with leukemia may experience abdominal swelling resulting from an accumulation of leukemia cells in the abdomen. Joint swelling may result from an accumulation of leukemia cells in the joint. Swollen lymph nodes are often seen in leukemia and result from the body attempting to fight the illness.
CN: Physiological integrity; CNS: Physiological adaptation; CL: Analyze; DIFFICULTY: Moderate

76. The nurse is preparing a child newly diagnosed with leukemia for a spinal tap. The parents state, "Why is the health care provider doing this? What is the **best** response by the nurse?
1. It will rule out meningitis.
2. It will decrease intracranial pressure (ICP).
3. It will aid in classification of the leukemia.
4. It will assess for central nervous system infiltration.

76. 4. A spinal tap is performed to assess for central nervous system infiltration. A spinal tap can be done to rule out meningitis, but this isn't the reason for the test on a child with leukemia. A spinal tap doesn't decrease ICP or aid in the classification of the leukemia.
CN: Physiological integrity; CNS: Physiological adaptation; CL: Apply; DIFFICULTY: Difficult

77. For which test would the nurse expect to prepare a client with leukemia before initiation of therapy to evaluate the ability to metabolize chemotherapeutic agents?
1. Lumbar puncture
2. Liver function studies
3. Complete blood count (CBC)
4. Peripheral blood smear

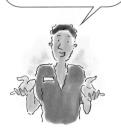

A client is suspected of having leukemia. What tests should you expect to be ordered?

77. 2. Liver and kidney function studies are done before initiation of chemotherapy to evaluate the child's ability to metabolize the chemotherapeutic agents. A lumbar puncture is performed to assess for central nervous system infiltration. A CBC is performed to assess for anemia. A peripheral blood smear is done to assess the level of immature white blood cells (blastocytes).
CN: Physiological integrity; CNS: Pharmacological therapies; CL: Apply; DIFFICULTY: Challenge

78. When reinforcing education for an adolescent with iron deficiency anemia about diet choices, which menu selection by the adolescent indicates that more instruction is necessary?
1. Caesar salad and pretzels
2. Cheeseburger and milkshake
3. Red beans and rice with sausage
4. Egg sandwich and snack peanuts

78. 1. Caesar salad and pretzels aren't foods high in iron and protein. Meats (especially organ meats), eggs, and nuts have high protein and iron.
CN: Physiological integrity; CNS: Basic care and comfort; CL: Analyze; DIFFICULTY: Challenge

79. A nurse is discussing with a parent the discharge plan for a child on methotrexate. The parent asks the nurse how the drug works. Which statement by the nurse is **most** accurate?
1. "The drug interferes with the use of folic acid by cancer cells."
2. "The drug keeps the cancer cell wall from forming."
3. "The drug makes the cancer cells ineffective by massing them together."
4. "The drug interferes with mitochondrial activity."

79. 1. Methotrexate is an antimetabolite and antifolate. It prevents folic acid from being used to create nucleic acid. As a result, it interferes with mitosis, which prevents the cancer cells from multiplying. It doesn't interfere with the cell wall, cause massing of the cells, or interfere with mitochondrial activity.
CN: Physiological integrity; CNS: Pharmacological therapies; CL: Apply; DIFFICULTY: Difficult

80. Which medication, administered as prophylaxis against pneumocystis pneumonia (PCP), does the nurse anticipate reinforcing education about for a child with leukemia?
1. Sulfamethoxazole-trimethoprim
2. Oral nystatin suspension
3. Prednisone
4. Vincristine sulfate PFS

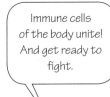

Immune cells of the body unite! And get ready to fight.

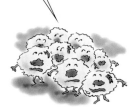

80. 1. The most common cause of death from leukemia is overwhelming infection. Pneumocystis pneumonia infection is lethal to a child with leukemia. As prophylaxis against pneumocystis pneumonia, continuous low dosages of sulfamethoxazole-trimethoprim are usually prescribed. Oral nystatin suspension would be indicated for the treatment of thrush. Prednisone isn't an antibiotic and increases susceptibility to infection. Vincristine sulfate is an antineoplastic agent.
CN: Physiological integrity; CNS: Pharmacological therapies; CL: Apply; DIFFICULTY: Moderate

81. A child is admitted to the pediatric unit with an unknown mass in the lower left abdomen. Which action should be the nurse's **priority**?
1. Obtain the history of the illness.
2. Place a "Do Not Palpate Abdomen" sign over the child's bed.
3. Obtain a complete set of vital signs.
4. Schedule a hemoglobin and hematocrit test for early morning.

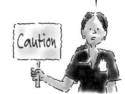

The priority in question #81 is to "first do no harm."

82. A client reports nausea and vomiting as a side effect of radiation and chemotherapy. When is the **best** time for the nurse to administer antiemetics?
1. 30 minutes before initiation of therapy
2. With the administration of therapy
3. Immediately after nausea begins
4. When therapy is completed

83. The nurse is caring for a client who has painful mouth ulcers resulting from chemotherapy treatments. Which nursing actions will be beneficial in promoting comfort for this client? Select all that apply.
1. Use lemon glycerin swabs.
2. Administer milk of magnesia.
3. Provide a bland, moist, soft diet.
4. Frequently wash the mouth with alcohol-based mouthwash.
5. Drink from a straw.

84. A parent of a child receiving the antineoplastic drug procarbazine indicates an understanding of the child's dietary requirements when which statement is made?
1. "I'll decrease his spicy food intake."
2. "I'll decrease his fluid intake."
3. "I'll include foods such as liver."
4. "I'll keep him away from cheese and pepperoni pizza."

85. The nurse is reinforcing education for a client who has hemorrhagic cystitis caused by bladder irritation from chemotherapeutic medications. Which suggestions can the nurse make to prevent this occurrence?
1. Giving antacids
2. Giving antibiotics
3. Restricting fluid intake
4. Increasing fluid intake

81. 2. The nurse must take measures to prevent palpation of the mass, if possible. If the mass is a malignant tumor, a do-not-palpate warning will help prevent trauma and rupture of the suspected tumor capsule. Rupture of the tumor capsule may cause seeding of cancer cells throughout the abdomen. Obtaining the history and vital signs and scheduling laboratory work are important but not the priority.
CN: Physiological integrity; CNS: Physiological adaptation; CL: Analyze; DIFFICULTY: Moderate

82. 1. Antiemetics are most beneficial if given before the onset of nausea and vomiting. To calculate the optimum time for administration, the first dose is given 30 minutes to 1 hour before nausea is expected, and then every 2, 4, or 6 hours for approximately 24 hours after chemotherapy. If the antiemetic were given with the medication or after the medication, it could lose its maximum effectiveness when needed.
CN: Physiological integrity; CNS: Pharmacological therapies; CL: Apply; DIFFICULTY: Easy

83. 3, 5. Oral ulcers are red, eroded, and painful. Providing a bland, moist, soft diet will make chewing and swallowing less painful. Drinking from a straw will prevent liquids from irritating the ulcerated areas. The use of lemon glycerin swabs and milk of magnesia should be avoided. Glycerin, a trihydric alcohol, absorbs water and dries the membranes. Milk of magnesia also has a drying effect because unabsorbed magnesium salts exert an osmotic pressure on tissue fluids. Many children also find the taste unpleasant. Frequent mouthwashes consisting of ½ tsp of salt plus ½ tsp of baking soda dissolved in an 8-oz glass of water are recommended.
CN: Physiological integrity; CNS: Basic care and comfort; CL: Apply; DIFFICULTY: Difficult

84. 4. Procarbazine has monoamine oxidatory activity. Foods high in tyramine, such as cheese and pepperoni, should be avoided. There's no chemotherapeutic or physiologic reason to restrict spicy foods. Increased fluid intake is essential to prevent calculi formation. Liver should be avoided because it contains tyramine, which can cause tremors, palpitations, and increased blood pressure.
CN: Physiological integrity; CNS: Pharmacological therapies; CL: Analyze; DIFFICULTY: Moderate

85. 4. Sterile hemorrhagic cystitis is an adverse effect of chemical irritation of the bladder from cyclophosphamide. It can be prevented by liberal fluid intake (at least 1½ times the recommended daily fluid requirement). Antacids aren't indicated for treatment. Antibiotics don't aid in the prevention of sterile hemorrhagic cystitis. Restricting fluids would only increase the risk of developing cystitis.
CN: Physiological integrity; CNS: Reduction of risk potential; CL: Apply; DIFFICULTY: Moderate

86. Which nursing action helps prepare the parent and child for alopecia, a common adverse effect of several chemotherapeutic agents?
1. Introduce the idea of a wig after hair loss occurs.
2. Explain that hair begins to regrow in 6 to 9 months.
3. Stress that hair loss during a second treatment with the same medication will be more severe.
4. Explain that, as hair thins, keeping it clean, short, and fluffy may camouflage partial baldness.

86. 4. The nurse must prepare parents and children for possible hair loss. Cutting the hair short lessens the impact of seeing large quantities of hair on bed linens and clothing. Sometimes, keeping the hair short and fuller can make a wig unnecessary. A child should be encouraged to pick out a wig similar to his own hair style and color before the hair falls out, to foster adjustment to hair loss. Hair regrows in 3 to 6 months. Hair loss during a second treatment with the same medication is usually less severe.
CN: Psychosocial integrity; CNS: None; CL: Apply;
DIFFICULTY: Challenge

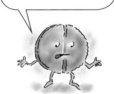

Remember to "select all that apply" in question #87.

87. The school nurse is conducting registration for a first-grader. Which immunizations should the school nurse verify that the child has had before entering school? Select all that apply.
1. Hepatitis B series
2. Diphtheria-tetanus-pertussis series
3. *Haemophilus influenzae* type b series
4. Varicella zoster
5. Pneumonia vaccine
6. Inactivated polio vaccine

87. 1, 2, 3, 6. Hepatitis B series, diphtheria-tetanus-pertussis series, *H. influenzae* type b series, and inactivated polio vaccine are immunizations that the child should receive before entering first grade. The varicella zoster vaccine is administered only if the child hasn't had chickenpox. Pneumonia vaccine isn't required or routinely given to children.
CN: Health promotion and maintenance; CNS: None; CL: Apply;
DIFFICULTY: Challenge

If bleeding is an issue for you, then you'd better steer clear of me.

88. The parents of a child diagnosed with leukemia have stated that they'll give aspirin to their child for pain relief. Which statement by the nurse about aspirin would be most accurate?
1. "It's contraindicated because it decreases platelet production."
2. "It's contraindicated because it promotes bleeding tendencies."
3. "It's not a strong enough analgesic."
4. "It decreases the effects of methotrexate."

88. 2. Aspirin would be contraindicated because it promotes bleeding. Aspirin use has also been associated with Reye syndrome in children. For home use, acetaminophen is recommended for mild to moderate pain. Aspirin enhances the effects of methotrexate and has no effect on platelet production. Nonopioid analgesia has been effective for mild to moderate pain in children with leukemia.
CN: Physiological integrity; CNS: Pharmacological therapies;
CL: Apply; DIFFICULTY: Easy

89. The nurse is preparing a school-age child for a bone marrow biopsy to rule out leukemia. The nurse explains that the sample will be taken from the anterior iliac crest. Identify this area.

89. A bone marrow biopsy may be taken from the anterior or posterior iliac crests, as shown. A bone marrow biopsy may also be taken from the sternum, vertebral spinous process, rib, or tibia.

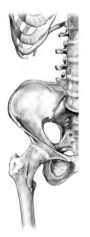

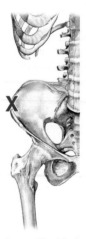

CN: Physiological integrity; CNS: Physiological adaptation;
CL: Apply; DIFFICULTY: Difficult

90. A child is admitted to the unit with a diagnosis of hemophilia. When assisting with development of the care plan, what facts about the disease should the nurse keep in mind? Select all that apply.
1. Hemophilia is a sex-linked genetic disorder.
2. Bleeding occurs most commonly in the joints.
3. The most common treatments include pressure and ice.
4. Hemophilia can be caused by a retrovirus.
5. Administration of whole blood is generally effective in stopping bleeding episodes.

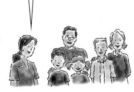

Genetics is a big deal. It not only determines our hair color and mannerisms, but what diseases we're likely to get.

90. 1, 2. Hemophilia is a sex-linked genetic disorder, and bleeding episodes most commonly occur in joints, such as the knee or elbow. Pressure and ice may be helpful, but these interventions don't have any effect on clotting factors in the blood, so bleeding may resume as soon as these interventions stop. Hemophilia isn't caused by a retrovirus. Administration of clotting factors VIII and IX (not whole blood) is the treatment of choice.
CN: Safe, effective care environment; CNS: Coordinated care; CL: Analyze; DIFFICULTY: Difficult

91. The nurse is meeting with a 17 year-old who has recently tested positive for HIV. The client states, "What information will be disclosed to others." What information can be provided by the nurse?
1. "You will need to disclose information to your teachers."
2. "Your employers have a legal right to know your HIV status."
3. "In some jurisdictions laws may require you share this information with future sexual partners."
4. "You will be legally required to locate all past sexual contacts to inform them of your status."

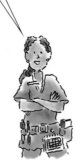

Well done, grasshopper. You are now ready to advance to the next level.

91. 3. Most jurisdictions have laws requiring an HIV positive person to share their status with a contact prior to sexual activity. Sharing a positive HIV status is an obvious area of concern for a client. Studies have shown that those who disclose their status to friends and family experience a greater source of support and benefit from it. Disclosures to teachers, employers, friends and family is voluntary and not a requirement. Disclosures of a positive HIV status to past contacts is a courtesy and while recommended is not required.
CN: Safe, effective care environment; CNS: Management of care; CL: Apply; DIFFICULTY: Challenge

92. The health care provider has recommended a diet rich in folic acid for the client with sickle cell anemia. Which food selections are appropriate for inclusion? Select all that apply.
1. Peas
2. String cheese
3. Orange juice
4. Bananas
5. Kale

92. 1, 3, 5. Folic acid is associated with red blood cell production. Folic acid is encouraged in the diet for individuals with sickle cell anemia. Sources of folic acid include peas, legumes, citrus fruits, and leafy green vegetables. String cheese and bananas are not considered good sources of folic acid.
CN: Physiological integrity; CNS: Physiological adaptation; CL: Apply; DIFFICULTY: Challenge

93. The health care provider has prescribed hydroxyurea for a client with sickle cell anemia. When reinforcing education to this client and family what information should be included? Select all that apply.
1. "This medication may initially cause nausea and vomiting."
2. "If you forget to take a dose of this medication take it when you remember it."
3. "Do not double doses of this medication."
4. "If you feel excessively fatigued or weak contact your health care provider."
5. "Report any darkening of your skin or fingernails to your health care provider."

93. 1, 2, 3, 4. Hydroxyurea may be prescribed for the client with sickle cell anemia. This medication is used to prevent the frequency of crisis episodes. The medication is administered orally. It may initially cause nausea and vomiting. If a dose is missed it should be taken when realized. If the dose is recalled at the time the next is due do not double up on the dosages. The medication may have adverse effects that require immediate notification of the health care provider, such as excessive weakness or fatigue. Darkening of the skin and fingernails is a side effect of the medication and does not require notification of the health care provider.
CN: Physiological integrity; CNS: Pharmacological therapies, CL: Apply; DIFFICULTY: Difficult

Chapter 28

Respiratory Disorders

From the simple otitis media to the uncommon and dangerous epiglottitis, this chapter covers a wide variety of respiratory disorders in children. So, take a deep breath and go for it!

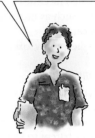

Asthma

Lung disease that inflames and narrows the airways

Key signs and symptoms
- Diaphoresis
- Dyspnea
- Prolonged expiration with an expiratory wheeze; in severe distress, inspiratory wheeze
- Unequal or decreased breath sounds
- Use of accessory muscles

Key test results
- Oxygen saturation via pulse oximetry may show decreased oxygen saturation
- Arterial blood gas measurement may show increased partial pressure of arterial carbon dioxide from respiratory acidosis

Key treatments
- Short-acting bronchodilator: albuterol
- Chromone derivative: cromolyn sodium
- Long-acting bronchodilator: salmeterol, formoterol
- Leukotriene modifiers: montelukast, zafirlukast
- Inhaled glucocorticoids: fluticasone, budesonide, flunisolide

Key interventions
- Monitor respiratory and cardiovascular status
- Monitor vital signs during an acute attack
- Allow the child to sit upright to ease breathing; provide moist oxygen, if necessary
- Monitor for alterations in vital signs (especially cardiac stimulation and hypotension)

Bronchiolitis

Infection of the bronchioles usually caused by a viral infection and usually found in children under 2 years of age

Key signs and symptoms
- Sternal retractions
- Tachypnea

Key test results
- Bronchial mucus culture shows respiratory syncytial virus

Key treatments
- Humidified oxygen
- IV fluids

Key interventions
- Monitor vital signs and pulse oximetry
- Monitor respiratory and cardiovascular status
- Administer humidified oxygen therapy

Bronchopulmonary dysplasia

Chronic bronchial tube and lung disease that affects infants who have been on a ventilator

Key signs and symptoms
- Crackles, rhonchi, wheezes
- Dyspnea
- Sternal retractions

Key test results
- Chest x-ray reveals pulmonary changes (bronchiolar metaplasia and interstitial fibrosis)

Key treatments
- Chest physiotherapy
- Continued ventilatory support and oxygen
- Bronchodilators such as albuterol

Key interventions
- Monitor respiratory and cardiovascular status
- Monitor vital signs, pulse oximetry, and intake and output

Some respiratory disorders are treated with oxygen therapy.

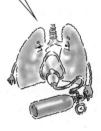

Croup

Upper respiratory tract viral infection that causes a barking cough

Key signs and symptoms
- Barking, brassy cough or hoarseness
- Inspiratory stridor with varying degrees of respiratory distress
- Temperature of 103.5° F (39.7° C) or higher

Bronchiolitis is usually found in children under 2 years of age.

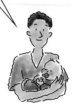

Key test results
- Laryngoscopy may reveal inflammation and obstruction in epiglottis and laryngeal areas
- Neck x-ray shows areas of upper airway narrowing and edema in subglottic folds

Key treatments
- Cool humidification during sleep with a cool mist tent or room humidifier
- Inhaled racemic epinephrine and corticosteroids such as methylprednisolone sodium succinate
- Tracheostomy, oxygen administration

Key interventions
- Monitor vital signs and pulse oximetry
- Administer oxygen therapy and maintain the child in a cool mist tent, if needed
- Allow parent to hold the child

Cystic fibrosis
Inherited disease that causes thick, sticky mucus to form in the lungs, pancreas and other organs

Key signs and symptoms
- History of a chronic, productive cough and recurrent respiratory infections, often due to *Pseudomonas* infections
- Parents report salty taste on the child's skin
- History of poor weight gain and growth, intestinal blockage, foul-smelling, greasy stools

Key test results
- Sweat test using pilocarpine iontophoresis is positive
- Newborn screening test may reveal cystic fibrosis
- Sputum cystic fibrosis respiratory screen reveals bacterial or fungal lung infection

Key treatments
- Chest physiotherapy
- Oral pancreatic enzyme replacement
- Antibiotics: tobramycin, azithromycin
- Bronchodilators
- Mucolytics: dornase alfa

Key interventions
- Monitor respiratory and cardiovascular status

- Administer pancreatic enzymes with meals and snacks
- Encourage breathing exercises and perform chest physiotherapy two to four times a day

Epiglottitis
Acute inflammation of the epiglottis; an emergency that may result in death if not treated quickly

Key signs and symptoms
- Difficult and painful swallowing
- Increased drooling
- Restlessness
- Stridor

Key test results
- Lateral neck x-ray shows enlarged epiglottis

Key treatments
- Emergency endotracheal intubation or tracheotomy
- Oxygen therapy or cool mist tent
- 10-day course of parenteral antibiotics

Key interventions
- Monitor vital signs and pulse oximetry
- Monitor respiratory and cardiovascular status
- Defer inspection of the throat until the arrival of emergency personnel and supplies

Sudden infant death syndrome (SIDS)
Sudden and unexpected death of an infant younger than 1 year of age

Key signs and symptoms
- Death takes place during sleep without noise or struggle

Key test results
- Autopsy is the only way to diagnose SIDS

Key treatments
- Emotional and other support for the parents

Key interventions
- Let parents touch, hold, and rock the infant
- Reinforce the fact that the death wasn't the parents' fault

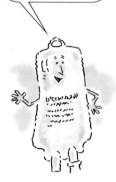
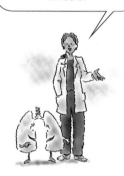
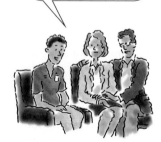

Respiratory questions, answers, and rationales

1. The nurse is reinforcing education for a parent about newborn care and how to prevent SIDS (sudden infant death syndrome). Which statement made by the parent would indicate an understanding of SIDS?
1. SIDS is caused by cardiac dysrhythmias
2. SIDS is caused by apnea of prematurity
3. SIDS is an unexplained death of an infant
4. SIDS is always found in premature infants

2. While teaching a class to new parents, which child does the nurse correctly identify as having an increased risk of sudden infant death syndrome (SIDS)?
1. Premature infant with low birth weight
2. A healthy 2-year-old
3. Infant hospitalized for fever
4. Firstborn child

3. A 6-week-old infant who isn't breathing is brought to the emergency department; a preliminary diagnosis of sudden infant death syndrome (SIDS) is made to the parents. Which intervention should the nurse take **first**?
1. Call their spiritual advisor.
2. Explain the etiology of SIDS.
3. Allow them to see their infant.
4. Collect the infant's belongings and give them to the parents.

4. A client who has just delivered a full term baby tells the nurse that sudden infant death syndrome (SIDS) is a big fear. When educating the mother about SIDS which factor does the nurse identify as being associated with SIDS?
1. Breast-feeding the infant
2. Gestational age of 42 weeks
3. Immunizations
4. Low birth weight

5. An infant is brought to the emergency department and pronounced dead with the preliminary finding of sudden infant death syndrome (SIDS). Which question to the parents is **most** appropriate?
1. "Did you hear the infant cry out?"
2. "Was the infant's head buried in a blanket?"
3. "Were any of the siblings jealous of the new baby?"
4. "How did the infant look when you found him?"

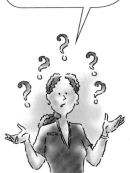

What should the nurse do first, in this case?

1. 3. SIDS can best be defined as the sudden death of an infant younger than age 1 that remains unexplained after autopsy. Apnea of prematurity occurs in infants less than 32 weeks' gestation who have periodic breathing lapses for 20 seconds or more. Apparent life-threatening events usually have some combination of apnea, color change, marked change in muscle tone, choking, or gagging.
CN: Physiological integrity; CNS: Physiological adaptation; CL: Apply; DIFFICULTY: Easy

2. 1. Premature infants, especially those with low birth weight, have an increased risk for SIDS. Infants with apnea, central nervous system disorders, or respiratory disorders also have a higher risk of SIDS. Peak age for SIDS is 2 to 4 months. Hospitalization for fever doesn't affect risk for SIDS. There's an increased risk of SIDS in subsequent siblings of two or more SIDS victims.
CN: Physiological integrity; CNS: Reduction of risk potential; CL: Analyze; DIFFICULTY: Easy

3. 3. The parents need time with their infant to assist with the grieving process. Calling their pastor and collecting the infant's belongings are also important steps in the care plan but aren't priorities. The parents will be too upset to understand an explanation of SIDS at this time.
CN: Psychosocial integrity; CNS: None; CL: Apply; DIFFICULTY: Easy

4. 4. Prematurity, low birth weight, maternal smoking, and multiple births are all risk factors for SIDS. Breast-feeding and a gestational age of 42 weeks aren't related to SIDS. Immunizations have been disproved to be associated with the disorder.
CN: Physiological integrity; CNS: Reduction of risk potential; CL: Apply; DIFFICULTY: Easy

5. 4. During the initial history in the emergency department, only factual questions should be asked of the parents whose child has died of SIDS. The other questions imply blame, guilt, or neglect.
CN: Physiological integrity; CNS: Physiological adaptation; CL: Apply; DIFFICULTY: Easy

6. Which intervention should be included in the care plan for children with an increased risk of sudden infant death syndrome (SIDS)?
1. Pulmonary function testing at regular intervals
2. Home apnea monitoring
3. Pulse oximetry while sleeping
4. Chest x-ray at age 1 month

7. Which reaction is usually exhibited first by the family of an infant who has died from sudden infant death syndrome (SIDS)?
1. Feelings of blame or guilt
2. Acceptance of the diagnosis
3. Requests for the infant's belongings
4. Questions regarding the etiology of the diagnosis

8. The parents of an infant who just died from sudden infant death syndrome (SIDS) are angry at God and refuse to see any members of the clergy. Which process **best** defines this situation?
1. Ineffective cooping
2. Spiritual distress
3. Complicated grieving
4. Chronic sorrow

9. Which plan is **most** appropriate for a discharge home visit to parents who lost an infant to sudden infant death syndrome (SIDS)?
1. One visit in 2 weeks
2. No visit is necessary
3. As soon after death as possible
4. One visit with parents only, no siblings

10. A few days after the death of an infant from sudden infant death syndrome (SIDS), the nurse making a home visit notices that the parents are disorganized in their thought patterns. What is the **best** action for the nurse?
1. Realize that this is a normal process for the impact phase of crisis.
2. Instruct the parents that this is not normal and they should try to accept the situation.
3. Inform the parents that many parents go through this but it is not a healthy behavior.
4. Tell the parents that they need to go on with their life as there is nothing they can do now.

> Which is most likely to be the first response of the family?

6. 2. A home apnea monitor is recommended for infants with an increased risk of SIDS. Diagnostic tests, such as pulmonary function tests, pulse oximetry, and chest x-rays, can't diagnose the risk of surviving or dying from SIDS.
CN: Physiological integrity; CNS: Reduction of risk potential; CL: Apply; DIFFICULTY: Easy

7. 1. During the first few moments, the parents usually are in shock and have overwhelming feelings of blame or guilt. Acceptance of the diagnosis and questions regarding the etiology may not occur until the parents have had time to see the child. The infant's belongings are usually packaged for the family to take home, but some parents may see this as a painful reminder of their deceased child.
CN: Psychosocial integrity; CNS: None; CL: Apply; DIFFICULTY: Easy

8. 2. The defining characteristic of spiritual distress includes anger and refusal to interact with spiritual leaders. While anger is part of the grieving process, there's no indication that the parents aren't coping effectively or are experiencing complicated grieving. Chronic sorrow, as the name implies, occurs over a period of time and may be cyclical. These are not nursing diagnoses but appropriate feelings that parents experience after such a horrible event.
CN: Psychosocial integrity; CNS: None; CL: Analyze; DIFFICULTY: Moderate

9. 3. When parents return home, a visit is necessary as soon after the death as possible. The nurse should assess what the parents have been told, what they think happened, and how they've explained this to the other siblings. Not all of these issues will be resolved in one visit. The number of visits and a plan for intervention must be flexible. The needs of the siblings must always be considered.
CN: Psychosocial integrity; CNS: None; CL: Apply; DIFFICULTY: Easy

10. 1. Within a day or two of the infant's death, the parents enter the impact phase of crisis, which consists of disorganized thoughts in which they can't deal with the crisis in concrete terms. This is a normal reaction at this time. Informing the parents that it is not a healthy behavior is untrue and will only add to the parents feeling worse. Telling them to go on with their life would be very distressing and not compassionate or therapeutic.
CN: Psychosocial integrity; CNS: None; CL: Apply; DIFFICULTY: Easy

11. When reinforcing discharge education for a parent and newborn, which statement made by the parent indicates a need for further instruction?
1. I will place my baby in a supine position when napping
2. I will place my baby in a prone position when napping
3. I know the importance of correct positioning when my baby is napping
4. It is acceptable to let my baby lay prone when playing only with supervision

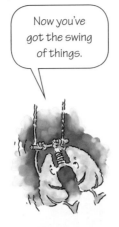

Now you've got the swing of things.

12. Which activity should be recommended for long-term support of parents who have lost an infant due to sudden infant death syndrome (SIDS)?
1. Attending support groups
2. Attending church regularly
3. Attending counseling sessions
4. Discussing feelings with family and friends

13. Which nursing intervention is **best** to help a 2-year-old child adapt to a hospitalization?
1. Allow the child to have favorite toys.
2. Allow the child to play with equipment used on him.
3. Explain procedures in simple terms.
4. Ask one or both parents to stay with the child.

14. A 2-year-old child comes to the emergency department with inspiratory stridor and a barking cough. What is the **highest priority** action by the nurse?
1. Administer IV antibiotics.
2. Provide oxygen by facemask.
3. Establish and maintain the airway.
4. Ask the mother to go to the waiting room.

15. Which action is the **best** intervention for parents to take if their child is experiencing an episode of "midnight croup" or acute spasmodic laryngitis?
1. Give warm liquids.
2. Raise the heat on the thermostat.
3. Provide humidified air with cool mist.
4. Take the child into the bathroom with a cold, running shower.

11. 2. The American Academy of Pediatrics endorses placing infants only face-up in their cribs as a way to reduce the risk of sudden infant death syndrome (SIDS). The side-lying position promotes gastric emptying but the infant might roll to a prone position, predisposing him to SIDS. Placing infants on their stomachs is thought to make an attack of apnea harder to fight off, as it may restrict respiratory muscles, but exactly how the sleeping position predisposes a child to SIDS is still unclear. It is, however, acceptable to allow the infant on his stomach while awake and playing with supervision.
CN: Health promotion and maintenance; CNS: None; CL: Apply; DIFFICULTY: Easy

12. 1. The best support will come from parents who have had the same experience. Attending church and discussing feelings with family and friends can offer support, but they may not understand the experience. Counseling sessions are usually a short-term support.
CN: Psychosocial integrity; CNS: None; CL: Apply; DIFFICULTY: Easy

13. 4. The most important factor in helping a child cope with new and strange surroundings is to encourage feelings of security by having the parents present—the hallmark of family-centered care. Placing the child's favorite toys in the room provides distraction and allows the child to have something of his own, but it may not alleviate fears. Allowing the child to play with the equipment may pose a safety hazard and isn't appropriate. Explaining procedures in simple terms is important but a 2-year-old has limited understanding.
CN: Psychosocial integrity; CNS: None; CL: Apply; DIFFICULTY: Moderate

14. 3. The initial priority is to establish and maintain the airway. Edema and accumulation of secretions may contribute to airway obstruction. Antibiotics aren't indicated for viral illnesses. Oxygen should be administered by tent as soon as possible to decrease the child's distress. Allowing the child to stay with the mother reduces anxiety and distress.
CN: Physiological integrity; CNS: Physiological adaptation; CL: Apply; DIFFICULTY: Easy

15. 3. High humidity with cool mist, such as from a cool mist humidifier, provides the most (and safest form of) relief. Cool liquids would be best for the child. If unable to take liquid, the child needs emergency care. Raising the heat on the thermostat will result in dry, warm air, which may cause secretions to adhere to the airway wall. A warm, running shower provides a mist that may be helpful to moisten and decrease the viscosity of airway secretions and may also decrease laryngeal spasm.
CN: Physiological integrity; CNS: Physiological adaptation; CL: Apply; DIFFICULTY: Challenge

16. A child is admitted with a diagnosis of croup. Which characteristic signs would the nurse monitor in this client? Select all that apply.
  1. "Barking" cough
  2. Temperature in normal range
  3. Low heart rate
  4. Severe respiratory distress
  5. Increased heart rate

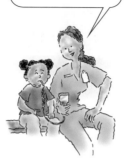

Croup is associated with an upper respiratory infection, resulting in a high-grade fever.

16. 1, 5. A resonant cough described as "barking" is the most characteristic sign of croup. Usually the heart rate is rapid. The child may present with a low-grade or high fever depending on whether the etiologic agent is viral or bacterial. The child may have varying degrees of respiratory distress related to swelling or obstruction.
CN: Physiological integrity; CNS: Physiological adaptation; CL: Apply; DIFFICULTY: Challenge

17. A child has been diagnosed with croup and is experiencing increased respiratory distress. What would the nurse expect to see in this child?
  1. A barking cough
  2. Intercostal retractions
  3. Clubbing of the fingers
  4. Increased anteroposterior chest diameter

17. 2. Intercostal retractions occur as the child's breathing becomes more labored and the use of other muscles is necessary to draw air into the lungs. A barking cough occurs in a child with croup and in itself isn't a sign that the condition is worsening. Clubbing of the fingers and a change in chest diameter occur with chronic respiratory conditions.
CN: Physiological integrity; CNS: Physiological adaptation; CL: Analyze; DIFFICULTY: Moderate

18. The nurse identifies which goal to be a high **priority** for a young client with ineffective airway clearance?
  1. Reduce the child's anxiety.
  2. Maintain a patent airway.
  3. Provide adequate oral fluids.
  4. Administer medications as ordered.

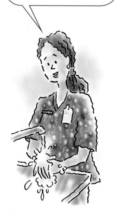

Protect yourself and your clients from infection by washing your hands frequently, observing your facility's protocols.

18. 2. The most important goal is to maintain a patent airway. Reducing anxiety and administering medications will follow after the airway is secure. The child shouldn't be allowed to eat or drink anything to avoid the risk of aspiration.
CN: Physiological integrity; CNS: Physiological adaptation; CL: Apply; DIFFICULTY: Easy

19. When obtaining data on a 2-year old child with croup in respiratory distress, which finding would the nurse expect to observe **first**?
  1. Capillary refill time less than 3 seconds
  2. Low temperature
  3. Grunting or head bobbing
  4. Respiratory rate of 28 breaths/minute

19. 3. Grunting or head bobbing is seen in a child in respiratory distress. Capillary refill time of less than 3 seconds and a respiratory rate of 28 breaths/minute are normal findings. The child's temperature may be elevated if infection is present.
CN: Physiological integrity; CNS: Physiological adaptation; CL: Apply; DIFFICULTY: Challenge

20. The nurse is caring for a child with a respiratory infection. Which precaution should the nurse take to adhere to infection control measures?
  1. Enforce handwashing.
  2. Place the child in isolation.
  3. Educate the child on the use of tissues.
  4. Provide a roommate in the same room.

20. 1. Handwashing helps prevent the spread of infections. Ill children should be placed in separate rooms if possible but don't need to be isolated. Educating children on the proper use of tissues is important, but the key is tissue disposal and handwashing after use.
CN: Health promotion and maintenance; CNS: None; CL: Apply; DIFFICULTY: Challenge

21. The nurse is reinforcing education for a parent regarding the best time to administer a nebulizer treatment to a child with croup. Which statement made by the parent indicates an understanding of the teaching?
  1. Any time is fine since the croup is still present
  2. During playtime would be best
  3. During naptime
  4. After the child eats but not before

21. 3. The nurse should administer nebulizer treatments at prescribed intervals and only certain times are appropriate. Administering treatment during naptime allows for as little disruption as possible. Administering treatment during playtime disrupts the child's daily pattern. A child should be given a treatment before eating so the airway will be open and the work of eating will be decreased. Parents are usually helpful when administering treatments. The child can sit on the parent's lap to help decrease anxiety or fear.
CN: Physiological integrity; CNS: Pharmacological therapies; CL: Apply; DIFFICULTY: Moderate

22. A parent brings a child to the ED reporting difficulty swallowing, increased drooling, restlessness, and stridor. The position of comfort is observed to be tripod-sitting position. What does the nurse suspect may be occurring?
1. Asthma
2. Epiglottitis
3. Bronchiolitis
4. Croup

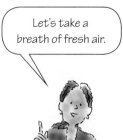

Let's take a breath of fresh air.

22. **2.** Epiglottitis is associated with difficult swallowing, increased drooling, restlessness, stridor and tripod sitting position Asthma is accompanied dyspnea, fatigue, wheezing, decreased breath sounds and use of accessory muscles. Bronchiolitis normally is diagnosed by a cough, sternal retractions, thick mucous, and elevated temperature. Croup is identifies with a barking cough, crackles and/or decreased breath sounds, increased dyspnea and inspiratory stridor.
CN: Physiological integrity; CNS: Physiological adaptation;
CL: Analyze; DIFFICULTY: Difficult

23. Which intervention is **most** important to explain to parents during the recovery stages of croup?
1. Limit oral fluid intake.
2. Recognize signs of respiratory distress.
3. Provide three nutritious meals per day.
4. Allow the child to go to the playground.

23. **2.** Although most children with croup recover without complications, the parents should be able to recognize signs and symptoms of respiratory distress and know how to access emergency services. Oral fluids should be encouraged because fluids help to thin secretions. Although nutrition is important, frequent small nutritious snacks are usually more appealing than an entire meal. Children should have optimal rest and engage in quiet play. A comfortable environment free of noxious stimuli lessens respiratory distress.
CN: Physiological integrity; CNS: Physiological adaptation;
CL: Apply; DIFFICULTY: Easy

24. The nurse is obtaining data on a child with suspected epiglottitis. Which findings would the nurse expect to observe in this child? Select all that apply.
1. Decreased secretions
2. Drooling
3. High fever
4. Spontaneous cough
5. Tripod position

Tripods aren't just for cameras.

24. **2, 3, 5.** Drooling is common due to the pain of swallowing, excessive secretions, and sore throat. The child usually has a high fever and the absence of a spontaneous cough. The classic picture is the child in a tripod position with mouth open and tongue protruding.
CN: Physiological integrity; CNS: Physiological adaptation;
CL: Apply; DIFFICULTY: Difficult

25. Which strategy would be **best** to include when assisting with planning care for a child with acute epiglottitis?
1. Encourage oral fluids for hydration.
2. Maintain the child in semi-Fowler's position.
3. Administer IV antibiotic therapy.
4. Maintain respiratory isolation for 48 hours.

25. **3.** The etiologic agent for epiglottitis is usually bacterial; therefore, the treatment consists of IV antibiotic therapy. The child shouldn't be allowed anything by mouth during the initial phases of the infection to prevent aspiration. The child should be placed in Fowler's position or any position that provides the most comfort and security. Respiratory isolation isn't required.
CN: Physiological integrity; CNS: Physiological adaptation;
CL: Apply; DIFFICULTY: Challenge

26. A 2-year-old child is found on the floor next to a toy chest. After first determining unresponsiveness and calling for help, which step should be taken next?
1. Start mouth-to-mouth resuscitation.
2. Begin chest compressions.
3. Check for a pulse.
4. Open the airway.

26. **3.** According to the 2015 American Heart Association CPR guidelines, the sequence is C-A-B (chest compressions-airway-breathing). Initially check the child for a pulse. If no pulse is detected, perform chest compressions (30 as a single rescuer). Next, open the airway by using the head-tilt, chin-lift maneuver, and if a single rescuer, give two rescue breaths.
CN: Physiological integrity; CNS: Physiological adaptation;
CL: Apply; DIFFICULTY: Challenge

27. A 10-month-old infant is found in respiratory arrest, and cardiopulmonary resuscitation is started. Which site is best to check for a pulse?

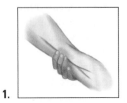
1.

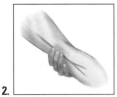
2.

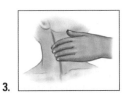
3.

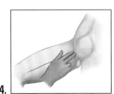
4.

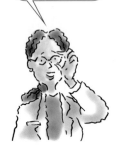

If you arm yourself with knowledge, I'm sure you'll be able to answer question #27.

27. 1. Palpation of the brachial artery is recommended. The short, chubby neck of infants makes rapid location of the carotid artery difficult. After age 1, the carotid would be used. The femoral pulse, often palpated in a hospital setting, may be difficult to assess because of the infant's position, fat folds, and clothing. The radial pulse isn't a good indicator of central artery perfusion.
CN: Physiological integrity; CNS: Physiological adaptation; CL: Apply; DIFFICULTY: Moderate

28. The nurse is caring for a child with a diagnosis of croup. What advice should the nurse give to the parent when concern is expressed about the child waking at night due to the cough?
1. Call 911 for assistance.
2. Immediately take the child to an ambulatory care center.
3. Take the child to the bathroom, shut the door, and turn on a hot shower.
4. Administer another dose of medication.

28. 3. Steam from the shower will decrease laryngeal spasms, so taking the child to the bathroom and turning on a hot shower should help. It is not necessary to call 911 each time a child has a coughing episode with croup. Driving the child to a patient care center would be dangerous if something more serious happened on the way. If the child is coughing he would not be able to do a breathing treatment successfully.
CN: Physiological integrity; CNS: Physiological adaptation; CL: Apply; DIFFICULTY: Easy

29. A nurse observes a parent in a class performing chest compressions on a simulated 2-year-old child. The nurse knows the parent is doing compressions correctly when observing compressions to be approximately how many inches in depth?
1. 1 in (2.5 cm)
2. 1½ in (3.8 cm)
3. 2 in (5 cm)
4. 2½ in (6.4 cm)

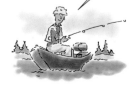

Be patient. The answer will come to you.

29. 3. The chest compressions should compress at least one-third of the anteroposterior diameter of the chest or approximately 2 in (5 cm). For infants, compress 1½ in (3.8 cm), and compress at least 2 in (5 cm) for adults.
CN: Physiological integrity; CNS: Physiological adaptation; CL: Apply; DIFFICULTY: Difficult

30. A nurse rescuer knows that chest compressions must be coordinated with ventilations. Which ratio should the nurse rescuer use for a 3-year-old child?
1. 15 compressions to one ventilation
2. 15 compressions to two ventilations
3. 30 compressions to one ventilation
4. 30 compressions to two ventilations

30. 4. A single rescuer should use a ratio of 30 chest compressions to two ventilations (30:2) for children ages 1 year to the onset of adolescence. Ratios of 15:2 are indicated if there are two rescuers. Ratios of 15:1 and 30:1 won't provide optimal compression and ventilation.
CN: Physiological integrity; CNS: Physiological adaptation; CL: Apply; DIFFICULTY: Moderate

31. A 10-month-old child is found choking and soon becomes unconscious. Which intervention should the nurse attempt **first** after opening the airway?
1. Look inside the infant's mouth for a foreign object.
2. Give five back blows and five chest thrusts.
3. Attempt a blind finger sweep.
4. Attempt rescue breathing.

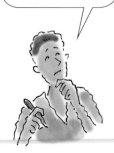

Hmm. Those words "after opening the airway" seem important.

31. 1. After the airway is open, the nurse should check for a foreign object and remove it with a finger sweep if it can be visualized. After this step, rescue breathing should be attempted. If ventilation is unsuccessful, the nurse should then give five back blows and five chest thrusts in an attempt to dislodge the object. Blind finger sweeps should never be performed because this may push the object farther back into the airway.
CN: Physiological integrity; CNS: Physiological adaptation; CL: Apply; DIFFICULTY: Moderate

32. A nursing student is learning how to perform chest compressions on a young child. Which statements made by the student would indicate a need for further education? Select all that apply.
   1. I should use the heels of both hands.
   2. I should only use the heel of one hand.
   3. I should use the index and middle fingers.
   4. It does not matter what fingers or hands you use.
   5. The rules are too complicated.

32. 1, 3, 4, 5. The heel of one hand is recommended for performing chest compressions on children between ages 1 and 8. Two hands are used for adult cardiopulmonary resuscitation. Chest thrusts administered with the middle and third fingers, and in some cases the thumbs of each hand, are used on infants younger than age 1. It does matter which fingers or hands one uses and the rules are very simple to follow; everyone should be familiar with them.
CN: Physiological integrity; CNS: Physiological adaptation; CL: Apply; DIFFICULTY: Difficult

33. A 3-year-old child who is unable to make a sound and is cyanotic and lethargic is brought to the emergency department. The parent states that the child swallowed a penny. Which should the nurse do **first**?
   1. Give 100% oxygen.
   2. Administer five back blows.
   3. Attempt a blind finger sweep.
   4. Administer abdominal thrusts.

33. 4. A child between ages 1 and 8 should receive abdominal thrusts to help dislodge the object. Blind finger sweeps should never be performed because this could push the object farther back into the airway. Administering 100% oxygen won't help if the airway is occluded. Infants younger than age 1 should receive back blows before chest thrusts.
CN: Physiological integrity; CNS: Physiological adaptation; CL: Apply; DIFFICULTY: Challenge

34. A 7-month-old child is diagnosed with otitis media; the health care provider orders amoxicillin 40 mg/kg/day to be administered three times per day. The child weighs 9 kg. How many milligrams of amoxicillin should the child receive per dose? Record your answer using a whole number.

_____ mg

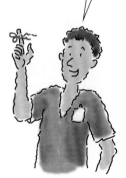

Remember— you are looking for the number of milligrams per dose.

34. 120.
The child should receive 120 mg per dose. Use the following equations:

$$40\frac{mg}{kg} / day \times 9\,kg = 360\,mg / day$$

$$360\,mg / 3\,doses = 120\,mg / dose$$

CN: Physiological integrity; CNS: Pharmacological therapies; CL: Analyze; DIFFICULTY: Difficult

35. A 2-year-old child is diagnosed with epiglottitis. Ampicillin is ordered 50 mg/kg/day in six divided doses. The client weighs 12 kg. How many milligrams of ampicillin is given per dose? Record your answer using a whole number.

_____ mg

35. 100.
The child should receive 100 mg per dose. Use the following equations:

$$50\,mg \times 12\,kg = 600\,mg / day$$

$$600\,mg / 6\,doses = 100\,mg / dose$$

CN: Physiological integrity; CNS: Pharmacological therapies; CL: Analyze; DIFFICULTY: Moderate

36. A 3-year-old child is receiving ampicillin for acute epiglottitis. Which sign would lead the nurse to suspect that the child is experiencing a common adverse effect of this drug?
   1. Constipation
   2. Generalized rash
   3. Increased appetite
   4. Low-grade temperature

36. 2. Some children with epiglottitis may develop an erythematous or maculopapular rash after 3 to 14 days of therapy; however, this complication doesn't necessitate discontinuing the drug. Nausea, vomiting, epigastric pain, diarrhea, and respiratory symptoms of anaphylaxis are adverse effects that may necessitate discontinuation of the drug.
CN: Physiological integrity; CNS: Pharmacological therapies; CL: Apply; DIFFICULTY: Easy

37. A 3-year-old child is given a preliminary diagnosis of acute epiglottitis. Which nursing intervention is appropriate?
1. Obtain a throat culture immediately.
2. Place the child in a side-lying position.
3. Don't attempt to visualize the epiglottis.
4. Use a tongue depressor to look inside the throat.

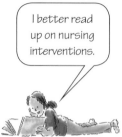

I better read up on nursing interventions.

37. 3. The nurse shouldn't attempt to visualize the epiglottis. The use of tongue blades or throat culture swabs may cause the epiglottis to spasm and totally occlude the airway. Throat inspection should be attempted only when immediate intubation or tracheostomy can be performed, in the event of further or complete obstruction. The child should always remain in the position that provides the most comfort and security and ease of breathing.
CN: Physiological integrity; CNS: Physiological adaptation; CL: Apply; DIFFICULTY: Difficult

38. Administration of which childhood vaccination assists in decreasing a child's incidence of developing epiglottitis?
1. Diphtheria vaccine
2. Haemophilus influenzae type B (Hib) vaccine
3. Measles vaccine
4. Inactivated polio vaccine (IPV)

38. 2. Epiglottitis is caused by the bacterial agent *H. influenzae.* The American Academy of Pediatrics recommends that beginning at age 2 months, children receive the Hib conjugate vaccine. A decline in the incidence of epiglottitis has been seen as a result of this vaccination regimen. The diphtheria vaccine, measles vaccine, and IPV are preventive for those diseases, not epiglottitis.
CN: Health promotion and maintenance; CNS: None; CL: Apply; DIFFICULTY: Moderate

39. In addition to an increasing respiratory rate, which sign in a 3-year-old child with acute epiglottitis indicates that respiratory distress is increasing?
1. Progressive, barking cough
2. Increasing irritability
3. Increasing heart rate
4. Productive cough

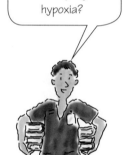

Which answer is an early sign of hypoxia?

39. 3. Increasing heart rate is an early sign of hypoxia. A progressive, barking cough is characteristic of spasmodic croup. A child in respiratory distress will be irritable and restless. As distress increases, the child will become lethargic related to the work of breathing and impending respiratory failure. A productive cough shows that secretions are moving and the child can effectively clear them.
CN: Physiological integrity; CNS: Physiological adaptation; CL: Apply; DIFFICULTY: Difficult

40. While examining a child with acute epiglottitis, the nurse should have which item available?
1. Cool mist tent
2. Intubation equipment
3. Tongue depressors
4. Viral culture medium

40. 2. Emergency intubation equipment should be at the bedside to secure the airway if the examination precipitates further or complete obstruction occurs. Tongue depressors are contraindicated and may cause the epiglottis to spasm. Cool mist tents and viral culture medium are recommended for the treatment and diagnosis of croup.
CN: Physiological integrity; CNS: Physiological adaptation; CL: Apply; DIFFICULTY: Moderate

41. What's the **best** way for a nurse to position a 3-year-old child with right lower lobe pneumonia?
1. Right side-lying
2. Left side-lying
3. Supine
4. Prone

41. 2. The child with right lower lobe pneumonia should be placed on the left side. This places the unaffected left lung in a position that allows gravity to promote blood flow through the healthy lung tissue and improve gas exchange. Placing the child on the right side, back, or stomach doesn't promote circulation to the unaffected lung.
CN: Physiological integrity; CNS: Physiological adaptation; CL: Apply; DIFFICULTY: Moderate

42. A 2-year-old child is brought to the emergency department in respiratory distress. The child is drooling, sitting upright, and leaning forward with the chin thrust out, mouth open, and tongue protruding. Which nursing action is **most** appropriate?
1. Check the child's gag reflex with a tongue blade.
2. Allow the child to cry to keep the lungs expanded.
3. Check the airway for a foreign body obstruction.
4. Support the child in an upright position on the parent's lap.

Float like a butterfly, sting like a bee. Hang in there!

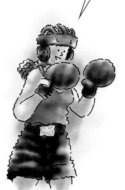

42. 4. The classic signs of epiglottitis are drooling, sitting upright, and leaning forward with the chin thrust out, mouth open, and tongue protruding. The child should be kept in an upright position to ease the work of breathing, to avoid aspiration of secretions, and to help ease obstruction of the airway by the swollen epiglottis. Placing the child on the lap of a parent may help reduce the child's anxiety. The gag reflex of a child with epiglottitis should never be checked unless emergency personnel and equipment are immediately available to perform a tracheotomy (in the event that the airway becomes obstructed by the swollen epiglottis). Crying and inspecting the airway for a foreign body may also cause complete airway obstruction.
CN: Physiological integrity; CNS: Reduction of risk potential; CL: Apply; DIFFICULTY: Challenge

43. The arterial blood gas analysis of a child with asthma shows a pH of 7.30, Pa_{CO_2} of 56 mm Hg, and HCO_3– of 25 mEq/L. The nurse determines that the child has which condition?
1. Metabolic acidosis
2. Metabolic alkalosis
3. Respiratory acidosis
4. Respiratory alkalosis

43. 3. Respiratory acidosis is an acid-base disturbance characterized by excess CO_2 in the blood, indicated by a Pa_{CO_2} greater than 45 mm Hg. The pH level is usually below the normal range of 7.36 to 7.45. The HCO_3– level is normal in the acute stage and elevated in the chronic stage.
CN: Physiological integrity; CNS: Physiological adaptation; CL: Analyze; DIFFICULTY: Moderate

44. When caring for a child with increased laryngotracheal edema and early signs of impending airway obstruction, the nurse should observe for which warning sign?
1. Decreased heart and respiratory rates and a high peak flow rate
2. Increased heart and respiratory rates, retractions, and restlessness
3. Decreased blood pressure
4. Increased temperature

44. 2. Increased heart and respiratory rates, retractions, and restlessness are classic indicators of hypoxia. The heart and respiratory rates increase to enable increased oxygenation. Accessory breathing muscles are used, causing retractions in substernal, suprasternal, and intercostal areas. Reduced oxygen to the brain causes restlessness initially and altered level of consciousness later. A decrease in heart and respiratory rates would be a late, ominous sign of decompensation. Peak flow rate is a test used in asthma. A decrease, not increase, in peak flow is diagnostic of disease. A drop in blood pressure would be a late sign of hypoxia. An increase in temperature is more indicative of infection or inflammation than respiratory distress.
CN: Physiological integrity; CNS: Physiological adaptation; CL: Apply; DIFFICULTY: Easy

45. Which nursing action would relieve respiratory distress and dyspnea in a 2-year-old child with laryngotracheobronchitis (croup)?
1. Stimulate the child to stay awake.
2. Provide an atmosphere of cool mist, high humidity.
3. Offer frequent, oral feedings.
4. Administer frequent sedatives.

Looks like a trip to the rainforest might be in order.

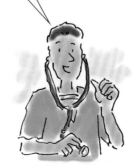

45. 2. An atmosphere of cool mist, high humidity reduces mucosal edema and prevents drying of secretions, thus helping to maintain an open airway. Keeping the child calm, not stimulated, helps to reduce oxygen need. Oral feedings may need to be withheld in a child experiencing respiratory distress because eating may interfere with the ability to breathe. Sedation is generally contraindicated because it may cause respiratory depression and mask anxiety, a sign of respiratory distress.
CN: Physiological integrity; CNS: Physiological adaptation; CL: Apply; DIFFICULTY: Easy

46. Which strategy is recommended when caring for an infant with bronchopulmonary dysplasia?
1. Provide frequent playful stimuli.
2. Decrease oxygen during feedings.
3. Place the infant on a set schedule.
4. Place the infant in an open crib.

46. 3. Timing care activities with rest periods to avoid fatigue and to decrease respiratory effort is essential. Early stimulation activities are recommended, but the infant will have limited tolerance for them because of the illness. Oxygen is usually increased during feedings to help decrease respiratory and energy requirements. Thermoregulation is important because both hypothermia and hyperthermia will increase oxygen consumption and may increase oxygen requirements. These infants are usually maintained on warmer beds or in Isolettes.
CN: Safe, effective care environment; CNS: Coordinated care; CL: Apply; DIFFICULTY: Difficult

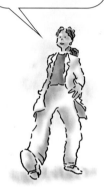

Great job! You've taken a great step forward.

47. Which problem does the nurse identify as the **high priority** for an infant with bronchopulmonary dysplasia?
1. Imbalanced nutrition
2. Effective breast-feeding
3. Impaired gas exchange
4. Imbalanced fluid volume

47. 3. The infant will have impaired gas exchange related to retention of carbon dioxide and borderline oxygenation secondary to fibrosis of the lungs. Although the infant may require increased caloric intake and may have excess fluid volume, the other problems aren't the priority.
CN: Safe, effective care environment; CNS: Coordinated care; CL: Analyze; DIFFICULTY: Easy

48. Which intervention is most appropriate for helping parents cope with a child newly diagnosed with bronchopulmonary dysplasia?
1. Educate them on cardiopulmonary resuscitation.
2. Refer them to support groups.
3. Help parents identify necessary lifestyle changes.
4. Evaluate and assess parents' stress and anxiety levels.

48. 4. The emotional impact of bronchopulmonary dysplasia is clearly a crisis situation. The parents are experiencing grief and sorrow over the loss of a "healthy" child. The other strategies are more appropriate for long-term intervention.
CN: Psychosocial integrity; CNS: None; CL: Apply; DIFFICULTY: Difficult

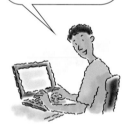

Which intervention is best for improving gas exchange?

49. The care plan for an infant with bronchopulmonary dysplasia identifies impaired gas exchange as a high priority. Which nursing action would be the **most** appropriate for the nurse to include?
1. Provide chest physiotherapy.
2. Provide enteral feedings.
3. Provide appropriate age-related activities.
4. Promote bonding between parents and child.

49. 1. All of these activities are appropriate to include in the care of a child with bronchopulmonary dysplasia; however, providing chest physiotherapy is the nursing action that addresses impairment of gas exchange.
CN: Safe, effective care environment; CNS: Coordinated care; CL: Analyze; DIFFICULTY: Moderate

50. Theophylline is ordered for a 1-year-old infant with bronchopulmonary dysplasia. The recommended dosage is 24 mg/kg/day. The child weighs 10 kg. How many milligrams should be given per dose when administered 4 times per day? Record your answer using a whole number.

_____ mg

50. 60.
The child should receive 60 mg/dose. Use the following equations:

$$24 \text{ mg} / \text{kg} \times 10 \text{ kg} = 240 \text{ mg} / \text{day}$$

$$240 \text{ mg} / 4 \text{ doses} = 60 \text{ mg} / \text{dose}$$

CN: Physiological integrity; CNS: Pharmacological therapies; CL: Analyze; DIFFICULTY: Moderate

CN: Client needs category   CNS: Client needs subcategory   CL: Cognitive level

51. An infant with bronchopulmonary dysplasia requires frequent, prolonged rest periods. Which sign does the nurse recognize indicates overstimulation?
1. Increased alertness
2. Good eye contact
3. Cyanosis
4. Lethargy

52. At discharge, which parental care outcome should be anticipated for a child with bronchopulmonary dysplasia?
1. Reports increased levels of stress
2. Only makes safe decisions with professional assistance
3. Participates in routine, but not complex, caretaking activities
4. Verbalizes the causes, risks, therapy options, and nursing care

53. The nurse is caring for a client with bronchopulmonary dysplasia. Which characteristic will the nurse observe in the early stage of the disease?
1. Clubbing of the fingers
2. Barrel chest
3. Cyanosis
4. Dyspnea with exertion

54. The nurse is caring for a child with bronchopulmonary dysplasia. The child is showing signs of increased fluid in the lungs due to disruption of the alveolar-capillary membrane and is prescribed furosemide. For which adverse effect should the nurse monitor?
1. Hypercalcemia
2. Hyperkalemia
3. Hypernatremia
4. Irregular heart rhythm

55. A child is to receive furosemide 4 mg/kg/day in one daily dose. The child weighs 20 kg. How many milligrams should the nurse administer in each dose? Record your answer using a whole number.

_____ mg

56. A 2-year-old child with bronchopulmonary dysplasia is placed on furosemide once per day. The nurse is educating the parents on foods that are rich in potassium. Which food should the nurse recommend?
1. Apples
2. Oranges
3. Peaches
4. Raisins

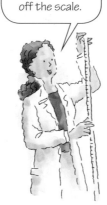

Impressive. Your performance is off the scale.

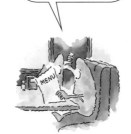

I have a sudden craving for some potassium. What should I pick?

51. 3. Signs of overstimulation in an infant with chronic respiratory dysfunction include cyanosis, avoidance of eye contact, vomiting, diaphoresis, or falling asleep. The child may also become irritable and show signs of respiratory distress.
CN: Psychosocial integrity; CNS: None; CL: Apply; DIFFICULTY: Challenge

52. 4. The parents should understand the causes, risks, therapy options, and care of their infant by the time of discharge. Asking the parents to verbalize this information is the only way to assess their understanding. The parents should report decreased levels of stress, be capable of making decisions independently, and participate in routine and complex care.
CN: Physiological integrity; CNS: Basic care and comfort; CL: Analyze; DIFFICULTY: Moderate

53. 4. Stage I can be characterized by early interstitial changes and resembles respiratory distress syndrome. Stage III shows signs of the beginning of chronic disease with interstitial edema, signs of emphysema, and pulmonary hypertension. Stage IV shows interstitial fibrosis and hyperexpansion on chest x-ray. Clubbing of the fingers, barrel chest, and cyanosis would be observed in the later stage of the disease.
CN: Physiological integrity; CNS: Physiological adaptation; CL: Analyze; DIFFICULTY: Moderate

54. 4. An irregular heart rhythm and muscle cramps are adverse effects of hypokalemia and hypocalcemia, not hypercalcemia or hyperkalemia. Diuretics cause volume depletion by inhibiting reabsorption of sodium and chloride. Hypocalcemia is related to the urinary excretion of calcium. Hypokalemia can occur with excessive fluid loss or as part of contraction alkalosis.
CN: Physiological integrity; CNS: Pharmacological therapies; CL: Apply; DIFFICULTY: Difficult

55. 80.
The child should receive 80 mg per dose. Use the following equation:

$$4 \text{ mg} / \text{kg} \times 20 \text{ kg} = 80 \text{ mg}$$

CN: Physiological integrity; CNS: Pharmacological therapies; CL: Analyze; DIFFICULTY: Easy

56. 4. Raisins, dates, figs, and prunes are among the highest potassium-rich foods. They average 17 to 20 mEq of potassium. Apples, oranges, and peaches have very low amounts of potassium. They average 3 to 4 mEq.
CN: Physiological integrity; CNS: Pharmacological therapies; CL: Apply; DIFFICULTY: Difficult

CN: Client needs category   CNS: Client needs subcategory   CL: Cognitive level

57. The nurse is caring for an infant with bronchopulmonary dysplasia. When would the nurse anticipate that tracheostomy tube placement would be indicated for this infant?
1. Increased risk of tracheomalacia
2. Prolonged dependence on the ventilator
3. Need to allow for gastrostomy tube feedings
4. Increased signs of respiratory distress

58. A 1-year-old infant with bronchopulmonary dysplasia has just received a tracheostomy. Which intervention by the nurse is appropriate?
1. Keep extra tracheostomy tubes at the bedside.
2. Secure ties at the side of the neck.
3. Change the tracheostomy tube 2 weeks after surgery.
4. Secure the tracheostomy ties tightly to prevent dislodgment of the tube.

59. An 11-month-old infant with bronchopulmonary dysplasia and a tracheostomy experiences a decline in oxygen saturation from 97% to 88%. The infant appears anxious and the heart rate is 180 beats/minute. Which intervention is **most** appropriate?
1. Change the tracheostomy tube.
2. Suction the tracheostomy tube.
3. Obtain an arterial blood gas (ABG) level.
4. Increase the oxygen flow rate.

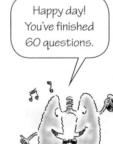

Happy day! You've finished 60 questions.

60. Which nursing intervention is **most** appropriate when suctioning thick secretions through a tracheostomy tube from a 2-year-old child?
1. Hypoventilate the child before suctioning.
2. Repeat the suctioning process for two intervals.
3. Insert the catheter 1 to 2 cm below the tracheostomy tube.
4. Inject a small amount of normal saline solution into the tube before suctioning.

61. A child comes to the emergency department (ED) with sneezing and itching of the eyes and nose. What should the nurse suspect?
1. A cold
2. An allergy
3. Pneumonia
4. Asthma

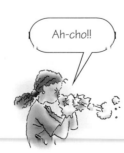

Ah-cho!!

57. 2. Tracheostomy may be required after a child has been dependent on a ventilator and can't wean from it. Tracheomalacia can be a complication of prolonged tracheal intubation, not a condition that necessitates a tracheostomy. The need for gastrostomy feedings wouldn't necessitate putting in a tracheostomy tube. Increased signs of respiratory distress may indicate the need for endotracheal intubation and mechanical ventilation, not tracheostomy.
CN: Physiological integrity; CNS: Physiological adaptation; CL: Apply; DIFFICULTY: Challenge

58. 1. Extra tracheostomy tubes should be kept at the bedside in case of an emergency, including one size smaller in case the appropriate size doesn't fit due to edema. The ties should be placed securely but should allow some space (the width of a pinky finger) in order to prevent excessive pressure or skin breakdown. The first tracheostomy tube change is usually performed by the health care provider after 7 days. Ties are placed at the back of the neck.
CN: Physiological integrity; CNS: Physiological adaptation; CL: Apply; DIFFICULTY: Moderate

59. 2. Tracheostomy tubes, particularly in small children, require frequent suctioning to remove mucus plugs and excessive secretions. The tracheostomy tube can be changed if suctioning is unsuccessful. Obtaining an ABG level may be beneficial if oxygen saturation remains low and the child appears to be in respiratory distress. Increasing the oxygen flow rate will only help if the airway is patent.
CN: Physiological integrity; CNS: Physiological adaptation; CL: Apply; DIFFICULTY: Easy

60. 4. Injecting a small amount of normal saline solution helps to loosen secretions for easier aspiration but should not be done routinely. Preservative-free normal saline solution should be used. The child should be *hyperventilated* before and after suctioning to prevent hypoxia. The suctioning process should be repeated until the trachea is clear. The catheter should be inserted 0.5 cm beyond the tracheostomy tube. If the catheter is inserted too far, it will irritate the carina and may cause blood-tinged secretions.
CN: Physiological integrity; CNS: Physiological adaptation; CL: Apply; DIFFICULTY: Difficult

61. 2. Allergies elicit consistent bouts of sneezing, are seldom accompanied by fever, and tend to cause itching of the eyes and nose. A cold is accompanied by fever and is characterized by sporadic sneezing. Pneumonia is accompanied by fever and chest pain and coughs. Asthma is associated with chest tightness and wheezing.
CN: Health promotion and maintenance; CNS: None; CL: Apply; DIFFICULTY: Easy

62. The nurse is caring for a child with asthma. Which symptom would cause the **most** concern if observed in the child?
1. Exercise intolerance
2. Diaphoresis
3. Cough
4. Diminished breath sounds bilaterally

62. 4. Diminished breath sounds are an indication that the child is in distress and not exchanging air adequately; this is an immediate concern. The nurse would anticipate that the child may have exercise intolerance and be fatigued easily prior to an asthma attack. Diaphoresis is not an indication of asthma and may be caused by other factors. Cough is not a concern at this time, because the child is still able to clear the airway.
CN: Physiological integrity; CNS: Physiological adaptation;
CL: **Analyze**; DIFFICULTY: Easy

63. A 2-year-old child has been diagnosed with asthma. The parents ask about the **most** common asthma triggers. What is the nurse's response?
1. Weather
2. Peanut butter
3. The cat next door
4. One parent with asthma

63. 1. Excessively cold air, wet or humid changes in weather and seasons, and air pollution are some of the most common asthma triggers. Food allergens are rarely responsible for airway reactions in children. Household pets are a trigger. Evidence suggests that asthma is partly hereditary in nature, but heredity isn't an allergen.
CN: Physiological integrity; CNS: Physiological adaptation;
CL: **Apply**; DIFFICULTY: Easy

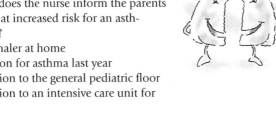

Uh oh. Trigger alert!

You really know your stuff. That helps me breathe a little easier.

64. When obtaining data from a child with asthma, which finding does the nurse determine correlates with the disorder?
1. Stridor
2. Rhonchi
3. Rales
4. Wheezing

64. 4. Asthma frequently occurs with wheezing and coughing. Airway inflammation and edema increase mucus production. Other signs include dyspnea, tachycardia, and tachypnea. Stridor is heard in croup. Rhonchi and rales are not as common in asthma as is wheezing.
CN: Physiological integrity; CNS: Physiological adaptation;
CL: **Apply**; DIFFICULTY: Easy

65. Which factor does the nurse inform the parents will place a child at increased risk for an asthma-related death?
1. Use of an inhaler at home
2. One admission for asthma last year
3. Prior admission to the general pediatric floor
4. Prior admission to an intensive care unit for asthma

65. 4. Asthma results in varying degrees of respiratory distress. A prior admission to an intensive care unit marks an increased severity and need of immediate therapy. Two or more hospitalizations for asthma, a recent hospitalization or emergency department visit in the past month, or three or more emergency department visits in the past year puts a child at high risk for asthma-related death. Although current use of systemic steroids would also be a risk factor, not all inhalers contain steroids.
CN: Physiological integrity; CNS: Reduction of risk potential;
CL: **Apply**; DIFFICULTY: Easy

66. A child is seen in the emergency department (ED) with severe chest tightness and wheezing. The parents inform the nurse that these symptoms have been constant and bronchodilators do not help. Which condition does the nurse suspect?
1. Asthma
2. Status asthmaticus
3. Pneumonia
4. Bronchitis

66. 2. Status asthmaticus can best be described as constant attacks unrelieved by bronchodilators. Moderate asthma is characterized by several attacks per month. Mild asthma is less than six attacks per year. Little or no response to bronchodilators occurs in severe asthma. Pneumonia symptoms include crackles in the affected lung. Bronchitis may display with diffuse wheezing that clears with bronchodilators and steroid use. Chest tightness may occur with bronchitis, but it is not severe and may be related to the discomfort of coughing.
CN: Physiological integrity; CNS: Physiological adaptation;
CL: **Apply**; DIFFICULTY: Difficult

67. A 2-year-old child with status asthmaticus is admitted to the pediatric unit and begins to receive continuous treatment with albuterol, given by nebulizer. The nurse should observe for which adverse reaction?
1. Bradycardia
2. Lethargy
3. Tachycardia
4. Tachypnea

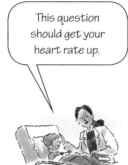

This question should get your heart rate up.

67. 3. Albuterol is a rapid-acting bronchodilator. Common adverse effects include tachycardia, nervousness, tremors, insomnia, irritability, and headache.

CN: Physiological integrity; CNS: Pharmacological therapies; CL: Apply; DIFFICULTY: Moderate

68. A 10-year-old child is admitted with asthma. The health care provider orders an aminophylline infusion. A loading dose of 6 mg/kg is ordered. The client weighs 30 kg. How many milligrams of aminophylline is contained in the loading dose? Record your answer using a whole number.

_____ mg

68. 180.
The child should receive 180 mg for the loading dose. Use the following equation:

$$6\,mg\,/\,kg \times 30\,kg = 180\,mg$$

CN: Physiological integrity; CNS: Pharmacological therapies; CL: Apply; DIFFICULTY: Easy

69. Which complication should the nurse monitor for that may be seen in a child receiving mechanical ventilation?
1. Pneumothorax
2. High cardiac output
3. Polycythemia
4. Hypovolemia

69. 1. Mechanical ventilation can cause barotrauma, as occurs with pneumothorax. A child receiving mechanical ventilation must be carefully monitored. Mechanical ventilation decreases, not increases, cardiac output. Polycythemia is the result of chronic hypoxia, not mechanical ventilation. Mechanical ventilation can cause fluid overload, not dehydration.

CN: Physiological integrity; CNS: Physiological adaptation; CL: Apply; DIFFICULTY: Moderate

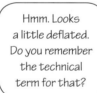

Hmm. Looks a little deflated. Do you remember the technical term for that?

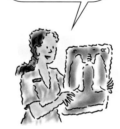

70. The nurse is reviewing diagnostic test results for a child admitted with asthma. Which finding on the chest x-ray results does the nurse determine is characteristic of this disorder?
1. Atelectasis
2. Hemothorax
3. Infiltrates
4. Pneumothoraces

70. 1. Hyperexpansion, atelectasis, and a flattened diaphragm are typical x-ray findings for a child with asthma. Air becomes trapped behind the narrowed airways and the residual capacity rises, leading to hyperinflation. Hypoxemia results from areas of the lung not being well perfused. A hemothorax isn't a finding related to asthma. Infiltrates and pneumothoraces are uncommon.

CN: Physiological integrity; CNS: Physiological adaptation; CL: Analyze; DIFFICULTY: Moderate

71. The nurse is caring for a child with atelectasis as a result of status asthmaticus. Which nursing action is a **priority** for this child?
1. Perform chest physiotherapy.
2. Increase IV fluids.
3. Administer oxygen.
4. Obtain arterial blood gas (ABG) levels.

71. 1. Chest physiotherapy and incentive spirometry help to enhance the clearance of mucus and open the alveoli. Although not the most important intervention, giving IV and oral fluids is recommended to help liquefy and thin secretions. Administration of oxygen won't provide enough pressure to open the alveoli. Obtaining ABG levels isn't necessary unless the client has signs of hypoxemia.

CN: Physiological integrity; CNS: Physiological adaptation; CL: Apply; DIFFICULTY: Challenge

72. The parents of a 10-year-old child recently diagnosed with asthma ask if the child can continue to play sports. Which response is **most** appropriate?
1. "Sports don't cause asthma attacks."
2. "You should limit activities to quiet play."
3. "It's okay to play some sports but swimming isn't recommended."
4. "Physical activity and sports are encouraged as long as the asthma is under control."

73. A child with thoracic water-seal drainage is on the elevator. The transport aide has placed the drainage system on the stretcher. Which action should the nurse on the elevator take **first**?
1. Assist the aide in placing the drainage system lower than the child's chest.
2. Report the incident to the registered nurse when the aide returns to the unit.
3. Clamp the drainage tubing with a hemostat.
4. Immediately take the child's respiratory and pulse rates.

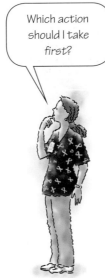

Which action should I take first?

74. Which nursing intervention is appropriate to correct dehydration for a 2-year-old child with asthma?
1. Give warm liquids.
2. Give cold juice or ice pops.
3. Provide three meals and three snacks.
4. Provide small, frequent meals and snacks.

75. The nurse is reinforcing education for parents of a child being discharged with asthma. Which teaching point decreases allergens in the home?
1. Covering floors with carpeting
2. Designating the basement as the play area
3. Dusting and cleaning the house thoroughly twice a month
4. Using foam rubber pillows and synthetic blankets

76. The nurse on the pediatric unit is caring for a child with asthma. When assisting the health care team to develop a plan of care, which problem should the team be sure to address?
1. Imbalanced nutrition
2. Excess fluid volume
3. Activity intolerance
4. Constipation

72. 4. Participation in sports is encouraged but should be evaluated on an individual basis as long as the asthma is under control. Exercise-induced asthma is an example of the airway hyperactivity common to asthmatics. Exclusion from sports or activities may hamper peer interaction. Swimming is well tolerated because of the type of breathing involved and the moisture in the air.
CN: Physiological integrity; CNS: Physiological adaptation; CL: Apply; DIFFICULTY: Easy

73. 1. The drainage device must be kept below the level of the chest to maintain straight gravity drainage. Placing it on the stretcher may cause a backflow of drainage into the thoracic cavity, which could collapse the partially expanded lung. Reporting the incident is indicated, but the immediate safety of the child takes priority. Clamping the tubing would place the child at risk for a tension pneumothorax. After the drainage system has been properly repositioned, the child's respiratory and pulse rates may be taken.
CN: Physiological integrity; CNS: Basic care and comfort; CL: Apply; DIFFICULTY: Easy

74. 1. Liquids are best tolerated if they're warm. Cold liquids may cause bronchospasm and should be avoided. Dehydration should be corrected slowly. Overhydration may increase interstitial pulmonary fluid and exacerbate small airway obstruction. Small, frequent meals should be provided to avoid abdominal distention that may interfere with diaphragm excursion, but these won't correct the dehydration.
CN: Physiological integrity; CNS: Physiological adaptation; CL: Apply; DIFFICULTY: Challenge

75. 4. Bedding should be free from allergens and have nonallergenic covers. Unnecessary rugs should be removed, and floors should be bare and mopped a few times per week to reduce dust. Basements or cellars should be avoided to lessen the child's exposure to molds and mildew. Dusting and cleaning should occur daily or at least weekly.
CN: Physiological integrity; CNS: Physiological adaptation; CL: Apply; DIFFICULTY: Challenge

76. 3. Ineffective oxygen supply and demand may lead to activity intolerance. The nurse should promote rest and encourage developmentally appropriate activities. Nutrition may be decreased, not increased, due to respiratory distress and GI upset. Dehydration is common due to diaphoresis, insensible water loss, and hyperventilation. Medications given to treat asthma may cause nausea, vomiting, and diarrhea, not constipation.
CN: Physiological integrity; CNS: Physiological adaptation; CL: Apply; DIFFICULTY: Easy

77. A nurse is explaining bronchiolitis to the parents of an infant admitted with the condition. Which statement made by the parents demonstrates an understanding of the disorder?
 1. "It is caused by inflammation and obstruction of the bronchioles."
 2. "My child probably has an airway obstruction from aspiration of a solid object."
 3. "It is an inflammation of the pulmonary parenchyma."
 4. "My child is highly contagious and has a crouplike disease."

78. A 2-month-old infant is given a preliminary diagnosis of bronchiolitis. Which symptom would the nurse expect to find?
 1. Bradycardia
 2. Increased appetite
 3. Wheezing on auscultation
 4. No signs of an upper respiratory infection

79. A nurse is caring for a child diagnosed with bronchiolitis. Which symptom would cause the nurse the **most** concern?
 1. The presence of thick mucus
 2. An elevated temperature of 100.6° F (38.1° C)
 3. Severe sternal retractions
 4. Oxygenation saturation of 97%

80. A child comes to the emergency department (ER) with symptoms of asthma and the health care provider begins treatment. The nurse is requested to obtain a sputum culture. What is the **best** explanation for the test in this situation?
 1. It will identify the causative agent of the asthma attack.
 2. It will rule out a respiratory infection.
 3. It will complete the protocol for asthma treatment.
 4. It will identify any risk factors associated with asthma.

81. Which precaution should a nurse caring for a 2-month-old infant with respiratory syncytial virus (RSV) take to prevent the spread of infection?
 1. Wear gloves only.
 2. Wear gown, gloves, and mask.
 3. No precautions are required; the virus isn't contagious.
 4. Proper hand washing between clients only

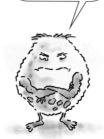

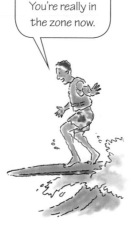

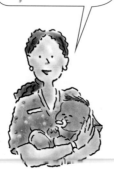

77. 1. Bronchiolitis is an infection of the bronchioles, causing the mucosa to become edematous, inflamed, and full of mucus. Lower airway obstruction from a solid object is a form of foreign body aspiration. Pneumonia is characterized by inflammation of the pulmonary parenchyma. Croup syndromes are generally upper airway infections or obstructions.
CN: Physiological integrity; CNS: Physiological adaptation; CL: Apply; DIFFICULTY: Easy

78. 3. In bronchiolitis, the bronchioles become narrowed and edematous, which can cause wheezing. These infants typically have a 2- to 3-day history of an upper respiratory infection and feeding difficulties with loss of appetite, due to nasal congestion and increased work of breathing. This combination leads to respiratory distress with tachypnea and tachycardia.
CN: Physiological integrity; CNS: Physiological adaptation; CL: Apply; DIFFICULTY: Easy

79. 3. Bronchiolitis is a lower respiratory infection and is characterized by possible air trapping, tachypnea, thick mucus, and sternal retraction. A child with severe sternal retraction has more difficulty breathing; therefore, not enough air is getting into the lungs. This needs to be a high priority and needs to be monitored closely.
CN: Physiological integrity; CNS: Physiological adaptation; CL: Analyze; DIFFICULTY: Easy

80. 2. When a client has asthma it is appropriate to do a sputum analysis to rule out a respiratory infection. It is not part of the protocol for asthma treatment and it will not identify risk factors or agents that precipitated an asthma attack.
CN: Physiological integrity; CNS: Physiological adaptation; CL: Apply; DIFFICULTY: Moderate

81. 2. RSV is highly contagious and is spread through direct contact with infectious secretions via hands, droplets, and fomites. Gown, gloves, and mask should be worn for care of the infant to prevent the spread of infection, in addition to proper hand washing between clients.
CN: Safe, effective care environment; CNS: Safety and infection control; CL: Apply; DIFFICULTY: Easy

82. Which child would be at increased risk for a respiratory syncytial virus (RSV) infection?
1. 2-month-old child managed at home
2. 2-month-old child with bronchopulmonary dysplasia
3. 3-month-old child requiring low-flow oxygen
4. 2-year-old child

83. Which problem would the nurse expect to find on the care plan of a 10-month-old infant to promote coping during hospitalization?
1. Self-care deficit
2. Powerlessness
3. Boredom
4. Anxiety

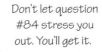
Don't let question #84 stress you out. You'll get it.

84. A client has respiratory syncytial virus (RSV). Which prescribed medication does the nurse anticipate administering?
1. Albuterol
2. Aminophylline
3. Cromolyn sodium
4. Ribavirin

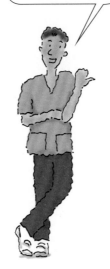

85. Which intervention is **most** important when the nurse is monitoring dehydration in an infant with bronchiolitis?
1. Measurement of intake and output
2. Blood levels every 4 hours
3. Urinalysis every 8 hours
4. Weighing each diaper

86. When assisting with the development of the care plan of the child with bronchiolitis, which problem should the nurse determine is a **priority**?
1. Nutritional deficiency
2. Lack of diversional activities
3. Impaired gas exchange
4. Social isolation

Ouch! I think he just broke our gas exchange.

82. 2. Infants with cardiac or pulmonary conditions are at highest risk for RSV. Because of their underlying conditions, they're more likely to require mechanical ventilation. Many infants can be managed at home; few require hospitalization. A 3-month-old on low-flow oxygen has some risks of progression but isn't at high risk. A 2-year-old child has built up the immune system and can tolerate the infection without major problems.
CN: Physiological integrity; CNS: Reduction of risk potential; CL: Apply; DIFFICULTY: Easy

83. 4. Attachment is critical in infancy, and prolonged separation has been well documented as a risk factor that compromises normal infant development. Being separated from parents can cause high anxiety. Self-care deficit wouldn't be an issue for a 10-month-old. Powerlessness is a concern after the toddler stage, when a child develops autonomy and independence. Boredom won't be an issue until the acute phase of the illness has passed. Providing diversion for infants is easily accomplished by the use of age-appropriate toys and play activities.
CN: Safe, effective care environment; CNS: Coordinated care; CL: Apply; DIFFICULTY: Easy

84. 4. Ribavirin is an antiviral agent sometimes used to reduce the severity of bronchiolitis caused by RSV in high-risk clients. It is used rarely due to its potential for teratogenic effects. Aminophylline and albuterol are bronchodilators and haven't been proven effective in treating viral bronchiolitis. Cromolyn sodium is an inhaled anti-inflammatory agent.
CN: Physiological integrity; CNS: Pharmacological therapies; CL: Apply; DIFFICULTY: Moderate

85. 1. Accurate measurement of intake and output is essential to assess for dehydration. Blood levels may be obtained daily or every other day. A urinalysis every 8 hours isn't necessary. Urine specific gravities are recommended but can be obtained with diaper changes. Weighing diapers is a way of measuring output only.
CN: Physiological integrity; CNS: Physiological adaptation; CL: Apply; DIFFICULTY: Challenge

86. 3. Infants with bronchiolitis will have impaired gas exchange related to bronchiolar obstruction, atelectasis, and hyperinflation. Nutrition may be seen as less than body requirements. If respiratory distress is present, these infants should have nothing by mouth and fluids given IV only. Deficient diversional activity and social isolation usually aren't priorities. These infants are too uncomfortable to respond to social stimuli and need quiet, soothing activities that minimize energy.
CN: Physiological integrity; CNS: Physiological adaptation; CL: Apply; DIFFICULTY: Easy

87. The nurse is discharging an infant who has been treated in the hospital for bronchiolitis. Which education should the nurse be sure to provide to the parents?

1. Place the child in a prone position for comfort.
2. Use warm mist to replace insensible fluid loss.
3. Recognize signs of increasing respiratory distress.
4. Engage the child in many activities to prevent developmental delay.

87. 3. It's essential for parents to be able to recognize signs of increasing respiratory distress and know how to count the respiratory rate. The child should be positioned with the head of the bed elevated for comfort and to facilitate removal of secretions. Use of cool mist may help to replace insensible fluid loss. Quiet play activities are required only as the child's energy level permits. These infants show clinical improvement in 3 to 4 days; therefore, developmental delay isn't an issue.
CN: Physiological integrity; CNS: Physiological adaptation; CL: Apply; DIFFICULTY: Easy

88. The nurse is reinforcing education about treatments for the parents of a child diagnosed with pneumonia. What does the nurse identify as the **best** action to help in promoting a clear airway?

1. Dietary changes
2. Oxygen therapy
3. Chest physiotherapy
4. Antipyretics

88. 3. Pneumonia is an inflammation of the pulmonary parenchyma and ventilation decreases as secretions thicken. The most effective treatment to promote a clear airway is chest physiotherapy, including postural drainage, coughing, and deep breathing as well as incentive spirometry. Dietary changes, especially forcing fluids, will help but chest physiotherapy, coughing and deep breathing will be more effective. Oxygen therapy will help to increase oxygen saturation but does not work well if the bronchioles are blocked with mucus or constricted. Antipyretics will decrease a fever but has nothing to do with opening the airways.
CN: Physiological integrity; CNS: Physiological adaptation; CL: Analyze; DIFFICULTY: Easy

89. The nurse is caring for a client with bacterial pneumonia and performs a sputum culture. Which organism does the nurse expect the culture to identify as the causative agent?

1. Mycoplasma
2. Parainfluenza virus
3. Pneumococci
4. Respiratory syncytial virus (RSV)

89. 3. Pneumococcal pneumonia is the most common causative agent, accounting for about 90% of bacterial pneumonia. Mycoplasma is a causative agent for primary atypical pneumonia. Parainfluenza virus and RSV account for viral pneumonia.
CN: Physiological integrity; CNS: Physiological adaptation; CL: Apply; DIFFICULTY: Easy

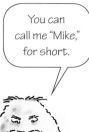
You can call me "Mike," for short.

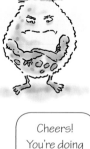
Cheers! You're doing great.

90. The nurse is caring for an 8-year-old child admitted with pneumonia. Based on the child's age, which type of pneumonia would the nurse suspect?

1. Enteric bacilli
2. Mycoplasma pneumonia
3. Staphylococcal pneumonia
4. Streptococcal pneumonia

90. 2. Mycoplasma pneumonia is a primary atypical pneumonia seen in children between ages 5 and 12. Streptococcal pneumonia, enteric bacilli, and staphylococcal pneumonia are mostly seen in children in the 3-month to 5-year age group.
CN: Physiological integrity; CNS: Physiological adaptation; CL: Apply; DIFFICULTY: Challenge

91. A child is diagnosed with tuberculosis (TB). When reinforcing education for the parents about care of the child, which statement made by the parent would indicate a need for further instruction?

1. "As long as I keep a surgical mask on I will not get TB."
2. "I understand that tuberculosis is highly contagious."
3. "I am willing to follow the rigid medication regimen."
4. "Increasing calories will be important at this time."

91. 1. Tuberculosis is highly contagious. To prevent the spread of infection a negative pressure room is needed and the nurse needs to wear an N95 medical mask when around the child while contagious. A regular surgical mask is not effective. A rigid medication regimen is required. Increasing calories, including carbohydrates, proteins, and vitamins, is important during care for TB.
CN: Physiological integrity; CNS: Physiological adaptation; CL: Apply; DIFFICULTY: Moderate

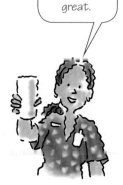

92. The nurse knows to monitor a child with a diagnosis of pertussis for the development of which sign or symptom?
1. Barking cough
2. Whooping cough
3. Abrupt, high fever
4. Inspiratory stridor

92. 2. Pertussis is characterized by consistent short, rapid coughs followed by a sudden inspiration with a high-pitched whooping sound. A barking cough and inspiratory stridor are noted with croup. Pertussis usually is accompanied by a low-grade fever.
CN: Physiological integrity; CNS: Physiological adaptation; CL: Apply; DIFFICULTY: Easy

93. A child comes to the clinic with symptoms of TB. Which test should the nurse expect to perform on this client?
1. Chest x-ray
2. Sputum specimen
3. Tuberculin test
4. Urine culture

93. 2. A sputum culture is the definitive test for TB in children. The tuberculin test is the most accurate, but not necessarily the most reliable, test for TB in children. X-rays usually appear normal in children with TB. Stool culture, not urine culture, and gastric washings will show positive results on acid-fast smears but aren't specific for *Mycobacterium tuberculosis*.
CN: Physiological integrity; CNS: Physiological adaptation; CL: Apply; DIFFICULTY: Difficult

94. The nurse is teaching parents about preventing aspiration in their child. Which activity is recommended to prevent foreign body aspiration during meals?
1. Insist that children are seated.
2. Give children toys to play with.
3. Allow children to watch television.
4. Allow children to eat in a separate room.

94. 1. Children should remain seated while eating. The risk of aspiration increases if children are running, jumping, or talking with food in their mouth. Toys and television are a dangerous distraction to toddlers and young children and should be avoided. Children need constant supervision and should be monitored while eating snacks and meals.
CN: Safe, effective care environment; CNS: Safety and infection control; CL: Apply; DIFFICULTY: Easy

95. A 2-year-old child was brought to the emergency department after aspirating a foreign body. After removal, what should the nurse recommended to the parents to prevent aspiration?
1. Cut hot dogs in half.
2. Limit popcorn and peanuts.
3. Cut grapes into small pieces.
4. Limit hard candy to special occasions.

95. 3. Grapes, hot dogs, and sausage should be cut into many small pieces. Hard candy, raisins, popcorn, and peanuts should be avoided for children age 4 and younger.
CN: Physiological integrity; CNS: Reduction of risk potential; CL: Apply; DIFFICULTY: Moderate

96. A child is admitted with a possible tracheal foreign body. Which findings would the nurse observe that indicates this may have occurred?
1. Cough, dyspnea, and drooling
2. Cough, stridor, and changes in phonation
3. Expiratory wheeze and inspiratory stridor
4. Cough, asymmetric breath sounds, and wheeze

96. 3. Expiratory and inspiratory noise indicates that the foreign body is in the trachea. Cough, dyspnea, drooling, and gagging indicate supraglottic obstruction. A cough with stridor and changes in phonation occurs if the foreign body is in the larynx. Asymmetric breath sounds indicate that the object may be located in the bronchi.
CN: Physiological integrity; CNS: Physiological adaptation; CL: Apply; DIFFICULTY: Difficult

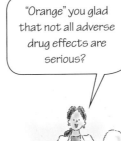

"Orange" you glad that not all adverse drug effects are serious?

97. Which adverse effect can be expected by the parents of a 2-year-old child who has been started on rifampin after testing positive for tuberculosis?
1. Hyperactivity
2. Orange body secretions
3. Decreased bilirubin levels
4. Decreased levels of liver enzymes

97. 2. Rifampin and its metabolites will turn urine, feces, sputum, tears, and sweat an orange color. This isn't a serious adverse effect. Rifampin may also cause GI upset, headache, drowsiness, dizziness, vision disturbances, and fever. Liver enzyme and bilirubin levels increase because of hepatic metabolism of the drug. Parents should be taught the signs and symptoms of hepatitis and hyperbilirubinemia, such as jaundice of the sclera or skin.
CN: Physiological integrity; CNS: Pharmacological therapies; CL: Apply; DIFFICULTY: Moderate

CN: Client needs category   CNS: Client needs subcategory   CL: Cognitive level

98. A child comes to the emergency department (ED) with a cough and difficulty breathing. The parents inform the nurse that the child may have swallowed a crayon. Which diagnostic test should the nurse prepare the parents and child for?
1. Bronchoscopy
2. Chest x-ray
3. Fluoroscopy
4. Lateral neck x-ray

98. 1. Bronchoscopy can give a definitive diagnosis of the presence of foreign bodies and is also the best choice for removal of the object with direct visualization. Chest x-ray and lateral neck x-ray may also be used but findings vary. Some films may appear normal or show changes such as inflammation related to the presence of the foreign body. Fluoroscopy is valuable in detecting and localizing foreign bodies in the bronchi.
CN: Physiological integrity; CNS: Physiological adaptation; CL: Apply; DIFFICULTY: Challenge

99. Which nursing intervention is **most** appropriate for a child with cystic fibrosis who is having difficulty clearing secretions?
1. Perform chest physiotherapy four times per day.
2. Administer pancreatic enzymes with meals.
3. Provide oxygen by nasal cannula at all times.
4. Provide a high-calorie, high-protein diet at each meal.

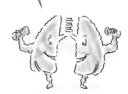

I just love chest PT. It makes me feel so strong and healthy.

99. 1. Chest physiotherapy should be performed to mobilize secretions so they can be more easily cleared. Pancreatic enzymes should be administered with meals to aid in digestion. Administering oxygen may improve oxygenation but won't help clear secretions. A high-calorie, high-protein diet is important for normal growth and development, but it won't aid in clearing secretions.
CN: Physiological integrity; CNS: Reduction of risk potential; CL: Apply; DIFFICULTY: Moderate

100. Which statement by the parent of a 16-month-old child with cystic fibrosis should alert a nurse to investigate further?
1. "My child is not walking yet."
2. "My child is saying a few words and short phrases."
3. "My child doesn't interact with other 16-month-olds."
4. "My child cries when I leave the room."

100. 1. A toddler should be walking by 15 months. At 10 months, an infant holds on to furniture while walking, walks with support at 11 months, and takes first steps at 12 months. By 12 months, a child can say a few words, with more words and short phrases being added each month. A child at 16 months engages in solitary play and has little interaction with other children. Separation anxiety is common in toddlers.
CN: Health promotion and maintenance; CNS: None; CL: Apply; DIFFICULTY: Easy

101. A nurse is obtaining data on a newborn with a possible diagnosis of cystic fibrosis. Which sign does the nurse recognize as an early indicator of the disease?
1. Constipation
2. Decreased appetite
3. Hyperalbuminemia
4. Meconium ileus

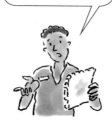

Enzymes help promote digestion. So, when would be a logical time to take them?

101. 4. Meconium ileus is a common early sign of cystic fibrosis. Thick, mucilaginous meconium blocks the lumen of the small intestine, causing intestinal obstruction, abdominal distention, and vomiting. Large-volume, loose, frequent, foul-smelling stools are common. The undigested food is excreted, increasing the bulk of feces. These infants may have an increased appetite related to poor absorption from the intestine. Hypoalbuminemia is a common result from the decreased absorption of protein.
CN: Physiological integrity; CNS: Physiological adaptation; CL: Apply; DIFFICULTY: Moderate

102. A nurse is caring for a child with cystic fibrosis. The parents ask the nurse if any foods make it worse. Which diet should the nurse include when reinforcing dietary education?
1. Fat-restricted diet
2. High-calorie diet
3. Low-protein diet
4. Sodium-restricted diet

102. 2. A well-balanced, high-calorie, high-protein diet is recommended for a child with cystic fibrosis due to impaired intestinal absorption. Fat restriction isn't required because digestion and absorption of fat in the intestine are impaired. The child usually increases enzyme intake when high-fat foods are eaten. Low-sodium foods can lead to hyponatremia; therefore, high-salt foods are recommended, especially during hot weather or when the child has a fever.
CN: Physiological integrity; CNS: Basic care and comfort; CL: Apply; DIFFICULTY: Moderate

103. The nurse is reinforcing education about the administration of pancreatic enzymes to the child and parents. Which statement by the parents indicates the education was effective?
1. Capsules may not be opened.
2. Microcapsules can be crushed.
3. Encourage eating throughout the day.
4. Administer enzymes at each meal and with snacks.

103. 4. Enzymes are administered with each feeding, meal, and snack to optimize absorption of the nutrients consumed. Microcapsules shouldn't be crushed due to the enteric coating. Regular capsules may be opened and the contents mixed with a small amount of applesauce or other nonalkaline food. Eating throughout the day should be discouraged. Three meals and two or three snacks per day are recommended.
CN: Physiological integrity; CNS: Physiological adaptation; CL: Apply; DIFFICULTY: Easy

104. The nurse is caring for a child with cystic fibrosis. Ranitidine 4 mg/kg/day every 12 hours is ordered. The child weighs 20 kg. How many milligrams per dose should the nurse give the child? Record your answer using a whole number.

_____ mg

104. 40.
The child should receive 40 mg per dose. Use the following equations:
$$20 \text{ kg} \times 4 \text{ mg} / \text{kg} = 80 \text{ mg}$$
$$24 \text{ hours} / 12 \text{ hours} = 2 \text{ doses}$$
$$80 \text{ mg} / 2 \text{ doses} = 40 \text{ mg}$$
CN: Physiological integrity; CNS: Pharmacological therapies; CL: Apply; DIFFICULTY: Difficult

105. Which nursing intervention is appropriate for care of the child with cystic fibrosis?
1. Decrease exercise and limit physical activity.
2. Administer cough suppressants and antihistamines.
3. Administer chest physiotherapy two to four times per day.
4. Administer bronchodilator or nebulizer treatments after chest physiotherapy.

105. 3. Chest physiotherapy is recommended two to four times per day to help loosen and move secretions to facilitate expectoration. Exercise and physical activity are recommended to stimulate mucus secretion and to establish a good habitual breathing pattern. Cough suppressants and antihistamines are contraindicated. The goal is for the child to be able to cough and expectorate mucus secretions. Bronchodilator or nebulizer treatments are given before chest physiotherapy to help open the bronchi for easier expectoration.
CN: Safe, effective care environment; CNS: Coordinated care; CL: Apply; DIFFICULTY: Challenge

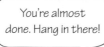
Cystic fibrosis is all in the genes.

106. Which statement is appropriate for the nurse to make to the parents of a child with cystic fibrosis who are planning to have a second child?
1. Genetic counseling is recommended.
2. There's a 50% chance that the child will be normal.
3. There's a 50% chance that the child will be affected.
4. There's a 25% chance that the child will only be a carrier.

106. 1. Genetic counseling should be recommended. Cystic fibrosis is an autosomal-recessive disease. Therefore, there's a 25% chance of the child having the disease, a 25% chance of the child being normal, and a 50% chance of the child being a carrier.
CN: Health promotion and maintenance; CNS: None; CL: Apply; DIFFICULTY: Moderate

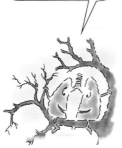
You're almost done. Hang in there!

107. A 3-year-old child is admitted with pneumonia and exhibits a productive cough and difficulty breathing. The parents inform the nurse of a poor appetite and inactivity. Which interventions would be included in the care plan to improve airway clearance? Select all that apply.
1. Restrict fluid intake.
2. Perform chest physiotherapy as ordered.
3. Encourage coughing and deep breathing.
4. Keep the head of the bed flat.
5. Perform postural drainage.
6. Maintain humidification with a cool mist humidifier.

107. 2, 3, 5, 6. Chest physiotherapy and postural drainage work together to break up congestion and drain secretions. Coughing and deep breathing are also effective to remove congestion. A cool mist humidifier helps loosen thick mucus and relax airway passages. Fluids should be encouraged, not restricted. The child should be placed in semi-Fowler's or high Fowler's position to facilitate breathing and promote optimal lung expansion.
CN: Physiological integrity; CNS: Physiological adaptation; CL: Apply; DIFFICULTY: Moderate

CN: Client needs category   CNS: Client needs subcategory   CL: Cognitive level

108. A nurse is educating the parents of a 5-year-old child admitted to the pediatric unit with cystic fibrosis. Which statement concerning steatorrheic stools is **most** accurate?

1. They're black and tarry.
2. They're frothy, foul-smelling, and fatty.
3. They're clay-colored.
4. They're orange or green.

109. A nurse is caring for a 17-year-old female with cystic fibrosis who has been admitted to the hospital for treatment of a recurrent lung infection. The adolescent has many questions about her future and the consequences of her disease. Which statements about the course of cystic fibrosis are accurate? Select all that apply.

1. Breast development is frequently delayed.
2. The adolescent is at risk for developing diabetes.
3. Pregnancy and birth aren't affected.
4. Normal sexual relationships can be expected.
5. Only males carry the gene for the disease.
6. By age 20, the client should be able to decrease the frequency of respiratory treatment.

110. Ceftazidime has been ordered for a child with cystic fibrosis. The order states to give 40 mg/kg every 8 hours. The child is 2 years old and weighs 38½ lb. How many milligrams should the nurse administer in each dose? Record your answer using a whole number.

_____ mg

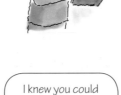

Put on your math cap. Time to crunch some numbers.

111. A nurse is preparing to administer the first dose of tobramycin to an adolescent with cystic fibrosis. The order is for 3 mg/kg IV daily in three divided doses. The client weighs 110 lb. How many milligrams should the nurse administer per dose? Record your answer using a whole number.

_____ mg

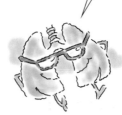

I knew you could do it. Congrats!

108. 2. Children with cystic fibrosis have an abnormal electrolyte transport system in the cells that eventually blocks the pancreas, preventing the secretion of enzymes that digest certain foods such as protein and fats. This results in foul-smelling, fatty stool. Black, tarry stool is observed in clients who have upper GI bleeding, are on iron medications, or who consume diets high in red meat and dark-green vegetables. Clay-colored stool indicates possible bile obstruction. Orange or green stool may indicate intestinal infection.

CN: Physiological integrity; CNS: Physiological adaptation; CL: Apply; DIFFICULTY: Easy

109. 1, 2, 4. Cystic fibrosis delays growth and the onset of puberty. Children with cystic fibrosis tend to be smaller-than-average size and develop secondary sexual characteristics later in life. In addition, clients with cystic fibrosis are at risk for developing diabetes because the pancreatic duct becomes obstructed as pancreatic tissue is damaged. Adolescents with cystic fibrosis can expect to have normal sexual relationships, but fertility may be affected because of changes in mucous membranes. Both males and females carry the gene for cystic fibrosis. Pulmonary disease commonly progresses as the adolescent ages, requiring additional respiratory treatment, not less.

CN: Physiological integrity; CNS: Physiological adaptation; CL: Analyze; DIFFICULTY: Difficult

110. 233.
The child should receive 233 mg per dose. Use the following equations:

$$38.5 \text{ lb} / 2.2 \text{ kg} = 17.5 \text{ kg (1 lb equals 2.2 kg)}$$

$$40 \text{ mg} / \text{kg} \times 17.5 \text{ kg} = 700 \text{ mg}$$

$$24 \text{ hours} / 8 \text{ hours} = 3 \text{ doses}$$

$$700 \text{ mg} / 3 \text{ doses} = 233 \text{ mg}$$

CN: Physiological integrity; CNS: Pharmacological therapies; CL: Apply; DIFFICULTY: Difficult

111. 50.
To perform this dosage calculation, the nurse should first convert the adolescent's weight to kilograms using this formula:

$$1 \text{ kg} / 2.2 \text{ lb} = X \text{ kg} / 110 \text{ lb}$$

$$2.2 X = 110$$

$$X = 50 \text{ kg}$$

Then the nurse should calculate the adolescent's daily dose using this formula:

$$50 \text{ kg} \times 3 \text{ mg} / \text{kg} = 150 \text{ mg}$$

Finally, the nurse should calculate the divided dose:

$$150 \text{ mg} \div 3 \text{ doses} = 50 \text{ mg} / \text{dose}$$

CN: Physiological integrity; CNS: Pharmacological therapies; CL: Apply; DIFFICULTY: Moderate

Chapter 29

Neurosensory Disorders

Pediatric neurosensory refresher

Attention deficit hyperactivity disorder

Displaying signs of inattentiveness, hyperactivity, and impulsivity; often, difficulty staying on task or concentrating for long periods of time

Key signs and symptoms
- Decreased attention span
- Difficulty organizing tasks and activities
- Easily distracted

Key test results
- Complete psychological, medical, and neurologic evaluations rule out other problems

Key treatments
- Behavioral modification and psychological therapy
- Amphetamines: methylphenidate, dextro-amphetamine sulfate, amphetamine sulfate, and amphetamine aspartate

Key interventions
- Give one simple instruction at a time
- Provide consistency in child's daily routine
- Reduce environmental stimuli
- Praise child for accomplishments

Cerebral palsy

Non-progressive brain disorder that is often associated with spasticity and difficulty with posture; usually occurs due to some type of brain injury during pregnancy or early childhood; symptoms can range from mild to severe, and may or may not be associated with intellectual disorders

Key signs and symptoms
- Abnormal muscle tone and coordination (most common associated problem)
- Difficulty sucking or keeping a nipple or food in mouth
- Infrequent voluntary movement, or arm or leg tremors with voluntary movement
- Legs crossed when lifted from behind

Key test results
- Neuroimaging studies determine site of brain impairment
- Cytogenic studies (genetic evaluation of the child and other family members) rule out other potential causes
- Metabolic studies rule out other causes

Key treatments
- Braces or splints and special appliances (such as adapted eating utensils and a low toilet seat with arms) to help child perform activities independently
- Range-of-motion (ROM) exercises to minimize contractures
- Muscle relaxants or neurosurgery to decrease spasticity, if appropriate

Key interventions
- Assist with locomotion, communication, and educational opportunities
- Divide tasks into small steps
- Perform ROM exercises if child is spastic

Down syndrome

Genetic disorder, Trisomy 21, in which there are distinct physical manifestations, as well as some degree of cognitive disorder; the severity of the disorder is often not known until the child stops meeting developmental milestones

Key signs and symptoms
- Flat, broad forehead
- Mild to moderate retardation
- Short stature with pudgy hands
- Small head with slow brain growth
- Small jaw
- Upward slanting eyes
- Transverse palmar creases

Key test results
- Amniocentesis allows prenatal diagnosis

Key treatments
- Treatment for coexisting conditions— congenital heart problems, visual defects, or hypothyroidism

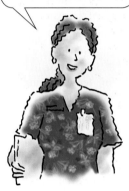

Here are three Web sites for more information about neurosensory disorders in children: *www.chadd.org* (Children and Adults with Attention-Deficit Hyperactivity Disorder), *www.ndss.org* (National Down Syndrome Society), and *www.spinabifidaassociation.org* (Spina Bifida Association of America).

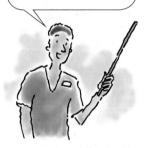

I'm sure you'll have no problem staying focused on these disorders. Let's dive in.

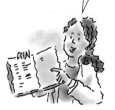

Can you remember the key signs and symptoms of Down syndrome?

Key interventions
- Provide activities appropriate for the child's mental rather than chronological age
- Set realistic, reachable, short-term goals; break tasks into small steps
- Provide stimulation and communicate at a level appropriate to the child's mental age rather than chronologic age

Hydrocephalus

Dysfunction between cerebrospinal fluid production and absorption, resulting in increased fluid within the ventricles of the brain, which leads to increased intracranial pressure; may be fatal if not treated promptly; may be congenital or acquired

Key signs and symptoms
- High-pitched cry
- Rapid increase in head circumference and full, tense, bulging fontanels (before cranial sutures close)

Key test results
- Skull x-ray shows thinning of the skull with separation of the sutures and widening of fontanels

Key treatments
- Ventriculoperitoneal shunt insertion to allow cerebrospinal fluid (CSF) to drain from the lateral ventricle in the brain
- Anticonvulsants: carbamazepine, phenobarbital, diazepam, phenytoin

Key interventions
- Monitor vital signs and intake and output
- Monitor neurologic status
- After shunt is inserted, don't lay child on the side of the body where it's located
- Lay the child flat
- If the caudal end of the shunt must be externalized because of infection, keep the bag at ear level

Meningitis

Infection and inflammation of the meninges surrounding the brain and spinal cord; may be caused by viruses, bacteria, and other organisms; bacterial meningitis is highly contagious; viral meningitis is not

Key signs and symptoms
- Nuchal rigidity that may progress to opisthotonos (severe posturing with arched back and head thrown backwards)
- Positive Brudzinski sign (flexion of the knees and hips in response to passive neck flexion)
- Positive Kernig sign (inability to extend leg when hip and knee are flexed)
- Bulging anterior fontanel

Key test results
- Lumbar puncture shows increased CSF pressure, cloudy color, increased white blood cell count and protein level, and decreased glucose level if the meningitis is caused by bacteria

Key treatments
- Airborne precautions should be maintained until at least 24 hours of effective antibiotic therapy have elapsed; continued precautions recommended for meningitis caused by *Haemophilus influenzae or Neisseria meningitidis*
- Seizure precautions
- Analgesics to treat pain of meningeal irritation
- Corticosteroids such as dexamethasone
- Parenteral antibiotics: ceftazidime, ceftriaxone; possibly intraventricular administration of antibiotics

Key interventions
- Monitor vital signs and intake and output
- Monitor child's neurologic status frequently
- Examine young infant for bulging fontanels and measure head circumference

Otitis media

Infection of the middle part of the ear that causes pain; repeated ear infections may lead to hearing loss

Key signs and symptoms
Acute suppurative otitis media
- Fever (mild to very high)
- Severe, deep, throbbing pain (from pressure behind the tympanic membrane)
- Pain that suddenly stops (if tympanic membrane ruptures)
- Signs of upper respiratory tract infection (sneezing, coughing)

Acute secretory otitis media
- Popping, crackling, or clicking sounds on swallowing or with jaw movement
- Sensation of fullness in the ear

Chronic otitis media
- Cholesteatoma (cystlike mass in the middle ear)
- Decreased or absent tympanic membrane mobility
- Painless, purulent discharge in chronic suppurative otitis media

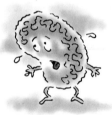

What are the possible causes of brain inflammation?

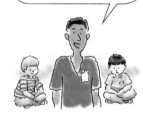

Remember—bacterial meningitis is highly contagious. Observe airborne precautions for 24 hours after starting antibiotics.

Key test results

Acute suppurative otitis media
- Otoscopy reveals obscured or distorted bony landmarks of the tympanic membrane

Acute secretory otitis media
- Otoscopy reveals clear or amber fluid behind the tympanic membrane and tympanic membrane retraction, which causes the bony landmarks to appear more prominent; if hemorrhage into the middle ear has occurred, as in barotrauma, the tympanic membrane appears blue-black

Chronic otitis media
- Otoscopy shows thickening, sometimes scarring, and decreased mobility of the tympanic membrane

Key treatments

Acute suppurative otitis media
- Myringotomy for children with severe, painful bulging of the tympanic membrane
- Antibiotic therapy, usually amoxicillin

Acute secretory otitis media
- Inflation of the eustachian tube by performing Valsalva maneuver several times a day, which may be the only treatment required
- Nasopharyngeal decongestant therapy

Chronic otitis media
- Elimination of eustachian tube obstruction
- Excision of cholesteatoma
- Mastoidectomy
- Antibiotic therapy, usually amoxicillin

Key interventions
- Watch for and report headache, fever, severe pain, or disorientation
- Instruct parents not to feed their infant in a supine position or put him to bed with a bottle
- After myringotomy, maintain drainage flow; place sterile cotton loosely in the external ear and change cotton frequently
- After tympanoplasty, reinforce dressings and observe for excessive bleeding from the ear canal
- Warn the child against blowing his nose or getting the ear wet when bathing

Seizure disorders

Abnormal movements or behaviors, resulting from unusual electrical activity in the brain; there are many different types of seizures; all can produce unusual symptoms

Key signs and symptoms
- Aura just before the seizure's onset (reports of unusual tastes, feelings, or odors)
- Eyes deviating to a particular side or blinking

- Usually unresponsive during tonic-clonic muscular contractions; may experience incontinence
- Irregular breathing with spasms

Key test results
- EEG results help differentiate epileptic from nonepileptic seizures; each seizure has a characteristic EEG tracing

Key treatments
- IV diazepam or lorazepam
- Phenobarbital or fosphenytoin
- Phenytoin or carbamazepine to keep neuron excitability below the seizure threshold

Key interventions
- Monitor neurologic status
- Stay with the child during a seizure
- Move the child to a flat surface
- Place the child on his side to allow saliva to drain out
- Don't try to interrupt the seizure

Spina bifida

Neural tube defect that occurs from the time of brain and neural tube formation. It can range from mild, such as spina bifida occulta, to a myelomeningocele with permanent neurological dysfunction

Key signs and symptoms

Spina bifida occulta
- Dimple on the skin over the spinal defect
- No neurologic dysfunction (usually), except occasional foot weakness or bowel and bladder disturbances

Meningocele
- No neurologic dysfunction (usually)
- Saclike structure protruding over the spine

Myelomeningocele
- Permanent neurologic dysfunction (paralysis below the spinal defect, bowel and bladder incontinence)

Key test results
- Amniocentesis reveals neural tube defect
- Elevated alpha-fetoprotein levels in mother's blood may indicate the presence of a neural tube defect
- Acetylcholinesterase measurement can be used to confirm diagnosis
- Ultrasound may detect spina bifida prenatally

Key interventions
- Teach parents how to cope with their infant's physical problems

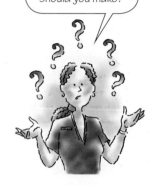

A pediatric client is diagnosed with otitis media. What interventions should you make?

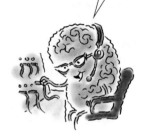

I'm sorry—we're having an electrical disturbance; I can't make your connection at the moment.

- Teach parents how to recognize early signs of complications, such as hydrocephalus, pressure ulcers, and urinary tract infections
- Before surgery:
  ○ watch for signs of hydrocephalus; measure head circumference daily; be sure to mark the spot where the measurement was made
  ○ watch for signs of meningeal irritation, such as fever and nuchal rigidity
- After surgery:
  ○ watch for hydrocephalus, which commonly follows surgery; measure the infant's head circumference as ordered

Reye syndrome

Complication that occurs when recovering from a viral illness with concurrent aspirin use to reduce fever/body aches; starts with an accumulation of fat in the liver and other organs, and increased pressure in the brain; syndrome goes through several phases, and is considered a medical emergency

Key signs and symptoms
- Vomiting, listlessness
- Disorientation confusion
- Convulsions
- Coma

Key test results
- Elevated SGOT and SGPT in the absence of jaundice

Key interventions
- Early recognition
- Maintain airway and brain oxygenation
- ICU placement with intubation

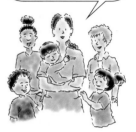

Teach parents and family members how to recognize signs of Reye syndrome.

thePoint® You can download tables of drug information to help you prepare for the NCLEX®! View Generic Drug Names, Drug Classifications, Drug Actions, and Nursing Implications for the drugs discussed in this refresher at **http://thePoint.lww.com**.

Neurosensory questions, answers, and rationales

1. A child presents to the clinic for a follow up after starting methylphenidate for attention deficit hyperactivity disorder. Which findings would indicate to the nurse that the medication is helping the child?
1. Improved manners during mealtimes
2. Able to concentrate for longer periods of time
3. Grades in school have gone up to A's and B's rather than C's and D's
4. Fewer outbursts and less defiant behavior

2. Which complications should the nurse be **most** concerned about in the first 12 hours of life for a neonate born with a myelomeningocele?
1. Infection
2. Constipation
3. Impaired physical mobility
4. Delayed growth and development

3. Which conditions would the nurse expect when measuring the head circumference of a neonate with possible hydrocephalus? Select all that apply.
1. Bulging fontanel
2. Depressed fontanel
3. Eyes rotated downward
4. High-pitched cry
5. Increased interest in feeding
6. Increased irritability

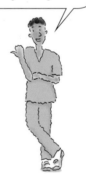

If you concentrate hard enough on question #1, I'm sure you'll get it right.

1. 2. The purpose of the medication is to increase the ability of the child to concentrate; consequently, some of the other behaviors might be observed. The purpose of the stimulant in a child with ADHD is to actually calm the child.
CN: Physiological integrity; CNS: Pharmacological therapies; CL: Analyze; DIFFICULTY: Moderate

2. 1. All of these complications are a potential for a child with a myelomeningocele. However, during the first 12 hours of life, the most life-threatening event would be an infection. The other potential complications will be addressed as the child develops.
CN: Physiological integrity; CNS: Reduction of risk potential; CL: Apply; DIFFICULTY: Easy

3. 1, 3, 4. Hydrocephalus is caused by an alteration in circulation of the cerebrospinal fluid (CSF). CSF volume increases, causing the fontanel to bulge. This also causes an increase in intracranial pressure. This increase in pressure causes the neonate's eyes to deviate downward (the "setting sun sign"), and the neonate's cry becomes high-pitched.
CN: Physiological integrity; CNS: None; CL: Apply; DIFFICULTY: Moderate

4. Which nursing action should be included in the care plan for a child following shunt insertion on the right side of the head to relieve hydrocephalus?
1. Place the child flat in bed on the right side.
2. Place the child flat in bed on the left side.
3. Place the child in a semi-Fowler's position.
4. Place the child in an upright position.

5. Which nursing action is appropriate to prevent injury when a child has a seizure?
1. Inserting a nasogastric tube to prevent emesis
2. Restraining the extremities with a pillow or blanket
3. Inserting a tongue blade to prevent injury to the tongue
4. Padding the side rails of the bed to protect the child from injury

6. The nurse is caring for a child with a seizure disorder. Which nursing actions are appropriate to prevent injury when the child is having a seizure? Select all that apply.
1. Lower the bed to the lowest position.
2. Turn the child to the side.
3. Place pillows or blankets against the side rails.
4. Monitor the child for signs of airway obstruction.
5. Insert a padded tongue blade into the mouth to maintain the airway.

7. A parent brings a 12-week-old infant to the emergency department and says the child has had a seizure. While the nurse is obtaining a history, the parent says the child was running out of formula, so the parent stretched the formula by adding three times the normal amount of water. Electrolyte and blood glucose levels are drawn on the infant. The nurse would expect which laboratory value?
1. Blood glucose: 120 mg/dL
2. Chloride: 104 mmol/L
3. Potassium: 4 mmol/L
4. Sodium: 125 mmol/L

8. Which statement by the parent of a child with cerebral palsy indicates that a nurse's education has been successful?
1. "My child's muscles will get stronger."
2. "My child's condition will get progressively worse."
3. "My child will have low intelligence."
4. "My child will need continual therapy to maintain functioning."

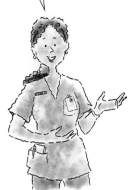

Seizures can produce violent, uncontrollable movements in the client. How can we best help protect them?

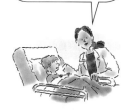

The hospital can be a scary place, especially for kids. Take time comfort your clients and calm their fears.

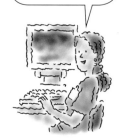

In other words, which statement is *true* in question #8?

4. 2. The child should be placed flat in bed to avoid rapid decompression of cerebrospinal fluid (CSF) and on the left side (or on his back) to avoid occlusion of the shunt and blockage of the drainage of CSF. Placing the child in a semi-Fowler's or upright position may cause a dangerously rapid decompression of CSF.
CN: Physiological integrity; CNS: Reduction of risk potential; CL: Apply; DIFFICULTY: Challenge

5. 4. A child having a seizure could fall out of bed and cause injury, including the side rails of the bed. Padding the side rails helps to protect the child. Attempts to insert anything into the child's mouth may cause injury. Attempting to restrain the child will not stop seizures. In fact, tactile stimulation may increase the seizure activity; therefore, it must be limited as much as possible.
CN: Safe, effective care environment; CNS: Safety and infection control; CL: Apply; DIFFICULTY: Easy

6. 1, 2, 3, 4. When a child has a seizure the most important aspects of care include airway maintenance and safety. Lowering the bed, turning the child to the side, and placing pillows against the side rails will ensure the child does not incur further injury during the seizure. Monitoring for signs of an obstructed airway are important to ensure patency. It is no longer recommended to put anything into the child's mouth as this can cause airway obstruction and possible injury to the oral cavity.
CN: Physiological integrity; CNS: Reduction of risk potential; CL: Apply; DIFFICULTY: Moderate

7. 4. Diluting formula differently from the recommendation alters the infant's electrolyte levels. Normal serum sodium for an infant is 135 to 145 mmol/L. When formula is diluted, the sodium in it is also diluted and will decrease the infant's sodium level. Hyponatremia is one of the causes of seizures in infants. The other laboratory values are all within normal limits.
CN: Physiological integrity; CNS: Physiological adaptation; CL: Analyze; DIFFICULTY: Moderate

8. 4. The child with cerebral palsy needs continual treatment and therapy to maintain or improve functioning. Without therapy, muscles will get progressively weaker and more spastic. Although some children with cerebral palsy have an intellectual disability, many have normal intelligence.
CN: Health promotion and maintenance; CNS: None; CL: Analyze; DIFFICULTY: Easy

CN: Client needs category CNS: Client needs subcategory CL: Cognitive level

9. A neonate is diagnosed with bacterial meningitis. For which **priority** signs and symptoms will the nurse monitor? Select all that apply.
1. Hypothermia
2. Irritability
3. Nuchal rigidity
4. Hyperthermia
5. Poor feeding

9. **1, 2, 4.** The clinical appearance of a neonate with meningitis is different from that of a child or an adult. The neonate may be either hypothermic or hyperthermic. The irritation to the meninges causes the neonate to be irritable and to have a decreased appetite. The child may be pale and mottled with a bulging, full fontanel. Normal neonates have positive Babinski reflexes and Moro embrace. Older children and adults with meningitis have headaches, nuchal rigidity, and hyperthermia as clinical manifestations. Developmental delays, if present, would appear when the child is older.
CN: Physiological integrity; CNS: Physiological adaptation; CL: Apply; DIFFICULTY: Difficult

10. Which behavior demonstrated by a 6-year-old would help the nurse recognize a learning disability as opposed to attention deficit hyperactivity disorder?
1. The child reverses letters and words while reading.
2. The child is easily distracted and reacts impulsively.
3. The child is always getting into fights during recess.
4. The child has a difficult time reading a chapter book.

10. **1.** Children who reverse letters and words while reading have dyslexia. Two of the most common characteristics of children with ADHD include inattention and impulsiveness. Although aggressiveness may be common in children with ADHD, it isn't a characteristic that will aid in the diagnosis of this disorder. Six-year-old children aren't usually cognitively ready to read a chapter book.
CN: Health promotion and maintenance; CNS: None; CL: Apply; DIFFICULTY: Moderate

11. A child is taking methylphenidate 20 mg twice a day for attention deficit hyperactivity disorder. Available from the pharmacy is methylphenidate 40 mg/tablet. How many tablets should the child take per dose? Record your answer using one decimal place.

_____ tablets

Get ready to crunch some numbers—it's another math question.

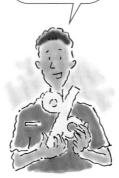

11. **0.5.**
The correct formula to calculate a drug dose is:

$$\frac{\text{Dose on hand}}{\text{Quantity on hand}} = \frac{\text{Dose desired}}{X}$$

The child is taking 20 mg, which is the dose desired. The pharmacy has available 40-mg tablets, which is the dose on hand.

$$\frac{40 \text{ mg}}{1 \text{ tablet}} = \frac{20 \text{ mg}}{X}$$

$$X = 0.5 \text{ tablets}$$

CN: Physiological integrity; CNS: Pharmacological therapies; CL: Analyze; DIFFICULTY: Easy

12. A nurse is educating the parents of an 18-month-old infant diagnosed with bilateral otitis media about the prescribed medication amoxicillin and clavulanate potassium. Which statement by the parents indicates the education has been effective?
1. "It can cause diarrhea."
2. "It can cause headache."
3. "It can cause petechiae."
4. "It can cause a rash."

12. **1.** Diarrhea is a common adverse effect of amoxicillin/clavulanate potassium suspension. Red rash and petechiae occur less commonly. Headache isn't a common adverse effect of amoxicillin/clavulanate potassium and would be difficult to determine in an 18-month-old infant.
CN: Physiological integrity; CNS: Pharmacological therapies; CL: Analyze; DIFFICULTY: Moderate

13. A 1-year-old child is brought to the emergency department with a mild respiratory infection and a temperature of 101.3° F (38.5° C). Otitis media is diagnosed. Which sign would the nurse also expect to find?
1. Excessive drooling
2. Tugging on the ears
3. High-pitched, barking cough
4. Pearl-gray tympanic membrane

14. A nurse is educating the parents of a 10-month-old infant on the correct method for instilling eardrops prescribed for the infant when discharged. Which statement by the parents indicates understanding?
1. "We should pull the earlobe upward."
2. "We should pull the earlobe up and back."
3. "We should pull the earlobe down and back."
4. "We should pull the earlobe down and forward."

15. A child is diagnosed as having right chronic otitis media. After the child returns from surgery for myringotomy and placement of ear tubes, which intervention is appropriate?
1. Apply gauze dressings.
2. Position the child on the left side.
3. Position the child on the right side.
4. Apply warm compresses to both ears.

16. A child is diagnosed with chronic otitis media. Which statement made by the mother indicates an understanding of this condition?
1. "I need to be sure the baby is dressed warmly."
2. "I must be sure he gets all of his DTaP vaccinations."
3. "I'll tell my relatives they can't smoke around the baby."
4. "I'll give him Tylenol once a day every week."

17. Which finding of otoscopy would the nurse identify as suggestive of acute otitis media?
1. Pearl-gray tympanic membrane
2. Red tympanic membrane
3. Dull-gray membrane with fluid behind the eardrum
4. Bright-red or yellow bulging or retracted tympanic membrane

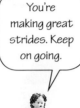

You're making great strides. Keep on going.

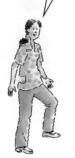

13. 2. Tugging on the ears is a common sign for a child with ear pain. Pearl-gray tympanic membranes are a normal finding. Excessive drooling and a high-pitched, barking cough indicate croup. A child with otitis media usually exhibits a discolored tympanic membrane (bright red, yellow, or dull gray).
CN: Physiological integrity; CNS: Physiological adaptation; CL: Apply; DIFFICULTY: Easy

14. 3. For infants, the parents should understand that they should gently pull the earlobe down and back to visualize the external auditory canal. For children older than age 3 and for adults, the earlobe is gently pulled slightly up and back.
CN: Physiological integrity; CNS: Pharmacological therapies; CL: Analyze; DIFFICULTY: Easy

15. 3. The child should be positioned on the right side to facilitate drainage. The left side isn't an area of concern for drainage. Gauze dressings aren't necessary after surgery. Some health care providers may prefer a loose, cotton wick. Warm compresses may help to facilitate drainage only when used on the affected ear.
CN: Physiological integrity; CNS: Physiological adaptation; CL: Apply; DIFFICULTY: Challenge

16. 3. Eliminating tobacco smoke and other allergens from the environment can help prevent otitis media. No extra clothing is needed. Diphtheria, tetanus, and pertussis aren't causes of otitis media. Tylenol should only be given when indicated for fever or pain.
CN: Health promotion and maintenance; CNS: None; CL: Analyze; DIFFICULTY: Moderate

17. 4. With acute otitis media, the tympanic membrane may present as bright-red or yellow, bulging or retracted. A pearl-gray tympanic membrane is a normal finding. A red tympanic membrane isn't diagnostic for acute otitis media. A dull-gray membrane with fluid is consistent with subacute or chronic otitis media.
CN: Physiological integrity; CNS: Physiological adaptation; CL: Understand; DIFFICULTY: Moderate

18. Which statement by the parent of a child with otitis media indicates an understanding of the nurse's discharge instructions about the use of antibiotics?
1. "I'll give my child the full course of antibiotics."
2. "I'll stop the antibiotics when my child no longer has ear pain."
3. "I'll give the antibiotics when my child has ear pain."
4. "I'll put antibiotics in the affected ear."

19. A young child has had multiple ear infections and is brought to the clinic screaming and holding the right ear. Which most common complication related to acute otitis media does the nurse expect this client is experiencing?
1. Eardrum perforation
2. Hearing loss
3. Meningitis
4. Tympanosclerosis

20. A nurse is educating the parents of a 1-year-old infant with otitis media. Which statement regarding predisposing factors for otitis media would be **most** accurate for the nurse to make?
1. "The cartilage lining is overdeveloped."
2. "A sitting position contributes to the pooling of fluid."
3. "Humoral defense mechanisms decrease the risk of infection."
4. "Eustachian tubes are short, wide, and straight and lie in a horizontal plane."

21. Parents report that their school-age child has been reprimanded for daydreaming during class. This is a new behavior, and the child's grades are dropping. The nurse should suspect which problem?
1. The child may have a hearing problem and needs to have his ears checked.
2. The child may have a learning disability and needs referral to the special education department.
3. The child may have attention deficit hyperactivity disorder (ADHD) and needs medication.
4. The child may be having absence seizures and needs to see his primary health care provider for evaluation.

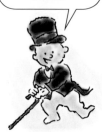
Thanks for the antibiotics. My ear ache is all gone, and I feel like a million bucks!

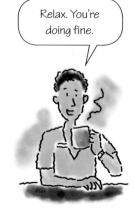
Relax. You're doing fine.

18. 1. Antibiotics should be given for the fully prescribed course of therapy, regardless of whether the child still has symptoms. Antibiotics are taken at prescribed intervals and not for episodes of ear pain. Oral antibiotics are used to treat otitis media.
CN: Physiological integrity; CNS: Pharmacological therapies; CL: Apply; DIFFICULTY: Easy

19. 1. Eardrum perforation is the most common complication of acute otitis media as the exudate accumulates and pressure increases. Hearing loss in most cases is conductive in nature and mild in severity but is less common than eardrum perforation. Hearing tests aren't usually performed during episodes of otitis media. Meningitis and tympanosclerosis are possible but uncommon when adequate antibiotic therapy is implemented.
CN: Physiological integrity; CNS: Physiological adaptation; CL: Apply; DIFFICULTY: Easy

20. 4. In an infant or child, the eustachian tubes are short, wide, and straight and lie in a horizontal plane, allowing them to be more easily blocked by conditions such as large adenoids and infections. Until the eustachian tubes change in size and angle, children are more susceptible to otitis media. Cartilage lining is underdeveloped, making the tubes more distensible and more likely to open inappropriately. The usual lying-down position of infants contributes to the pooling of fluid, such as formula in the pharyngeal cavity. Immature humoral defense mechanisms increase the risk of infection.
CN: Physiological integrity; CNS: Physiological adaptation; CL: Analyze; DIFFICULTY: Easy

21. 4. Absence seizures are commonly misinterpreted as daydreaming. The child loses awareness but no alteration in motor activity is exhibited. A mild hearing problem usually is exhibited as leaning forward, talking louder, listening to louder TV and music than usual, and a repetitive "what?" from the child. There isn't enough information in the question scenario to indicate a learning disability. ADHD is characterized by episodes of hyperactivity, not quiet daydreaming.
CN: Physiological integrity; CNS: Physiological adaptation; CL: Apply; DIFFICULTY: Moderate

22. A 2-year-old child is admitted to the pediatric unit with the diagnosis of bacterial meningitis. Which nursing action would be appropriate for the nurse to perform **first**?
1. Obtain a urine specimen.
2. Draw ordered laboratory tests.
3. Place the toddler in respiratory isolation.
4. Explain the treatment plan to the parents.

23. A 10-month-old infant with bacterial meningitis was just started on antibiotic therapy. Which nursing action is especially important in this situation?
1. Wear a mask while providing care.
2. Flex the child's neck every 4 hours to maintain range of motion.
3. Administer oral gentamicin.
4. Encourage the child to drink 3,000 mL of fluid per day.

24. A 2-month-old infant is brought to the well-baby clinic for a first checkup. On initial measurements, the nurse notes the infant's head circumference is at the 95th percentile. Which action would the nurse take **first**?
1. Obtain vital signs.
2. Measure the head again.
3. Observe neurologic signs.
4. Notify the primary health care provider.

25. A preschool-age child has just been admitted to the pediatric unit with a diagnosis of bacterial meningitis. The nurse would include which recommendation in the nursing plan?
1. Take vital signs every 4 hours.
2. Monitor temperature every 4 hours.
3. Decrease environmental stimulation.
4. Encourage the parents to hold the child.

26. A child has just returned to the pediatric unit following ventriculoperitoneal shunt placement for hydrocephalus. Which intervention would the nurse perform **first**?
1. Monitor intake and output.
2. Place the child on the side opposite the shunt.
3. Offer fluids because the child has a dry mouth.
4. Administer pain medication by mouth as ordered.

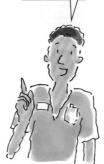
Keep in mind that bacterial meningitis is an airborne infection.

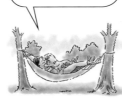
Our brains need a break, too. Remember to get up and walk around occasionally.

22. 3. Nurses should take necessary precautions to protect themselves and others from possible infection from the bacterial organism causing meningitis. The affected child should immediately be placed in respiratory isolation; then the parents can be informed about the treatment plan. This should be done before laboratory tests are performed.
CN: Safe, effective care environment; CNS: Safety and infection control; CL: Apply; DIFFICULTY: Moderate

23. 1. With bacterial meningitis, respiratory isolation must be maintained for at least 24 hours after beginning antibiotic therapy. Wearing a mask is an important part of respiratory isolation. Moving the child's head to maintain range of motion would cause pain because the meninges are inflamed. Gentamicin is never administered orally. Encouraging 3,000 mL of fluid would cause overhydration in a 10-month-old infant and place them at risk for increased intracranial pressure.
CN: Safe, effective care environment; CNS: Safety and infection control; CL: Apply; DIFFICULTY: Moderate

24. 2. Whenever there's a question about vital signs or assessment data, the first logical step is to reassess and determine if an error has been made initially. In this case, measuring the head again would be the priority. Notifying the primary health care provider and assessing neurologic and vital signs are important and would follow the head reassessment, if warranted.
CN: Health promotion and maintenance; CNS: None; CL: Analyze; DIFFICULTY: Difficult

25. 3. A child with the diagnosis of meningitis is much more comfortable with decreased environmental stimuli. Noise and bright lights stimulate the child and can be irritating, causing the child to cry, in turn increasing intracranial pressure. Vital signs would be taken initially every hour and temperature monitored every 2 hours. Children with bacterial meningitis are usually much more comfortable if allowed to lie flat because this position doesn't cause increased meningeal irritation.
CN: Physiological integrity; CNS: Physiological adaptation; CL: Apply; DIFFICULTY: Moderate

26. 2. Following shunt placement surgery, the child should be placed on the side opposite the surgical site to prevent pressure on the shunt valve. Intake and output will be monitored, but that isn't the priority nursing intervention. Many children are nauseated after a general anesthetic, and ice chips or clear liquids would be introduced if the nurse determines the child is nauseated. Pain medication should initially be administered by an IV route postoperatively.
CN: Physiological integrity; CNS: Basic care and comfort; CL: Apply; DIFFICULTY: Moderate

CN: Client needs category   CNS: Client needs subcategory   CL: Cognitive level

27. An otherwise healthy 18-month-old child with a history of febrile seizures is in the well-child clinic. Which statement by the parent would indicate to the nurse that additional education is needed?
1. "I have ibuprofen available in case it's needed."
2. "My child will likely outgrow these seizures by age 5."
3. "I always keep phenobarbital with me in case of a fever."
4. "The most likely time for a seizure is when the fever is rising."

28. When checking a 5-month-old infant, which symptom would alert the nurse that the infant needs further follow-up?
1. Absent grasp reflex
2. Rolls from back to side
3. Balances head when sitting
4. Presence of Moro embrace reflex

29. An adolescent is started on valproic acid to treat seizures. Which statement should be included when educating the adolescent?
1. "This medication has no adverse effects."
2. "A common adverse effect is weight gain."
3. "Drowsiness and irritability commonly occur."
4. "Early morning dosing is recommended to decrease insomnia."

30. Which statement by the nurse to a parent regarding cerebral palsy would be accurate?
1. "Cerebral palsy is a condition that runs in families."
2. "Cerebral palsy means there will be many disabilities."
3. "Cerebral palsy is a condition that doesn't get worse."
4. "Cerebral palsy occurs because of too much oxygen to the brain."

31. Which nursing action should be included in the care plan to promote comfort in a 4-year-old child hospitalized with meningitis?
1. Avoid making noise when in the child's room.
2. Rock the child frequently.
3. Let the child's 2-year-old brother stay in the room.
4. Keep the lights on brightly so that he can see his mother.

32. A 6-month-old infant is admitted with a diagnosis of bacterial meningitis. The nurse would place the infant in which room?
1. A room with a 12-month-old infant with a urinary tract infection
2. A room with an 8-month-old infant with failure to thrive
3. A private room near the nurses' station
4. A two-bed room in the middle of the hall

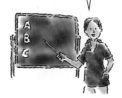

Make sure the parents of pediatric clients understand the purpose of their medications.

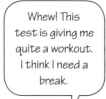

Whew! This test is giving me quite a workout. I think I need a break.

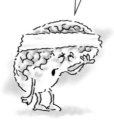

27. 3. Antiepileptics, such as phenobarbital, are administered to children with prolonged seizures or neurologic abnormalities. Ibuprofen, not phenobarbital, is given for fever. Febrile seizures usually occur after age 6 months and are unusual after age 5. Treatment is to decrease the temperature because seizures occur as the temperature rises.
CN: Health promotion and maintenance; CNS: None; CL: Apply; DIFFICULTY: Moderate

28. 4. Moro embrace reflex should be absent at 4 months. Grasp reflex begins to fade at 2 months and should be absent at 3 months. A 4-month-old infant should be able to roll from back to side and balance the head when sitting.
CN: Health promotion and maintenance; CNS: None; CL: Apply; DIFFICULTY: Challenge

29. 2. Weight gain is a common adverse effect of valproic acid. Drowsiness and irritability are adverse effects more commonly associated with phenobarbital. Felbamate more commonly causes insomnia.
CN: Physiological integrity; CNS: Pharmacological therapies; CL: Apply; DIFFICULTY: Challenge

30. 3. By definition, cerebral palsy is a nonprogressive neuromuscular disorder. It can be mild or quite severe and is believed to be the result of a hypoxic event during pregnancy or the birth process. Cerebral palsy doesn't run in families.
CN: Physiological integrity; CNS: Basic care and comfort; CL: Apply; DIFFICULTY: Difficult

31. 1. Meningeal irritation may cause seizures and heightens a child's sensitivity to all stimuli, including noise, lights, movement, and touch. Frequent rocking, presence of a younger sibling, and bright lights would increase stimulation.
CN: Physiological integrity; CNS: Basic care and comfort; CL: Apply; DIFFICULTY: Easy

32. 3. A child who has the diagnosis of bacterial meningitis is considered contagious and will need to be placed in a private room until receiving IV antibiotics for 24 hours. Additionally, bacterial meningitis can be quite serious; therefore, the child should be placed near the nurses' station for close monitoring and easier access in case of a crisis.
CN: Safe, effective care environment; CNS: Safety and infection control; CL: Apply; DIFFICULTY: Easy

33. In caring for a child immediately after a head injury, the nurse notes a blood pressure of 110/60 mm Hg, a heart rate of 78 beats/minute, dilated and nonreactive pupils, minimal response to pain, and slow response to name. Which symptom would cause the nurse the **most** concern?
1. Vital signs
2. Nonreactive pupils
3. Slow response to name
4. Minimal response to pain

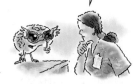

Sometimes symptoms are hidden and have to be discovered.

33. 2. Dilated and nonreactive pupils indicate that anoxia or ischemia of the brain has occurred. If the pupils are also fixed (don't move), then herniation of the brain through the tentorium has occurred. The vital signs are normal. Slow response to name can be normal after a head injury. Minimal response to pain is an indication of the child's level of consciousness.
CN: Physiological integrity; CNS: Basic care and comfort; CL: Apply; DIFFICULTY: Easy

34. An older child has a craniotomy for removal of a brain tumor. Which statement would be appropriate for the nurse to say to the parents?
1. "Your child really had a close call."
2. "I'm sure your child will be back to normal soon."
3. "I'm so glad to hear your child doesn't have cancer."
4. "What has the health care provider told you about the tumor?"

34. 4. When comforting parents, it's best to first ascertain what the health care provider has told them about the tumor. Since the outcome of the surgery isn't known, it would be inappropriate to indicate that the child had a close call. Usually after a craniotomy, it takes several weeks or longer before the child is back to normal. Final pathology results won't be available for several days, so refrain from making premature statements about the tumor and malignancy.
CN: Psychosocial integrity; CNS: None; CL: Apply; DIFFICULTY: Easy

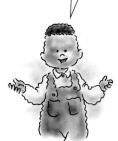

Check out what I can do. Impressive, huh?

35. Which developmental milestone would the nurse expect an 11-month-old infant to have achieved?
1. Sitting independently
2. Walking independently
3. Building a tower of four cubes
4. Turning a doorknob

35. 1. Infants typically sit independently, without support, by age 8 months. Walking independently may be accomplished as late as age 15 months and still be within the normal range. Few infants walk independently by age 11 months. Building a tower of three or four blocks is a milestone of an 18-month-old. Turning a doorknob is a milestone of a 24-month-old.
CN: Health promotion and maintenance; CNS: None; CL: Apply; DIFFICULTY: Easy

36. What's the nurse's **priority** when caring for a 10-month-old infant with meningitis?
1. Maintain an adequate airway.
2. Maintain fluid and electrolyte balance.
3. Control seizures.
4. Control hyperthermia.

36. 1. Maintaining an adequate airway is always a top priority. Maintaining fluid and electrolyte balance and controlling seizures and hyperthermia are all important, but maintaining an adequate airway takes priority.
CN: Physiological integrity; CNS: Reduction of risk potential; CL: Apply; DIFFICULTY: Moderate

37. Which intervention prevents a 17-month-old child with spastic cerebral palsy from going into a scissoring position?
1. Keep the child in leg braces 23 hours per day.
2. Let the child lie down as much as possible.
3. Try to keep the child as quiet as possible.
4. Place the child on the hip.

37. 4. To interrupt the scissoring position, flex the knees and hips. Placing the child with spastic cerebral palsy on the hip is an easy way to stop this common spastic positioning. This child needs stimulation and movement to reach the goal of development to the fullest potential. Wearing leg braces 23 hours per day is inappropriate and doesn't allow the child to move freely. Trying to keep the child quiet and lying flat are inappropriate measures.
CN: Physiological integrity; CNS: Basic care and comfort; CL: Apply; DIFFICULTY: Difficult

38. The parent of a child with a ventriculoperitoneal shunt calls the nurse stating, "my child has a temperature of 101.2° F (38.4° C), a blood pressure of 108/68 mm Hg, and a pulse of 100 beats/minute." The child is lethargic and vomited the night before. Other children in the family have had similar symptoms. Which nursing intervention is **most** appropriate?

1. Provide symptomatic treatment.
2. Advise the parent that this is a viral infection.
3. Consult the primary health care provider.
4. Tell the parent to bring the child to the primary health care provider's office.

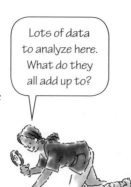

Lots of data to analyze here. What do they all add up to?

38. 4. One of the complications of a ventriculoperitoneal shunt is a shunt infection. Shunt infections can have similar symptoms as a viral infection, so it's best to have the child examined. These symptoms may be due to the same viral infection that the siblings have, but it's better to rule out a shunt infection because it can progress quickly to a very serious illness.

CN: Physiological integrity; CNS: Basic care and comfort;

CL: Apply; DIFFICULTY: Easy

39. The parent of a 10-year-old child with attention deficit hyperactivity disorder (ADHD) says her spouse won't allow their child to take more than 5 mg of methylphenidate every morning. The child isn't doing better in school. Which recommendation would the nurse make to the parent?

1. Sneak the medication to the child anyway.
2. Put the child in charge of administering the medication.
3. Bring the child's parent to the clinic to discuss the medication.
4. Ask the school nurse to give the child the rest of the medication.

39. 3. Bringing the parent to the clinic for an educational session about the medication should assist him in understanding why it's necessary for the child to receive the full dose. The parent should be included in the treatment as much as possible. A nurse shouldn't advise dishonesty to a client or family. Putting a 10-year-old in charge of medication is inappropriate. School nurses can only administer medications as per health care provider prescriptions.

CN: Physiological integrity; CNS: Pharmacological therapies;

CL: Apply; DIFFICULTY: Easy

40. A hospitalized child is to receive 75 mg of acetaminophen for fever control. How much will the nurse administer if the acetaminophen concentration is 40 mg per 0.4 mL? Record your answer using two decimal places.

_____ mL

40. 0.75.
Use the following equations:

$$\frac{\text{Dose on hand}}{\text{Quantity on hand}} = \frac{\text{Dose desired}}{X}$$

$$\frac{40 \text{ mg}}{0.4 \text{ mL}} = \frac{75 \text{ mg}}{X}$$

$$X = 0.75 \text{ mL}$$

CN: Physiological integrity; CNS: Pharmacological therapies;

CL: Apply; DIFFICULTY: Easy

41. The nurse is observing an infant who may have acute bacterial meningitis. Which finding should the nurse anticipate?

1. Flat fontanel
2. Irritability, fever, and vomiting
3. Jaundice, drowsiness, and refusal to eat
4. Negative Kernig sign

41. 2. Findings associated with acute bacterial meningitis may include irritability, fever, and vomiting along with seizure activity. Fontanels would be bulging as intracranial pressure rises, and Kernig sign would be present due to meningeal irritation. Jaundice, drowsiness, and refusal to eat indicate a GI disturbance rather than meningitis.

CN: Physiological integrity; CNS: Physiological adaptation;

CL: Apply; DIFFICULTY: Moderate

42. The nurse is preparing a toddler for a lumbar puncture. For this procedure, the nurse should place the child in which position?

1. Lying prone, with the neck flexed
2. Sitting up, with the back straight
3. Lying on one side, with the back curved
4. Lying prone, with the feet higher than the head

42. 3. Lumbar puncture involves placing a needle between the lumbar vertebrae into the subarachnoid space. For this procedure, the nurse should position the client on one side with the back curved; curving the back maximizes the space between the lumbar vertebrae, facilitating needle insertion. Prone and seated positions don't achieve maximum separation of the vertebrae.

CN: Physiological integrity; CNS: Reduction of risk potential;

CL: Apply; DIFFICULTY: Easy

43. A nurse notes the chart entry below concerning a school-age child who has had a brain tumor removed. Which nursing action should be performed **first**?

Progress notes	
	Pupils equal and reactive to light; motor
	strength equal; aware of name, date, but not
	location. Reporting headache.
	—*S. Jones, L.P.N 10/14/16 1300 QI*

1. Provide medication for the headache.
2. Immediately notify the primary health care provider.
3. Check what the child's level of consciousness has been.
4. Call the child's parents to come and sit at the child's bedside.

44. Parents bring a toddler age 19 months to the clinic for a regular checkup. When palpating the toddler's fontanels, what should the nurse expect to find?
1. Closed anterior fontanel and open posterior fontanel
2. Open anterior fontanel and closed posterior fontanel
3. Closed anterior and posterior fontanels
4. Open anterior and posterior fontanels

45. A 10-year-old child with a concussion is admitted to the pediatric unit. The nurse would place this child in a room with which roommate?
1. A 6-year-old child with osteomyelitis
2. An 8-year-old child with gastroenteritis
3. A 10-year-old child with rheumatic fever
4. A 12-year-old child with a fractured femur

46. A nurse is caring for a child with spina bifida. The child's parent asks the nurse what they did to cause the birth defect. Which statement would be the nurse's **best** response?
1. "Older age at conception is one of the major causes of the defect."
2. "It's a common complication of amniocentesis."
3. "It has been linked to maternal alcohol consumption during pregnancy."
4. "The cause is unknown and there are many environmental factors that may contribute to it."

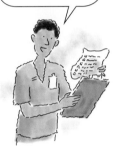

What's the priority intervention in question #43?

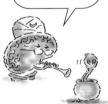

Brains and hard work are irresistible.

43. **3.** When there's an abnormality in current assessment data, it's vital to determine what the client's previous status was. Determine whether the status has changed or remained the same. Providing medication for the headache would be done after ascertaining the previous level of consciousness. Contacting the primary health care provider and the child's parents isn't necessary before a final assessment has been made.
CN: Physiological integrity; CNS: Physiological adaptation; CL: Apply; DIFFICULTY: Easy

44. **3.** By age 18 months, the child's anterior and posterior fontanels should be closed. The diamond-shaped anterior fontanel normally closes between ages 9 and 18 months. The triangular posterior fontanel normally closes between ages 2 and 3 months.
CN: Health promotion and maintenance; CNS: None; CL: Apply; DIFFICULTY: Moderate

45. **4.** A child with a concussion should be placed with a roommate who's free from infection and close to the child's age. Osteomyelitis, gastroenteritis, and rheumatic fever involve infection.
CN: Safe, effective care environment; CNS: Coordinated care; CL: Apply; DIFFICULTY: Easy

46. **4.** There is no one known cause of spina bifida, but scientists believe that it's linked to hereditary and environmental factors. Neural tube defects, including spina bifida, have been strongly linked to low dietary intake of folic acid. Maternal age doesn't impact spina bifida. An amniocentesis is performed to help diagnose spina bifida in utero but doesn't cause the disorder. Maternal alcohol intake during pregnancy has been linked to intellectual disability, craniofacial defects, and cardiac abnormalities but not spina bifida.
CN: Physiological integrity; CNS: Physiological adaptation; CL: Apply; DIFFICULTY: Easy

47. An 11-year-old child with a head injury has been in the hospital 2 weeks while receiving therapy. The child sometimes makes inappropriate statements, and occasionally has combative and violent outbursts. When questioned about this behavior, what is the **best** response by the nurse?

1. "Your child probably didn't receive enough discipline growing up and is throwing tantrums."
2. "Your child needs to be restrained during these episodes."
3. "This is a stage of healing for your child."
4. "Your child will need to be on life-long medication to control temper tantrums."

48. A child is being treated for an increase in intracranial pressure (ICP) and is now reporting severe headaches. When discussing this with the parents, the nurse should base the response based on which associated factor?

1. Cervical hyperextension
2. Stretching of the meninges
3. Cerebral ischemia related to altered circulation
4. Reflex spasm of the neck extensors to splint the neck against cervical flexion

49. The nurse at a family health clinic is educating a group of parents about normal infant development. Which patterns of communication should the nurse tell parents to expect from an infant at age 1?

1. Squeals and makes pleasure sound
2. Understands "no" and other simple commands
3. Uses speechlike rhythm when talking with an adult
4. Uses multisyllabic babbling

50. A nurse is assessing a 3-year-old child with nuchal rigidity. Which sign would be documented on the chart to support this condition?

1. Positive Kernig sign
2. Negative Brudzinski sign
3. Positive Homans sign
4. Negative Kernig sign

51. When assisting with the plan of care for a 9-year-old with Down syndrome, which statement should a nurse keep in mind?

1. Nursing interventions should be planned at a 9-year-old developmental level.
2. Nursing interventions should be planned at a 7-year-old developmental level.
3. The nurse should assess the child's developmental level before planning interventions.
4. The developmental level of the child is not important in planning care.

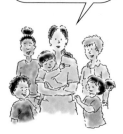

Nurses need to know how to communicate with kids of all ages.

47. 3. Clients with head injuries may pass through eight stages during their recovery. Stage 1, marked by unresponsiveness, is the worst stage. Stage 8, characterized by purposeful, appropriate behavior, is the final stage of healing. This child is somewhere between stage 4 (confused, agitated behavior) and stage 6 (confused, appropriate behavior) because sometimes the child can answer appropriately but at other times becomes confused and angry, resorting to violent behavior. Restraining the child is inappropriate and can increase intracranial pressure. The other responses are inappropriate.
CN: Health promotion and maintenance; CNS: None;
CL: Apply; DIFFICULTY: Easy

48. 2. The mechanism producing the headache that accompanies increased ICP may be the stretching of the meninges and pain fibers associated with blood vessels. Cerebral ischemia occurs because of vascular obstruction and decreased perfusion of the brain tissue. With nuchal rigidity, cervical flexion is painful due to the stretching of the inflamed meninges; the pain triggers a reflex spasm of the neck extensors to splint the area against further cervical flexion. It occurs in response to the pain; it doesn't cause it.
CN: Physiological integrity; CNS: Physiological adaptation;
CL: Apply; DIFFICULTY: Challenge

49. 2. At age 1, most babies understand the word "no" and other simple commands. Children at this age also learn one or two other words. Babies squeal, make pleasure sounds, and use multisyllabic babbling at age 3 to 6 months. Using speechlike rhythm when talking with an adult usually occurs between ages 6 to 9 months.
CN: Health promotion and maintenance; CNS: None;
CL: Remember; DIFFICULTY: Moderate

50. 1. A positive Kernig sign indicates nuchal rigidity, caused by an irritative lesion of the subarachnoid space. A positive Brudzinski sign also is indicative of the condition. A positive Homans sign may indicate venous inflammation of the lower leg. Negative signs mean that the condition is not present.
CN: Physiological integrity; CNS: Physiological adaptation;
CL: Apply; DIFFICULTY: Moderate

51. 3. Before developing a care plan, the nurse should assess the child's developmental level and plan care at that level. The nurse shouldn't plan care geared toward the child's chronologic age without first assessing the child. The nurse shouldn't assume that the child is at a lower developmental level without assessment. The child's developmental age is important in planning care.
CN: Health promotion and maintenance; CNS: None; CL: Apply;
DIFFICULTY: Easy

CN: Client needs category   CNS: Client needs subcategory   CL: Cognitive level

52. The nurse is collecting data from a child who may have a seizure disorder. Which behaviors indicate to the nurse that the child may be having an absence seizure?
  1. Sudden, momentary loss of muscle tone, with a brief loss of consciousness
  2. Muscle tone maintained and child frozen in position
  3. Brief, sudden contracture of a muscle or muscle group
  4. Minimal or no alteration in muscle tone, with a brief loss of consciousness

52. **4.** Absence seizures are characterized as generalized seizures and consist of a brief loss of responsiveness with minimal or no alteration in muscle tone. They may go unrecognized because the child's behavior changes very little. A sudden loss of muscle tone describes atonic seizures. A frozen position describes the appearance of someone having akinetic seizures. A brief, sudden contraction of muscles describes a myoclonic seizure.
CN: Physiological integrity; CNS: Physiological adaptation; CL: Remember; DIFFICULTY: Difficult

53. A child with a diagnosis of meningococcal meningitis develops sudden signs of sepsis and a purpuric rash over both lower extremities. The primary health care provider should be notified immediately because these signs could be indicative of which complication?
  1. A severe allergic reaction to the antibiotic regimen with impending anaphylaxis
  2. Onset of the syndrome of inappropriate antidiuretic hormone (SIADH)
  3. Fulminant meningococcemia (Waterhouse-Friderichsen syndrome)
  4. Adhesive arachnoiditis

53. **3.** Meningococcemia is a serious complication usually associated with meningococcal infection. When onset is severe, sudden, and rapid (fulminant), it's known as Waterhouse-Friderichsen syndrome. Anaphylactic shock would need to be differentiated from septic shock. SIADH can be an acute complication but wouldn't be accompanied by the purpuric rash. Adhesive arachnoiditis occurs in the chronic phase of the disease and leads to obstruction of the flow of cerebrospinal fluid.
CN: Physiological integrity; CNS: Reduction of risk potential; CL: Apply; DIFFICULTY: Challenge

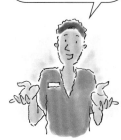

Which intervention in question #54 would be most effective in alleviating pain and fear?

54. To alleviate a child's pain and fear of lumbar puncture, which intervention should the nurse perform?
  1. Sedate the child with fentanyl.
  2. Apply a topical anesthetic to the skin 5 to 10 minutes before the puncture.
  3. Ask a parent to hold the child in her lap during the procedure.
  4. Tell the child to inhale small amounts of nitrous oxide gas before the puncture.

54. **1.** Sedation with fentanyl or other drugs can alleviate the pain and fear associated with a lumbar puncture. Fentanyl can be administered IV, IM, or patch. A topical anesthetic can be applied instead, but it should be done 30 minutes to 1 hour before the procedure to be fully effective. Asking a parent to hold a child in the lap increases the risk of neurologic injury due to the inability to assume and maintain the proper anatomical position required for a safe lumbar puncture. Use of nitrous oxide gas isn't recommended.
CN: Physiological integrity; CNS: Basic care and comfort; CL: Apply; DIFFICULTY: Difficult

55. The nurse should anticipate that antibiotic therapy to treat meningitis will be instituted immediately after which event?
  1. Admission to the nursing unit
  2. Initiation of IV therapy
  3. Identification of the causative organism
  4. Collection of cerebrospinal fluid (CSF) and blood for culture

55. **4.** Antibiotic therapy should always begin immediately after the collection of CSF and blood cultures. After the specific organism is identified, bacteria-specific antibiotics can be administered if the initial choice of antibiotic therapy isn't appropriate. It is not appropriate to begin antibiotic therapy upon admission to the unit or at the initiation of IV.
CN: Physiological integrity; CNS: Pharmacological therapies; CL: Apply; DIFFICULTY: Challenge

56. Which description of the complications of bacterial meningitis is **most** accurate?
1. Complications occur most often when the disease is contracted during the first 2 months of life.
2. Complications occur most often in children with meningococcal meningitis.
3. Complications primarily involve the fourth ventricle of the brain.
4. Complications most commonly involve the facial nerve, leading to facial paralysis.

57. A 1-month-old infant is admitted to the pediatric unit and diagnosed with bacterial meningitis. Which findings by the nurse support the diagnosis?
1. Hemorrhagic rash, first appearing as petechiae
2. Photophobia, diarrhea, increased appetite
3. Fever, change in feeding pattern, vomiting, or diarrhea
4. Fever, lethargy, and purpura or large necrotic patches

58. The nurse is caring for a child with meningitis. Which goal will the nurse recognize may be **most** difficult to achieve?
1. Protecting self and others from possible infection
2. Avoiding actions that increase discomfort, such as lifting the head
3. Keeping environmental stimuli to a minimum, such as reduced light and noise
4. Maintaining IV infusion to administer adequate antimicrobial therapy

59. The nurse is obtaining data from a 1-month-old infant during a routine examination at a family health center. Which method does the nurse use to test for Babinski sign?
1. Raise the child's leg with the knee flexed and then extend the child's leg at the knee to determine if resistance is noted.
2. With the knee flexed, dorsiflex the foot to determine if there's pain in the calf of the leg.
3. Flex the child's head while he's in a supine position to determine if the knees or hips flex involuntarily.
4. Stroke the bottom of the foot to determine if there's fanning and dorsiflexion of the big toe.

60. The clinical manifestations of acute bacterial meningitis are dependent on which factor?
1. Age of the child
2. Length of the prodromal period
3. Time span from bacterial invasion to onset of symptoms
4. Degree of elevation of cerebrospinal fluid (CSF) glucose compared to serum glucose level

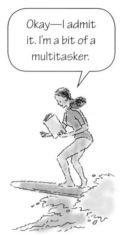

Okay—I admit it. I'm a bit of a multitasker.

56. 1. Infants younger than age 2 months with bacterial meningitis commonly have such complications as hearing loss, impaired vision, seizures, and cardiac and renal abnormalities. Complications are seen less commonly among children diagnosed with meningococcal meningitis. Complications aren't isolated to the fourth ventricle of the brain. The facial nerve isn't commonly affected.
CN: Physiological integrity; CNS: Physiological adaptation; CL: Understand; DIFFICULTY: Difficult

57. 3. Fever, change in feeding patterns, vomiting, and diarrhea are commonly observed in children with bacterial meningitis. Hemorrhagic rashes, petechiae, photophobia, fever, lethargy, and purpura are common manifestations in older children with meningitis.
CN: Physiological integrity; CNS: Physiological adaptation; CL: Apply; DIFFICULTY: Moderate

58. 4. One of the most difficult problems in the nursing care of children with meningitis is maintaining the IV infusion for the length of time needed to provide adequate therapy. All of the other options are important aspects in the provision of care for the child with meningitis, but they're secondary to antimicrobial therapy.
CN: Physiological integrity; CNS: Basic care and comfort; CL: Apply; DIFFICULTY: Difficult

59. 4. To test for Babinski sign, stroke the bottom of the foot to determine if there's fanning and dorsiflexion of the big toe. Raising the child's leg with the knee flexed and then extending the leg at the knee to determine resistance are noted tests for Kernig sign. Dorsiflexion of the foot with the knee flexed to determine if there's pain in the calf of the leg tests for Homans sign. Flexing the child's head while he's in a supine position to determine if the knees or hips flex involuntarily tests for Brudzinski sign.
CN: Physiological integrity; CNS: Physiological adaptation; CL: Remember; DIFFICULTY: Easy

60. 1. Clinical manifestations of acute bacterial meningitis depend largely on the age of the child. Clinical manifestations are neither dependent on the prodromal (initial) period of the disease nor the time from invasion of the host to the onset of symptoms. The glucose level of the CSF is reduced, not elevated, in bacterial meningitis.
CN: Physiological integrity; CNS: Physiological adaptation; CL: Understand; DIFFICULTY: Difficult

61. Parents of a child with a history of closed-head injury asks the nurse why their child would begin having seizures without warning. Which response by the nurse is the **most** accurate?
1. "Clonic seizure activity is usually interpreted as falling."
2. "It's not unusual to develop seizures after a head injury because of brain trauma."
3. "Focal discharge in the brain may lead to absence seizures that go unnoticed."
4. "The brain needs multiple stimuli before it manifests as a seizure."

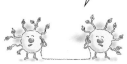

I'm feeling a little hyperexcitable today. How about you?

62. Which nursing data should be given the **highest priority** for a child with clinical findings related to tubercular meningitis?
1. Onset and character of fever
2. Degree and extent of nuchal rigidity
3. Signs of increased intracranial pressure (ICP)
4. Occurrence of urine and fecal contamination

63. Parent and client education should stress which rule in relation to the differences in bio-availability of different forms of phenytoin?
1. Use the cheapest formulation the pharmacy has on hand at the time of refill.
2. Shop around to get the least expensive formulation.
3. There's no difference between one formulation and another, regardless of price.
4. Avoid switching formulations without the primary health care provider's approval.

64. Which behavioral responses to pain would a nurse observe from an infant younger than age 1?
1. Localized withdrawal and resistance of the entire body
2. Passive resistance, clenching fists, and holding body rigid
3. Reflex withdrawal to stimulus and facial grimacing
4. Low frustration level and striking out physically

65. The parents of a child with a history of seizures who has been taking phenytoin ask the nurse why it's difficult to maintain therapeutic plasma levels of this medication. Which statement by the nurse would be **most** accurate?
1. "A drop in the plasma drug level will lead to a toxic state."
2. "The capacity to metabolize the drug becomes overwhelmed over time."
3. "Small increments in dosage lead to sharp increases in plasma drug levels."
4. "Large increments in dosage lead to a more rapid, stabilizing therapeutic effect."

61. 2. Stimuli from an earlier injury may eventually elicit seizure activity, a process known as kindling. Atonic seizures, not clonic seizures, are commonly accompanied by falling. Focal seizures are partial seizures; absence seizures are generalized seizures. Focal seizures don't lead to absence seizures. The epileptogenic focus consists of a group of hyperexcitable neurons responsible for initiating synchronous, high-frequency discharges that lead to a seizure and don't need multiple stimuli.
CN: Physiological integrity; CNS: Physiological adaptation; CL: Apply; DIFFICULTY: Easy

62. 3. Assessment of fever and evaluation of nuchal rigidity are important aspects of care, but assessment for signs of increasing ICP should be the highest priority due to the life-threatening implications. Urinary and fecal incontinence can occur in a child who's ill from nearly any cause but doesn't pose a great danger to life.
CN: Physiological integrity; CNS: Reduction of risk potential; CL: Apply; DIFFICULTY: Moderate

63. 4. Differences in bioavailability of phenytoin exist among different formulations (tablets and capsules) and among the same formulations produced by different manufacturers. Children shouldn't be switched from one formulation to another or from one brand to another without primary health care provider approval and supervision.
CN: Physiological integrity; CNS: Pharmacological therapies; CL: Apply; DIFFICULTY: Easy

64. 3. Infants younger than age 1 become irritable and exhibit reflex withdrawal to the painful stimulus. Facial grimacing also occurs. Localized withdrawal is experienced by toddlers ages 1 to 3 in response to pain. The nurse would observe passive resistance in school-age children. Preschoolers show a low frustration level and strike out physically.
CN: Physiological integrity; CNS: Physiological adaptation; CL: Understand; DIFFICULTY: Moderate

65. 3. Within the therapeutic range for phenytoin, small increments in dosage produce sharp increases in plasma drug levels. The capacity of the liver to metabolize phenytoin is affected by slight changes in the dosage of the drug, not necessarily the length of time the client has been taking the drug. Large increments in dosage will greatly increase plasma levels, leading to drug toxicity.
CN: Physiological integrity; CNS: Pharmacological therapies; CL: Apply; DIFFICULTY: Moderate

CN: Client needs category   CNS: Client needs subcategory   CL: Cognitive level

66. During the trial period to determine the efficacy of an anticonvulsant drug, which caution should be explained to the parents?
   1. Plasma levels of the drug will be monitored on a daily basis.
   2. Drug dosage will be adjusted depending on the frequency of seizure activity.
   3. The drug must be discontinued immediately if even the slightest problem occurs.
   4. The child shouldn't participate in activities that could be hazardous if a seizure occurs.

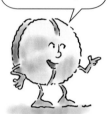

A trial period will help make sure I am working.

66. 4. Until seizure control is certain, children who experience convulsions shouldn't participate in activities (such as riding a bicycle) that could be hazardous if a seizure were to occur. Plasma levels need to be monitored periodically over the course of drug therapy; daily monitoring isn't necessary. Dosage changes are usually based on plasma drug levels as well as seizure control. Anticonvulsant drugs should be withdrawn over a period of 6 weeks to several months, never immediately, as doing so could precipitate status epilepticus.
CN: Physiological integrity; CNS: Pharmacological therapies; CL: Apply; DIFFICULTY: Moderate

67. To detect complications as early as possible in a child with meningitis who's receiving IV fluids, monitoring for which condition should be the nurse's **priority**?
   1. Cerebral edema
   2. Renal failure
   3. Left-sided heart failure
   4. Cardiogenic shock

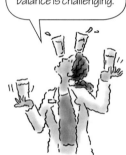

Man ... maintaining fluid balance is challenging.

67. 1. The child with meningitis is already at increased risk for cerebral edema and increased intracranial pressure due to inflammation of the meningeal membranes; therefore, the nurse should carefully monitor fluid intake and output to avoid fluid volume overload. Renal failure and cardiogenic shock aren't complications of IV therapy. The child with a healthy heart wouldn't be expected to develop left-sided heart failure.
CN: Physiological integrity; CNS: Pharmacological therapies; CL: Apply; DIFFICULTY: Easy

68. Which instruction should be included in parent and client education specifically related to anticonvulsant drug efficacy?
   1. The child should wear a medical identification bracelet.
   2. Maintain a seizure frequency chart.
   3. Avoid potentially hazardous activities.
   4. Discontinue the drug immediately if adverse effects are suspected.

68. 2. Ongoing evaluation of therapeutic effects can be accomplished by maintaining a frequency chart that indicates the date, time, and nature of the child's seizure activity. These data may be helpful in making dosage alterations and specific drug selection. Wearing a medical identification bracelet and avoiding hazardous activities are ways to minimize danger related to seizure activity, but these factors don't affect drug efficacy. Anticonvulsant drugs should never be discontinued abruptly due to the potential for development of status epilepticus.
CN: Physiological integrity; CNS: Pharmacological therapies; CL: Apply; DIFFICULTY: Difficult

69. A 13-year-old with structural scoliosis has Cotrel-Dubousset rods inserted. Which position would be **best** during the postoperative period?
   1. Supine in bed
   2. Side-lying
   3. Semi-Fowler's
   4. High Fowler's

What position would you want to be in after having rods put in your back?

69. 1. After placement of Cotrel-Dubousset rods, the child must remain flat in bed. The gatch on a manual bed should be taped, and electric beds should be unplugged to prevent the child from raising the head or foot of the bed. Other positions, such as the side-lying, semi-Fowler's, and high Fowler's positions, could prove damaging because the rods won't be able to maintain the spine in a straight position.
CN: Physiological integrity; CNS: Reduction of risk potential; CL: Apply; DIFFICULTY: Moderate

70. The parents of a child newly diagnosed with seizures ask the nurse at what time seizure activity is most likely to occur. Which response by the nurse would be **most** accurate?
1. "During the rapid eye movement (REM) stage of sleep."
2. "During long periods of excitement."
3. "While falling asleep and on awakening."
4. "While eating, particularly if the child is hurried."

71. When educating the family of a child with seizures, it's appropriate to tell them to call emergency medical services in the event of a seizure if which complication occurs?
1. Continuous vomiting for 30 minutes after the seizure
2. Stereotypic or automatous body movements during onset
3. Lack of expression, pallor, or flushing of the face during the seizure
4. Unilateral or bilateral posturing of one or more extremities during onset

72. Identifying factors that trigger seizure activity could lead to which alteration in the child's environment or activities of daily living?
1. Avoid striped wallpaper and ceiling fans.
2. Let the child sleep alone to prevent sleep interruption.
3. Include extended periods of intense physical activity daily.
4. Allow the child to drink soda only between noon and 5 p.m.

73. Which nursing intervention would be included to support the goal of avoiding injury, respiratory distress, or aspiration during a seizure?
1. Position the child with the head hyperextended.
2. Place a hand under the child's head for support.
3. Use pillows to prop the child into the sitting position.
4. Work a padded tongue blade or small plastic airway between the teeth.

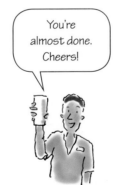

You're almost done. Cheers!

74. Which diagnostic measure is **most** accurate in detecting neural tube defects?
1. Flat plate of the lower abdomen after the 23rd week of gestation
2. Significant level of alpha-fetoprotein present in amniotic fluid
3. Amniocentesis for lecithin-sphingomyelin (L/S) ratio
4. Presence of high maternal levels of albumin after 12th week of gestation

70. 3. Falling asleep or awakening from sleep are periods of functional instability of the brain; seizure activity is more likely to occur during these times. Eating quickly, excitement without undo fatigue, and REM sleep haven't been identified as contributing factors.
CN: Physiological integrity; CNS: Physiological adaptation;
CL: Apply; DIFFICULTY: Challenge

71. 1. Continuous vomiting after a seizure has ended can be a sign of an acute problem and indicates that the child requires an immediate medical evaluation. All of the other body responses to seizure are normally present in various types of seizure activity and don't require immediate medical evaluation.
CN: Physiological integrity; CNS: Reduction of risk potential;
CL: Apply; DIFFICULTY: Easy

72. 1. Striped wallpaper and ceiling fans can be triggers to seizure activity if the child is photosensitive. Sleep interruption hasn't been identified as a triggering factor. Avoidance of fatigue can reduce seizure activity; therefore, intense physical activity for extended periods of time should be avoided. Restricting caffeine intake by using caffeine-free soda is a dietary modification that may prevent seizures.
CN: Physiological integrity; CNS: Physiological adaptation;
CL: Apply; DIFFICULTY: Moderate

73. 2. Placing a hand or a small cushion or blanket under the child's head will help prevent injury. Position the child with the head in midline, not hyperextended, to promote a good airway and adequate ventilation. Don't attempt to prop the child up into a sitting position but ease to the floor to prevent falling and possible injury. Don't put anything in the child's mouth because it could cause infection or obstruct the airway.
CN: Physiological integrity; CNS: Reduction of risk potential;
CL: Apply; DIFFICULTY: Moderate

74. 2. Screening for significant levels of alpha-fetoprotein is 90% effective in detecting neural tube defects. Prenatal screening includes a combination of maternal serum and amniotic fluid levels, amniocentesis, amniography, and ultrasonography and has been relatively successful in diagnosing the defect. Flat plate x-rays of the abdomen, L/S ratio, and maternal serum albumin levels aren't diagnostic for neural tube defect.
CN: Health promotion and maintenance; CNS: None;
CL: Understand; DIFFICULTY: Moderate

CN: Client needs category   CNS: Client needs subcategory   CL: Cognitive level

75. A nurse is reinforcing education for the parents of a child who has been diagnosed with spina bifida. Which statement by the parents would indicate an understanding of spina bifida?
1. "It has little influence on the intellectual and perceptual abilities of the child."
2. "It's a simple neurologic defect that's completely corrected surgically within 1 to 2 days after birth."
3. "Its presence indicates that many areas of the central nervous system (CNS) may not develop or function adequately."
4. "It's a complex neurologic disability that involves a collaborative health team effort for the entire first year of life."

75. 3. When a spinal cord lesion exists at birth, it commonly leads to altered development or function of other areas of the CNS. Spina bifida is a complex neurologic defect that heavily impacts the physical, cognitive, and psychosocial development of the child and involves collaborative, lifelong management due to the chronicity and multiplicity of the problems involved.
CN: Physiological integrity; CNS: Physiological adaptation; CL: Apply; DIFFICULTY: Moderate

76. The nurse is caring for a child with spina bifida. Which complication should the nurse observe for related to the muscle activity or inactivity of the lower extremities?
1. Clubfoot
2. Hip extension
3. Ankylosis of the knee
4. Abduction and external rotation of the hip

76. 1. The type and extent of deformity in the lower extremities of a child with spina bifida depends on the muscles that are active or inactive. Passive positioning in utero may result in deformities of the feet, such as equinovarus (clubfoot), knee flexion and extension contractures, and hip flexion with adduction and internal rotation leading to subluxation or dislocation of the hip.
CN: Physiological integrity; CNS: Physiological adaptation; CL: Apply; DIFFICULTY: Challenge

77. A nurse notes that a 4-year-old child with cerebral palsy has a weight at the 30th percentile and a height at the 60th percentile. Which teaching information is appropriate for this child and parents?
1. The child should eat fewer calories.
2. The child's weight and height are within the normal range.
3. The child needs to increase his daily caloric intake.
4. The child is small for his age and will remain so through adolescence.

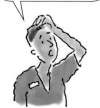

What's the normal percentile range for weight and height?

77. 2. The weight and height are between the 25th and 75th percentiles, so the child is considered within normal range.
CN: Health promotion and maintenance; CNS: None; CL: Apply; DIFFICULTY: Challenge

78. Infants with myelomeningocele must be closely observed for manifestations of Chiari II malformation. Which finding would indicate this manifestation?
1. Rapidly progressing scoliosis
2. Changes in urologic functioning
3. Back pain below the site of the sac closure
4. Respiratory stridor, apneic periods, and difficulty swallowing

78. 4. Children with a myelomeningocele have a 90% chance of having a Chiari II malformation. This may lead to respiratory function problems, such as respiratory stridor associated with paralysis of the vocal cords, apneic episodes of unknown cause, difficulty swallowing, and an abnormal gag reflex. Scoliosis and urologic function changes occur with myelomeningocele, but these complications aren't specifically related to Chiari II malformation. Lower back pain doesn't occur because the infant has a loss of sensory function below the level of the cord defect.
CN: Physiological integrity; CNS: Reduction of risk potential; CL: Apply; DIFFICULTY: Moderate

79. The nurse is preparing to administer antibiotic eardrops to a 2-year-old child with an infection of the external auditory canal. The order reads, "2 gtts right ear t.i.d." Which steps should the nurse take to administer this medication? Select all that apply.
1. Wash hands and arrange supplies at the bedside.
2. Warm the medication to body temperature.
3. Lay the child on the right side with the left ear facing up.
4. Examine the client's ear canal for drainage.
5. Gently pull the pinna up and back and instill the drops into the external ear canal.

80. The nurse is caring for a 1-month-old infant who fell from the changing table during a diaper change. Which signs and symptoms of increased intracranial pressure (ICP) is the nurse likely to assess in this child? Select all that apply.
1. Bulging fontanels
2. Decreased blood pressure
3. Increased pulse
4. High-pitched cry
5. Headache
6. Irritability

81. An 11-month-old is diagnosed with an ear infection. Because it's his second ear infection, the mother asks why children experience more ear infections than adults. The nurse shows the mother a diagram of the ear and explains the differences in anatomy. Identify the portion of the infant's ear that allows fluid to stagnate and act as a medium for bacteria.

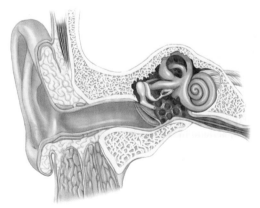

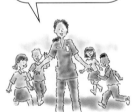

Good job! You're done. Now go out and play.

79. 1, 2, 4. The nurse should prepare to instill the eardrops by washing hands, gathering the supplies, and arranging the supplies at the bedside. To avoid adverse effects resulting from eardrops that are too cold (such as vertigo, nausea, and pain), the medication should be warmed to body temperature in a bowl of warm water. The temperature of the drops should be tested by placing a drop on the wrist. Before instilling the drops, the ear canal should be examined for drainage that may reduce the medication's effectiveness. The child should be placed on the left side with the right ear facing up. For an infant or a child younger than age 3, gently pull the auricle down and back because the ear canal is straighter in children of this age group.
CN: Physiological integrity; CNS: Pharmacological therapies; CL: Apply; DIFFICULTY: Challenge

80. 1, 4, 6. Signs and symptoms of increased ICP in a 1-month-old infant include full, tense, bulging fontanels; a high-pitched cry; and irritability. With increased ICP, blood pressure rises while heart rate (pulse) falls. The infant may have a headache, but the nurse can't assess this finding in an infant.
CN: Physiological integrity; CNS: Physiological adaptation; CL: Analyze; DIFFICULTY: Challenge

81.
The eustachian tube in an infant is shorter and wider than in an adult or older child. It also slants horizontally. Because of these anatomical features, nasopharyngeal secretions can enter the middle ear more easily, stagnate, and cause infections.

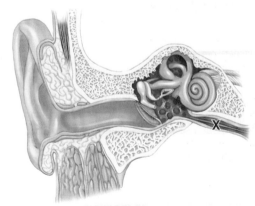

CN: Health promotion and maintenance; CNS: None; CL: Understand; DIFFICULTY: Moderate

Chapter 30

Musculoskeletal Disorders

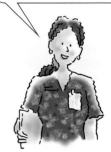

Challenge yourself with these questions on musculoskeletal system disorders in children. I'm betting you'll have a blast!

Pediatric musculoskeletal refresher

Clubfoot

Abnormality of the foot, which is usually congenital, in which the tendons are shorter than normal

Key signs and symptoms
- Can't be corrected manually (distinguishes true clubfoot from apparent clubfoot)

Key test results
- X-rays show superimposition of the talus and calcaneus and a ladderlike appearance of the metatarsals

Key treatments
- Correcting deformity with a series of casts or surgical correction
- Maintaining correction until foot gains normal muscle balance
- Observing foot closely for several years to prevent foot deformity from recurring

Key interventions
- Ensure that shoes fit correctly
- Prepare for surgery, if necessary

Developmental hip dysplasia

Dislocation or instability of the hip at birth, which may result in hip dysplasia

Key signs and symptoms
- Affected side exhibits an increased number of folds on posterior thigh when child is supine with knees bent
- Appearance of shortened limb on affected side when child is supine
- Restricted abduction of hips

Key test results
- Barlow sign: A click is felt when the infant is placed supine with hips flexed 90 degrees and when the knees are fully flexed and the hip is brought into midabduction
- Ortolani click: Can be felt by the fingers at the hip area as the femur head snaps out of and back into the acetabulum; it's also palpable during examination with the child's legs flexed and abducted.

- Positive Trendelenburg test: When child stands on the affected leg, the opposite pelvis dips to maintain erect posture.

Key treatments
- Hip spica cast or corrective surgery for older children
- Bryant traction
- Casting or a Pavlik harness to keep the hips and knees flexed and the hips abducted for at least 3 months

Key interventions
- Give reassurance that early, prompt treatment will probably result in complete correction
- Assure parents that the child will adjust to restricted movement and return to normal sleeping, eating, and playing in a few days

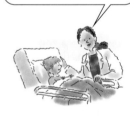

Be sure to use appropriate precautions when moving a client who is being treated for a musculoskeletal injury or disorder.

Duchenne muscular dystrophy

Incurable inherited disorder that involves muscle weakness and wasting, which progresses rapidly

Key signs and symptoms
- Eventual muscle weakness and wasting
- Gowers sign (use of hands to push self up from floor)
- Pelvic girdle weakness, indicated by waddling gait and falling

Key test results
- Electromyography typically demonstrates short, weak bursts of electrical activity in affected muscles
- Muscle biopsy shows variation in the size of muscle fibers and, in later stages, shows fat and connective tissue deposits, with no dystrophin

Key treatments
- Physical therapy
- Surgery to correct contractures
- Use of such devices as splints, braces, trapeze bars, overhead slings, and a wheelchair to help preserve mobility

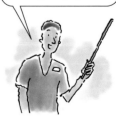

What key signs and symptoms would you expect to see in Duchenne muscular dystrophy?

Key interventions

- Perform range-of-motion exercises
- If respiratory involvement occurs, encourage:
  - coughing
  - deep-breathing exercises
  - diaphragmatic breathing
- Encourage adequate fluid intake
- Increase dietary fiber
- Obtain an order for a stool softener

Fractures

Complete or incomplete break of a bone

Key signs and symptoms

- Loss of motor function
- Muscle spasm
- Pain or tenderness
- Skeletal deformity
- Swelling

Key test results

- X-rays may be used to confirm location and extent of fracture

Key treatments

- Casting
- Reduction and immobilization of the fracture
- Surgery: open reduction and external fixation of the fracture

Key interventions

- Keep child in proper body alignment
- Provide support above and below fracture site when moving the child
- Elevate the fracture above the level of the heart
- Apply ice to the fracture to promote vasoconstriction
- Monitor pulses distal to the fracture every 2 to 4 hours
- Monitor color, temperature, and capillary refill

Juvenile rheumatoid arthritis

Most common form of arthritis in children; long-term (chronic) disease resulting in joint pain and swelling which may or may not resolve in adulthood

Key signs and symptoms

- Inflammation around joints
- Stiffness, pain, and guarding of affected joints

Key test results

- Hematology studies reveal:
  - elevated erythrocyte sedimentation rate
  - positive antinuclear antibody test
  - presence of rheumatoid factor

Key treatments

- Heat therapy: warm compresses, baths
- Splint application

Key interventions

- Monitor joints for deformity

Scoliosis

Abnormal lateral curvature of the spine

Key signs and symptoms

- Disappearance of the curve in the spinal column
- Nonstructural scoliosis
- When child bends at the waist to touch the toes, the curve in the spinal column disappears

Structural scoliosis

- Failure of the spinal curve to straighten; asymmetry of the hips, ribs, shoulders, and shoulder blades when the child bends forward with the knees straight and the arms hanging down toward the feet

Key test results

- X-rays may aid diagnosis

Key treatments

- Nonstructural scoliosis: postural exercises, shoe lifts
- Structural scoliosis: steel rods, prolonged bracing, spinal fusion

Key interventions

- After spinal fusion and insertion of rods:
  - turn the child by logrolling only
  - maintain the child in correct body alignment
  - maintain the bed in a flat position

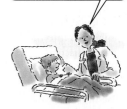

Your client with juvenile rheumatoid arthritis reports joint pain and swelling. What's a good treatment?

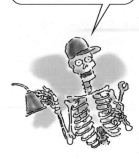

What are some devices in the care provider's "toolbox" that might be used to treat musculoskeletal disorders?

Musculoskeletal questions, answers, and rationales

1. The parents of a neonate diagnosed with clubfoot ask the nurse to explain *talipes varus*. The nurse would describe this as which condition?
1. Inversion of the foot
2. Eversion of the foot
3. Plantar flexion
4. Dorsiflexion

2. Which observation by a nurse indicates that an 18-month-old in Bryant traction is properly positioned?
1. The hips are resting on the bed.
2. The hips are slightly elevated off the bed.
3. The hips are elevated above the level of the heart.
4. The hips are resting on a pillow.

3. The parent of a child who is scheduled to start corticosteroid therapy for a diagnosis of juvenile rheumatoid arthritis asks the how the child will need to take the medication. What is the **best** response by the nurse? Select all that apply.
1. Oral
2. Subcutaneously
3. Injection into the joint
4. Intermuscular
5. Topical

4. The nurse is reinforcing education for the parent of a neonate with clubfoot. Which information should the nurse include?
1. It's hereditary.
2. More girls than boys are affected.
3. More boys than girls are affected.
4. It occurs once in every 500 births.

5. A nurse is assisting with the education of the parents of a 3-month-old infant who has severe torticollis, with the head rotated to the left and side bent to the right. Which statement by the parents indicates that the education has been effective?
1. "It involves shortening of the left upper trapezius."
2. "It involves shortening of the right middle trapezius."
3. "It involves shortening of the left sternocleidomastoid."
4. "It involves shortening of the right sternocleidomastoid."

6. A 9-month-old infant has torticollis with rotation of the head to the left and side bending to the right. Placing the infant in which position would be **most** effective for developing muscle lengthening?
1. Prone
2. Supine
3. Left side-lying
4. Right side-lying

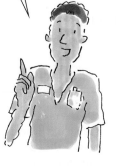

Remember— more than one answer may be right in question #3.

1. 1. Talipes varus is an inversion of the foot. Talipes valgus is an eversion of the foot. Talipes equinus is plantar flexion of the foot and talipes calcaneus is dorsiflexion of the foot.
CN: Physiological integrity; CNS: Physiological adaptation;
CL: Apply; DIFFICULTY: Moderate

2. 2. In Bryant traction, the child's hips should be slightly elevated off the bed at a 15-degree angle. They shouldn't be resting on the bed or on a pillow and shouldn't be elevated above the level of the heart.
CN: Physiological integrity; CNS: Basic care and comfort;
CL: Apply; DIFFICULTY: Moderate

3. 1, 3. This medication has the possibility to be given orally or by injection directly into the joint to control symptoms of juvenile rheumatoid arthritis.
CN: Physiological integrity; CNS: Pharmacological therapies;
CL: Apply; DIFFICULTY: Difficult

4. 3. Boys are affected twice as often as girls. It isn't known if the condition is hereditary. It occurs once in every 1,000 births.
CN: Physiological integrity; CNS: Physiological adaptation;
CL: Apply; DIFFICULTY: Difficult

5. 4. The right sternocleidomastoid is shortened when the head rotates left. The left upper trapezius isn't shortened. The middle trapezius isn't affected, and the left sternocleidomastoid is lengthened.
CN: Physiological integrity; CNS: Physiological adaptation; CL: Apply; DIFFICULTY: Difficult

6. 3. The left side lying position will assist with lengthening of the muscles because this position makes it easier to stretch the sternocleidomastoid and upper trapezius. No other positions will assist in increasing muscle length.
CN: Physiological integrity; CNS: Reduction of risk potential;
CL: Apply; DIFFICULTY: Difficult

CN: Client needs category   CNS: Client needs subcategory   CL: Cognitive level

7. A nurse is preparing to give an IM injection into the left leg of a 2-year-old client. Place an "X" on the area where the nurse will administer this injection.

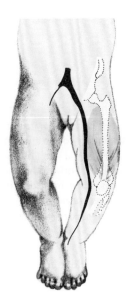

7. The nurse should administer this IM injection in the vastus lateralis, located in the child's thigh. To give the injection, the nurse should first divide the distance between the greater trochanter and the knee joints into quadrants and then inject in the center of the upper quadrant.

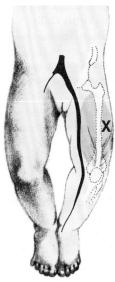

CN: Physiological integrity; CNS: Pharmacological therapies; CL: **Apply**; DIFFICULTY: Moderate

8. The parents of a child newly diagnosed with scoliosis ask the nurse to describe this condition. Which response provides an accurate definition?
1. An increase in the lumbar lordosis
2. A decrease in the thoracic kyphosis
3. Lateral curves in the spinal column described as right or left concavities
4. Lateral curves in the spinal column described as right or left convexities

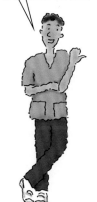

Which data would indicate neurovascular compromise due to the cast?

8. 4. Scoliosis is defined as "S" curves along the longitudinal axis of the body. Curves are defined by their convexity, not their concavity. Lordosis and kyphosis describe a person's back in the frontal plane.
CN: Physiological integrity; CNS: Physiological adaptation; CL: Understand; DIFFICULTY: Challenge

9. A nurse is caring for a child who received a hip spica cast 24 hours ago for hip dysplasia. Which data obtained by the nurse should be immediately reported to the charge nurse?
1. SpO$_2$ of 97%
2. Absent pedal pulses
3. Capillary refill is less than 3 seconds
4. Urinary output of 35 mL/hr

9. 2. Neurovascular compromise is an assessment that would need to be reported immediately due to swelling within the confined space of the cast. All the other assessment data is within normal limits.
CN: Safe, effective care environment; CNS: Coordinated care; CL: Analyze; DIFFICULTY: Easy

10. The Milwaukee brace is commonly used in the treatment of scoliosis. Which position **best** describes the placement of the pressure rods?
1. Laterally on the convex portion of the curve
2. Laterally on the concave portion of the curve
3. Posteriorly on the convex portion of the curve
4. Posteriorly along the spinal column at the exact level of the curve

10. 1. Lateral pressure applied to the convex portion of the curve helps best to reduce the curvature. Pressure pads applied posteriorly help maintain erect posture. Pressure applied to the concave portion of the curve will increase the lordosis.
CN: Physiological integrity; CNS: Reduction of risk potential; CL: Understand; DIFFICULTY: Difficult

CN: Client needs category CNS: Client needs subcategory CL: Cognitive level

11. A child with juvenile rheumatoid arthritis comes to the outpatient infusion clinic to receive his first infusion of etanercept. The parents want to know about **serious** potential adverse side effects of the medication. What is the **best** response by the nurse? Select all that apply.
1. The child may develop an infection.
2. The child may experience chills.
3. There is a potential to develop malignant tumors.
4. The child may have a sore throat.
5. The child may experience nausea.

12. When gathering data from a child, which observation would alert the nurse that the child may be developing scoliosis?
1. Scapula winging
2. Forward head posture
3. Raised right iliac crest
4. Forward flexion of the cervical spine

13. The nurse is reinforcing education for strengthening the muscles of a child diagnosed with clubfoot (talipes equinovarus) to the parents. The nurse knows education has been effective when the parents state that which muscle group is important for their child to strengthen?
1. Evertors
2. Invertors
3. Plantar flexors
4. Plantar fascia musculature

14. A nurse is caring for a 15-year-old who sustained a fracture of the femur 24 hours ago. Which finding should alert the nurse to an early complication?
1. Pain
2. Local swelling
3. Loss of function
4. Dyspnea

15. Which statement made by an adolescent with scoliosis indicates that the instruction received is understood?
1. "I will have to wear a brace for several years."
2. "I can put on the brace after I get home from school."
3. "I should avoid any exercise that will stretch my spine."
4. "I can remove the brace at night."

16. Which observation by a nurse indicates proper fit of crutches in a client?
1. The crutches fit snugly under the axilla.
2. The crutches end 2 in (5 cm) below the axilla.
3. The elbow is flexed 60 degrees.
4. The elbow is flexed 90 degrees.

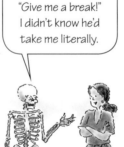

So I said to him, "Give me a break!" I didn't know he'd take me literally.

11. 1, 3. Clients who are treated with etanercept are at an increased risk of serious infection and also are at a greater risk of malignancies, specifically lymphoma. Chills, nausea and sore throat are common side effects of etanercept.
CN: Physiological integrity; CNS: Pharmacological therapies; CL: Apply; DIFFICULTY: Difficult

12. 3. A raised iliac crest may be a warning sign of some curvature secondary to the attachment of the pelvis to the spine. Scapula winging could be caused by muscle paralysis. Forward head posture isn't a result of scoliosis. Forward flexion isn't indicative of lateral curves in the spine.
CN: Physiological integrity; CNS: Physiological adaptation; CL: Analyze; DIFFICULTY: Moderate

13. 1. Because the foot is held in inversion, it's important to strengthen the evertors to counter the inversion present in the foot. Invertor is incorrect because the child's foot is already held in the inversion position. Plantar musculature and plantar flexors aren't correct because the foot is already in a plantar flexed position.
CN: Physiological integrity; CNS: Reduction of risk potential; CL: Analyze; DIFFICULTY: Challenge

14. 4. After the fracture of a long bone such as the femur, the client is at risk for fat embolism. Clinical manifestations included dyspnea, hypoxia, tachypnea, tachycardia, and chest pain. Pain, local swelling, and loss of function are all typical findings after a fracture.
CN: Physiological integrity; CNS: Reduction of risk potential; CL: Analyze; DIFFICULTY: Moderate

15. 1. A brace worn to correct scoliosis must be worn for several years to correct the spinal deformity. The child must wear the brace all day, even during school and sleep. Exercises are commonly prescribed to be performed several times per day to stretch and strengthen back muscles. The brace should only be removed for 1 hour each day while bathing.
CN: Physiological integrity; CNS: Basic care and comfort; CL: Analyze; DIFFICULTY: Moderate

16. 2. The crutches should end 2 in (5 cm) below the axilla, and the elbow should be flexed 20 to 30 degrees.
CN: Physiological integrity; CNS: Basic care and comfort; CL: Apply; DIFFICULTY: Moderate

CN: Client needs category   CNS: Client needs subcategory   CL: Cognitive level

17. A child has just returned to the room with a cast on the leg after open reduction of a fractured femur. What's the **most** appropriate action for a nurse to take when a 6 cm by 10 cm area of blood is noted on the cast?
1. Tape gauze pads over the bloody area.
2. Mark the bloody drainage and monitor hourly.
3. Assess vital signs.
4. Call the health care provider.

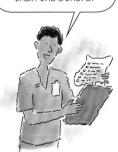

One of these actions is more vital than the others.

17. 3. The most appropriate action for the nurse is to assess the child's vital signs for evidence of hemorrhage, such as tachycardia and hypotension. After the assessments, the health care provider should be notified with the findings. Gauze pads may be placed over the bloody drainage after the child has been assessed and the health care provider notified. The size of the bloody drainage should be monitored after the assessment and health care provider notification.
CN: Physiological integrity; CNS: Reduction of risk potential; CL: Apply; DIFFICULTY: Difficult

18. Which nursing intervention may assist a 3-month-old client diagnosed with torticollis with elongation of the muscle?
1. Have the child lie supine
2. Gentle massage
3. Range-of-motion exercises
4. Have the child lie on the side

18. 4. Side-lying opposite the affected side may help elongate shortened muscles. Lying supine and gentle massage won't assist with elongation of muscles. Range-of-motion exercises won't assist with shortened muscles unless they're performed in specific patterns and with stretching.
CN: Health promotion and maintenance; CNS: None; CL: Apply; DIFFICULTY: Difficult

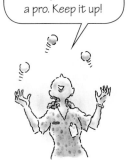

You're juggling these questions like a pro. Keep it up!

19. A physical therapist has instructed the nursing staff in range-of-motion exercises for an infant with torticollis. Which intervention should the nurses perform if they feel uncomfortable performing stretches that result in the infant's crying and grimacing?
1. Check the primary health care provider's orders.
2. Call the primary health care provider.
3. Call the physical therapist.
4. Discontinue the exercises.

19. 3. The only cure for the torticollis is exercise or surgery. The physical therapist is the expert in exercise and should be called for assistance in this situation. The primary health care provider would be called only if there was concern over the orders written or an abnormal development in the child.
CN: Physiological integrity; CNS: Physiological adaptation; CL: Apply; DIFFICULTY: Moderate

20. A nurse is caring for a child with severe scoliosis. Which complication should the nurse closely monitor for?
1. Increased vital capacity
2. Increased oxygen uptake
3. Diminished vital capacity
4. Decreased residual volume

20. 3. Scoliosis of greater than 60 degrees can shift organs and decrease ability of the ribs to expand, thus decreasing vital capacity. An increase in vital capacity or oxygen uptake wouldn't occur secondary to a decrease in chest expansion. Residual volume would increase secondary to decreased ability of the lungs to expel air.
CN: Physiological integrity; CNS: Physiological adaptation; CL: Apply; DIFFICULTY: Moderate

21. A client has developed a right torticollis with side bending to the right and rotation to the left. Which exercises may assist in reduction of the torticollis?
1. Rotation exercises to the right
2. Rotation exercises to the left
3. Cervical extension exercises
4. Cervical flexion exercises

21. 1. Performing rotation exercises to the right will help increase the length of the shortened right sternocleidomastoid. Rotation to the left will exacerbate the torticollis, as the head is already rotated in that direction. Cervical extension exercises won't lengthen tightened muscles. Cervical flexion will shorten the muscles further.
CN: Physiological integrity; CNS: Reduction of risk potential; CL: Apply; DIFFICULTY: Difficult

22. A 4-year-old child is diagnosed with thoracic scoliosis secondary to cerebral palsy. Which condition should the nurse monitor for that may be a contributing factor to scoliosis?
1. Hypotonia
2. Intellectual disability
3. Increased thoracic kyphosis
4. Autonomic dysreflexia

23. A child with muscular dystrophy is admitted to the hospital with reports of chest pain. The EKG showed cardiac muscle damage. Which cardiac medications does the nurse anticipate administering? Select all that apply.
1. Benazepril
2. Enalapril
3. Metoprolol
4. Amlodipine
5. Nifedipine

24. During a scoliosis screening, a school nurse examines a child and notes there is a raised right iliac crest. The nurse should notify the child's parents and suggest further screening for which condition?
1. Forward head posture
2. Leg length discrepancy
3. Increased lumbar lordosis
4. Increased thoracic kyphosis

25. A school nurse is performing a scoliosis screening on a group of students. Which student would **most** commonly develop this condition?
1. A 7-year-old girl
2. A 7-year-old boy
3. A 13-year-old girl
4. A 13-year-old boy

26. The nurse is caring for a child with a Harrington rod placement. Which data gathered by the nurse would be of **greatest** concern 2 days postoperatively?
1. Fever of 99.5° F (37.5° C)
2. Reports of pain along the incision
3. Urine output less than 30 mL/hr
4. Hypoactive bowel sounds

27. When gathering data from a child suspected of having scoliosis, what structures will the nurse focus on during the screening process? Select all that apply.
1. Thoracic spine
2. Lumbar spine
3. Acromion processes
4. Posterior superior iliac spines
5. Cervical spine

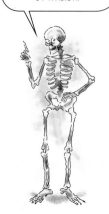

Sometimes poor muscle tone can throw your whole skeleton out of whack.

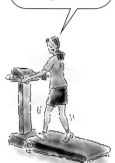

Nursing is an endurance sport. Pace yourself!

22. 1. Cerebral palsy is usually associated with some degree of hypotonia or hypertonia. Poor muscle tone may result in scoliosis. Intellectual disability isn't a cause of scoliosis. Increased thoracic kyphosis won't result in scoliosis. Autonomic dysreflexia occurs in spinal cord injury and involves abnormal muscle spasms secondary to abnormal inhibitory neurons present during stretch reflexes.
CN: Physiological integrity; CNS: Physiological adaptation; CL: Apply; DIFFICULTY: Challenge

23. 1, 2, 3. When cardiac muscle damage in relation the muscular dystrophy has occurred the health care provider would likely order ACE inhibitors (benazepril, enalapril) or beta blockers (metoprolol). Calcium channel blockers (amlodipine, nifedipine) would not be ordered as first line treatment for cardiac muscle damage.
CN: Physiological integrity; CNS: Pharmacological therapies; CL: Analyze; DIFFICULTY: Difficult

24. 2. A raised iliac crest may be indicative of a leg length discrepancy or a curvature in the lumbar spine. It isn't indicative of forward head posture, lumbar lordosis, or thoracic kyphosis.
CN: Health promotion and maintenance; CNS: None; CL: Apply; DIFFICULTY: Moderate

25. 3. Scoliosis is eight times more prevalent in adolescent girls than boys. Peak incidence is between ages 8 and 15. Therefore, a 13-year-old girl is at the highest risk. Seven-year-old boys and girls are at lower risk.
CN: Physiological integrity; CNS: Physiological adaptation; CL: Analyze; DIFFICULTY: Moderate

26. 3. Due to extensive blood loss during surgery and possible renal hypoperfusion, decreased urine output could indicate decreased renal function and this symptom is of greatest concern. A fever of 99.5° F is of concern but may be due to decreased chest expansion secondary to anesthesia, surgery, and pain. A paralytic ileus is common after Harrington rod placement surgery, and the child may have a nasogastric tube for the first 48 hours.
CN: Physiological integrity; CNS: Reduction of risk potential; CL: Apply; DIFFICULTY: Moderate

27. 1, 2, 5. Thoracic, lumbar and cervical areas of the spine are the best bony landmarks to identify when attempting to screen for scoliosis because they show lateral deviation of the column. Abnormalities in the acromion processes and posterior superior iliac spines are not indicative of scoliosis.
CN: Physiological integrity; CNS: Physiological adaptation; CL: Apply; DIFFICULTY: Moderate

CN: Client needs category   CNS: Client needs subcategory   CL: Cognitive level

28. The nurse is caring for a child with clubfoot (talipes equinovarus). What intervention does the nurse prepare to assist with?
1. Traction
2. Serial casting
3. Short leg braces
4. Inversion range-of-motion exercises

29. When performing stretches with a child who has scoliosis, which technique should be used?
1. Slow and sustained
2. Gradual, until a change in muscle length is seen
3. Quick movements to the end range of pain
4. Slow movements for brief, 3- to 4-second periods

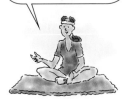

When come it comes to stretching, be sure to educate proper technique for the client.

30. A health care provider has prescribed oral prednisone for a child diagnosed with Duchenne muscular dystrophy. The parents ask the nurse what is the benefit of this medication. Which responses would be the **best**? Select all that apply.
1. Prednisone can strengthen the bones.
2. Prednisone can improve muscle strength.
3. Prednisone can stop the progression of the disease.
4. Prednisone can delay the progression of the disease.
5. Prednisone can decrease depression.

31. The nurse would expect a child's suspected developmental dysplasia of the hip (DDH) to be confirmed by which diagnostic technique?
1. X-ray
2. Positive Ortolani sign
3. Positive Trendelenburg gait
4. Audible clicking with adduction

32. The health care provider has ordered a child with juvenile rheumatoid arthritis to receive an intravenous infusion of methylprednisolone sodium succinate. The child weighs 22.5 kg. The order reads to administer 10 mg/kg over 1 hour. The vial comes in 100 mg/mL. How many milliliters would the nurse infuse? Record your answer using two decimal places.

_____ mL

33. Which activity in a child with muscular dystrophy should a nurse anticipate difficulty with **first**?
1. Breathing
2. Sitting
3. Standing
4. Swallowing

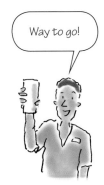

Way to go!

28. 2. Serial casting is the treatment of choice when attempting to change the length of soft tissue. Traction isn't a treatment option. Corrective shoes are used instead of short leg braces. Inversion exercises won't help; eversion exercises will.
CN: Physiological integrity; CNS: Reduction of risk potential; CL: Apply; DIFFICULTY: Difficult

29. 1. Stretches should be slow and sustained. It's difficult to see changes in muscle length. Stretches shouldn't be performed with quick movements and should be performed for longer than a few seconds.
CN: Health promotion and maintenance; CNS: None; CL: Apply; DIFFICULTY: Moderate

30. 2, 4. Prednisone's benefits for the child with Duchenne muscular dystrophy are that it can delay the progression of the disease and also improve muscle strength. Prednisone will not stop the progression of the disease nor will it strengthen the bones; in fact, it weakens the bones. Prednisone has been shown to possibly increase depression, not decrease it.
CN: Physiological integrity; CNS: Pharmacological therapies; CL: Apply; DIFFICULTY: Difficult

31. 1. X-ray will confirm the diagnosis of DDH. All of the other diagnostic techniques are positive signs of DDH, but only the x-ray will confirm the diagnosis.
CN: Physiological integrity; CNS: Physiological adaptation; CL: Apply; DIFFICULTY: Moderate

32. 2.25.

$$10 \text{ mg} (22.5 \text{ kg}) = 225 \text{ mg}$$
$$225 \text{ mg}/100 \text{ mg} = 2.25 \times 1 \text{ mL} = 2.25 \text{ mL}$$

CN: Physiological integrity; CNS: Pharmacological therapies; CL: Apply; DIFFICULTY: Challenge

33. 3. Muscular dystrophy usually affects postural muscles of the hip and shoulder first. Swallowing and breathing are usually affected last. Sitting may be affected, but a child would have difficulty standing before having difficulty sitting.
CN: Physiological integrity; CNS: Physiological adaptation; CL: Apply; DIFFICULTY: Moderate

34. Which observation by the nurse indicates that the parent of a neonate with developmental dysplasia of the hip understands the discharge education?
1. A folded towel is placed between the infant's legs.
2. The infant is wearing three diapers.
3. The infant is tightly swaddled in a blanket.
4. The infant is placed in the prone position to sleep.

35. The nurse is trying to weigh a 3-year-old child who's irritable and refuses to stand on the scale. What's the **best** way to obtain an accurate weight?
1. Ask the parent to approximate the weight.
2. Ask the parent to hold the child and record the combined weight.
3. Weigh the parent and child and subtract the parent's weight from the combined weight.
4. Obtain the admission weight and add 2 oz per day.

36. A young child sustains a dislocated hip as well as a subcapital fracture. Which complication is of greatest concern?
1. Avascular necrosis
2. Postoperative infection
3. Hemorrhage during surgery
4. Poor postoperative ambulation

37. In a child with developmental dysplasia of the hip (DDH), which position of the femur is accurate in relation to the acetabulum?
1. Anterior
2. Inferior
3. Posterior
4. Superior

38. The nurse is reinforcing education about muscular dystrophy for the parents of a child newly diagnosed with the disease. When asked about what the disease is, what should the nurse respond?
1. A demyelinating disease
2. Lesions of the brain cortex
3. Upper motor neuron lesions
4. Degeneration of muscle fibers

39. When a child is suspected of having muscular dystrophy, a nurse should expect which muscles to be affected **first**?
1. Muscles of the hip
2. Muscles of the foot
3. Muscles of the hand
4. Muscles of respiration

In DDH, the head of the femur is *in front of* the acetabulum. Can you remember the medical term for this?

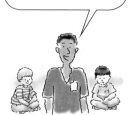

34. 2. Placing several diapers on the infant will keep the hips abducted. A towel placed between the legs is not enough to abduct the hips. Swaddling the infant tightly straightens the legs and doesn't allow the hips to abduct. Placing the infant in a prone position won't keep the hips abducted and isn't recommended due to the increased risk of sudden infant death syndrome.
CN: Physiologic integrity; CNS: Basic care and comfort; CL: Apply; DIFFICULTY: Challenge

35. 3. Subtracting the parent's weight from the combined weight will yield the child's weight. Weight is an important parameter used in calculating drug dosages based on kilograms per body weight. It also provides the most accurate information about the child's fluid balance. For these reasons, weight should never be approximated. Adding a couple of ounces per day to the admission weight would be inaccurate.
CN: Health promotion and maintenance; CNS: None; CL: Apply; DIFFICULTY: Easy

36. 1. Avascular necrosis is common with fractures to the subcapital region secondary to possible compromise of blood supply to the femoral head. Postoperative infection is always a concern but not a priority at first. Hemorrhage shouldn't occur. Poor postoperative ambulation is of concern but not as much as the possibility of avascular necrosis.
CN: Physiological integrity; CNS: Reduction of risk potential; CL: Analyze; DIFFICULTY: Difficult

37. 1. The head of the femur is anterior to the acetabulum in DDH. All of the other positions are incorrect.
CN: Physiological integrity; CNS: Physiological adaptation; CL: Apply; DIFFICULTY: Difficult

38. 4. Degeneration of muscle fibers with progressive weakness and wasting best describes muscular dystrophy. Demyelination of myelin sheaths is a description of multiple sclerosis. Lesions within the brain cortex and the upper motor neurons suggest a neurologic, not a muscular, disease.
CN: Physiological integrity; CNS: Physiological adaptation; CL: Apply; DIFFICULTY: Easy

39. 1. Positional muscles of the hip and shoulder are affected first. Progression later advances to muscles of the foot and hand. Involuntary muscles, such as the muscles of respiration, are affected last.
CN: Physiological integrity; CNS: Physiological adaptation; CL: Understand; DIFFICULTY: Moderate

40. The nurse is caring for a child with suspected muscular dystrophy. For which diagnostic test will the nurse prepare the child?
1. X-ray
2. Muscle biopsy
3. EEG
4. Assessment of ambulation

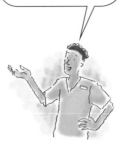

Which diagnostic test will reveal the degeneration of muscle fibers?

41. The nurse is reviewing the laboratory tests of a child diagnosed with muscular dystrophy. Which laboratory test does the nurse observe that would help diagnose this condition?
1. Bilirubin
2. Creatinine
3. Serum potassium
4. Sodium

42. The nurse is preparing for an admission of a child with muscular dystrophy. What form of the disorder should the nurse research to understand care?
1. Duchenne
2. Becker
3. Limb-girdle
4. Myotonic

43. Which condition would alert the nurse that a child may be suffering from muscular dystrophy?
1. Hypertonia of extremities
2. Increased lumbar lordosis
3. Upper extremity spasticity
4. Hyperactive lower extremity reflexes

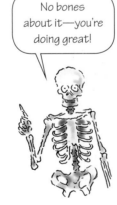

No bones about it—you're doing great!

44. The health care provider has ordered for a child with an open femur fracture morphine sulfate 10 mg PO times one dose. The elixir on hand is 100 mg/5 mL. How many milliliters will the nurse administer? Record your answer using one decimal place.

_____ mL

45. A child with muscular dystrophy has lost complete control of the lower extremities. There is some strength bilaterally in the upper extremities but poor trunk control. Which mechanism would be the **most** important to have on the wheelchair?
1. Anti-tip device
2. Extended brakes
3. Headrest support
4. Wheelchair belt

40. 2. A muscle biopsy shows the degeneration of muscle fibers and infiltration of fatty tissue. It's used for diagnostic confirmation of muscular dystrophy. X-ray is best for identifying an osseous deformity. Ambulation assessment alone wouldn't diagnose this child's disorder. EEG wouldn't be appropriate in this case.
CN: Health promotion and maintenance; CNS: None; CL: Apply;
DIFFICULTY: Moderate

41. 2. Creatinine is a by-product of muscle metabolism as the muscle hypertrophies; it aids in the diagnosis of muscular dystrophy. Bilirubin is a by-product of liver function. Potassium and sodium levels can change due to various factors that don't indicate muscular dystrophy.
CN: Health promotion and maintenance; CNS: None; CL: Analyze;
DIFFICULTY: Challenge

42. 1. Duchenne accounts for 50% of all cases of muscular dystrophy. It affects cardiac and respiratory muscles as well as all voluntary muscles.
CN: Physiological integrity; CNS: Physiological adaptation;
CL: Analyze; DIFFICULTY: Moderate

43. 2. An increased lumbar lordosis would be seen in a child suffering from muscular dystrophy secondary to paralysis of lower lumbar postural muscles. Increased lower extremity support may also be seen. Hypertonia isn't seen in muscular dystrophy. Upper extremity spasticity isn't seen because this disease isn't caused by upper motor neuron lesions. Hyperactive reflexes aren't indications of muscular dystrophy.
CN: Physiological integrity; CNS: Physiological adaptation;
CL: Analyze; DIFFICULTY: Difficult

44. 0.5.

$$10 \text{ mg}/100 \text{ mg} = 0.1$$
$$0.1 \times 5 \text{ mL} = 0.5 \text{ mL}$$

CN: Physiological integrity; CNS: Pharmacological therapies;
CL: Apply; DIFFICULTY: Challenge

45. 4. Since the child has poor trunk control, a belt will prevent falling out of the wheelchair. Anti-tip devices, headrest supports, and extended brakes are all important options but aren't the most important mechanisms in this situation.
CN: Safe, effective care environment; CNS: Safety and infection control; CL: Apply; DIFFICULTY: Moderate

46. When assessing a 2-year-old child with a history of muscular dystrophy, the nurse observes that the child's legs appear to be held together and the knees are touching. The nurse suspects contraction of which muscles?
1. Hip abductors
2. Hip adductors
3. Hip extensors
4. Hip flexors

47. A child diagnosed with muscular dystrophy is hospitalized secondary to a fall and is scheduled for surgery and skeletal traction. The nurse is preparing to administer an opioid analgesic. What life threatening side effect would the nurse want to monitor for?
1. Lethargy
2. Confusion
3. Respiratory depression
4. Dizziness

48. Which problem should the nurse address that is **most** commonly encountered by an adolescent female that is diagnosed with scoliosis?
1. Respiratory distress
2. Poor self-esteem
3. Poor appetite
4. Renal difficulty

49. A nurse is examining the progress record of a client with femur fractures who has had bilateral leg skeletal traction applied. The nurse reinforces education of the child on performing Kegel exercises. What is the **most** important purpose of these exercises?
1. To strengthen the child's arms so that she can better use the trapeze to lift up for bedpan placement and removal
2. To strengthen the child's calf muscles so that she's less likely to get leg cramps
3. To distract the child
4. To maintain good perineal muscle tone by tightening the pubococcygeus muscle

50. A child has developed difficulty ambulating and tends to walk on the toes. Which surgical technique does the nurse prepare the child for that will be beneficial?
1. Adductor release
2. Hamstring release
3. Plantar fascia release
4. Achilles tendon release

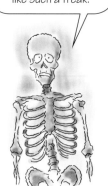

My scoliosis has really got me all bent out of shape. I feel like such a freak.

46. 2. The child's hip adductors are in a shortened position. The abductors are in a lengthened position. This position isn't indicative of hip flexor or hip extensor shortening.
CN: Physiological integrity; CNS: Physiological adaptation; CL: Apply; DIFFICULTY: Moderate

47. 3. Respiratory depression is the life threatening side effect the nurse should monitor for. Lethargy, confusion and dizziness should be monitored for but are non-life threatening for the client.
CN: Physiological integrity; CNS: Pharmacological therapies; CL: Apply; DIFFICULTY: Easy

48. 2. Poor self-esteem is a major issue with many adolescents, but the use of orthopedic appliances such as those used to treat scoliosis make this issue much more significant for teens with scoliosis. Although respiratory distress and poor appetite may surface, they aren't as common as self-esteem problems. Renal problems aren't usually an issue in adolescents with scoliosis.
CN: Health promotion and maintenance; CNS: None; CL: Apply; DIFFICULTY: Easy

49. 4. Because there's no evidence of a urinary tract infection, Kegel exercises are the appropriate intervention. Kegel exercises involve tightening the perineal muscles to help strengthen the pubococcygeus muscle and increase its elasticity. This helps to keep the child from becoming incontinent. None of the other interventions is related to Kegel exercises.
CN: Physiological integrity; CNS: Basic care and comfort; CL: Apply; DIFFICULTY: Easy

50. 4. A shortened Achilles tendon may cause a child to walk on the toes. A release of the tendon may assist the child in walking. An adductor release is commonly performed if the legs are held together. A plantar fascia release won't help a tight Achilles tendon, and a hamstring release is done only when there's a knee flexion contracture.
CN: Physiological integrity; CNS: Reduction of risk potential; CL: Apply; DIFFICULTY: Moderate

51. The parents of a child with muscular dystrophy ask the nurse what causes this condition. What is the best response by the nurse?
1. Gene mutation
2. Chromosomal aberration
3. Unknown nongenetic origin
4. Genetic and environmental factors

52. A nurse is assessing the lower extremity strength of a child diagnosed with muscular dystrophy. Which muscle group would be the **most** important to assess when planning actions to maintain maximum lower extremity function?
1. Gastrocnemius
2. Gluteus maximus
3. Hamstrings
4. Quadriceps

53. Which strategy does the nurse reinforce education regarding, that would be the first choice in attempting to maximize function in a child with muscular dystrophy?
1. Long leg braces
2. Motorized wheelchair
3. Manual wheelchair
4. Walker

54. A child with muscular dystrophy is having increased difficulty getting out of the chair at school. Which recommendation may the nurse make to assist the child?
1. A seat cushion
2. Long leg braces
3. Powered wheelchair
4. Removable armrests on wheelchair

55. What finding when the nurse gathers data that would be expected while palpating the muscles of a child with muscular dystrophy?
1. Soft on palpation
2. Firm or woody on palpation
3. Extremely hard on palpation
4. No muscle consistency on palpation

56. How would the nurse **best** describe *Gowers sign* to the parents of a child with muscular dystrophy?
1. A transfer technique
2. A waddling-type gait
3. The pelvis position during gait
4. Muscle twitching present during a quick stretch

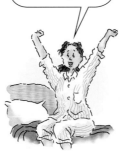

Wake up! We still have a lot of questions to get through.

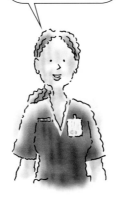

Muscular dystrophy involves infiltration of connective tissue and fatty tissue into the muscle. So, on palpation, how would the muscles feel?

51. 1. Muscular dystrophy is a result of a gene mutation. It isn't caused by a chromosome aberration or environmental factors. It's genetic and there is a known origin of the disease.
CN: Physiological integrity; CNS: Physiological adaptation; CL: Apply; DIFFICULTY: Difficult

52. 2. Gluteus maximus is the strongest muscle in the body and is important for standing as well as for transfers. All of the named muscles are important, but the maintenance of the gluteus maximus will enable maximum function.
CN: Health promotion and maintenance; CNS: None; CL: Apply; DIFFICULTY: Difficult

53. 1. Long leg braces are functional assistive devices that provide increased independence and increased use of upper and lower body strength. Wheelchairs, both motorized and manual, provide less independence and less use of upper and lower body strength. Walkers are functional assistive devices that provide less independence than braces.
CN: Physiological integrity; CNS: Basic care and comfort; CL: Apply; DIFFICULTY: Moderate

54. 1. A seat cushion will put the hip extensors at an advantage and make it somewhat easier to get up. Long leg braces wouldn't be the first choice. A powered wheelchair wouldn't assist with the transfer. Removable armrests have no bearing on assisting the client.
CN: Physiological integrity; CNS: Basic care and comfort; CL: Apply; DIFFICULTY: Moderate

55. 2. Muscles will usually be firm on palpation secondary to the infiltration of fatty tissue and connective tissue into the muscle. The muscles won't be soft secondary to the infiltration and won't be hard upon palpation. There's some consistency to the muscle, although in advanced stages atrophy is present.
CN: Physiological integrity; CNS: Physiological adaptation; CL: Analyze; DIFFICULTY: Difficult

56. 1. Gowers sign is a description of a transfer technique present during some phases of muscular dystrophy. The child turns on the side or abdomen, extends the knees, and pushes on the torso to an upright position by walking the hands up the legs. The child's gait is unrelated to the presence of Gowers sign. Muscle twitching present after a quick stretch is termed clonus.
CN: Physiological integrity; CNS: Physiological adaptation; CL: Analyze; DIFFICULTY: Difficult

57. The nurses should instruct a wheelchair-bound children with muscular dystrophy in which exercises to best prevent skin breakdown?

1. Wheelchair push-ups
2. Leaning side-to-side
3. Leaning forward
4. Gluteal sets

57. 1. Wheelchair push-ups will alleviate the most pressure to the buttocks. Leaning side-to-side will help but not as much as wheelchair push-ups. Gluteal sets won't help with pressure relief.

CN: Health promotion and maintenance; CNS: None; CL: Apply; DIFFICULTY: Challenge

58. The parents of a child newly diagnosed with pseudohypertrophic muscular dystrophy ask the nurse to describe this disease. The nurse's best response would be?

1. Increased muscle hypertrophy secondary to increased hormone production
2. Increased muscle hypertrophy secondary to fat infiltration
3. Decreased muscle secondary to muscle degeneration
4. Decreased muscle mass secondary to disease

58. 2. Pseudohypertrophic muscular dystrophy, also known as Duchenne muscular dystrophy, is present secondary to fat infiltration. Increased muscle mass is called hypertrophy and is related to increased work of muscles, not hormone production. Pseudohypertrophy isn't due to muscle degeneration or decreased muscle mass.

CN: Physiological integrity; CNS: Physiological adaptation; CL: Apply; DIFFICULTY: Difficult

59. A toddler is hospitalized for treatment of multiple injuries. The parents state that the injuries occurred when their child fell down the stairs. However, inconsistencies between the history and physical findings suggest child abuse. What should the nurse do next?

1. Refer the parents to Parents Anonymous.
2. Prepare the child for foster care placement.
3. Prevent the parents from seeing their child.
4. Report the incident to proper authorities.

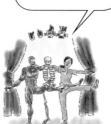

Get out there and break a leg— or at least sprain an ankle.

59. 4. The law requires the nurse to report all cases of suspected child abuse. Therefore, the nurse's first action should be to report this incident. After the authorities have been notified, steps can be taken toward protective custody, if appropriate, when the child is medically stable. Later, the nurse can refer the parents to Parents Anonymous, if needed. The nurse should give the parents opportunities to visit and help care for their child. During these visits, she can reinforce positive parenting behaviors.

CN: Safe, effective care environment; CNS: Coordinated care; CL: Apply; DIFFICULTY: Easy

60. A child with bilateral fractured femurs is scheduled for a double hip spica cast and says to the nurse, "Only 3 more months, and I can go home." Further investigation reveals that the child and family believe hospitalization is required until the cast comes off. What should the nurse explain to the family?

1. May be hospitalized 2 to 4 months.
2. Will go home 2 to 4 days after casting.
3. Will go home 1 week after casting.
4. Will go home as soon as she can move.

60. 2. The double hip spica cast will dry fairly rapidly with the use of fiberglass casting material. The time spent in the hospital after casting, typically 2 to 4 days, will be for educating the child and family about home care and for evaluating the child's skin integrity and neurovascular status before discharge. The time frames in the other options given are inaccurate for application of a double hip spica cast.

CN: Health promotion and maintenance; CNS: None; CL: Apply; DIFFICULTY: Difficult

61. An adolescent admitted with a fractured femur had an open reduction and internal fixation 2 days ago and is currently in traction and asks the nurse what would happen if a terrorist decided to bomb the hospital. What's the nurse's best response?

1. "I wouldn't worry about that. Spend your energy on getting well and going home."
2. "We have plans to call your parents and take care of you if there's a problem."
3. "What do you think might happen if terrorists attacked?"
4. "That's silly thinking. Why would anyone bomb a hospital?"

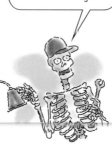

Fractured femur? No problem. You just need to gather the right tools for the job.

61. 3. Something prompted the child to ask such a question, and the nurse needs to take advantage of this opportunity to further explore his concerns and fears. Telling the child to concentrate on getting well discounts the feelings and may actually increase anxiety. Telling the child that parents would be called doesn't provide reassurance or help build a therapeutic relationship that can promote health and wellness. Telling the child thinking silly is dismissive and ridicules the child for asking the question.

CN: Psychosocial integrity; CNS: None; CL: Analyze; DIFFICULTY: Moderate

62. The nurse receives a report on a child admitted with severe muscular dystrophy and is receiving corticosteroids. The nurse understands that side effects may include: Select all that apply.
1. Weight gain.
2. Blurred vision.
3. Weakened bones.
4. Restlessness.
5. Loss of peripheral vision

63. Which finding should alert a nurse to a potential complication in a client with a cast following fracture of the radius?
1. Discomfort occurs at the site of the break.
2. Fingers are pink and warm.
3. Swelling is reduced with cast elevation.
4. Pain occurs over a bony prominence.

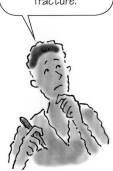

You're looking for something that would be unusual, not typical signs and symptoms of a fracture.

64. The parents of a child newly diagnosed with developmental dysplasia of the hip (DDH) ask the nurse how their child developed this condition. The nurse explains that the *greatest number* of cases are caused by which condition?
1. Dislocation
2. Subluxation
3. Acetabular dysplasia
4. Dislocation with fracture

65. Which finding would the nurse expect in a child with developmental dysplasia of the hip (DDH)?
1. Ligamentum teres is shortened.
2. Femoral head has lost contact with the acetabulum and is displaced inferiorly.
3. Femoral head has lost contact with the acetabulum and is displaced posteriorly.
4. Femoral head is in contact with acetabulum, but there's a noted capsular rupture.

66. The licensed practical nurse (LPN) is assigned to care for a 4-year-old child who had a Harrington rod inserted the day before and notices the client is receiving antibiotics by a syringe pump. The nurse is IV certified, but uncomfortable because they are unfamiliar with the equipment. What would be the **best** course of action?
1. Request another assignment.
2. Refuse the assignment for safety reasons.
3. Request in-service education for use of the syringe pump.
4. Read through the unit policy and procedure manual.

62. 1, 2, 3, 4. Weight gain, blurred vision, weakened bones and restlessness are all possible side effects. Loss of peripheral vision is not a possible side effect.
CN: Physiological integrity; CNS: Pharmacological therapies; CL: Apply; DIFFICULTY: Difficult

63. 4. Pain over a bony prominence, such as in the wrist or elbows, signals an impending pressure ulcer and requires prompt attention. Pain or discomfort at the site of the fracture is expected and is relieved by analgesics. Warm and pink fingers are an expected finding. Swelling may be relieved by elevation of the extremity. Swelling that isn't relieved by elevation of the affected limb should be reported to the health care provider.
CN: Physiological integrity; CNS: Reduction of risk potential; CL: Apply; DIFFICULTY: Moderate

64. 2. Studies show that subluxation accounts for the greatest number of cases of DDH.
CN: Physiological integrity; CNS: Physiological adaptation; CL: Apply; DIFFICULTY: Difficult

65. 3. In DDH, the femoral head loses contact with the acetabulum and is displaced posteriorly, not inferiorly, and the ligamentum teres is lengthened.
CN: Physiological integrity; CNS: Physiological adaptation; CL: Apply; DIFFICULTY: Difficult

66. 3. Using this piece of equipment is within the LPN's scope of practice, so it's inappropriate to refuse the assignment. Reading the policy and procedure manual is a good first step but not sufficient to ensure that they will be rendering safe care. Although requesting another assignment, it is best to request in-service education; the nurse is taking responsibility for the lack of experience in order to care for the child in a safe manner.
CN: Safe, effective care environment; CNS: Safety and infection control; CL: Analyze; DIFFICULTY: Moderate

CN: Client needs category   CNS: Client needs subcategory   CL: Cognitive level

67. The nurse is caring for a child with a hip spica cast which has become soiled. What is the appropriate action by the nurse?
1. Clean with damp cloth and dry cleanser.
2. Clean with soap and water.
3. Don't do anything.
4. Change the cast.

68. The nurse is providing care to a child in a hip spica cast who needs to be toileted. What position should the child be assisted into?
1. Supine
2. Sitting in a toilet chair
3. Shoulder lower than buttocks
4. Buttocks lower than shoulder

69. Which intervention should a nurse perform in a 4-year-old child in Buck traction?
1. Provide daily pin site care.
2. Release weights for 1 hour each day.
3. Change the child's position every 4 hours.
4. Unwrap the elastic bandage every shift to assess the skin.

70. The nurse is reinforcing education to the parents of a child with developmental hip dysplasia. The nurse recognizes that the family needs further education when they are observed placing the child in what position that may cause further complications?
1. Hip abduction.
2. Knee extension.
3. External rotation.
4. Internal rotation.

71. The health care provider has ordered sulfasalazine for a child with juvenile rheumatoid arthritis. The nurse questions the order when readings that the client has an allergy to what medication?
1. Alazopram
2. Naproxen
3. Sulfamethoxazole-trimethoprim
4. Penicillin

72. A toddler is immobilized with traction to the legs. Which play activity would be appropriate for this child?
1. Pounding board
2. Tinker toys
3. Pull toy
4. Board games

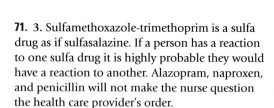

Read the question again. I'm sure the light bulb will come on.

67. **1.** A damp cloth is best to use rather than water. Water will break down the cast. Changing the cast isn't practical. If nothing is done, the cast will give off an odor.
CN: Physiological integrity; CNS: Basic care and comfort;
CL: Apply; DIFFICULTY: Moderate

68. **4.** The buttocks need to be lowered to toilet the child. This will keep the cast from being soiled. Supine positioning will soil the cast. The child can't use a toilet chair while in a hip spica cast.
CN: Physiological integrity; CNS: Basic care and comfort;
CL: Apply; DIFFICULTY: Moderate

69. **1.** Buck traction is a form of skeletal traction which pulls directly on the skeleton using a pin placed into the bone. Pin site care involves cleaning the insertion sites to reduce the risk of infection and observing the site for signs and symptoms of infection. Weights should hang freely and shouldn't be released. The child's position should be changed every 2 hours to prevent skin breakdown. Elastic bandages are used in skin traction, not skeletal traction.
CN: Physiological integrity; CNS: Basic care and comfort;
CL: Apply; DIFFICULTY: Moderate

70. **4.** Internal rotation increases the risk of hip dislocation. Abduction, external rotation, and knee extension won't increase the risk of dislocation.
CN: Health promotion and maintenance; CNS: None; CL: Apply;
DIFFICULTY: Challenge

71. **3.** Sulfamethoxazole-trimethoprim is a sulfa drug as if sulfasalazine. If a person has a reaction to one sulfa drug it is highly probable they would have a reaction to another. Alazopram, naproxen, and penicillin will not make the nurse question the health care provider's order.
CN: Physiological integrity; CNS: Pharmacological therapies;
CL: Analyze; DIFFICULTY: Challenge

72. **1.** A pounding board is appropriate for an immobilized toddler because it promotes physical development and provides an acceptable energy outlet. Toys with small parts, such as tinker toys, aren't suitable because a toddler may swallow the parts. A pull toy is suitable for most toddlers but not for one who's immobilized. Board games are usually too advanced for the developmental skills of a toddler.
CN: Health promotion and maintenance; CNS: None; CL: Apply;
DIFFICULTY: Difficult

CN: Client needs category   CNS: Client needs subcategory   CL: Cognitive level

73. The nurse would expect to see which activity level prescribed for a client immediately after a spinal fusion?
1. Supine bed rest
2. No weight bearing
3. No restriction
4. Limited weight bearing

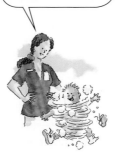

Working with pediatric clients comes with its own set of challenges.

73. **1.** After a spinal fusion, the child is usually placed on bed rest and ordered to lie flat. In 2 to 4 days, the child is allowed to sit up in and get out of bed. Other activities are gradually reintroduced. CN: Physiological integrity; CNS: Basic care and comfort; CL: Analyze; DIFFICULTY: Moderate

74. Which intervention would a nurse expect to use to prevent venous stasis after skeletal traction application?
1. Bed rest only
2. Convoluted foam mattress
3. Vigorous pulmonary care
4. Antiembolism stockings or an intermittent compression device

74. **4.** To prevent venous stasis after skeletal traction application, antiembolism stockings or an intermittent compression device are used on the unaffected leg. Convoluted foam mattresses and pulmonary care don't prevent venous stasis. Bed rest can *cause* venous stasis. CN: Health promotion and maintenance; CNS: None; CL: Apply; DIFFICULTY: Easy

75. A school nurse suspects that a 13-year-old has structural scoliosis. Asking the child to perform which maneuver would be the nurse's **priority** when assessing for this condition?
1. The child bends over and touches toes while the nurse observes from behind.
2. The child stands sideways while the nurse observes the profile.
3. The child assumes a knee-chest position on the examination table.
4. The child arches the back while the nurse observes from behind.

75. **1.** As the child bends over, the curvature of the spine is more apparent. The scapula on one side becomes more prominent, and the opposite side hollows. Scoliosis can't be properly assessed from the side or the front. The knee-chest position is used for lumbar puncture, not assessment. CN: Health promotion and maintenance; CNS: None; CL: Apply; DIFFICULTY: Easy

76. At the scene of a trauma, which nursing intervention is appropriate for a child with a suspected fracture?
1. Never move the child.
2. Sit the child up to facilitate breathing.
3. Move the child to a safe place immediately.
4. Immobilize the extremity and then move the child to a safe place.

76. **4.** At the scene of a trauma, the nurse should immobilize the extremity of a child with a suspected fracture and then move him to safety. If the child is already in a safe place, don't attempt to move them. Never try to sit the child up; this could make the fracture worse. CN: Safe, effective care environment; CNS: Safety and infection control; CL: Apply; DIFFICULTY: Easy

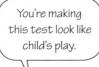

You're making this test look like child's play.

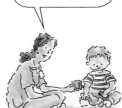

77. Which statement should the nurse include in the education plan for the parents of a child about to undergo a fracture reduction?
1. "All fractures can be reduced."
2. "Fracture reduction restores alignment."
3. "Undisplaced fractures may be reduced."
4. "Fracture reduction is usually performed with minimal discomfort."

77. **2.** Fracture reduction restores alignment. Some fractures, such as undisplaced fractures, can't be reduced. Fracture reduction is usually painful. CN: Physiological integrity; CNS: Reduction of risk potential; CL: Apply; DIFFICULTY: Moderate

78. A child in skeletal traction for a fracture of the right femur reports new and constant left calf pain. Also, the nurse notes that the child's left calf is 1 inch larger than the right and that there is nonpitting edema below the left knee. The nurse knows these signs are **most** consistent with which condition?
1. A fat emboli
2. An infection
3. A pulmonary embolism
4. Deep vein thrombosis (DVT)

78. **4.** Constant unilateral leg pain and significant edema should lead the nurse to suspect DVT. Symptoms of fat emboli include restlessness, tachypnea, and tachycardia and are more common in long-bone injuries. It's unlikely that an infection would occur on the side opposite the fracture without cause. Tachycardia, chest pain, and shortness of breath may be symptoms of a pulmonary embolism. CN: Physiological integrity; CNS: Reduction of risk potential; CL: Analyze; DIFFICULTY: Easy

CN: Client needs category   CNS: Client needs subcategory   CL: Cognitive level

79. When providing care for a child in traction, which intervention is a **priority**?
1. Assessing pin sites every shift and as needed
2. Ensuring that the rope knots catch on the pulley
3. Adding and removing weights per the child's or parent's request
4. Placing all joints through range of motion every shift

80. After assisting the primary health care provider in applying a cast, the nurse should include which intervention in immediate cast care?
1. Rest the cast on the bedside table.
2. Dispose of the plaster water in the sink.
3. Support the cast with the palms of the hand.
4. Wait until the cast dries before cleaning surrounding skin.

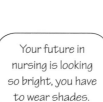

Your future in nursing is looking so bright, you have to wear shades.

81. The parents of a child who just had a synthetic cast applied ask the nurse how long it takes for the cast to dry. Which response by the nurse is the **most** accurate?
1. Immediately
2. 20 minutes
3. 45 minutes
4. 2 hours

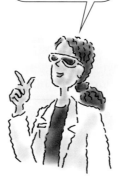

82. Which nursing intervention should be taken if, as the cast is drying, the child reports heat from the cast?
1. Remove the cast immediately.
2. Notify the primary health care provider.
3. Assess the child for other signs of infection.
4. Explain to the child that this is a normal sensation.

83. Which nursing intervention can **best** prevent foot drop in a casted leg?
1. Encourage bed rest.
2. Support the foot with 45 degrees of flexion.
3. Support the foot with 90 degrees of flexion.
4. Place a stocking on the foot to provide warmth.

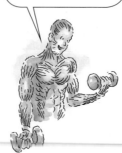

Tell your client to take it easy with the weight bearing after a fracture.

84. A nurse determines that an adolescent with a fractured left femur understands the instructions to perform only touch-down weight bearing when making what statement?
1. "I will place full weight on my left leg."
2. "I will place about 30% to 50% of my weight on my left leg."
3. "I will keep my left leg off the floor."
4. "I will allow my left leg to touch the floor without placing weight on it."

79. 1. Nursing care for a child in traction may include assessing pin sites every shift and as needed and ensuring that the knots in the rope don't catch on the pulley. Weights should be added and removed per the primary health care provider's order, and all joints, except those immediately proximal and distal to the fracture, should be placed through range of motion every shift.
CN: Physiological integrity; CNS: Basic care and comfort; CL: Apply; DIFFICULTY: Moderate

80. 3. After a cast has been applied, it should be immediately supported with the palms of the nurse's hands. Later, the nurse should dispose of the plaster water in a sink with a plaster trap or in a garbage bag. Then the nurse should clean the surrounding skin before the cast dries, and make sure that the cast isn't resting on a hard or sharp surface.
CN: Safe, effective care environment; CNS: Coordinated care; CL: Apply; DIFFICULTY: Challenge

81. 2. Synthetic casts take about 20 minutes to set.
CN: Safe, effective care environment; CNS: Coordinated care; CL: Apply; DIFFICULTY: Moderate

82. 4. Normally, as the cast is drying, the child may report heat from the cast. The nurse should offer reassurance that this is a normal sensation. Notifying the primary health care provider or removing the cast is unnecessary. Heat from a newly applied cast isn't a sign of infection.
CN: Safe, effective care environment; CNS: Coordinated care; CL: Apply; DIFFICULTY: Moderate

83. 3. To prevent foot drop in a casted leg, the foot should be supported with 90 degrees of flexion. Bed rest can cause foot drop. Keeping the extremity warm won't prevent foot drop.
CN: Health promotion and maintenance; CNS: None; CL: Apply; DIFFICULTY: Challenge

84. 4. Touch-down weight bearing allows the child to put no weight on the extremity, but the child may touch the floor with the affected extremity. Full weight bearing allows the child to bear all of his weight on the affected extremity. Partial weight bearing allows for only 30% to 50% weight bearing on the affected extremity. Non-weight bearing means bearing no weight on the extremity, and it must remain elevated.
CN: Physiological integrity; CNS: Basic care and comfort; CL: Apply; DIFFICULTY: Easy

85. The nurse suspects that a child with juvenile rheumatoid arthritis has presented with ibuprofen toxicity. Which laboratory tests dies the nurse expect the health care provider will order? Select all that apply.
1. Liver function panel
2. BUN
3. Creatinine
4. Blood cultures
5. Cerebrospinal fluid cultures (CSF)

85. 1, 2, 3. The health care provider would order liver function panel, BUN and creatinine in addition the other tests to determine ibuprofen toxicity. There is no need to order blood cultures and CSF cultures because there is no evidence of infection.
CN: Physiological integrity; CNS: Pharmacological therapies; CL: Apply; DIFFICULTY: Moderate

86. The nurse is collecting data for a child with developmental dysplasia of the hip (DDH). Which data obtained is **most** significant?
1. Mother's activity during the third trimester
2. Breech presentation at birth
3. Infant's serum calcium level at birth
4. Apgar score of 4 at 1 minute and 6 at 5 minutes

86. 2. Breech presentation is a factor commonly associated with DDH. The mother's activity during the third trimester, the infant's serum calcium level at birth, and Apgar scores have no bearing on DDH.
CN: Health promotion and maintenance; CNS: None; CL: Apply; DIFFICULTY: Easy

87. When assisting in discharge planning for a child with Duchenne muscular dystrophy what should the nurse be sure to include regarding the diet?
1. Low calorie, high protein, and high fiber
2. Low calorie, high protein, and low fiber
3. High calorie, high protein, and restricted fluids
4. High calorie, high protein, and high fiber

87. 1. A child with Duchenne muscular dystrophy is prone to constipation and obesity, so dietary intake should include a diet low in calories, high in protein, and high in fiber. Adequate fluid intake should also be encouraged.
CN: Physiological integrity; CNS: Basic care and comfort; CL: Apply; DIFFICULTY: Challenge

88. A nurse is educating the parents of a child with structural scoliosis who has been fitted for a Milwaukee brace. The parents ask how many hours per day the child should wear the brace. Which statement is **most** accurate?
1. 8 hours per day
2. 12 hours per day
3. 23 hours per day
4. 24 hours per day

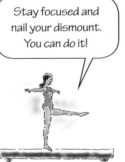

Stay focused and nail your dismount. You can do it!

88. 3. The Milwaukee brace can be removed only 1 hour per day for bathing and hygiene; otherwise, it must remain in place. Wearing the brace for 8 or 12 hours per day isn't enough time to provide the necessary correction. Wearing the brace 24 hours per day doesn't allow for bathing or skin integrity checks.
CN: Physiological integrity; CNS: Reduction of risk potential; CL: Apply; DIFFICULTY: Difficult

89. Which is the **best** strategy for a nurse to educate an adolescent about preventing sports-related injuries?
1. Warming up
2. Pacing activity
3. Building strength
4. Moderating intensity

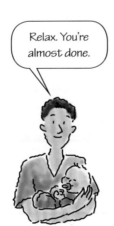

Relax. You're almost done.

89. 1. To prevent sports-related injuries, the nurse should teach the adolescent that the best prevention is warming up. Pacing activity, building strength, and using moderate intensity are other helpful, injury-prevention measures.
CN: Health promotion and maintenance; CNS: None; CL: Apply; DIFFICULTY: Easy

90. Which activity should the nurse discuss with the client that may be most therapeutic for a child who's allowed full activity after repair of a clubfoot?
1. Playing catch
2. Standing
3. Swimming
4. Walking

90. 4. Walking will stimulate all of the involved muscles and help with strengthening. All of the other activities are good exercises, but walking is the best choice.
CN: Physiological integrity; CNS: Physiological adaptation; CL: Apply; DIFFICULTY: Challenge

91. A client is taking high doses of methotrexate for juvenile rheumatoid arthritis which drug class would be contraindicated?
1. NSAIDS
2. ACE inhibitors
3. Corticosteroids
4. Beta blockers

91. 1. NSAIDS would be contraindicated because methotrexate decreases platelet levels and adding NSAIDS would possibly cause hematologic toxicity. All other medications would not cause adverse side effects to the client if used with methotrexate.
CN: Physiological integrity; CNS: Pharmacological therapies; CL: Apply; DIFFICULTY: Moderate

CN: Client needs category   CNS: Client needs subcategory   CL: Cognitive level

92. An adolescent suffers a broken leg as a result of a car accident and is taken to the emergency department and a plaster cast is applied. Before discharge, the nurse provides the child with instructions regarding cast care. Which instructions are **most** appropriate? Select all that apply:

1. Support the wet cast with pillows until it dries.
2. Use a hair dryer to speed the drying process.
3. Use the fingertips when moving the wet cast.
4. Apply powder to the inside of the cast after it dries.
5. Notify the health care provider if itching occurs under the cast.
6. Avoid putting straws or hangers inside the cast.

92. 1, 6. Supporting the wet cast with pillows prevents the cast from changing shape and interfering with the alignment of the fractured bone. The nurse should instruct the client not to place sharp objects, such as straws or hangers, down the inside of the cast if itching occurs to avoid the risk of impairing the skin and causing infection. Using a hair dryer isn't advised because it dries the cast unevenly, can burn the tissue, and can crack the cast, causing poor alignment to the injured bone. The palms, not the fingertips, should be used when handling the wet cast because fingertips can dent the cast, thus causing pressure points that can affect the skin's integrity. Powder shouldn't be used because it can cake under the cast. Itching is a common occurrence with casts because the skin cells can't slough as they normally would and the dry skin causes itching. The health care provider isn't usually called for this problem.

CN: Physiological integrity; CNS: Basic care and comfort; CL: Apply; DIFFICULTY: Difficult

93. The nurse is observing the chest of a child who has been diagnosed with a pectus excavatum. Which graphic depicts this abnormality?

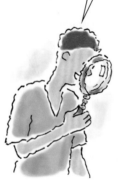

Pectus excavatum—do you remember what that condition looks like?

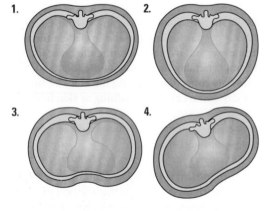

1. 2. 3. 4.

93. 3. Pectus excavatum is an indentation of the lower portion of the sternum. Option 1 shows a normal chest. Options 2 shows a barrel chest contour. Option 4 shows a thoracic scoliosis chest contour.

CN: Physiological integrity; CNS: Physiological adaptation; CL: Apply; DIFFICULTY: Moderate

94. The health care provider orders methylprednisolone sodium 1.5 mg/kg for a child weighing 51 kg. Methylprednisolone sodium is available as 125 mg/2 mL. How many milliliters must the nurse administer? Record your answer using two decimal places.

_____ mL

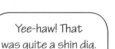

Yee-haw! That was quite a shin dig. Well done, partner.

94. 1.22.

$$1.5 \text{ mg/kg} \times 51 \text{ kg} = 76.5 \text{ mg}.$$
$$76.5 \text{ mg} \div 125 \text{ mg/2 mL} = 1.224 \text{ mL}.$$

In pediatric doses, it is rounded to the nearest hundredth, which would make the answer 1.22 mL.

CN: Physiological integrity; CNS: Pharmacological therapies; CL: Apply; DIFFICULTY: Difficult

95. A child has a fractured femur. The health care provider orders morphine sulfate 0.15 mg/kg/dose IV every 4 hours prn pain. The child weighs 50 kg. Morphine sulfate is supplied 2 mg/mL. How many milligrams may the child receive per day? Record your answer using a whole number.

_____ mg

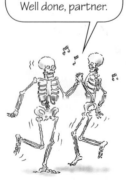

95. 45.

$$.15 \text{ mg/kg/dose} \times 50 \text{ kg} = 7.5 \text{ mg/dose}.$$
$$7.5 \text{ mg/dose} \times 6 \text{ doses/day} = 45 \text{ mg/day}.$$

CN: Physiological integrity; CNS: Pharmacological therapies; CL: Apply; DIFFICULTY: Difficult

Chapter 31

Gastrointestinal Disorders

Pediatric gastrointestinal refresher

Accidental poisoning

Ingestion of a toxic substance, which over-whelms the body's ability to clear or detoxify the substance

Key treatments

- Prevention:
  o educating parents and those who care for children about poisoning hazards
  o keeping child safety locks on cabinets
  o keeping hazardous chemicals and medications out of the reach of children
  o teaching parents or those who care for children to place the number for Poison Control near the phones for ease of access
- Always treat the child first by stopping further exposure to the substance and stabilizing the child

Acetaminophen poisoning

Ingestion of a toxic amount of acetaminophen, which occurs in an 8-hour period or less

Key signs and symptoms

- Diaphoresis, pallor, and hypothermia (2 to 4 hours)
- Slow-weak pulse (24 to 36 hours)
- Nausea and vomiting (2 to 4 hours)
- Right upper quadrant pain (48 hours)

Key test results

- Serum aspartate aminotransferase (AST) and serum alanine aminotransferase (ALT) levels (liver necrosis occurs in 2 to 5 days) become elevated soon after ingestion; BUN and creatinine
- Acetaminophen levels are greatly elevated

Key treatments

- Gastric lavage and induced vomiting
- N-acetylcysteine antidote: most effective in 8 to 10 hours; must be given within 24 hours; administer orally every 4 hours × 72 hours or IV × 3 doses

Key interventions

- Monitor cardiovascular, respiratory, renal, and GI status

- Monitor vital signs, intake and output, and maintain hydration status
- Monitor lab results for liver and kidney function

Corrosive agent poisoning

Ingestion of substances containing hydrocarbon (e.g., drain or oven cleaner, bleach, or battery acid) that adversely affect the body's systems

Key signs and symptoms

- Burning in the mouth and throat
- White, swollen mucous membranes
- Vomiting

Key test results

- Inspection of the face, mouth, and oropharynx
- Urine and serum blood analysis
- Chest x-ray

Key treatments

- Gastric lavage and activated charcoal
- IV fluids

Key interventions

- Monitor respiratory, cardiovascular, neurologic, GI, and renal status
- Assess vital signs, face, mouth, and oropharynx
- Do not induce vomiting
- Administer IV fluids and oral fluids when indicated
- Provide comfort measures for the child and supportive measures for the parents

Hydrocarbon poisoning

Ingestion of substances containing hydrocarbon (e.g., kerosene, turpentine, or gasoline) that adversely affect the body's systems

Key signs and symptoms

- Burning in the mouth and throat
- Choking and gagging
- CNS depression

Key test results

- Urine and serum blood analysis
- Chest x-ray and EEG, if indicated

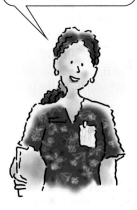

I'll bet that when you started nursing school, you had no idea kids could be subject to so many GI disorders. I know I didn't. This chapter tests you on the most common ones. Good luck!

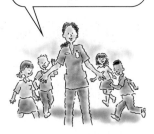

Poisoning is preventable. Encourage parents to keep all medications in a locked cabinet.

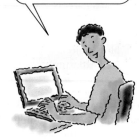

What interventions would you make for a client who consumed drain cleaner?

Key treatments
- Gastric lavage and activated charcoal
- IV fluids

Key interventions
- Monitor respiratory, cardiovascular, neurologic, GI, and renal status
- Assess vital signs
- Administer IV fluids and oral fluids when indicated
- Provide comfort measures for the child and supportive measures for the parents

Lead poisoning

Ingestion of lead or lead-containing products that build up in the body over a period of time

Key signs and symptoms
- Impaired growth and clumsiness
- Developmental regression and irritability
- Neurologic involvement

Key test results
- Blood lead levels above 9 micrograms per deciliter is considered elevated
- Erythrocyte protoporphyrin (EP) level
- Complete blood count (CBC) and long bone X-Rays (may reveal radiopaque material "lead lines")

Key treatments
- Chelation therapy (dimercaprol, calcium disodium edetate, succimer, and deferoxamine)
- IV fluids and hydration

Key interventions
- Neurologic assessment, physical examination, biophysical measurements (height, weight, head circumference if indicated)
- Provide for hydration (IV or oral) and a diet high in calcium and iron
- Rotate injection sites for chelation therapy
- Educate parents to wash the child's hands, toys, and to frequently remove lead dust
- Teach parents about sources of lead (flaking paint, crumbling plaster, pottery with lead glaze, lead solder in pipes, and other sources)
- Teach parents about reading labels on toy packaging for possible lead contents
- Screen and monitor young children who place objects in their mouth (toddlers) for lead exposure/poisoning

Salicylate poisoning

Ingestion of a toxic amount of salicylate that builds up in the system over a period of time

Key signs and symptoms
- High fever from the stimulation of carbohydrate metabolism
- Petechiae and bleeding tendency

Key test results
- Prothrombin time is prolonged
- Serum salicylate levels are elevated

Key treatments
- Gastric lavage and activated charcoal
- IV fluids
- Sodium bicarbonate and Vitamin K
- Peritoneal dialysis for severe cases

Key interventions
- Monitor respiratory, cardiovascular, GI, renal, and neurologic status
- Assess vital signs and urine pH
- Administer oral and IV fluids
- Provide comfort measures

Appendicitis

Inflammation of the appendix that results from a blockage of the organ and causes infection and pus accumulation

Key signs and symptoms
- Periumbilical pain that radiates to the right lower abdomen (McBurney's point) and rebound tenderness.
- Low grade fever and elevated WBC count
- Nausea, and vomiting
- Sudden cessation of pain (indicates rupture)

Key test results
- Hematology shows moderately elevated white blood cell count
- Ultrasound or CT of the abdomen shows a distended or enlarged appendix

Key treatments
- Appendectomy

Key interventions
- Assess and monitor vital signs, abdomen, GI status, and pain
- Avoid laxatives and applying heat to the area
- Perform preoperative care and teaching appropriate for child's developmental level
  - involve the parents as appropriate
  - assess parents' and child's understanding
- Provide postoperative care by assessing vital signs, cardiac, respiratory, and abdominal status
  - position right side-lying or semi-Fowler's if surgery is post-rupture
  - provide pain relief and teach use of patient-controlled analgesia pump (PCA) as indicated
  - encourage deep breathing, coughing, and use of incentive spirometer or other age appropriate devices as indicated
  - teach incisional splinting, change positions slowly, and promote early ambulation

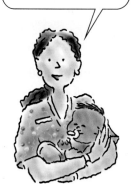

Be sure parents understand the sources of lead poisoning, such as flaking paint, and how to address them.

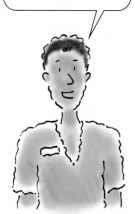

A client is suspected of having acute appendicitis. What signs should you look for?

- maintain nothing-by-mouth (NPO) status until bowel sounds return postoperatively and then advance diet as tolerated
- Monitor for postoperative complications:
  - atelectasis (dyspnea, cyanosis)
  - bleeding/hemorrhage (decreased blood pressure, increased pulse rate, cool, clammy skin)
  - peritonitis (rigid abdomen and guarding)
  - fluid and electrolyte disturbances
  - paralytic ileus (absence of bowel sounds, inability to pass gas or stool, and abdominal distention)
  - infection (redness, swelling, or abnormal drainage or order from the incision)

Celiac disease

Intolerance to gluten (protein found in wheat, rye, oats, and barley)

Key signs and symptoms

- Generalized malnutrition and failure to thrive due to protein and carbohydrate malabsorption
- Steatorrhea and chronic diarrhea due to fat malabsorption
- Weight and height below normal for age-group

Key test results

- Immunologic assay screen is positive for celiac disease
- Bowel biopsy

Key treatments

- Gluten-free diet-avoid wheat, rye, oats, and barley
- Vitamin supplementation (fat soluble vitamins A, D, E, and K)

Key interventions

- Monitor and plot growth and development using appropriate forms such as growth charts
- Give small, frequent meals avoiding wheat, rye, oats, and barley; substitute corn and rice for wheat, rye, oats, and barley
- Teach parents to read labels to identify foods containing hidden wheat, rye, oats, and barley

Cleft lip and palate

Congenital malformation, which causes fissure(s) that involve any of these facial or mouth structures: lip, nasal septum, anterior maxilla, and soft and hard palate

Key signs and symptoms

- Cleft lip is obvious at birth (with or without cleft palate): ranges from simple notch on upper lip to complete cleft from lip edge

to floor of the nostril, on either side of the midline but rarely along the midline itself
- Cleft palate without cleft lip may not be detected until mouth examination or observation of feeding difficulties

Key test results

- Prenatal ultrasound may indicate severe defects
- Physical examination of the face, lips, and palate (soft and hard) reveals the deformity

Key treatments

- Cheiloplasty performed between 2 and 3 months of age to unite lip and gum edges in anticipation of teeth eruption
- Cleft palate repair surgery
  - scheduled at between 12 and 18 months to allow for growth of palate and to be done before infant develops speech patterns
  - infant must be free from ear and respiratory infections

Key interventions

- Visualize the face, lips, nose, and gums, and palpate the soft and hard palate for deformities at birth
- Use interventions that encourage a positive view of the child and that facilitate parent-infant bonding
- Assess infant's ability to suck and swallow at birth
  - keep suction equipment and bulb syringe at bedside
- Monitor intake and output and weigh daily
- Before cleft lip repair surgery
  - assess for signs and symptoms of ear or respiratory infection
  - be alert for respiratory distress while feeding and hold the infant when feeding
  - maintain adequate nutrition by feeding small amounts in an upright position; feed utilizing special nipples and feeders, burp frequently, and promote sucking between meals
  - provide information to the parents and allow time for verbalization of feelings
- After cleft lip repair surgery
  - maintain airway, observe for distress, and position infant to prevent aspiration
  - keep infant's hands away from the mouth by using restraints or pinning the sleeves to the shirt; use adhesive strips to hold the suture line in place
  - clean the suture line after each feeding by as ordered
  - provide soothing measures (rocking, cuddling), age-appropriate activities, and minimize crying
  - administer pain medications and antibiotics as ordered

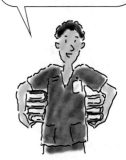

You have a client who has diarrhea after eating wheat or rye bread or oatmeal. What condition should you suspect?

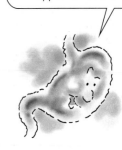

Dietary intolerances can be managed with ingredient substitutions and vitamin supplementation.

- After cleft palate repair surgery
  - place a suction set-up and endotracheal tray at the bedside and position the toddler on the abdomen or side
  - anticipate edema and a reduction in airway clearance from palate closure and assess for signs of altered oxygenation
  - teach parents to keep hard or pointed objects (utensils, straws, frozen dessert sticks) away from the mouth and to monitor for signs of infection (infection increases the chance of increased scaring)
  - provide referrals to speech therapy and orthodontists as needed

Esophageal atresia and tracheoesophageal fistula

Malformation of the esophagus that results in a blind pouch or an opening between the esophagus and trachea

Key signs and symptoms

Esophageal atresia
- Excessive salivation and drooling due to inability to pass food through the esophagus

Tracheoesophageal fistula
- Choking, coughing, and intermittent cyanosis caused by secretions, or during feeding due to secretions, or food that goes through the fistula into the trachea

Key test results

- Abdominal x-ray reveals a stomach filled with air
- NG tube insertion does not yield gastric aspirate when verifying placement
- Radiologic visualization of the tube does not reveal it in the stomach (curls in the blind pouch)
- Neonates are fed first with a few sips of sterile water to detect these anomalies and to prevent aspiration of formula or breast milk into the lungs

Key treatments

- Surgical correction by ligating the tracheo-esophageal fistula and reanastomosing the esophageal ends; in many cases, done in stages
- Transport to neonatal intensive care (NICU) when possible
- Antibiotic therapy started early because of aspiration

Key interventions

- Before surgery
  - monitor respiratory status, cardiac and GI systems; monitor vital signs

  - manage secretions with nasal and oral suctioning; position to promote airway drainage and to prevent aspiration
  - administer antibiotics and other medications as prescribed
  - manage the gastrostomy tube and facilitate drainage; weigh daily and monitor I&O.
- After surgery
  - monitor respiratory, cardiac, and GI status; position to prevent aspiration; and manage secretions with suctioning
  - provide care of the incision; maintain total parenteral nutrition (TPN) until gastrostomy or oral feedings are tolerated (check for cloudy fluid color, agitate the bag periodically, use a 10 micron filter, is greater than 10% glucose concentration administered only through a central line); weigh daily and monitor I&O
  - Monitor for postoperative complications (respiratory difficulty, aspiration, bleeding, infection, and fluid balance and electrolyte disturbances)
  - Teach parents soothing techniques, positioning, CPR, care of the incision, signs and symptoms to report, and when to follow up postoperatively

Failure to thrive

When a child's current weight or rate of weight gain is much lower than that of other children of similar age and gender

Key signs and symptoms

- Altered body posture (child is stiff or floppy and does not cuddle)
- Avoids eye contact
- Disparities between chronologic age and height, weight, and head circumference
- History of insufficient stimulation and inadequate parental knowledge of child development

Key test results

- Growth chart analysis and Denver Developmental Screening (Ages and Stages)
- Complete blood count (CBC), chemistry panel, and hormone studies in older children

Key treatments

- High-calorie diet
- Parental counseling
- Vitamin and mineral supplements

Key interventions

- Assign care to the same team of caregivers when possible
- Provide adequate food and fluid intake and interact appropriately with the child

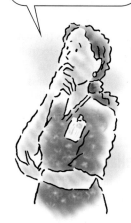

Esophageal atresia … tracheoesophageal fistula—what do these terms mean?

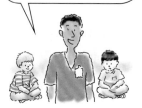

Don't be alarmed by the term "failure to thrive"—it usually just means a child is not gaining as much weight as needed.

- Provide the child with visual and auditory stimulation
- When caring for child in parent's presence, act as role model for effective parenting skills
- Demonstrate comfort measures and show the mother how to hold infant in the en-face position

Gastroenteritis

Increase in the frequency of liquid stool expulsion

Key signs and symptoms
- Increase in fluid content, frequency, and volume of stool
- Weight loss (1 g of weight equals 1 mL of body fluid)

Key test results
- Serum electrolytes, complete blood count, blood cultures, and stool cultures
- History becomes important because antibiotic use, diet (lactose intolerance), travel, and exposure to contagious illnesses can also cause diarrhea

Key treatments
- IV therapy to correct fluid and electrolyte imbalances and antidiarrheal medications
- Correction of the underlying problem

Key interventions
- Assess vital signs, weight, skin, and for signs of dehydration (poor skin turgor [tenting of skin when pinched], sunken eye sockets, sunken fontanels, absence of tears, dry mouth, decreased urine output)
- Administer IV rehydration therapy as ordered, weigh daily, and maintain strict intake and output
- Monitor laboratory results and observe for signs of electrolyte imbalance (deep breathing, listlessness, and other changes in level of consciousness)
- Maintain nothing by mouth (NPO) status until reintroduction of oral food is ordered
- Introduce clear liquids slowly and frequently in small amounts using over-the-counter oral rehydration fluid; avoid apple juice or juices high in sugar
- Administer antidiarrheal medications as ordered
- Report bloody stools, continued weight loss, physiologic changes in condition, decreased urinary output, bloody stool, persistent diarrhea, changes in level of consciousness

Intestinal obstruction

Partial or complete obstruction of the small or large intestine resulting from intussusception, Hirschsprung disease, other mechanical blockage by a foreign object, or a volvulus

Key signs and symptoms
- Complete small-bowel obstruction:
  - bowel contents are propelled toward mouth (instead of rectum) by vigorous peristaltic waves causing vomiting
  - persistent epigastric or periumbilical pain
- Partial large-bowel obstruction:
  - leakage of liquid stool around the obstruction (common) resulting in soiling or reports of diarrhea
- Hirschsprung's disease:
  - abdominal distention is common in all age groups
  - neonate signs and symptoms: failure to pass first meconium stool within 24-48 hours, refusal to eat, and vomiting bile
  - infant signs and symptoms: failure to thrive, constipation, vomiting and diarrhea
  - older children signs and symptons: ribbon-like stool, palpable fecal mass, visible peristalsis, and malnourished appearance
- Intussusception:
  - sudden onset of acute abdominal pain
  - stools with mucous and blood that resemble currant jelly
  - palpable "sausage" mass in the right upper quadrant of the abdomen and/or a tender distended abdomen

Key test results
- With large-bowel obstruction, barium enema reveals a distended, air-filled colon
- With sigmoid volvulus, barium enema reveals a closed loop of sigmoid with extreme distention or the presence of an intussusception
- X-rays confirm the diagnosis
- Abdominal films show the presence and location of intestinal gas or fluid
- Abdominal ultrasound to determine presence of intussusception (telescoping of the intestines into itself)
- Full thickness and/or rectal biopsies to determine presence of Hirschsprung disease, which is an absence of ganglion (nerve) cells in the colon

Key treatments
- IV therapy to correct fluid and electrolyte imbalances
- Laparoscopic surgery or open abdominal surgery to correct the underlying problem

Ugh. I'm feeling a little ... obstructed. What should I do?

- Surgical reduction (if inflating the bowel with air or administering a barium enema is not successful)
- Proton pump inhibitors (omeprazole), histamine-2 (H$_2$) receptor antagonist (ranitidine), and antibiotics for intussusception
- Analgesics and antibiotics for Hirschsprung disease

Key interventions

- Monitor vital signs, respiratory and cardiovascular status
- Observe child closely for signs of shock (pallor, rapid pulse, and hypotension)
- Monitor for fluid and electrolyte disturbances
- Maintain strict I&O
- Weigh daily
- Position child side lying with head elevated to prevent aspiration during vomiting episodes
- Stay alert for signs and symptoms of:
  - metabolic alkalosis (changes in sensorium; slow, shallow respirations; hypertonic muscles; tetany)
  - metabolic acidosis (dyspnea on exertion; disorientation; deep, rapid breathing; weakness; malaise)
- Document characteristics, amount of emesis, and behaviors during vomiting episodes
- Provide meticulous oral care after vomiting
- Watch for signs and symptoms of secondary infection
- Provide preoperative and postoperative care as indicated

Pyloric stenosis

Narrowing of the pylorus, the opening from the stomach into the small intestine

Key signs and symptoms

- Projectile vomiting during or shortly after feedings
- Hunger immediately after vomiting and possible olive shaped mass in the right upper quadrant of the abdomen
- Peristaltic wave moves from right to left when lying flat
- Failure to gain weight/signs of dehydration

Key test results

- Ultrasound of the abdomen reveals hypertrophied sphincter

Key treatments

- Pyloromyotomy performed by laparoscopy

Key interventions

- Provide small, frequent, thickened feedings with the head of the bed elevated
- Burp frequently
- Position child on the right side or with head slightly elevated to prevent aspiration
- Weigh daily and monitor intake and output
- Maintain NPO status and document amount and characteristics of emesis along with the behaviors observed
- Maintain IV fluid replacement and monitor for fluid and electrolyte disturbances
- Perform preoperative teaching and encourage parents to verbalize feelings
- Provide postoperative care, maintain NG tube placement (verify) and patency, and maintain NPO status until bowel sounds return

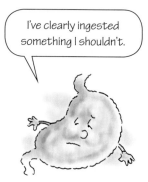

I've clearly ingested something I shouldn't.

thePoint® You can download tables of drug information to help you prepare for the NCLEX®! View Generic Drug Names, Drug Classifications, Drug Actions, and Nursing Implications for the drugs discussed in this refresher at **http://thePoint.lww.com**.

Gastrointestinal questions, answers, and rationales

1. The nurse evaluates the outcomes of care for a child with celiac disease. Which finding indicates that the child is meeting the goal of care?
   1. The child's growth is appropriate for both height and weight.
   2. The child verbalizes the importance of maintaining good health.
   3. The parents and the child meet a peer with celiac disease for support.
   4. The parents and child follow the prescribed dietary restrictions.

1. 1. Because celiac disease is a disease that involves protein and carbohydrate malabsorption, the child is at risk for failure to thrive. The main goal of care is to promote a normal growth pattern for the child. Following the prescribed diet is a way to reach the goal of maintaining the child's growth. Stressing good health and meeting a peer with celiac disease are also important nursing considerations but would come after maintaining normal growth patterns.
CN: Physiological integrity; CNS: Reduction of risk potential; CL: Analyze; DIFFICULTY: Challenge

2. Which interventions should the nurse perform when caring for an adolescent client who is receiving total parenteral nutrition (TPN)? Select all that apply.
1. Inspect the central line insertion site
2. Monitor the client's vital signs
3. Agitate the IV bag frequently
4. Monitor the client's visitors
5. Assess blood glucose levels
6. Observe the fluid's clarity

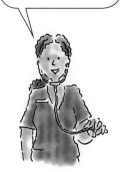

No, "total parenteral nutrition" doesn't mean that the parents are the only ones feeding the client.

2. **1, 2, 3, 5, 6.** The high sugar content of TPN solutions increases the possibility of bacteria growth in the bag and tubing and can raise the blood glucose levels. This increases the client's risk for infection. Crystallization of the mixture can occur in the bag. The nurse should assess for elevated temperature, inspect the central line insertion site for signs of infection, inspect the TPN mixture for clarity, and assess blood glucose levels. TPN should not be stopped abruptly or infused rapidly. Special tubing is used that contains an in-line filter to remove bacteria and particulate material. Monitoring visitors does not apply to the care for TPN but for clients with compromised immune functioning.
CN: Physiological integrity; CNS: Pharmacological therapies; CL: Apply; DIFFICULTY: Difficult

3. Which food items selected by a child with celiac disease would cause the nurse to intervene? Select all that apply.
1. Corn flakes cereal, skim milk, and a banana
2. A bologna, lettuce, and tomato sandwich
3. Sliced cheese, sausage and vegetable pizza
4. A wheat tortilla with southwestern chicken and rice
5. Steamed broccoli florets with a grilled pork chop
6. Sliced strawberries with a tossed green salad

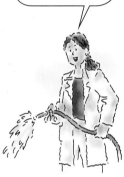

Watery stool may be a sign of celiac disease.

3. **1, 2, 3, 4.** Sources of gluten found in wheat, rye, barley, and oats should be avoided. Rice and corn are suitable substitutes because they don't contain gluten. Pizza, lunch meat, and cereal contain gluten and, when broken down, can't be digested by people with celiac disease. The remaining dietary choices do not contain gluten.
CN: Physiological integrity; CNS: Reduction of risk potential; CL: Apply; DIFFICULTY: Difficult

4. A nurse interviewing the parents of a child diagnosed with celiac disease would expect them to report which characteristic?
1. "Our child's behavior has not changed."
2. "There are no problems with weight gain."
3. "Playing is our child's favorite way to pass the time."
4. "Our child has 5 to 6 oily looking stools a day."

4. **4.** Diarrhea is common due to the child's inability to absorb the protein gluten and fat. Profuse watery diarrhea is usually a sign of celiac crisis. Behavior changes, such as irritability, uncooperativeness, and apathy are common, and they usually aren't pleasant. Poor weight gain would be a symptom of celiac disease because impaired absorption leads to malnutrition.
CN: Physiological integrity; CNS: Physiological adaptation; CL: Analyze; DIFFICULTY: Easy

5. To help promote a normal life for children with celiac disease, which intervention should the parents use?
1. Treat the child differently from other siblings.
2. Focus on restrictions that make them feel different.
3. Introduce the child to a peer with celiac disease.
4. Don't allow the child to express doubt about following dietary restrictions.

5. **3.** Introducing the child to a peer with celiac disease will let this child know he isn't alone. It will show the child how other people live a normal life with similar restrictions. Instead of focusing on restrictions that makes the child feel different, the parents should focus on ways the child can be normal. They should treat the child no differently from other siblings but set appropriate limits. Allow the child with celiac disease to express feelings about dietary restrictions.
CN: Psychosocial integrity; CNS: None; CL: Apply; DIFFICULTY: Easy

6. Which data collected by the nurse would **best** evaluate the effectiveness of nutritional therapy on a child with celiac disease?
1. Vital signs
2. Appearance, size, and number of stools
3. Blood urea nitrogen (BUN) and serum creatinine levels
4. Intake and output

6. **2.** The fat, bulky, foul-smelling stools should be gone when a child with celiac disease follows a gluten-free diet. Vital signs, BUN and serum creatinine levels, and intake and output aren't affected by a gluten-free diet.
CN: Physiological integrity; CNS: Basic care and comfort; CL: Analyze; DIFFICULTY: Moderate

7. Which finding should the nurse expect to see in a child with celiac disease who has started a prescribed diet?
1. Increased diarrhea
2. Foul-smelling stools
3. Improved appetite
4. Weight loss

8. To prevent trauma to the suture line of an infant who underwent cleft lip repair, the nurse would perform which intervention?
1. Placing mittens on the infant's hands
2. Maintaining arm restraints
3. Not allowing the parents to touch the infant
4. Removing the lip device from the infant after surgery

9. Which intervention should the nurse use to prevent tissue infection after cleft palate and lip repair?
1. Keep the suture line moist at all times.
2. Allow the infant to suck on a pacifier.
3. Rinse the infant's mouth after each feeding.
4. Feed the infant with a catheter-tipped syringe.

10. Which nursing intervention should be used when feeding an infant with cleft palate?
1. Burp the infant often.
2. Limit the amount the infant eats.
3. Feed the infant at scheduled times.
4. Remove the nipple if the infant is making loud noises.

11. Which nursing intervention has the **highest priority** in the care of an infant during the first 24 hours after surgery for cleft lip?
1. Carefully clean the suture line after feedings using sterile technique.
2. Position the infant in the prone position after feedings.
3. Allow the infant to cry to promote lung expansion.
4. Provide the infant with a pacifier to satisfy the urge to suck.

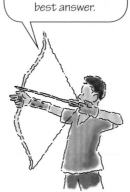

If you aim at nothing, you'll hit it every time. Keep your sights set on the best answer.

7. 3. Within a day or two of starting their diet, most children show improved appetite and reduction or disappearance of diarrhea. Steatorrhea (fatty, oily, foul-smelling stool) disappearance and weight gain are good indicators that the child's ability to absorb nutrients is improving.
CN: Physiological integrity; CNS: Physiological adaptation; CL: Apply; DIFFICULTY: Moderate

8. 2. Arm restraints are used to prevent the infant from rubbing the sutures. Mittens alone won't prevent the infant from rubbing the suture line. Parental contact will increase the infant's comfort. The lip device shouldn't be removed.
CN: Physiological integrity; CNS: Reduction of risk potential; CL: Analyze; DIFFICULTY: Challenge

9. 3. To prevent formula buildup around the suture line, the infant's mouth is usually rinsed. The sutures should be kept clean and dry. Placing objects in the mouth is generally avoided after surgery. Infants are fed by mouth using a catheter-tipped, plunger-type syringe.
CN: Physiological integrity; CNS: Physiological adaptation; CL: Apply; DIFFICULTY: Moderate

10. 1. Infants with cleft lip and palate have a tendency to swallow an excessive amount of air, so they need burping often. The amount of formula they eat at each feeding is the same as an infant without cleft lip or palate, and scheduled feedings aren't necessary. Loud noises are common when these infants eat.
CN: Physiological integrity; CNS: Physiological adaptation; CL: Apply; DIFFICULTY: Moderate

11. 1. The suture line must be cleaned after each feeding to reduce the risk of infection, which could adversely affect the healing and cosmetic results. The incision should be cleaned carefully so the sutures are not disrupted. A sterile solution should be used to reduce the risk of infection. The infant should not be placed on his abdomen in the prone position because this puts pressure on the incision and may affect healing. Anticipatory care should be provided to reduce the risk of the infant crying, which puts pressure on the incision. Pacifiers and other firm objects should not be placed in the infant's mouth because they can disrupt the suture line.
CN: Physiological integrity; CNS: Reduction of risk potential; CL: Apply; DIFFICULTY: Easy

12. Which nursing intervention is essential in the care of an infant with cleft lip and palate?
1. Discourage breast-feeding.
2. Hold the infant flat while feeding.
3. Involve the parents in the infant's care.
4. Use a normal nursery nipple for feedings.

12. 3. The sooner the parents become involved, the quicker they can determine the method of feeding best suited for them and the infant. Breast-feeding, like bottle-feeding, may be difficult but can be facilitated if the mother intends to breast-feed. Sometimes, especially if the cleft is not severe, breast-feeding may be easier because the human nipple conforms to the shape of the infant's mouth. Feedings are usually given in the upright position to prevent formula from coming through the nose. Various special nipples have been devised for infants with cleft lip or palate; a normal nursery nipple is not effective.

CN: Physiological integrity; CNS: Physiological adaptation; CL: Apply; DIFFICULTY: Easy

13. The nurse is educating the parents of an infant undergoing repair for a cleft lip. Which instructions should the nurse give? Select all that apply.
1. Offer a pacifier as needed.
2. Lay the infant on his back to sleep.
3. Sit the infant up for each feeding.
4. Loosen the arm restraints every 4 hours.
5. Clean the suture line after each feeding by dabbing it with saline solution.
6. Give the infant extra care and support.

13. 2, 3, 5, 6. An infant with a repaired cleft lip should be put to sleep on the back to prevent trauma to the surgery site. The infant should be fed in the upright position with a syringe and attached tubing to prevent stress to the suture line from sucking. To prevent crusts and scarring, the suture line should be cleaned after each feeding by dabbing it with half-strength hydrogen peroxide or saline solution. The infant should receive extra care and support since emotional needs cannot be met by sucking. Extra care and support may also prevent crying, which stresses the suture line. Pacifiers shouldn't be used during the healing process because they stress the suture line. Arm restraints are used to keep the infant's hands away from the mouth and should be loosened every 2 hours.

CN: Physiological integrity; CNS: Reduction of risk potential; CL: Apply; DIFFICULTY: Difficult

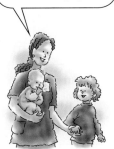

Congenital defects in infants, such as cleft palate, can be upsetting to the family. Stay optimistic and be encouraging.

14. The parents of an infant born with cleft lip and palate are seeing their child for the first time. Which nursing action will assist with facilitating parent-infant bonding?
1. Point out the infant's positive features when providing care.
2. Discuss the parent's feelings of irritation with how the infant eats.
3. Recognize the parent's ambivalence in caring for an infant with this defect.
4. Allow the parents to share their feeling of dissatisfaction with the infant's appearance.

14. 1. To relieve the parents' anxiety, positive aspects of the infant's physical appearance need to be emphasized. Showing optimism toward surgical correction and showing a photograph of possible cosmetic improvements may be helpful. The other responses are inappropriate.

CN: Psychosocial integrity; CNS: None; CL: Apply; DIFFICULTY: Moderate

15. The parents of a child who has cleft palate repair should be educated about which potential long-term complication?
1. Deviated septum
2. Recurring tonsillitis
3. Tooth decay
4. Hearing loss

15. 4. Improper draining of the middle ear causes recurrent otitis media and scarring of the tympanic membrane, which lead to varying degrees of hearing loss. The septum remains intact with c left palate repair. Cleft palate does not cause problems with the tonsils. Improper tooth alignment, not tooth decay, is common.

CN: Physiological adaptation; CNS: Reduction of risk potential; CL: Analyze; DIFFICULTY: Difficult

16. The parent of a neonate born with a cleft lip and palate prepares to feed the child for the first time. Which parent education should the nurse complete as a **priority** of care before the parent attempts the first feeding?
1. Methods of burping the neonate
2. How to clean the neonate's mouth
3. Proper positioning of the neonate
4. How to lay the neonate down

16. 3. When neonates are held in the upright position, the formula is less likely to leak out the nose or mouth. Neonates need to be burped frequently after feeding. There is no need to clean the mouth before eating and the infant should be positioned after feeding to prevent aspiration. After surgical repair, the mouth is cleaned at the suture site to prevent infection. The bottle should be prepared using a special nipple or feeding device.
CN: Physiological integrity; CNS: Physiological adaptation;
CL: Apply; DIFFICULTY: Easy

17. Which **priority** intervention should the nurse perform when caring for an infant who returns from surgery after repair of a cleft palate?
1. Offer a pacifier for comfort.
2. Position the infant on the side.
3. Suction all secretions from the mouth and nose.
4. Remove the arm restraints placed on the infant after surgery.

17. 2. The infant should be positioned on the side to allow oral secretions to drain from the mouth so suctioning is not necessary. Pacifiers should not be used because they can damage the suture line. Arm restraints should be kept on to protect the suture line. The restraints should be removed periodically to allow the infant full range of motion during this time. Only one restraint should be removed at a time, and the infant should be closely supervised.
CN: Physiological integrity; CNS: Reduction of risk potential;
CL: Apply; DIFFICULTY: Challenge

18. The nurse prepares to teach the parents of a child who had had surgical repair of a cleft palate. Which instruction should the nurse include in the discharge education to the parents?
1. Continue a normal diet.
2. Continue using arm restraints at home.
3. Avoid allowing the child to drink from a cup.
4. Teach good mouth care and proper brushing.

"Oto" relates to the ears and hearing, and "laryngo" relates to the larynx—areas that are affected by cleft lip and palate.

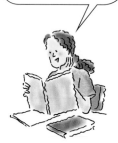

18. 2. Arm restraints are also used at home to keep the child's hands away from the mouth until the palate is healed. A soft diet is recommended. No food harder than mashed potatoes can be eaten. Fluids are best taken from a cup. Proper mouth care is encouraged after the palate is healed.
CN: Physiological integrity; CNS: Physiological adaptation;
CL: Apply; DIFFICULTY: Challenge

19. The nurse would explain to the parents of a newborn with a cleft lip and palate that they will need to schedule an appointment with which specialist?
1. Cardiologist
2. Neurologist
3. Nutritionist
4. Otolaryngologist

19. 4. An appointment with an otolaryngologist is important because ear infections are common in the neonate with a cleft lip and palate, along with hearing loss. Brain and cardiac function are usually normal. A nutritionist is not needed unless the neonate becomes malnourished.
CN: Safe, effective care environment; CNS: Coordinated care;
CL: Apply; DIFFICULTY: Easy

You're doing udderly awesome! Seriously, you must be dairy smart. Okay—I think I've milked this joke for all it's worth.

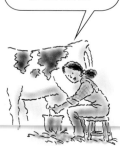

20. After an infant with a cleft lip has surgical repair and heals, the parents can expect to see which result?
1. Malaligned teeth
2. A larger upper lip
3. Distortion of the jaw
4. Minimal scarring

20. 4. If there is no trauma or infection to the site, healing occurs with little scar formation. There may be some inflammation right after surgery, but after healing, the lip is a normal size. No jaw malformation occurs with cleft lip repair.
CN: Physiological integrity; CNS: Physiological adaptation;
CL: Apply; DIFFICULTY: Easy

21. The nurse assesses a neonate with esophageal atresia for signs of dehydration. Which finding should the nurse expect to see?
1. Bulging of the eyeballs
2. A sunken anterior fontanel
3. Increase in the neonate's weight
4. Brisk return of the skin when pinched

21. 2. A sunken anterior fontanel is a sign of dehydration in the neonate whose fontanel has not yet closed. Bulging eyeballs and weight gain are signs of overhydration. Skin that returns quickly when pinched is a sign of adequate hydration.
CN: Physiological integrity; CNS: Reduction of risk potential;
CL: Apply; DIFFICULTY: Easy

CN: Client needs category   CNS: Client needs subcategory   CL: Cognitive level

22. Which assessment finding in a neonate born with esophageal atresia indicates to the nurse that the neonate needs suctioning?
  1. Cyanosis of the skin
  2. Reduced gag reflex
  3. Inadequate swallow reflex
  4. Reduced saliva production

23. The nurse is caring for a neonate suspected of having esophageal atresia. Which data collected by the nurse will correlate with this diagnosis?
  1. Decreased breath sounds
  2. Absent bowel sounds
  3. Inability to tolerate feeding
  4. Inability to aspirate gastric contents

24. Which intervention should the nurse expect to perform when caring for a neonate diagnosed with a tracheoesophageal fistula?
  1. Initiating antibiotic therapy
  2. Keeping the neonate lying flat
  3. Providing continuing feedings
  4. Removing the esophageal catheter

When aspiration pneumonia is a threat, I'm your guy.

25. Which intervention should the nurse perform **first** when caring for a neonate suspected of having tracheoesophageal fistula or esophageal atresia?
  1. Administer oxygen
  2. Inform the parents
  3. Lay the neonate in a radiant warmer.
  4. Report the suspicion to the health care provider

26. A nurse assigned to care for a neonate following the surgical repair of a tracheoesophageal fistula should prioritize nursing care interventions to prevent which postoperative complication?
  1. Atelectasis
  2. Choking
  3. Swelling
  4. Infection

22. 1. Cyanosis occurs when fluid from the blind pouch is aspirated into the trachea, requiring suctioning. Increased saliva production is common, along with choking, coughing, and sneezing. The ability to swallow is not affected by this disorder.
CN: Physiological integrity; CNS: Physiological adaptation; CL: Analyze; DIFFICULTY: Moderate

23. 4. In a neonate suspected of having esophageal atresia, a catheter will meet resistance and not reach the stomach because the esophagus is blocked. The neonate will not be able to aspirate gastric contents. If the esophagus is patent, the catheter will pass unobstructed to the stomach. Breath sounds and bowel sounds are not affected in esophageal atresia. The neonate who does not tolerate feedings might have any number of other conditions.
CN: Physiological integrity; CNS: Physiological adaptation; CL: Apply; DIFFICULTY: Challenge

24. 1. Antibiotic therapy is started for the neonate with a tracheoesophageal fistula because aspiration pneumonia is inevitable and appears early. The neonate's head is usually kept in an upright position to prevent aspiration. IV fluids are started, and the neonate is not allowed any oral intake. The catheter is left in the upper esophageal pouch to easily remove fluid that collects there.
CN: Safe, effective care environment; CNS: Coordinated care; CL: Apply; DIFFICULTY: Difficult

25. 4. Inform the health care provider when tracheoesophageal fistula or esophageal atresia is suspected so that immediate diagnostic tests can be done to confirm the diagnosis and surgical correction can begin. Oxygen should be given only after notifying the health care provider, except in the case of an emergency. It is not the nurse's responsibility to inform the parents of the suspected finding. By the time tracheoesophageal fistula or esophageal atresia is suspected, the neonate would have already been placed in an Isolette or a radiant warmer.
CN: Physiological integrity; CNS: Physiological adaptation; CL: Apply; DIFFICULTY: Challenge

26. 1. Respiratory complications (atelectasis) are a threat to the neonate's life preoperatively and postoperatively due to the continual risk of aspiration. Choking is more likely to occur preoperatively, although careful attention is paid postoperatively when neonates begin to eat to make sure they can swallow without choking. Vocal cord damage is not common after this repair. The neonate is generally given antibiotics preoperatively to prevent infection.
CN: Physiological integrity; CNS: Physiological adaptation; CL: Apply; DIFFICULTY: Difficult

27. Which initial sign should the nurse anticipate seeing in a neonate suspected of having esophageal atresia with a distal tracheoesophageal fistula?
1. Abdominal distention
2. Decreased oral secretions
3. Normal respiratory effort
4. A scaphoid abdomen

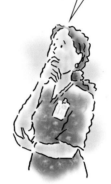

Hmm. I think the key word in this question is "immediately."

28. A neonate returns from the operating room after surgical repair of a tracheoesophageal fistula and esophageal atresia. Which intervention should the nurse perform **immediately**?
1. Maintain a patent airway.
2. Start feedings right away.
3. Let the parents hold the neonate right away.
4. Suction the trachea and stop when resistance is met.

29. Before discharging a neonate with a repaired tracheoesophageal fistula and esophageal atresia, the nurse would give the parents or caregivers instructions in which area?
1. Giving antibiotics
2. Preventing infection
3. Positioning techniques
4. Giving solid food

30. A nurse is reviewing the following progress note entry in a neonate's chart and suspects the neonate has which structural defect?

Progress notes	
9/29/16	4-day-old neonate male admitted with
1300	coughing, choking, and sneezing following
	feedings. Neonate's mother states, "He seems
	edto have a lot of saliva in his mouth and
	drools quite a bit."
	— S. Jones, L.P.N

1. Cleft lip
2. Cleft palate
3. Gastroschisis
4. Tracheoesophageal fistula

Your gastrointestinal system works hard for you round the clock. Be sure to give it high-quality fuel.

31. When assessing a neonate, the nurse notes visible peristaltic waves across the epigastrium. Which condition should the nurse suspect in this neonate?
1. Hypertrophic pyloric stenosis
2. Imperforate anus
3. Intussusception
4. Short-gut syndrome

27. 1. Crying may force air into the stomach, causing distention. Secretions in a client with this condition may be more visible, though normal in quantity, due to the client's inability to swallow effectively. Respiratory effort is usually more difficult. When no distal fistula is present, the abdomen will appear scaphoid.
CN: Physiological integrity; CNS: Physiological adaptation; CL: Apply; DIFFICULTY: Moderate

28. 1. Maintaining a patent airway is essential until sedation from surgery for repair of a tracheoesophageal fistula and esophageal atresia wears off. Feedings usually aren't started for at least 48 hours after surgery. Parents are encouraged to participate in the neonate's care but not immediately after surgery. Tracheal suctioning should be done only with a premeasured catheter to avoid injury to the surgical site.
CN: Physiological integrity; CNS: Physiological adaptation; CL: Apply; DIFFICULTY: Easy

29. 3. Positioning instructions should be given during hospitalization and before the neonate returns home. Antibiotics are usually discontinued before discharge. Preventing infection, especially at the operative sites, is a responsibility of the nurse postoperatively. For optimal effective respiration and because gastroesophageal reflux is a common complication, solid food usually isn't started until liquid feedings are tolerated and isn't given during the neonatal period.
CN: Physiological integrity; CNS: Basic care and comfort; CL: Apply; DIFFICULTY: Challenge

30. 4. Because of an ineffective swallow, saliva and secretions appear in the mouth and around the lips of the neonate with a tracheoesophageal fistula and esophageal atresia. Coughing, choking, and sneezing occur for the same reason and usually after an attempt at eating. Cleft lip and palate don't produce excessive salivation. None of these symptoms occurs with gastroschisis.
CN: Physiological integrity; CNS: Physiological adaptation; CL: Analyze; DIFFICULTY: Difficult

31. 1. The diagnosis of pyloric stenosis can be established from a finding of hypertrophic pyloric stenosis. Imperforate anus, intussusception, and short-gut syndrome are diagnosed by other symptoms.
CN: Physiological integrity; CNS: Physiological adaptation; CL: Analyze; DIFFICULTY: Moderate

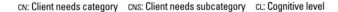

CN: Client needs category   CNS: Client needs subcategory   CL: Cognitive level

32. Which nursing intervention takes the **highest priority** during the first 24 hours following surgical repair of esophageal atresia and tracheoesophageal fistula?
1. Perform daily weights
2. Monitor for excessive secretions
3. Encourage maternal-infant bonding
4. Provide gastrostomy feedings

32. 2. The nursing intervention that takes the highest priority for the first postoperative day is monitoring for excessive secretions (airway clearance). The nurse must assess the infant's airway for the buildup of mucus and other secretions. The nurse must also carefully monitor the infant's respiratory status and keep suction equipment and a laryngoscope immediately available. Although the other nursing interventions are important in the immediate postoperative period, they do not take the highest priority.
CN: Safe, effective care environment; CNS: Coordinated care;
CL: Analyze; DIFFICULTY: Easy

33. Which nursing action helps verify that a nasogastric (NG) tube is properly positioned in a child's stomach?
1. Invert the tube into a glass of water and observe for bubbling.
2. Examine the aspirate with a pH test strip.
3. Clamp the tube for 10 minutes and listen with a stethoscope for increased peristalsis.
4. Instill 30 mL of normal saline solution and observe the child's response.

33. 2. To verify positioning of an NG tube, the gastric aspirate should be tested with a pH test strip. Probability of gastric placement is increased if the aspirate has a typical gastric fluid appearance (grassy green, clear and colorless with mucus shreds, or brown) and the pH is ≤7.0. Inverting the tube into a glass of water and observing for bubbling would be done to verify that an NG tube is in the respiratory tract. Clamping the tube and listening for increased peristalsis provides no information on the location of the tube. If the tube is in the respiratory tract, instilling normal saline causes respiratory distress.
CN: Physiological integrity; CNS: Reduction of risk potential;
CL: Understand; DIFFICULTY: Easy

34. The nurse caring for an infant with pyloric stenosis should be alert for which classic sign or symptom?
1. Loss of appetite
2. Chronic diarrhea
3. Projectile vomiting
4. Excessive drooling

This pyloric stenosis is killing me. I feel like I'm going to hurl.

34. 3. The obstruction seen in pyloric stenosis doesn't allow food to pass through to the duodenum. The classic sign of projectile vomiting occurs when the stomach becomes full, and the infant vomits for relief. Drooling would not be a finding in a child with pyloric stenosis but rather in a child with tracheoesophageal fistula. Chronic hunger is commonly seen. There's no diarrhea because food doesn't pass the stomach.
CN: Physiological integrity; CNS: Physiological adaptation;
CL: Analyze; DIFFICULTY: Easy

35. The mother of an infant with pyloric stenosis expresses feelings of guilt and fear that she may have caused her child's condition. Which response by the nurse is accurate?
1. "The cause of pyloric stenosis is unknown."
2. "The cause of pyloric stenosis is believed to be hereditary."
3. "Pyloric stenosis is typically caused by poor nutrition in pregnancy."
4. "Pyloric stenosis is directly related to poor muscle development in the stomach."

35. 1. The cause of the narrowing of the pyloric musculature is unknown. A hereditary link hasn't been established. Poor nutrition in pregnancy and poor muscle development in the stomach may relate to this defect, but they haven't been established as a definitive cause.
CN: Physiological integrity; CNS: Physiological adaptation;
CL: Analyze; DIFFICULTY: Challenge

36. A nurse admits an infant diagnosed with pyloric stenosis. Which nursing intervention should the nurse complete **first**?
1. Weigh the infant
2. Check urine specific gravity
3. Place an IV catheter
4. Change the infant and weigh the diaper

36. 1. Weighing the infant diagnosed with pyloric stenosis would be done first so that a baseline weight can be established and weight changes can be assessed. After a baseline weight is obtained, an IV catheter can be placed because oral feedings generally aren't given. These infants are usually dehydrated, so while checking the diaper and specific gravity are important tools to help assess their status, they aren't the first priority.
CN: Physiological integrity; CNS: Physiological adaptation; CL: Apply; DIFFICULTY: Moderate

37. The nurse completes the feeding for an infant with pyloric stenosis. In which position should the nurse place the infant after the feeding?
1. Prone without elevation
2. Supine in Fowler position
3. Left lateral in semi-Fowler position
4. Right lateral in high Fowler position

37. 4. Positioning the infant diagnosed with pyloric stenosis slightly on his right side in high Fowler position will help facilitate gastric emptying. The other positions won't facilitate gastric emptying and may cause the infant to vomit.
CN: Physiological integrity; CNS: Physiological adaptation; CL: Apply; DIFFICULTY: Moderate

38. When preparing to feed an infant with pyloric stenosis, which intervention should the nurse give **highest priority**?
1. Give feedings quickly.
2. Burp the infant frequently.
3. Discourage parental participation.
4. Discontinue feedings if the infant vomits.

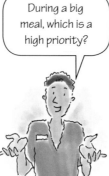

During a big meal, which is a high priority?

38. 2. Infants with pyloric stenosis usually swallow a lot of air from sucking on their hands and fingers because of their intense hunger (feedings aren't easily tolerated). Burping often lessens gastric distention and increases the likelihood the infant will retain the feeding. Feedings are given slowly with the infant lying in a semiupright position. Parental participation should be encouraged and allowed to the extent possible. Record the type, amount, and character of the vomit as well as its relation to the feeding. The amount of feeding volume lost is usually refed.
CN: Physiological integrity; CNS: Physiological adaptation; CL: Apply; DIFFICULTY: Challenge

39. Which common symptom would the nurse expect in an infant up to 48 hours after surgical repair of pyloric stenosis?
1. Dysuria
2. Oral aversion
3. Scaphoid abdomen
4. Vomiting

39. 4. Even with successful surgery for pyloric stenosis, most infants experience some vomiting during the first 24 to 48 hours after surgery. Dysuria isn't a complication with this surgical procedure. Oral aversion doesn't occur because these infants may be fed until surgery. Scaphoid abdomen isn't characteristic of pyloric stenosis. The abdomen may appear distended, not scaphoid.
CN: Physiological integrity; CNS: Physiological adaptation; CL: Analyze; DIFFICULTY: Moderate

40. Which intervention should the nurse perform to help prevent vomiting in an infant diagnosed with pyloric stenosis?
1. Hold the infant for 1 hour after feeding.
2. Handle the infant minimally after feedings.
3. Space out feedings and give large amounts.
4. Lay the infant prone with the head of the bed elevated.

40. 2. Minimal handling, especially after a feeding, will help prevent vomiting. Holding the infant would provide too much stimulation, increasing the risk of vomiting. Feedings are given frequently and slowly in small amounts. An infant should be positioned in semi-Fowler position and slightly on the right side after a feeding.
CN: Physiological integrity; CNS: Physiological adaptation; CL: Apply; DIFFICULTY: Moderate

41. Which nursing intervention provides the **best** support to the parents of an infant diagnosed with pyloric stenosis?
1. Keep the parents informed of the infant's progress.
2. Provide all care for the infant, even when the parents visit.
3. Tell the parents to minimize handling of the infant at all times.
4. Tell the health care provider to keep the parents informed of the infant's progress.

41. 1. Keeping the parents informed of their child's progress will decrease their anxiety. The nurse should encourage the parents to be involved with the infant's care. Telling the parents to minimize handling of the infant isn't appropriate because parent-child contact is important. The health care provider is responsible for updating the parents on the infant's medical condition, and the nurse is responsible for updating the parents on the day-to-day activities of the infant and his improvement with the day's activities.
CN: Psychosocial integrity; CNS: None; CL: Analyze; DIFFICULTY: Easy

42. Which symptom would the nurse **most** likely find in an infant diagnosed with pyloric stenosis?
1. Slow response to stimuli
2. Irregular heart rate
3. Dryness of the lips
4. Low body temperature

42. 3. Dry lips and skin are signs of dehydration, which is common in infants with pyloric stenosis. These infants are constantly hungry due to their inability to retain feedings. A slow response to stimuli, dysrhythmias, and hypothermia are not clinical findings with pyloric stenosis.
CN: Physiological integrity; CNS: Physiological adaptation; CL: Apply; DIFFICULTY: Moderate

43. Which finding should the nurse anticipate when assessing an infant diagnosed with pyloric stenosis?
1. Decreased bowel sounds
2. Irregular heart murmur
3. Normal respiratory effort
4. Increased bowel sounds

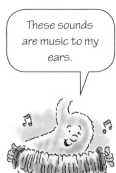

These sounds are music to my ears.

43. 1. Bowel sounds decrease in an infant with pyloric stenosis because food can't pass into the intestines. Normal respiratory effort is adversely affected due to the abdominal distention that pushes the diaphragm up into the pleural cavity. Heart murmurs may be present but aren't directly associated with pyloric stenosis.
CN: Physiological integrity; CNS: Physiological adaptation; CL: Analyze; DIFFICULTY: Moderate

44. The nurse admits a child who has a suspected bowel obstruction. Which assessment finding should the nurse anticipate in this child? Select all that apply.
1. Abdominal distention
2. Hyperactive bowel sounds
3. Low grade fever
4. Abdominal pain
5. Vomiting

44. 1, 4, 5. Children with a bowel obstruction may have various symptoms depending on the cause of the obstruction. General assessment finding include abdominal pain, abdominal distention, diarrheal stool leakage around the obstruction, soiling, nausea, and vomiting. A low-grade fever may or may not be present depending on symptoms of dehydration. Bowel sounds are usually hypoactive.
CN: Physiological integrity; CNS: Physiological adaptation; CL: Apply; DIFFICULTY: Difficult

45. Which nursing intervention takes **priority** when caring for a child who has been poisoned?
1. Stabilize the child
2. Notify the parents
3. Identify the poison
4. Determine when it occurred

45. 1. Stabilization and the initial emergency treatment of the child (such as respiratory assistance, circulatory support, or control of seizures) will prevent further damage to the body from the poison. If the parents didn't bring the child in, they can be notified as soon as the child is stabilized or treated. Although identification of the poison is crucial and should begin at the same time as the stabilization of the child, the assessment of airway, breathing, and circulation should occur first. Determining when the poisoning took place is an important consideration, but emergency stabilization and treatment are most important.
CN: Physiological integrity; CNS: Physiological adaptation; CL: Apply; DIFFICULTY: Challenge

46. A preschooler is brought to the emergency department after ingesting a large amount of liquid acetaminophen. Which assessment finding should the nurse anticipate in this child?
1. Bradycardia
2. Hypertension
3. Tachypnea
4. Tinnitus

47. A nurse admits a child that has been treated in the emergency department after ingesting drain cleaner. Which interventions should the nurse include in this child's plan of care? Select all that apply.
1. Evaluate vital signs for subtle changes.
2. Assess the child's ability to speak.
3. Monitor for fluid balance disturbances.
4. Assess for swelling of the tongue.
5. Position the child flat in bed.

48. A parent brings a child to the clinic after ingestion of a poisonous substance. Which **priority** action should the nurse take?
1. Induce vomiting with syrup of ipecac.
2. Notify the health care provider immediately.
3. Give large amounts of water to drink.
4. Assess the child for additional symptoms.

49. A parent brings a child to the emergency department after ingesting a poisonous hydrocarbon., What is a **priority** nursing action?
1. Induce vomiting.
2. Keep the child calm and relaxed.
3. Scold the child for the wrongdoing.
4. Keep the parents away from the child.

50. The nurse caring for a child with an extreme case of salicylate poisoning should prepare the child for which treatment?
1. Gastric lavage
2. Hypothermia blankets
3. Peritoneal dialysis
4. Vitamin K injection

You're doing great. Keep riding that wave!

46. 1. A weak-slow pulse (bradycardia), diaphoresis, pallor, hypothermia, nausea and vomiting, and right upper quadrant pain are all signs of acetaminophen poisoning. The other conditions are not associated with acetaminophen ingestion.
CN: Physiological integrity; CNS: Physiological adaptation; CL: Apply; DIFFICULTY: Difficult

47. 1, 2, 4. Subtle changes in vital signs can indicate changes in oxygenation in children. Assessing the ability to speak and for tongue swelling helps to determine airway compromise and patency. Fluid balance disturbances do not commonly occur after drain cleaner ingestion. The child should be positioned semi-Fowler's or high Fowler's to maintain airway patency and to prevent aspiration if the child is vomiting.
CN: Physiological integrity; CNS: Physiological adaptation; CL: Analyze; DIFFICULTY: Challenge

48. 2. Notify the health care provider first so that appropriate care is initiated. Inducing vomiting is important but is contraindicated with some poisons. Only small amounts of water are recommended so the poison is confined to the smallest volume. Large amounts of water will let the poison pass the pylorus. The small intestines absorb fluid rapidly, increasing the risk of toxicity.
CN: Physiological integrity; CNS: Physiological adaptation; CL: Apply; DIFFICULTY: Moderate

49. 2. Keeping the child calm and relaxed will help prevent vomiting in a child who has ingested poisonous hydrocarbons. If vomiting occurs, there's a great chance the esophagus will be damaged from regurgitation of the gastric poison. Additionally, the risk of chemical pneumonitis exists if vomiting occurs. Scolding the child may upset him. The parents should remain with the child to help keep him calm.
CN: Physiological integrity; CNS: Physiological adaptation; CL: Apply; DIFFICULTY: Challenge

50. 3. Peritoneal dialysis is usually reserved for cases of life-threatening salicylism. Gastric lavage is the immediate treatment for salicylate poisoning because the stomach contents and salicylates will move from the stomach to the remainder of the GI tract, where vomiting will no longer result in the removal of the poison. Hypothermia blankets may be used to reduce the possibility of seizures. Vitamin K may be used to decrease bleeding tendencies but only if evidence of this exists.
CN: Physiological integrity; CNS: Physiological adaptation; CL: Analyze; DIFFICULTY: Challenge

51. When a child has been poisoned, identifying the ingested poison is an important treatment goal. Which action would help determine which poison was ingested?
1. Call the local poison control center.
2. Ask the child.
3. Ask the parents.
4. Save all evidence of poison.

52. A nurse is reinforcing the education about salicylate poisoning to a parent. Which education information by the nurse is the **most** important?
1. Identify the salicylate overdose level.
2. Educate children on the hazards of ingesting nonfood items.
3. Decrease the child's curiosity by educating parents about keeping aspirin and drugs in clear view.
4. Teach parents to keep large amounts of drugs on hand but out of reach of children.

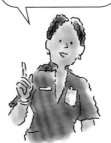

Only one of these interventions would actually help prevent poisoning.

53. A nurse is aware that which condition is the **most** likely to develop as a result of an acute overdose of acetaminophen?
1. Brain damage
2. Heart failure
3. Hepatic damage
4. Kidney damage

54. A child is diagnosed with acetaminophen poisoning. Which sign would the nurse expect when assessing the client 12 to 24 hours after ingestion?
1. Hyperthermia
2. Increased urine output
3. Profuse sweating
4. Rapid pulse

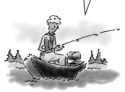

Fishing for the right answer takes time. Be patient and keep at it.

55. A nurse is evaluating the effectiveness of therapy with acetylcysteine in a child with acetaminophen poisoning. Which laboratory values would be **most** important for the nurse to monitor?
1. Serum alanine aminotransferase (ALT)
2. Serum calcium levels
3. Prothrombin time (PT)
4. Serum glucose levels

51. 4. Saving all evidence of poison (container, vomitus, urine) will help determine which drug was ingested and how much. Calling the local poison control center may help get information on specific poisons or determine if a certain household placed a call; rarely can they help determine which poison has been ingested. Asking the child may help, but the child may fear punishment and may not be honest about the incident. The parent may be helpful in some instances but not if the parent wasn't present when the ingestion occurred.
CN: Physiological integrity; CNS: Reduction of risk potential;
CL: Apply; DIFFICULTY: Moderate

52. 2. Educating children on the hazards of ingesting nonfood items will help prevent ingestion of poisonous substances. Identifying the overdose level won't prevent it from occurring. Aspirin and drugs should be kept out of the sight and reach of children. Parents should be warned about keeping large amounts of drugs on hand.
CN: Health promotion and maintenance; CNS: None; CL: Analyze;
DIFFICULTY: Moderate

53. 3. The damage to the hepatic system isn't from acetaminophen but from one of its metabolites. This metabolite binds to liver cells in large quantities. Brain damage, heart failure, and kidney damage may develop later but not initially.
CN: Physiological integrity; CNS: Physiological adaptation;
CL: Apply; DIFFICULTY: Challenge

54. 3. During the first 12 to 24 hours, profuse sweating is a significant sign of acetaminophen poisoning. Weak pulse, hypothermia, and decreased urine output are also common findings.
CN: Physiological integrity; CNS: Physiological adaptation;
CL: Analyze; DIFFICULTY: Challenge

55. 1. Acetaminophen poisoning damages the liver, leading to elevated ALT and AST levels. After therapy with acetylcysteine is started, these liver enzyme levels should begin to decrease. Serum calcium levels may fall following chelation therapy in children with lead poisoning. Because PT is elevated and blood glucose levels are reduced with salicylate poisoning, the nurse should observe that the PT and blood glucose levels return to normal after treatment is initiated.
CN: Physiological integrity; CNS: Reduction of risk potential;
CL: Analyze; DIFFICULTY: Easy

56. The ingestion of substances containing lead is mostly influenced by which **risk** factor?
1. Child's age
2. Child's gender
3. Child's nationality
4. A parent with the same habit

56. 1. The highest risk of lead poisoning occurs in young children who tend to put things in their mouths. In older homes that contain lead-based paint, paint chips may be eaten directly by the child, or they may cling to toys or hands that are then put into the child's mouth. Poisoning isn't gender-related. Blacks have a higher incidence of lead poisoning, but it can happen in any race. Children of low socioeconomic status are more likely to eat lead-based paint chips. Most parents don't eat lead-based paint on purpose.
CN: Health promotion and maintenance; CNS: None; CL: Understand; DIFFICULTY: Easy

57. An infant is admitted to the hospital with gastroenteritis. Which nursing intervention takes **priority** in the infant's plan of care?
1. Observing for signs of pain
2. Introducing oral feedings as indicated
3. Monitoring for decreased urine output
4. Assessing the infant's skin turgor

57. 3. Monitoring for decreased urinary output is a priority. If urinary output decreases while the child is receiving treatment for gastroenteritis it should be reported to the health care provider. Young children with gastroenteritis are at high risk for developing a fluid volume deficit. Their intestinal mucosa allows for more fluid and electrolytes to be lost when they have gastroenteritis. The main goal of the health care team should be to rehydrate the infant. The other nursing interventions are important, but decreased urine output (indicates deficient fluid volume) is the most life threatening.
CN: Physiological integrity; CNS: Physiological adaptation; CL: Apply; DIFFICULTY: Challenge

58. The nurse explains to the parent of a child with lead poisoning that x-rays are necessary. What is the **best** response by the nurse when the parent questions the necessity of the x-ray?,
1. Lead is initially absorbed by bone.
2. Lead is initially stored in the brain and will cause dementia.
3. Lead is initially stored in the kidney and will cause renal failure.
4. Lead is initially stored in the liver and will cause cirrhosis

58. 1. Ingested lead is initially absorbed by bone. If chronic ingestion occurs, then the hematologic, renal, and central nervous systems are affected.
CN: Physiological integrity; CNS: Physiological adaptation; CL: Apply; DIFFICULTY: Difficult

59. When monitoring a child with lead poisoning, the nurse should be alert for which condition that commonly appears **first**?
1. Anemia
2. Diarrhea
3. Overeating
4. Paralysis

Lead poisoning really does a number on red blood cells.

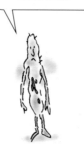

59. 1. Lead is dangerously toxic to the biosynthesis of heme. The reduced heme molecule in red blood cells causes anemia. Constipation (not diarrhea) and a poor appetite and vomiting (not overeating) are signs of lead poisoning. Paralysis may occur as toxic damage to the brain progresses, but it isn't an initial sign.
CN: Physiological integrity; CNS: Physiological adaptation; CL: Analyze; DIFFICULTY: Challenge

60. The nurse is gathering data from a child suspected of ingesting paint chips from an old home. Which system does the nurse closely monitor for serious effects?
1. Central nervous system (CNS)
2. Hematologic system
3. Renal system
4. Respiratory system

60. 1. Damage that occurs to the CNS after lead poisoning is difficult to repair. Damage to the renal and hematologic systems can be reversed if treated early. The respiratory system is not affected until coma and death occur.
CN: Physiological integrity; CNS: Physiological adaptation; CL: Understand; DIFFICULTY: Moderate

CN: Client needs category   CNS: Client needs subcategory   CL: Cognitive level

61. Which nursing outcome would be **most** important for a child with lead poisoning who must undergo chelation therapy?
1. Prepare the child for complete bed rest.
2. Prepare the child for IV fluid therapy.
3. Prepare the child for an extended hospital stay.
4. Prepare the child for a large number of injections.

61. 4. Chelation therapy involves receiving a large number of injections in a relatively short period. It is traumatic to most children, and they need some preparation for the treatment. The other listed components of the treatment plan are important but not as likely to cause the same anxiety as multiple injections. Receiving IV fluid isn't as traumatizing as multiple injections. Physical activity is usually limited so as to not aggravate the painful injection sites.

CN: Physiological integrity; CNS: Physiological adaptation; CL: Apply; DIFFICULTY: Challenge

62. A child is admitted to the floor after being treated in the emergency department with gastric lavage for ingestion of a bottle of acetaminophen. The nurse has orders to administer N-acetylcysteine 140 mg/kg stat. The child weighs 15 pounds. The package label reads 2 gram in 40 mL of a 5% solution. How many mL should the nurse prepare to administer? Record your answer using one decimal place.

_____ mL

62. 38.1.
Convert child's weight to kg (1 kg = 2.2 lb)

$$15\,lb / 2.2 = 6.8\,kilograms$$

Multiply child's weight in kilograms × 140 mg/kg

$$6.8\,kilograms \times 140\,mg/kg = 952\,mg$$
$$of\ N\ acetylcysteine$$

Convert 2 grams to mg by multiplying by 1,000 (1 gram = 1,000 mg)

$$2\,grams \times 1,000\,mg / gram = 2,000\,mg$$

Use the formula Dose desired/Dose on hand × Form of the drug

$$952\,mg / 2,000\,mg \times 40\,mL = 38.1\,mL$$
$$administered$$

CN: Physiological integrity; CNS: Pharmacological therapies; CL: Apply; DIFFICULTY: Difficult

63. A nurse is caring for a 5-year-old child who exhibits signs of lead poisoning. The nurse should assess the child for which signs?
1. Nausea, vomiting, seizures, and coma
2. Jaundice, confusion, and coagulation abnormalities
3. Insomnia, weight loss, diarrhea, and gingivitis
4. General fatigue, difficulty concentrating, tremors, and headache

63. 4. Signs and symptoms of lead poisoning depend on the degree of toxicity. General fatigue, difficulty concentrating, tremors, and headache indicate moderate toxicity. Nausea, vomiting, seizures, and coma are observed in salicylate and iron poisoning. Jaundice, confusion, and coagulation abnormalities are observed in acetaminophen poisoning. Insomnia, weight loss, diarrhea, and gingivitis are observed in mercury poisoning.

CN: Physiological integrity; CNS: Physiological adaptation; CL: Analyze; DIFFICULTY: Challenge

In question #64, look for the best intervention.

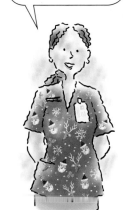

64. Which nursing intervention is the **best** way to help reduce the occurrence of poisoning in children?
1. Teach parents to put child locks on doors and cabinets.
2. Provide education to those who care for children.
3. Identify children who are at risk of poisoning.
4. Teach parents to read toy labels.

64. 2. Educating those who care for children about poisoning is the best way to reduce the occurrence of poisoning. Identifying high-risk groups will help but won't reduce poisoning. Reading toy labels will help to identify toys that may contain lead and may help reduce lead exposure.

CN: Health promotion and maintenance; CNS: None; CL: Apply; DIFFICULTY: Difficult

CN: Client needs category   CNS: Client needs subcategory   CL: Cognitive level

65. Which condition should the nurse closely monitor that may occur during chelation therapy in a child with lead poisoning?
1. Hypercalcemia
2. Hypocalcemia
3. Hyperglycemia
4. Hypoglycemia

65. 2. A calcium chelating agent is used for the treatment of lead poisoning, so calcium is removed from the body with the lead. Hypocalcemia, not hypercalcemia, occurs. Hyperglycemia and hypoglycemia don't occur as a result of chelation therapy.
CN: Physiological integrity; CNS: Physiological adaptation;
CL: Analyze; DIFFICULTY: Moderate

66. Which symptom should the nurse assess for in a child suspected of having acute appendicitis?
1. Reports pain in epigastric area
2. Decreased heart rate
3. Elevated temperature
4. Pain descending to the lower left quadrant

66. 3. Elevated temperature (fever), abdominal pain, and tenderness are the first symptoms of appendicitis. Tachycardia, not bradycardia, is seen. Pain can be generalized or periumbilical. It usually descends to the lower right quadrant, not to the left and not to the legs.
CN: Physiological integrity; CNS: Physiological adaptation;
CL: Apply; DIFFICULTY: Difficult

67. Which advice should a nurse give over the phone to the parent of a 7-year-old child with right lower abdominal pain, fever, and vomiting?
1. "Give prune juice to relieve constipation."
2. "Test for rebound tenderness in the left lower abdominal quadrant."
3. "Encourage fluids to prevent dehydration."
4. "Seek immediate emergency medical care."

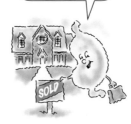

Keeping your gastrointestinal system healthy is always a good investment.

67. 4. The parent of a child with abdominal pain, fever, and vomiting (the cardinal signs of appendicitis) should be urged to seek immediate emergency care to reduce the risk of complications from potential appendix rupture. Prune juice has laxative effects and shouldn't be given because laxatives increase the risk of rupture of the appendix. Testing for rebound tenderness may elicit McBurney's sign in the right lower quadrant (an indication of appendicitis); however, the nurse shouldn't rely on the parent's findings. The child should be given nothing by mouth in case surgery is needed.
CN: Physiological integrity; CNS: Reduction of risk potential;
CL: Apply; DIFFICULTY: Easy

68. Which nursing intervention is important for the nurse to perform preoperatively for a child with appendicitis?
1. Give clear fluids.
2. Apply heat to the abdomen.
3. Maintain complete bed rest.
4. Administer an enema, if ordered.

68. 3. Bed rest will prevent aggravating the condition. Clients with appendicitis aren't allowed anything by mouth. Cold applications are placed on the abdomen, as heat would increase blood flow to the area and possibly spread infection. Enemas may aggravate appendicitis.
CN: Physiological integrity; CNS: Physiological adaptation;
CL: Apply; DIFFICULTY: Moderate

69. Postoperative nursing care of a child with peritonitis from a ruptured appendix would include which intervention?
1. Give a liquid-only diet.
2. Give oral antibiotics for 7 to 10 days.
3. Position the child on his left side.
4. Give parenteral antibiotics for 7 to 10 days.

69. 4. Parenteral antibiotics are used for 7 to 10 days postoperatively to help prevent the spread of peritonitis infection. The child is kept on IV fluids and isn't allowed anything by mouth. Oral antibiotics may continue after the parenteral antibiotics are discontinued. The child is positioned on his right side after surgery.
CN: Physiological integrity; CNS: Physiological adaptation;
CL: Apply; DIFFICULTY: Moderate

70. After surgical repair of a ruptured appendix, which position would be **most** appropriate for the nurse to place the child?
1. High Fowler position
2. Left side-lying
3. Semi-Fowler position
4. Supine with knees flexed

71. The nurse assesses the laboratory results for a 9-year-old child hospitalized with severe vomiting and diarrhea. Which serum potassium level would the nurse expect to see in this child?
1. 4.5 to 7.2 mmol/L
2. 4.7 to 6.0 mmol/L
3. 2.5 to 3.4 mmol/L
4. 3.5 to 5.8 mmol/L

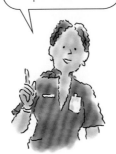

Severe vomiting and diarrhea can lead to a loss of potassium.

72. A neonate is suspected of having a tracheo-esophageal fistula type III/C. Which sign should the nurse expect to see on the initial assessment?
1. Excessive drooling
2. Distended abdomen
3. Mottling of the skin
4. Slow respiratory rate

73. A 5-year-old child is admitted with diarrhea and vomiting for the past 2 days. Vital signs are temperature, 98.8° F (37.1° C); pulse, 132 beats/minute; respirations, 28 breaths/minute; and blood pressure, 88/56 mm Hg. The nurse notes poor skin turgor, dry mucous membranes, and tearless crying. Which intervention should the nurse perform next in this child's care?
1. Obtain a stool specimen, complete blood count (CBC), and blood chemistries.
2. Implement nothing-by-mouth (NPO) status and start an IV.
3. Begin offering an oral electrolyte solution.
4. Obtain a blood culture and sensitivity test.

70. 3. Semi-Fowler or right side-lying positions after surgery for a ruptured appendix will facilitate drainage from the peritoneal cavity and prevents the formation of a subdiaphragmatic abscess. High Fowler, left side-lying, and supine positions will not facilitate drainage from the peritoneal cavity.
CN: Physiological integrity; CNS: Physiological adaptation; CL: Apply; DIFFICULTY: Difficult

71. 3. Potassium is lost through diarrhea and is expected to be low normal or low. A level below 3.5 mmol/L should be expected with severe diarrhea. The normal potassium level in children ranges from 3.5 to 5.8 mmol/L. Levels of 4.5 to 7.2 mmol/L are observed in premature infants. Potassium levels of 3.7 to 5.2 mmol/L are observed in full-term infants. Potassium levels of 3.5 to 5.5 mmol/L are usually seen in adults.
CN: Physiological integrity; CNS: Reduction of risk potential; CL: Remember; DIFFICULTY: Challenge

72. 1. In type III/C tracheoesophageal fistula, the proximal end of the esophagus ends in a blind pouch and a fistula connects the distal end of the esophagus to the trachea. Saliva will pool in this pouch and cause the child to drool. Because the distal end of the esophagus is connected to the trachea, the neonate cannot vomit, but can aspirate, and stomach acid may go into the lungs through this fistula, causing pneumonitis. Mottling is a net-like, reddish-blue discoloration of the skin usually due to vascular contraction in response to hypothermia. Tachypnea may be present but not bradypnea (slow respiratory rate).
CN: Physiological integrity; CNS: Physiological adaptation; CL: Apply; DIFFICULTY: Moderate

73. 2. This child shows signs of severe dehydration and should be put on NPO status in order to rest the bowel. An IV should be started immediately to begin the rehydration process. A stool specimen; HCT, CBC, and chemistries; and IV antibiotics may be ordered, but they aren't the priority intervention. There's no reason to suspect that the child will need a blood culture at this time because the temperature isn't elevated.
CN: Physiological integrity; CNS: Basic care and comfort; CL: Analyze; DIFFICULTY: Challenge

74. When assessing a client suspected of having pyloric stenosis, which finding should the nurse expect?
1. An "olive" mass in the right upper quadrant
2. An "olive" mass in the left upper quadrant
3. A "sausage" mass in the right upper quadrant
4. A "sausage" mass in the left upper quadrant

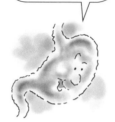

Yuck! I never did like olives and sausages.

74. 1. Pyloric stenosis involves hypertrophy of the circular muscle fibers of the pylorus. This hypertrophy is palpable as an "olive" mass in the right upper quadrant of the abdomen. A "sausage" mass is palpable in the right upper quadrant in children with intussusception. A "sausage" mass in the left upper quadrant doesn't indicate pyloric stenosis.
CN: Physiological integrity; CNS: Physiological adaptation; CL: Analyze; DIFFICULTY: Moderate

75. The nurse caring for an infant with pyloric stenosis would expect which laboratory values?
1. pH, 7.30; chloride, 120 mEq/L
2. pH, 7.38; chloride, 110 mEq/L
3. pH, 7.43; chloride, 100 mEq/L
4. pH, 7.49; chloride, 90 mEq/L

75. 4. Infants with pyloric stenosis vomit hydrochloric acid. This causes them to become alkalotic and hypochloremic. Normal serum pH is 7.35 to 7.45; levels above 7.45 represent alkalosis. The normal serum chloride level is 99 to 111 mEq/L; levels below 99 mEq/L represent hypochloremia.
CN: Physiological integrity; CNS: Physiological adaptation; CL: Apply; DIFFICULTY: Challenge

76. A 13-month-old is admitted to the pediatric unit with a diagnosis of gastroenteritis. The toddler has experienced vomiting and diarrhea for the past 3 days, and laboratory tests reveal that the child is dehydrated. Which nursing interventions are correct to prevent further dehydration? Select all that apply.
1. Encourage the child to eat a balanced diet.
2. Give clear liquids in small amounts.
3. Give milk in small amounts.
4. Encourage the child to eat non-salty soups and broths.
5. Monitor the IV solution per the health care provider's order.
6. Withhold all solid food and liquids until the symptoms pass.

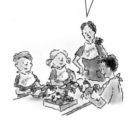

Nothing makes me crabbier than a bad case of gastroenteritis.

76. 2, 4, 5. A child experiencing nausea and vomiting won't be able to tolerate a regular diet. The child should be given sips of clear liquids, and the diet should be advanced as tolerated. Unsalted soups and broths are appropriate clear liquids. IV fluids should be monitored to maintain the fluid status and help to rehydrate the child. Milk shouldn't be given because it can worsen the child's diarrhea. Solid foods may be withheld throughout the acute phase, but clear fluids should be encouraged in small amounts (3 to 4 tablespoons every half hour).
CN: Physiological integrity; CNS: Basic care and comfort; CL: Apply; DIFFICULTY: Difficult

77. Which nursing intervention has the **highest priority** in the care of a 1-month-old infant admitted with projectile vomiting after feeding?
1. Providing small, frequent, thickened feedings
2. Positioning child on the right side
3. Promoting breast-feeding
4. Weighing the infant daily

77. 2. Projectile vomiting in infants is a sign of pyloric stenosis, a condition that requires surgical correction. Positioning aspiration is a priority before and after surgical intervention. This is accomplished by positioning the infant on his right side or by elevating the head of the bassinette or crib slightly. Providing thickened and small, frequent feedings is a correct choice but is not a priority over airway clearance. Promoting breast-feeding is also a correct choice but is not a priority in this situation. Fluid and electrolyte imbalances can occur because of the vomiting, and the nurse should monitor for this by weighing the infant and monitoring for signs and symptoms of electrolyte imbalance; however, maintaining a patent airway takes priority.
CN: Physiological integrity; CNS: Reduction of risk potential; CL: Analyze; DIFFICULTY: Moderate

78. A nurse is assigned the care of a child who is prescribed activated charcoal dosing 1 gram/kg orally via NG tube once. The child weighs 51 pounds. The package insert reads, dilute 20-30 grams in 240 mL of water. How many grams of activated charcoal should the nurse administer to the child? Record your answer using a whole number.

_____ g

78. 23.

Convert child's weight to kilograms
(2.2 lb = 1 kg):

$$51\,\text{lb} \div 2.2\,\text{lb} / \text{kg} = 23.13\,\text{kg}.$$

Multiply child's weight in kilograms by the dose:

$$23.13\,\text{kg} \times 1\,\text{gram} / \text{kg} = 23.13\,\text{grams of}$$
activated charcoal

CN: Physiological integrity; CNS: Pharmacological therapies;
CL: Apply; DIFFICULTY: Difficult

79. Which medication should the nurse prepare to administer for a child with confirmed ingestion of a toxic amount of acetaminophen?
1. Sodium bicarbonate
2. Dimercaprol
3. Acetylcysteine
4. Syrup of Ipecac

79. 3. N-acetylcysteine is the antidote for acetaminophen overdose. Sodium bicarbonate is given for salicylate poisoning to correct the metabolic acidosis. Dimercaprol and deferoxamine are given for lead poisoning.

CN: Physiological integrity; CNS: Pharmacological therapies;
CL: Apply; DIFFICULTY: Moderate

80. Which interventions should the nurse perform when evaluating a child for a suspected ingestion of household bleach? Select all that apply.
1. Obtain a complete set of vital signs
2. Inspect the mouth and oropharynx
3. Administer activated charcoal
4. Monitor respiratory status
5. Offer oral fluids
6. Induce vomiting

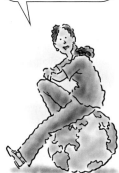

Congrats— you finished the chapter! You're on top of the world.

80. 1, 2. Inspection of the face, mouth, and oropharynx gathers assessment data to support to a suspected ingestion of bleach. The mucous membranes, lips, and oropharynx will have a white appearance. Obtaining a complete set of vital signs provides additional data for the assessment (opening the mouth to get an oral temperature depending on the age of the child is an ideal time to inspect the oral cavity). Monitoring respiratory status is important; however, there is nothing in the question that indicates the child is having trouble breathing and gathering data that assists in confirming bleach ingestion should be completed first. Administering activated charcoal and offering oral fluids are treatment interventions, not evaluations. Inducing vomiting is an incorrect treatment for the ingestion of a corrosive agent (suspected or confirmed).

CN: Physiological integrity; CNS: Physiological adaptation;
CL: Apply; DIFFICULTY: Challenge

Chapter 32

Endocrine Disorders

Pediatric endocrine refresher

Diabetes mellitus type 1

Chronic metabolic syndrome that is auto-immune in origin. Destruction of the beta cells of the pancreas results in lack of insulin production

Key signs and symptoms
- Polydipsia
- Polyphagia
- Polyuria
- Insidious onset with lethargy, weakness, and weight loss
- If left untreated, ketoacidosis will develop

Key test results
- Fasting plasma glucose level (no calorie intake for at least 8 hours) is greater than or equal to 126 mg/dL
- Plasma glucose value in the 2-hour sample of the oral glucose tolerance test is greater than or equal to 200 mg/dL; this test should be performed after a loading dose of 75 g of anhydrous glucose
- A random plasma glucose value (obtained without regard to the time of the child's last food intake) greater than or equal to 200 mg/dL accompanied by symptoms of diabetes indicates diabetes
- Glycosylated hemoglobin (HbA1c): 6%-9% represents good control, values greater than 12% indicate poor control

Key treatments
- Well-balanced diet that meets growth and development needs while distributing food intake so that the diet aids metabolic control; should be individualized in accordance with the child's ethnicity, age, sex, weight, activity level, family economics and personal preference
- Precise insulin administration
- Regular exercise

Key interventions
- Monitor vital signs, intake and output, and blood glucose
- Provide appropriate treatment for hyperglycemia and hypoglycemia

- Teach the child and parents about:
  - adhering to the prescribed treatment program
  - monitoring blood glucose levels at home
  - rotating injection sites
  - preventing, recognizing, and treating hypoglycemia and hyperglycemia at home

Hypothyroidism

Deficiency in hormone secretions of the thyroid gland

Key signs and symptoms

Untreated hypothyroidism in infants
- Hoarse crying
- Persistent jaundice
- Puffy face and swollen tongue
- Sluggish, sleeps a lot, floppy when handled
- If left untreated, irreversible mental retardation and physical disabilities result

Untreated hypothyroidism in older children
- Stunted growth (short stature)
- Cognitive impairment
- Weight gain

Key test results
- Radioimmunoassay confirms hypothyroidism with low triiodothyronine and thyroxine levels
- Screening test for hypothyroidism is mandatory in the U.S. and is performed at birth

Key treatments
- Oral thyroid hormone (thyroxine)
- Supplemental vitamin D to prevent rickets from rapid bone growth

Key interventions
- During early management of infantile hypothyroidism, monitor blood pressure and pulse rate and report hypertension and tachycardia immediately (normal infant heart rate is approximately 120 beats/minute)

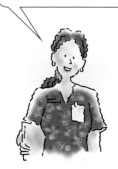

Caring for a child with an endocrine system disorder can be overwhelming. To get started on the right track, check out the Web site of the Juvenile Diabetes Research Foundation at www.jdrf.org/. Go for it!

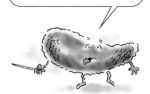

When it comes to diabetes mellitus type 1, remember the three poly's: -dipsia, -phagia, and -uria.

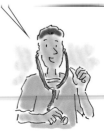

Hypothyroidism means low (hypo) hormone secretions from the thyroid gland.

- Check axillary temperature every 2 to 4 hours; keep infant warm and skin moist
- If infant's tongue is unusually large, position on his side and observe frequently
- Teach child and parents to recognize signs of supplemental thyroid hormone overdose (rapid pulse rate, irritability, insomnia, fever, sweating, weight loss)

Diabetes insipidus

Insufficient antidiuretic hormone (ADH) secreted by the pituitary gland, resulting in excretion of copious volumes of urine

Key signs and symptoms

- Polydipsia (consumption of 4 to 40 L/day)
- Polyuria (greater than 5 L/day of dilute urine)
- Dehydration
- Infant: Irritability, poor feeding, failure to grow, high fevers

Key test results

- Urine chemistry shows:
  - urine specific gravity less than 1.005
  - osmolality 50 to 200 mOsm/kg
  - decreased urine pH
  - decreased sodium and potassium levels

Key treatments

- IV therapy: hydration (when first diagnosed, intake and output must be matched milliliter to milliliter to prevent dehydration), electrolyte replacement
- Synthetic drugs with ADH activity that reduce urine output: desmopressin acetate nasal solution or lypressin nasal spray

Key interventions

- Monitor fluid balance and daily weight
- Monitor and record vital signs, intake and output (urine output should be measured every hour when first diagnosed), urine specific gravity (check every 1 to 2 hours when first diagnosed), and laboratory studies

- Maintain IV fluid
- Teach family about medication: signs and symptoms of disorder which indicate a need for desmopressin acetate, and signs and symptoms of overdosage (decreased urine output, headache, fluid retention, weight gain)

Growth hormone deficiency (idiopathic hypopituitarism or idiopathic growth hormone failure)

Diminished secretion of growth hormone by the pituitary gland

Key signs and symptoms

- Short stature but proportional height and weight
- Delayed epiphyseal closure

Key test results

- Decreased growth hormone levels (peak < 10 ng/mL on stimulation test)
- Insulin-like growth factor 1 (IGF-1)
- Bone-age radiographs of the hand

Key treatments

- Recombinant human growth hormone replacement by subcutaneous injection usually daily at bedtime
- Growth hormone therapy lasts until the conclusion of growth during late puberty

Key interventions

- Accurate measurement, documentation, and interpretation of height
- Family teaching regarding medication administration (technique for administration, site selection and rotation, administer at bedtime)
- Child 10 years of age or older can learn to self-administer the drug
- Promote positive body image

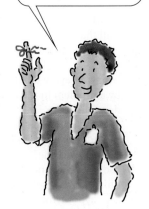

Remember—polyuria means "much urine"; that is, you have to pee a lot.

Endocrine questions, answers, and rationales

1. The nurse explains the causes of hypothyroidism to the parents of a newly diagnosed infant. The nurse recognizes that further education is needed when the parents ask which question? Select all that apply.
1. "So, hypothyroidism can be only temporary, right?"
2. "Are you saying that hypothyroidism is caused by a problem in the way the thyroid gland develops?"
3. "Do you mean that hypothyroidism may be caused by a problem in the way the body makes thyroxine?"
4. "So, this is a condition that will always require thyroid replacement therapy for life?"
5. "So, hypothyroidism can be treated by exposing our baby to a special light, right?"

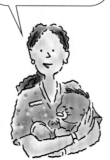

In question #1, you're looking for incorrect statements from the parents.

2. An infant with hypothyroidism is receiving oral thyroid hormone. Which assessment finding should alert a nurse to a potential overdose?
1. Tachycardia, irritability, and diaphoresis
2. Bradycardia, excessive sleepiness, and dry, scaly skin
3. Bradycardia, irritability, and cool extremities
4. Tachycardia, cool extremities, and irritability

3. When a nurse is educating parents of a neonate newly diagnosed with hypothyroidism, which statement should be included?
1. A large goiter in a neonate doesn't present a problem.
2. Preterm neonates usually aren't affected by hypothyroidism.
3. Usually, the neonate exhibits obvious signs of hypothyroidism.
4. The severity of the disorder depends on the amount of thyroid tissue present.

4. When collecting data on an infant, which condition would alert the nurse to a **subtle** sign of hypothyroidism? Select all that apply.
1. Diarrhea
2. Lethargy
3. Severe jaundice
4. Poor feeding
5. Tachycardia

1. 4, 5. Congenital hypothyroidism can be permanent or transient and may result from a defective thyroid gland or an enzymatic defect in thyroxine synthesis. Phototherapy is not used to treat physiologic jaundice and indicates that the parents need more information. Thyroid replacement therapy can be a life-long treatment. However, because some congenital hypothyroidism is transient, the child is reevaluated at age 3 for continued need for thyroid replacement.
CN: Health promotion and maintenance; CNS: None; CL: Analyze; DIFFICULTY: Challenge

2. 1. Clinical manifestations of thyroid hormone overdose in an infant include tachycardia, irritability, and diaphoresis. Bradycardia; excessive sleepiness; dry, scaly skin; and cool extremities are manifestations of hypothyroidism or inadequate hormone replacement (underdosage).
CN: Physiological integrity; CNS: Pharmacological therapies; CL: Apply; DIFFICULTY: Easy

3. 4. The severity of hypothyroidism depends on the amount of thyroid tissue present. The more thyroid tissue present, the less severe the disorder. Usually, the neonate doesn't exhibit obvious signs of the disorder because of maternal circulation. A large goiter in a neonate could possibly occlude the airway and lead to obstruction. Preterm neonates are usually affected by hypothyroidism as a result of hypothalamic and pituitary immaturity.
CN: Physiological integrity; CNS: Physiological adaptation; CL: Apply; DIFFICULTY: Moderate

4. 2, 4. Subtle signs of hypothyroidism that may be seen shortly after birth include lethargy, poor feeding, prolonged jaundice, respiratory difficulty, cyanosis, constipation, and bradycardia. Diarrhea in the neonate isn't normal and isn't associated with this disorder. Severe jaundice needs immediate attention by the health care provider and isn't a subtle sign. Tachycardia typically occurs in hyperthyroidism, not hypothyroidism.
CN: Physiological integrity; CNS: Physiological adaptation; CL: Apply; DIFFICULTY: Difficult

5. Which results would indicate to the nurse the possibility that a neonate has congenital hypothyroidism?
1. High thyroxine (T₄) level and low thyroid-stimulating hormone (TSH) level
2. Low T₄ level and high TSH level
3. Normal TSH level and high T₄ level
4. Normal T₄ level and low TSH level

6. When observing a neonate with congenital hypothyroidism, the nurse would be alert for which complication as the **most** serious consequence of this condition?
1. Anemia
2. Cyanosis
3. Retarded bone age
4. Delayed central nervous system (CNS) development

7. When counseling parents of a neonate with congenital hypothyroidism, the nurse emphasizes that the severity of the intellectual deficit is related to which parameter?
1. Duration of the condition before treatment
2. Degree of hypothermia
3. Cranial malformations
4. Thyroxine (T₄) level at diagnosis

8. Which statement should the nurse include in an explanation of the diagnostic evaluation of neonates for congenital hypothyroidism?
1. Tests are mandatory in all states.
2. An arterial blood test is preferred.
3. Tests shouldn't be performed until after discharge.
4. Blood tests should be done after the first month of life.

9. The nurse is reinforcing education with parents about therapeutic management of their neonate diagnosed with congenital hypothyroidism. Which response by a parent would indicate the need for further education?
1. "My baby will need regular measurements of his thyroxine levels."
2. "Treatment involves lifelong thyroid hormone replacement therapy."
3. "Treatment should begin as soon as possible after diagnosis is made."
4. "As my baby grows, his thyroid gland will mature and he won't need medications."

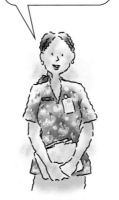

Don't be nervous when answering question #6. It will come to you.

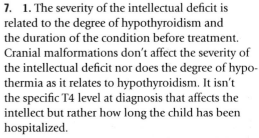

One step at a time ... you can do it!

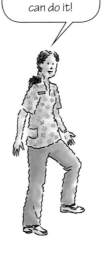

5. 2. Screening results that show a low T₄ level and a high TSH level indicate congenital hypothyroidism and the need for further tests to determine the cause of the disease.
CN: Physiological integrity; CNS: Reduction of risk potential; CL: Analyze; DIFFICULTY: Moderate

6. 4. The most serious consequence of congenital hypothyroidism is delayed development of the CNS, which leads to severe intellectual disability. The other complications of congenital hypothyroidism occur but aren't the most serious consequences.
CN: Physiological integrity; CNS: Physiological adaptation; CL: Apply; DIFFICULTY: Moderate

7. 1. The severity of the intellectual deficit is related to the degree of hypothyroidism and the duration of the condition before treatment. Cranial malformations don't affect the severity of the intellectual deficit nor does the degree of hypothermia as it relates to hypothyroidism. It isn't the specific T4 level at diagnosis that affects the intellect but rather how long the child has been hospitalized.
CN: Health promotion and maintenance; CNS: None; CL: Apply; DIFFICULTY: Challenge

8. 1. Heel stick blood tests are mandatory in all states and are usually done on neonates between ages 2 and 6 days. Typically, specimens are taken before the neonate is discharged from the hospital; the test is included with other tests that screen the neonate for errors of metabolism.
CN: Health promotion and maintenance; CNS: None; CL: Apply; DIFFICULTY: Difficult

9. 4. Treatment involves lifelong thyroid hormone replacement therapy that begins as soon as possible after diagnosis. The goal of treatment is to abolish all signs of hypothyroidism and to reestablish normal physical and mental development. The drug of choice is synthetic levothyroxine. Regular measurements of thyroxine levels are important in ensuring optimal treatment.
CN: Physiological integrity; CNS: Physiological adaptation; CL: Analyze; DIFFICULTY: Easy

10. Which comment made by the parent of a neonate at a 2-week office visit should alert the nurse to suspect congenital hypothyroidism?
1. "My baby is unusually quiet and good."
2. "My baby seems to study my face during feeding time."
3. "After feedings, my baby pulls the legs up and cries."
4. "My baby seems to be a yellowish color."

11. Which statement should be included when reinforcing education with a parent about giving levothyroxine to the neonate after a diagnosis of hypothyroidism is made? Select all that apply.
1. Administer in the morning, at the same time each day.
2. The drug has a bitter taste.
3. The pill shouldn't be crushed.
4. Never put the medication in formula or juice.
5. If a dose is missed, double the dose the next day.

12. When reinforcing education with the parents about signs that indicate levothyroxine overdose, which comment by a parent indicates the need for further education?
1. "Irritability is a sign of overdose."
2. "If my baby's heartbeat is fast, I should count it."
3. "If my baby loses weight, I should be concerned."
4. "I shouldn't worry if my baby doesn't sleep very much."

13. A nurse should recognize that exophthalmos may occur in children with which condition?
1. Hypothyroidism
2. Hyperthyroidism
3. Hypoparathyroidism
4. Hyperparathyroidism

14. The nurse is assessing a child with juvenile hypothyroidism. Which common clinical finding would the nurse **most** likely observe? Select all that apply.
1. Accelerated growth
2. Diarrhea
3. Dry skin
4. Fatigue
5. Insomnia

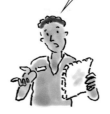

With question #11, it's all about the timing.

10. 1. Parental remarks about an unusually "quiet and good" neonate, together with any of the early physical manifestations, should lead to a suspicion of hypothyroidism, which requires a referral for specific tests. The normal neonate likes looking at the human face and should show this interest at age 2 weeks. If the neonate is pulling the legs up and crying after feedings, the neonate might be showing signs of colic. If a neonate begins to look yellow in color, hyperbilirubinemia may be the cause.
CN: Health promotion and maintenance; CNS: None; CL: Analyze;
DIFFICULTY: Difficult

11. 1, 5. Levothyroxine should be administered daily at a consistent time. Morning is the ideal time. If a dose is missed, twice the dose should be given the next day. The importance of compliance with the drug regimen must be emphasized in order for the neonate to achieve normal growth and development. Because the drug is flavorless, it can be crushed and added to formula or breast milk.
CN: Physiological integrity; CNS: Pharmacological therapies;
CL: Analyze; DIFFICULTY: Difficult

12. 4. Parents need to be aware of signs indicating overdose, such as insomnia, rapid pulse, dyspnea, irritability, fever, sweating, and weight loss. The parents are given acceptable parameters for the heart rate and weight loss or gain. If the baby is experiencing a heart rate or weight loss outside of the acceptable parameters, the health care provider should be called.
CN: Physiological integrity; CNS: Pharmacological therapies;
CL: Analyze; DIFFICULTY: Moderate

13. 2. Exophthalmos occurs when there's an overproduction of thyroid hormone. Protruding eyeballs should alert the primary health care provider to follow up with further testing.
CN: Health promotion and maintenance; CNS: None; CL: Apply;
DIFFICULTY: Moderate

14. 3, 4. Children with hypothyroidism have dry skin, fatigue, constipation, and dry, brittle hair. The other clinical findings aren't evident in children with juvenile hypothyroidism.
CN: Health promotion and maintenance; CNS: None; CL: Apply;
DIFFICULTY: Difficult

15. A nurse is observing an infant with thyroid hormone deficiency. Which signs would the nurse commonly observe?
1. Tachycardia, profuse perspiration, and diarrhea
2. Lethargy, feeding difficulties, and constipation
3. Hypertonia, small fontanels, and moist skin
4. Dermatitis, dry skin, and round face

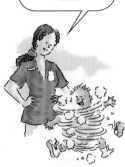

No problem with lethargy here.

15. **2.** Hypothyroidism results from inadequate thyroid production to meet an infant's needs. Clinical signs include feeding difficulties, prolonged physiologic jaundice, lethargy, and constipation.
CN: Physiological integrity; CNS: Physiological adaptation; CL: Analyze; DIFFICULTY: Easy

16. When counseling parents of a neonate with congenital hypothyroidism, the nurse should encourage which action?
1. Seek professional genetic counseling.
2. Retrace the family tree for others born with this condition.
3. Talk to relatives who have gone through a similar experience.
4. Wait until the neonate is 1 year of age before obtaining counseling.

16. **1.** Seeking professional genetic counseling is the best option for parents who have a neonate with a genetic disorder such as congenital hypothyroidism. Retracing the family tree and talking to relatives won't help the parents to become better educated about the disorder. Education about the disorder should occur as soon as the parents are ready so they'll understand the genetic implications for future children.
CN: Health promotion and maintenance; CNS: None; CL: Apply; DIFFICULTY: Moderate

17. Which symptoms would lead the nurse to suspect possible hypoglycemia? Select all that apply.
1. Irritability
2. Drowsiness
3. Headache
4. Abdominal pain
5. Nausea and vomiting
6. Hunger

Uh oh. Looks like another breakdown in insulin production.

17. **1, 3, 6.** Signs of hypoglycemia include irritability, shaky feeling, hunger, headache, and dizziness. Drowsiness, abdominal pain, nausea, and vomiting are signs of *hyper*glycemia.
CN: Physiological integrity; CNS: Physiological adaptation; CL: Apply; DIFFICULTY: Difficult

18. When children are more physically active, which change in the management of the child with diabetes should the nurse expect?
1. Increased food intake
2. Decreased food intake
3. Decreased risk of insulin shock
4. Increased risk of hyperglycemia

18. **1.** If a child is more active at one time of the day than another, food or insulin should be altered to meet the child's activity pattern. Food intake should be increased when a child with diabetes is more physically active. There would be an increased risk of insulin shock if the child didn't take in more food, and the child would become hypoglycemic, not hyperglycemic.
CN: Physiological integrity; CNS: Reduction of risk potential; CL: Apply; DIFFICULTY: Easy

19. The nurse is participating in a care planning conference for an adolescent client recently diagnosed with diabetes mellitus type 1. Which characteristics of adolescents does the nurse identify that should be taken into consideration when planning client education and care? Select all that apply.
1. Desire to be an individual
2. Desire to be like peers
3. Preoccupation with future plans
4. Ability to educate peers about the seriousness of the disease
5. Desire to become independent of parents

19. **2, 5.** Adolescents appear to have the most difficulty adjusting to diabetes. Adolescence is a time when being "perfect" and being like one's peers are emphasized, and having diabetes means the adolescent is different. One of the tasks of adolescents is to become independent from their parents and develop decision making skills.
CN: Safe, effective care environment; CNS: Coordinated care; CL: Apply; DIFFICULTY: Challenge

20. An adolescent with diabetes tells the community nurse they recently started drinking alcohol on the weekends. Which action would be **most** appropriate for the nurse to take?
1. Recommend referral to counseling.
2. Make the adolescent promise to stop drinking.
3. Discuss with the adolescent why he has started drinking.
4. Educate the adolescent about the effects of alcohol on diabetes.

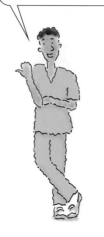

The words "most appropriate" are key to getting question #20 right.

21. A nurse is reinforcing education about type 1 diabetes with an adolescent who has the disease. Which instruction by the nurse about how to prevent hypoglycemia would be **most** appropriate for the adolescent?
1. "Limit participation in planned exercise activities that involve competition."
2. "Carry crackers or fruit to eat before or during periods of increased activity."
3. "Increase the insulin dosage before planned or unplanned strenuous exercise."
4. "Check your blood glucose level before exercising, and eat a protein snack if the level is elevated."

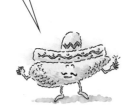

Muy Bueno! You really know your endocrine disorders.

22. The nurse is working with a 2-year-old child who has been admitted with a new diagnosis of diabetes mellitus. Which signs would the nurse expect to observe in the child? Select all that apply.
1. Increased appetite
2. Seizure
3. Decreased fluid intake
4. Weight loss
5. Frequent urination

23. Which statement made by the nurse to the client and parents about diabetic ketoacidosis is **most** accurate?
1. "It's a normal outcome of diabetes."
2. "It's a life-threatening situation."
3. "It's a situation that can easily be treated at home."
4. "It's a situation that's best treated in the pediatrician's office."

20. 4. The adolescent must be taught the effects of alcohol on diabetes. Ingestion of alcohol inhibits the release of glycogen from the liver, resulting in hypoglycemia. Teens who drink alcohol may become hypoglycemic. Manifesting behaviors that are similar to intoxication include shakiness, combativeness, slurred speech, and loss of consciousness. Recommending that the teen see a counselor is a good option, but should first be taught about the effects of alcohol consumption. The nurse can't stop an adolescent from doing something if the teenager doesn't understand why it's wrong. Discussing the reason for the adolescent's drinking should be left up to the counselor.
CN: Health promotion and maintenance; CNS: None;
CL: Apply; DIFFICULTY: Easy

21. 2. Hypoglycemia can usually be prevented if an adolescent with diabetes eats more food before or during exercise. Because exercise with adolescents isn't commonly planned, carrying additional carbohydrate foods such as crackers or fruit is a good preventive measure.
CN: Health promotion and maintenance; CNS: None;
CL: Apply; DIFFICULTY: Easy

22. 1, 4, 5. Polyphagia, polyuria, polydipsia, and weight loss are cardinal signs of diabetes. Other signs include irritability, shortened attention span, lowered frustration tolerance, fatigue, dry skin, blurred vision, sores that are slow to heal, and flushed skin. If on initial presentation the child was in diabetic ketoacidosis, signs and symptoms would include fruity odor to the breath, Kussmaul respirations, and stupor.
CN: Health promotion and maintenance; CNS: None;
CL: Apply; DIFFICULTY: Difficult

23. 2. Diabetic ketoacidosis, the most complete state of insulin deficiency, is a life-threatening situation. The child should be admitted to an intensive care facility for management, which consists of rapid assessment, adequate insulin to reduce the elevated blood glucose level, fluids to overcome dehydration, and electrolyte replacement (especially potassium).
CN: Physiological integrity; CNS: Physiological adaptation;
CL: Apply; DIFFICULTY: Easy

24. Which guideline is appropriate when reinforcing education about insulin injections with an 11-year-old child recently diagnosed with diabetes?

1. The parents don't need to be involved in learning this procedure.
2. Self-injection techniques aren't usually taught until the child reaches age 16.
3. At age 11, the child should be old enough to give most of his own injections.
4. Self-injection techniques should be taught only when the child can reach all injection sites.

25. The nurse is preparing a mixed insulin injection of 15 units of humulin N and 5 units of humulin R for a child with type 1 diabetes. In which order should the nurse perform these steps?

1. Wipe the stoppers of both vials of insulin with alcohol.
2. Inject 5 units of air into the humulin R vial.
3. Draw up 5 units of humulin R.
4. Draw up 15 units of humulin N.
5. Inject 15 units of air into the vial of humulin N.
6. Gently roll the bottle of humulin N in the hands.
7. Draw up 20 units of air into the insulin syringe.

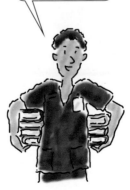

Question #25 is about putting the steps in the right order.

24. 3. The parents must supervise and manage the child's therapeutic program, but the child should assume responsibility for self-management as soon as he can. Children can learn to collect their own blood for glucose testing at a relatively young age (4 to 5 years), and most can check their blood glucose level and administer insulin at all injection sites by about age 9. Some children can do it earlier.

CN: Health promotion and maintenance; CNS: None;
CL: Apply; DIFFICULTY: Moderate

25.

6. Gently roll the bottle of humulin N in the hands.
1. Wipe the stoppers of both vials of insulin with alcohol.
7. Draw up 20 units of air into the insulin syringe.
5. Inject 15 units of air into the vial of humulin N.
2. Inject 5 units of air into the humulin R vial.
3. Draw up 5 units of humulin R.
4. Draw up 15 units of humulin N.

Mixing insulins begins with washing the hands, followed by gently rolling the vial of humulin N (cloudy insulin). The intermediate acing insulin can precipitate, therefore it must be mixed well before drawing up. Wipe the stoppers of both vials of insulin with alcohol. Twenty units of air is drawn into the insulin syringe — first 15 units of air is injected into the humulin N vial and then 5 units of air is injected into the humulin R vial. Without removing the needle from the humulin R vial, it is inverted and 5 units of humulin R is drawn up. The needle is then inserted in the topper of the humulin N vial and the vial is inverted and 15 units of humulin N is drawn up. The regular insulin (humulin R) is drawn up first to prevent contamination of the regular insulin vial with the intermediate acting insulin (humulin N). The mnemonic "clear to cloudy" helps to remember to draw up the regular insulin first. The humulin N is drawn up to the 20 unit marking, as the 15 units are added to 5 units of humulin R drawn up initially.

CN: Physiological integrity; CNS: Pharmacological therapies;
CL: Apply; DIFFICULTY: Moderate

26. A child has experienced symptoms of hypoglycemia and has eaten sugar cubes. The nurse expects to follow this rapid-releasing sugar with which food?
1. Fruit juices
2. Six glasses of water
3. Foods that are high in protein
4. Complex carbohydrates and protein

26. 4. When a child exhibits signs of hypoglycemia, most cases can be treated with a simple concentrated sugar, such as honey or sugar cubes, that can be held in the mouth for a short time. This will elevate the blood glucose level and alleviate the symptoms. The simpler the carbohydrate, the more rapidly it will be absorbed. A complex carbohydrate and protein, such as a slice of bread or a cracker spread with peanut butter, should follow the rapid-releasing sugar, or the child may become hypoglycemic again.
CN: Health promotion and maintenance; CNS: None; CL: Apply; DIFFICULTY: Moderate

27. A child with type 1 diabetes reports to the nurse about feeling shaky. The nurse observes the child's skin to be pale and sweaty. Which action should the nurse initiate **immediately**?
1. Give supplemental insulin.
2. Give the child a glucose tablet to eat.
3. Administer glucagon subcutaneously.
4. Offer the child a complex carbohydrate snack.

27. 2. Shakiness and pale, sweaty skin are symptoms of hypoglycemia. Rapid treatment involves giving the alert child a glucose tablet (4 mg dextrose) or, if unavailable, a glass of glucose-containing liquid. Either would be followed by a complex carbohydrate snack and protein. Giving supplemental insulin is contraindicated because that would lower the blood glucose even more. Glucagon would be given only if there were a risk of aspiration with oral glucose, such as if the child was semiconscious.
CN: Safe, effective care environment; CNS: Coordinated care; CL: Apply; DIFFICULTY: Challenge

28. The parents of a child diagnosed with diabetes ask the nurse about maintaining metabolic control during a minor illness with loss of appetite. Which nursing response is appropriate?
1. "Decrease the child's insulin by one-half of the usual dose during the course of the illness."
2. "Call your health care provider to arrange hospitalization."
3. "Give increased amounts of clear liquids to prevent dehydration."
4. "Substitute calorie-containing liquids for uneaten solid food."

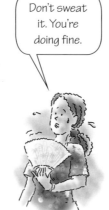

Don't sweat it. You're doing fine.

28. 4. Calorie-containing liquids can help maintain more normal blood glucose levels as well as decrease the danger of dehydration. The child with diabetes should always take *at least* the usual dose of insulin during an illness, based on more frequent blood glucose checks. During an illness that involves vomiting or loss of appetite, NPH insulin may be lowered by 25% to 30% to avoid hyperglycemia, and regular insulin is given according to home glucose monitoring results. Minor illnesses usually don't require hospitalization. Giving increased amounts of clear liquids may prevent dehydration, but the child with diabetes should try to maintain caloric intake during illness.
CN: Safe, effective care environment; CNS: Coordinated care; CL: Apply; DIFFICULTY: Moderate

29. To increase the adolescent's adherence with treatment for diabetes, the nurse should attempt which strategy?
1. Provide for a special diet in the high school cafeteria.
2. Clarify the adolescent's values to promote involvement in care.
3. Identify energy requirements for participation in sports activities.
4. Educate the adolescent about long-term consequences of poor metabolic control.

29. 2. Adolescent adherence with diabetes management may be hampered by "dependence versus independence" conflicts and ego development. Helping the adolescent clarify personal values fosters compliance. Providing for a special meal in the school cafeteria isn't feasible and doesn't guarantee that the adolescent would eat it. The question doesn't provide sufficient information about the adolescent's sports activity. An adolescent is usually concerned only with the present, not the future.
CN: Health promotion and maintenance; CNS: None; CL: Apply; DIFFICULTY: Challenge

30. The parent of a child with diabetes asks a nurse why blood glucose monitoring is needed. The nurse should base the reply on which premise?
1. This is an easier method of testing.
2. This is a less expensive method of testing.
3. This allows children the ability to better manage their diabetes.
4. This gives children a greater sense of control over their diabetes.

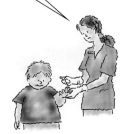

Teaching kids about their conditions and how to manage them can be empowering.

30. 3. Blood glucose monitoring improves diabetes management and is used successfully by children from the onset of their diabetes. By testing their own blood, children can change their insulin regimen to maintain their glucose level in the normoglycemic range of 60 to 100 mg/dL. This allows them to better manage their diabetes.
CN: Health promotion and maintenance; CNS: None; CL: Apply; DIFFICULTY: Moderate

31. Which criteria would the nurse use to measure good metabolic control in a child with diabetes?
1. Fewer than eight episodes of severe hyperglycemia in a month
2. Infrequent occurrences of mild hypoglycemic reactions
3. Hemoglobin A1c values less than 12%
4. Growth below the 15th percentile

31. 2. Criteria for good metabolic control generally include few episodes of hypoglycemia or hyperglycemia, hemoglobin A1c values less than 8%, and normal growth and development.
CN: Health promotion and maintenance; CNS: None; CL: Apply; DIFFICULTY: Moderate

32. The nurse is participating a discharge planning conference for a school-age child with newly diagnosed diabetes mellitus. The parents express concern about the accommodations needed when the child returns to school. Which recommendations does the nurse expect the team to make? Select all that apply.
1. A schedule for blood glucose testing with target ranges and interventions.
2. A written plan for the school to follow regarding insulin administration.
3. Home schooling to decrease the risk of complications.
4. No participation in physical education or recess.
5. Education for appropriate school staff about care that will be rendered.

32. 1, 2, 5. It is important for the parents to feel confident that the child will be safe in the school environment. The school care plan should include a schedule for when blood glucose testing should be done, what the target ranges are, and any interventions that are to be done for low or high blood sugars. If the child is to receive insulin injections at school those orders should be specified. It is important for proper education of the school personnel who will be providing care at school. Home schooling is not recommended. It is important to keep the child's life as normal as possible. Regular exercise is an important part of the child's treatment plan, so recess and PE are not restricted.
CN: Safe, effective care environment; CNS: Coordinated care; CL: Analyze; DIFFICULTY: Challenge

33. The nurse is reinforcing education regarding hypoglycemia. The nurse should inform the client and parents that which condition could possibly cause hypoglycemia? Select all that apply.
1. Too little insulin
2. Mild illness with fever
3. Skipping a meal
4. Excessive exercise without a carbohydrate snack
5. Eating ice cream and cake to celebrate a birthday

33. 3, 4. Excessive exercise without a carbohydrate snack could cause hypoglycemia. Skipping a meal can also result in hypoglycemia. The other conditions cause *hyper*glycemia.
CN: Health promotion and maintenance; CNS: None; CL: Apply; DIFFICULTY: Easy

34. Which assessment tool provides the **best** reflection of glycemic control of a child with diabetes during the preceding 2 to 3 months?
1. Fasting glucose level
2. Oral glucose tolerance test
3. Glycosylated hemoglobin level
4. The client's record of glucose monitoring

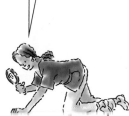

Looking for a clue to answer question #34? Focus on "2 to 3 months."

34. 3. A glycosylated hemoglobin level provides an overview of a person's blood glucose level over the previous 2 to 3 months. Glycosylated hemoglobin values are reported as a percentage of the total hemoglobin to which glucose is bound, within an erythrocyte. The time frame is based on the fact that the usual life span of an erythrocyte is 2 to 3 months; a random blood sample, therefore, will theoretically give samples of erythrocytes for this same period. The other assessment factors won't provide a true picture of the person's blood glucose level over the previous 2 to 3 months.
CN: Health promotion and maintenance; CNS: None; CL: Apply; DIFFICULTY: Moderate

35. An older child has received diet instruction as part of the treatment plan for type 1 diabetes. Which statement by the older child indicates to the nurse the need for additional instruction?
1. "I will need a bedtime snack because I take an evening dose of NPH insulin."
2. "I can eat whatever I want as long as I cover the calories with sufficient insulin."
3. "I can have an occasional low-calorie drink as long as I include it in my meal plan."
4. "I should eat meals as scheduled, even if I'm not hungry, to prevent hypoglycemia."

36. A child with diabetes is brought by the parents to the emergency department. The nurse observes a flushed face, drowsiness, and detects a fruity odor to the breath. The parents report that the child has become progressively worse over the course of the day. The nurse suspects that the child is experiencing which condition? Select all that apply.
1. Hyperglycemia
2. Insulin overdose
3. Somogyi phenomenon
4. Ketoacidosis
5. Hypoglycemia

37. An adolescent with diabetes is learning to mix regular insulin and NPH insulin in the same syringe. Which action, if performed by the teen, would indicate the need for further instruction?
1. Withdraws the NPH insulin first
2. Injects air into the NPH insulin bottle first
3. After drawing up the first insulin, removes air bubbles from the syringe
4. Injects an amount of air equal to the desired dose of insulin

38. Which sign or symptom would a nurse commonly observe **first** in an infant with diabetes insipidus?
1. Dehydration
2. Inability to be aroused
3. Extreme hunger relieved by frequent feedings of milk
4. Irritability relieved with feedings of water but not milk

39. When collecting data on a child for possible diabetes insipidus, a nurse should recognize which condition as a sign of this disorder? Select all that apply.
1. Hyponatremia
2. Jaundice
3. Dehydration
4. Polyuria
5. Excessive thirst relieved by water
6. Hypochloremia

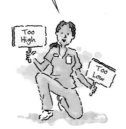

Remember: *hyper* means "too high" and *hypo* means "too low."

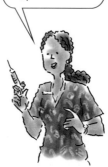

The order of withdrawal is important when mixing different types of insulin.

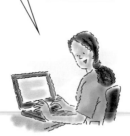

Water—and the lack of it—is central to the answers in question #39.

35. 2. The goal of diet therapy in diabetes is to attain and maintain ideal body weight. Each child with diabetes will be prescribed a specific caloric intake and insulin regimen to help accomplish this goal.
CN: Physiological integrity; CNS: Basic care and comfort;
CL: Analyze; DIFFICULTY: Easy

36. 1, 4. In ketoacidosis, the blood glucose is markedly elevated. The child's skin is dry, and the face is flushed. The breath has a fruity odor. Insulin overdose produces hypoglycemia. Hypoglycemia is characterized by irritability, pallor, sweating, reports of hunger, and weakness. Somogyi phenomenon is rebound hyperglycemia in clients requiring fairly large doses of insulin. Hypoglycemia during the night with marked hyperglycemia in the morning is suggestive of Somogyi phenomenon.
CN: Physiological integrity; CNS: Physiological adaptation;
CL: Analyze; DIFFICULTY: Challenge

37. 1. Regular insulin is *always* withdrawn first so it won't become contaminated with NPH insulin. The adolescent with diabetes is instructed to inject air into the NPH insulin bottle equal to the amount of insulin to be withdrawn, because there will be regular insulin in the syringe and there will be an inability to inject air when withdrawing the NPH. It's necessary to remove the air bubbles from the syringe to ensure a correct dosage before drawing up the second insulin.
CN: Physiological integrity; CNS: Pharmacological therapies;
CL: Apply; DIFFICULTY: Easy

38. 4. An initial symptom of diabetes insipidus in an infant is irritability relieved with feedings of water but not milk. Dehydration and the inability to be aroused are late signs.
CN: Health promotion and maintenance; CNS: None; CL: Apply;
DIFFICULTY: Difficult

39. 3, 4, 5. The cardinal signs of diabetes insipidus are polyuria and polydipsia. Dehydration occurs as a result of the excessive urine output. Hypernatremia, not hyponatremia, occurs with diabetes insipidus. Jaundice occurs because of abnormal bilirubin metabolism, not diabetes insipidus. Hyperchloremia, not hypochloremia, occurs with diabetes insipidus.
CN: Physiological integrity; CNS: Physiological adaptation;
CL: Apply; DIFFICULTY: Easy

40. The nurse is reinforcing education about home care with the parents of a child diagnosed with type 1 diabetes. The nurse determines the education has been successful when the parent makes which of the following statements? Select all that apply.

1. "We can dispose of used lancets and insulin syringes in a puncture-proof container such as a bleach bottle."
2. "I will be sure my child wears a Medic Alert bracelet."
3. "I should limit my child's exercise to prevent hypoglycemia."
4. "As long as my child takes insulin as ordered, there is no need to perform routine blood glucose checks."
5. "My child should receive immunizations for influenza and pneumonia."

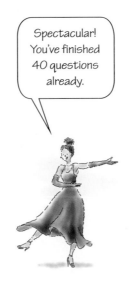

Spectacular! You've finished 40 questions already.

40. 1, 2, 5. Used lancets and syringes should be disposed of in a red biohazard container or a narrow, open, opaque, nonpierceable container like a bleach bottle. A Medic Alert bracelet identifying the child as a diabetic will be helpful in case of emergency. Prevention of influenza and pneumonia through immunization is important for the child's glycemic control and health. Exercise and regular monitoring of blood glucose levels are important components of the treatment program.
CN: Safe, effective care environment; CNS: Safety and infection control; CL: Analyze; DIFFICULTY: Moderate

41. A nurse is assisting parents to understand when treatments of growth hormone replacement will end. Which statement should be included?

1. "The dosage of growth hormone will decrease as the child's age increases."
2. "The dosage of growth hormone will increase as the time of epiphyseal closure nears."
3. "After giving growth hormone replacement for 1 year, the dose will be tapered."
4. "Growth hormone replacement can't be abruptly stopped. Decreasing growth hormone replacement must be spread out over several months."

41. 2. Dosage of growth hormone is increased as the time of epiphyseal closure nears in order to gain the most growth from the growth hormone. The medication is then stopped. There's no tapering of the dose.
CN: Physiological integrity; CNS: Pharmacological therapies; CL: Apply; DIFFICULTY: Challenge

42. The nurse is reinforcing education with an infant's parents about diabetes insipidus. When explaining the diagnostic test that's used, the nurse knows that which comment by the parents indicates an understanding of the diagnostic test?

1. "Fluids will be offered every 2 hours."
2. "My infant's fluid intake will be restricted."
3. "I won't change anything about my infant's intake."
4. "Formula will be restricted, but glucose water is OK."

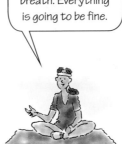

Feeling stressed? Close your eyes and take a deep breath. Everything is going to be fine.

42. 2. The simplest test used to diagnose diabetes insipidus is restriction of oral fluids and observation of consequent changes in urine volume and concentration. A weight loss of 3% to 5% indicates severe dehydration, and the test should be terminated at this point. This test is done in the hospital, and the infant is watched closely.
CN: Health promotion and maintenance; CNS: None; CL: Analyze; DIFFICULTY: Moderate

43. A nurse should anticipate which physiologic response in an infant being tested for diabetes insipidus?

1. Increase in urine output
2. Decrease in urine output
3. No effect on urine output
4. Increase in urine specific gravity

43. 3. In diabetes insipidus, fluid restriction for diagnostic testing has little or no effect on urine formation, but it causes weight loss from dehydration.
CN: Physiological integrity; CNS: Physiological adaptation; CL: Apply; DIFFICULTY: Challenge

44. In reinforcing education with the parents of an infant diagnosed with diabetes insipidus, the nurse should include which treatment?
1. The need for blood products
2. Antihypertensive medications
3. Hormone replacement
4. Fluid restrictions

45. An infant has a positive test result for diabetes insipidus. The nurse should anticipate the health care provider will order a test dose of which medication?
1. Human placental lactogen
2. Glucose
3. Corticotropin
4. Aqueous vasopressin

46. When providing information about treatment of diabetes insipidus to parents, a nurse explains the use of nasal spray and injections. Which indication might deter a parent from choosing nasal spray treatment?
1. Applications must be repeated every 8 to 12 hours.
2. Applications must be repeated every 2 to 4 hours.
3. Nasal sprays can't be used on infants.
4. Measurements are too difficult.

47. When reinforcing education with parents of an infant newly diagnosed with diabetes insipidus, which statement by the parent indicates an appropriate understanding of this condition?
1. "When my infant stabilizes, I won't have to worry about giving hormone medication."
2. "I don't have to measure the amount of fluid intake that I give my infant."
3. "I realize that treatment for diabetes insipidus is lifelong."
4. "My infant will outgrow this condition."

48. A child presents in the emergency department after being hit in the head by a baseball. The child begins to excrete extremely large amounts of urine and becomes dehydrated. Which condition does the nurse suspect the child has developed?
1. Diabetes mellitus
2. Diabetes insipidus
3. Syndrome of inappropriate ADH secretion
4. Parathyroid hypofunction

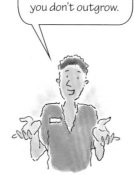

Unfortunately, diabetes insipidus is a condition that you don't outgrow.

44. 3. The usual treatment for diabetes insipidus is hormone replacement with vasopressin or desmopressin acetate. Blood products shouldn't be needed. Hypertension isn't associated with this condition, and fluids shouldn't be restricted.
CN: Physiological integrity; CNS: Pharmacological therapies; CL: Apply; DIFFICULTY: Moderate

45. 4. If the fluid restriction test is positive, the child should be given a test dose of injected aqueous vasopressin, which should alleviate the polyuria and polydipsia. Unresponsiveness to exogenous vasopressin usually indicates nephrogenic diabetes insipidus. The other medications are used to determine other types of endocrine disorders.
CN: Physiological integrity; CNS: Pharmacological therapies; CL: Apply; DIFFICULTY: Moderate

46. 1. Applications of nasal spray used to treat diabetes insipidus must be repeated every 8 to 12 hours; injections, although quite painful, last for 48 to 72 hours. The nasal spray must be timed for adequate night sleep. Nasal sprays have been used on infants with diabetes insipidus and are dispensed in premeasured intranasal inhalers, eliminating the need for measuring doses.
CN: Physiological integrity; CNS: Pharmacological therapies; CL: Analyze; DIFFICULTY: Challenge

47. 3. Diabetes insipidus requires lifelong treatment. The amount of fluid intake is important and must be measured with the infant's output to monitor the medication regimen. The infant won't outgrow this condition.
CN: Safe, effective care environment; CNS: Coordinated care; CL: Analyze; DIFFICULTY: Easy

48. 2. Diabetes insipidus is the principal disorder caused by posterior pituitary hypofunction. The disorder results from hyposecretion of antidiuretic hormone, producing a state of uncontrolled diuresis. Diabetes insipidus can be acquired as the result of a head injury or tumor.
CN: Health promotion and maintenance; CNS: None; CL: Apply; DIFFICULTY: Moderate

49. A nurse is reinforcing education about an injectable drug to treat diabetes insipidus with the parents of an infant diagnosed with the disorder. Which statement made by the parent would indicate the need for further education?

1. "I must hold the medication under warm running water for 10 to 15 minutes before administering it."
2. "The medication must be shaken vigorously before being drawn up into the syringe."
3. "Small, brown particles must be seen in the suspension."
4. "I will store this medication in the refrigerator."

50. Which assessment finding would alert the nurse to change the intranasal route for vasopressin administration?

1. Mucous membrane irritation
2. Severe coughing
3. Nosebleeds
4. Pneumonia

51. After the nurse has discussed the causes of diabetes insipidus with the parents of a neonate, which statement made by a parent indicates the need for further education?

1. "This condition could be familial or congenital."
2. "Drinking alcohol during my pregnancy caused this condition."
3. "My child might have a tumor that's causing these symptoms."
4. "An infection such as meningitis may be the reason my child has diabetes insipidus."

Can you spot which statement by the parent is incorrect in question #51?

52. The nurse should include which in-home management instruction for a child who's receiving desmopressin acetate for symptomatic control of diabetes insipidus?

1. Give desmopressin acetate only when urine output begins to decrease.
2. Clean skin with alcohol before applying the desmopressin acetate dermal patch.
3. Increase the desmopressin acetate dose if polyuria occurs just before the next scheduled dose.
4. Call the health care provider for an alternate route of desmopressin acetate when the child has an upper respiratory infection (URI) or allergic rhinitis.

49. 4. The medication should be stored at room temperature. When giving injectable vasopressin, it must be thoroughly resuspended in the oil by being held under warm running water for 10 to 15 minutes and shaken vigorously before being drawn into the syringe. If this isn't done, the oil may be injected minus the drug. Small, brown particles, which indicate drug dispersion, must be seen in the suspension.

CN: Physiological integrity; CNS: Pharmacological therapies; CL: Analyze; DIFFICULTY: Difficult

50. 1. Mucous membrane irritation caused by a cold or allergy renders the intranasal route of medication administration unreliable. Severe coughing, pneumonia, or nosebleeds shouldn't interfere with the intranasal route of vasopressin administration.

CN: Physiological integrity; CNS: Pharmacological therapies; CL: Apply; DIFFICULTY: Challenge

51. 2. Drinking alcohol during pregnancy can lead to a neonate born with fetal alcohol syndrome but has no known effect on diabetes insipidus. The other statements regarding diabetes insipidus are correct.

CN: Physiological integrity; CNS: Physiological adaptation; CL: Apply; DIFFICULTY: Difficult

52. 4. Excessive nasal mucus associated with URI or allergic rhinitis may interfere with desmopressin acetate absorption because it's given intranasally. Parents should be instructed to contact the health care provider for advice in altering the hormone dose during times when nasal mucus may be increased. To avoid overmedicating the child, the desmopressin acetate dose should remain unchanged, even if there's polyuria just before the next dose.

CN: Safe, effective care environment; CNS: Coordinated care; CL: Apply; DIFFICULTY: Moderate

53. A nurse is caring for a child with suspected hypopituitarism. Which sign or symptom of this condition would the nurse most commonly observe? Select all that apply.
1. Sleep disturbance
2. Polyuria
3. Delay in tooth development
4. Polydipsia
5. Short stature

54. Which statement made to the nurse by the parents of a child with hypopituitarism would indicate the need for further education?
1. "This disorder may be familial."
2. "There's no genetic basis for this disorder."
3. "This disorder may be secondary to hypothalamic deficiency."
4. "There may be other disorders related to pituitary hormone deficiencies."

55. A nurse is educating a class of fifth-graders on personal health. Which statement related to growth should be included?
1. "There's nothing that you can do to influence your growth."
2. "Intensive physical activity that begins before puberty might stunt growth."
3. "Children who are short in stature also have parents who are short in stature."
4. "Because this is a time of tremendous growth, being concerned about calorie intake isn't important."

56. While reinforcing education with the parents of a child of short stature, the nurse discusses familial short stature. Which statement by the nurse about this condition is **most** accurate?
1. "It occurs in children who are members of a very large family with limited resources."
2. "It occurs in children who have no siblings, and in kids who moved a great deal during their early childhood."
3. "It occurs in children with delayed linear growth and skeletal and sexual maturation that's behind that of peers."
4. "It occurs in children who have ancestors with adult height in the lower percentiles and whose height during childhood is appropriate."

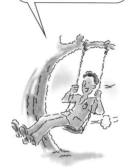

Now you've got some momentum! Keep pumping those legs.

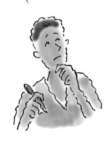

The words "most accurate" in question #56 are important. That means that answers that are "partly accurate" may not be right.

53. 3, 5. The most common sign in most instances of hypopituitarism is short stature. Delayed tooth development may also be seen. Sleep disturbance may indicate thyrotoxicosis. Polydipsia and polyuria may be indications of diabetes or diabetes insipidus.
CN: Physiological integrity; CNS: Physiological adaptation; CL: Apply; DIFFICULTY: Moderate

54. 2. There's a higher-than-average occurrence of hypopituitarism in some families, which indicates a possible genetic cause. The cause of idiopathic growth hormone deficiency is unknown. The condition is typically associated with other pituitary hormone deficiencies, such as deficiencies of thyroid-stimulating hormone and corticotropin, and thus may be secondary to hypothalamic deficiency.
CN: Psychosocial integrity; CNS: None; CL: Apply; DIFFICULTY: Moderate

55. 2. Intensive physical activity (greater than 18 hours per week) that begins before puberty may stunt growth so that the child doesn't reach full adult height. During the school-age years, growth slows and doesn't accelerate again until adolescence. Children who are short in stature don't necessarily have parents who are short in stature. Nutrition and environment influence a child's growth.
CN: Health promotion and maintenance; CNS: None; CL: Apply; DIFFICULTY: Difficult

56. 4. Familial short stature refers to otherwise healthy children who have ancestors with adult height in the lower percentiles and whose height during childhood is appropriate for genetic background. Children with delayed linear growth and delayed skeletal and sexual maturation (behind that of their peers) are said to have constitutional growth delay. Children who are members of very large families with limited resources, or who have no siblings, don't fit the description of familial short stature.
CN: Physiological integrity; CNS: Physiological adaptation; CL: Apply; DIFFICULTY: Challenge

57. When collecting data from a 2-year-old child, which finding would indicate to the nurse the possibility of growth hormone deficiency?
1. The child had normal growth during the first year of life but showed a slowed growth curve below the 3rd percentile for the second year of life.
2. The child fell below the 5th percentile for growth during the first year of life but, at this checkup, only falls below the 50th percentile.
3. There has been a steady decline in growth over the 2 years of this infant's life that has accelerated during the past 6 months.
4. There was delayed growth below the 5th percentile for the first and second years of life.

57. 1. Children with growth hormone deficiency generally grow normally during the first year and then follow a slowed growth curve that's below the 3rd percentile. Growth consistently below the 5th percentile may be an indication of failure to thrive.
CN: Health promotion and maintenance; CNS: None; CL: Apply; DIFFICULTY: Difficult

> No signs of growth hormone deficiency here.

58. A nurse is collecting data on a child with growth hormone deficiency. Which characteristic would the nurse **most** commonly observe?
1. Decreased weight with no change in height
2. Decreased weight with increased height
3. Increased weight with decreased height
4. Increased weight with increased height

58. 3. Height may be retarded more than weight because, with good nutrition, children with growth hormone deficiency can become overweight or even obese. Their well-nourished appearance is an important diagnostic clue to differentiation from other disorders, such as failure to thrive.
CN: Physiological integrity; CNS: Physiological adaptation; CL: Apply; DIFFICULTY: Moderate

59. The nurse should find which characteristic during observations of a child with growth hormone deficiency? Select all that apply.
1. Normal skeletal proportions
2. Abnormal skeletal proportions
3. Child appearing older than his age
4. Difficulty keeping up with peers in play
5. Failure to show age appropriate signs of puberty
6. Longer than normal upper extremities

59. 1, 4, 5. Skeletal proportions are normal for the age, but children with growth hormone deficiency appear younger than their chronological age. Their classmates appear to be growing faster than they do. They may have difficulty keeping up with other children of the same age in play. Parents report they are not outgrowing their clothes and shoes. There is failure to show signs of sexual development by 13 years of age in females and 15 years of age in males. However, later in life, premature aging is evident.
CN: Physiological integrity; CNS: Physiological adaptation; CL: Apply; DIFFICULTY: Challenge

> Well, bless my beta cells … there's no deficiency in your knowledge of endocrine disorders.

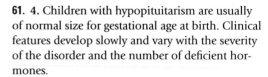

60. When counseling the parents of a child with growth hormone deficiency, the nurse should encourage which sport? Select all that apply.
1. Swimming
2. Basketball
3. Field hockey
4. Football
5. Gymnastics

60. 1, 5. Children with growth hormone deficiency can be no less active than other children if directed to size-appropriate sports, such as gymnastics, swimming, wrestling, or soccer.
CN: Health promotion and maintenance; CNS: None; CL: Apply; DIFFICULTY: Moderate

61. The parents of a child diagnosed with hypopituitarism tells the nurse they feel guilty because they should have recognized this disorder. Which statement by the nurse about children with hypopituitarism would be the most helpful?"
1. "They're usually large for gestational age at birth."
2. "They're usually small for gestational age at birth."
3. "They usually exhibit signs of this disorder soon after birth."
4. "They're usually of normal size for gestational age at birth."

61. 4. Children with hypopituitarism are usually of normal size for gestational age at birth. Clinical features develop slowly and vary with the severity of the disorder and the number of deficient hormones.
CN: Physiological integrity; CNS: Physiological adaptation; CL: Apply; DIFFICULTY: Moderate

62. When plotting height and weight on a growth chart, which observation by the nurse would indicate that a 4-year-old child has a growth hormone deficiency?
1. Upward shift of 1 percentile or more
2. Upward shift of 5 percentiles or more
3. Downward shift of 2 percentiles or more
4. Downward shift of 1 percentile or more

63. When collecting data about a child with suspected growth hormone deficiency, the nurse is asked to measure the child's height and plot it on a growth chart. What are **priority** actions of the nurse? Select all that apply.
1. Remove the child's shoes and any hair ornaments prior to measurement.
2. Have the child stand on a carpeted floor with only the shoulders against the wall.
3. Measure either the height or the length, whichever is easier.
4. Use the height as reported by the parent if the child is uncooperative.
5. Select the appropriate growth chart based on gender and age.

64. In explaining to parents the social behavior of children with hypopituitarism, a nurse should recognize which statement as a need for further education?
1. "I realize that my child might have school anxiety and low self-esteem."
2. "Because my child is of short stature, people expect less of my child than of his peers."
3. "Because of my child's short stature, my child may not be pushed to perform at chronologic age by others."
4. "My child's vocabulary is very well developed, so even though short in stature, no one will treat my child differently."

65. A single parent of a school-age child recently diagnosed with a growth hormone deficiency comments that the prescribed treatment plan seems very complicated. What is the **best** response from the nurse?
1. "Everyone feels that way at first."
2. "This must be a stressful time for you."
3. "Don't worry, it will get easier with time."
4. "I can teach you anything you need to know."

66. A nurse is reinforcing education to parents who are planning to give growth hormone to their child at home. What is the best time to administer growth hormone in order to achieve optimal dosing?
1. At bedtime
2. After dinner
3. In the middle of the day
4. First thing in the morning

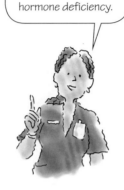

Accuracy counts when measuring the height of a client with growth hormone deficiency.

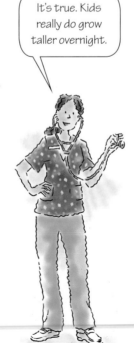

It's true. Kids really do grow taller overnight.

62. 3. When the health care provider evaluates the results of plotting height and weight, upward or downward shifts of 2 percentiles or more in children older than age 3 may indicate a growth abnormality.
CN: Health promotion and maintenance; CNS: None; CL: Analyze; DIFFICULTY: Easy

63. 1, 5. To accurately measure the child's height, remove the shoes, all hair ornaments, and bulky clothing. The child should stand on the uncarpeted surface with the feet flat and together. The head, back, buttocks, and heel should be flat against the wall. Use a flat headpiece to form a right angle with the wall and lower the headpiece until it firmly touches the crown of the head. For accuracy the nurse cannot use a reported value. Use a gender- and age-appropriate chart so that growth can be properly reported.
CN: Health promotion and maintenance; CNS: None; CL: Apply; DIFFICULTY: Difficult

64. 4. Height discrepancy has been significantly correlated with emotional adjustment problems and may be a valuable predictor of the extent to which children with growth hormone delays will have trouble with anxiety, social skills, and positive self-esteem. Also, academic problems aren't uncommon. These children aren't usually pushed to perform at their chronologic age but are typically subjected to juvenilization (related to an infantile or childish manner).
CN: Psychosocial integrity; CNS: None; CL: Apply; DIFFICULTY: Moderate

65. 2. The single parent appears to be overwhelmed trying to deal with the child's diagnosis and treatment plan. The best response is for the nurse to acknowledge the parent's stress. The other responses do not do that.
CN: Psychosocial integrity; CNS: None; CL: Analyze; DIFFICULTY: Challenge

66. 1. Optimal dosing is usually achieved when growth hormone is administered at bedtime. Pituitary release of growth hormone occurs during the first 45 to 90 minutes after the onset of sleep, so normal physiologic release is mimicked with bedtime dosing.
CN: Physiological integrity; CNS: Pharmacological therapies; CL: Apply; DIFFICULTY: Challenge

67. The parents of a child who's going through testing for hypopituitarism ask the nurse what test results they should expect. The nurse's response should be based on which factor?
1. Measurement of growth hormone will occur only one time.
2. Growth hormone levels are decreased after strenuous exercise.
3. There will be increased overnight urinary growth hormone concentration.
4. Growth hormone levels are elevated 45 to 90 minutes following the onset of sleep.

67. 4. Growth hormone levels are elevated 45 to 90 minutes following the onset of sleep. Low growth hormone levels following the onset of sleep indicate the need for further evaluation. Exercise is a natural and benign stimulus for growth hormone release, and elevated levels can be detected after 20 minutes of strenuous exercise in normal children. Also, growth hormone levels need to be checked frequently related to the type of therapy instituted.
CN: Physiological integrity; CNS: Physiological adaptation; CL: Apply; DIFFICULTY: Moderate

68. Which comment made by a parent to the nurse would indicate the possibility of hypopituitarism in a child?
1. "I can pass down my child's clothes to the younger sibling."
2. "Usually my child wears out clothes before the size changes."
3. "I have to buy larger sized clothes for my child about every 2 months."
4. "I have to buy larger shirts more frequently than larger pants for my child."

68. 2. Parents of children with hypopituitarism usually comment that the child wears out clothes before growing out of them or that, if the clothing fits the body, it's typically too long in the sleeves or legs.
CN: Physiological integrity; CNS: Physiological adaptation; CL: Apply; DIFFICULTY: Moderate

69. Which method is considered the definitive treatment for hypopituitarism due to growth hormone deficiency?
1. Treatment with desmopressin acetate
2. Replacement of antidiuretic hormone
3. Treatment with testosterone or estrogen
4. Replacement with biosynthetic growth hormone

69. 4. The definitive treatment of growth hormone deficiency is replacement of growth hormone; it is successful in 80% of affected children. Desmopressin acetate is used to treat diabetes insipidus. Antidiuretic hormone deficiency causes diabetes insipidus and isn't related to hypopituitarism. Testosterone or estrogen may be given during adolescence for normal sexual maturation but neither is the definitive treatment for hypopituitarism.
CN: Physiological integrity; CNS: Pharmacological therapies; CL: Apply; DIFFICULTY: Moderate

70. In educating parents of a child with hypopituitarism about realistic expectations of height for their child, who's successfully responding to growth hormone replacement, a nurse should include which statement?
1. "Your child will never reach a normal adult height."
2. "Your child will attain the eventual adult height at a faster rate."
3. "Your child will attain the eventual adult height at a slower rate."
4. "The rate of your child's growth will be the same as children without this disorder."

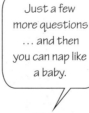

Just a few more questions … and then you can nap like a baby.

70. 3. Even when hormone replacement is successful, children with hypopituitarism attain their eventual adult height at a slower rate than their peers do; therefore, they need assistance in setting realistic expectations regarding height improvement.
CN: Health promotion and maintenance; CNS: None; CL: Apply; DIFFICULTY: Easy

71. The nurse is collecting data from a school-age child recently diagnosed with growth hormone deficiency. Which finding would lead the nurse to suspect the child had been physically abused?
1. Bruises and scrapes on both knees
2. Small circular burns on the back
3. A small soft tissue injury on the forehead
4. Scratches on the forearms

71. 2. Of the injuries described, circular burns to the back were the only injuries that could not have occurred inadvertently during play or been self-inflicted by the child.
CN: Psychosocial integrity; CNS: None; CL: Apply; DIFFICULTY: Easy

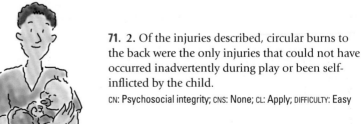

72. Which statement made by a parent of a child with short stature would indicate to the nurse the need for further education?
1. "Obtaining blood studies won't aid in proper diagnosis."
2. "A history of my child's growth patterns should be discussed."
3. "X-rays should be included in my child's diagnostic procedures."
4. "A family history is important information for me to share with my health care provider."

73. Which metabolic alteration characteristic might the nurse expect to be associated with growth hormone deficiency?
1. Galactosemia
2. Homocystinuria
3. Hyperglycemia
4. Hypoglycemia

74. When collecting data on a neonate diagnosed with diabetes insipidus, which finding would indicate the need for intervention?
1. Edema
2. Increased head circumference
3. Weight gain
4. Weight loss

75. A child is admitted to the medical-surgical unit reporting weight loss and lack of energy. The child's ears and cheeks are flushed, and the nurse observes an acetone odor to the client's breath. The blood glucose level is 325 mg/dL. The blood pressure is 104/60 mm Hg, pulse is 88 beats/minute, and respirations are 16 breaths/minute. Which does the nurse expect the health care provider to order first?
1. Subcutaneous administration of glucagon
2. Administration of regular insulin by continuous infusion pump
3. Administration of regular insulin subcutaneously every 4 hours as needed by sliding scale insulin
4. Administration of IV fluids in boluses of 20 mL/kg

76. In a child with diabetes insipidus, a nurse could expect which characteristics of the urine?
1. Pale; specific gravity less than 1.006
2. Concentrated; specific gravity less than 1.006
3. Concentrated; specific gravity less than 1.030
4. Pale; specific gravity more than 1.030

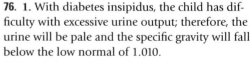
When urine output is increased, urine is more diluted, and thus pale.

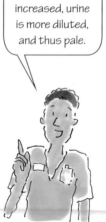

72. 1. A complete diagnostic evaluation should include a family history, a history of the child's growth patterns and previous health status, physical examination, physical evaluation, radiographic survey, and endocrine studies that may involve blood samples.
CN: Physiological integrity; CNS: Reduction of risk potential;
CL: Apply; DIFFICULTY: Easy

73. 4. The development of hypoglycemia is a characteristic finding related to growth hormone deficiency. Galactosemia is a rare autosomal recessive disorder with an inborn error of carbohydrate metabolism. Homocystinuria is an indication of amino acid transport or metabolism problems. Hyperglycemia isn't a problem in hypopituitarism.
CN: Physiological integrity; CNS: Physiological adaptation;
CL: Understand; DIFFICULTY: Difficult

74. 4. Diabetes insipidus usually appears gradually. Weight loss from a large loss of fluid occurs. A normal neonate should gain weight as they grow. There should be an increase in head circumference with treatment. Edema isn't evident in the neonate with diabetes insipidus.
CN: Physiological integrity; CNS: Reduction of risk potential;
CL: Apply; difficulty: Moderate

75. 2. Weight loss, lack of energy, acetone odor to the breath, and a blood glucose level of 325 mg/dL indicate diabetic ketoacidosis. Insulin is given by continuous infusion pump at a rate not to exceed a decrease in blood sugar greater than 100 mg/dL/hour. Faster reduction of hypoglycemia could be related to the development of cerebral edema. Glucagon is administered for mild hypoglycemia. Sliding scale insulin isn't as effective as the administration of insulin by continuous infusion pump in the treatment of diabetic ketoacidosis. Administration of IV fluids in boluses of 20 mL/kg is recommended for the treatment of shock.
CN: Physiological integrity; CNS: Physiological adaptation;
CL: Apply; DIFFICULTY: Moderate

76. 1. With diabetes insipidus, the child has difficulty with excessive urine output; therefore, the urine will be pale and the specific gravity will fall below the low normal of 1.010.
CN: Physiological integrity; CNS: Physiological adaptation;
CL: Analyze; DIFFICULTY: Moderate

CN: Client needs category   CNS: Client needs subcategory   CL: Cognitive level

77. In a child with diabetes insipidus, which characteristic would **most** likely be present in the child's health history?
1. Delayed closure of the fontanels, coarse hair, and hypoglycemia in the morning
2. Gradual onset of personality changes, lethargy, and blurred vision
3. Vomiting early in the morning, headache, and decreased thirst
4. Abrupt onset of polyuria, nocturia, and polydipsia

77. 4. Diabetes insipidus is characterized by deficient secretion of antidiuretic hormone leading to diuresis. Most children with this disorder experience an abrupt onset of symptoms, including polyuria, nocturia, and polydipsia. The other findings are symptoms of pituitary hyperfunction.
CN: Physiological integrity; CNS: Physiological adaptation; CL: **Apply**; DIFFICULTY: **Easy**

78. A child is on fluid restriction before diagnostic testing for diabetes insipidus. Which condition would indicate to the nurse the need to discontinue fluid restriction?
1. Weight gain of 3% to 5%
2. Weight loss of 3% to 5%
3. Increase in urine output
4. Generalized edema

78. 2. A weight loss of 3% to 5% indicates significant dehydration and requires termination of fluid restriction. Weight gain would be a good sign. Generalized edema doesn't occur with fluid restriction nor does increased urine output.
CN: Physiological integrity; CNS: Physiological adaptation; CL: **Analyze**; DIFFICULTY: **Moderate**

That's it! I think you got that one right.

SNAP

79. When a child with diabetes insipidus has a viral illness that includes congestion, nausea, and vomiting, the nurse should instruct the parents to take which action?
1. Make no changes in the medication regimen.
2. Give medications only once per day.
3. Obtain an alternate route for desmopressin acetate administration.
4. Give medication 1 hour after vomiting has occurred.

79. 3. For a child with diabetes insipidus who has a viral illness, an alternate route for administration of desmopressin acetate would be needed for absorption due to nasal congestion. The other actions need to be ordered by a health care provider.
CN: Physiological integrity; CNS: Pharmacological therapies; CL: **Apply**; DIFFICULTY: **Moderate**

80. The nurse is educating a client on how to draw up NPH insulin into an insulin syringe. The dose is 40 units. The client draws up the insulin using the correct technique. Which syringe shows that the client drew up the correct dose?

80. 4. Option 4 correctly shows 40 units of insulin drawn into the syringe. All of the other options show incorrect drug amounts (option 1 shows 50 units, option 2 shows 30 units, and option 3 shows 25 units).
CN: Physiological integrity; CNS: Pharmacological therapies; CL: **Apply**; DIFFICULTY: **Easy**

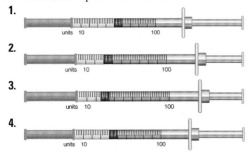

1.
units 10   100

2.
units 10   100

3.
units 10   100

4.
units 10   100

81. When providing care for a school-age child with diabetes insipidus, the nurse recognizes that which behavior might be difficult related to this child's growth and development?
1. Taking the medication at school
2. Taking the medication before bedtime
3. Letting the parent administer medication
4. Self-administering vasopressin injection before school starts

81. 1. Anything that singles out a child and makes him feel different from peers will result in possible nonadherence with the medical regimen. It's important for the nurse to help the child schedule medication times for when not in school.
CN: Health promotion and maintenance; CNS: None; CL: **Apply**; DIFFICULTY: **Moderate**

82. A nurse is caring for a neonate with congenital hypothyroidism. Which assessment finding should the nurse anticipate observing in the neonate?
1. Hyperreflexia
2. Long forehead
3. Puffy eyelids
4. Small tongue

83. Which nursing objective is **most** important when working with neonates who are suspected of having congenital hypothyroidism?
1. Early identification
2. Promoting bonding
3. Allowing rooming-in with the mother
4. Encouraging fluid intake

84. The nurse cares for an infant receiving inadequate treatment for congenital hypothyroidism. Which signs or symptoms should the nurse expect to observe?
1. Irritability and jitteriness
2. Fatigue and sleepiness
3. Increased appetite
4. Diarrhea

85. When the parents of an infant diagnosed with hypothyroidism have been taught to count the pulse, which intervention should the nurse teach them in case they obtain a high pulse rate?
1. Allow the infant to take a nap and then give the medication.
2. Withhold the medication and give a double dose the next day.
3. Withhold the medication and call the health care provider.
4. Give the medication and then consult the health care provider.

86. Which signs and symptoms would the health care team most commonly use as a basis for determining appropriate priorities and interventions for a child with type 1 diabetes? Select all that apply.
1. Polyuria
2. Weakness
3. Abdominal pain
4. Weight loss
5. Postprandial nausea
6. Orthostatic hypertension

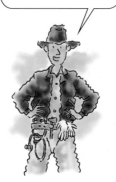

Time to break out your assessment tools. We have some assessing to do.

82. 3. Assessment findings for a neonate with congenital hypothyroidism include depressed nasal bridge, short forehead, puffy eyelids, and large tongue; thick, dry, mottled skin that feels cold to the touch; coarse, dry, lusterless hair; abdominal distention; umbilical hernia; hyporeflexia; bradycardia; hypothermia; hypotension; anemia; and wide cranial sutures.
CN: Physiological integrity; CNS: Physiological adaptation; CL: Apply; DIFFICULTY: Moderate

83. 1. The most important nursing objective is early identification of the disorder. Nurses caring for neonates must be certain that screening is performed, especially in neonates who are preterm, discharged early, or born at home. Promoting bonding, allowing rooming-in, and encouraging fluid intake are all important but are less critical than early identification.
CN: Physiological integrity; CNS: Basic care and comfort; CL: Apply; DIFFICULTY: Easy

84. 2. Signs of inadequate treatment in an infant with congenital hypothyroidism are fatigue, sleepiness, decreased appetite, and constipation.
CN: Physiological integrity; CNS: Reduction of risk potential; CL: Apply; DIFFICULTY: Easy

85. 3. If parents have been taught to count the pulse of an infant diagnosed with hypothyroidism, they should be instructed to withhold the dose and consult their health care provider if the pulse rate is above a certain value.
CN: Physiological integrity; CNS: Reduction of risk potential; CL: Apply; DIFFICULTY: Easy

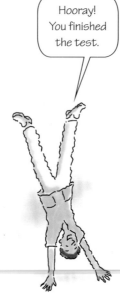

Hooray! You finished the test.

86. 1, 2, 4, 5. Polyuria, weakness, weight loss, and postprandial nausea are commonly seen in diabetes. The health care team would plan care to manage these signs and symptoms. Abdominal pain isn't a symptom of type 1 diabetes, and orthostatic *hypo*tension rather than orthostatic hypertension would be a significant finding.
CN: Safe, effective care environment; CNS: Coordinated care; CL: Analyze; DIFFICULTY: Difficult

Chapter 33

Genitourinary Disorders

Pediatric genitourinary refresher

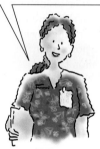

This chapter covers altered patterns of urinary elimination in children and includes glomerulonephritis, hypospadias, and—oh, a whole lot of other plumbing problems ... er, genitourinary disorders. Let's roll up our sleeves and get to work.

Glomerulonephritis (acute poststreptococcal glomerulonephritis)

Kidney disorder characterized by inflammatory injury in the glomerulus. Acute poststreptococcal glomerulonephritis occurs as an immune reaction to a group A beta-hemolytic streptococcal infection of the skin or throat

Key signs and symptoms
- Hematuria
- Edema abrupt onset, mild periorbital or lower extremities
- Hypertension
- Proteinuria
- Usually young school-age child

Key test results
- Urinalysis: RBC's, casts, small amounts of protein (0-3+)
- Altered electrolytes, elevated blood urea nitrogen (BUN) and creatinine levels
- Elevated ASO titer or streptozyme, decreased serum complement level

Key treatments
- Supportive
- Antihypertensives and diuretics; antibiotic treatment for active streptococcal infection
- Low salt diet
- Possible fluid restrictions

Key interventions
- Bed rest
- Strict intake and output (I&O)
- Frequent blood pressure monitoring
- Daily weight measurement
- Test urine frequently for protein and hematuria

Hypospadias and epispadias

Hypospadias
Congenital defect in which the urinary meatus is located on the underside of the shaft of the penis; may be accompanied by chordee, a downward curvature of the penis from a fibrous band of tissue

Epispadias
Congenital defect in which the urinary meatus is on the upper surface of the penis

Key signs and symptoms
- Altered angle of urination
- Meatus terminating at some point along lateral fusion line (hypospadias), ranging from the perineum to the distal penile shaft
- Meatus terminating on the upper surface of the penis (epispadias)

Key test results
- Observation confirms aberrant placement of the meatus; therefore, diagnostic testing isn't necessary

Key treatments
- Avoid circumcision (the foreskin may be needed later during surgical repair)
- Analgesics: morphine or acetaminophen for postoperative pain relief
- Antispasmodic agent: propantheline prescribed postoperatively
- Surgery
- Meatotomy (surgical procedure in which the urethra is extended into a normal position); may initially be performed to restore normal urinary function
- When the child is age 12 to 18 months, surgery to release the adherent chordee (fibrous band that causes the penis to curve downward)
- Surgery possibly delayed until age 4 if repair is to be extensive
- Indwelling urinary catheter or suprapubic urinary catheter postoperatively

Key interventions
- Keep the area clean
- Encourage parents to express feelings and concerns about changes in the child's body appearance or function; provide accurate information and answer questions thoroughly
- Instruct parents in hygiene of uncircumcised penis
- Postoperative care
- Monitor for signs of infection

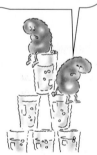

"Whoa!" It is important to achieve and maintain appropriate fluid balance.

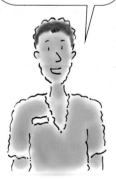

You can't just call a spadias a spadias. There are different types—like "hypospadias" and "epispadias."

- Leave the dressing in place for several days
- Take care to avoid pressure on the child's catheter and avoid kinking the catheter

Nephrotic syndrome (nephrosis)

Different types of kidney conditions distinguished by the presence of marked protein, edema, and hypoalbuminemia: idiopathic nephrosis is the most common type

Key signs and symptoms

- Severe proteinuria: frothy urine
- Edema: insidious onset, massive edema from shift into interstitial spaces, worsens during the day
- Hypovolemia
- Pallor, fatigue
- Usually toddler or preschool-age child

Key test results

- Protein in urine (3+ to 4+), possible microscopic hematuria
- Hypoalbuminemia (less than 2.5 g/dL), elevated cholesterol and triglyceride, hemoglobin, hematocrit, and platelet levels

Key treatments

- Prednisone to initiate remission (0 to trace protein in the urine for 5 to 7 days)
- Diuretics, possible albumin administration
- Diet with no added salt

Key interventions

- Prevent infection and skin breakdown
- Monitor vital signs (temperature) every 4 to 8 hours.
- Assess weight daily
- Assess edema and condition of the skin every 4 to 8 hours
- Strict intake and output (I&O)
- Adhere to "no added salt" diet and fluid restriction if ordered; teach child and parents about no added salt diet

Nephroblastoma (Wilms tumor)

Rare kidney cancer that primarily affects children. Most often occurs in one kidney, though sometimes found in both kidneys

Key signs and symptoms

- Associated congenital anomalies—microcephaly, intellectual disability, genitourinary tract problems
- Nontender mass, usually midline near the liver; usually detected by the parent while bathing or dressing the child

Key test results

- Excretory urography reveals a mass displacing the normal kidney structure

- Computed tomography (CT) scan or sonography reveals metastasis

Key treatments

- Nephrectomy within 24 to 48 hours of diagnosis because these tumors metastasize quickly
- Radiation therapy (following surgery)
- Chemotherapy (following surgery) with dactinomycin, doxorubicin, or vincristine

Key interventions

- Monitor vital signs and intake and output
- Don't palpate the abdomen, and prevent others from doing so
- Handle and bathe the child carefully, and loosen clothing around the abdomen
- Prepare the child and family members for a nephrectomy within 24 to 48 hours of diagnosis
- After nephrectomy:
  ○ monitor urine output and report output less than 30 mL/hour
  ○ assist with turning, coughing, and deep breathing
  ○ encourage early ambulation
  ○ provide pain medications, as necessary
  ○ monitor postoperative dressings for signs of bleeding
  ○ use aseptic technique for dressing changes

Urinary tract infection

Infection in any structure of the urinary tract, especially the urethra and bladder

Key signs and symptoms

- Frequent urge to void with pain or burning on urination
- Lethargy
- Low-grade fever
- Urine that's cloudy and foul-smelling

Key test results

- Clean-catch urine culture yields large amounts of bacteria

Key treatments

- Cranberry juice to acidify urine
- Forced fluids to flush infection from the urinary tract
- Antibiotics: sulfamethoxazole-trimethoprim or ampicillin to prevent glomerulonephritis

Key interventions

- Monitor intake and output
- Evaluate toileting habits for proper front-to-back wiping and proper hand washing

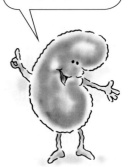

I kidney you not—this chapter will be easy. Just go with the flow.

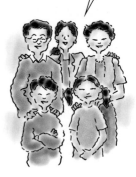

When a nephrectomy is required, educate the whole family on what to expect.

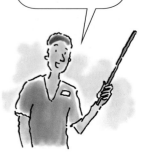

What are the signs of a urinary tract infection?

- Assist the child when necessary to ensure that the perineal area is clean after elimination
- Encourage increased intake of fluids and cranberry juice
- Force fluids to achieve urine output of more than 2 L/day; however, discourage intake greater than 3 L/day
- Teach the child and parents about:
  ○ refrigerating or culturing a urine specimen within 30 minutes of collection to prevent overgrowth of bacteria
  ○ completing the prescribed antibiotic therapy, even after symptoms subside
  ○ long-term follow-up care for high-risk children

Sexually transmitted infections (STIs)

Diverse group of infections spread through sexual activity with an infected person. Besides AIDS, the five most common STIs are chlamydia, gonorrhea, syphilis, genital herpes, and genital warts

Key signs and symptoms

- Sores or lesions on the genitals or in the oral or rectal area
- Pain or burning on urination
- Discharge from the penis
- Unusual or foul-smelling vaginal discharge
- Pain during sex
- Sore, swollen lymph nodes, particularly in the groin, but sometimes more widespread
- Lower abdominal pain
- Rash over the trunk, hands, or feet

Key test results

- Culture of discharge from penis/vagina/rectum or oral cavity (gonorrhea, chlamydia)
- Scraping of lesion (genital herpes)
- Blood test (syphilis, HIV)

Key treatments

- Gonorrhea and chlamydia: oral or injectable antibiotics, partners should also be treated
- Gonorrhea: ceftriaxone 250 mg IM and azithromycin 1g PO in a single dose
- Chlamydia: azithromycin 1g in a single dose or doxycycline BID x 7 days
- Genital herpes: antiviral drugs (acyclovir, valacyclovir, famciclovir)
- Syphilis: benzathine penicillin G
- Genital warts: cryotherapy, trichloroacetic acid (TCA) or bichloroacetic acid application

Key interventions

- Gather health information, sexual history, and allergy history
- Maintain non-judgmental attitude
- Teach methods for preventing STIs
- Provide specific education that is appropriate for the particular STI

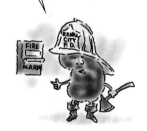

"Sound the alarm!" Some genitourinary disorders can cause serious complications.

thePoint® You can download tables of drug information to help you prepare for the NCLEX®! View Generic Drug Names, Drug Classifications, Drug Actions, and Nursing Implications for the drugs discussed in this refresher at **http://thePoint.lww.com**.

Genitourinary questions, answers, and rationales

1. The nurse is caring for a 20 kg child being treated for acute glomerulonephritis (AGN). Which of the following data collected by the nurse indicates improvement in the child's condition? Select all that apply.
1. A weight loss of 1 kg
2. Decreased urinary output over the last 24 hours
3. Demonstrates no periorbital, facial, or body edema
4. A fluid intake of more than 2,000 mL in 24 hours
5. An increased blood pressure

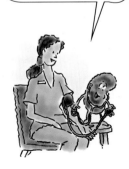

Hey—looks like you're back up to normal. The treatment must be working.

1. 1, 3. Weight loss indicates improvement in the condition. Weight gain is an early indication of excess fluid and occurs prior to visible edema. Diuretics cause excretion of excess fluid by preventing resorption of water and sodium. Sodium and water retention leads to edema. Increased urine output, not decreased output, and lack of edema indicates improved fluid balance and improvement in the condition. Normal fluid intake in a 20 kg child would be approximately 1,500 mL/day, not 2,000 mL/day. Often children with AGN are on a fluid restriction initially. Blood pressure drops as the child's condition improves.
CN: Health promotion and maintenance; CNS: None; CL: Analyze; DIFFICULTY: Difficult

2. When caring for a child with acute glomerulonephritis, which nursing action would be a **priority**? Select all that apply.
1. Measure daily weight.
2. Increase oral fluid intake.
3. Provide sodium supplements.
4. Monitor the child for signs of hypokalemia.
5. Assess for periorbital or dependent edema.

3. A child has been diagnosed with acute glomerulonephritis. Based on the results of the routine urinalysis below, which component is **most** consistent with this diagnosis?

Laboratory results	
Urinalysis	
Color:	Straw
Appearance:	Clear
Specific gravity:	1.032
pH:	5.5
Protein:	Negative
Blood:	Negative
RBC casts:	Present
Crystals:	Negative

1. Specific gravity
2. Protein
3. Blood
4. Red blood cell (RBC) casts

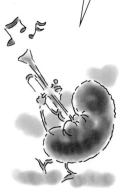

You're off to a great start! Let me toot my horn for you.

4. Which statement by the nurse would be the best response to parents who want to know the first indication that their child's acute glomerulonephritis is improving?
1. Urine output will increase.
2. Urine will be protein-free.
3. Blood pressure will stabilize.
4. The child will have more energy.

5. A nurse is taking frequent blood pressure readings on a child diagnosed with acute glomerulonephritis. The parents ask the nurse why this is necessary. When implementing nursing care, which teaching statement by the nurse is **most** accurate?
1. "Blood pressure fluctuations are a sign that the condition has become chronic."
2. "Blood pressure fluctuations are a common adverse effect of antibiotic therapy."
3. "Hypotension leading to sudden shock can develop at any time."
4. "Acute hypertension must be anticipated and identified."

2. 1, 5. The child with acute glomerulonephritis should be monitored for fluid imbalance, which is done through daily weights. Sodium and water retention leads to edema. Weight gain is an early sign of fluid retention. Increasing oral intake, providing sodium supplements, and monitoring for hypokalemia aren't part of the therapeutic management of acute glomerulonephritis.
CN: Physiological integrity; CNS: Physiological adaptation; CL: Apply; DIFFICULTY: Challenge

3. 4. Urinalysis findings consistent with acute glomerulonephritis include the presence of RBC casts. In addition, a specific gravity less than 1.030, proteinuria, and hematuria would also be findings consistent with acute glomerulonephritis. The presence of crystals in the urine typically indicates a congenital metabolic problem.
CN: Physiological integrity; CNS: Physiological adaptation; CL: Apply; DIFFICULTY: Moderate

4. 1. One of the first signs of improvement during the acute phase of glomerulonephritis is an increase in urine output. It will take time for the urine to be protein-free. Antihypertensive drugs may be needed to stabilize blood pressure. Children generally don't have much energy during the acute phase of this disease.
CN: Physiological integrity; CNS: Physiological adaptation; CL: Analyze; DIFFICULTY: Moderate

5. 4. Regular measurement of vital signs, including blood pressure, body weight, and intake and output, is essential to monitor the progress of acute glomerulonephritis and to detect complications that may appear at any time during the course of the disease. Hypertension is more likely to occur with glomerulonephritis than hypotension and should be anticipated. Blood pressure fluctuations don't indicate that the condition has become chronic and aren't common adverse reactions to antibiotic therapy.
CN: Physiological integrity; CNS: Physiological adaptation; CL: Apply; DIFFICULTY: Moderate

CN: Client needs category   CNS: Client needs subcategory   CL: Cognitive level

6. When evaluating the urinalysis report of a child with acute glomerulonephritis, the nurse would expect which result?
1. Proteinuria and decreased specific gravity
2. Bacteriuria and increased specific gravity
3. Hematuria and proteinuria
4. Bacteriuria and hematuria

7. Which statement regarding acute glomerulonephritis indicates that the parents of a child with this diagnosis understand the education provided by the nurse?
1. "This disease occurs after a urinary tract infection."
2. "This disease is associated with renal vascular disorders."
3. "This disease occurs after a streptococcal infection."
4. "This disease is associated with structural anomalies of the genitourinary tract."

8. When obtaining a child's daily weight, the nurse notes that the child has lost 6 lb (2.7 kg) after 3 days of hospitalization for acute glomerulonephritis. This is **most** likely the result of which factor?
1. Poor appetite
2. Reduction of edema
3. Decreased salt intake
4. Restriction to bed rest

9. The nurse is reinforcing education about antihypertensive therapy with the parents of a child with glomerulonephritis. Which statement made by the parent indicates that further teaching is required?
1. "My child will need to take antihypertensive drugs for the rest of his life."
2. "I should be sure to keep my child's regular appointments."
3. "I should watch my child for dizziness and lightheadedness."
4. "I will administer the medication at the same time each day."

10. The nurse is evaluating a group of children for acute glomerulonephritis. Which child would be **most** likely to develop the disease?
1. A child who had pneumonia a month ago
2. A child who was bitten by a brown spider
3. A child who shows no signs of periorbital edema
4. A child who had a streptococcal infection 2 weeks ago

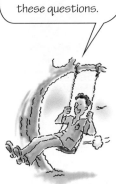

Hang on tight! We're flying through these questions.

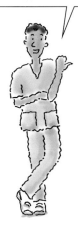

"Further teaching is required" is code for "the parent doesn't know what they're talking about."

6. 3. Urinalysis during the acute phase of glomerulonephritis characteristically shows hematuria, proteinuria, and increased specific gravity.
CN: Physiological integrity; CNS: Physiological adaptation; CL: Analyze; DIFFICULTY: Moderate

7. 3. Acute glomerulonephritis is an immune-complex disease that occurs as a by-product of an antecedent streptococcal infection. Certain strains of the infection are usually beta-hemolytic streptococci.
CN: Physiological integrity; CNS: Physiological adaptation; CL: Analyze; DIFFICULTY: Moderate

8. 2. When edema is reduced, the child will lose weight. This should normally occur after treatment for acute glomerulonephritis has been followed for several days. It will take longer for the child's appetite to improve, but this shouldn't lead to such a dramatic weight loss in a child this age.
CN: Physiological integrity; CNS: Physiological adaptation; CL: Apply; DIFFICULTY: Moderate

9. 1. The child will be weaned off the antihypertensive drugs as blood pressure decreases and the condition improves. Regular appointments should be kept to monitor the child's blood pressure. Blood pressure should be rechecked a week after the antihypertensive has been discontinued. Dizziness and lightheadedness can be a side effect. A daily antihypertensive should be given at the same time each day (as close to every 24 hours as possible).
CN: Physiological integrity; CNS: Pharmacological therapies; CL: Apply; DIFFICULTY: Easy

10. 4. A latent period of 10 to 14 days occurs between the streptococcal infection of the throat or skin and the onset of clinical manifestations. The peak incidence of disease corresponds to the incidence of streptococcal infections. Pneumonia isn't a precursor to glomerulonephritis nor is a bite from a brown spider. A sign of periorbital edema would lead the nurse to investigate the possibility of glomerulonephritis, especially if reported to be worse in the morning.
CN: Health promotion and maintenance; CNS: None; CL: Analyze; DIFFICULTY: Easy

CN: Client needs category   CNS: Client needs subcategory   CL: Cognitive level

11. A nurse should make which dietary recommendation to a child who has been newly diagnosed with acute glomerulonephritis?
1. Reduce calories.
2. Increase potassium.
3. Severely restrict sodium.
4. Moderately restrict sodium.

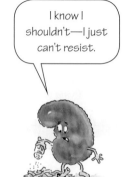

I know I shouldn't—I just can't resist.

12. The nurse is collecting data on a child with acute glomerulonephritis. Which finding would be of **immediate** concern to the nurse?
1. Cola-colored urine
2. Blurred vision
3. Albumin in the urine
4. Peripheral edema

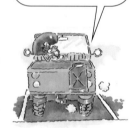

Treat your kidneys well, and they'll keep you trucking for many years to come.

13. Which comment made by a parent would indicate to the nurse the need for further education about acute glomerulonephritis complications?
1. "Dizziness is expected, and I should have my child lie down."
2. "I should let the nurse know every time my child urinates."
3. "I need to ask my child if he has a headache."
4. "I should encourage quiet play activities."

14. A previously toilet-trained 4-year-old child begins wetting the bed after being hospitalized. Which statement should a nurse make to the parents?
1. "Children commonly show regressive behavior when hospitalized."
2. "Your child is just acting out to make you feel bad."
3. "Sometimes 4-year-olds still have accidents."
4. "Let's try cutting back on fluids and see whether that helps."

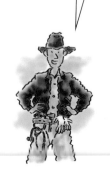

Assessing pediatric clients can be an adventure. Make sure you're fully equipped before you enter that exam room.

15. Which action is a nursing **priority** for a child with acute glomerulonephritis? Select all that apply.
1. Assess blood pressure every 4 hours.
2. Check urine specific gravity every 8 hours.
3. Encourage daily fluid intake of 3,500 L.
4. Weigh every morning.
5. Provide a 2,500 mg sodium diet.

11. 4. Moderate sodium restriction with a diet that has no added salt after cooking is usually effective. Reduced calorie consumption and increased potassium consumption aren't necessary because of the decrease in urine output. Severe sodium restriction isn't needed and will make it more difficult to ensure adequate nutrition.
CN: Physiological integrity; CNS: Basic care and comfort; CL: Apply; DIFFICULTY: Challenge

12. 2. Visual disturbances can be an indication of rising blood pressure and should be investigated. Presence of albumin in the urine, red blood cells (causing the cola-colored urine), and peripheral edema are common symptoms in acute glomerulonephritis.
CN: Physiological integrity; CNS: Reduction of risk potential; CL: Analyze; DIFFICULTY: Difficult

13. 1. Dizziness and headache are signs of encephalopathy, not glomerulonephritis, and must be reported to the nurse. Hypertensive encephalopathy, acute cardiac decompensation, and acute renal failure are the major complications that tend to develop during the acute phase of glomerulonephritis. In order to maintain an accurate intake and output record, the parent should let the nurse know when the child urinates. Quiet play is encouraged to avoid overstressing the kidneys.
CN: Physiological integrity; CNS: Reduction of risk potential; CL: Apply; DIFFICULTY: Difficult

14. 1. Young children may exhibit regressive behaviors when they're under stress, such as occurs with hospitalization. The child may be acting out, but more likely, this is not voluntary bed-wetting. Four-year-olds should be fully toilet trained. Restricting fluids as a first step in a hospitalized child isn't appropriate; other causes of enuresis should be considered first.
CN: Psychosocial integrity; CNS: None; CL: Apply; DIFFICULTY: Easy

15. 1, 4. Because hypertension is a complication of acute glomerulonephritis, the nurse should check the child's blood pressure every 4 hours. An increase in weight is the first sign of fluid retention, so the child should be weighed daily. The urine specific gravity should also be monitored, but it isn't as high a priority as monitoring the blood pressure. The child may be placed on fluid or sodium restrictions.
CN: Physiological integrity; CNS: Reduction of risk potential; CL: Apply; DIFFICULTY: Difficult

16. When instructing an 8-year-old child about obtaining a clean-catch urine specimen, which information should be included by the nurse?
1. Collect the specimen right after a nap.
2. Discard the first voided specimen of the day.
3. Collect the specimen at the beginning of urination.
4. You don't need to wash your perineal area before collecting the specimen.

16. 2. When collecting a clean-catch urine specimen, the first voided specimen of the day should never be used because of urinary stasis; this also applies after a nap. The specimen should be collected midstream, not at the beginning of urination. Washing the perineal area before collecting a specimen is important to make sure there are no contaminants from the skin in the specimen.
CN: Physiological integrity; CNS: Reduction of risk potential; CL: Apply; DIFFICULTY: Moderate

17. The nurse is reinforcing education with the parents about the treatment of acute glomerulonephritis. Which statement made by the parents reflects an understanding of the teaching?
1. "All children who have signs of glomerulonephritis are hospitalized for approximately 1 week."
2. "Parents should expect children to have a normal energy level during the acute phase."
3. "Children who have normal blood pressure and a satisfactory urine output can generally be treated at home."
4. "Children with gross hematuria and significant oliguria should be brought to the health care provider's office about every 2 days for monitoring."

17. 3. Children who have normal blood pressure and a satisfactory urine output can generally be treated at home. Those with gross hematuria and significant oliguria will probably be hospitalized for monitoring. Parents should expect children to have decreased energy during the acute phase of the disease.
CN: Physiological integrity; CNS: Reduction of risk potential; CL: Apply; DIFFICULTY: Moderate

18. The nurse is caring for a child diagnosed with acute glomerulonephritis? Which food choices would be appropriate for a child with this diagnosis? Select all that apply.
1. Turkey sandwich with mayonnaise
2. Canned soup and crackers
3. Hot dog with ketchup and mustard
4. Tuna salad in a pita
5. Garden salad with grilled chicken
6. Apple with peanut butter

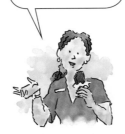

Did somebody mention food? I feel hungry all of a sudden.

18. 1, 4, 5, 6. Foods that are high in sodium should be eliminated from the child's diet. Such snacks as pretzels and potato chips should be discouraged. Because hot dogs contain a great deal of sodium, they should be eliminated from the child's diet. Canned foods and crackers are also high in sodium. Processed foods and restaurant foods typically contain large amounts of sodium. Any other foods that the child likes should be encouraged
CN: Physiological integrity; CNS: Basic care and comfort; CL: Apply; DIFFICULTY: Challenge

19. After the acute phase of glomerulonephritis is over, which discharge instructions should the nurse include to the child's parents?
1. Every 6 months, a cystogram will be needed for evaluation of progress.
2. Weekly visits to the health care provider may be needed for evaluation.
3. It will be acceptable to keep the regular yearly checkup appointment for the next evaluation.
4. There's no need to worry about further evaluations by the health care provider related to this disease.

19. 2. Weekly or monthly visits to the health care provider will be needed for evaluation of improvement and will usually involve the collection of a urine specimen for urinalysis. A cystogram isn't helpful in determining the progression of this disease; it's used to review the anatomical structures of the urinary tract.
CN: Physiological integrity; CNS: Reduction of risk potential; CL: Apply; DIFFICULTY: Moderate

20. Which therapy should the nurse expect to incorporate into the care of the child with acute glomerulonephritis?
1. Antibiotic therapy
2. Dialysis therapy
3. Diuretic therapy
4. Play therapy

21. The nurse is preparing to administer penicillin VK to a 25 kg child with acute glomerulonephritis. The health care provider has ordered penicillin VK 500 mg by mouth every 8 hours. The recommended dose (from the drug literature) is 50 to 75 mg/kg/day by mouth every 6 to 8 hours. After reviewing the information, the nurse draws which conclusion?
1. The ordered dosage is larger than the maximum dosage recommended by the drug literature.
2. The ordered dosage is smaller than the minimum dosage recommended by the drug literature.
3. The dose is safe to give and falls within the safe dose range for this child.
4. It is not the nurse's responsibility to question the health care provider's orders.

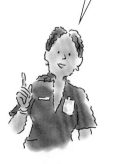

Careful. It's important to be accurate when calculating dosages. Your client's safety depends on it.

22. The nurse is preparing to administer penicillin VK 0.5 g to a child with glomerulonephritis. The nurse has available an oral solution of penicillin VK 250 mg/5 mL. How many milliliters should the nurse administer with each dose? Record your answer using a whole number.

_____ mL

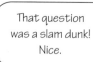

That question was a slam dunk! Nice.

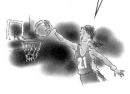

23. The nurse is caring for an infant with hypospadias. Which anomaly, which commonly accompanies this condition, would the nurse obtain data for in the infant? Select all that apply.
1. Undescended testes
2. Chordee
3. Ambiguous genitalia
4. Umbilical hernias
5. Inguinal hernias

20. 4. Play therapy is a very important aspect of care to help the child understand what's happening to him. It allows the child to express concerns and fears, to avoid night terrors and regression in the stage of growth and development. Antibiotic and diuretic therapies aren't routine treatments for acute glomerulonephritis. Dialysis therapy is appropriate for renal failure.
CN: Health promotion and maintenance; CNS: None;
CL: Apply; DIFFICULTY: Difficult

21. 3. The calculated safe dosage range for this child is 1,250 to 1,875 mg per day. The child will be receiving 1,500 mg per day (500 mg x 3 doses/day) which is within the recommended range, so it is safe to administer.
CN: Physiological integrity; CNS: Pharmacological therapies;
CL: Analyze; DIFFICULTY: Challenge

22. 10.
The correct formula to calculate a drug dose is:

$$\frac{\text{Dose on hand}}{\text{Quantity on hand}} = \frac{\text{Dose desired}}{X}$$

The health care provider prescribes 0.5 g, which is the dose desired. The nurse has available 250 mg/5 mL, which is the dose on hand.

$$\frac{250 \text{ mg}}{5 \text{ mL}} = \frac{0.5 \text{ g}}{X}$$

$$\frac{250 \text{ mg}}{5 \text{ mL}} = \frac{500 \text{ mg}}{X}$$

$$250X = 2500 \text{ mL}$$

$$X = 10 \text{ mL}$$

CN: Physiological integrity; CNS: Pharmacological therapies;
CL: Apply; DIFFICULTY: Moderate

23. 1, 2. Because undescended testes may also be present in hypospadias, the small penis may appear to be an enlarged clitoris. This shouldn't be mistaken for ambiguous genitalia. If there's any doubt, more tests should be performed. Chordee, or ventral curvature of the penis, results from the replacement of normal skin with a fibrous band of tissue. It usually accompanies more severe forms of hypospadias. Hernias don't generally accompany hypospadias.
CN: Physiological integrity; CNS: Reduction of risk potential;
CL: Apply; DIFFICULTY: Challenge

24. The nurse is reinforcing education about surgery with the parent of an infant with hypospadias. Which statement by the parent indicates an understanding of the education?
1. "Early surgery is to prevent separation anxiety."
2. "Doing the surgery in infancy helps prevent urinary complications."
3. "Infants are more accepting of hospitalization, so the surgery is done then."
4. "The surgery is done while the child is an infant to promote development of normal body image."

24. 4. Whenever there are defects of the genitourinary tract, surgery should be performed early to promote development of a normal body image, not acceptance of hospitalization. A child with normal emotional development shows separation anxiety at 7 to 9 months. Within a few months, he understands the mother's permanence, and anxiety diminishes. Hypospadias doesn't put the child at a greater risk for urinary complications.
CN: Physiological integrity; CNS: Reduction of risk potential; CL: Apply; DIFFICULTY: Challenge

25. A child is undergoing hypospadias repair. Which statement made by the child's parents about the principal objective of surgical correction implies a need for further education?
1. "The purpose is to improve the physical appearance of the genitalia for psychological reasons."
2. "The purpose is to enhance the child's ability to void in the standing position."
3. "The purpose is to decrease the chances of urinary tract infections."
4. "The purpose is to preserve a sexually adequate organ."

25. 3. A child with hypospadias isn't at greater risk for urinary tract infections. The principal objectives of surgical corrections are to enhance the child's ability to void in the standing position with a straight stream, to improve the physical appearance of the genitalia for psychological reasons, and to preserve a sexually adequate organ.
CN: Physiological integrity; CNS: Reduction of risk potential; CL: Apply; DIFFICULTY: Difficult

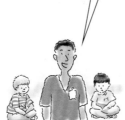

Remember the body part where hypospadias occurs? Keep that in mind when answering question #26.

26. The nurse should counsel parents to postpone which action until after their son's hypospadias has been repaired?
1. Circumcision
2. Phototherapy
3. Getting hepatitis B vaccine
4. Checking blood for inborn errors of metabolism

26. 1. Circumcision shouldn't be performed until after the hypospadias has been repaired. The foreskin might be needed to help in the repair of hypospadias. None of the other actions has any bearing on the repair of hypospadias.
CN: Physiological integrity; CNS: Reduction of risk potential; CL: Apply; DIFFICULTY: Easy

27. Which nursing intervention should be included in the care plan for a male infant following surgical repair of hypospadias?
1. Sterile dressing changes every 4 hours
2. Frequent inspection of the tip of the penis
3. Removal of the urethral stent or catheter on the second postoperative day
4. Urethral catheterization if voiding doesn't occur over an 8-hour period

27. 2. Following hypospadias repair, a pressure dressing is applied to the penis to reduce bleeding and tissue swelling. The penile tip should then be assessed frequently for signs of circulatory impairment. The dressing around the penis shouldn't be changed as frequently as every 4 hours. The health care provider will determine when the urethral stent/ catheter will be removed. There is no need to limit fluid intake; in fact, fluids should be encouraged.
CN: Physiological integrity; CNS: Basic care and comfort; CL: Apply; DIFFICULTY: Moderate

28. When explaining to the parents the optimal time for repair of hypospadias, the nurse should indicate which as the age of choice?
1. 1 week
2. 6 to 18 months
3. 2 years
4. 4 years

28. 2. The preferred time for surgical repair is ages 6 to 18 months, before the child has developed body image and castration anxiety. Surgical repair of hypospadias as early as age 3 months has been successful, but with a high incidence of complications.
CN: Physiological integrity; CNS: Reduction of risk potential; CL: Apply; DIFFICULTY: Easy

29. After a nurse has provided discharge education to the parents of a child with hypospadias, which statement by the parent indicates that additional education is needed?
1. "I'll need to learn irrigation techniques."
2. "I should bathe my child in the tub daily."
3. "Proper catheter care helps prevent infection."
4. "It's important to keep the catheter free of kinks and blockages."

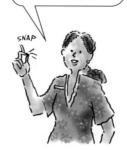

That was easy. I think you're getting the hang of this.

SNAP

30. When providing discharge instructions to parents of an older child who has had hypospadias repair, which activity should be encouraged?
1. Riding a bicycle
2. Playing in sandboxes
3. Increased fluid intake
4. Playing with the family pet

31. The parent of a neonate born with hypospadias is sharing feelings of guilt about this anomaly with a nurse. What is the **best** response by the nurse?
1. "You should not feel guilty; there is nothing you could have done."
2. "Maybe you need to talk to a specialist to see if it is hereditary."
3. "It is a waste of time to worry; you need to concentrate on taking care of your baby."
4. "Do you want to talk about how you have been feeling?"

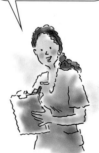

The long and the short of it is that you need to know the right dimensions to calculate body surface area.

32. The nurse is preparing to calculate the safe dose range of a chemotherapy drug for a child with Wilms tumor. The drug is ordered in mg/m². What information does the nurse need in order to calculate the body surface area (m²) of the child? Select all that apply.
1. The child's blood type.
2. The child's weight.
3. The child's height.
4. The child's white blood cell count (WBC).
5. The child's birth weight.

33. A 1-year-old underwent hypospadias repair yesterday; he has a urethral catheter in place and an IV. Which rationale is appropriate for administering propantheline on an as-needed basis?
1. To decrease the chance of infection at the suture line
2. To decrease the number of organisms in the urine
3. To prevent bladder spasms while the catheter is present
4. To increase urine flow from the kidney to the ureters

29. 2. A tub bath should be avoided to prevent infection until the stent has been removed. Parents are taught to care for the indwelling catheter or stent and how to perform irrigation techniques if indicated. They need to know how to empty the urine bag and how to avoid kinking, twisting, or blockage of the catheter or stent.
CN: Physiological integrity; CNS: Reduction of risk potential; CL: Analyze; DIFFICULTY: Easy

30. 3. The family is advised to encourage the child to increase fluid intake. Playing in sand boxes, riding bicycles, and engaging in potentially rough activities (e.g., playing with the family pet) are avoided until allowed by the surgeon.
CN: Physiological integrity; CNS: Reduction of risk potential; CL: Apply; DIFFICULTY: Easy

31. 4. The nurse should encourage the parent to talk about how she has been feeling and allow her to be heard. This defect isn't hereditary nor is it carried by an autosomal recessive gene. The other two options belittle the parent's feelings.
CN: Psychosocial integrity; CNS: None; CL: Apply; DIFFICULTY: Easy

32. 2, 3. Body surface area is calculated using a pediatric nomogram or by a formula. Both of these methods require knowledge of the height and weight of the child.
CN: Physiological adaptation; CNS: Pharmacological therapies; CL: Apply; DIFFICULTY: Moderate

33. 3. Propantheline is an antispasmodic that works effectively on children. It prevents bladder spasms while the catheter is in place. It isn't an antibiotic and therefore won't decrease the chance of infection or the number of organisms in the urine. The drug has no diuretic effect and won't increase urine flow.
CN: Physiological integrity; CNS: Pharmacological therapies; CL: Apply; DIFFICULTY: Moderate

34. Which intervention by the nurse would be **most** helpful when discussing hypospadias with the parents of an infant with this defect?
1. Refer the parents to a counselor.
2. Be there to listen to the parents' concerns.
3. Notify the health care provider and have him talk to the parents.
4. Suggest a support group of other parents who have gone through this experience.

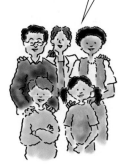

When working with pediatric clients, remember to care for the whole family.

35. The nurse is collecting data on a 6-year old child. The child reports dysuria and urgency. The parent reports that the child has recently had some enuresis. The nurse recognizes these as signs and symptoms of which condition?
1. Nephrotic syndrome
2. Urinary tract infection
3. Acute glomerulonephritis
4. Obstructive uropathy

36. The difference between hypospadias and epispadias is defined by which characteristic?
1. Epispadias defects can only occur in males.
2. The difference between the defects is the length of the urethra.
3. Hypospadias is an abnormal opening on the ventral side of the penis; epispadias is an abnormal opening on the dorsal side.
4. Hypospadias is an abnormal opening on the dorsal side of the penis; epispadias is an abnormal opening on the ventral side.

37. The nurse is reinforcing education with the parent of a child with nephrosis who will be discharged on prednisone. In discussing prevention of infection, which statements by the parent would indicate a need for further teaching? Select all that apply.
1. "I will contact my child's pediatrician if she runs a fever or reports a sore throat."
2. "All members of the family should wash our hands frequently, especially after using the bathroom."
3. "I should keep my child away from people who are sick."
4. "I need to keep my house clean and prepare and store food properly."
5. "My child should be allowed to play with pets to help her develop a healthy immune system."
6. "My child should receive all routine childhood immunizations.

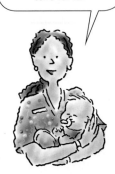

Make sure your client's parents have an accurate understanding of the condition and how to care for it.

34. 2. The nurse must recognize that parents are going to grieve the loss of the normal child when they have a neonate born with a birth defect. Initially, the parents need to have a nurse who will listen to their concerns for their neonate's health. Suggesting a support group or referring the parents to a counselor might be helpful but not initially. The health care provider will need to spend time with the parents to discuss surgery, but the nurse is in the best position to allow the parents to vent their grief and anger initially.
CN: Psychosocial integrity; CNS: None; CL: Apply; DIFFICULTY: Moderate

35. 2. Frequency and urgency can lead to enuresis. All are symptoms of urinary tract infection.
CN: Physiological integrity; CNS: Physiological adaptation; CL: Apply; DIFFICULTY: Easy

36. 3. Hypospadias results from the incomplete closure of the urethral folds along the ventral surface of the developing penis. Epispadias results when the urinary meatus is on the dorsal surface of the penis. Epispadias defects can occur in males and females. The difference is where the opening of the urinary meatus is located, not the urethra's length.
CN: Physiological integrity; CNS: Physiological adaptation; CL: Understand; DIFFICULTY: Challenge

37. 5, 6. Family members should be up-to-date on immunizations to prevent exposing the child; the immunocompromised child should not receive live-virus immunization. Immunocompromised children should not be around pets. Any signs and symptoms of infections should be reported for prompt treatment. Proper handwashing is the first line of defense against infection. The child should not be around anyone who is sick, especially someone with chicken pox or measles. Environmental cleanliness and handling and storing food properly decreases bacteria.
CN: Safe, effective care environment; CNS: Safety and infection control; CL: Analyze; DIFFICULTY: Difficult

38. When a nurse is educating a parent on how to care for the son's penis after hypospadias repair with a skin graft, which statement made by the parent would indicate the need for further education?
1. "My infant will be able to take baths after the repair has healed."
2. "I'll change the dressing around his penis daily."
3. "I'll make sure I change my infant's diaper often."
4. "If there's a color change in his penis, I'll notify my health care provider."

38. 2. Dressing changes after a hypospadias repair with a skin graft are generally performed by the health care provider, but they aren't performed every day because the skin graft needs time to heal and adhere to the penis. Changing the infant's diapers usually helps keep the penis dry. Baths aren't given until postoperative healing has taken place. If the penis color changes, it might be evidence of circulation problems and should be reported to the health care provider.
CN: Physiological integrity; CNS: Reduction of risk potential;
CL: Analyze: DIFFICULTY: Moderate

39. The nurse is preparing the parents of an infant with hypospadias for surgery. Which statement made by the parents would indicate the need for further education?
1. "Skin grafting might be involved in my infant's repair."
2. "After surgery, my infant's penis will look perfectly normal."
3. "Surgical repair may need to be performed in several stages."
4. "My infant will probably be in some pain after the surgery and might need to take some medication for relief."

39. 2. It's important to stress to the parents that even after a repair of hypospadias the outcome isn't a completely "normal-looking" penis. The goals of surgery are to allow the child to void from the tip of his penis, void with a straight stream, and stand up while voiding.
CN: Psychosocial integrity; CNS: None;
CL: Apply: DIFFICULTY: Moderate

40. Which data collected by the nurse would indicate to the health care provider the need for a staged repair of a hypospadias rather than a single repair?
1. Chordee is present with the hypospadias.
2. The urinary meatus opens close to the scrotum.
3. The urinary meatus is just below the tip of the penis.
4. The infant had been circumcised before the defect was discovered.

40. 2. Increased surgical experience and improvements in technique have reduced the number of staged procedures applied to hypospadias defects; however, a staged procedure is indicated in particularly severe defects, such as the urinary meatus opening close to the scrotum, with marked deficits of available skin for mobilization of flaps. If an infant has a relatively minor hypospadias or has been circumcised, the repair can still occur in one stage. Having chordee present doesn't require a staged hypospadias repair.
CN: Physiological integrity; CNS: Physiological adaptation;
CL: Analyze; DIFFICULTY: Difficult

41. A nurse is preparing a presentation to a group of female adolescents about pelvic inflammatory disease (PID). Which statement **best** reflects the focus of preventive education needs for this age group?
1. Poor hygiene practices increase the risk of PID.
2. The use of hormonal contraceptives decreases the risk of PID.
3. There are long-term complications related to reproductive tract infections.
4. There are risks of defects in future infants born to adolescents with PID.

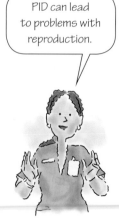

PID can lead to problems with reproduction.

41. 3. Long-term complications of PID include abscess formation in the fallopian tubes and adhesion formation leading to an increased risk of ectopic pregnancy or infertility. PID isn't prevented by proper personal hygiene or by any form of contraception, even though some forms of contraception, such as the male or female condom, do help to decrease the incidence. PID does not increase the risk of birth defects in infants born to adolescents with PID.
CN: Health promotion and maintenance; CNS: None CL: Apply;
DIFFICULTY: Moderate

42. The nurse is reinforcing education with an adolescent diagnosed with chlamydia. Which statement by the adolescent indicates a correct understanding of the teaching?
1. "The preferred treatment for chlamydia is oral penicillin."
2. "I can stop taking my doxycycline after the discharge goes away."
3. "My sexual partners will also need to be treated."
4. "Since I have had chlamydia I am immune to it in the future."

43. The nurse is participating in a staff education workshop about preventing STDs in adolescents. Which statements by the nurse would indicate an understanding of the prevention strategies? Select all that apply.
1. "I should maintain a non-judgmental attitude when dealing with adolescents that are sexually active."
2. "It is important to educate adolescents about the specific behaviors that put them at risk for STDs."
3. "Being in a mutually monogamous relationship will decrease the risk of STDs for adolescents."
4. "Parents will need to be notified and give consent for an adolescent to be tested and treated for STDs."
5. "Abstinence is the only strategy for preventing STDs that should be discussed with adolescents because it is 100% effective."
6. "Adolescents who choose to be sexually active should be encouraged to use condoms correctly and consistently when having oral, vaginal, and anal sex."

44. Before an adolescent with syphilis can be treated, the nurse must determine which factor?
1. Portal of entry
2. Size of the chancre
3. Names of sexual contacts
4. Existence of medication allergies

45. After the nurse has completed discharge education, which statement made by the female adolescent treated for a sexually transmitted disease would indicate that discharge instructions were understood?
1. "I don't need those condoms because I'm not allergic to penicillin, and I'll come for a shot at the first sign of infection."
2. "I will notify my sex partners and not have unprotected sex from now on."
3. "I will be careful not to have intercourse with someone who isn't clean."
4. "I don't think it will happen to me again."

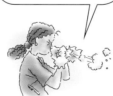

Achoo! Excuse me … I think I'm allergic to question #44.

42. 3. Sexual partners will need to be treated to prevent reinfection. The treatment of choice is doxycycline or azithromycin. When doxycycline is prescribed, the dosage is 100 mg by mouth, twice a day for 7 days. It is important to complete the full course of therapy even if symptoms subside. No immunity is conferred by exposure; it is possible to be infected multiple times if precautions are not taken.
CN: Health promotion and maintenance; CNS: None;
CL: Apply; DIFFICULTY: Easy

43. 1, 2, 3, 6. Many adolescents are reluctant to seek care because of concerns about judgmental attitudes of health care providers and confidentiality. Most states have laws that allow minors to receive STD and pregnancy services without the consent/knowledge of the parents. Abstinence is the only 100% effective strategy, but it is not the only strategy that should be discussed. Knowledge of specific behaviors that increase the risk of STDs, engaging in a mutually monogamous relationship, and correct and consistent condom use also reduce the risk of contracting STDs.
CN: Safe, effective care environment; CNS: Coordinated care;
CL: Analyze; DIFFICULTY: Challenge

44. 4. The treatment of choice for syphilis is penicillin; clients allergic to penicillin must be given another antibiotic. The other information isn't necessary before treatment can begin.
CN: Health promotion and maintenance; CNS: None; CL: Apply;
DIFFICULTY: Easy

45. 2. Goal achievement is indicated by the female adolescent's ability to describe preventive behaviors and health practices. The other statements indicate that she doesn't understand the need to take preventive measures.
CN: Health promotion and maintenance; CNS: None; CL: Analyze;
DIFFICULTY: Easy

46. Which technique should the nurse consider when she's discussing sex and sexual activities with adolescents?
1. Break down all the information into scientific terminology.
2. Refer adolescents to their parents for sexual information.
3. Only answer questions that are asked; don't present any other content.
4. Present sexual information using the proper terminology and in a straightforward manner.

47. An adolescent has been diagnosed with gonorrhea. The health care provider has ordered ceftriaxone 250 mg to be administered prior to discharge from the clinic. Before preparing and administering the medication, which data should the nurse collect from the client? Select all that apply.
1. Allergy to penicillin
2. Previous history of treatment for gonorrhea
3. Allergy to cephalosporins
4. Names of sexual partners
5. Sites of sexual penetration

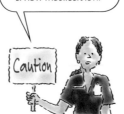

Collecting pertinent information is always a good idea before administering a new medication.

Caution

48. Which statement should the nurse include when educating an adolescent about gonorrhea?
1. It is caused by *Treponema pallidum*.
2. Treatment of sexual partners is an essential part of treatment.
3. It is usually treated by multidose administration of penicillin.
4. It may be contracted through contact with a contaminated toilet seat.

49. When planning sex education and contraceptive education for adolescents, which factor should the nurse consider?
1. Neither sexual activity nor contraception requires planning.
2. Most teenagers today are knowledgeable about reproduction.
3. Most teenagers use pregnancy as a way to rebel against their parents.
4. Most teenagers are open about contraception but inconsistently use birth control.

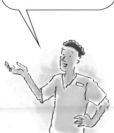

Only one answer to question #50 prevents STIs. Which one is it?

50. A sexually active teenager seeks counseling from the school nurse about prevention of sexually transmitted diseases (STDs). Which contraceptive measure should the nurse recommend?
1. Rhythm method
2. Withdrawal method
3. Prophylactic antibiotic use
4. Condom and spermicide use

CN: Client needs category   CNS: Client needs subcategory   CL: Cognitive level

46. 4. Although many adolescents have received sex education from parents and school throughout childhood, they aren't always adequately prepared for the impact of puberty. A large portion of their knowledge is acquired from peers, television, movies, and magazines. Consequently, much of the sex information they have is incomplete, inaccurate, riddled with cultural and moral values, and not very helpful. The public perceives nurses as having authoritative information and being willing to take time with adolescents and their parents. To be effective teachers, nurses need to be honest and open with sexual information.
CN: Health promotion and maintenance; CNS: None;
CL: Apply; DIFFICULTY: Easy

47. 1, 3. Ceftriaxone is a third generation cephalosporin and should not be administered if the client has an allergy to cephalosporins. Cephalosporins are also contraindicated if there has been a previous anaphylactic reaction to penicillin. The other information may be collected, but it does not relate to preparation or administration of the ceftriaxone.
CN: Physiological integrity; CNS: Pharmacological therapies;
CL: Analyze; DIFFICULTY: Challenge

48. 2. Adolescents should be taught that treatment is needed for all sexual partners. *Treponema pallidum* is the causative organism of syphilis, not gonorrhea. The medication of choice is a single dose of IM ceftriaxone in males and a single oral dose of cefixime in females. Gonorrhea can't be contracted from a contaminated toilet seat.
CN: Health promotion and maintenance; CNS: None;
CL: Apply; DIFFICULTY: Easy

49. 4. Most teenagers today are very open about discussing contraception and sexuality, but they may get caught up in the moment of sexuality and forget about birth control measures. Adolescents receive most of their information on reproduction and sexuality from their peers, who generally don't have correct information. Teenagers generally become pregnant because they fail to use birth control for reasons other than rebelling against their parents. Contraception should always be part of sex education and requires planning.
CN: Health promotion and maintenance; CNS: None; CL: Analyze;
DIFFICULTY: Easy

50. 4. Prevention of STDs is the primary concern of health care professionals. Barrier contraceptive methods, such as condoms with the addition of spermicide, seem to offer the best protection for preventing STDs and their serious complications. The other contraceptive choices don't prevent the transmission of an STD. Antibiotics can't be taken throughout the life span.
CN: Health promotion and maintenance; CNS: None; CL: Apply;
DIFFICULTY: Easy

51. The nurse understands that which developmental rationale explains risk-taking behavior in adolescents?
 1. Adolescents are concrete thinkers and concentrate only on what's happening at that time.
 2. Belief in their own invulnerability persuades adolescents that they can take risks safely.
 3. Risk of parents' anger and disappointment usually deters adolescents from risky behavior.
 4. Peer pressure usually doesn't play an important part in an adolescent's decision to become sexually active.

51. 2. Understanding the growth and development of adolescents helps the nurse recognize that teenagers feel they are invulnerable and can take risks safely. Peer pressure plays an important role in risk-taking behaviors, more so than fear of parents' anger or disappointment. Adolescents can and do think about the future but are willing to take risks that more mature adults might not take.
CN: Health promotion and maintenance; CNS: None; CL: Analyze; DIFFICULTY: Moderate

52. The nurse is preparing to administer 250 mg of ceftriaxone IM to an adolescent with a diagnosis of gonorrhea. Available is a vial of ceftriaxone 1 g powder for reconstitution. Instructions are to dilute with 3.6 mL of sterile water, 0.9% sodium chloride, or 1% lidocaine to make a solution of 1 g ceftriaxone per 4 mL of solution. How many milliliters would the nurse administer? Record your answer using a whole number.

_____ mL

52. 1.
The correct formula to calculate a drug dose is:

$$\frac{4 \text{ mL}}{1 \text{ g}} \times \frac{1 \text{ g}}{1,000 \text{ mg}} \times 250 \text{ mg} = 1 \text{ mL}$$

CN: Physiological integrity; CNS: Pharmacological therapies; CL: Apply; DIFFICULTY: Difficult

53. Which statement by an adolescent would alert the nurse that more education about sexually transmitted disease (STD) is needed?
 1. "You always know when you've got gonorrhea."
 2. "The most common STD in kids my age is chlamydia infection."
 3. "Most of the girls who have chlamydia don't even know it."
 4. "If you have symptoms of gonorrhea, they can show up a day or a couple of weeks after you got the infection to begin with."

53. 1. Gonorrhea can occur with or without symptoms. There are four main forms of the disease: asymptomatic, uncomplicated symptomatic, complicated symptomatic, and disseminated disease. All of the other statements by the adolescent about STIs are accurate.
CN: Health promotion and maintenance; CNS: None; CL: Apply; DIFFICULTY: Easy

54. Which statement describes primary prevention of sexually transmitted diseases (STDs) by avoiding exposure?
 1. The least accepted and most difficult approach
 2. The least expensive and most effective approach
 3. The most expensive and least effective approach
 4. The most difficult and most time-consuming approach

54. 2. Primary prevention of STDs by avoiding exposure is the least expensive and most effective approach. The nurse can play a role in offering this education to young people before they initiate sexual intercourse.
CN: Safe, effective care environment; CNS: Safety and infection control; CL: Apply; DIFFICULTY: Easy

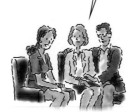

Be sure to explain all potential drug interactions to clients before discharge.

55. Which statement is important for the nurse to include in discharge education for the adolescent who's taking metronidazole to treat trichomoniasis?
 1. Sexual intercourse should stop.
 2. Alcohol shouldn't be consumed.
 3. Milk products should be avoided.
 4. Exposure to sunlight should be limited.

55. 2. While taking metronidazole to treat trichomoniasis, adolescents shouldn't consume alcohol for at least 3 days following the last dose because the drug is similar to disulfiram and may lead to a psychotic reaction. Milk and sunlight have no effect on the adolescent while taking this medication. Sexual intercourse need not be avoided.
CN: Physiological integrity; CNS: Pharmacological therapies; CL: Apply; DIFFICULTY: Moderate

CN: Client needs category   CNS: Client needs subcategory   CL: Cognitive level

56. When educating an adolescent group about the human immunodeficiency virus (HIV) which fact is it important for the nurse to include?
1. The incidence of HIV in the adolescent population has declined since 1995.
2. The virus can be spread through many routes, including sexual contact.
3. Knowledge about HIV spread and transmission has led to a decrease in the spread of the virus among adolescents.
4. About 50% of all new HIV infections in the United States occur in people younger than age 22.

57. When planning a program to educate adolescents about acquired immunodeficiency syndrome (AIDS), which action might lead to better acceptance of the program?
1. Survey the community to evaluate the level of education.
2. Obtain peer educators to provide information about AIDS.
3. Set up clinics in community centers and supply condoms readily.
4. Invite health care providers to host workshops in community centers.

58. Which adolescent would the nurse consider at greater risk for developing acquired immunodeficiency syndrome (AIDS)?
1. A teen who lives in crowded housing with poor ventilation
2. A young, sexually active client with multiple partners
3. A homeless adolescent who lives in a shelter
4. A young, sexually active teen with one partner

59. When collecting data from an adolescent with pelvic inflammatory disease (PID), which signs and symptoms should the nurse expect to see?
1. A hard, painless, red defined lesion
2. Small vesicles on the genital area with itching
3. Cervical discharge with redness and edema
4. Lower abdominal pain and urinary tract symptoms

60. After a nurse reinforces education with an adolescent about syphilis, which statement by the adolescent indicates the need for further education?
1. "The disease is divided into four stages: primary, secondary, latent, and tertiary."
2. "Affected persons are most infectious during the first year."
3. "Syphilis is easily treated with penicillin or doxycycline."
4. "Syphilis is rarely transmitted sexually."

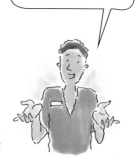

If you can remember how AIDS is transmitted, question #58 will be easy.

56. 2. HIV can be spread through many routes, including sexual contact and contact with infected blood or other body fluids. The incidence of HIV in the adolescent population has *increased* since 1995, even though more information about the virus is targeted to reach the adolescent population. Only about 25% of all new HIV infections in the United States occur in people younger than age 22.
CN: Health promotion and maintenance; CNS: None; CL: Apply; DIFFICULTY: Moderate

57. 2. Peer education programs have shown that teens are more likely to pose questions to peer educators than to adults, and that peer education can change personal attitudes and the perception of the risk of HIV infection. The other approaches would be helpful but wouldn't necessarily make the outreach program more successful.
CN: Health promotion and maintenance; CNS: None; CL: Analyze; DIFFICULTY: Moderate

58. 2. The younger the client when sexual activity begins, the higher the incidence of human immunodeficiency virus and AIDS. Also, the more sexual partners, the higher the incidence of HIV and AIDS. Neither crowded living environments nor homeless environments by themselves lead to an increase in the incidence of AIDS.
CN: Health promotion and maintenance; CNS: None; CL: Analyze; DIFFICULTY: Easy

59. 4. PID is an infection of the upper female genital tract most commonly caused by sexually transmitted infections. Initial symptoms in the adolescent may be generalized, with fever, abdominal pain, urinary tract symptoms, and vague, influenza-like symptoms. Small vesicles on the genital area with itching indicate herpes genitalis. Cervical discharge with redness and edema indicates chlamydia. A hard, painless, red defined lesion indicates syphilis.
CN: Physiological integrity; CNS: Physiological adaptation; CL: Apply; DIFFICULTY: Easy

60. 4. About 95% of the cases of syphilis are transmitted sexually. There are four stages to syphilis, although some people may only experience the first three stages. Affected persons are most contagious in the first year of the disease. The drug of choice for treating syphilis is penicillin or doxycycline.
CN: Health promotion and maintenance; CNS: none; CL: Analyze; DIFFICULTY: Moderate

CN: Client needs category   CNS: Client needs subcategory   CL: Cognitive level

61. In educating a group of parents about monitoring for urinary tract infection (UTI) in preschoolers, which symptom would indicate that a child needs to be evaluated?
  1. Voids only twice in any 6-hour period
  2. Exhibits incontinence after being toilet trained
  3. Has difficulty sitting still for more than a 30-minute period of time
  4. Urine smells strongly of ammonia after standing for more than 2 hours

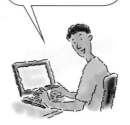

UTIs can make urination painful—so a lot of kids will hold it as long as they can.

61. 2. A child who exhibits incontinence after being toilet trained should be evaluated for UTI. Most urine smells strongly of ammonia after standing for more than 2 hours, so this doesn't necessarily indicate UTI. The other symptoms aren't reasons for parents to suspect problems with their child's urinary system.
CN: Health promotion and maintenance; CNS: None; CL: Apply;
DIFFICULTY: Moderate

62. The nurse is reinforcing education with the parents of a child with a recurrent urinary tract infection (UTI). Which statement should the nurse include?
  1. Antibiotics should be discontinued 48 hours after symptoms subside.
  2. Recurrent symptoms should be treated by renewing the antibiotic prescription.
  3. Complicated UTIs are related to poor perineal hygiene practice.
  4. Follow-up urine cultures are necessary to detect recurrent infections and antibiotic effectiveness.

62. 4. A routine follow-up urine specimen is usually obtained 2 or 3 days after the completion of the antibiotic treatment. All of the antibiotic should be taken as ordered and not stopped when symptoms disappear. If recurrent symptoms appear, a urine culture should be obtained to see whether the infection is resistant to antibiotics. Simple, not complicated, UTIs are generally caused by poor perineal hygiene.
CN: Health promotion and maintenance; CNS: None; CL: Apply;
DIFFICULTY: Moderate

63. Which instructions should a nurse include in the education plan for the parents of a child receiving sulfamethoxazole-trimethoprim for a repeated urinary tract infection with *Escherichia coli*?
  1. "For the drug to be effective, keep your child's urine acidic by having him drink at least a quart of cranberry juice per day."
  2. "Make sure your child takes the medication for 10 days even if his symptoms improve in a few days."
  3. "Return to the clinic in 3 days for another urine culture."
  4. "Give your child two pills each day, but keep the rest of the pills to give if the symptoms reappear within 2 weeks."

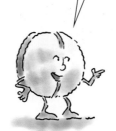

No syringe for me. I go straight down the hatch.

63. 2. Discharge instructions for parents of children receiving an anti-infective medication should include taking all of the prescribed medication for the prescribed time. The child won't need to have a culture repeated until the medication is completed. Drinking highly acidic juices, such as cranberry juice, may help maintain urinary health but won't get rid of an infection already present.
CN: Physiological integrity; CNS: Pharmacological therapies;
CL: Apply; DIFFICULTY: Easy

64. A nurse is monitoring a child with vesicoureteral reflux. Which condition should the nurse be alert for as a potential complication?
  1. Glomerulonephritis
  2. Hemolytic uremia syndrome
  3. Nephrotic syndrome
  4. Renal damage

64. 4. Reflux of urine into the ureters and then back into the bladder after voiding sets up the child for a urinary tract infection, which can lead to renal damage due to scarring of the parenchyma. Glomerulonephritis is an autoimmune reaction to a beta-hemolytic streptococcal infection. Eighty percent of nephrotic syndrome cases are idiopathic. Hemolytic uremia syndrome may be the result of genetic factors.
CN: Health promotion and maintenance; CNS: None;
CL: Analyze; DIFFICULTY: Difficult

65. A nurse reviewing a child's clean-voided urine specimen results understands that which of the following data indicates a urinary tract infection (UTI)?
1. A specific gravity of 1.020
2. Cloudy color without odor
3. A large amount of casts present
4. 100,000 bacterial colonies per milliliter

65. 4. The diagnosis of UTI is determined by the detection of bacteria in the urine. Infected urine usually contains more than 100,000 colonies/mL, often of a single organism. The urine is usually cloudy, hazy, and may have strands of mucus. It also has a foul, fishy odor even when fresh. Casts and increased specific gravity aren't specific to UTI.

CN: Physiological integrity; CNS: Physiological adaptation;
CL: Apply; DIFFICULTY: Moderate

66. A nurse is reinforcing education with the parents of a child with a urinary tract infection. Which factor should the nurse indicate contributes to urinary tract infection? Select all that apply.
1. Increased fluid intake
2. Short urethra
3. Ingestion of highly acidic juices
4. Constipation
5. Infrequent emptying of the bladder

66. 2, 4, 5. A short urethra contributes to infection because bacteria have to travel a shorter distance to the urinary tract. The risk of infection is higher in women than men because women have shorter urethras (0.75 in [1.9 cm] in young women, 1½ in [3.8 cm] in mature women, 7¾ in [19.7 cm] in adult men). Urinary stasis contributes to bacterial growth. Constipation increases the risk of UTI. Increased fluid intake helps flush the urinary tract system, and frequent emptying of the bladder decreases the risk of urinary tract infection. Drinking highly acidic juices, such as cranberry juice, may help maintain urinary health. In addition to being acidic, cranberry juice is a healthy choice because studies suggest it helps prevent the bacteria from attaching to the bladder wall.

CN: Health promotion and maintenance; CNS: None;
CL: Apply; DIFFICULTY: Moderate

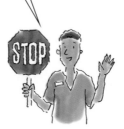

Hold up, there, partner. Remember to look for the *most* accurate answer in question #67.

67. The parent of a female child asks the nurse why the child seems to have so many urinary tract infections (UTIs). Which response by the nurse would be the **most** accurate?
1. Vaginal secretions are too acidic.
2. Girls can't be protected by circumcision like boys can.
3. The urethra is in close proximity to the anus.
4. Girls touch their genitalia more often than boys do.

67. 3. Girls are especially at risk for bacterial invasion of the urinary tract because of basic anatomical differences; the urethra is shorter and closer to the anus. Vaginal secretions are normally acidic, which decreases the risk of infection. Circumcision doesn't protect boys from UTIs. There's no documented research that supports that girls touch their genitalia more often than boys do.

CN: Health promotion and maintenance; CNS: None;
CL: Apply; DIFFICULTY: Easy

68. Which intervention should a nurse recommend to parents of young girls to help prevent urinary tract infections (UTIs)?
1. Limit bathing as much as possible.
2. Increase fluids and decrease salt intake.
3. Dress the child in cotton underpants.
4. Educate the child about cleaning her perineum from back to front.

68. 3. Cotton is a more breathable fabric than nylon and allows for dampness to be absorbed from the perineum. Dressing the child in cotton underpants helps prevent UTIs. Increasing fluids would be helpful, but decreasing salt isn't necessary. Bathing shouldn't be limited; however, the use of bubble bath or whirlpool baths should be avoided. If the child has frequent UTIs, taking a bath should be discouraged and taking a shower encouraged. The perineum should always be cleaned from *front to back*.

CN: Health promotion and maintenance; CNS: None;
CL: Apply; DIFFICULTY: Moderate

69. A child has been sent to the school nurse for wetting her pants three times in the past 2 days. The nurse should recommend that this child be evaluated for which complication?
1. School phobia
2. Emotional trauma
3. Urinary tract infection
4. Structural defect of the urinary tract

69. 3. Frequent urinary incontinence should be evaluated by the health care provider, and the nurse's first action should be to check the urine for infection. Children exhibit signs of school phobia by reporting an ailment before school starts and getting better after they're allowed to miss school. After infection, structural defect, and diabetes have been ruled out, emotional trauma should be investigated.
CN: Health promotion and maintenance; CNS: None; CL: Apply; DIFFICULTY: Moderate

70. The nurse is caring for a 21 kg child with a urinary tract infection. The health care provider has ordered amoxicillin 750 mg by mouth every 8 hours. The recommended pediatric dosage is 40 to 90 mg/kg/day in two to three divided doses. Which action should the nurse take?
1. Administer the medication in 4 ounces of juice.
2. Do not begin the antibiotic therapy until the culture and sensitivity results are final.
3. Hold the medication and notify the health care provider that the dose exceeds the recommended range.
4. Administer the medication by injection if the child is uncooperative and refuses the oral medication.

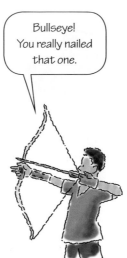

Bullseye! You really nailed that one.

70. 3. The nurse should notify the health care provider that the ordered dosage exceeds the recommended range for this child, which is 280 to 630 mg/dose.

$$\frac{40\text{ mg}}{\text{kg/day}} \times \frac{1\text{ day}}{3\text{ doses}} \times 21\text{ kg} = \frac{840}{3} = 280\text{mg/dose}$$

$$\frac{90\text{ mg}}{\text{kg/day}} \times \frac{1\text{ day}}{3\text{ doses}} \times 21\text{ kg} = \frac{1,890}{3} = 630\text{mg/dose}$$

Oral medication is not diluted in large volumes. Antimicrobial therapy is started after the cultures are collected, not until the results are obtained. The nurse cannot change the route without a health care provider's order.
CN: Physiological integrity; CNS: Pharmacological therapies; CL: Analyze; DIFFICULTY: Easy

71. The nurse is caring for a child with a urinary tract infection. The health care provider has ordered cephalexin 125 mg by mouth every 8 hours. Cephalexin is available 250 mg per 5 mL. How many milliliters should the nurse administer per dose? Record your answer using one decimal place.

_____ mL

71. 2.5.
The correct formula to calculate a drug dose is:

$$\frac{5\text{ mL}}{250\text{ mg}} = \frac{125\text{ mg}}{\text{dose}} = \frac{625}{250} = 2.5\text{ mL}$$

CN: Physiological integrity; CNS: Pharmacological therapies; CL: Apply; DIFFICULTY: Moderate

72. When evaluating infants and young toddlers for signs of urinary tract infections (UTIs), a nurse should know that which symptom would be **most** common?
1. Abdominal pain
2. Feeding problems
3. Frequency
4. Urgency

72. 2. In infants and children younger than age 2, the signs of UTI are characteristically nonspecific, and feeding problems are usually the first indication. Symptoms more nearly resemble GI tract disorders. Abdominal pain, urgency, and frequency are signs that would be observed in the older child with a UTI.
CN: Physiological integrity; CNS: Pharmacological therapies; CL: Apply; DIFFICULTY: Challenge

73. When obtaining a urine specimen for culture and sensitivity, the nurse should identify that which method of collection yields the **most** accurate results?
1. Bagged urine specimen
2. Clean-catch urine specimen
3. First-voided urine specimen
4. Catheterized urine specimen

73. 4. The most accurate tests of bacterial content are suprapubic aspiration (for children younger than age 2) and properly performed bladder catheterization. The other methods of obtaining a specimen have a high incidence of contamination not related to infection.
CN: Physiological integrity; CNS: Basic care and comfort; CL: Apply; DIFFICULTY: Challenge

74. After collecting a urine specimen, which action by the nurse is **most** appropriate?
1. Take the specimen to the laboratory immediately.
2. Send the specimen to the laboratory on the scheduled run.
3. Take the specimen to the laboratory on the nurse's next break.
4. Keep the specimen in the refrigerator until it can be taken to the laboratory.

75. When reinforcing education about fluid intake with the parents of a child with a urinary tract infection (UTI), which statement by a parent would indicate the need for further education?
1. "I should encourage my child to drink about 50 mL per pound of body weight daily."
2. "Clear liquids should be the primary liquids that my child drinks."
3. "I should offer my child carbonated beverages about every 2 hours."
4. "My child should avoid drinking caffeinated beverages."

76. Which treatment should the nurse anticipate in a child who has a history of recurrent urinary tract infections (UTIs)?
1. Frequent catheterizations
2. Prophylactic antibiotics
3. Limited activities
4. Surgical intervention

77. When reinforcing education with parents about administering medications to children for recurrent urinary tract infections, which instructions should the nurse include?
1. The medication should be given first thing in the morning.
2. The medication should be given right before bedtime.
3. The medication is generally given four times per day.
4. It doesn't matter when the medication is given.

78. A nurse is reinforcing education with a group of parents about urinary tract infections (UTIs). The nurse knows the education has been effective when the parents state which of the following has the greatest impact on the potential for progressive renal injury after UTIs?
1. A school-age child who must get permission to go to the bathroom
2. An adolescent female who has started menstruation
3. Children who participate in competitive sports
4. Infections occurring in young infants and toddlers

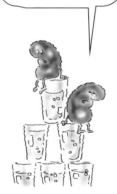

Whoa. This is a lot of water to process. It makes my nephrons hurt just thinking about it.

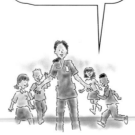

I believe the children are our future. Teach them well about avoiding UTIs.

74. 1. Care of urine specimens obtained for culture is an important nursing goal related to diagnosis. Specimens should be taken to the laboratory for culture immediately. If the culture is delayed, the specimen can be placed in the refrigerator, but storage can result in a loss of formed elements, such as blood cells and casts.
CN: Physiological integrity; CNS: Basic care and comfort; CL: Apply; DIFFICULTY: Moderate

75. 3. Carbonated or caffeinated beverages are avoided because of their potentially irritating effect on the bladder mucosa. Adequate fluid intake is always indicated during an acute UTI. It's recommended that a person drinks approximately 50 mL/lb of body weight daily. The child should primarily drink clear liquids.
CN: Physiological integrity; CNS: Basic care and comfort; CL: Analyze; DIFFICULTY: Easy

76. 2. Children who experience recurrent UTI may require antibiotic therapy for months or years. Recurrent UTI would be investigated for anatomic abnormalities and surgical intervention may be indicated, but the child would also be placed on antibiotics before the tests. The child's activities aren't limited. Frequent catheterization predisposes a child to infection.
CN: Physiological integrity; CNS: Physiological adaptation; CL: Apply; DIFFICULTY: Easy

77. 2. Medication is commonly administered once per day, and the parents are advised to give the antibiotic before sleep because it is the longest period without voiding.
CN: Physiological integrity; CNS: Pharmacological therapies; CL: Apply; DIFFICULTY: Challenge

78. 4. The hazard of progressive renal injury is greatest when infection occurs in young children, especially those under age 2. The first two situations might lead to a simple UTI that would need to be treated. Competitive sports have no impact on UTI.
CN: Health promotion and maintenance; CNS: None; CL: Apply; DIFFICULTY: Moderate

79. Which statement should the nurse make to help parents understand the recovery period after a child has had surgery to remove a Wilms tumor?

1. "Children will easily lie in bed and restrict their activities."
2. "Recovery is usually fast in spite of the abdominal incision."
3. "Recovery usually takes a great deal of time because of the large incision."
4. "Parents need to perform the child's activities of daily living for about 2 weeks after surgery."

80. The nurse is caring for a child who has had a nephrectomy after diagnosis of a Wilms tumor. The nurse has assessed the child's pain and is preparing to administer an oral opiate. Which method is the **best** choice for administering the medication?

1. A plastic one ounce calibrated medicine cup.
2. A teaspoon.
3. An oral syringe.
4. An injectable syringe with the needle removed.

81. When gathering data on a preschool child, which observation indicates that a child has a potential Wilms tumor?

1. Pain in the abdomen
2. Fever greater than 104° F (40° C)
3. Decreased blood pressure
4. Swelling within the abdomen

82. When reinforcing education with parents about administering sulfamethoxazole-trimethoprim to a child for treatment of a urinary tract infection, the nurse should include which instructions?

1. Give the medication with food.
2. Give the medication with water.
3. Give the medication with a cola beverage.
4. Give the medication one hour after a meal.

83. When the nurse is reinforcing education about the diagnosis of Wilms tumor to parents, which statement by a parent would indicate the need for further education?

1. "Wilms tumor usually involves both kidneys."
2. "Wilms tumor is slightly more common in the left kidney."
3. "Wilms tumor is staged during surgery for treatment planning."
4. "Wilms tumor stays encapsulated for an extended time."

79. 2. Children generally recover very quickly from surgery to remove a Wilms tumor, even though they may have a large abdominal incision. Children like to get back into the normalcy of being a child, which is through play. Parents need to encourage their children to do as much for themselves as possible, although some regression is expected.

CN: Psychosocial integrity; CNS: None; CL: Analyze; DIFFICULTY: Moderate

80. 3. The most accurate and safest way to administer the medication is using an oral syringe.

CN: Physiological integrity; CNS: Pharmacological therapies; CL: Apply; DIFFICULTY: Moderate

81. 4. The most common initial sign of Wilms tumor is a swelling or mass within the abdomen. The mass is characteristically firm, nontender, confined to one side, and deep within the flank. A high fever isn't an initial sign of Wilms tumor. Blood pressure is characteristically increased, not decreased.

CN: Physiological integrity; CNS: Physiological adaptation; CL: Apply; DIFFICULTY: Moderate

82. 2. When giving sulfamethoxazole-trimethoprim, the medication should be administered with a full glass of water on an empty stomach. If nausea and vomiting occur, giving the drug with food may decrease gastric distress. Carbonated beverages should be avoided because they irritate the bladder.

CN: Physiological integrity; CNS: Pharmacological therapies; CL: Apply; DIFFICULTY: Challenge

83. 1. Wilms tumor usually involves only one kidney, and is usually staged during surgery so that an effective course of treatment can be established. Wilms tumor has a slightly higher occurrence in the left kidney, and it stays encapsulated for an extended time.

CN: Physiological integrity; CNS: Physiological adaptation; CL: Apply; DIFFICULTY: Difficult

84. Parents ask the nurse about the prognosis of their child diagnosed with Wilms tumor. The nurse should base the response on which factor?
1. Usually, children with Wilms tumor need only surgical intervention.
2. Survival rates for Wilms tumor are the lowest among childhood cancers.
3. Survival rates for Wilms tumor are the highest among childhood cancers.
4. Children with localized tumor have only a 30% chance of cure with multimodal therapy.

85. If both kidneys are involved with Wilms tumor, the nurse should expect that treatment before surgery might include which method?
1. Peritoneal dialysis
2. Abdominal gavage
3. Radiation and chemotherapy
4. Antibiotics and IV fluid therapy

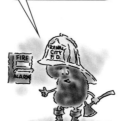

Wilms tumor is a true renal emergency. It requires a heavy-duty response.

86. When caring for the child with Wilms tumor preoperatively, which nursing intervention would be **most** important?
1. Avoid abdominal palpation.
2. Closely monitor arterial blood gas (ABG) values.
3. Prepare the child and family for long-term dialysis.
4. Prepare the child and family for renal transplantation.

87. A child is scheduled for surgery to remove a Wilms tumor from one kidney. The parents ask the nurse what treatment, if any, they should expect after their child recovers from surgery. Which response would be **most** accurate?
1. "Chemotherapy may be necessary."
2. "Kidney transplant is indicated eventually."
3. "No additional treatments are usually necessary."
4. "Chemotherapy with or without radiation therapy is indicated."

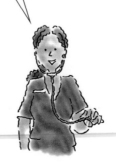

What substance is most likely to show up in your urine if you have nephrotic syndrome?

88. A toddler is admitted to the hospital with nephrotic syndrome. The nurse carefully monitors the toddler's fluid intake and output and checks urine specimens regularly with a reagent strip. Which finding is the nurse **most** likely to report?
1. Proteinuria
2. Glucosuria
3. Ketonuria
4. Polyuria

84. 3. Survival rates for Wilms tumor are the highest among childhood cancers. Usually, children with Wilms tumor who have a stage I or II localized tumor have a 90% chance of cure with multimodal therapy.
CN: Physiological integrity; CNS: Physiological adaptation;
CL: Apply; DIFFICULTY: Moderate

85. 3. If both kidneys are involved, the child may be treated with radiation therapy or chemotherapy preoperatively to shrink the tumor, allowing more conservative surgery. Peritoneal dialysis would be needed only if the kidneys weren't functioning. Abdominal gavage isn't indicated. Antibiotics aren't needed because Wilms tumor isn't an infection.
CN: Physiological integrity; CNS: Reduction of risk potential;
CL: Apply; DIFFICULTY: Moderate

86. 1. After the diagnosis of Wilms tumor is made, the abdomen shouldn't be palpated. Palpation of the tumor might lead to rupture, which would cause the cancerous cells to spread throughout the abdomen. ABG values shouldn't be affected. If surgery is successful, there won't be a need for long-term dialysis or renal transplantation.
CN: Physiological integrity; CNS: Reduction of risk potential;
CL: Apply; DIFFICULTY: Moderate

87. 4. Because radiation therapy and chemotherapy are usually begun immediately after surgery, parents need an explanation of what to expect. Kidney transplant isn't usually necessary.
CN: Physiological integrity; CNS: Physiological adaptation;
CL: Apply; DIFFICULTY: Difficult

88. 1. In nephrotic syndrome, the glomerular membrane of the kidneys becomes permeable to proteins. This results in massive proteinuria, which the nurse can detect with a reagent strip. Nephrotic syndrome typically doesn't cause glucosuria or ketonuria. Because the syndrome causes fluids to shift from plasma to interstitial spaces, it's more likely to decrease urine output than to cause polyuria (excessive urine output).
CN: Physiological integrity; CNS: Reduction of risk potential;
CL: Apply; DIFFICULTY: Moderate

89. The nurse is reinforcing education about surgery with the parents of a child with Wilms tumor. Which statement by the nurse **best** explains the role of surgery for Wilms tumor?
  1. "Surgery is not indicated in children with Wilms tumor."
  2. "Surgery is usually performed within 24 to 48 hours of admission."
  3. "Surgery is the least favorable therapy for the treatment of Wilms tumor."
  4. "Surgery will be delayed until the child's overall health status improves."

90. A 3-year-old child has had surgery to remove a Wilms tumor. Which action should the nurse take **first** when the parent asks for pain medication for the child?
  1. Get the pain medication ready for administration.
  2. Assess the child's pain using a pain scale of 1 to 10.
  3. Assess the child's pain using a smiley face pain scale.
  4. Check for the last time pain medication was administered.

91. The nurse is caring for a child diagnosed with Wilms tumor. Because of the parents' religious beliefs, they choose not to treat the child. Which statement by the nurse to a colleague indicates the need for further discussion?
  1. "I know this is a lot of information for them to absorb in a short period of time."
  2. "I don't think parents have the legal right to make these kinds of decisions."
  3. "These parents just don't understand how easily treatable a Wilms tumor is."
  4. "I think the parents are in shock."

92. A child with nephrotic syndrome develops generalized edema as a result of nephrosis. In updating the plan of care, which goal would be included in the care plan to prevent complications of edema?
  1. Continually support the scrotum.
  2. Change the child's position every 2 hours.
  3. The child's skin will remain intact during hospitalization.
  4. Maintain continuous bed rest.

93. A child with a Wilms tumor has had surgery to remove a kidney and has received chemotherapy. The nurse should include which instructions at discharge?
  1. Avoid contact sports.
  2. Decrease fluid intake.
  3. Decrease sodium intake.
  4. Avoid contact with other children.

Can you spot the statement that is incorrect in question #91?

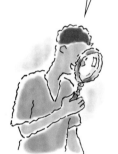

89. 2. Surgery is the preferred treatment and is scheduled as soon as possible after confirmation of a renal mass, usually within 24 to 48 hours of admission, to make sure the encapsulated tumor remains intact.

CN: Physiological integrity; CNS: Physiological adaptation; CL: Understand; DIFFICULTY: Moderate

90. 3. The first action by the nurse should be to assess the child for pain. A 3-year-old child is too young to use a pain scale from 0 to 10 but can easily use the smiley face pain scale. After assessing the pain, the nurse should then investigate the time the pain medication was last given and administer the medication accordingly.

CN: Physiological integrity; CNS: Pharmacological therapies; CL: Apply; DIFFICULTY: Challenge

91. 2. Parents *do* have the legal right to make decisions regarding the health issues for their child. Religion plays an important role in many people's lives, and decisions about surgery and treatment for cancer are sometimes made that scientifically don't make sense to the health care provider. The parents are probably in a state of shock because a lot of information has been given, and this is a cancer that requires decisions to be made quickly, especially surgical intervention.

CN: Safe, effective care environment; CNS: Coordinated care; CL: Analyze; DIFFICULTY: Moderate

92. 3. The child's skin remaining intact during hospitalization is the only option written as a goal. The other options are interventions recommended to maintain skin integrity, not goals.

CN: Safe, effective care environment; CNS: Coordinated care; CL: Apply; DIFFICULTY: Challenge

93. 1. Because the child is left with only one kidney, certain precautions, such as avoiding contact sports, are recommended to prevent injury to the remaining kidney. Decreasing fluid intake isn't indicated; fluid intake is essential for renal function. The child's sodium intake shouldn't be reduced. Avoiding other children is unnecessary, will make the child feel self-conscious, and may lead to regressive behavior.

CN: Physiological integrity; CNS: Reduction of risk potential; CL: Apply; DIFFICULTY: Moderate

94. The nurse is reinforcing education with a parent of a preschool-age child with nephrosis who will be discharged on prednisone. Which statement by the parent indicates that the teaching has been effective? Select all that apply.
1. "My child should not receive any immunizations with live vaccines while on prednisone."
2. "Prednisone will prevent my child's kidneys from becoming infected."
3. "While on prednisone my child will be more susceptible to infections."
4. "Prednisone should never be discontinued abruptly."
5. "My child's appetite will be decreased and he may lose weight while taking the prednisone."

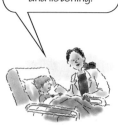

Effective teaching requires both careful speaking and listening.

94. 1, 3, 4. Anyone receiving a systemic corticosteroid in high doses for longer than 2 weeks should wait at least 3 months before receiving a live-virus vaccine. Corticosteroids suppress the immune response, should not be discontinued abruptly due to the risk of acute adrenocortical crisis, and do not convey any infective protection. An initial weight gain may occur do to an increase in appetite.
CN: Physiological integrity; CNS: Pharmacological therapies; CL: Apply; DIFFICULTY: Moderate

95. In providing psychosocial care to a 6-year-old child who has had abdominal surgery for Wilms tumor, which activity initiated by the nurse would be the **most** appropriate?
1. Allow the child to watch a 2-hour movie without interruptions.
2. Give the child a puzzle with five pieces to encourage him to move while in bed.
3. Tell the child that medication can be given so that he feels no pain.
4. Provide the child with supplies and ask him to draw how he feels.

95. 4. A movie is a good diversion, but giving supplies and encouraging the child to draw his feelings is a better outlet. Many procedures have been performed on this child since admission. The nurse probably can't give enough pain medication so that a child who has had surgery will feel no pain. A puzzle with only five pieces is too basic for a 6-year-old and wouldn't hold his interest.
CN: Psychosocial integrity; CNS: None; CL: Apply; DIFFICULTY: Easy

96. When caring for a child after removal of a Wilms tumor, which finding would indicate the need to notify the health care provider?
1. Fever of 100° F (37.8° C)
2. Absence of bowel sounds
3. Slight congestion in the lungs
4. Reports of pain when moving

96. 2. After tumor removal, the child is at risk for intestinal obstruction. GI abnormalities require notification of the health care provider. A slight fever following surgery isn't uncommon; slight congestion in the lungs and reports of pain are not uncommon either.
CN: Physiological integrity; CNS: Reduction of risk potential; CL: Apply; DIFFICULTY: Moderate

97. The nurse is conducting a follow-up phone call with the parent of a child with nephrosis who was recently discharged. Which statement by the parent indicates the discharge instructions are being followed correctly? Select all that apply.
1. "I am administering my child's prednisone once a day, every day."
2. "I am keeping my child out of school indefinitely."
3. "I am weighing my child every morning and keeping a logbook."
4. "If my child's morning urine has 2+ protein for 2 days in a row, I will call the health care provider."
5. "My child is scheduled for his MMR vaccine next week."

97. 1, 3, 4. Initial therapy with prednisone is 60 mg/m²/day for 4 weeks. A single daily dose has fewer side effects. The child should avoid people who are ill, but there is no need to keep the child from school. Daily weights and urine protein checks should be measured and logged. Parents should notify the health care provider if the urine is 2+ for protein for 2 days in a row. A child on prednisone should not receive a live-virus vaccine like MMR.
CN: Safe, effective care environment; CNS: Coordinated care; CL: Analyze; DIFFICULTY: Moderate

98. The nurse is reinforcing education with parents about Wilms tumor. Which statement made by a parent would indicate the need for further education?
1. "My child could have inherited this disease."
2. "Wilms tumor can be associated with other congenital anomalies."
3. "This disease could have been a result of trauma to the baby in utero."
4. "There's no method to identify gene carriers of Wilms tumor."

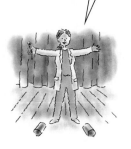

What a performance! You're really killing it on this test.

98. 3. Wilms tumor isn't a result of trauma to the fetus in utero. Wilms tumor can be genetically inherited and is associated with other congenital anomalies. There is, however, no method to identify gene carriers of Wilms tumor at this time.
CN: Psychosocial integrity; CNS: None;
CL: Apply; DIFFICULTY: Difficult

99. A 6-year-old child's indwelling urinary catheter was removed at 6 a.m. At noon, the child still has not voided, appears uncomfortable, and the nurse palpates slight bladder distention. Which action should the nurse take **first**?
1. Insert a straight catheter, as ordered, for urine retention.
2. Consult the health care provider about replacing the indwelling urinary catheter.
3. Wait awhile longer to see whether the child can void on his own.
4. Turn on the water faucet and provide privacy.

99. 4. Urine retention can result from many factors, including stress and use of opiates. Initially, the nurse should use independent nursing actions, such as providing the client with privacy, placing him in a sitting or standing position to enlist the aid of gravity and increase intra-abdominal pressure, and turning on the water faucet. If these measures are unsuccessful and the health care provider has left standing orders for straight catheterization, the nurse can proceed with the catheterization. Consulting the health care provider would involve the use of a dependent nursing action; independent actions should be attempted first. Waiting longer will only increase the child's distention and pain.
CN: Physiological integrity; CNS: Basic care and comfort;
CL: Apply; DIFFICULTY: Moderate

100. When describing enuresis to a child's parents, which statements would the nurse include in the description? Select all that apply.
1. The child may experience involuntary urination after age 5.
2. Episodes primarily occur when the child is awake and playing.
3. The child may suffer deep feelings of shame and may withdraw from peers because of ridicule.
4. The condition may respond to tricyclic antidepressants and antidiuretics.
5. The condition may become permanent without appropriate intervention.

100. 1, 3, 4. Enuresis is a condition in which there is involuntary urination after age 5. It generally occurs while the child is sleeping. There can be long-lasting emotional trauma resulting from peer ridicule and feelings of shame and embarrassment. The condition may be treated with the use of tricyclic antidepressants and antidiuretics. With support and understanding, the condition generally resolves in time.
CN: Physiological integrity; CNS: Physiological adaptation;
CL: Analyze; DIFFICULTY: Difficult

101. A parent reports that her 6-year-old girl recently started wetting the bed and running a low-grade fever. A urinalysis is positive for bacteria and protein. A diagnosis of a urinary tract infection (UTI) is made, and the child is prescribed antibiotics. Which interventions are appropriate? Select all that apply.
1. Limit fluids for the next few days to decrease the frequency of urination.
2. Assess the parent's understanding of UTI and its causes.
3. Instruct the parent to administer the antibiotic as prescribed—even if the symptoms diminish.
4. Provide instructions solely to the parent, not the child.
5. Discourage taking bubble baths.
6. Advise wiping from the back to the front after voiding and defecation.

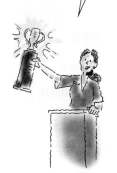

Outstanding! You really aced this test.

101. 2, 3, 5. Assessing the parent's understanding of UTI and its causes provides the nurse with a baseline for education. The full course of antibiotics must be given to eradicate the organism and prevent recurrence, even if the child's signs and symptoms decrease. Bubble baths can irritate the vulva and urethra and contribute to the development of a UTI. Fluids should be encouraged, not limited, in order to prevent urinary stasis and help flush the organism out of the urinary tract. Instructions should be given to the child at her level of understanding to help her better understand the treatment and promote compliance. The child should wipe from the *front to the back*, not back to front, to minimize the risk of contamination after elimination.
CN: Health promotion and maintenance; CNS: None; CL: Apply;
DIFFICULTY: Easy

Chapter 34

Integumentary Disorders

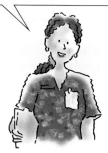

Skin diseases in children and teens are common and varied. This chapter covers common and uncommon skin disorders among these populations.

Pediatric integumentary refresher

Acne vulgaris

Overactive sebaceous glands that become plugged and inflamed

Key signs and symptoms

- Closed comedo or whitehead: acne plug not protruding from the follicle and covered by the epidermis
- Inflammation and characteristic acne pustules, papules or, in severe forms, acne cysts or abscesses (caused by rupture or leakage of an enlarged plug into the dermis)
- Open comedo or blackhead: acne plug protruding from the follicle and not covered by the epidermis

Key treatments

- Exposure to ultraviolet light (but never when a photosensitizing agent, such as tretinoin, is being used)
- Oral isotretinoin limited to those with nodulocystic or recalcitrant acne who don't respond to conventional therapy
- Systemic therapy: usually tetracycline to decrease bacterial growth; alternatively, erythromycin (tetracycline contraindicated during pregnancy and childhood because it discolors developing teeth)
- Topical medications: benzoyl peroxide, clindamycin, or erythromycin and benzoyl peroxide antibacterial agents, alone or in combination with tretinoin (retinoic acid), or a keratolytic

Key interventions

- Identify predisposing factors
- Instruct adolescent using tretinoin to apply it at least 30 minutes after washing the face and at least 1 hour before bedtime; warn against using it around the eyes or lips; after treatments, skin should look pink and dry
- Advise adolescent to avoid exposure to sunlight or to use a sunblock; if prescribed regimen includes tretinoin and benzoyl peroxide, tell adolescent to use one preparation in the morning and the other at night

- Instruct adolescent to take tetracycline on an empty stomach and not to take it with antacids or milk
- Tell adolescent who's taking isotretinoin to avoid vitamin A supplements; discuss how to deal with the dry skin and mucous membranes that usually occur during treatment; the female should use 2 forms of birth control
- Offer emotional support to the adolescent who's insecure about his appearance

Burns

Injuries to the tissues caused by heat, friction, chemical, electricity, or radiation

Key signs and symptoms

First-degree burn (partial thickness of skin)
- Dry, painful, red skin with edema
- Sunburn appearance

Second-degree burn (partial thickness of skin)
- Moist, weeping blisters with edema
- Severe pain

Third-degree burn (full thickness of skin)
- Avascular site without blanching or pain
- Dry, pale, leathery skin

Key test results

- Many burn facilities use the Lund-Browder chart (body surface area chart that accounts for age) to determine the extent of injury

Key treatments

- IV fluids to prevent and treat shock; urine output maintained at 1 to 2 mL/kg
- Protective isolation, depending on burn severity
- Tetanus toxoid according to child's immunization status

Key interventions

- Stop the burning in an emergency situation
- Maintain a patent airway in the immediate postburn phase

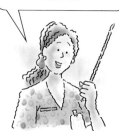

Tell your clients who are on tretinoin to make like a vampire and avoid the sun.

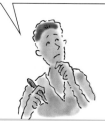

Hmm. A sunburn would be which degree of burn?

- Monitor vital signs and intake and output
- Prevent heat loss
- Analgesia for pain

Contact dermatitis

Irritation of the skin due to contact between the skin and a substance

Key signs and symptoms

- Characteristic bright red, maculopapular rash in the diaper area

Key treatments

- Cleaning affected area with mild soap and water
- Leaving affected area open to air

Key interventions

- Keep the diaper area clean and dry

Head lice

Tiny insects that live on the scalp

Key signs and symptoms

- Pruritus of the scalp
- White flecks attached to the hair shafts

Key test results

- Examination reveals lice eggs, which look like white flecks, firmly attached to hair shafts near the base

Key treatments

- Pyrethrin or permethrin shampoos, or lindane in resistant cases

Key interventions

- Explain the need to wash bed linens, hats, combs, brushes, and anything else that comes in contact with the hair

Impetigo

Acute, contagious staphylococcal or streptococcal skin disease

Key signs and symptoms

- Macular rash progressing to a papular and vesicular rash, which oozes and forms a moist, honey-colored crust

Key treatments

- Washing affected area with disinfectant soap

Key interventions

- Apply antibiotic ointment
- Wash the area three times daily with antiseptic soap

Rashes

Change of the skin which affects its color, appearance, or texture

Key signs and symptoms

Papular rash
- Raised solid lesions with color changes in circumscribed areas

Pustular rash
- Vesicles and bullae that fill with purulent exudate

Vesicular rash
- Small, raised, circumscribed lesions filled with clear fluid

Key test results

- Aspirate from lesions may reveal cause
- Patch test may identify cause

Key treatments

- Antibacterial, antifungal, or antiviral agent (depending on cause)
- Antihistamines if the rash is the result of an allergy

Key interventions

- Maintain standard precautions to prevent the spread of infection
- Teach sanitary techniques
- Cover weeping lesions

Scabies

Contagious, itchy skin condition caused by mites

Key signs and symptoms

- Linear black burrows between fingers and toes and in palms, axillae, and groin

Key test results

- Drop of mineral oil placed over the burrow, followed by superficial scraping and examination of expressed material under a microscope, may reveal ova or mite feces

Key treatments

- Application of permethrin

Key interventions

- Teach the child and parents to apply permethrin from the neck down covering the entire body, wait 15 minutes before dressing, and avoid bathing for 8 to 12 hours
- Explain the need to change bed linens, towels, and clothing after bathing and lotion application

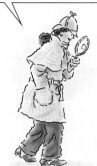

Your client has a bright red, maculopapular rash in the diaper area. What condition should you suspect?

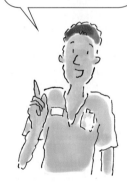

And coming in at number 1 on our top-ten list of least popular pets is ... you guessed it ... head lice.

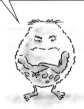

Hi. My name is scabies. I get under people's skin—literally.

Lyme disease

Inflammatory disease which is transmitted to humans via the deer tick

Key signs and symptoms

- Bull's eye rash is a classic symptom.
- Possible flu-like symptoms (e.g., fever, fatigue, headache)
- If not treated, can affect the heart and nervous system

Key test results

- Enzyme-linked immunosorbent assay test (ELISA)
- Western blot test

Key treatments

- Amoxicillin in children younger than 8 and doxycycline in children 8 and older, unless allergies make them contra-indicated

Key interventions

- DEET is an effective tick repellent but should be used on the child's clothes instead of the skin
- If child is outdoors often, long sleeves and pants should be worn and hair pulled back or under a hat

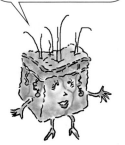

The skin's layers are the body's first line of defense against the outside world.

thePoint® You can download tables of drug information to help you prepare for the NCLEX®! View Generic Drug Names, Drug Classifications, Drug Actions, and Nursing Implications for the drugs discussed in this refresher at **http://thePoint.lww.com**.

Integumentary questions, answers, and rationales

1. A 3-year-old child gets a burn at the angle of the mouth from chewing on an electrical cord. Which finding should the nurse expect to observe 10 days after the injury?
   1. Normal granular tissue
   2. Contracture of the injury site
   3. Ulceration with serous drainage
   4. Profuse bleeding from the injury site

Yes— unfortunately, kids sometimes chew on electrical cords. That's why we have ERs.

2. The nurse is caring for a child in the burn unit who sustained partial thickness burns to the lower extremities. What does the nurse determine the nutritional needs of this child will be?
   1. The child needs 100 cal/kg during hospitalization.
   2. The hypermetabolic state after a burn injury can lead to poor healing if not corrected.
   3. Caloric needs can be lowered by controlling environmental temperature.
   4. Maintaining a hypermetabolic rate will lower the child's risk of infection.

3. An 18-month-old child is admitted to the hospital with full-thickness burns to the anterior chest. The parent asks how the burn will heal. Which statement would the nurse incorporate in the response?
   1. "Surgical closure and grafting are usually needed."
   2. "Healing takes 10 to 12 days, with little or no scarring."
   3. "Pigment will return to the injured area."
   4. "Healing can take up to 6 weeks, with a high incidence of scarring."

1. 4. Ten days after oral burns from electrical cords, the eschar falls off, exposing arteries and veins. There will be profuse bleeding from the injury site. Burns to the oral cavity heal rapidly but with contractures and scarring. Although contractures are likely, they aren't seen 10 days postinjury.
CN: Physiological integrity; CNS: Physiological adaptation;
CL: Apply; DIFFICULTY: Challenge

2. 2. A burn injury causes a hypermetabolic state leading to protein and lipid catabolism, which affects wound healing. Caloric intake should be 1½ to 2 times the basal metabolic rate, with a minimum of 1.5 to 2 g/kg of body weight of protein daily. High metabolic rates increase the risk of infection. Keeping the temperature within a normal range lets the body function efficiently and use calories for healing and normal physiologic processes. If the temperature is too warm or too cold, energy must be used for warming or cooling, taking energy away from tissue repair.
CN: Physiological integrity; CNS: Basic care and comfort;
CL: Understand; DIFFICULTY: Moderate

3. 1. Full-thickness burns usually need surgical closure and grafting for complete healing. Deep partial-thickness burns heal in 6 weeks, with scarring. Healing in 10 to 12 days with little or no scarring is associated with superficial partial-thickness burns. With superficial partial-thickness burns, pigment is expected to return to the injured area after healing.
CN: Physiological integrity; CNS: Physiological adaptation;
CL: Apply; DIFFICULTY: Challenge

4. A 7-year-old child is brought to the emergency department with burns to the back of the head and the back of the right thigh. According to the Lund-Browder classifications, what percentage of body surface area is affected and should be recorded?
1. 9.5%
2. 9.75%
3. 8.5%
4. 9%

5. Which finding would the nurse associate with a deep partial-thickness burn in a 9-year-old child?
1. Erythema and pain
2. Minimal damage to the epidermis
3. Necrosis through all layers of skin
4. Tissue necrosis through most of the dermis

6. When talking with the parents of a child with erythema infectiosum (fifth disease), the nurse should include which statement?
1. There's a possible reappearance of the rash for up to 1 week.
2. Isolation of high-risk contacts should be avoided for 4 to 10 days.
3. Pregnant women are at risk for fetal death if infected with fifth disease.
4. Children with fifth disease are contagious only while the rash is present.

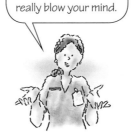

If you think fifth disease sounds bad, sixth, seventh, and eighth diseases will really blow your mind.

7. A 4-year-old child is admitted to the burn unit with a circumferential burn to the left forearm. Which finding would alert the nurse to a potential complication that should be reported to the health care provider?
1. Numbness of fingers
2. +2 radial and ulnar pulses
3. Full range of motion and no pain
4. Bilateral capillary refill less than 2 seconds

8. Parents are concerned that their 3-year-old child has been exposed to erythema infectiosum (fifth disease). Which characteristic finding would the nurse explain to the parents they should monitor for?
1. A fine, erythematous rash with a sandpaper-like texture
2. Intense redness of both cheeks that may spread to the extremities
3. Low-grade fever, followed by vesicular lesions of the trunk, face, and scalp
4. A 3- to 5-day history of sustained fever, followed by a diffuse erythematous maculopapular rash

4. 2. The back of the head in a 7-year-old is 5.5%. The back of the right thigh is 4.25%. Therefore, the total body surface area affected is 9.75%.
CN: Physiological integrity; CNS: Physiological adaptation; CL: Apply; DIFFICULTY: Difficult

5. 4. A client with a deep partial-thickness burn will have tissue necrosis to the epidermis and dermis layers. Necrosis through all skin layers is seen with full-thickness injuries. Erythema and pain are characteristic of superficial injury. With deep burns, the nerve fibers are destroyed and the client won't feel pain in the affected area. Superficial burns present with slight epidermal damage.
CN: Physiological integrity; CNS: Physiological adaptation; CL: Apply; DIFFICULTY: Moderate

6. 3. There's a 3% to 5% risk of fetal death from hydrops fetalis if a pregnant woman is exposed during the first trimester. The cutaneous eruption of fifth disease can reappear for up to 4 months. A child with fifth disease is contagious during the first stage, not after the rash, when symptoms of headache, body aches, fever, and chills are present. The child should be isolated from pregnant women, immunocompromised clients, and clients with chronic anemia for up to 2 weeks.
CN: Safe, effective care environment; CNS: Safety and infection control; CL: Apply; DIFFICULTY: Moderate

7. 1. Circumferential burns can compromise blood flow to an extremity, causing numbness. Capillary refill less than 2 seconds indicates a normal vascular blood flow. Absence of pain and full range of motion imply good tissue oxygenation from intact circulation. +2 pulses indicate normal circulation.
CN: Physiological integrity; CNS: Physiological adaptation; CL: Analyze; DIFFICULTY: Easy

8. 2. The classic symptoms of erythema infectiosum begin with intense redness of both cheeks. An erythematous rash after a fever is characteristic of roseola. Children with varicella typically have vesicular lesions of the trunk, face, and scalp after a low-grade fever. An erythematous rash with a sandpaper-like texture is associated with scarlet fever, which is a bacterial infection.
CN: Physiological integrity; CNS: Physiological adaptation; CL: Apply; DIFFICULTY: Moderate

CN: Client needs category   CNS: Client needs subcategory   CL: Cognitive level

9. A family that recently went camping brings their child to the clinic with a report of a rash after a tick bite. Which finding should the nurse expect to see in a child with Lyme disease?
1. Erythematous rash surrounding a necrotic lesion
2. Bright rash with red outer border circling the bite site
3. Onset of a diffuse rash over the entire body 2 months after exposure
4. A linear rash of papules and vesicles that occurs 1 to 3 days after exposure

10. When reviewing medication instructions to an adolescent prescribed doxycycline, what should the nurse reinforce to the client to avoid? Select all that apply.
1. Taking with antacids
2. Taking birth control
3. Taking on an empty stomach
4. Taking with milk
5. Taking with food

11. When reinforcing education for the parents of a child with Kawasaki disease, which information should the nurse be sure to include?
1. It's highly contagious.
2. It's an afebrile condition with cardiac involvement.
3. It usually occurs in children older than age 5.
4. Prolonged fever, with peeling of the fingers and toes, are the initial symptoms.

12. A 22 lb (10 kg) child is diagnosed with Kawasaki disease and started on gamma globulin therapy. The health care provider orders an IV infusion of gamma globulin, 2 g/kg, to run over 12 hours. How many grams should the nurse give the client? Record your answer using a whole number.

_____ g

13. Parents are concerned because their child was exposed to varicella in day care. Which statement by the nurse would be **most** accurate?
1. "The rash is nonvesicular."
2. "The treatment of choice is aspirin."
3. "Varicella has an incubation period of 5 to 10 days."
4. "A child is no longer contagious once the rash has crusted over."

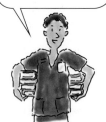

Doxycycline does not play well with others.

9. 2. A bull's-eye rash is a classic symptom of Lyme disease. In Lyme disease, the rash is located primarily at the site of the bite and occurs almost immediately, not 2 months after exposure. Necrotic, painful rashes are associated with the bite of a brown recluse spider. A linear, papular, vesicular rash indicates exposure to the leaves of poison ivy.
CN: Physiological integrity; CNS: Physiological adaptation; CL: Apply; DIFFICULTY: Easy

10. 1, 4, 5. Contraindications for tetracycline use are taking with antacids, milk, food and pregnancy. The client should be instructed to take doxycycline on an empty stomach and to take her birth control to avoid pregnancy.
CN: Physiological integrity; CNS: Pharmacological therapies; CL: Apply; DIFFICULTY: Difficult

11. 4. To be diagnosed with Kawasaki disease, the child must have a fever for 5 days or more, plus at least four of these symptoms: bilateral conjunctivitis, changes in the oral mucosa, changes in the peripheral extremities, rash, and lymphadenopathy. Kawasaki disease is more likely to occur in children younger than age 5. It isn't contagious.
CN: Physiological integrity; CNS: Physiological adaptation; CL: Apply; DIFFICULTY: Moderate

12. 20.
To calculate the dose, use the child's weight in kilograms.

$$2\,g \times 10 = 20\,g$$

CN: Physiological integrity; CNS: Pharmacological therapies; CL: Apply; DIFFICULTY: Moderate

13. 4. When every varicella lesion is crusted over, the child is no longer considered contagious. The incubation period is 10 to 20 days. Use of aspirin has been associated with Reye syndrome and is contraindicated in varicella. The rash is typically a maculopapular vesicular rash.
CN: Physiological integrity; CNS: Physiological adaptation; CL: Apply; DIFFICULTY: Challenge

14. The parents of a child diagnosed with varicella ask the nurse what medications may be used to treat this virus. What would be the nurse's **best** answer? Select all that apply.
1. Rimantadine
2. Valcyclovir
3. Oseltamivir
4. Acyclovir
5. Zanamivir

15. Which statement would be appropriate when discussing frostbite with the parents of a child brought to the emergency department after an extended period of sledding?
1. The skin is white.
2. The skin looks deeply flushed and red.
3. Frostbite is helped by rubbing to increase circulation.
4. Gradual rewarming of the extremities with hot water is needed.

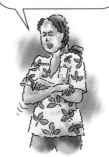

Grrr! My roommate keeps the thermostat so low I worry about getting frostbite.

16. A parent brings a child to the health care provider's office because the child reports pain, redness, and tenderness of the left index finger. The child is diagnosed with paronychia. Which organism is the **most** likely cause of this superficial abscess of the cuticle?
1. *Borrelia burgdorferi*
2. *Escherichia coli*
3. *Pseudomonas* species
4. *Staphylococcus* species

17. The nurse is reinforcing education about the treatment for paronychia. What would the nurse be sure to review with the parents?
1. Give warm soaks.
2. Splint and put ice on the affected finger.
3. Allow the infection to resolve without treatment.
4. Admit the child to the hospital for IV antibiotic therapy.

18. The nurse is obtaining data from a child who is suspected of having a scabies infestation. What finding by the nurse would correlate with this diagnosis?
1. Diffuse, pruritic wheals
2. Oval, white dots stuck to the hair shafts
3. Pain, erythema, and edema with an embedded stinger
4. Pruritic papules, pustules, and linear burrows of the finger and toe webs

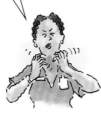

Scabies really is as horrible as it sounds.

19. An infant is being treated with antibiotic therapy for otitis media and develops an erythematous, fine, raised rash in the groin and suprapubic area. Which explanation would the nurse suspect?
1. The infant most likely has candidiasis.
2. The brand of diapers should be changed.
3. An over-the-counter diaper remedy is best to use.
4. The antibiotic therapy must be stopped immediately.

14. 2, 4. In varicella, the medications used are acyclovir or valcyclovir. Rimantadine, zanamivir, and oseltamivir are used to treat influenza.
CN: Physiological integrity; CNS: Physiological adaptation;
CL: Apply; DIFFICULTY: Difficult

15. 1. Signs and symptoms of frostbite include tingling, numbness, burning sensation, and white skin. Treatment includes very gentle handling of the affected area. Rubbing is contraindicated as it can damage fragile tissue. Gradual rewarming by exposure to hot water can lead to more tissue damage.
CN: Physiological integrity; CNS: Physiological adaptation;
CL: Apply; DIFFICULTY: Difficult

16. 4. Paronychia is a localized infection of the nail bed caused by either staphylococci or streptococci. *B. burgdorferi* is responsible for Lyme disease. *E. coli* is associated with urinary tract infections. *Pseudomonas* species are associated with ecthyma.
CN: Physiological integrity; CNS: Physiological adaptation;
CL: Understand; DIFFICULTY: Moderate

17. 1. Giving warm soaks is the treatment of choice for paronychia. Splinting and icing aren't indicated. Untreated, the local abscess can spread beneath the nail bed, a condition called secondary lymphangitis. IV antibiotic therapy isn't needed if the abscess is kept from spreading.
CN: Physiological integrity; CNS: Physiological adaptation;
CL: Apply; DIFFICULTY: Moderate

18. 4. Pruritic papules, vesicles, and linear burrows are diagnostic for scabies. Urticaria is associated with an allergic reaction of diffuse pruritic wheals. Nits, seen as white oval dots, are characteristic of head lice. Bites from honeybees are associated with a stinger, pain, and erythema.
CN: Physiological integrity; CNS: Physiological adaptation;
CL: Apply; DIFFICULTY: Easy

19. 1. Candidiasis, caused by yeastlike fungi, can occur with the use of antibiotics. Changing the brand of diapers or suggesting that the parent use an over-the-counter remedy would be appropriate for treating diaper rash, not candidiasis. The treatment for candidiasis is topical nystatin ointment. Antibiotic therapy shouldn't be stopped.
CN: Physiological integrity; CNS: Physiological adaptation;
CL: Analyze; DIFFICULTY: Challenge

20. The parent of a 5-month-old infant is planning a trip to the beach and asks for advice about sunscreen. Which instruction would the nurse incorporate into the education plan?
   1. The sun protection factor (SPF) of the sunscreen should be at least 10.
   2. Sunscreen is applied to the exposed areas of the skin.
   3. Sunscreen shouldn't be applied to infants younger than age 6 months.
   4. Sunscreen needs to be applied heavily only once, 30 minutes before going out in the sun.

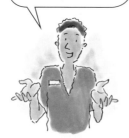

Note the client's age in question #20. It's important.

21. The nurse is performing a dressing change when there's an overhead page announcing the hospital code for a security situation. What would be the **most** appropriate initial course of action?
   1. Close the door to the room and stay with the child.
   2. Immediately report to the site of the security alert to demonstrate a show of force.
   3. Reassure the child as the dressing is completed; then report to the charge nurse.
   4. Reassure the child and report to the charge nurse.

22. The skin in the diaper area of a 6-month-old infant is excoriated and red. Which instructions would the nurse give to the parent?
   1. Change the diaper more often.
   2. Apply talcum powder with diaper changes.
   3. Wash the area vigorously with each diaper change.
   4. Decrease the infant's fluid intake to decrease saturating diapers.

Increasing the frequency of diaper changes can help prevent diaper rash. Speaking of which …

23. A 9-year-old child is being discharged from the hospital after severe urticaria caused by an allergy to nuts. Which instructions would be included in discharge education for the child's parents?
   1. Use emollient lotions and baths.
   2. Apply topical steroids to the lesions as needed.
   3. Apply over-the-counter products such as diphenhydramine.
   4. Instruct parents and child on how to use an epinephrine administration kit.

24. The nurse is reinforcing education about treatment options for the parent of a child with lice. Which adverse effect would the nurse teach regarding lindane shampoo?
   1. Lindane causes alopecia.
   2. Lindane causes hypertension.
   3. Lindane is associated with seizures.
   4. Lindane increases liver function test (LFT) results.

Way to go! You're running a good race.

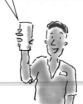

20. 3. Sunscreen isn't recommended for use in infants younger than age 6 months. These children should be dressed in cool, light clothes and kept in the shade. On children older than age 6 months, sunscreen should be applied evenly throughout the day and each time the child is in the water. The SPF for children should be 15 or greater. Sunscreen should be applied to all areas of the skin.
CN: Health promotion and maintenance; CNS: None;
CL: Apply; DIFFICULTY: Moderate

21. 3. A security alert notifies everyone in the hospital that there may be a dangerous situation occurring that indicates a trained show of force. The nurse should complete the dressing change, reassure the child, and then report to the charge nurse for further instructions. Simply closing the door and remaining with the child would not appropriately address the security situation and could potentially place the nurse and child in danger. The nurse shouldn't leave the room with the child's wound uncovered nor would it be appropriate to leave the room without first reassuring the child.
CN: Safe, effective care environment; CNS: Safety and infection control; CL: Analyze; DIFFICULTY: Challenge

22. 1. Simply decreasing the amount of time the skin comes in contact with wet, soiled diapers will help heal the irritation. Talcum is contraindicated in children because of the risks associated with inhalation of the fine powder. Gentle cleaning of the irritated skin should be encouraged. Infants shouldn't have fluid intake restrictions.
CN: Safe, effective care environment; CNS: Safety and infection control; CL: Apply; DIFFICULTY: Easy

23. 4. Children who have urticaria in response to nuts, seafood, or bee stings should be warned about the possibility of anaphylactic reactions to future exposure. The use of epinephrine pens should be taught to the parents and to older children. Other treatment choices, such as emollients, topical steroids, and diphenhydramine, are for the treatment of mild urticaria.
CN: Physiological integrity; CNS: Reduction of risk potential; CL: Apply; DIFFICULTY: Easy

24. 3. Lindane is associated with seizures after absorption with topical use. Alopecia, hypertension, and increased LFT results aren't associated with the use of lindane.
CN: Physiological integrity; CNS: Pharmacological therapies; CL: Apply; DIFFICULTY: Moderate

CN: Client needs category   CNS: Client needs subcategory   CL: Cognitive level

25. A 5-year-old is admitted to the emergency department with a broken clavicle. The nurse notices bruises in various stages of healing on the torso and extremities. The parent enters the room and angrily demands to take the child home. Which action is **most** appropriate?
1. Inform the parent that the child has a broken bone and can't leave.
2. Ask the parent whether it is known how the child received the bruises.
3. Step out of the room, notify the charge nurse, and then call security.
4. Take the child out of the room and call security.

26. Which instructions would the nurse include for the parents about the treatment of head lice?
1. The treatment should be repeated in 7 to 12 days.
2. Treatment should be repeated every day for 1 week.
3. If treated with a shampoo, combing to remove eggs isn't necessary.
4. All contacts with the infested child should be treated even without evidence of infestation.

27. The parents of a 4-year-old report that their child has been scratching the rectum recently. About which infestation or condition will the nurse reinforce education?
1. Anal fissure
2. Lice
3. Pinworms
4. Scabies

28. When examining a preschool-age child, the nurse finds multiple contusions over the body. Which statement indicates the findings that should be documented?
1. Contusions confined to one body area are typically suspicious.
2. All lesions, including location, shape, and color, should be documented.
3. Natural injuries usually have straight linear lines, while injuries from abuse have multiple curved lines.
4. The depth, location, and amount of bleeding that initially occurs is constant, but the sequence of color change is variable.

29. The parent asks the nurse how many clear cellophane tape tests will the child need to have to detect pinworm infestation at virtually 100% accuracy. Which response by the nurse would be **best**?
1. One
2. Three
3. Five
4. Ten

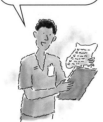

Don't try to worm your way out of answering question #27.

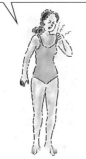

Of course, sunscreen is optional . . . as long as you don't mind frying your skin, feeling excruciating pain, and risking skin cancer.

25. 3. In order to ensure the nurse's safety as well as the safety of the child, the best course of action would be to leave the room and immediately notify the charge nurse, and then call security. The nurse wouldn't want to further anger the parent and create the potential for violence by taking the child out of the room. Asking for personal information and telling the parent the child cannot be taken is an inappropriate action.
CN: Psychosocial integrity; CNS: None; CL: Apply;
DIFFICULTY: Moderate

26. 1. Treatment for head lice should be repeated in 7 to 12 days to ensure that all eggs are killed. Combing the hair thoroughly is necessary to remove the lice eggs. People exposed to head lice should be examined to assess the presence of infestation before treatment.
CN: Physiological integrity; CNS: Physiological adaptation;
CL: Apply; DIFFICULTY: Challenge

27. 3. The clinical sign of pinworms is perianal itching that increases at night. Anal fissures are associated with rectal bleeding and pain with bowel movements. Lice are infestations of the hair. Scabies are associated with a pruritic rash characterized as linear burrows of the webs of the fingers and toes.
CN: Physiological integrity; CNS: Physiological adaptation;
CL: Analyze; DIFFICULTY: Easy

28. 2. An accurate, precise examination must be properly substantiated as a legal document. Contusions that result from falls are typically confined to a single body area and are considered a reasonable finding of a child still learning to walk. Injuries from normal falls are usually not linear in nature. Bleeding can cause variations, but color change is consistent.
CN: Psychosocial integrity; CNS: None; CL: Apply;
DIFFICULTY: Easy

29. 3. Detection is virtually 100% accurate with five tests. Three tests should detect infestations at about 90% accuracy. One test is only 50% accurate. Ten tests aren't necessary.
CN: Physiological integrity; CNS: Reduction of risk potential;
CL: Apply; DIFFICULTY: Challenge

CN: Client needs category   CNS: Client needs subcategory   CL: Cognitive level

30. Each member of the family of a child diagnosed with pinworms is prescribed a single dose of mebendazole. Which statement would the nurse incorporate into the education plan?
1. The drug may stain the feces red.
2. The dose may be repeated in 2 weeks.
3. Fever and rash are common adverse effects.
4. The medicine will kill the eggs in about 48 hours.

31. A large dog bit the hand of a child. The nurse would expect to find which type of injury?
1. Abrasion
2. Crush injury
3. Fracture
4. Puncture wound

32. The nurse understands that bites from dogs heighten the risk of infection. Which intervention should be done to help prevent infection in a child that has been bitten?
1. Give the rabies vaccine.
2. Give antibiotics immediately.
3. Clean and irrigate the wounds.
4. Nothing; bites from dogs have a low incidence of infection.

33. When collecting data from a 6-year-old child who has a 20% deep partial-thickness (second-degree) burn of the arms and trunk, the nurse determines that the child has damage to what layers of skin?
1. Epidermis
2. Epidermis and part of the dermis
3. Epidermis and all of the dermis
4. Dermis and subcutaneous tissue

34. A child is brought to the health care provider's office for multiple scratches and bites from a kitten and is being evaluated for cat-scratch disease. While collecting data, which symptom would the nurse expect to find with cat-scratch disease?
1. Abdominal pain
2. Adenitis
3. Fever
4. Pruritus

35. In which child population would the nurse be alert for giardiasis, the most common parasitic intestinal infection in the United States?
1. Children riding a school bus
2. Children playing on a playground
3. Children attending a sporting event
4. Children attending group day care or nursery school

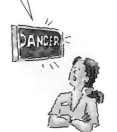

All those bacteria that live in a dog's mouth can enter the body when a client is bitten.

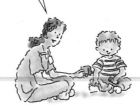

Sometimes kids pick up more than toys when they're in day care.

30. 2. Mebendazole is effective against the adult worms only (not eggs), so treatment should be repeated in 2 weeks to eradicate any emerging parasites. Staining the feces isn't associated with mebendazole. Common adverse effects of mebendazole are reports of headaches and abdominal pain.
CN: Physiological integrity; CNS: Pharmacological therapies; CL: Apply; DIFFICULTY: Moderate

31. 2. Although the bite of a large dog can exert pressure of 150 to 400 lb per square inch, the bite causes crush injuries, not fractures. Abrasions are associated with friction injuries. Puncture wounds are associated with bites of smaller animals such as cats.
CN: Physiological integrity; CNS: Physiological adaptation; CL: Apply; DIFFICULTY: Challenge

32. 3. Not every dog bite requires antibiotic therapy, but cleaning the wound is necessary for all injuries involving a break in the skin. Rabies vaccine is used if the dog is suspected of having rabies. The infection rate for dog bites has been reported to be as high as 50%.
CN: Physiological integrity; CNS: Reduction of risk potential; CL: Apply; DIFFICULTY: Moderate

33. 2. A deep partial-thickness burn affects the epidermis and part of the dermis. A superficial partial-thickness (first-degree) burn affects the epidermis only. A full-thickness (third-degree) burn involves epidermis and all of the dermis as well as nerves and blood vessels in the skin.
CN: Physiological integrity; CNS: Physiological adaptation; CL: Apply; DIFFICULTY: Moderate

34. 2. Adenitis (inflammation of a gland or lymph node) is the primary feature of cat-scratch disease. Although low-grade fever has been associated with cat-scratch disease, it's present only 25% of the time. Pruritus and abdominal pain aren't symptoms of cat-scratch disease.
CN: Physiological integrity; CNS: Physiological adaptation; CL: Analyze; DIFFICULTY: Difficult

35. 4. The most common intestinal parasitic infection in the United States is giardiasis, prevalent among children attending group day care or nursery school. Playgrounds, sporting events, and school buses don't present unusual risk of giardiasis.
CN: Safe, effective care environment; CNS: Safety and infection control; CL: Understand; DIFFICULTY: Challenge

CN: Client needs category   CNS: Client needs subcategory   CL: Cognitive level

36. Which finding should the nurse expect to observe if a child has papules?
1. Palpable elevated masses
2. Loss of the epidermal layer
3. Fluid-filled elevations of the skin
4. Nonpalpable, flat changes in skin color

36. 1. Papules are palpable elevated up to 0.5 cm. Nodules and tumors are elevated more than 0.5 cm. Erosions are characterized as loss of the epidermal layer. Fluid-filled lesions are vesicles and pustules. Macules and patches are described as nonpalpable, flat changes in skin color.
CN: Health promotion and maintenance; CNS: None; CL: Apply; DIFFICULTY: Challenge

37. When collecting data on a child diagnosed with impetigo, which symptom would the nurse identify as the primary manifestation?
1. Lesion filled with pus
2. Superficial area of localized edema
3. Serous-filled lesion less than 0.5 cm
4. Serous-filled lesion greater than 0.5 cm

37. 1. Pustules, the primary lesions with impetigo, are pus-filled lesions, such as acne and impetigo. Bullae are serous-filled lesions greater than 0.5 cm in diameter. A wheal is a superficial area of localized edema. Vesicles are serous-filled lesions up to 0.5 cm in diameter.
CN: Physiological integrity; CNS: Physiological adaptation; CL: Apply; DIFFICULTY: Difficult

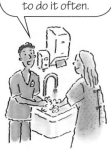

Hand washing is basic maintenance for your integument. Teach your clients to do it often.

38. A child is brought to the health care provider's office for treatment of a rash. Many petechiae are seen over the entire body. The nurse would suspect which condition?
1. Bleeding disorder
2. Scabies
3. Varicella
4. Vomiting

38. 1. Petechiae are caused by blood outside a vessel, associated with low platelet counts and bleeding disorders. Petechiae aren't found with varicella disease or scabies. Petechiae can be associated with vomiting, but in this case, they would be present on the face, not the entire body.
CN: Physiological integrity; CNS: Physiological adaptation; CL: Analyze; DIFFICULTY: Moderate

39. A child fell at camp and sustained a bruise to the thigh. Which description would accurately describe the bruise after 1 week?
1. Resolved
2. Reddish blue
3. Greenish yellow
4. Dark blue to bluish brown

39. 3. After 7 to 10 days, the bruise becomes greenish yellow. Resolution can take up to 2 weeks. Initially after a fall, a bruise has a reddish-blue discoloration, followed by dark blue to bluish brown at days 1 to 3.
CN: Physiological integrity; CNS: Physiological adaptation; CL: Apply; DIFFICULTY: Moderate

40. A 5-year-old child sustained third-degree burns to the right upper extremity after tipping over a frying pan. Which skin structures would the nurse include when explaining a third-degree burn to the child's parent?
1. Epidermis only
2. Epidermis and dermis
3. All skin layers and nerve endings
4. Skin layers, nerve endings, muscles, tendons, and bone

40. 3. A third-degree burn involves all of the skin layers and the nerve endings. First-degree burns involve only the epidermis. Second-degree burns affect the epidermis and dermis. Fourth-degree burns involve all skin layers, nerve endings, muscles, tendons, and bone.
CN: Physiological integrity; CNS: Physiological adaptation; CL: Apply; DIFFICULTY: Moderate

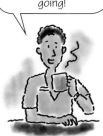

Hey—you've finished 40 questions. Nice going!

41. The nurse is gathering data from a child suspected of being a victim of abuse. What observation by the nurse would lead to this suspicion?
1. Multiple contusions of the shins
2. Contusions of the back and buttocks
3. Contusions at the same stages of healing
4. Large contusion and hematoma of the forehead

41. 2. Contusions of the back and buttocks are highly suggestive of abuse related to punishment. Contusions at various stages of healing are red flags to potential abuse. Contusions of the shins and forehead are usually related to an active toddler falling and bumping into objects.
CN: Psychosocial integrity; CNS: None; CL: Analyze; DIFFICULTY: Easy

42. Which statement would the nurse include when reinforcing education for a parent about salmon patches (stork bites)?
1. "They're benign and usually fade in adult life."
2. "They're usually associated with syndromes of the neonate."
3. "They can cause mild hypertrophy of the muscle associated with the lesion."
4. "They're treatable with laser pulse surgery in late adolescence and adulthood."

43. When inspecting a neonate, the nurse observes a blue-black macular lesion over the lower lumbar sacral region. What does the nurse interpret this finding as?
1. Café au lait spots.
2. Mongolian spots.
3. Nevus of Ota.
4. Stork bites.

44. The nurse is caring for a child who has experienced vomiting and diarrhea for 2 days. Which finding would alert the nurse that the child is experiencing severe dehydration?
1. Gray skin and decreased tears
2. Capillary refill less than 2 seconds
3. Mottling and tenting of the skin
4. Pale skin with dry mucous membranes

45. Clindamycin is being prescribed for a child diagnosed with severe acne. The nurse is reinforcing medication education and is sure to include which adverse effects? Select al that apply.
1. Diarrhea
2. Gram-negative folliculitis
3. Teratogenesis
4. Vaginal candidiasis
5. Constipation

46. The nurse is reinforcing education to a group of adolescents on acne. Which statement by an adolescent would show that the teaching has been effective?
1. "Diet is a cause of acne."
2. "Gender is a cause of acne."
3. "Poor hygiene is a cause of acne."
4. "Hormonal changes are a cause of acne."

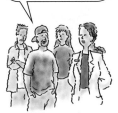

Word on the street is you're completely owning this test. Let me see your swagger.

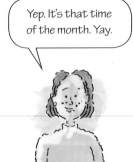

Yep. It's that time of the month. Yay.

42. 1. Salmon patches occur over the back of the neck in 40% of neonates and are harmless, needing no intervention. Laser pulse surgery isn't recommended for salmon patches because they typically fade on their own in adulthood. Port-wine stains are associated with Sturge-Weber syndrome. Port-wine stains found on the face or extremities may be associated with soft tissue and bone hypertrophy.
CN: Health promotion and maintenance; CNS: None; CL: Apply; DIFFICULTY: Easy

43. 2. Mongolian spots are large, blue-black macular lesions generally located over the lumbosacral areas, buttocks, and limbs. Café au lait spots occur between ages 2 and 16, not in infancy. Nevus of Ota is found surrounding the eyes. Stork bites, or salmon patches, occur at the neck and hairline area.
CN: Health promotion and maintenance; CNS: None; CL: Analyze; DIFFICULTY: Easy

44. 3. Severe dehydration is associated with mottling and tenting of the skin. Malnutrition is characterized by gray skin. Capillary refill less than 2 seconds is normal. Pale skin with dry mucous membranes is a sign of *mild* dehydration.
CN: Physiological integrity; CNS: Physiological adaptation; CL: Apply; DIFFICULTY: Challenge

45. 1, 2. Clindamycin is associated with both diarrhea and gram-negative folliculitis. Isotretinoin has been associated with severe birth defects. Most female clients are prescribed oral contraceptives while taking isotretinoin. Tetracycline is associated with yeast infections. Diarrhea is an adverse side effect of clindamycin, not constipation.
CN: Physiological integrity; CNS: Pharmacological therapies; CL: Apply; DIFFICULTY: Difficult

46. 4. Acne is caused by hormonal changes in sebaceous gland anatomy and the biochemistry of the glands. These changes lead to a blockage in the follicular canal and cause an inflammatory response. Diet, hygiene, and the adolescent's gender don't cause acne.
CN: Health promotion and maintenance; CNS: None; CL: Apply; DIFFICULTY: Easy

47. While caring for a 2-day-old neonate, a nurse notices the left side of the neonate reddens for 2 to 3 minutes. What does this finding suggest?
   1. Contact dermatitis
   2. Environmental conditions
   3. Harlequin color change
   4. Hypercyanotic event

47. 3. Harlequin color change is a benign disorder related to the immaturity of the hypothalamic centers that control the tone of peripheral blood vessels. A newborn who has been lying on its side may appear reddened on the dependent side. The color fades on position change. Contact dermatitis isn't short-lived. Changes in environmental conditions can cause diffuse bilateral mottling of the skin. Tet spells are associated with tetralogy of Fallot and cause cyanotic changes.
CN: Health promotion and maintenance; CNS: None; CL: Apply;
DIFFICULTY: Moderate

48. When educating a client about tetracycline for severe inflammatory acne, which instructions must be given?
   1. Take the drug with or without meals.
   2. Take the drug with milk and milk products.
   3. Take the drug on an empty stomach with small amounts of water.
   4. Take the drug 1 hour before or 2 hours after meals with large amounts of water.

48. 4. Tetracycline must be taken on an empty stomach to increase absorption and with ample water to avoid esophageal irritation. Milk products impede absorption.
CN: Physiological integrity; CNS: Pharmacological therapies;
CL: Apply; DIFFICULTY: Moderate

49. When advising parents about the prevention of burns from tap water, which instructions should be given?
   1. Set the water-heater temperature at 130° F (54.4° C) or less.
   2. Run the hot water first, then adjust the temperature with cold water.
   3. Before you put your infant in the tub, test the water with your hand.
   4. Supervise an infant in the bathroom, only leaving him for a few seconds if needed.

49. 3. Instruct the parents to fill the tub with water first, then test all of the water in the tub with their hand for hot spots. The cold water should be run first and then adjusted with hot water. Water heaters should be set at 120° F (48.9° C). Never leave an infant alone in the bathroom, even for a second.
CN: Physiological integrity; CNS: Reduction of risk potential;
CL: Apply; DIFFICULTY: Easy

50. A 14-year-old adolescent is brought to the hospital with smoke inhalation because of a house fire. What is the nurse's **priority** intervention for this adolescent?
   1. Check the oral mucous membranes.
   2. Check for any burned areas.
   3. Obtain a medical history.
   4. Ensure a patent airway.

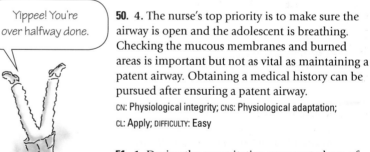

Yippee! You're over halfway done.

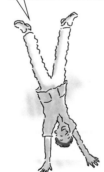

50. 4. The nurse's top priority is to make sure the airway is open and the adolescent is breathing. Checking the mucous membranes and burned areas is important but not as vital as maintaining a patent airway. Obtaining a medical history can be pursued after ensuring a patent airway.
CN: Physiological integrity; CNS: Physiological adaptation;
CL: Apply; DIFFICULTY: Easy

51. A 13-year-old has received third-degree burns over 20% of the body. When observing this client 72 hours after the burn, which finding should the nurse expect?
   1. Increased urine output
   2. Severe peripheral edema
   3. Respiratory distress
   4. Absent bowel sounds

51. 1. During the resuscitative-emergent phase of a burn, fluids shift back into the interstitial space, resulting in the onset of diuresis. Edema resolves during the emergent phase, when fluid shifts back to the intravascular space. Respiratory rate increases during the first few hours as a result of edema. When edema resolves, respirations return to normal. Absent bowel sounds occur in the initial stage.
CN: Physiological integrity; CNS: Physiological adaptation;
CL: Apply; DIFFICULTY: Challenge

52. A 15-month-old child is diagnosed with pedic-ulosis of the eyebrows. Which intervention would the nurse expect to be included in the treatment?
1. Using lindane
2. Using petroleum jelly
3. Shaving the eyebrows
4. Doing nothing; no treatment is needed

52. 2. Pediculosis must be treated. Petroleum jelly should be applied twice daily for 8 days, followed by manual removal of nits. Lindane is contraindi-cated because of the risk of seizures. The eyebrow should never be shaved because of the uncertainty of hair return.
CN: Physiological integrity; CNS: Physiological adaptation;
CL: Apply; DIFFICULTY: Difficult

53. A child is diagnosed with Kawasaki disease. Which changes in the mouth area would the nurse observe with this disorder? Select all that apply.
1. Swollen lymph nodes in the neck
2. Tonsillar exudate
3. Vesicular lesions
4. Dry, cracked lips; strawberry tongue
5. Swollen red feet and hands

53. 1, 4, 5. Oral changes associated with Kawasaki disease include a reddened pharynx; red, dry fissured lips and strawberry tongue; swollen lymph nodes in the neck, and swollen red feet and hands. Koplik spots are consistent with measles. Tonsillar exudate is consistent with pharyngitis caused by group A beta-hemolytic streptococci. Vesicular lesions are associated with coxsackievirus.
CN: Physiological integrity; CNS: Physiological adaptation;
CL: Analyze; DIFFICULTY: Easy

54. The nurse is weighing a 3-month-old infant of Mediterranean descent during a routine examina-tion in a family health center. The nurse docu-ments the bluish discoloration of the skin on the lower back as which condition?
1. Milia
2. Mongolian spots
3. Lanugo
4. Vernix caseosa

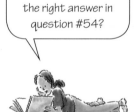

Can you spot the right answer in question #54?

54. 2. Bluish discolorations of the skin, which are common in babies of black, Native American, and Mediterranean races, are called Mongolian spots. Pinpoint pimples caused by obstruction of seba-ceous glands are called milia. The fine hair cover-ing the body of a neonate is called lanugo. Vernix caseosa is a cheese-like substance that covers the skin of a neonate.
CN: Health promotion and maintenance; CNS: None; CL: Apply;
DIFFICULTY: Easy

55. Topical treatment with 2.5% hydrocortisone is prescribed for a 6-month-old infant with eczema. The nurse advises the parent to use the cream for no more than 1 week based on which rationale?
1. The drug loses its efficacy after prolonged use.
2. Excessive use can have adverse effects, such as skin atrophy and fragility.
3. If no improvement is seen, a stronger concen-tration will be prescribed.
4. If no improvement is seen after 1 week, an antibiotic will be prescribed.

55. 2. Hydrocortisone cream should be used for brief periods to decrease adverse effects such as atrophy of the skin. The drug doesn't lose efficacy after prolonged use. A stronger concentration may not be prescribed if no improvement is seen. An antibiotic would be inappropriate in this instance.
CN: Physiological integrity; CNS: Pharmacological therapies;
CL: Apply; DIFFICULTY: Moderate

56. A 1-year-old infant is hospitalized with a diag-nosis of eczema. Which signs and symptoms does the nurse expect to observe?
1. Exudative, crusty, papulovesicular, erythema-tous lesions on the cheeks, scalp, forehead, and arms
2. Erythematous, dry, scaly, papular, thickened, well-circumscribed, and lichenified pruritic lesions on the wrists, hands, and neck
3. Large, thickened, lichenified plaques on the face, neck, and back
4. Erythematous papules with oozing, crusting, and edema

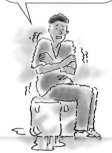

Brain freeze? Move on to another question and return to this one later, once your brain has thawed out.

56. 1. Exudative, crusty, papulovesicular, erythe-matous lesions on the cheeks, scalp, forehead, and arms are observed in children ages 2 months to 2 years with a diagnosis of eczema. Erythematous, dry, scaly, well-circumscribed, papular, thickened, lichenified, pruritic lesions on the wrists, hands, and neck are observed in children with eczema ages 2 years to puberty. In adolescents with eczema, lesions on the face, neck, and back consist of large plaques that are thickened and lichenified. Erythematous papules with oozing, crusting, and edema are characteristic of contact dermatitis.
CN: Physiological integrity; CNS: Physiological adaptation;
CL: Understand; DIFFICULTY: Challenge

57. A 4-year-old child had a subungual hemorrhage of the toe after a jar fell on the foot. Which statement regarding the rationale for using electrocautery to treat the injury is **most** accurate?
1. It's used to prevent loss of nail growth.
2. It's used to prevent loss of the nail.
3. It's used to relieve pain and reduce the risk of infection.
4. It's used to prevent permanent discoloration of the nail bed.

58. The nurse is caring for a 12-year-old child with a diagnosis of eczema. Which nursing intervention is appropriate for this child?
1. Administer antibiotics as prescribed.
2. Administer antifungals as ordered.
3. Administer tepid baths and pat dry or air-dry the affected areas.
4. Administer hot baths and use moisturizers immediately after the bath.

59. A 9-year-old child is brought to the emergency department with extensive burns received in a restaurant fire. What's the **most** important aspect of caring for this child?
1. Administer antibiotics to prevent superimposed infections.
2. Conduct wound management.
3. Administer liquids orally to replace fluid.
4. Administer frequent small meals to support nutritional requirements.

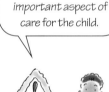

Question #59 is asking for the *most* important aspect of care for the child.

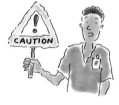

60. The parent of a 4-month-old infant asks about the strawberry hemangioma on the cheek. Which statement would the nurse include when responding to the mother?
1. "The lesion will continue to grow for 3 years, then need surgical removal."
2. "If the lesion continues to enlarge, referral to a pediatric oncologist is warranted."
3. "Surgery is indicated before age 12 months if the diameter of the lesion is greater than 3 cm."
4. "The lesion will continue to grow until age 12 months, then begin to resolve by age 2 to 3 years."

You know—next time I think I'll just use sunscreen.

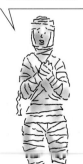

61. A 3-year-old child is being discharged from the emergency department after receiving three sutures for a scalp laceration. The nurse should tell the family to return for suture removal in how many days?
1. 1 to 3 days
2. 5 to 7 days
3. 8 to 10 days
4. 10 to 14 days

57. 3. The hematoma is treated with electrocautery to relieve pain and reduce the risk of infection. Electrocautery doesn't prevent the loss of the nail. The discoloration seen with subungual hemorrhage is from the collection of blood under the nail bed. It isn't permanent and doesn't affect nail growth.
CN: Physiological integrity; CNS: Physiological adaptation; CL: Apply; DIFFICULTY: Moderate

58. 3. Tepid baths and moisturizers are indicated to keep the infected areas clean and minimize itching. Antibiotics are given only when superimposed infection is present. Antifungals aren't usually administered in the treatment of eczema. Hot baths can exacerbate the condition and increase itching.
CN: Physiological integrity; CNS: Physiological adaptation; CL: Apply; DIFFICULTY: Easy

59. 2. The most important aspect of caring for a burned child is wound management. The goals of wound care are to speed debridement, protect granulation tissue and new grafts, and conserve body heat and fluids. Antibiotics aren't always administered prophylactically. Fluids are administered IV according to the child's body weight to replace volume. Enteral feedings, rather than meals, are initiated within the first 24 hours after the burn to support the child's increased nutritional requirements.
CN: Physiological integrity; CNS: Physiological adaptation; CL: Apply; DIFFICULTY: Difficult

60. 4. Hemangiomas are rapidly growing vascular lesions that reach maximum growth by age 1 year. The growth period is then followed by an involution period of 6 to 12 months. Lesions show complete involution by age 2 or 3 years. These benign lesions don't need surgical or oncologic referrals.
CN: Health promotion and maintenance; CNS: None; CL: Apply; DIFFICULTY: Moderate

61. 2. The recommended healing time for a scalp laceration is 5 to 7 days. Sutures need longer than 1 to 3 days to form an effective bond. Sutures of the fingertips and feet need 8 to 10 days, and 10 to 14 days is the recommended healing time for extensor surfaces of the knees and elbows.
CN: Physiological integrity; CNS: Physiological adaptation; CL: Apply; DIFFICULTY: Moderate

62. The nurse is reinforcing education for a 17-year-old who'll be discharged on how to change a sterile dressing on the right leg. During the education session, the nurse observes redness, swelling, and induration at the wound site. What does this indicate to the nurse?
1. Infection
2. Dehiscence
3. Hemorrhage
4. Evisceration

62. 1. Infection produces such signs as redness, swelling, induration, warmth, and, possibly, drainage. Dehiscence may cause unexplained fever and tachycardia, unusual wound pain, prolonged paralytic ileus, and separation of the surgical incision. Hemorrhage can result in increased pulse and respiratory rate, decreased blood pressure, restlessness, thirst, and cold, clammy skin. Evisceration produces visible protrusion of organs, usually through an incision.

CN: Physiological integrity; CNS: Physiological adaptation;
CL: Analyze; DIFFICULTY: Easy

63. When being examined, a 6-year-old child is noted to have a papulovesicular eruption on the left anterior lateral chest, with reports of pain and tenderness of the lesion. The nurse interprets this finding as which condition?
1. Contusion
2. Herpes zoster
3. Scabies
4. Varicella

63. 2. Herpes zoster is caused by the varicella zoster virus. It has papulovesicular lesions that erupt along a dermatome, usually with hyperesthesia, pain, and tenderness. Contusions aren't found with papulovesicular lesions. Scabies appear as linear burrows of the fingers and toes caused by a mite. The papulovesicular lesions of varicella are distributed over the entire trunk, face, and scalp and don't follow a dermatome.

CN: Physiological integrity; CNS: Physiological adaptation;
CL: Analyze; DIFFICULTY: Difficult

64. During an examination of a 5-month-old infant, a flat, dull pink, macular lesion is noted on the infant's forehead. The nurse suspects which condition?
1. Cavernous hemangioma
2. Nevus flammeus
3. Salmon patch
4. Strawberry hemangioma

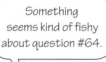

Something seems kind of fishy about question #64.

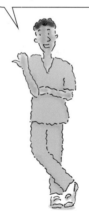

64. 3. Salmon patches are common vascular lesions in infants. They appear as flat, dull-pink, macular lesions in various regions of the face and head. When they appear on the nape of the neck, they're commonly called *stork bites*. These lesions fade by the first year of life. Nevus flammeus, or port-wine stains, are reddish purple lesions that don't fade. Strawberry and cavernous hemangiomas are raised lesions.

CN: Physiological integrity; CNS: Physiological adaptation;
CL: Analyze; DIFFICULTY: Challenge

65. The nurse is caring for a 15-year-old who has suffered third degree burns to 30% total burn surface area (TBSA). The health care provider has order morphine 0.5 mg by mouth every 3 to 4 hours as needed for pain. The elixir comes in 2 mg/1 mL. How many milliliters would the nurse give? Record your answer using two decimal places.

_____ mL

65. 0.25.
The correct formula to calculate a drug dose is:

$$\frac{\text{Dose on hand}}{\text{Quantity on hand}} = \frac{\text{Dose desired}}{X}$$

The health care provider prescribes 0.5 mg, which is the dose desired. The elixir is 2 mg/1 mL, which is the dose/quantity on hand.

$$\frac{2\text{ mg}}{1\text{ mL}} = \frac{0.5\text{ mg}}{X}$$

$$X = 0.25\text{ mL}$$

CN: Physiological integrity; CNS: Pharmacological Therapies;
CL: Apply; DIFFICULTY: Moderate

66. A child's parents ask for advice on the use of an insect repellent that contains DEET. Which statement would the nurse incorporate in the response?
1. "Spray the child's clothing instead of the skin."
2. "The repellent works better as the temperature increases."
3. "The repellent isn't effective against the ticks responsible for Lyme disease."
4. "Apply insect repellent as you would sunscreen, with frequent applications during the day."

66. **1.** DEET spray has been approved for use on children. It should be used sparingly on all skin surfaces. By concentrating the spray on clothing and camping equipment, the adverse effects and potential toxic buildup are significantly reduced. Repellent is lost to evaporation, wind, heat, and perspiration. Each 10° F increase in temperature leads to as much as a 50% reduction in protection time. DEET is very effective as a tick repellent.
CN: Physiological integrity; CNS: Reduction of risk potential; CL: Apply; DIFFICULTY: Moderate

67. A nurse is reinforcing education for a parent about a DEET-containing insect repellent to use on a child. Which concentration should the parent use on the child's skin for optimal results?
1. 10%
2. 15%
3. 20%
4. 30%

67. **1.** The highest concentration of DEET approved by the Food and Drug Administration for children is 10%. Because of thinner skin and a greater surface-area-to-mass ratio in children, parents should use DEET products sparingly.
CN: Physiological integrity; CNS: Reduction of risk potential; CL: Understand; DIFFICULTY: Difficult

68. Which statement about warts would the nurse incorporate when assisting with a community health education program on common skin problems?
1. "Cutting the wart is the preferred treatment for children."
2. "No treatment exists that specifically kills the wart virus."
3. "Warts are caused by a virus affecting the inner layer of skin."
4. "Warts are harmless and usually last 2 to 4 years if untreated."

68. **2.** The goal of treatment is to kill the skin that contains the wart virus. Cutting the wart is likely to spread the virus. The virus that causes warts affects the outer layer of the skin. Warts are harmless and last 1 to 2 years if untreated.
CN: Health promotion and maintenance; CNS: None; CL: Apply; DIFFICULTY: Challenge

69. The 2-year-old child has been diagnosed with cellulitis. The health care provider has order the client to get ceftriaxone 50 mg IM. The pharmacy sends 100 mg/2 mL. The nurse will administer the medication in the vastus lateralis. How many milliliters should be administered? Record your answer using a whole number.

_____ mL

How should we tackle this dosage calculation? Setting up an equation sounds like a good idea.

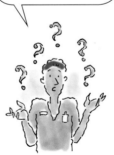

69. **1.**
The correct formula to calculate a drug dose is:

$$\frac{\text{Dose on hand}}{\text{Quantity on hand}} = \frac{\text{Dose desired}}{X}$$

The health care provider prescribes 50 mg, which is the dose desired. The pharmacy delivers 100 mg/2 mL, which is the dose/quantity on hand.

$$\frac{100 \text{ mg}}{2 \text{ mL}} = \frac{50 \text{ mg}}{X}$$

$$X = 1 \text{ mL}$$

CN: Health promotion and maintenance; CNS: None; CL: Apply; DIFFICULTY: Moderate

70. When collecting data on a child with cellulitis, which symptoms would the nurse expect to find?
1. Pale, irritated, and cold to touch
2. Vesicular blisters at the site of the injury
3. Fever, edema, tenderness, and warmth at the site
4. Swelling and redness with well-defined borders

70. **3.** Cellulitis is a deep, locally diffuse infection of the skin. It's associated with redness, fever, edema, tenderness, and warmth at the site of the injury. Vesicular blisters suggest impetigo. Cellulitis has no well-defined borders.
CN: Physiological integrity; CNS: Physiological adaptation; CL: Analysis; DIFFICULTY: Moderate

CN: Client needs category   CNS: Client needs subcategory   CL: Cognitive level

71. The nurse is working in a pediatric emergency department. Which client would be seen first?
1. 2-year-old with cellulitis to the finger
2. 4-year-old with pinworms
3. 3-month-old with oral candidiasis
4. 5-year-old with orbital cellulitis

71. 4. The 5-year-old with orbital cellulitis should be seen first because significant damage to the optic nerve can occur, causing permanent vision problems or total loss of vision.
CN: Physiological integrity; CNS: Physiological adaptation;
CL: Analysis; DIFFICULTY: Easy

72. A child has a desquamative rash of the hands and feet. Which additional finding should the nurse expect to observe with this rash?
1. Peeling skin
2. Thin, reddened layers of epidermis
3. Thick skin with deep, visible burrows
4. Thinning skin that may appear translucent

72. 1. Desquamation is characteristic in diseases such as Stevens-Johnson syndrome. Scaling is described as thin, reddened layers of epidermis. Thickening of the skin with burrows is defined as lichenification. Thinning skin is best described as atrophy of the skin.
CN: Physiological integrity; CNS: Physiological adaptation;
CL: Apply; DIFFICULTY: Challenge

73. Which instructions would the nurse include for the parents of a child who is to receive nystatin oral solution?
1. "Give the solution immediately after feedings."
2. "Give the solution immediately before feedings."
3. "Mix the solution with small amounts of the feeding."
4. "Give half the solution before and half the solution after the feeding."

73. 1. Nystatin oral solution should be swabbed onto the mouth after feedings to allow for optimal contact with mucous membranes. Administering nystatin before meals or with meals doesn't allow the best contact with the mucous membranes.
CN: Physiological integrity; CNS: Pharmacological therapies;
CL: Apply; DIFFICULTY: Moderate

74. An infant is examined and found to have a petechial rash. How will the nurse document this rash?
1. Purple, macular lesions larger than 1 cm in diameter.
2. Purple to brown bruises, macular or papular, of various sizes.
3. A collection of blood from ruptured blood vessels and larger than 1 cm in diameter.
4. Pinpoint, pink to purple, nonblanching, macular lesions that are 1 to 3 mm in diameter.

74. 4. Petechiae are small pinpoint, pink to purple, macular lesions 1 to 3 mm in diameter. Purple, macular lesions greater than 1 cm in diameter are defined as purpura. A bruise is defined as ecchymosis. A hematoma is a collection of blood.
CN: Physiological integrity; CNS: Physiological adaptation;
CL: Apply; DIFFICULTY: Easy

75. A child has a red rash in a circular shape on the legs. The lesions aren't connected. Which classification is the **most** appropriate for this rash?
1. A linear rash
2. A diffuse rash
3. An annular rash
4. A confluent rash

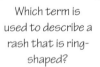

Which term is used to describe a rash that is ring-shaped?

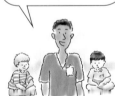

75. 3. An annular rash is ring-shaped. Linear rashes are lesions arranged in a line. A diffuse rash usually has scattered, widely distributed lesions. Confluent rash has lesions that are touching or adjacent to each other.
CN: Physiological integrity; CNS: Physiological adaptation;
CL: Remember; DIFFICULTY: Moderate

76. Parents report that their teenager is losing hair in small, round areas on the scalp. The nurse interprets this as suggesting which condition?
1. Alopecia
2. Amblyopia
3. Exotropia
4. Seborrhea dermatitis

76. 1. Alopecia is the correct term for thinning hair loss. Amblyopia and exotropia are eye disorders. Seborrhea dermatitis is cradle cap and occurs in infants.
CN: Physiological integrity; CNS: Physiological adaptation;
CL: Apply; DIFFICULTY: Easy

77. When inspecting the palms of a child, with which rash would the nurse expect to find no changes?
1. Coxsackievirus
2. Measles
3. Rocky Mountain spotted fever
4. Syphilis

78. A parent of a toddler diagnosed with atopic dermatitis is concerned about how the child acquired the disease. The nurse should explain that atopic dermatitis is caused by which condition?
1. Fungal infection
2. Hereditary disorder
3. Sex-linked disorder
4. Viral infection

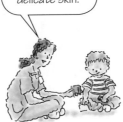

Babies and toddlers have particularly delicate skin.

79. The parent of a 6-month-old infant with atopic dermatitis asks for advice on bathing the child. Which instructions or information should the nurse give to the parent?
1. Bathe the infant twice daily.
2. Bathe the infant every other day.
3. Use bubble baths to decrease itching.
4. The frequency of the infant's baths isn't important in atopic dermatitis.

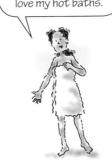

I'm so glad I don't have dermatitis—I love my hot baths.

80. Discharge instructions for a child with atopic dermatitis include keeping the fingernails cut short. Which rationale should the nurse give for this intervention?
1. To prevent infection of the nail bed
2. To prevent the spread of the disorder
3. To prevent the child from causing a corneal abrasion
4. To reduce breaks in skin from scratching that may lead to secondary bacterial infections

81. The nurse is caring for an 11-year-old child with cerebral palsy who has a pressure ulcer on the sacrum. When reinforcing education for the parent about dietary intake, which foods should the nurse plan to emphasize?
1. Legumes and cheese
2. Whole grain products
3. Fruits and vegetables
4. Lean meats and low-fat milk

82. A 10-year-old child being treated for common warts asks about the cause. The nurse would reveal which virus as the cause?
1. Coxsackievirus
2. Human herpesvirus (HHV)
3. Human immunodeficiency virus (HIV)
4. Human papillomavirus (HPV)

77. 2. The rash in measles occurs on the face, trunk, and extremities. Rocky Mountain spotted fever, syphilis, and coxsackievirus present with changes on the palms and soles.
CN: Physiological integrity; CNS: Physiological adaptation;
CL: Analysis; DIFFICULTY: Difficult

78. 2. Atopic dermatitis is a hereditary disorder associated with a family history of asthma, allergic rhinitis, or atopic dermatitis. Fungal and viral infections don't cause atopic dermatitis.
CN: Physiological integrity; CNS: Physiological adaptation;
CL: Apply; DIFFICULTY: Challenge

79. 2. Bathing removes lipoprotein complexes that hold water in the stratum corneum and increase water loss. Decreasing bathing to every other day can help prevent the removal of lipoprotein complexes. Soap and bubble bath should be used sparingly while bathing the child.
CN: Physiological integrity; CNS: Basic care and comfort;
CL: Apply; DIFFICULTY: Easy

80. 4. Keeping fingernails cut short will prevent breaks in the skin when a child scratches. Cutting fingernails too short or cutting the skin around the nail can increase the risk of infection. Atopic dermatitis can be found in various areas of the skin but isn't spread from one area to another. Keeping fingernails short is a good way to reduce corneal abrasions but doesn't apply to atopic dermatitis
CN: Physiological integrity; CNS: Physiological adaptation;
CL: Apply; DIFFICULTY: Easy

81. 4. Although the child should eat a balanced diet with foods from all food groups, the diet should emphasize foods that supply complete protein, such as lean meats and low-fat milk. Protein helps build and repair body tissue, which promotes healing. Legumes provide incomplete protein. Cheese contains complete protein but also fat, which should be limited to 30% or less of caloric intake. Whole grain products supply incomplete proteins and carbohydrates. Fruits and vegetables provide mainly carbohydrates.
CN: Physiological integrity; CNS: Basic care and comfort;
CL: Apply; DIFFICULTY: Moderate

82. 4. HPV is responsible for various forms of warts. Coxsackievirus is associated with hand-foot-and-mouth disease. HHV is associated with varicella and herpes zoster. HIV infections aren't associated with epithelial tumors known as warts.
CN: Physiological integrity; CNS: Physiological adaptation;
CL: Understand; DIFFICULTY: Moderate

83. A nurse is explaining treatment to the parents of a child with hypertrophic scarring. Which method would be the **best** for controlling this condition?

1. Compression garments
2. Moisturizing creams
3. Physiotherapy
4. Splints

84. A 6-year-old child has had a recent diagnosis of Lyme disease. Which medication would the nurse expect the health care provider to order if the child has an allergy to penicillin?

1. Amoxicillin
2. Cefuroxime
3. Doxycycline
4. Clindamycin

85. A neonate is examined and noted to have bruising on the scalp, along with diffuse swelling of the soft tissue that crosses over the suture line. How would the nurse document this finding?

1. Caput succedaneum
2. Cephalohematoma
3. Craniotabes
4. Hydrocephalus

86. An adolescent reports feet that itch, sweat a lot, and have a foul odor. The nurse suspects which condition?

1. Candidiasis
2. Tinea corporis
3. Tinea pedis
4. Molluscum contagiosum

87. A child has a healed wound from a traumatic injury. A keloid has formed over the wound. Which finding **best** supports the wound description? Select all that apply.

1. Pink, thickened and smooth
2. Linear depressions of the skin
3. Rubbery in nature
4. Depressed vesicular lesion
5. Evulsion with eschar

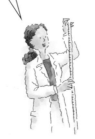

They say beauty is only skin deep. In that case, this chapter is gorgeous.

How can I have athlete's foot when I'm not even an athlete? No fair.

83. 1. Compression garments are worn for up to 1 year to control hypertrophic scarring. Moisturizing creams help decrease hyperpigmentation. Physiotherapy and splints help keep joints and limbs supple.
CN: Physiological integrity; CNS: Physiological adaptation; CL: Apply; DIFFICULTY: Challenge

84. 2. In a child less than 8 years of age the treatment would be amoxicillin, unless the child has an allergy to penicillin; in that case, cefuroxime would be used. In a child older than 8 the treatment would be doxycycline, unless the client has a tetracycline allergy; in that case, the health care provider would prescribe amoxicillin or cefuroxime.
CN: Physiological integrity; CNS: Pharmacological therapies; CL: Apply; DIFFICULTY: Difficult

85. 1. Caput succedaneum originates from trauma to the neonate while descending through the birth canal. It's usually a benign injury that spontaneously resolves over time. Cephalohematoma is a collection of blood in the periosteum of the scalp that doesn't cross over the suture line. Craniotabes is the thinning of the bone of the scalp. Hydrocephalus is an increased volume of cerebrospinal fluid (CSF) or the obstruction of the flow of the CSF and isn't related to soft-tissue swelling.
CN: Physiological integrity; CNS: Physiological adaptation; CL: Analysis; DIFFICULTY: Challenge

86. 3. Tinea pedis is a superficial fungal infection on the feet, commonly called *athlete's foot*. Candidiasis is a fungal infection of the skin or mucous membranes commonly found in the oral, vaginal, and intestinal mucosal tissue. Tinea corporis, or ringworm, is a flat, scaling, papular lesion with raised borders. Molluscum contagiosum is a viral skin infection with lesions that are small, red papules.
CN: Physiological integrity; CNS: Physiological adaptation; CL: Analysis; DIFFICULTY: Easy

87. 1, 3. Keloids are an exaggerated connective tissue response to skin injury and can be described as pink, thickened, smooth, and rubbery in nature. Striae are linear depressions of the skin. An erosion is a depressed vesicular lesion. Evulsion with eschar formation is characteristic of a stage IV pressure ulcer.
CN: Physiological integrity; CNS: Physiological adaptation; CL: Apply; DIFFICULTY: Moderate

88. An infant's parent gives a history of poor feeding for a few days. The nurse observes white plaques in the infant's mouth with an erythematous base. The plaques stick to the mucous membranes tightly and bleed when scraped. The nurse would suspect which condition?
1. Chickenpox
2. Herpes lesions
3. Measles
4. Oral candidiasis

89. A child was found unconscious at home and brought to the emergency department by the fire and rescue unit. While collecting data, the nurse observes cherry-red mucous membranes, nail beds, and skin. Which cause is the **most** likely explanation for the child's condition?
1. Aspirin ingestion
2. Carbon monoxide poisoning
3. Hydrocarbon ingestion
4. Spider bite

90. The nurse observes a ring-shaped rash that has a red raised border and a clearer center on the upper arm. The client asks the nurse what kind of rash it is. What is the **best** response by the nurse?
1. Tinea capitis
2. Tinea corporis
3. Tinea cruris
4. Tinea pedis

91. A teenager asks advice about getting a tattoo. Which statements made by the nurse about tattoos are correct? Select all that apply.
1. Human immunodeficiency virus (HIV) is a possible risk factor.
2. Hepatitis C is a possible risk factor.
3. Tattoos are not easily removed with laser surgery.
4. Allergic response to pigments is a possible risk factor.
5. Hepatitis A is a possible risk factor.

92. The nurse is observing a 6-year-old child with a spiny projection from the skin suspended from a narrow stalk on the forehead. Which condition would the nurse suspect?
1. Filiform wart
2. Flat wart
3. Plantar wart
4. Venereal warts

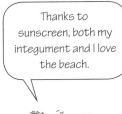
Thanks to sunscreen, both my integument and I love the beach.
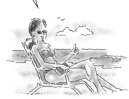

88. 4. Oral candidiasis, or *thrush,* is a painful inflammation that can affect the tongue, soft and hard palates, and buccal mucosa. Chickenpox, or *varicella,* causes open ulcerations of the mucous membranes. Herpes lesions are usually vesicular ulcerations of the oral mucosa around the lips. Measles that form Koplik spots can be identified as pinpoint, white, elevated lesions.
CN: Physiological integrity; CNS: Physiological adaptation; CL: Apply; DIFFICULTY: Easy

89. 2. Cherry-red skin changes are seen when a child has been exposed to high levels of carbon monoxide. Nausea and vomiting and pale skin are symptoms of aspirin ingestion. A hydrocarbon or petroleum ingestion usually results in respiratory symptoms and tachycardia. Spider-bite reactions are usually localized to the area of the bite.
CN: Physiological integrity; CNS: Physiological adaptation; CL: Apply; DIFFICULTY: Easy

90. 2. Tinea corporis describes fungal infections of the body. Tinea capitis describes fungal infections of the scalp. Tinea cruris is used to describe fungal infections of the inner thigh and inguinal creases. Tinea pedis is the term for fungal infections of the foot.
CN: Physiological integrity; CNS: Physiological adaptation; CL: Apply; DIFFICULTY: Moderate

91. 1, 2, 3, 4. Because of the moderate amount of bleeding with a tattoo, both hepatitis C and HIV are potential risks if proper techniques aren't followed. Allergic reactions have been seen when establishments don't use pigments approved by the U.S. Food and Drug Administration for tattoo coloring. The removal of tattoos isn't easily done, and most people are left with a significant scar. The cost is expensive and not covered by insurance. Hepatitis A is not a possible risk factor of tattoos.
CN: Health promotion and maintenance; CNS: None; CL: Remember; DIFFICULTY: Difficult

92. 1. Filiform warts are long, spiny projections from the skin surface. Flat warts are flat-topped, smooth-surfaced lesions. Plantar warts are rough papules, commonly found on the soles of the feet. Venereal warts appear on the genital mucosa and are confluent papules with rough surfaces.
CN: Physiological integrity; CNS: Physiological adaptation; CL: Apply; DIFFICULTY: Moderate

93. A 15-kg toddler is started on amoxicillin and clavulanate therapy, 200 mg/5 mL, for cellulitis. The dose is 40 mg/kg over 24 hours given three times daily. How many milliliters per dose will the nurse administer? Record your answer using a whole number.

_____ mL

94. A 4-year-old child has a tick embedded in the scalp. Which method should the nurse use to remove the tick?
1. Burn the tick at the skin surface.
2. Surgically remove the tick.
3. Grasp the tick with tweezers and apply slow, outward pressure.
4. Grasp the tick with tweezers and quickly pull the tick out.

95. An infant with hives is prescribed diphenhydramine 5 mg/kg over 24 hours in divided doses every 6 hours. The child weighs 8 kg. How many milligrams should be given with each dose? Record you answer using a whole number.

_____ mg

96. An 8-year-old child arrives at the emergency department with chemical burns to both legs. Which nursing action should the nurse perform **first**?
1. Dilute the burns.
2. Apply sterile dressings.
3. Apply topical antibiotics.
4. Debride and graft the burns

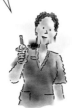

The key to question #96 is the word first.

93. 5.
The dose is first calculated by multiplying the weight and the milligrams and then dividing into three even doses.

$$weight \times mg = X\,mg$$

$$15\,kg \times 40\,mg = 600\,mg$$

$$\frac{total\,mg}{number\,of\,does} = X\,mg\,per\,dose$$

The milligrams are then used to determine the milliliters based on the concentration of the medicine.

$$\frac{600\,mg}{3} = 200\,mg\,per\,dose$$

The concentration is 200 mg in every 5 mL.
CN: Physiological integrity; CNS: Pharmacological therapies; CL: Apply; DIFFICULTY: Difficult

94. 3. Applying gentle outward pressure prevents injuring the skin and leaving parts of the tick in the skin. Surgical removal is indicated if portions of the tick remain in the skin. Burning the tick and quickly pulling the tick out may injure the skin and should be avoided.
CN: Physiological integrity; CNS: Physiological adaptation; CL: Apply; DIFFICULTY: Easy

95. 10.
Multiplying 5 mg by the weight (8 kg) gives the amount of milligrams for 24 hours.

$$5\,mg \times 8\,kg = 40\,mg$$

Divide this by the number of doses per day (4), giving milligrams/dose.

$$\frac{40\,mg}{4\,doses} = 10\,mg/dose$$

CN: Physiological integrity; CNS: Pharmacological therapies; CL: Apply; DIFFICULTY: Difficult

96. 1. Diluting the chemical is the first treatment. It will help remove the chemical and stop the burning process. The remaining treatments are initiated after dilution.
CN: Physiological integrity; CNS: Physiological adaptation; CL: Analysis; DIFFICULTY: Moderate

97. A 14-year-old diagnosed with acne vulgaris asks what causes it. Which factors should the nurse identify for this client? Select all that apply.
1. Chocolates and sweets
2. Increased hormone levels
3. Growth of anaerobic bacteria
4. Caffeine
5. Heredity
6. Fatty foods

97. 2, 3, 5. Acne vulgaris is characterized by the appearance of comedones (blackheads and white-heads). Comedones develop for various reasons, including increased hormone levels, heredity, irritation or application of irritating substances (such as cosmetics), and growth of anaerobic bacteria. A direct relationship between acne vulgaris and consumption of chocolates, caffeine, or fatty foods hasn't been established.
CN: Physiological integrity; CNS: Physiological adaptation; CL: Apply; DIFFICULTY: Difficult

98. A 7-year-old child is admitted to the hospital for treatment of facial cellulitis. Which interventions would help this child cope with the insertion of a peripheral IV line? Select all that apply.
1. Explain the procedure to the child immediately before the procedure.
2. Apply a topical anesthetic to the IV site before the procedure.
3. Ask the child which hand he uses for drawing.
4. Explain the procedure to the child using abstract terms.
5. Avoid letting the child see the equipment to be used in the procedure.
6. Tell the child that the procedure won't hurt.

98. 2, 3. Topical anesthetics reduce the pain of a venipuncture. The cream should be applied about 1 hour before the procedure and requires a health care provider's order. Asking which hand the child draws with helps to identify the dominant hand. The IV should be inserted into the opposite extremity so that the child can continue to play and to do homework with a minimum amount of disruption. Younger school-age children don't have the capability for abstract thinking. The procedure should be explained using simple words. Definitions of unfamiliar terms should be provided. The child should have the procedure explained to him well before it takes place so that he has time to ask questions. Although the topical anesthetic will relieve some pain, there's usually some discomfort involved in venipuncture, so the child shouldn't be told otherwise.
CN: Psychosocial integrity; CNS: None; CL: Apply; DIFFICULTY: Challenge

99. A child has been admitted with a papular rash. Which illustration depicts this type of rash?

1.
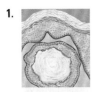

2.
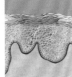

3.
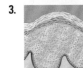

4.
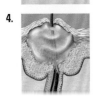

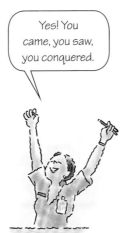
Yes! You came, you saw, you conquered.

99. 3. A papular rash manifests with solid, raised lesions that are usually less than 1 cm in diameter. Option 2 depicts a small, discolored spot or patch on the skin called a macule. Option 4 depicts a pustule, which is a small, pus-filled lesion (a follicular pustule if it contains a hair). Option 1 depicts a cyst, which is a closed sac in or under the skin that contains fluid or semi-solid material.
CN: Physiological integrity; CNS: Physiological adaptation; CL: Apply; DIFFICULTY: Moderate

Chapter 35

Concepts of Management & Supervision

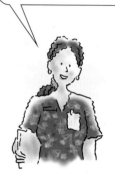

Knowing key concepts of management and supervision is just as important as your clinical knowledge for a successful nursing career. Test your knowledge of these concepts with the following questions.

Management refresher

Nurse-manager role

- Assumes 24–hour accountability for the nursing care delivered in a specific nursing area

Management styles

- Autocratic: decisions made with little or no staff input; manager doesn't delegate responsibility; staff dependence is fostered; the autocratic leader excels in times of crisis
- Laissez-faire: little direction, structure, or support provided by manager; manager abdicates responsibility and decision making when possible; staff development isn't facilitated; there's little interest in achieving the goals necessary for adequate client care
- Democratic: staff members are encouraged to participate in decision making when possible; most decisions are made by the group; staff development is encouraged; responsibilities are carefully delegated and feedback is given to staff members to encourage professional growth
- Participative: problems are identified by the manager and presented to the staff with possible solutions; staff members are encouraged to provide input but the manager makes the decision; negotiation is the key; manager encourages staff advancement

Delegation

- Involves entrusting a task to another staff member
- Helps free the nurse of tasks that can be completed successfully by someone else
- Prepares staff member for career advancement

Discharge planning and client teaching

- Should be initiated on admission
- For clients with planned admissions, teaching should begin before hospitalization
- Should take into account cultural and developmental needs

Clinical pathways

- Multidisciplinary guidelines for client care
- Documentation tool for nurses and other health care providers
- Provides sequences of multidisciplinary interventions that incorporate education, consultation, discharge planning, medications, nutrition, diagnostic testing, activities, treatments, and therapeutic modalities

Quality management

- System used to continually assess and evaluate the effectiveness of client care

Disaster management plan

- Must be able to be implemented quickly
- Must include measures to control resources, establish and maintain communication within the facility and with neighboring responders, protect as many lives as possible, protect property, provide resources for the community, help the facility and staff recover after the disaster

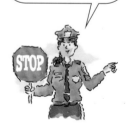

I think you might be on the wrong clinical pathway.

Concepts of management & supervision questions, answers, and rationales

1. The nursing instructor informs the student nurse about proper procedures for administering medications. Which statement made by the student demonstrates that education provided by the instructor was understood? Select all that apply.
 ✓ 1. "I will be sure to check for the right dose of medication."
 2. "I need to be sure that it is the right health care provider who prescribed it."
 ✓ 3. "I will ask the client the name and date of birth while checking the name bracelet."
 ✓ 4. "I will check to ensure that the medication is the right one."
 5. "I need to be sure I am giving the medication for the right reason."

2. The nurse is caring for a client diagnosed with left-sided cerebrovascular accident (CVA), with expressive aphasia and right-sided weakness. When administering care for this client, which intervention should the nurse delegate to unlicensed assistive personnel (UAP)?
 1. Accompany the client to speech therapy.
 2. Perform active range-of-motion (ROM) exercises for the client's upper extremities.
 3. Begin educating the client on simple sign language phrases.
 ✓ 4. Turn and position the client every 2 hours.

3. A nurse finds a suicidal client trying to hang with a belt. In order to preserve self-esteem and safety, what action should the nurse take?
 1. Place the client in seclusion with checks every 30 minutes.
 • 2. Assign a nursing staff member to remain with the client at all times.
 3. Make the client stay with the group at all times.
 4. Refuse to let the client in his room.

4. While discussing a client's care with unlicensed assistive personnel (UAP), the nurse detects an odor of alcohol on the breath. Which action should the nurse take?
 1. Monitor the UAP closely to determine whether performance is impaired.
 2. Tell the UAP to leave the unit immediately.
 3. Report observations to the nurse manager.
 4. Warn the UAP about losing certification.

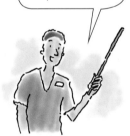

Which of these interventions is most appropriate for a nursing assistant to perform?

1. 1, 3, 4. Before administering medication, the nurse should make sure it is the right client by checking the identification band, checking the health care provider's order for dosage and frequency, checking that the medication is ordered for the right route, and making sure the medication is administered at the right time. The right reason, right health care provider, and right quantity aren't part of the medication administration process.
CN: Physiological integrity; CNS: Pharmacological therapies; CL: Apply; DIFFICULTY: Challenge

2. 4. Unlicensed assistive personnel (UAP) are taught proper positioning skills, although this activity should still be supervised. It isn't necessary to accompany the client to speech therapy and would take the UAP off the unit, reducing available help. Not all UAP are taught to perform active ROM exercises. It wouldn't be necessary to teach the client sign language, as the speech therapist will be working with the client to help learn to speak again, if it is possible.
CN: Safe, effective care environment; CNS: Coordinated care; CL: Analyze; DIFFICULTY: Easy

3. 2. Implementing a one-on-one staff-to-client ratio is the nurse's highest priority. This allows the client to maintain his self-esteem and keeps him safe. Seclusion may damage the client's self-esteem. Forcing the client to stay with the group or refusing to let him in his room doesn't guarantee safety.
CN: Safe, effective care environment; CNS: Coordinated care; CL: Apply; DIFFICULTY: Easy

4. 3. The nurse is obligated to report suspected substance abuse. Allowing the UAP to continue to work could jeopardize client care. It isn't the practical nurse's role to decide that the UAP must leave the unit immediately. Warning the UAP that she could lose her certification doesn't address the issue sufficiently.
CN: Safe, effective care environment; CNS: Coordinated care; CL: Apply; DIFFICULTY: Easy

5. New evacuation procedures are being developed for the unit by a task committee at the long-term care facility, but have not been approved. A bomb threat has occurred in the facility. Which action is appropriate by the nurse?

1. Tell staff members to use whatever procedures they feel are best.
2. Ask staff members to quickly meet among themselves and decide what procedures to follow.
3. Tell staff members to assemble in the staff lounge to quickly offer their opinions about what to do.
4. Determine that the procedures currently in place must be followed.

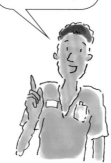

Now here's a situation I know you can manage.

6. The unlicensed assistive personnel (UAP) reports to the nurse that a client became short of breath while being bathed, but is breathing better now. Which action should the nurse take **first**?

1. Instruct UAP to observe the client for further shortness of breath.
2. Check the client and gather subjective and objective data related to shortness of breath.
3. Call the health care provider about the client's episode of shortness of breath.
4. Instruct UAP to complete the bath after the client rests.

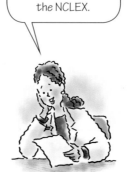

I wish I could delegate taking the NCLEX.

7. A nurse manager can appropriately delegate which task?

1. Scheduling staff assignments for the next month
2. Terminating unlicensed assistive personnel (UAP) for insubordination
3. Deciding on salary increases for licensed practical nurses after they complete orientation
4. Telling a staff nurse to initiate disciplinary action against one of her peers

8. The nurse is concerned about another nurse's relationship with the members of a family and their ill preschooler. Which behavior should be brought to the attention of the nurse-manager?

1. The nurse attempts to influence the family's decisions by presenting their own thoughts and opinions.
2. The nurse keeps communication channels open among the family, physician, and other health care providers.
3. The nurse works with the family members to find ways to decrease their dependence on health care providers.
4. The nurse has developed education skills to instruct the family members so they can accomplish tasks independently.

5. 4. In an emergency situation, the nurse manager must determine the best course of action for the safety and welfare of clients and staff. In this particular situation, there's no time for hesitation. Allowing staff members to do whatever they think best will cause confusion and inefficient client evacuation, because following different procedures won't allow them to function effectively as a team during this crisis. A meeting among the staff members and the nurse-manager wastes valuable time during a life-or-death crisis.
CN: Safe, effective care environment; CNS: Coordinated care; CL: Analyze; DIFFICULTY: Easy

6. 2. The nurse must assess the client to determine what caused the episode and obtain a pulse oximetry reading, if indicated. Instructing the UAP to observe the client for further shortness of breath would be appropriate after the nurse has checked the client. It wouldn't be necessary at this time to call the health care provider about the client's episode of shortness of breath since the client's breathing has improved, but the health care provider should be informed in a timely manner, and this should be documented. After checking the client, the nurse may ask the UAP to complete the bath after allowing the client to rest.
CN: Safe, effective care environment; CNS: Coordinated care; CL: Apply; DIFFICULTY: Easy

7. 1. Scheduling tasks may be safely and appropriately delegated. Termination, disciplinary action, and salary increases shouldn't be delegated to staff that don't have the authority to make such decisions.
CN: Safe, effective care environment; CNS: Coordinated care; CL: Understand; DIFFICULTY: Easy

8. 1. When a nurse attempts to influence a family's decision with their own opinions and values, the situation becomes one of inappropriate intrusion and a nontherapeutic relationship develops. When a nurse keeps communication channels open, works with family members to decrease their dependence on health care providers, and instructs family members so they can accomplish tasks independently, an appropriate therapeutic relationship has been developed.
CN: Safe, effective care environment; CNS: Coordinated care; CL: Analyze; DIFFICULTY: Difficult

CN: Client needs category   CNS: Client needs subcategory   CL: Cognitive level

9. A nurse manager is appropriately using an autocratic method of leading the team. Which situation does the staff nurse determine demonstrates this form of leadership?
1. Directing staff activities if a client has a cardiac arrest
2. Planning vacation time for staff
3. Evaluating a new medication administration process
4. Identifying the strengths and weaknesses of a client education video

10. A client is admitted for pneumonia secondary to human immunodeficiency virus (HIV). The nurse asks unlicensed assistive personnel (UAP) to give the client a bed bath. The UAP is hesitant to bathe the client for fear that they will contract the virus. Which statements would be **most** appropriate for the nurse to include in the response? Select all that apply.
1. "As a nursing assistant, you should already know that there's little chance you will acquire HIV from bathing anyone."
2. "I know you're frightened, but by taking proper precautions, there's little to no risk of acquiring HIV."
3. "I'm in charge, and you need to follow through on this assignment."
4. "The use of personal protective equipment (PPE) may prevent the unintentional transmission of diseases in situations where you may come in contact with blood, body fluids, or secretions."
5. "If you don't bathe the child as I requested, I'll have to write up an incident report."

11. An unlicensed assistive personnel (UAP) frequently disappears from the floor without telling anyone and when returning to the floor, their clothing smells strongly of smoke. What steps should the nurse take to eliminate this behavior? Using the options below, place the steps in chronologic order.

| 1. Approach the UAP privately to discuss the issue |
| 2. Report the UAP to the charge nurse if the behavior remains unchanged. |
| 3. Keep notes with dates and times this behavior is observed. |
| 4. Try to work with the UAP to schedule daily breaks. |
| 5. Observe the UAP's behavior for signs of improvement. |

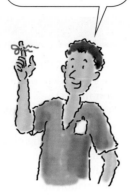

Remember— Reserve the autocratic leadership approach for critical decisions that must be made rapidly.

Congratulations! You managed this test amazingly well.

9. **1.** In a crisis situation, the nurse-manager should take command for the benefit of the client. Planning vacation time and evaluating procedures and client resources require staff input characteristic of a democratic or participative manager.
CN: Safe, effective care environment; CNS: Coordinated care; CL: Apply; DIFFICULTY: Moderate

10. **2, 4.** Recognizing that the UAP is frightened and then clarifying information about the use of personal protective equipment provides him with guidance and education to alleviate his fears. Telling the UAP that he should already know there's little chance of acquiring HIV by bathing someone is demeaning and doesn't encourage the UAP to take appropriate precautions. Statements such as "I'm in charge" or "I'll have to write up an incident report" are threatening and don't address the UAP's fears.
CN: Safe, effective care environment; CNS: Coordinated care; CL: Analyze; DIFFICULTY: Challenge

11.

| 3. Keep notes with dates and times this behavior is observed. |
| 1. Approach the UAP privately to discuss the issue. |
| 4. Try to work with the UAP to schedule daily breaks. |
| 5. Observe the UAP's behavior for signs of improvement. |
| 2. Report the UAP to the charge nurse if the behavior remains unchanged. |

Keeping notes listing dates and times that the inappropriate behavior is observed will be helpful to verify facts. Then approach the UAP privately and confidentially to discuss the issue. Work to schedule defined break times. The UAP should contact the nurse before leaving the unit. Observe the UAP behavior for signs of improvement, and bring the issue to the attention of the charge nurse for further action if the behavior continues.
CN: Safe, effective care environment; CNS: Coordinated care; CL: Analyze; DIFFICULTY: Moderate

CN: Client needs category   CNS: Client needs subcategory   CL: Cognitive level

Chapter 36

Ethical & Legal Issues

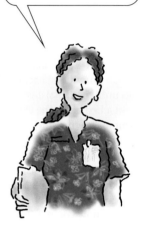

Ethical and legal issues are a daily challenge in nursing practice. Ace them on the NCLEX, and you'll be able to face each challenge with confidence! Let's go!

Ethical and legal refresher

Nurse practice acts

- State laws that are instrumental in defining the scope of nursing practice in order to protect the public
- Most important law affecting your nursing practice
- One for each state
- Designed to protect nurse and public by defining legal scope of practice and excluding untrained or unlicensed individuals from practicing nursing
- Outline conditions and requirements for licensure, such as passing NCLEX-PN examination
- All states require completion of a board of nursing-approved education program; your state may have additional requirements, including:
  - good moral character
  - good physical and mental health
  - minimum age
  - fluency in English
  - absence of drug or alcohol addiction.

Informed consent

- Agreement to do something or to allow something to happen only after all the relevant facts are disclosed
- The client's right to be adequately informed about a proposed treatment or procedure
- Responsibility for obtaining informed consent rests with the person who will perform the treatment or procedure (usually the health care provider)
- The client should be told that he has a right to refuse the treatment or procedure without having other care or support withdrawn, and that he can withdraw consent after giving it

Elements

- Description of the treatment or procedure
- Description of inherent risks and benefits that occur with frequency or regularity

(or specific consequences significant to the given client or his designated decision-maker)
- Explanation of the potential for death or serious harm (such as brain damage, stroke, paralysis, or disfiguring scars) or for discomforting adverse effects during or after the treatment or procedure
- Explanation and description of alternative treatments or procedures
- Name and qualifications of the person who will perform the treatment or procedure
- Discussion of possible consequences of not undergoing the treatment or procedure

Witnessing informed consent

- The client voluntarily consented
- The client's signature is authentic
- The client appears to be competent to give consent

Right to refuse treatment

- Any mentally competent adult may legally refuse treatment if he's fully informed about his medical condition and about the likely consequences of his refusal
- Some clients may refuse treatment on the grounds of freedom of religion

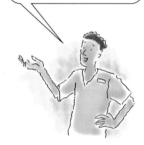

Consent must be informed and voluntary, and the client must be competent.

Advance directives

- Living will: an advance care document that specifies a client's wishes about medical care if he's unable to make the decision for himself (in some states, living wills don't address the issue of discontinuing artificial nutrition and hydration)
- Durable power of attorney for health care: a document in which the client designates a person to make medical decisions for him if he becomes incompetent (differs from the usual power of attorney, which requires the client's ongoing consent and deals only with financial issues)

Grounds for challenging a client's right to refuse treatment
- Client is incompetent
- Compelling reasons exist to overrule client's wishes

Living wills
- Living will laws generally include such provisions as:
  - who may execute a living will
  - witness and testator requirements
  - immunity from liability for following a living will's directives
  - documentation requirements
  - instructions on when and how the living will should be executed
  - under what circumstances the living will takes effect

Right to privacy
- Client has right of privacy regarding his health information
- Privacy law allows disclosure of personal health information when needed for client care

Medication administration
- One of the most important and, legally, one of the riskiest tasks a nurse performs

Five rights
1. Right drug
2. Right client
3. Right time
4. Right dosage
5. Right route

Negligence
- Failure to exercise the degree of care that a person of ordinary prudence would exercise under the same circumstances

Four criteria for negligence claim
- a person owed a duty to the person making the claim
- the duty was breached
- the breach resulted in injury to the person making the claim
- damages were a direct result of the negligence of the health care provider

Malpractice
- Specific type of negligence: a violation of professional duty or a failure to meet a standard of care or use the skills and knowledge of other professionals in similar circumstances

Documentation errors
- Complete, accurate, and timely documentation is crucial to the continuity of each client's care

Functions of well-documented record
- Reflects client care given
- Demonstrates results of treatment
- Helps plan and coordinate care contributed by each professional
- Allows interdisciplinary exchange of information about client
- Provides evidence of nurse's legal responsibilities toward client
- Demonstrates standards, rules, regulations, and laws of nursing practice
- Supplies information for analysis of cost-to-benefit reduction
- Reflects professional and ethical conduct and responsibility
- Furnishes information for continuing education, risk management, diagnosis-related group assignment and reimbursement, continuous quality improvement, case management monitoring, and research

Common documentation errors
- Omissions
- Personal opinions
- Vague entries
- Late entries
- Improper corrections
- Unauthorized entries
- Erroneous or vague abbreviations
- Illegible writing and lack of clarity

Abuse
- The nurse plays a crucial role in recognizing and reporting incidents of suspected abuse
- If the nurse detects evidence of apparent abuse, must pass the information along to appropriate authorities
- In many states, failure to report actual or suspected abuse constitutes a crime

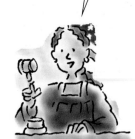

It would be malpractice to stop reading now.

Ethical & legal issues questions, answers, and rationales

1. A client with altered mental status fell out of bed while hospitalized and now the family wants to sue the facility. Which elements must be proven by the family's attorney in this case to result in a guilty verdict of professional negligence?
1. Duty, breach of duty, damages, and causation
2. Duty, damages, and causation
3. Duty, breach of duty, and damages
4. Breach of duty, damages, and causation

1. 1. Any professional negligence action must meet certain demands in order to be considered negligence and result in legal action. They're commonly known as the four D's: duty of the health care professional to provide care to the person making the claim; a dereliction (breach) of that duty; damages resulting from that breach of duty; and evidence that damages were directly due to negligence (causation).
CN: Safe, effective care environment; CNS: Coordinated care; CL: Understand; DIFFICULTY: Moderate

2. An older adult client has been admitted to the medical-surgical unit after surgery. While the nurse is off the floor, the client falls out of bed, resulting in a fracture of the right leg. The nurse finding the client states that the "side rails were left down and the bed was in the high position." Which charge is **most** appropriate for the nurse's actions?
1. Collective liability
2. Comparative negligence
3. Battery
4. Negligence

2. 4. Negligence is a general term that denotes conduct lacking in due care and is commonly interpreted as a deviation from the standard of care that a reasonable person would use in a particular set of circumstances. Collective liability stems from cooperation by several manufacturers in a wrongful activity that by its nature requires group participation. Comparative negligence is a defense that holds injured parties accountable for their fault in the injury. Battery involves harmful or unwarranted contact with the client.
CN: Safe, effective care environment; CNS: Safety and infection control; CL: Analyze; DIFFICULTY: Easy

3. The client refused an injection but the nurse administered it anyway. The client wants to sue the nurse. The attorney informs the client that this lawsuit must be filed within 2 years. What is this time frame called?
1. Discovery rule.
2. Statute of limitation.
3. Grace period.
4. Alternative dispute resolution.

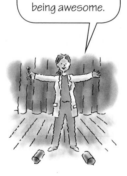

There's no statute of limitation on being awesome.

3. 2. Statute of limitation is the time interval during which a case must be filed; after this time, the injured party is barred from bringing the lawsuit. The statute of limitation typically gives clients 2 years from the time of discovery to file a lawsuit; however, this may vary from state to state. Statutes of limitation are set by state legislatures. Discovery rule is the term for the time the client discovers the injury. A grace period refers to any period specified in a contract during which payment is permitted without penalty, beyond the due date of the debt. Alternative dispute resolution refers to any means of settling disputes outside the courtroom setting.
CN: Safe, effective care environment; CNS: Safety and infection control; CL: Remember; DIFFICULTY: Moderate

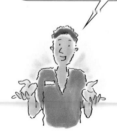

Don't let question #4 make you feel incompetent. There are many compelling reasons for you to succeed.

4. A client who is bleeding internally needs emergency surgery to stop the bleeding, but refuses treatment. Which of the following are grounds for challenging a client's right to refuse treatment? Select all that apply.
1. Client is incompetent.
2. The nurse disagrees with the client's decision.
3. Compelling reasons exist to overrule the client's wishes.
4. The treatment would be more cost efficient.
5. The health care provider does not want to be sued.

4. 1, 3. In order to challenge a client's right to refuse treatment either the client must be incompetent or there must be compelling reasons to overrule the client's wishes. Even if the nurse disagrees with the client's decision or the treatment might be more cost efficient the wishes of the client must be respected. The fact that the health care provider does not want to be sued should never interfere with care.
CN: Safe, effective care environment; CNS: Safety and infection control; CL: Apply; DIFFICULTY: Moderate

5. Nurses follow certain guidelines while caring for clients. Which of the following does the new nurse graduate correctly identify as defining the scope of nursing practice in order to protect the public?
1. Nursing process
2. Facilities' policies and procedures
3. Standards of Care
4. Nurse Practice Act

5. 4. The Nurse Practice Act is a series of statutes enacted by each state to outline the legal scope of nursing practice within that state. State boards of nursing oversee this statutory law. Nurse practice acts set educational requirements for the nurse, distinguish between nursing practice and medical practice, and define the scope of nursing practice. Nursing process is an organizational framework for nursing practice, encompassing all major steps a nurse takes when caring for a client. Facility policies govern the practice in that particular facility. Standards of Care are criteria that serve as a basis for comparison when evaluating the quality of nursing practice. Standards of Care are established by federal, state, professional, and accreditation organizations.
CN: Safe, effective care environment; CNS: Coordinated care; CL: Apply; DIFFICULTY: Easy

6. A client who's a member of the Jehovah's Witnesses refuses a blood transfusion based on religious beliefs and practices. Which ethical principle is the nurse following when honoring this client's wishes?
1. The right to die
2. Advance directive
3. The right to refuse treatment
4. Substituted judgment

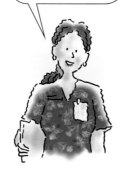

Never force a competent client to receive a treatment he or she doesn't want.

6. 3. The right to refuse treatment is grounded in the ethical principle of respect for autonomy of the individual. The client has the right to refuse treatment as long as he's competent and is made aware of the risks and complications associated with refusal of treatment. The right to die involves whether to initiate or withhold life-sustaining treatment for a client who is irreversibly comatose, vegetative, or suffering with end-stage terminal illness. Substituted judgment is an ethical principle used when the decision is made for an incapacitated client based on what's best for the client. An advance directive is a document used as a guideline for starting or continuing life-sustaining medical care of a client with a terminal disease or disability who can no longer indicate his own wishes.
CN: Safe, effective care environment; CNS: Coordinated care; CL: Apply; DIFFICULTY: Easy

7. A newly graduated nurse is working with the team that sets up organ donation. What is the **most** important concept this nurse must understand about organ or tissue donation before working with families?
1. It's done with a health care provider's approval and written order.
2. The individual requesting doesn't have to believe in the benefits of organ donation or support the process with a positive attitude.
3. The individual requesting is knowledgeable about the basics of organ and tissue donation and can educate the family members about brain death early in the organ donation process.
4. The family is offered an opportunity to speak with an organ procurement coordinator.

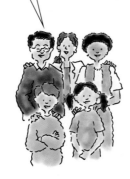

A big part of nursing is knowing when and to whom to refer a family for specialty assistance.

7. 4. The family should be offered an opportunity to speak with an organ procurement coordinator. An organ procurement coordinator is very knowledgeable about the organ donation process and dealing with grieving family members. Health care provider support in the process is desirable, but consent or written orders aren't necessary for a referral to the organ procurement organization. The individual requesting has to believe in the benefits of organ donation and support the process. Approaching the family should only occur when the family members are made aware of the client's condition and prognosis. Approaching a family member when he believes that there's still hope for recovery will only result in a negative outcome.
CN: Safe, effective care environment; CNS: Coordinated care; CL: Analyze; DIFFICULTY: Challenge

8. A nurse gives a client the wrong medication. After assessment of the client, the nurse completes an incident report. What is the next anticipated step?

1. The incident would be reported to the state board of nursing for disciplinary action.
2. The incident would be documented in the nurse's personnel file.
3. The medication error would result in the nurse being suspended and possibly terminated from employment at the facility.
4. The incident report would be used to promote quality care and risk management.

9. A well documented client record helps to ensure continuity of care. What is another function of the client record? Select all that apply.

1. Reflects client care given
2. Demonstrates results of treatment
3. Supplies information for analysis of cost-to-benefit reduction
4. Allows a secret way for only nurses and health care providers to follow the care
5. Reflects professional and ethical conduct

10. A nurse observes a coworker administering a medication several hours after it had been scheduled. When confronted, the coworker simply makes a dismissive joke and then charts the medication as given at the scheduled time. s What should the witnessing nurse do? Place the actions in ascending chronologic sequence. Use all the options.

1. Request a private meeting to discuss the incident.
2. Encourage the nurse to take responsibility for these actions.
3. Express concern and clearly inform the nurse the behavior is unethical.
4. Report the incident to the nurse-manager if resistance is noted.
5. Approach the coworker in a calm and professional manner.

8. **4.** Unusual occurrences and deviations from care are documented on incident reports. Incident reports are internal to the facility and are used to evaluate the care, determine potential risks, and identify possible system problems that could have contributed to the error. This type of error wouldn't result in suspension of the nurse or a report to the state board of nursing. Some facilities do trend and track the number of errors that take place on particular units (or by individual nurses) for educational purposes and as a way to improve the nursing process.

CN: Safe, effective care environment; CNS: Coordinated care; CL: Analyze; DIFFICULTY: Moderate

9. **1,2,3,5.** A well-documented record performs the following functions: reflects client care given; demonstrates results of treatment; helps plan and coordinate care contributed by each professional; allows interdisciplinary exchange of information about client; provides evidence of nurse's legal responsibilities toward client; demonstrates standards, rules, regulations, and laws of nursing practice; supplies information for analysis of cost-to- benefit reduction; reflects professional and ethical conduct and responsibility; furnishes information for continuing education, risk management, diagnosis-related group assignment and reimbursement, continuous quality improvement, case management monitoring, and research.

A well-documented client record is not secret for only nurses and health care providers as all member of the health care team are allowed to use the client record.

CN: Safe, effective care environment; CNS: Coordinated care; CL: Understand; DIFFICULTY: Difficult

10.

5. Approach the coworker in a calm and professional manner.
1. Request a private meeting to discuss the incident.
3. Express concern and clearly inform the nurse the behavior is unethical.
2. Encourage the nurse to take responsibility for these actions.
4. Report the incident to the nurse-manager if resistance is noted.

The nurse must maintain a calm and professional demeanor and talk with the coworker privately. It's important to discuss ethical concerns and encourage the coworker to take responsibility for these actions. The nurse-manager should be informed of the incident if resistance by the offending nurse is noted.

CN: Safe, effective care environment; CNS: Coordinated care; CL: Analyze; DIFFICULTY: Moderate

11. There are reports that morphine has been missing from the medication cart several times during the last 3 months. The nurse walks into the medication room and witnesses another nurse quickly slipping something into a pocket from the controlled substance drawer. Place the following steps in ascending chronologic sequence. Use all the options.

1.	If directed, fill out a confidential incident report describing what was seen.
2.	Approach the nurse-manager privately and discuss the matter.
3.	Do not share any observations with others on the unit.
4.	Continue to observe this nurse in question for signs of unusual behavior.
5.	Carefully review and document what was observed.

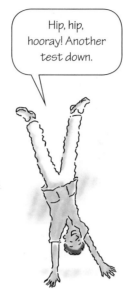

Hip, hip, hooray! Another test down.

11.

5.	Carefully review and document what was observed.
2.	Approach the nurse-manager privately and discuss the matter.
1.	If directed, fill out a confidential incident report describing what was seen.
3.	Do not share any observations with others on the unit.
4.	Continue to observe this nurse in question for signs of unusual behavior.

A premature conclusion shouldn't be drawn based on one suspicious incident. It's best to first review and carefully document in detail what was seen. Then speak with the nurse-manager privately and, if directed, fill out a confidential incident report describing what was observed. At this point, the charge nurse will follow through and investigate the situation further. It's important not to speak to others on the unit to maintain professionalism and to avoid spreading potentially unfounded rumors. The reporting nurse should remain alert for repeated suspicious behavior.

CN: Safe, effective care environment; CNS: Coordinated care; CL: Analyze; DIFFICULTY: Difficult

CN: Client needs category   CNS: Client needs subcategory   CL: Cognitive level

Comprehensive Test 1

This comprehensive test, the first of two, is just like the shortest NCLEX test: 85 questions. It's a great way to practice!

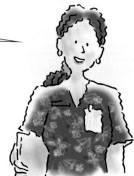

1. A victim of a motor vehicle crash with blunt chest trauma and no obvious signs of bleeding has a heart rate of 132 BPM, a blood pressure of 82/54 mm Hg, and muffled heart sounds. Which condition does the nurse suspect the client is experiencing?
1. Heart failure
2. Pneumothorax
3. Cardiac tamponade
4. Myocardial infarction (MI)

So, signs of shock + muffled heart sounds = what?

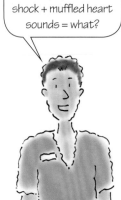

2. A client is experiencing cardiac tamponade after a chest trauma. Which type of shock will the nurse monitor for?
1. Anaphylactic
2. Cardiogenic
3. Hypovolemic
4. Septic

3. The nurse is caring for a client with cardiac tamponade. Which treatment would the nurse anticipate for this client?
1. Insertion of a stent
2. Infusion of dopamine
3. Blood transfusion
4. Pericardiocentesis

1. 3. Cardiac tamponade results in signs of obvious shock and muffled heart sounds. Heart failure results in inspiratory crackles, pulmonary edema, and jugular vein distention. Pneumothorax results in diminished breath sounds in the affected lung, respiratory distress, and tracheal displacement. In an MI, the client may report chest pain. An electrocardiogram could confirm changes consistent with an MI.
CN: Physiological integrity; CNS: Physiological adaptation;
CL: Analyze; DIFFICULTY: Moderate

2. 2. Fluid accumulates in the pericardial sac, hindering motion of the heart muscle and causing it to pump inefficiently, resulting in signs of cardiogenic shock. Anaphylactic and septic shock are types of distributive shock in which fluid is displaced from the capillaries and leaks into surrounding tissues. Hypovolemic shock involves the actual loss of fluid.
CN: Physiological integrity; CNS: Physiological adaptation;
CL: Apply; DIFFICULTY: Moderate

3. 4. Pericardiocentesis, or needle aspiration of the pericardial cavity, is done to relieve tamponade. An opening is created surgically if the client continues to have recurrent episodes of tamponade. Dopamine is used to restore blood pressure in normovolemic individuals. Blood transfusions may be given if the client is hypovolemic from blood loss.
CN: Physiological integrity; CNS: Physiological adaptation;
CL: Apply; DIFFICULTY: Moderate

4. The nurse is caring for a client suspected of having cardiac tamponade. Which diagnostic test will the nurse prepare the client for?
  1. Chest x-ray
  2. Echocardiography
  3. Electrocardiogram (ECG)
  4. Pulmonary artery pressure monitoring

5. A nurse is reinforcing education provided to a client about reducing risk factors for coronary artery disease. Which risk factor does the nurse inform the client is nonmodifiable?
  1. Age
  2. Hypertension
  3. Personality
  4. Smoking

6. A client states, "I am stressed by my job but enjoy the challenge. What is the **best** response by the nurse?
  1. "Switch job positions."
  2. "Take stress management classes."
  3. "Spend more time with your family."
  4. "Don't take your work home."

7. A client diagnosed with angina is being discharged from the hospital with a prescription for nitroglycerin. What should the nurse be sure to include in the discharge information?
  1. If chest pain is experienced, immediately call the rescue squad.
  2. If chest pain is experienced longer than 1 hour, take a nitroglycerin.
  3. Store the nitroglycerin in the bathroom medicine cabinet.
  4. If chest pain is experienced, take 1 tablet under the tongue every 5 minutes ×3.

8. A client with human immunodeficiency virus (HIV) is admitted to the hospital with flulike symptoms, dyspnea, and a cough. The client is placed on a 100% non-rebreather mask and arterial blood gases are drawn. Which results indicate the client needs intubation?
  1. Pa_{O_2}, 90 mm Hg; Pa_{CO_2}, 40 mm Hg
  2. Pa_{O_2}, 85 mm Hg; Pa_{CO_2}, 45 mm Hg
  3. Pa_{O_2}, 80 mm Hg; Pa_{CO_2}, 45 mm Hg
  4. Pa_{O_2}, 70 mm Hg; Pa_{CO_2}, 55 mm Hg

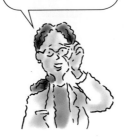

I keep looking for a way to "modify" my aging process but haven't had much luck.

4. 2. Echocardiography measures pericardial effusion and can detect signs of right ventricular and atrial compression. Chest x-rays show a slightly widened mediastinum and enlarged cardiac silhouette. An ECG can rule out other cardiac disorders. Pulmonary artery pressure monitoring shows increased right atrial or central venous pressure and right ventricular diastolic pressure.
CN: Physiological integrity; CNS: Reduction of risk potential; CL: Apply; DIFFICULTY: Challenge

5. 1. Age is a risk factor that can't be changed. Hypertension, type A personality, and smoking factors can be controlled.
CN: Health promotion and maintenance; CNS: None; CL: Understand; DIFFICULTY: Easy

6. 2. Stress management classes will educate the client on how to better manage the stress in his life, after identifying the factors that contribute to the stress. Alternatives may be found to leaving the job, which is enjoyable. Not spending enough time with family and not taking the job home haven't been identified as contributing factors to stress.
CN: Physiological integrity; CNS: Reduction of risk potential; CL: Apply; DIFFICULTY: Moderate

7. 4. It is important to inform the client to take 1 tablet under the tongue every 5 minutes ×3. If the pain is not relieved at this time the client should access the emergency medical system and go to the hospital. The client should not wait 1 hour to take the medication. The medication should not be stored in the bathroom medicine cabinet since the moisture may render the medication inactive. The client should take the nitroglycerin before immediately going to the hospital since the pain may be relieved by rest and nitroglycerin.
CN: Physiological integrity; CNS: Pharmacological therapies; CL: Analyze; DIFFICULTY: Easy

8. 4. A decreasing partial pressure of arterial oxygen (Pa_{O_2}) and an increasing partial pressure of arterial carbon dioxide (Pa_{CO_2}) indicate poor oxygen perfusion. Normal Pa_{O_2} levels are 80 to 100 mm Hg and normal Pa_{CO_2} levels are 35 to 45 mm Hg.
CN: Physiological integrity; CNS: Reduction of risk potential; CL: Analyze; DIFFICULTY: Easy

9. The nurse is discussing transmission of human immunodeficiency virus (HIV) to a group of high school students. Which substance does the nurse inform the students **most** commonly transmits the virus?
1. Blood
2. Feces
3. Saliva
4. Urine

10. A client with human immunodeficiency virus (HIV) has developed an opportunistic infection caused by a protozoa. Which infection does the nurse anticipate this client will be treated for?
1. Tuberculosis (TB)
2. Histoplasmosis
3. Kaposi sarcoma
4. *Pneumocystis jiroveci* infection

11. A client with acquired immunodeficiency syndrome (AIDS) is intubated and at risk for alteration in skin integrity from the endotracheal (ET) tube. Which nursing action would be beneficial in preventing this occurrence?
1. Using lubricant on the lips
2. Providing oral care every 2 hours
3. Suctioning the oral cavity every 2 hours
4. Repositioning the ET tube every 24 hours

12. A client requires the highest possible concentration of oxygen. Which delivery system will the nurse ensure the client receives?
1. Face tent
2. Venturi mask
3. Nasal cannula
4. Mask with reservoir bag

13. A client is refusing all medications and is having difficulty breathing, with a respiratory rate of 34 breaths/minute and anxiety. What is the **priority** nursing action?
1. Notify the health care provider of the status of this client.
2. Withhold the medication until the next scheduled dose.
3. Encourage the client to take medications.
4. Put the medicine in applesauce to give it without the client's knowledge.

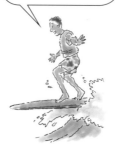

You're off to a great start! Ride that wave of momentum.

9. 1. HIV is most commonly transmitted by contact with infected blood. It exists in all body fluids, but transmission through feces, saliva, and urine is much less likely to occur.
CN: Safe, effective care environment; CNS: Safety and infection control; CL: Understand; DIFFICULTY: Easy

10. 4. *P. jiroveci* infection is caused by protozoa. TB is caused by bacteria. Histoplasmosis is a fungal infection. Kaposi sarcoma is a neoplasm.
CN: Physiological integrity; CNS: Physiological adaptation; CL: Apply; DIFFICULTY: Moderate

11. 4. Pressure causes skin breakdown. Repositioning the ET tube every 24 hours from one side of the mouth to the other (or to the center of the mouth) can relieve pressure. Extreme care must be taken to move the tube only laterally; it must not be pushed in or pulled out. The tape securing the tube must be changed daily. Two nurses should perform this procedure. Lubricant, oral care, and suctioning help keep skin clean and intact and reduce the risk of further infection; however, these actions do not prevent skin breakdown.
CN: Physiological integrity; CNS: Basic care and comfort; CL: Apply; DIFFICULTY: Difficult

12. 4. A mask with a reservoir bag administers 70% to 100% oxygen at flow rates of 8 to 10 L/minute. The nasal cannula maximum rate is 44% at 6 L/minute; the Venturi mask maximum rate is 24% to 55%; and a face tent maximum delivery is 22% to 34%.
CN: Physiological integrity; CNS: Physiological adaptation; CL: Understand; DIFFICULTY: Challenge

13. 1. Notifying the health care provider of the client's condition and refusal to take medications allows the health care provider to decide what alternatives should be instituted. Withholding a medication requires health care provider notification. Even if the client takes some of the medications, the health care provider still needs to be notified. Giving medications in applesauce without the client's knowledge destroys trust between the nurse and client. The reason the client believes the medications are making the condition worse needs to be explored.
CN: Physiological integrity; CNS: Pharmacological therapies; CL: Apply; DIFFICULTY: Easy

14. A nurse caring for a client with acquired immunodeficiency syndrome (AIDS) is working with a nursing student. The nurse notes the student doesn't attempt to suction or assist with care of the client. Which action is appropriate?
1. Talk to the student.
2. Talk to the nurse-manager.
3. Address a coworker with the concerns.
4. Seek advice from the student's instructor.

15. A client's spouse is upset over the client's condition, lack of improvement, and is feeling powerless. Which response by the nurse is **best**?
1. "Yes, you are powerless to do anything about your spouse."
2. "There is nothing that can be done."
3. "I understand what you are going through."
4. "Would you like to help with some comfort measures for your spouse?"

16. A client is admitted to the hospital with a diagnosis of respiratory failure. The client is intubated, placed on 100% FiO_2, and is coughing up copious secretions. Which intervention has **priority**?
1. Getting an x-ray
2. Suctioning the client
3. Restraining the client
4. Obtaining an arterial blood gas (ABG) analysis

17. A client with an endotracheal tube has copious, brown-tinged secretions. Which intervention is a **priority**?
1. Obtain a sputum specimen.
2. Instill saline to break up secretions.
3. Culture the specimen with a Culturette swab.
4. Obtain an order for a liquefying agent for the sputum.

18. A client's x-ray shows that an endotracheal (ET) tube is 0.75 in (2 cm) above the carina, and there are nodular lesions and patchy infiltrates in the upper lobe. Based on this report, the nurse can expect which conclusion?
1. The x-ray is inconclusive.
2. The client has a disease process going on.
3. The ET tube needs to be advanced.
4. The ET tube needs to be pulled back.

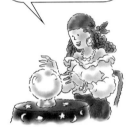

I see a fulfilling career in nursing ahead of you.

14. 1. The nurse should approach the student first to determine the student's feelings and experience in caring for a client with AIDS. The nurse-manager and coworkers aren't familiar with the student's abilities, but the instructor may be approached if the nurse can't communicate with the student.
CN: Safe, effective care environment; CNS: Coordinated care; CL: Analyze; DIFFICULTY: Easy

15. 4. The significant other expresses a need to help the client, and the nurse can encourage the client to do whatever he feels comfortable with, such as putting lubricant on lips, moist cloth on forehead, or lotion on skin. The nurse may not understand the situation, and agreeing with a person doesn't diminish powerlessness. There are many ways the significant other can assist.
CN: Psychosocial integrity; CNS: None; CL: Analyze; DIFFICULTY: Easy

16. 2. Suctioning the client is the priority because secretions can cut off the oxygen supply to the client and result in hypoxia. X-rays are the next priority; check placement of the endotracheal tube. Restraints are warranted only if the client is a threat to safety. After the client has acclimated to his ventilator settings, ABG levels can be drawn.
CN: Physiological integrity; CNS: Reduction of risk potential; CL: Analyze; DIFFICULTY: Easy

17. 1. Suspicious secretions should be obtained and sent for culture and sensitivity testing by using sterile technique. Saline would dilute the specimen. Swab Culturette are useful for wound cultures—not endotracheal cultures. Various liquefying agents are available to help break up secretions; respiratory therapists can usually recommend the right agent, but this isn't a priority.
CN: Safe, effective care environment; CNS: Safety and infection control; CL: Analyze; DIFFICULTY: Moderate

18. 2. The x-ray is conclusive and suggests tuberculosis. At 0.75 in (2 cm) above the carina, the ET tube is at an adequate level in the trachea and doesn't have to be advanced or pulled back.
CN: Physiological integrity; CNS: Reduction of risk potential; CL: Analyze; DIFFICULTY: Difficult

19. A client is admitted into the negative pressure room with suspected tuberculosis (TB). Which procedure does the nurse prepare the client for to affirm the diagnosis?
1. Chest x-ray
2. Tracheostomy
3. Bronchoscopy
4. Arterial blood gas (ABG) analysis

19. 3. Bronchoscopy can help diagnose TB and obtain specimens while clearing the bronchial tree of secretions. X-rays may be repeated periodically to determine lung and endotracheal tube status. Tracheostomy may be done if the client remains on the ventilator for a prolonged period. A change in condition or treatment may require an ABG analysis.

CN: Physiological integrity; CNS: Reduction of risk potential; CL: Apply; DIFFICULTY: Challenge

20. A client comes to the clinic and informs the nurse he may have been exposed to a family member with tuberculosis. The nurse administers the tuberculin skin test and 2 days later the test is positive. What does the nurse determine the results mean?
1. The client has active disease.
2. The client has a recent infection.
3. It will determine the extent of the infection.
4. The client has presence of infection at some point.

20. 4. A tuberculin skin test shows the presence of infection at some point; however, a positive skin test doesn't guarantee that an infection is currently present. Some people have false-positive results. Active disease may be viewed on a chest x-ray. Computed tomography scan or magnetic resonance imaging can evaluate the extent of lung damage.

CN: Safe, effective care environment; CNS: Safety and infection control; CL: Analyze; DIFFICULTY: Challenge

21. A nurse informs a client with tuberculosis that they will be considered infectious up until what time period after treatment is started?
1. 72 hours
2. 1 week
3. 2 weeks
4. 4 weeks

21. 4. After 4 weeks, tuberculosis is no longer infectious, but the client must continue to take the medication.

CN: Safe, effective care environment; CNS: Safety and infection control; CL: Apply; DIFFICULTY: Moderate

22. A client has been diagnosed with tuberculosis (TB). Which pharmacologic therapy does the nurse anticipate administering?
1. Theophylline
2. Penicillin intramuscular (IM)
3. Rifampin, isoniazid, and rifapentine
4. Aerosol treatments with pentamidine

I'm one tough bug. It takes an arsenal of meds to take me down.

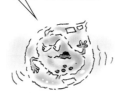

22. 3. Because TB has become resistant to many antibacterial agents, the initial treatment includes the use of multiple antitubercular or antibacterial drugs. The Centers for Disease Control and Prevention (CDC) recommends the use of rifampin, isoniazid, and rifapentine for use in treatment. Theophylline is a bronchodilator used to treat asthma and chronic obstructive pulmonary disease (COPD). Penicillins are used to treat *Staphylococcus aureus* infection—not TB. Pentamidine is used in the treatment of *Pneumocystis jiroveci* pneumonia.

CN: Physiological integrity; CNS: Pharmacological therapies; CL: Apply; DIFFICULTY: Moderate

23. A client with a diagnosis of tuberculosis (TB) is informed he will have to take medication for the treatment of the disease. How long does the nurse inform the client adherence with treatment will be required?
1. 2 to 4 months
2. 9 to 12 months
3. 18 to 24 months
4. More than 2 years

23. 2. Treatment for TB is usually continued for 9 to 12 months. Two to 4 months isn't adequate time for treatment to be successful. More than 2 years or 18 to 24 months are treatment times that are beyond therapeutic value.

CN: Physiological integrity; CNS: Pharmacological therapies; CL: Understand; DIFFICULTY: Moderate

24. A client is diagnosed with tuberculosis (TB). In addition to recommending skin testing of the family members, TB must be reported to which individual or agency?
1. Centers for Disease Control and Prevention (CDC)
2. Local health department
3. Infection-control nurse
4. Client's health care provider

24. **2.** The local health department must be informed of an outbreak of TB because it's a reportable disease. They, in turn, inform the CDC. The infection-control nurse or local health department may request that staff be tested if exposed. Generally, the client's family can inform his health care provider.
CN: Safe, effective care environment; CNS: Safety and infection control; CL: Apply; DIFFICULTY: Challenge

25. A client tells the nurse that tuberculosis medications are so expensive it is difficult to afford them. Which intervention by the nurse is **best**?
1. Refer the client to social services.
2. Tell the client to apply for Medicaid.
3. Refer the client to the local or county health department.
4. Tell the client to follow insurance rules and regulations.

25. **3.** The local and county health departments provide treatment and follow-up free of charge for all residents to ensure proper care. Social services can help seek alternative methods of payment and reimbursement but would probably first refer the client to the local and county health departments. Insurance can be an alternative source to help pay for treatment, but the client may not be insured or the policy may not cover prescriptions. Medicaid or medical assistance is another avenue for the client who can't afford medications, if qualifies.
CN: Safe, effective care environment; CNS: Coordinated care; CL: Analyze; DIFFICULTY: Challenge

26. The nurse is caring for a client at risk for skin impairment. Which intervention is **best** to decrease this client's risk?
1. Using a specialty mattress
2. Positioning the client in alignment
3. Repositioning the client every 4 hours
4. Massaging bony prominences every shift

26. **1.** Specialty beds having fluid, air, and convoluted foam mattresses can protect pressure areas on the client. Pressure areas on the client should be padded to prevent skin breakdown. Positioning the client in alignment is important, but pressure areas still need to be protected. The client should be turned every 2 hours. Massaging bony prominences causes friction and may irritate tissues.
CN: Physiological integrity; CNS: Reduction of risk potential; CL: Apply; DIFFICULTY: Moderate

27. A client admitted to the hospital with pneumonia has a history of Parkinson disease, which is progressively worsening. Which clinical manifestations does the nurse anticipate observing?
1. Impaired speech
2. Muscle flaccidity
3. Echolalia
4. Tremors in the fingers that increase with purposeful movement

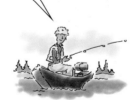

Having trouble with a question? Be patient. The answer will come to you.

27. **1.** In Parkinson disease, dysarthria (impaired speech) is due to a disturbance in muscle control. Muscle rigidity results in resistance to passive muscle stretching. The client may have a masklike appearance. Tremors should decrease with purposeful movement and sleep. Echolalia is repeating a word that is heard and is usually experienced by clients with schizophrenia.
CN: Physiological integrity; CNS: Physiological adaptation; CL: Apply; DIFFICULTY: Challenge

28. An older adult male client with Parkinson disease is frequently incontinent of urine. Which intervention by the nurse is appropriate?
1. Use adult briefs.
2. Apply a condom catheter.
3. Insert an indwelling urinary catheter.
4. Provide skin care every 4 hours.

28. **2.** A condom catheter uses a condom-type device to drain urine away from the client. Applying a brief on the client may keep urine away from the body but may also be demeaning if the client is alert or the family objects. Because the client with Parkinson disease is prone to urinary tract infections, an indwelling urinary catheter should be avoided because it may promote this. Skin care must be provided to prevent skin maceration and breakdown and should begin as soon as the client is incontinent.
CN: Physiological integrity; CNS: Basic care and comfort; CL: Analyze; DIFFICULTY: Difficult

CN: Client needs category   CNS: Client needs subcategory   CL: Cognitive level

29. Family members report to the nurse that they are exhausted and it is difficult taking care of a dependent family member. Which approach by the nurse is in the client's **best** interest?
1. Ask the client what he would like to do.
2. Tell the family members to discuss it among themselves.
3. Tell the family the client should go to a nursing care facility.
4. Call a family conference and ask social services for assistance.

30. A primigravida, in her second trimester with a history of rheumatic fever, tells a nurse her fingers feel tight and sometimes she feels as though her heart skips a beat. Which symptom indicates the client may be experiencing heart failure?
1. Clear breath sounds
2. A heart rate of 102 BPM
3. Bilateral crackles
4. Runs of paroxysmal atrial tachycardia

Listen up. The sounds I make can let you know when I'm in trouble.

31. A pregnant client is suspected of experiencing worsening mitral valve prolapse. Which diagnostic test should the nurse prepare the client for?
1. Stress test
2. Chest x-ray
3. Echocardiography
4. Cardiac catheterization

32. A nurse who is caring for a client in labor with a history of rheumatic heart disease should gather what data in order to determine fetal well-being?
1. Urinalysis
2. Fetal heart tones
3. Laboratory test results of the mother
4. Other signs and symptoms of the client

33. The nurse is obtaining subjective data from a client who is recently admitted to the hospital. What data does the nurse document as subjective?
1. CBC results
2. Vital signs
3. 2 × 2 cm sacral decubitus ulcer
4. Reports of nausea and abdominal pain

34. The nurse is caring for a pregnant client with cardiovascular disease. Which classification of medication may be used safely for the client?
1. Beta-blockers, including atenolol
2. Warfarin
3. Calcium channel antagonists
4. Diuretics

29. 4. A family conference with social services can enlighten the family to all prospects of care available to them. The client should supply input if possible, but this may not help solve the problems of exhaustion and care difficulties. The family may not be aware of alternative care measures for the client, so a discussion among themselves may not be helpful. The client may not qualify for a nursing care facility because of the need to meet stringent criteria.
CN: Safe, effective care environment; CNS: Coordinated care; CL: Analyze; DIFFICULTY: Moderate

30. 3. Crackles should alert the nurse to cardiovascular compromise and heart failure. Cardiac dysrhythmias (other than sinus tachycardia or paroxysmal atrial tachycardia) and persistent crackles at the bases are also symptoms of heart failure, not clear breath sounds.
CN: Health promotion and maintenance; CNS: None; CL: Analyze; DIFFICULTY: Challenge

31. 3. Echocardiography is less invasive than x-rays and other methods; it provides the information needed to determine cardiovascular disease, especially valvular disorders. Cardiac catheterization and stress tests may be postponed until after birth.
CN: Physiological integrity; CNS: Physiological adaptation; CL: Apply; DIFFICULTY: Easy

32. 2. Fetal heart tones show how the fetus is responding to the environment. Assessing other signs and symptoms of the mother, including laboratory test results and urinalysis, can only determine the effect on the mother, not the fetus.
CN: Health promotion and maintenance; CNS: None; CL: Apply; DIFFICULTY: Easy

33. 4. Subjective data, also known as symptoms or covert cues, include the client's own verbatim statements about health problems. Laboratory study results, physical assessment data, and diagnostic procedure reports are observable, perceptible, and measurable and can be verified and validated by others.
CN: Safe, effective care environment; CNS: Coordinated care; CL: Apply; DIFFICULTY: Easy

34. 3. Calcium channel antagonists may be used. Beta blockers are generally safe to use, but not atenolol since it causes growth retardation. Prophylactic antibiotics are reserved for clients susceptible to endocarditis. If anticoagulants are needed, heparin is the drug of choice—not warfarin. Diuretics should be used with extreme caution, if at all, because of the potential for causing uterine contractions.
CN: Physiological integrity; CNS: Pharmacological therapies; CL: Analyze; DIFFICULTY: Moderate

35. The nurse is assisting a client who is morbidly obese and diabetic with personal hygiene measures when the client states, "I've heard the nurses and others joking about me. Could you be my nurse tomorrow?" Which response by the nurse would be **most** appropriate?
1. "I can't promise that, but I'll make sure those nurses know how you feel."
2. "I'll check with the nurse-manager."
3. "I'll make sure the other nurses don't talk about you anymore."
4. "I'm going to report your concerns to my supervisor, and if I return I'll come see how you are."

35. 4. Telling the client that a supervisor will be made aware of the inappropriate comments acknowledges the client's feelings and indicates care and concern. It's best to go through the proper chain of command and inform the nursing supervisor of this situation. Telling the client that she'll make sure the others know how the client feels would only increase the client's embarrassment. Checking with the nurse-manager is incorrect because there's no assurance that a registry nurse will return to the institution. The registry nurse can't guarantee the other nurses won't talk about the client.
CN: Safe, effective care environment; CNS: Coordinated care; CL: Analyze; DIFFICULTY: Easy

36. After assessment of vital signs and application of an external monitor, which nursing intervention is a **priority** for a client with suspected placenta previa?
1. Insert an indwelling urinary catheter.
2. Plan for an immediate cesarean birth.
3. Place the client in Trendelenburg position.
4. Start IV catheters and obtain blood work.

36. 4. The priority nursing intervention for a client with suspected placenta previa is to draw blood for hemoglobin analysis, hematocrit, type, and cross-match and to insert IV catheters. Depending on the degree of bleeding and fetal maturity, a cesarean birth may be required. The nurse shouldn't attempt Trendelenburg positioning or urinary catheterization. The client may be placed on her left side.
CN: Physiological integrity; CNS: Reduction of risk potential; CL: Apply; DIFFICULTY: Challenge

37. A pregnant client with vaginal bleeding asks a nurse how the fetus is doing. Which response is **best**?
1. "I don't know for sure."
2. "I can't answer that question."
3. "It's too early to tell anything."
4. "I'll tell you what the monitors show."

37. 4. The client deserves a truthful answer and the nurse should be objective without giving opinions. Relating what the monitors show is objective and truthful. Vague answers may be misleading and aren't therapeutic.
CN: Psychosocial integrity; CNS: None; CL: Analyze; DIFFICULTY: Moderate

38. A client with placenta previa is hospitalized, and a cesarean birth is planned. In addition to the routine neonatal assessment, the neonate should be assessed for which condition?
1. Prematurity
2. Congenital anomalies
3. Respiratory distress
4. Aspiration pneumonia

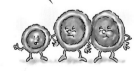

Wow. You guys are looking ancient. What are you, like 116 days old?

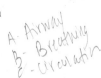

38. 3. Hypoxia, resulting in respiratory distress, is a potential risk due to decreased blood volume and prematurity. The age of maturity of the neonate can be determined through established maternal dates. Congenital anomalies aren't necessarily associated with placenta previa. Aspiration pneumonia isn't considered a threat unless the amniotic fluid is meconium-stained.
CN: Physiological integrity; CNS: Reduction of risk potential; CL: Apply; DIFFICULTY: Moderate

39. A nurse working in the triage area of an emergency department sees that several pediatric clients arrive simultaneously. Which child is treated first?
1. A crying 4-year-old child with a laceration on his scalp
2. A 3-year-old child with a barking cough and flushed appearance
3. A 3-year-old child with Down syndrome who's pale and asleep in his mother's arms
4. A 2-month-old infant with stridorous breath sounds, sitting up in his mother's arms and drooling

39. 4. The 2-month-old infant with the airway emergency should be treated first because of the risk of epiglottitis. The 3-year-old with the barking cough and fever should be suspected of having croup and should be seen promptly, as should the child with the laceration. The nurse would need to gather more information about the child with Down syndrome to determine the priority of care.
CN: Safe, effective care environment; CNS: Coordinated care; CL: Analyze; DIFFICULTY: Moderate

40. The nursing staff is developing a care plan for a client who's receiving palliative care for end-stage leukemia. The client is experiencing breakthrough pain, rated as a 5 on a pain scale of 1 to 10. Which action by the nurse should be included in the client's care plan?
1. Meet with the pain management team to devise a better plan to control pain.
2. Explain that pain relief may not be possible because she's receiving maximum doses of pain medications.
3. Assess whether the client is abusing the pain medications.
4. Provide nonpharmacologic pain measures only because maximum doses of pain medications are ineffective.

41. A 2-year-old child is being examined in the emergency department for epiglottitis. Which finding supports this diagnosis?
1. Mild fever
2. Clear speech
3. Tripod position
4. Gradual onset of symptoms

42. Which method is best when approaching a 2-year-old child to listen to breath sounds?
1. Tell the child it's time to listen to lungs now.
2. Tell the child to lie down while the nurse listens to his lungs.
3. Ask the caregiver to wait outside while the nurse listens to the lungs.
4. Ask the child if the nurse should listen to the front or the back of the chest first.

43. A pregnant client being seen in the clinic reports increasing leg cramps. Which response by the nurse is **most** appropriate?
1. "Have you asked the health care provider to prescribe a muscle relaxant for the cramps?"
2. "Sometimes gently stretching the legs helps relieve leg cramps."
3. "Relax! Everyone who's pregnant has leg cramps."
4. "Don't worry about them. They go away after you deliver."

44. A mother says a 2-year-old child is up to date with vaccines. Which immunization should be included?
1. Diphtheria-tetanus-pertussis (DTaP), inactivated poliovirus (IPV), measles-mumps-rubella (MMR), and pneumococcal vaccine (PCV)
2. DTaP, IPV, MMR, hepatitis B, Haemophilus influenzae type b (Hib), varicella, PCV, rotavirus (Rota), and influenza
3. DTaP, hepatitis B, and IPV
4. MMR, IPV, hepatitis B, and varicella

40. 1. Client comfort is top priority in palliative care. The nurse should meet with the pain management team to devise a plan to control the client's pain. Typically, palliative care doses are increased above the normal maximum doses to meet the client's needs. Clients who require opioids long term typically develop drug tolerance, so it's necessary to increase dosages. There's no need to assess the client for drug abuse. The nursing staff should also incorporate nonpharmacologic measures to relieve pain into the client's care plan, but they shouldn't be the only measures used to control pain.
CN: Physiological integrity; CNS: Basic care and comfort; CL: Apply; DIFFICULTY: Easy

41. 3. The tripod position (sitting up and leaning forward) facilitates breathing. Epiglottitis presents with a sudden onset of symptoms, high fever, and muffled speech. Additional symptoms are inspiratory stridor and drooling.
CN: Physiological integrity; CNS: Physiological adaptation; CL: Apply; DIFFICULTY: Challenge

42. 4. The 2-year-old child needs to feel in control, and asking if the chest should be listened to from the front or back best supports the child's independence. Giving the child no choice may encourage uncooperative behavior. The child should be allowed to remain in the tripod position to facilitate breathing. The caregiver should be allowed to remain with the child because fear of separation is common in 2-year-olds.
CN: Health promotion and maintenance; CNS: None; CL: Apply; DIFFICULTY: Moderate

43. 2. Leg cramps are a common discomfort of pregnancy. Gentle stretching may be effective in relieving the cramps. Typically, muscle relaxants aren't used for leg cramps associated with pregnancy. Telling the client to relax, not to worry, that every pregnant woman gets leg cramps, or that they go away after birth ignores the client's concern and dismisses the client's feelings.
CN: Physiological integrity; CNS: Basic care and comfort; CL: Analyze; DIFFICULTY: Easy

44. 2. By the age of 2, a child should have received the DTaP, IPV, MMR, hepatitis B, Hib, varicella, PCV, Rota, and influenza vaccines. The nurse should clarify this with the mother or caregiver.
CN: Safe, effective care environment; CNS: Safety and infection control; CL: Apply; DIFFICULTY: Moderate

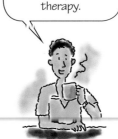

Feeling sleepy? Try some caffeine therapy.

CN: Client needs category   CNS: Client needs subcategory   CL: Cognitive level

windpipe inflam (handwritten)

45. A nurse is obtaining data on a child with epiglottitis. Which action by the nurse is appropriate?
1. Obtain a flashlight and tongue blade.
2. Obtain a sterile tongue blade and Culturette swab.
3. Ask the registered nurse to visualize the child's throat.
4. Wait for visualization to be done by the anesthesiologist.

46. The parent of a 2-year-old child with epiglottitis states "I have to leave to pick up another child from school." The 2-year-old child begins to cry and appears more stridorous. Which intervention by the nurse is **best**?
1. Ask the parent how long she may be gone.
2. Tell the 2-year-old everything will be all right.
3. Tell the 2-year-old that the nurse will stay with them.
4. Ask the parent if someone else can pick up the older child.

1/2 (handwritten)

47. A client is being treated for gastrointestinal bleeding. On his fifth day of hospitalization, the client begins to have tremors, is agitated, and is experiencing hallucinations. These signs suggest which condition?
1. Alcohol withdrawal
2. Allergic response
3. Alzheimer disease
4. Hypoxia

48. A client experiencing alcohol withdrawal reports seeing cockroaches on the ceiling. Which response by the nurse is appropriate?
1. Ask the client where they are being seen.
2. Ask the client if the cockroaches are still there.
3. Tell the client there are no cockroaches on the ceiling.
4. Tell the client it's dim in the room and turn on the overhead lights.

49. If a nurse suspects a client is experiencing alcohol withdrawal, which action is appropriate?
1. Verify it with family.
2. Inform social services.
3. Ask the client about drinking.
4. Tell the client everything will be all right.

45. 4. Direct visualization of the epiglottis can trigger a complete airway obstruction and should only be done in a controlled environment by an anesthesiologist or a health care provider skilled in pediatric intubation.
CN: Physiological integrity; CNS: Basic care and comfort; CL: Analyze; DIFFICULTY: Moderate

46. 4. Increased anxiety and agitation should be avoided in the child with epiglottitis to prevent airway obstruction. A 2-year-old child fears separation from parents, so the mother should be encouraged to stay. Other means of picking up the older child need to be found. The parent is the primary caregiver and important to the child for emotional and security reasons. Asking the parent how long she'll be gone isn't therapeutic because she shouldn't leave. A 2-year-old can't understand that all will be okay. The nurse offering to stay with the 2-year-old won't comfort the child as much as the parent being there.
CN: Health promotion and maintenance; CNS: None; CL: Analyze; DIFFICULTY: Moderate

47. 1. Tremors, agitation, and hallucinations are signs of alcohol withdrawal, which can occur within 12 hours after the last drink or even 7 to 10 days later depending on the severity of alcohol abuse. An allergic reaction would cause labored breathing, skin rash, or edema as primary symptoms. Alzheimer disease occurs in older individuals and has other psychosocial signs, such as a masklike face and altered mentation. Hypoxia would cause symptoms of respiratory distress.
CN: Psychosocial integrity; CNS: None; CL: Analyze; DIFFICULTY: Easy

48. 4. The nursing goal for a client with alcohol withdrawal is to try to reorient the client to reality and minimize distortions. Don't support the client's hallucinations or place the client on the defensive. Try to present reality gently without agitating the client.
CN: Psychosocial integrity; CNS: None; CL: Apply; DIFFICULTY: Challenge

49. 3. Confirming suspicions with the client is the most beneficial way to help in diagnosis and treatment of alcohol withdrawal. If the client isn't cooperative, verification can be sought with the family. Social services aren't required at this time but may be helpful in discharge planning. Giving false reassurance isn't therapeutic for the client.
CN: Psychosocial integrity; CNS: None; CL: Apply; DIFFICULTY: Easy

50. A client experiencing alcohol withdrawal reports itching everywhere from the bugs on the bed. Which action by the nurse is appropriate?
1. Examine the client's skin.
2. Ask what kind of bugs they are.
3. Tell the client there are no bugs on the bed.
4. Tell the client he is having tactile hallucinations.

51. A client with alcohol withdrawal is pulling at the central venous catheter saying "I am swatting the spiders crawling over me." Which intervention is appropriate?
1. Encourage the client to rest.
2. Protect the client from harm.
3. Tell the client there are no spiders.
4. Tell the client he is pulling the IV tubing.

52. A client who experienced alcohol withdrawal is no longer having hallucinations or tremors and states, "I would like to enter a rehabilitation facility to stop drinking." Which intervention is appropriate?
1. Ask about insurance.
2. Have the client discuss this with family members.
3. Refer the client to Alcoholics Anonymous (AA).
4. Promote participation in a treatment program.

53. A client with cirrhosis is admitted to the hospital in a hepatic coma. Which assessment would be the nurse's **priority**?
1. Perform a neurologic check.
2. Complete the client admission.
3. Orient the client to the environment.
4. Check airway, breathing, and circulation.

54. A client with cirrhosis is restless and at times tries to climb out of bed. Which intervention is **best** to promote safety?
1. Use leather restraints.
2. Use soft wrist restraints.
3. Use a vest restraint device.
4. Use a sheet tied across the client's chest.

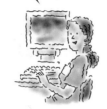

Woot woot! You've finished 50 questions already. Well done.

50. 1. Make sure the client doesn't have a rash, skin allergy, or something on the skin (such as food crumbs) causing discomfort. Reality should then be presented to the client gently without being derogatory. The nurse shouldn't support the client's hallucinations.
CN: Psychosocial integrity; CNS: None; CL: Apply; DIFFICULTY: Difficult

51. 2. During periods of alcohol withdrawal, the nurse must take necessary measures to protect the client from harming self, including preventing the dislodgment of the central venous catheter, which can cause a life-threatening embolus. Although encouraging the client to rest and presenting reality are important, the client may not heed the nurse's attempts to calm and reassure the client in this situation. Client safety is the priority.
CN: Psychosocial integrity; CNS: None; CL: Analyze; DIFFICULTY: Moderate

52. 4. The client should be encouraged to enter a facility if that's in the best interest. Arrangements can be made and discussed with the social services coordinator and health care provider as well as having social services discuss insurance concerns. The client can inform the family, and support should be encouraged. Referral to AA should be considered after rehabilitation takes place.
CN: Psychosocial integrity; CNS: None; CL: Apply; DIFFICULTY: Challenge

53. 4. Priorities for the client in a coma include checking the airway, breathing, and circulation. After these are assessed, a neurologic check is needed to determine status. General orientation and completing the admission may require the help of family members. The ability of the nurse to orient the client depends on the level of consciousness.
CN: Physiological integrity; CNS: Reduction of risk potential; CL: Apply; DIFFICULTY: Easy

54. 3. The client with cirrhosis may require gentle reminders not to get out of bed to prevent a fall. The vest restraint would help in this endeavor. Leather restraints are only warranted for extremely combative and unsafe clients. Soft wrist restraints may not stop the client from sitting up or trying to swing his legs over the bed rails. A sheet tied across the client's chest can hamper breathing or may asphyxiate the client if sliding down in the bed.
CN: Safe, effective care environment; CNS: Coordinated care; CL: Analyze; DIFFICULTY: Challenge

55. The nurse knows that which condition is consistent with a later stage of cirrhosis?
1. Constipation
2. Diarrhea
3. Hypoxia
4. Vomiting

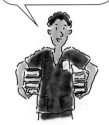

Check out that word "later" in question 55. It's important.

55. **3.** In the later stage of cirrhosis, fluid in the lungs and weak chest expansion can lead to hypoxia. Constipation, diarrhea, and vomiting are early signs and symptoms of cirrhosis.
CN: Physiological integrity; CNS: Physiological adaptation;
CL: Understand; DIFFICULTY: Moderate

56. A client with cirrhosis is jaundiced, edematous and experiencing severe itching with dryness. Which intervention is **best** to help the client?
1. Put mitts on the hands.
2. Use alcohol-free body lotion.
3. Lubricate the skin with baby oil.
4. Wash the skin with soap and water.

56. **2.** Alcohol-free body lotion applied to the skin is best to help relieve dryness and is absorbed without oiliness. Mitts may help keep the client from scratching skin open. Baby oil doesn't allow excretions through the skin and may block pores. Soap dries out the skin.
CN: Physiological integrity; CNS: Basic care and comfort;
CL: Apply; DIFFICULTY: Moderate

57. A client with a spinal cord injury sustained in a previous motorcycle accident is hospitalized for renal calculi. To reduce the client's risk for developing recurrent renal calculi, which instruction is correct?
1. Eat yogurt daily.
2. Drink cranberry juice.
3. Eat more fresh fruits and vegetables.
4. Increase the intake of dairy products.

57. **2.** Acid urine decreases the potential for renal calculi. Most renal calculi form in alkaline urine. Cranberries, prunes, and plums promote acidic urine. Yogurt helps restore pH balance to secretions in yeast infections. Fruits and vegetables increase fiber in the diet and promote alkaline urine. Dairy products may *contribute* to the formation of renal calculi.
CN: Physiological integrity; CNS: Reduction of risk potential;
CL: Apply; DIFFICULTY: Moderate

58. A client with a spinal cord injury states he has difficulty recognizing the symptoms of urinary tract infection (UTI) before it's too late. Which symptom is an early sign of UTI?
1. Lower back pain
2. Burning on urination
3. Frequency of urination
4. Fever and change in the clarity of urine

58. **4.** The client with a spinal cord injury should recognize fever and change in the clarity of urine as early signs of UTI. Lower back pain is a late sign. The client with a spinal cord injury may not experience burning or frequency of urination.
CN: Physiological integrity; CNS: Reduction of risk potential;
CL: Apply; DIFFICULTY: Difficult

59. A client tells a nurse that they boil urinary catheters to keep them sterile. Which question should the nurse ask?
1. "What technique do you use for sterilization?"
2. "What temperature are the catheters boiled at?"
3. "Why aren't prepackaged sterile catheters used?"
4. "Are the catheters dried and stored in a clean, dry place?"

59. **1.** The client should describe the procedure to make sure sterile technique is used. Water boils at 212° F (100° C), but the nurse should make sure the client is boiling the catheters for an appropriate amount of time. Catheters should be boiled just before use and allowed to cool before using. Prepackaged sterile catheters aren't necessary if the proper sterilization techniques are used.
CN: Physiological integrity; CNS: Reduction of risk potential;
CL: Analyze; DIFFICULTY: Difficult

60. A nurse approaches a client who recently had a colostomy and finds the client crying. Which action is appropriate?
1. Leave and come back another time.
2. Ask the client if there is pain or discomfort.
3. Tell the client vital signs need to be obtained.
4. Sit down with the client and offer to talk about anything.

60. **4.** Asking open-ended questions and appearing interested in what the client has to say will encourage verbalization of feelings. Leaving the client may cause feelings of unacceptance. Asking closed-ended questions won't encourage verbalization of feelings. Ignoring the client's present state isn't therapeutic for the client.
CN: Psychosocial integrity; CNS: None; CL: Apply; DIFFICULTY: Easy

61. After a review of colostomy care, a client states, "I don't know if I can care for myself at home without help." Which nursing intervention is **most** appropriate?
1. Review care with the client again.
2. Provide written instructions for the client.
3. Ask the client if there's anyone who can help.
4. Arrange for home health care to visit the client.

61. 4. Although all of these interventions may benefit the client, home health care should be contacted to ensure continuity of appropriate care after discharge from the hospital.
CN: Safe, effective care environment; CNS: Coordinated care;
CL: Apply; DIFFICULTY: Moderate

62. A client is experiencing mild diarrhea through the colostomy. Which instruction is correct?
1. Eat prunes.
2. Drink apple juice.
3. Increase lettuce intake.
4. Increase intake of bananas.

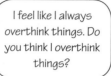

I feel like I always overthink things. Do you think I overthink things?

62. 4. Bananas help make formed stool and don't irritate the bowel. Apple juice and prunes can increase the frequency of diarrhea. Lettuce acts as a fiber and can increase the looseness of stool.
CN: Physiological integrity; CNS: Basic care and comfort;
CL: Apply; DIFFICULTY: Easy

63. A client reports a lot of gas in the colostomy bag. Which instruction is **best** to give this client?
1. Burp the bag.
2. Eat fewer beans.
3. Replace the bag.
4. Put a tiny hole in the top of the bag.

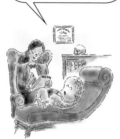

63. 1. Letting air out of the bag by opening it and burping it is the best solution. The client can be encouraged to note which foods are causing gas and to eat fewer gas-forming foods. Replacing the bag is costly. Putting a hole in the bag will cause fluids to leak out.
CN: Physiological integrity; CNS: Basic care and comfort;
CL: Apply; DIFFICULTY: Easy

64. A postpartum client recovering from spinal anesthesia with morphine reports that her nose itches. Which would the nurse suspect as the cause?
1. The client may be having a reaction to a material she encountered in the delivery room.
2. Postpartum itching is common after birth because of hormonal changes.
3. The client may be still be partially sedated and imagining this feeling.
4. The client is experiencing a common effect due to a morphine-based anesthetic.

64. 4. Morphine causes a relatively high incidence of itching when used in spinal anesthesia. The itching usually begins at the tip of the nose, possibly becoming more generalized. Antipruritics, such as diphenhydramine or hydroxyzine hydrochloride, may be prescribed after the use of morphine. Itching on the tip of the nose isn't typical of an allergic reaction nor is it caused by postpartum hormonal changes. The client is awake and speaking appropriately, so she is alert.
CN: Physiological integrity; CNS: Pharmacological therapies;
CL: Analyze; DIFFICULTY: Easy

65. A client recently diagnosed with pre-diabetes asks the nurse about the risk factors for developing diabetes. The nurse identifies which factor as the client's greatest risk for developing diabetes?
1. Obesity
2. Japanese descent
3. A great-grandparent with diabetes
4. Birth of a neonate weighing less than 9 lb

65. 1. Obesity is the risk factor that puts the client at greatest risk for developing diabetes. Other leading risk factors include birth of a neonate weighing more than 9 lb, a family history of diabetes (specifically a mother, father, or sibling), and Native American, Black, Asian, or Hispanic descent.
CN: Health promotion and maintenance; CNS: None; CL: Analyze;
DIFFICULTY: Easy

66. A client had gastric bypass surgery, is on nothing-by-mouth (NPO) status, and is in pain. The nurse gives morphine 4 mg as ordered. In 20 minutes, the client reports feeling nauseous. What would the nurse suspect as the **most** likely cause?
1. The surgery is causing nausea.
2. Being NPO, the increase in gastric secretions is precipitating this symptom.
3. Morphine, which was given for pain, has a tendency to cause nausea.
4. A reaction to blood still remaining in the mouth after extubation.

66. 3. Although gastric bypass surgery may precipitate some feelings of nausea, the timing of this symptom after the administration of morphine is suspicious. Most likely, this client is experiencing nausea as a very common adverse effect of the analgesic morphine. The status of being NPO wouldn't cause an increase in gastric secretions. It's possible that there may be some blood in the mouth after extubation, but the chances of this happening are minimal and less likely to be the cause of the client's nausea.
CN: Physiological integrity; CNS: Pharmacological therapies;
CL: Analyze; DIFFICULTY: Easy

CN: Client needs category   CNS: Client needs subcategory   CL: Cognitive level

67. A health care provider's order reads: amoxicillin 500 mg capsules × 2 PO now, followed by 500 mg PO every 6 hours. How many grams of amoxicillin will the nurse administer as the initial dose? Record your answer as a whole number.

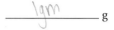

_____ g

68. A client with a family history of diabetes asks the nurse which measures can be practiced to decrease the chance of developing the disease. Which statement would be the nurse's **best** response?
  1. "Eat only poultry and fish."
  2. "Omit carbohydrates from your diet."
  3. "Start a moderate exercise program."
  4. "Check blood glucose levels every month."

69. An older adult client fractured a hip after a fall in the home and surgical correction is not an option due to comorbid factors. The client states to the nurse, "How will I ever get better?" Which response by the nurse is **best**?
  1. "You're doing fine."
  2. "What's your biggest concern right now?"
  3. "Just give it some time and you'll be okay."
  4. "You don't believe you're doing well?"

70. A client reports slipping on a throw rug while going to the bathroom at night. Which factor needs assessment?
  1. Home safety
  2. Client confusion
  3. Injury to the client's head
  4. Client has a urinary tract infection (UTI)

71. A client in her third trimester of pregnancy is having contractions 5 minutes apart that began suddenly. The nurse identifies that it's the client's seventh month. She's admitted directly to the obstetrics department. Which intervention has **priority**?
  1. Call the obstetrician.
  2. Time the contractions.
  3. Check fetal heart tones.
  4. Call the client's husband.

Keep your priorities in order when answering question #71. Which intervention should come first?

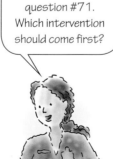

67. 1.
The order states the nurse is giving two 500 mg capsules now. This would equal a total of 1,000 mg (1 g) followed by 500 mg (0.5 g) every 6 hours. Therefore the correct answer is 1 g.
CN: Physiological integrity; CNS: Pharmacological therapies; CL: Analyze; DIFFICULTY: Easy

68. 3. Exercise and weight control are the goals in preventing and treating diabetes. Red meat can be eaten along with poultry and fish but should be limited because it contributes to cardiovascular disease. Complex carbohydrates, especially whole grains, are necessary for a healthy diet. Fiber intake of 14 g/1,000 kcal is recommended. Checking blood glucose levels will help monitor the development of diabetes but won't prevent or decrease the chance of it occurring.
CN: Physiological integrity; CNS: Reduction of risk potential; CL: Apply; DIFFICULTY: Easy

69. 2. Open-ended questions allow the client to control what is discussed and help the nurse determine care needs. Telling the client she is doing fine or that there is a need for more time doesn't encourage verbalizing concern. A reiteration of the client's concerns may not be helpful in encouraging the client to verbalize feelings.
CN: Health promotion and maintenance; CNS: None; CL: Understand; DIFFICULTY: Easy

70. 1. A safety assessment of the home can determine if changes need to be made to ensure the client doesn't fall again. The nurse might or might not determine if the client has experienced a head injury or confusion by asking how the injury occurred. Going to the bathroom at night isn't necessarily a sign of a UTI.
CN: Safe, effective care environment; CNS: Safety and infection control; CL: Apply; DIFFICULTY: Challenge

71. 3. The nurse should check fetal heart tones and assess the client's vital signs. The client should be placed on a monitor to check contractions and for continuous fetal monitoring. The obstetrician and husband should be notified as soon as possible.
CN: Health promotion and maintenance; CNS: None; CL: Apply; DIFFICULTY: Easy

72. The nurse is monitoring the following clients' vital signs. Which client's vital signs would be the **priority** to report to the health care provider?
1. A healthy male client who is undergoing elective surgery with a blood pressure of 120/72 mm Hg
2. A postoperative client with a pulse of 110 beats/minute on awakening in the morning
3. A healthy female client undergoing elective surgery with a blood pressure of 110/68 mm Hg
4. A client with a pulse of 120 beats/minute after 30 minutes of aerobic exercise in physical therapy

72. 2. The normal range for a pulse is 60 to 100 beats/minute and, in the morning, the rate is at its lowest. Blood pressures of 120/72 mm Hg for a healthy man and 110/68 mm Hg for a healthy woman are normal. Aerobic exercise increases the heart rate over the normal range of 60 to 100 beats/minute.
CN: Physiological integrity; CNS: Physiological adaptation; CL: Analyze; DIFFICULTY: Easy

73. A nurse is collecting data from a 40-year-old client preparing to undergo elective facial surgery and notes a pulse rate of 130 beats/minute with a regular rhythm. Which factor would be the most likely explanation for the tachycardia?
1. Age
2. Anxiety
3. Exercise
4. Pain

73. 2. Anxiety tends to increase heart rate, temperature, and respirations. The normal heart rate for a client this age is 60 to 100 beats/minute. Exercise will increase the heart rate but most likely wouldn't occur preoperatively. The client shouldn't be in any pain preoperatively.
CN: Physiological integrity; CNS: Physiological adaptation; CL: Apply; DIFFICULTY: Easy

74. A client on a psychiatric unit asks a nurse about the medications another client takes. Which response is **best**?
1. "How close are the two of you?"
2. "I can't give you that information. I must protect the client's privacy."
3. "Let me ask if it's OK for me to tell you about their condition and medications."
4. "The client is taking insulin for diabetes and digoxin for a heart condition."

74. 2. Revealing one client's medication to another client violates procedures of client confidentiality and directly violates the Health Insurance Portability and Accountability Act. Seeking the client's permission to release confidential information is an inappropriate action. Asking the client the nature of the relationship to the other client won't help the client understand the purpose of protecting confidentiality. Assuring the client that the facility has an obligation to protect not only confidentiality but that of others will provide the client with a sense of comfort.
CN: Safe, care environment; CNS: Coordinated care; CL: Apply; DIFFICULTY: Easy

75. The vital signs of a client are temperature, 98.6° F (37° C) orally; pulse, 80 beats/minute; and respirations, 30 breaths/minute. Which interpretation of these values is correct?
1. Pulse is above normal range.
2. Temperature is above normal range.
3. Respirations are above normal range.
4. Respirations and pulse are above normal range.

75. 3. Normal vital signs for an adult client are: temperature, 96.6° to 99° F (35.9° to 37.2° C); pulse, 60 to 100 beats/minute; respirations, 16 to 20 breaths/minute.
CN: Health promotion and maintenance; CNS: None; CL: Apply; DIFFICULTY: Easy

76. The nurse monitoring a client's pulse notes that it's easily palpable at 84 beats/minute and regular. Which term would the nurse use in charting the pulse assessment?
1. Dysrhythmia
2. Bradycardia
3. Regular
4. Tachycardia

76. 3. The pulse is regular when it's rhythmic, easily palpable, and between the rate of 60 and 100 beats/minute. Tachycardia is a heart rate faster than 100 beats/minute. Dysrhythmia is a heart rate with either irregular rate or rhythm. Bradycardia is a heart rate slower than 60 beats/minute.
CN: Health promotion and maintenance; CNS: None; CL: Apply; DIFFICULTY: Easy

77. The nurse is assessing a client's arterial pulses. Which graphic displays the appropriate site for palpating the dorsalis pedis pulse?

1.
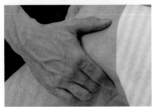
Femoral Pulse

2.
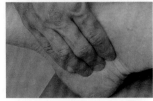
popliteal pulse

3.
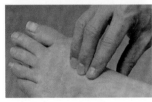
Posterior tibial pulse

4.
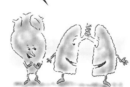
dorsalis pedis

77. 4. To palpate the dorsalis pedis pulse, the nurse places the fingers on the medial dorsum of the foot while the client points toes down. The first graphic shows palpation of the femoral pulse, located along the crease midway between the pubic bone and the anterior iliac crest. The second graphic shows palpation of the popliteal pulse in the popliteal fossa of the back of the knee. The third graphic shows palpation of the posterior tibial pulse, slightly below the malleolus of the ankle.
CN: Health promotion and maintenance; CNS: None; CL: Apply; DIFFICULTY: Easy

78. A client is determined to require tracheal suctioning. Which action is correct for the nurse performing this procedure? Select all that apply.
1. Apply suction during insertion of the catheter.
2. Limit suctioning to 10 to 15 seconds' duration.
3. Resterilize the suction catheter in alcohol after use.
4. Repeat suctioning intervals every 15 minutes until clear.
5. Pre-oxygenate prior to suctioning.

With his respiratory skills and my pumping power, our oxygen distribution system is second to none.

78. 2. The length of time a client should be able to tolerate the suction procedure is 10 to 15 seconds. Preoxygenation will help prevent hypoxia. Any longer may cause hypoxia. Suctioning during insertion can cause trauma to the mucosa and removes oxygen from the respiratory tract. Suction catheters are disposed of after each use and are cleaned in normal saline solution after each pass. Suctioning, with supplemental oxygen between suctions, is performed in a minimum of 1-minute intervals in order to allow the client to rest.
CN: Physiological integrity; CNS: Physiological adaptation; CL: Apply; DIFFICULTY: Difficult

79. The nurse is preparing to insert a nasogastric tube. In which position should the nurse place the client?
1. Fowler's
2. Prone
3. Side-lying
4. Supine

79. 1. The upright Fowler's position is more natural for swallowing and protects against aspiration. Positioning the client on the back, stomach, or side places the client at risk for aspiration if he should gag. It's also difficult to swallow in these positions.
CN: Physiological integrity; CNS: Basic care and comfort; CL: Understand; DIFFICULTY: Easy

80. The nurse is completing the intake and output record for a client who was restarted on his regular diet after being on nothing-by-mouth status for laboratory studies.

It reads: intake: 4 oz of cranberry juice, ½ cup of oatmeal, 2 slices of toast, 8 oz of black decaffeinated coffee, tuna fish sandwich, ½ cup of fruit-flavored gelatin, 1 cup of cream of mushroom soup, 6 oz of 1% milk, 16 oz of water. Output: 1,300 mL of urine

How many milliliters should the nurse document as the client's intake? Record the answer using a whole number.

_____1,380_____ mL

4oz (30)110
4oz (30)110
4oz (30)240
8oz (30)240
4oz (30)110

8oz (40)240
6 (30)180
16 (30)480
1,300 output

81. When caring for a client who sustained a chemical burn in the right eye, the nurse is preparing to irrigate the eye with sterile normal saline solution. Which steps are appropriate when performing the procedure? Select all that apply.
1. Tilt the client's head toward the left eye.
2. Place absorbent pads in the area of the client's shoulder.
3. Wash hands and put on gloves.
4. Place the irrigation syringe directly on the cornea.
5. Direct the solution onto the exposed conjunctival sac from the inner to outer canthus.
6. Irrigate the eye for 1 minute. 10 minutes

82. The nurse is caring for a client with peripheral vascular disease. When palpating for the dorsalis pedis pulse, where should the nurse place her fingers for location of the pulse?

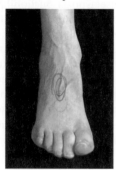

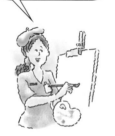

An eye for detail is a big asset in art and in test-taking.

80. 1,380.
There are 30 mL in each ounce and 240 mL in each cup. The fluid intake for this client includes 4 oz (120 mL) of cranberry juice, 8 oz (240 mL) of coffee, ½ cup (120 mL) of fruit-flavored gelatin, 1 cup (240 mL) of cream of mushroom soup, 6 oz (180 mL) of milk, and 16 oz (480 mL) of water, for a total of 1,380 mL.
CN: Physiological integrity; CNS: Basic care and comfort; CL: Apply; DIFFICULTY: Moderate

81. 2, 3, 5. The nurse should place absorbent pads on the client's shoulder area to prevent saturating the client's clothing and bed linens. The nurse should also wash hands and put on gloves to reduce the transmission of microorganisms. The solution should be directed from the inner to outer canthus of the eye to prevent contamination of the unaffected eye. The head should be tilted toward the affected (right) eye to facilitate drainage and to prevent irrigating solution from entering the left eye. The irrigation syringe should be held about 1 inch (2.5 cm) above the eye to prevent injury to the cornea. In a chemical exposure, the eye should be irrigated for at least 10 minutes.
CN: Physiological integrity; CNS: Reduction of risk potential; CL: Apply; DIFFICULTY: Challenge

82.

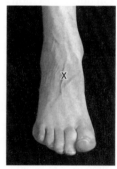

CN: Health promotion and maintenance; CNS: None; CL: Apply; DIFFICULTY: Moderate

83. The nurse is preparing to administer an iron dextran injection using the Z-track technique to minimize the risk of subcutaneous irritation and staining from the drug. Which drawing shows the correct technique for inserting the needle?

1.

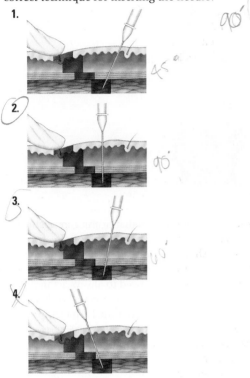

2.

3.

4.

83. **2.** The correct Z-track technique shows the skin surface pulled about ½ inch so the subcutaneous layers are moved out of alignment with the underlying muscle, allowing the needle to enter at a 90-degree angle. Option 1 is incorrect because the needle enters at a 45-degree angle. Option 3 is incorrect because the needle enters at a 60-degree angle. Option 4 is incorrect because the needle enters at a 120-degree angle.

CN: Physiological integrity; CNS: Pharmacological therapies; CL: Apply; DIFFICULTY: Easy

84. A client has sustained a severe burn to the face and neck. What is the **priority** intervention in the immediate burn phase?
1. Maintain a patent airway
2. Start IV fluids
3. Place ointment on the burned area
4. Obtain data regarding the fire

84. **1.** The priority intervention in a client with a burned face and chest is to ensure the patency of the airway. The nurse should follow the ABCDE of care of a burned client. A is airway, B is breathing, C is circulation, D is disability, and E is expose and examine. Starting IV fluids would occur after patency of airway and breathing. Obtaining data would be part of the secondary survey. Ointment should not be applied to a burn until after being prescribed by the health care provider.

CN: Safe, effective care environment; CNS: Coordinated care; CL: Analyze; DIFFICULTY: Easy

85. A client is scheduled for a surgical procedure for removal of a pancreatic tumor. The client states to the nurse, "I don't think I am going to live through the surgery. I am scared." What is the **best** response by the nurse?
1. "Well, it could happen. Not everyone makes it through surgery."
2. "If you feel like this, you should say goodbye to your family."
3. "Let's talk about your concerns and fears."
4. "When I had surgery, I felt the same way."

85. **4.** The client is expressing concerns and fears related to having a serious surgical procedure; the most therapeutic response the nurse can give is to let the client know that she is not alone and someone is present to talk to about the feelings being experienced. To tell the client that not everyone makes it through surgery is not addressing the fears that the client has, and can make the anxiety about the procedure worse. Stating the client should say goodbye to family also does not respond to the fears and lends finality to the situation. Discussing what the nurse felt when having surgery does not address the client's concern.

CN: Psychosocial integrity; CNS: None; CL: Apply; DIFFICULTY: Challenge

Comprehensive Test 2

This second comprehensive test is just like the longest NCLEX test: 205 questions. It's a great way to practice your endurance!

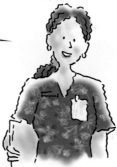

1. The nurse-manager asks a newly hired LPN if the facility's rules of ethical conduct are understood. Which statement by the LPN indicates the need for further education?
 1. "I make sure that I do everything in my client's best interest."
 2. "I maintain client confidentiality always."
 3. "I'll support the Patient Care Partnership."
 4. "I don't discuss advance directives unless the client initiates the conversation."

2. The nurse receives a medication order from a health care provider over the telephone. Which nursing intervention is a **priority** when receiving a telephone order?
 1. Inform the health care provider that the Nurse Practice Act prohibits taking medication orders over the telephone.
 2. Verify the order by repeating it back to the health care provider over the phone.
 3. Request that a second health care provider repeat the order to the nurse over the telephone.
 4. Insist that the health care provider sign the medication order within 1 hour.

3. Which task can a licensed practical nurse (LPN) safely delegate to unlicensed assistive personnel (UAP)?
 1. Applying a topical cream to a client's wound, as prescribed
 2. Performing wet-to-dry dressing changes every 8 hours
 3. Turning a client every 2 hours
 4. Documenting wound healing

1. 4. The law mandates that health care agencies ask all clients if they have an advance directive. Therefore, the nurse must address this question regardless of whether the client initiates a conversation about it. Nurses need to always act in the best interest of their clients, maintain confidentiality, and support the Patient Care Partnership.
CN: Safe, effective care environment; CNS: Coordinated care; CL: Analyze; DIFFICULTY: Easy

2. 2. When taking a medication order over the telephone, standard practice requires verbal verification of the order and the health care provider's written signature within 24 hours. The Nurse Practice Act doesn't prohibit taking medication orders over the telephone. Having a second health care provider repeat the order opens another avenue for misinterpretation and error. Insisting that the health care provider sign the order within 1 hour is unrealistic.
CN: Safe, effective care environment; CNS: Coordinated care; CL: Apply; DIFFICULTY: Easy

3. 3. The LPN can safely delegate the task of turning the client every 2 hours to the UAP. The nurse must administer all medications as prescribed; it isn't within the scope of practice for UAP to administer medication. The nurse must also perform prescribed dressing changes and document wound healing.
CN: Safe, effective care environment; CNS: Coordinated care; CL: Apply; DIFFICULTY: Easy

4. A client is provided two treatment options by the health care provider. During morning care, the client asks the nurse for an opinion about which treatment to undergo. Which response by the nurse is **most** appropriate?
1. "I'd choose the least painful option."
2. "I'd ask my health care provider to make the decision for me."
3. "Why are you asking me? I have no idea what's best for you!"
4. "It sounds like you need more time to make a decision. Would you like me to contact your health care provider for you?"

5. A client with type 1 diabetes tells a nurse in the clinic, "I sometimes skip my insulin dose in the morning so I won't gain back any of the weight I've lost." Which response would be appropriate for the nurse to make to this client?
1. "Oh, I didn't realize that holding off on insulin would keep the weight off!"
2. "You are worried about your weight? There are safer ways to prevent weight gain."
3. "Guess there is a good side to having diabetes!"
4. "Why bother to take any insulin? Hold off on it until you lose all the weight that you want."

6. A team conference has been called to discuss alternative treatment for a Jehovah's Witnesses client who has a hemoglobin level of 5.5 g/dL. Which fact regarding the religious beliefs of a Jehovah's Witness should be explained to the team during the conference?
1. A Jehovah's Witness is not allowed to take any medication.
2. Faith healing can be used as an alternative in this religious group.
3. Food high in iron can be eaten only to increase the blood count.
4. A Jehovah's Witness is forbidden from receiving blood products.

7. The health care provider prescribes 60 mEq of potassium chloride liquid as a one-time dose. The pharmacy supplies a liquid containing 20 mEq/15 mL. How many milliliters will the nurse administer? Record your answer using a whole number.

___45___ mL

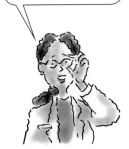

Sometimes the best intervention is to talk with your client.

4. 4. Even though the client is asking, the nurse shouldn't impose an opinion on the client. Instead, offer to contact the health care provider so more information can be provided; this will help the client make an informed decision. Offering opinions about the least painful option or that the health care provider's choice is best impose the nurse's opinion on the client. Brushing off the client's question with an angry retort is confrontational and offers the client no viable solution.
CN: Safe, effective care environment; CNS: Coordinated care; CL: Analyze; DIFFICULTY: Easy

5. 2. The nurse needs to ask the client more questions about his weight and begin instructing him in healthy ways to avoid gaining weight. Making references that connect withheld insulin to weight loss encourage the client not to take the prescribed medication, which would be dangerous to health. The comment that there's "a good side to diabetes" is incorrect and shouldn't be made.
CN: Safe, effective care environment; CNS: Coordinated care; CL: Apply; DIFFICULTY: Easy

6. 4. The administration of blood and blood products is forbidden in the Jehovah's Witnesses religion. A person who receives blood products can be excommunicated. A Jehovah's Witness is permitted to take medications and eat foods high in iron any time, not only when trying to increase the blood count. Faith healing isn't practiced in the Jehovah's Witnesses religion; therefore, it isn't appropriate to discuss this topic during the team conference.
CN: Safe, effective care environment; CNS: Coordinated care; CL: Apply; DIFFICULTY: Easy

7. 45.
The nurse can calculate the dose by setting up the following equation:

$$\frac{60 \text{ mEq}}{20 \text{ mEq}} = \frac{X \text{ mL}}{15 \text{ mL}}$$

Then cross multiply the fractions:

$$X \cdot 20 \text{ mEq} = 15 \text{ mL} \cdot 60 \text{ mEq}$$

Then solve for X:

$$X = 45 \text{ mL}$$

CN: Physiological integrity; CNS: Pharmacological therapies; CL: Analyze; DIFFICULTY: Easy

8. A client is in the bathroom when the nurse enters to give a prescribed medication. What is the appropriate action by the nurse?
1. Leave the medication at the client's bedside.
2. Tell the client to be sure to take the medication, and then leave it at the bedside.
3. Return shortly to the client's room and remain there until the client takes the medication.
4. Wait for the client to return to bed, and then leave the medication at the bedside.

8. **3.** The nurse should return shortly to the client's room and remain there until the client takes the medication to verify that it was taken as directed. The nurse should never leave medication at a client's bedside.
CN: Safe, effective care environment; CNS: Safety and infection control; CL: Apply; DIFFICULTY: Easy

9. The nurse is caring for an infant with suspected transposition of the great arteries (TGA). Which diagnostic test will the nurse prepare the infant and family for?
1. Blood cultures
2. Cardiac catheterization
3. Chest x-ray
4. Echocardiogram

9. **3.** Chest x-ray would be done first to visualize congenital heart diseases such as TGA. Blood cultures won't diagnose TGA. Cardiac catheterization and an echocardiogram would be done after TGA is seen on the chest x-ray.
CN: Health promotion and maintenance; CNS: None; CL: Apply; DIFFICULTY: Challenge

10. Four children, each 6 months of age, arrive at the clinic for diphtheria-pertussis-tetanus (DPT) immunization. Which child can safely be immunized at this time?
1. The child with a temperature of 103° F (39.4° C)
2. The child with a runny nose and cough
3. The child taking prednisone for the treatment of leukemia
4. The child with difficulty breathing after the last immunization

10. **2.** Children with cold symptoms can safely receive DPT immunization. Children with a temperature more than 102° F (38.9° C), serious reactions to previous immunizations, or those receiving immunosuppressive therapy shouldn't receive DPT immunization.
CN: Health promotion and maintenance; CNS: None; CL: Analyze; DIFFICULTY: Moderate

11. A nurse is reinforcing discharge instructions to the parents of a child who had a tonsillectomy. Which instruction is the **most** important?
1. The child should drink extra milk.
2. The child shouldn't drink from straws.
3. Orange juice should be given to provide pain control.
4. Rinse the mouth with salt water to provide pain relief.

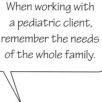

When working with a pediatric client, remember the needs of the whole family.

11. **2.** Straws and other sharp objects inserted into the mouth could disrupt the clot at the operative site. Extra milk wouldn't promote healing and may encourage mucus production. Although drinking orange juice and rinsing with salt water will irritate the tissue at the operative site, irritation doesn't pose the same level of danger as clot disruption.
CN: Physiological integrity; CNS: Basic care and comfort; CL: Apply; DIFFICULTY: Challenge

12. A 2-year-old child is diagnosed with bronchiolitis caused by respiratory syncytial virus (RSV). The client has an 8-year-old sibling. Which statement is correct?
1. RSV isn't highly communicable in infants.
2. RSV isn't communicable to older children and adults.
3. The 2-year-old client must be admitted to the hospital for isolation.
4. The siblings should be separated to prevent the spread of the infection.

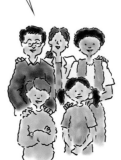

12. **4.** RSV is communicable among children and adults, so the siblings should be separated to prevent the spread of the infection. Older children and adults may have mild symptoms of the disorder. Hospitalization is indicated only for children who need oxygen and IV therapy.
CN: Safe, effective care environment; CNS: Safety and infection control; CL: Analyze; DIFFICULTY: Moderate

13. A child with asthma uses a peak expiratory flow meter in school. The results indicate the peak flow is in the yellow zone. Which intervention by the school nurse is appropriate?
  1. Follow the child's routine asthma treatment plan.
  2. Monitor for signs and symptoms of an acute attack and review the child's treatment plan.
  3. Call 911 and prepare for transport to the nearest emergency department.
  4. Call the child's parent to take the child to the family health care provider immediately.

14. Parents of a child with asthma are trying to identify possible allergens in their household. Which common inhaled allergen will be a **priority** for the parents to attempt to eliminate?
  1. Perfume
  2. Dust mites
  3. Passive smoke
  4. Dog or cat dander

15. A neonate was admitted to the pediatric unit with an unexpected congenital defect. What's the **best** way to involve the parents in the infant's care?
  1. Assume the parents have already been told how to care for their infant.
  2. Offer the parents opportunities to be involved with the infant's care while they adjust to this unexpected condition.
  3. Tell the parents that they'll be shown how to do everything for the infant one time before they take the child home.
  4. Don't show the parents how to care for the infant at this time.

16. The nurse is teaching child safety to the parents of a 6-month-old who's beginning to crawl. Which point should the nurse include in the education?
  1. Keeping furniture with sharp corners out of the area where the infant crawls
  2. Padding the infant's knees
  3. Allowing the infant to crawl on a blanket only
  4. Placing the infant in a baby walker instead of encouraging crawling

17. The nurse is reinforcing education for a parent about how to administer antibiotics at home to a toddler with acute otitis media. Which statement by the parent indicates that teaching has been successful?
  1. "I'll give the antibiotics for the full 10-day course of treatment."
  2. "I'll give the antibiotics until my child's ear pain is gone."
  3. "Whenever my child is cranky or pulls on an ear, I'll give a dose of antibiotics."
  4. "If the ear pain is gone, there's no need to see the health care provider for another examination of the ears."

13. 2. The routine treatment plan may be insufficient when the peak flow is in the yellow zone (50% to 80% of personal best). The child should be monitored to determine if an asthma attack is imminent and the treatment plan should be reviewed to see if revisions are needed. There's no immediate need to see the health care provider if the child is asymptomatic. This isn't an emergency situation.
CN: Physiological integrity; CNS: Reduction of risk potential; CL: Apply; DIFFICULTY: Moderate

14. 2. The household dust mite is the most commonly inhaled allergen that can cause an asthma attack. Perfume, passive smoke, and animal dander are allergens that can cause asthma attacks but aren't as common as dust mites.
CN: Safe, effective care environment; CNS: Safety and infection control; CL: Apply; DIFFICULTY: Moderate

15. 2. Many new parents need to grieve over the loss of a "normal" child. Adequate time and support should be given for the parents to adjust to the unexpected condition of their child. Never assume that the parents have already been educated about the infant's care or that they'll be able to learn everything they need to know after receiving instructions only once. The parents should be involved in the infant's care during hospitalization; this will help them learn and will instill confidence.
CN: Safe, effective care environment; CNS: Coordinated care; CL: Apply; DIFFICULTY: Easy

16. 1. Keeping furniture with sharp corners away from the infant who's beginning to crawl prevents injury. Padding the knees isn't necessary. An infant won't remain on a blanket when crawling. Baby walkers are dangerous and their use shouldn't be encouraged.
CN: Safe, effective care environment; CNS: Safety and infection control; CL: Apply; DIFFICULTY: Easy

17. 1. Antibiotics must be given for the full course of therapy, even if the child feels well; otherwise, the infection won't be eradicated. Antibiotics should be taken at prescribed intervals to maintain blood levels and not as needed for pain. A reexamination at the end of the course of antibiotics is necessary to confirm that the infection is resolved. If the infection is still present, additional antibiotic therapy will be prescribed.
CN: Physiological integrity; CNS: Pharmacological therapies; CL: Apply; DIFFICULTY: Easy

CN: Client needs category   CNS: Client needs subcategory   CL: Cognitive level

18. The nurse is reinforcing education about injury prevention to the parents of a toddler. Which instruction is appropriate for the nurse to tell the parents?
1. The toddler should wear a helmet when rollerblading.
2. Place locks on cabinets containing toxic substances.
3. Teach the toddler water safety.
4. Don't allow the toddler to use pillows when sleeping.

19. Parents of a 15-month-old are concerned that their child says "no" to everything. Which statement by the nurse would be an appropriate response?
1. "Place your child in an appropriate time-out."
2. "Ignore the behavior and the child will grow out of it."
3. "Explain to your child that saying 'no' all the time is inappropriate behavior."
4. "Saying 'no' is part of toddler development and is normal at this age."

20. The nurse is caring for a child with a fractured leg. The parents become concerned when visiting and notice the child sucking the thumb, a behavior previously given up. What does this behavior indicate?
1. The child is depressed.
2. The child is in pain.
3. The child wants attention.
4. The child is responding to stress.

21. The nurse is teaching a group of parents about normal toddler development. When talking about toddlers' play, the nurse should include which point?
1. They play with similar objects *nearby* other children rather than with them.
2. They become interactive with children around them.
3. They willingly share toys with other children.
4. They play with one toy for a long period because they have long attention spans.

22. Parents bring their 13-month-old toddler to the clinic. The toddler has erythema and small vesicles that ooze on the buttocks. Which instruction should the nurse give the parents?
1. Change diapers frequently and air-dry when possible.
2. Apply permethrin cream, leave it on for 8 hours, and then bathe the child.
3. Wash all bed linens and clothing with hot water.
4. Use cloth diapers and rubber pants until the rash heals.

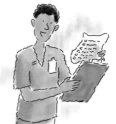

Dealing with mean clients makes me want to suck my thumb.

18. 2. All household cleaners and poisons should be secured with childproof locks. The toddler's curiosity and the ability to climb and open doors and drawers makes poisoning a concern in this age-group. Rollerblading isn't an appropriate activity for toddlers. Toddlers lack the cognitive development to understand water safety. (Note that rollerblading protection and teaching water safety are appropriate for school-age children.) Pillows shouldn't be placed in the crib of an infant to avoid suffocation; however, toddlers may use them.
CN: Safe, effective care environment; CNS: Safety and infection control; CL: Apply; DIFFICULTY: Easy

19. 4. Saying "no" is normal at this age. The child is attempting to exert independence. Punishing the child with a time-out is not appropriate because this is a normal stage of development. Ignoring the behavior is also inappropriate because the child needs to learn about limits. Children at this age may not understand all that they say because they repeat what they hear.
CN: Health promotion and maintenance; CNS: None; CL: Apply; DIFFICULTY: Easy

20. 4. Regression (reverting back to previously outgrown behaviors) is a common response to stressful situations. The nurse should reassure the parents that thumb sucking and other regressive behaviors should disappear after the stressful situation is resolved. Thumb sucking isn't a sign of depression or pain or an attention-seeking behavior.
CN: Psychosocial integrity; CNS: None; CL: Apply; DIFFICULTY: Easy

21. 1. During the toddler stage, children typically engage in parallel play with others. They play side by side, usually with similar objects, without actually interacting. Preschool-age children become interactive with other children and they have a better concept of sharing than toddlers do. Preschoolers may also play with toys for longer periods because they have longer attention spans than toddlers.
CN: Psychosocial integrity; CNS: None; CL: Apply; DIFFICULTY: Easy

22. 1. The child shows signs of diaper dermatitis. Therefore, the nurse should instruct the parent to change the child's diapers frequently, air-dry if possible, and avoid rubber pants. Permethrin cream and washing all bed linens and clothing with hot water are indicated for the treatment of scabies, not diaper dermatitis.
CN: Physiological integrity; CNS: Reduction of risk potential; CL: Apply; DIFFICULTY: Easy

CN: Client needs category   CNS: Client needs subcategory   CL: Cognitive level

23. A parent expresses concern over a toddler's eating habits, stating the toddler eats very little and consumes only a single type of food for weeks on end. Which instruction is **most** helpful?
1. This is normal toddler behavior.
2. This is indicative of an eating disorder.
3. The health care provider will assess for a nutrient deficiency.
4. The feeding pattern is a form of control and indicates a behavioral pattern.

24. When teaching the parents of a toddler with congenital heart disease, the nurse should explain all medical treatments and emphasize which instruction?
1. "Reduce your child's caloric intake to decrease cardiac demand."
2. "Relax discipline and limit-setting to prevent crying."
3. "Make sure your child avoids contact with small children to reduce overstimulation."
4. "Try to maintain your child's usual lifestyle to promote normal development."

25. Which complementary therapy might calm a 4-year-old who has separation anxiety when the child's parents leave the hospital?
1. Acupuncture
2. Acupressure
3. Music therapy
4. Aromatherapy

26. A child is to receive phenytoin, 5 mg/kg by mouth each day. When teaching the parents about the medication regimen, the nurse should use which approach?
1. Conduct brief education sessions, provide written materials during each visit, and repeat information as appropriate.
2. Ask the parents to spend an entire day at the facility so they can learn every detail about their child's care.
3. Call the parents at home and explain everything, allowing time for them to ask questions.
4. Send the parents the drug packaging insert so they can become familiar with the medication.

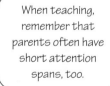
When teaching, remember that parents often have short attention spans, too.

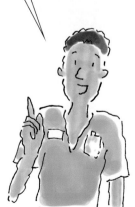

23. 1. Erratic eating is typical of toddlers. The physiologic need for food decreases at about age 18 months as growth declines from the rapid rate characteristic of infancy. The toddler also develops strong food and taste preferences, sometimes eating just one type of food for days or weeks and then switching to another. The child should not be forced to eat. Typically, the child switches to another food spontaneously after a while, correcting any nutritional imbalances. Parents may encourage the child to eat other foods by offering items from the various food groups at each meal. Erratic eating habits in toddlers are not characteristic of an eating disorder, a nutrient deficiency, or a behavioral problem.
CN: Health promotion and maintenance; CNS: None; CL: Analyze; DIFFICULTY: Easy

24. 4. Parents of a child with a congenital heart defect should treat the child normally and allow self-limited activity. Reducing the child's caloric intake wouldn't necessarily reduce cardiac demand. Altering disciplinary patterns and deliberately preventing crying or interactions with other children could foster maladaptive behaviors. Contact with peers promotes normal growth and development.
CN: Health promotion and maintenance; CNS: None; CL: Apply; DIFFICULTY: Easy

25. 3. Music therapy has proven effective in calming children. Acupuncture, acupressure, and aromatherapy aren't indicated for soothing children.
CN: Physiological integrity; CNS: Basic care and comfort; CL: Analyze; DIFFICULTY: Easy

26. 1. Effective teaching methods include providing simple instructions in short sessions, providing written materials, repeating information, and allowing time for questions. The other options are ineffective teaching strategies that may be overwhelming for the parents and frustrating for the nurse.
CN: Health promotion and maintenance; CNS: None; CL: Apply; DIFFICULTY: Easy

27. When administering medication to a pre-schooler at 9 a.m., which approach by the nurse is **best**?
1. "It's time for you to take your medicine right now."
2. "If you take your medicine now, you will go home sooner."
3. "Here is your medicine. Would you like apple juice or water after?"
4. "Do you want to take your morning medication now?"

28. The nurse is caring for a 4-year-old with a full-thickness burn. Before sending the child to hydrotherapy for a scheduled wound debridement, which nursing action is a **priority**?
1. Administer a fluid bolus of 500 mL
2. Initiate antibiotics as prescribed
3. Implement pain control measures
4. Provide high-protein drinks

29. A preschooler with a history of heart failure is prescribed digoxin. Which nursing intervention is most important to perform before administering this drug to a child?
1. Check apical heart rate for 1 minute
2. Obtain the child's blood pressure
3. Count the child's respiratory rate for 1 minute
4. Measure the child's urine output

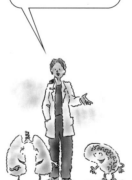

Morphine depresses the part of the brain that controls what essential function? Take a deep breath ... it will come to you.

30. The nurse is caring for a preschool-age child who sustained burns in a house fire. The child is prescribed morphine every 4 hours for pain. Which assessment parameter is **most** important when monitoring a child who's receiving morphine?
1. Pulse
2. Respirations
3. Temperature
4. Blood pressure

31. A preschool-age child scheduled for surgery in the morning is admitted to the facility for the first time. Which nursing action would ease the child's anxiety?
1. Beginning preoperative teaching as soon as possible
2. Explaining that the child will be "put to sleep" during the operation and will feel nothing
3. Having the child act out the surgical experience using dolls and medical equipment
4. Explaining preoperative and postoperative procedures step by step

27. 3. Involving the child by offering a choice promotes cooperation and permits the child to make appropriate choices, enhancing a sense of control. Telling a child to take the medicine "right now" could provoke a negative response. Promising that the child will go home sooner could decrease the child's trust in nurses and health care providers. Asking a question with a potential "no" response is not the best approach.
CN: Psychosocial integrity; CNS: None; CL: Apply; DIFFICULTY: Easy

28. 3. Because hydrotherapy is painful, the nurse should implement pain control measures before the treatment begins. Fluids and nutritional supplements can be given at any time and are not required specifically before hydrotherapy. Antibiotics should be administered according to a specified schedule without regard to treatment measures.
CN: Physiological integrity; CNS: Pharmacological therapies; CL: Apply; DIFFICULTY: Easy

29. 1. The child's apical pulse rate should be counted for 1 minute before digoxin administration. If the heart rate is below the specified rate in the health care provider's order (typically, 90 to 110 beats/minute for infants and young children), the dose should be withheld and the health care provider should be notified. Digoxin doesn't affect blood pressure, respiratory rate, or urine output.
CN: Physiological integrity; CNS: Pharmacological therapies; CL: Apply; DIFFICULTY: Easy

30. 2. Morphine depresses the brain's respiratory center; therefore, the nurse should assess the child's respirations to make sure breathing isn't compromised. Assessing for pulse, temperature, and blood pressure is also important but these measurements don't take priority over monitoring the child's respiratory status.
CN: Physiological integrity; CNS: Basic care and comfort; CL: Apply; DIFFICULTY: Easy

31. 3. Having the child act out the surgical experience using dolls and medical equipment would ease anxiety and give the nurse an opportunity to clarify the child's misconceptions. Preschoolers have a limited concept of time, so the nurse should provide preoperative teaching *just before* surgery rather than starting it as soon as possible; also, a delay between teaching and surgery may heighten anxiety by giving the child a chance to worry or fantasize. The nurse should avoid using such phrases as "put to sleep" because these may have a dual or negative meaning to a young child. Long explanations are inappropriate for the preschooler's developmental level and may increase anxiety.
CN: Psychosocial integrity; CNS: None; CL: Apply; DIFFICULTY: Easy

32. The nurse is evaluating a child with acute poststreptococcal glomerulonephritis (APSGN) for signs of improvement. Which early finding by the nurse would indicate that improvement is occurring?
1. Increased urine output
2. Increased appetite
3. Increased energy level
4. Decreased diarrhea

33. After collecting data on a newly admitted 5-year-old child, the nurse assists the team in making the nursing diagnosis of Parental Role Conflict related to child's hospitalization. Which defining characteristic would **most** suggest this diagnosis?
1. Supportive child-parent interaction (speaking, listening, touching, and eye-to-eye contact)
2. Parents' active participation in child's physical or emotional care
3. Parents' failure to use available support systems or agencies to assist in coping
4. Evidence of adaptation to parental role changes

34. The nurse is teaching a group of adolescent girls about personal hygiene. Which statement by an adolescent indicates the need for further education?
1. "It's important to bathe daily."
2. "It's unsafe to bathe during your period."
3. "I shouldn't share my razor with anyone."
4. "I shouldn't share my makeup with anyone."

35. To establish a good interview relationship with an adolescent, which strategy by the nurse is **most** appropriate?
1. Asking personal questions unrelated to the situation
2. Writing down everything the teen says
3. Asking open-ended questions
4. Discussing the nurse's own thoughts and feelings about the situation

36. How should the nurse proceed when discussing safe sexual practices with an adolescent?
1. Make sure the parent or legal guardian is present for the conversation.
2. Make sure the conversation remains within the confines of the adolescent's religious beliefs.
3. Assess the adolescent's level of knowledge and concerns.
4. Obtain an informed consent from the parent before initiating the discussion.

32. **1.** Increased urine output, a sign of improving kidney function, typically is the first sign that a child with APSGN is improving. Increased appetite, an increased energy level, and decreased diarrhea aren't specific to APSGN.
CN: Psychosocial integrity; CNS: None; CL: Apply; DIFFICULTY: Easy

33. **3.** A failure to use available support systems or agencies is one of the defining characteristics of this diagnosis. Supportive child-parent interaction, parents' active participation in the child's care, and evidence of adaptation to parental role changes don't suggest this diagnosis.
CN: Health Promotion and maintenance; CNS: None; CL: Analyze; DIFFICULTY: Easy

34. **2.** Although some religious and cultural beliefs prohibit bathing during menses, there's no physical basis for this practice. Bathing daily is important because of the physical changes that occur during adolescence, including menstruation. Sharing of razors should be avoided to prevent the transmission of blood-borne pathogens. Makeup shouldn't be shared because it may harbor bacteria.
CN: Health promotion and maintenance; CNS: None; CL: Analyze; DIFFICULTY: Easy

35. **3.** Open-ended questions allow the adolescent to share information and feelings. Asking personal questions not related to the situation jeopardizes the trust that must be established because the adolescent may feel as though he's being probed with unnecessary questions. Writing everything down during the interview can be a distraction and won't allow the nurse to observe how the adolescent behaves. Discussing the nurse's thoughts and feelings may bias the assessment and is inappropriate when interviewing any client.
CN: Psychosocial integrity; CNS: None; CL: Analyze; DIFFICULTY: Challenge

36. **3.** Before proceeding with a discussion about safe sexual practices, the nurse should assess the adolescent's current level of knowledge and any concerns he might have. The adolescent has the right to discuss sexuality issues without knowledge or consent of the parents. This discussion must remain confidential. The conversation doesn't have to remain within the confines of the adolescent's religious beliefs.
CN: Health promotion and maintenance; CNS: None; CL: Apply; DIFFICULTY: Easy

37. The nurse is gathering data from a female adolescent. Which statement made by the teen reveals an early indicator of anorexia nervosa?
1. "I have my menstrual period every 28 days."
2. "I go out to eat with my friends at least three times per week."
3. "I jog three times per day for a total of 5 hours per day."
4. "I try to maintain my weight around 115 lb, which is good for my height of 5 ft, 0 in.

38. A client has just undergone a bronchoscopy. Which **priority** nursing intervention will the nurse perform at this time?
1. Checking level of consciousness (LOC)
2. Checking airway patency
3. Recognizing personality changes
4. Evaluating intellectual ability

39. A client receiving long-term mechanical ventilation becomes very frustrated when trying to communicate. Which intervention should the nurse perform to assist the client?
1. Assure the client that everything will be all right and not to become upset.
2. Ask a family member to interpret what the client is trying to communicate.
3. Ask the health care provider to wean the client off the mechanical ventilator to allow the client to talk.
4. Ask the client to write, use a picture board, or spell words with an alphabet board.

40. After suctioning a tracheostomy, the nurse evaluates the client to determine the effectiveness of the suctioning. Which findings will the nurse document that indicates the airway is now patent?
1. A respiratory rate of 24 breaths/minute with accessory muscle use
2. Clear breath sounds and non-labored respirations
3. Increased pulse rate, rapid respirations, and cyanosis of the skin and nail beds
4. Restlessness, pallor, increased pulse and respiratory rates, and bubbling breath sounds

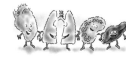

I love these organ recitals. Together we make some beautiful music.

37. 3. Excessive exercise, consumption of very small amounts of food, and food rituals are all signs of anorexia nervosa. Menstruation commonly stops, and the client's weight is below normal. Going out to eat with friends is a common adolescent social event and isn't a reliable indicator of anorexia nervosa. A weight of 115 lb (52 kg) is appropriate for someone who is 5 ft tall.
CN: Physiological integrity; CNS: Reduction of risk potential; CL: Analyze; DIFFICULTY: Easy

38. 2. After a bronchoscopy, checking the client's airway patency is the most important nursing intervention. After checking airway patency, the nurse should monitor the client's breathing and check vital signs every 15 minutes until they're stable. After these initial interventions, the nurse should check LOC. It isn't necessary to check for personality changes or intellectual ability at this time.
CN: Physiological integrity; CNS: Reduction of risk potential; CL: Apply; DIFFICULTY: Easy

39. 4. If the client uses an alternative method of communication, he will feel more in control and be less frustrated. Assuring the client that everything will be all right offers false reassurance. Telling the client not to be upset minimizes feelings. Neither of these methods helps the client to communicate. In a client with an endotracheal tube or tracheostomy tube, the family members are also likely to encounter difficulty interpreting the client's wishes. Making them responsible for interpreting the client's gestures may frustrate the family. The client may be weaned off a mechanical ventilator only when the physiologic parameters for weaning have been met.
CN: Psychosocial integrity; CNS: None; CL: Apply; DIFFICULTY: Easy

40. 2. Proper suctioning should produce a patent airway, as demonstrated by clear breath sounds and non-labored respirations. The other options suggest ineffective suctioning. A respiratory rate of 24 breaths/minute and accessory muscle use may indicate mild respiratory distress. Increased pulse rate, rapid respirations, and cyanosis are signs of hypoxia. Restlessness, pallor, increased pulse and respiratory rates, and bubbling breath sounds indicate respiratory secretion accumulation.
CN: Physiological integrity; CNS: Reduction of risk potential; CL: Apply; DIFFICULTY: Easy

H₂ ← COPD enlarge air spaces

41. A nurse, assigned to a client with emphysema, is providing shift report. Which nursing interventions would be appropriate to include? Select all that apply.

1. The nurse should reduce fluid intake to less than 850 mL per shift.
2. The nurse should teach diaphragmatic, pursed-lip breathing.
3. The nurse should administer low-flow oxygen.
4. The nurse should keep the client in a supine position as much as possible.
5. The nurse should encourage alternating activity with rest periods.
6. The nurse should teach the use of postural drainage and chest physiotherapy.

41. 2, 3, 5, 6. The nurse provides report on nursing interventions required for a client with emphysema. Diaphragmatic, pursed-lip breathing strengthens respiratory muscles and enhances oxygenation in clients with emphysema. Low-flow oxygen should be administered because a client with emphysema has chronic hypercapnia and a hypoxic respiratory drive. Alternating activity with rest allows the client to perform activities without excessive distress. If the client has difficulty mobilizing copious secretions, the nurse should teach the client and family members how to perform postural drainage and chest physiotherapy. Fluid intake should be increased to 3,000 mL/day, if not contraindicated, to liquefy secretions and facilitate their removal. The client should be placed in high Fowler's position to improve ventilation.
CN: Safe, effective care environment; CNS: Coordinated care; CL: Apply; DIFFICULTY: Difficult

42. A client comes to the emergency department with status asthmaticus. Based on the documentation note shown, the nurse suspects that the client has what abnormality?

Progress notes	
4/1/2017 1830	Pt. wheezing. RR 44, BP 140/90, P 104, T 98.4°F (36.9°C). ABG results show pH of 7.52, Pa_{CO_2} ↑ 30 mm Hg, HCO-3 26 mEq/L, and P_{O_2} 77 mm Hg. —C. Wynn, LPN

1. Respiratory acidosis
2. Respiratory alkalosis
3. Metabolic acidosis
4. Metabolic alkalosis

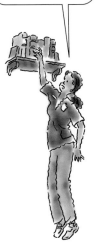

Hmm. Let's see … increased pH, decreased Pa_{CO_2} … which "osis" is that?

42. 2. Following review of the nursing documentation, the nurse notes respiratory alkalosis related to alveolar hyperventilation. Respiratory alkalosis is marked by an increase in pH to more than 7.45 and a concurrent decrease in partial pressure of arterial carbon dioxide (Pa_{CO_2}) to less than 35 mm Hg. Metabolic alkalosis shows the same increase in pH but also an increased bicarbonate level and normal Pa_{CO_2} (may be elevated also if compensatory mechanisms are working). Acidosis of any type means a low pH (below 7.35). Respiratory acidosis shows an elevated Pa_{CO_2} and a normal-to-high bicarbonate level. Metabolic acidosis is characterized by a decreased bicarbonate level and a normal-to-low Pa_{CO_2}.
CN: Physiological integrity; CNS: Physiological adaptation; CL: Analyze; DIFFICULTY: Moderate

43. The nurse is monitoring a client with the diagnosis of pulmonary edema. Which measurement can **best** be used to monitor the respiratory status of this client?

1. Arterial blood gas (ABG) analysis
2. Pulse oximetry
3. Skin color assessment
4. Lung sounds

43. 1. ABG analysis is the best measure for determining the extent of hypoxia caused by pulmonary edema and for monitoring the effects of therapy. The use of pulse oximetry is unreliable, especially in the case of severe vasoconstriction as is present in pulmonary edema. Although assessment of skin color and lung fields can be used to detect pulmonary changes, these options often are subject to interpretation by practitioners.
CN: Physiological integrity; CNS: Physiological adaptation; CL: Analysis; DIFFICULTY: Difficult

44. A nurse is verifying orders from a health care provider. Which diet will the nurse discuss with child and family related to a new diagnosis of celiac disease?
1. Low-fat diet
2. No-gluten diet
3. High-protein diet
4. No-phenylalanine diet

45. An adolescent client ingests a large number of acetaminophen tablets in an attempt to commit suicide. Which laboratory result is **most** consistent with an acetaminophen overdose?
1. Metabolic acidosis
2. Elevated liver enzyme levels
3. Increased serum creatinine level
4. Increased white blood cell (WBC) count

46. A client is undergoing a bedside thoracentesis. The nurse assists the client to an upright position with a table and pillow in front of him, supporting the arms. Which rationale does the nurse give to the client regarding this position?
1. Fluid will accumulate at the base of the lung.
2. There's less chance to injure lung tissue.
3. It allows for better expansion of the lung.
4. It's less painful for the client in this position.

47. The nurse is gathering data for an infant experiencing a sickle cell crisis. Which finding by the nurse is **most** significant to determine the state of hydration?
1. The infant has no bruises.
2. The infant has normal skin turgor.
3. The infant participates in exercise.
4. The infant maintains bladder control.

48. A nurse is caring for a client with dyspnea who has a resting respiratory rate of 44 breaths/minute and dusky nail beds. Arterial blood gases are obtained and the results are as follows: pH, 7.52; Pa_{O_2}, 50 mm Hg; Pa_{CO_2}, 28 mm Hg; HCO^-_3, 24 mEq/L. The nurse knows these results are consistent with which condition?
1. Metabolic acidosis
2. Metabolic alkalosis
3. Respiratory acidosis
4. Respiratory alkalosis

44. 2. The intestinal cells of individuals with celiac disease become inflamed when the child eats products containing gluten, such as wheat, rye, barley, or oats. The child with celiac disease needs normal amounts of fat and protein in the diet for growth and development. Omitting phenylalanine products would be appropriate for the client with phenylketonuria.
CN: Physiological integrity; CNS: Basic care and comfort; CL: Apply; DIFFICULTY: Easy

45. 2. Elevated liver enzyme levels, which could indicate liver damage, are associated with acetaminophen overdose. Metabolic acidosis isn't associated with acetaminophen overdose. An increased serum creatinine level may indicate renal damage. An increased WBC count indicates infection.
CN: Physiological integrity; CNS: Pharmacological therapies; CL: Apply; DIFFICULTY: Easy

46. 1. Fluids will drain and collect in the dependent positions. There's a risk of pneumothorax regardless of the client's position. The upright position doesn't allow for better expansion of the lung because the fluid in the pleural space is preventing this. Thoracentesis is done using local anesthesia, so it isn't painful.
CN: Physiological integrity; CNS: Physiological adaptation; CL: Analyze; DIFFICULTY: Challenge

47. 2. Normal skin turgor indicates the infant isn't severely dehydrated. Dehydration may cause sickle cell crisis or worsen a crisis. Bruising isn't associated with sickle cell crisis. Bed rest is preferable during a sickle cell crisis. Bladder control may be lost when oral or IV fluid intake is increased during a sickle cell crisis.
CN: Physiological integrity; CNS: Physiological adaptation; CL: Analyze; DIFFICULTY: Moderate

48. 4. A pH greater than 7.45 and a partial pressure of arterial carbon dioxide (Pa_{CO_2}) less than 35 mm Hg indicate respiratory alkalosis. A pH less than 7.35 and a bicarbonate (HCO^-_3) less than 22 mEq/L indicate metabolic acidosis. A pH greater than 7.45 and an HCO^-_3 greater than 24 mEq/L indicate metabolic alkalosis. A pH less than 7.35 and a Pa_{CO_2} greater than 45 mm Hg indicate respiratory acidosis.
CN: Physiological integrity; CNS: Reduction of risk potential; CL: Apply; DIFFICULTY: Moderate

49. A client with chronic alcohol use is admitted to the hospital for detoxification. Later that day, the blood pressure increases and the client is given lorazepam to prevent which complication?

1. Stroke
2. Seizure
3. Fainting
4. Anxiety reaction

50. Which action displayed by a grieving husband over his dying wife would cause the nurse to suggest counseling?

1. He takes out wedding pictures and memorabilia to show to the staff.
2. He refuses to acknowledge his wife's family and blames them for her current health problems.
3. He has already planned his wife's funeral.
4. He is planning to give away his wife's treasured items to family members.

51. A client exhibits signs of heightened anxiety. Which response by the nurse is **most** likely to reduce the client's anxiety?

1. "Everything will be fine. Don't worry."
2. "Read this manual and then ask me any questions you may have."
3. "Why don't you listen to the radio?"
4. "Let's talk about what is bothering you."

52. When discussing activities that are safe for the school-age child with hemophilia, which activities should the nurse encourage? Select all that apply.

1. Baseball
2. Cross-country running
3. Football
4. Swimming
5. Leisure walking

53. A nurse is caring for a client recently diagnosed with acute pancreatitis. Which statement indicates that a short-term goal of nursing care has been met?

1. The client denies abdominal pain.
2. The client doesn't report that he is overly thirsty.
3. The client denies pain at McBurney's point.
4. The client swallows liquids without coughing.

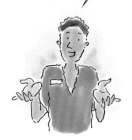

Many expressions of grief are normal. We're looking for ones that are excessive or exaggerated.

49. 2. During detoxification from alcohol, changes in the client's physiologic status, especially an increase in blood pressure, may indicate an increased risk for seizure. Clients are treated with benzodiazepines to prevent this occurrence. Stroke, fainting, and anxiety aren't the primary concerns when withdrawing from alcohol.
CN: Physiological integrity; CNS: Pharmacological therapies; CL: Apply; DIFFICULTY: Challenge

50. 2. Abnormal grief may manifest itself as exaggerated or excessive expressions of normal grief reactions, such as anger, sadness, or depression. It's therapeutic to review a person's life with loved ones. Funeral planning can be therapeutic because it allows the individual to do one last thing for his loved one. It's therapeutic to share treasured items with staff and other family members.
CN: Physiological integrity; CNS: None; CL: Apply; DIFFICULTY: Easy

51. 4. Anxiety may result from feelings of helplessness, isolation, or insecurity. This response helps reduce anxiety by encouraging the client to express feelings. The nurse should be supportive and develop goals together with the client to give the client some control over an anxiety-inducing situation. Because the other options ignore the client's feelings and block communication, they wouldn't reduce anxiety.
CN: Psychosocial integrity; CNS: None; CL: Apply; DIFFICULTY: Easy

52. 4, 5. Swimming is a noncontact sport with low risk of traumatic injury. Baseball, cross-country running, and football all involve a risk of trauma from falling, sliding, or contact. Leisure walking is a good low-impact activity that has a low risk of injury and promotes exercise.
CN: Physiological integrity; CNS: Physiological adaptation; CL: Apply; DIFFICULTY: Moderate

53. 1. Pancreatitis is accompanied by acute pain from autodigestion by pancreatic enzymes. When the client denies abdominal pain, the short-term goal of pain control is met. Clients with acute pancreatitis receive IV fluids and may not have a sensation of thirst. Pain at McBurney's point accompanies appendicitis. Clients with acute pancreatitis receive nothing by mouth during initial therapy.
CN: Physiological integrity; CNS: Physiological adaptation; CL: Apply; DIFFICULTY: Moderate

54. A health care provider prescribes acetaminophen gr X (10 grains) as necessary every 4 hours for pain for a client in a long-term care facility. How many milligrams of acetaminophen should the nurse give? Record your answer using a whole number.

_450_

_____ mg

55. A client stepped on a piece of sharp glass while walking barefoot and comes to the emergency department with a deep laceration on the bottom of the foot. Which question is the **most** important for the nurse to ask?
1. "Was the glass dirty?"
2. "Are you immune to tetanus?"
3. "When did you have your last tetanus shot?"
4. "How many diphtheria-tetanus-pertussis (DTaP) shots did you receive as a child?"

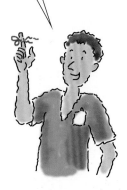

Remember to convert grains to milligrams.

56. A postmenopausal client asks a nurse how to prevent osteoporosis. Which response by the nurse is **best**?
1. "Take a multivitamin daily."
2. "After menopause, there's no way to prevent osteoporosis."
3. "Drink two glasses of milk each day and swim three times per week."
4. "Do weight-bearing exercises regularly."

57. A young adult client received her first chemotherapy treatment for breast cancer. Which statement by the client requires further exploration by the nurse?
1. "I'm thinking about joining a dance club."
2. "I don't think I'm going to work tomorrow."
3. "I don't care about the adverse effects of the drugs."
4. "I want to return to school for a college degree."

58. A client diagnosed with cardiomyopathy saw a posting on the Internet describing research about a new herbal treatment for the disorder. When the client asks about this research, which response is most appropriate?
1. "Herbs are commonly used to treat cardiomyopathy."
2. "Cardiomyopathy can be treated only by heart surgery."
3. "The Internet is a reliable source of research, verify the treatment."
4. "Research found on the Internet should be verified with a health care provider."

54. 650.
Use the following equation:

One grain = 65 mg; $10 \times 65 = 650$ mg.

CN: Physiological integrity; CNS: Pharmacological therapies; CL: Apply; DIFFICULTY: Difficult

55. 3. Questioning the client about the date of the last tetanus immunization is important because the booster immunization should be received every 10 years in adulthood (or at the time of the injury if the last booster immunization was given more than 5 years before the injury). Whether the client noticed dirt on the glass is immaterial because all deep lacerations require a tetanus immunization or booster. A client wouldn't know the tetanus immune status. DTaP immunizations in childhood don't give lifelong immunization to tetanus.
CN: Safe, effective care environment; CNS: Safety and infection control; CL: Apply; DIFFICULTY: Easy

56. 4. Weight-bearing exercises are recommended for the prevention of osteoporosis. Telling the client that there's no way to prevent osteoporosis would be an incorrect statement. A multivitamin doesn't provide adequate calcium for a postmenopausal woman, and calcium alone won't prevent osteoporosis. Two glasses of milk per day don't provide the daily requirements for adult women. Swimming isn't a weight-bearing exercise.
CN: Health promotion and maintenance; CNS: None; CL: Apply; DIFFICULTY: Moderate

57. 3. Adverse effects of chemotherapy may occur after treatment and should be discussed with the client because some can be treated, controlled, or prevented. The nurse needs to explore the client's meaning when she indicates apathy about the adverse effects of chemotherapy drugs. The client may feel poorly after chemotherapy and may want to take time off from work until she feels better. Joining social clubs and returning to school is typical behavior for a young adult.
CN: Psychosocial integrity; CNS: None; CL: Analyze; DIFFICULTY: Moderate

58. 4. Although the Internet contains some valid medical research, there's no control over the validity of information posted. The research should be discussed with a health care provider, who can verify the accuracy of the information. Herbs aren't standard treatment for cardiomyopathy. Cardiomyopathy is treatable with drugs or surgery.
CN: Psychosocial integrity; CNS: Coordinated care; CL: Apply; DIFFICULTY: Easy

CN: Client needs category   CNS: Client needs subcategory   CL: Cognitive level

59. A client is diagnosed with prehypertension. Which treatment option would **most** likely be included in the client's treatment plan?
1. Diuretics
2. Lifestyle modification instructions
3. Beta-adrenergic blockers
4. Angiotensin-converting enzyme (ACE) inhibitors

60. A client comes to the health care provider's office for a follow-up visit 4 weeks after suffering a myocardial infarction (MI). The nurse takes this opportunity to evaluate the client's knowledge of the prescribed cardiac rehabilitation program. Which evaluation statement suggests that the client needs more instruction?
1. "Client performs relaxation exercises three times per day to reduce stress."
2. "Client's 24-hour dietary recall reveals low intake of fat and cholesterol."
3. "Client verbalizes an understanding of the need to seek emergency help if the heart rate increases markedly while at rest."
4. "Client walks 4 miles (6.4 km) in 1 hour every day."

61. The nurse is caring for a client experiencing dyspnea, dependent edema, hepatomegaly, crackles, and jugular vein distention. Which condition should the nurse suspect?
1. Pulmonary embolism
2. Heart failure
3. Cardiac tamponade
4. Tension pneumothorax

62. The nurse is performing an electrocardiogram (ECG) for a client with chest pain. Which position will the nurse place the client in that will provide the best results?
1. Fowler's
2. Supine
3. Lateral
4. Prone

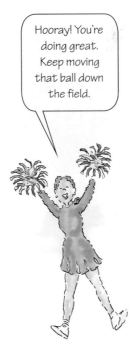

Hooray! You're doing great. Keep moving that ball down the field.

59. 2. Prehypertension signals the need for teaching about lifestyle modifications to prevent hypertension. Lifestyle modifications may include dietary changes, adopting relaxation techniques, regular exercise, smoking cessation, limiting intake of alcohol, and restricting sodium and saturated fat intake. Diuretics, beta-adrenergic blockers, and ACE inhibitors are used to treat hypertension.
CN: Health promotion and maintenance; CNS: None; CL: Apply; DIFFICULTY: Easy

60. 4. Four weeks after an MI, a client's walking program should aim for a goal of 2 miles (3.2 km) in less than 1 hour. Walking 4 miles (6.4 km) in 1 hour is excessive and may induce another MI by increasing the heart's oxygen demands. Therefore, this client requires appropriate exercise guidelines and precautions. The other options indicate understanding of the cardiac rehabilitation program. The client should reduce stress, which speeds the heart rate and thus increases myocardial oxygen demands. Reducing dietary fat and cholesterol intake helps lower the risk of atherosclerosis. A sudden rise in the heart rate while at rest warrants emergency medical attention because it may signal a life-threatening dysrhythmia and increase myocardial oxygen demands.
CN: Physiological integrity; CNS: Reduction of risk potential; CL: Apply; DIFFICULTY: Moderate

61. 2. A client with heart failure has decreased cardiac output caused by the heart's decreased pumping ability. A buildup of fluid occurs, causing dyspnea, dependent edema, hepatomegaly, crackles, and jugular vein distention. A client with pulmonary embolism experiences acute shortness of breath, pleuritic chest pain, hemoptysis, and fever. A client with cardiac tamponade experiences muffled heart sounds, hypotension, and elevated central venous pressure. A client with tension pneumothorax has a deviated trachea and absent breath sounds on the affected side as well as dyspnea and jugular vein distention.
CN: Physiological integrity; CNS: Physiological adaptation; CL: Apply; DIFFICULTY: Moderate

62. 2. The most appropriate position for a client undergoing an ECG is lying flat, as long as the client can tolerate being in a supine position. Otherwise, the client may be positioned with the head of the bed slightly elevated.
CN: Physiological integrity; CNS: Reduction of risk potential; CL: Apply; DIFFICULTY: Challenge

63. A nurse is caring for a client with a diagnosis of pericarditis. Which statement might indicate a violation of client confidentiality?
1. The nurse discussed the client's diagnosis with another nurse at shift report.
2. The nurse discussed the client's diagnosis with a family friend over the telephone.
3. The nurse discussed the client's medication therapy with the health care provider.
4. The nurse discussed the client's medication therapy with the hospital pharmacist.

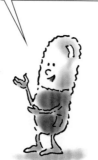

Be careful. I have a habit of getting wasted on potassium. Wait ... I mean wasting potassium.

64. The nurse administers furosemide to treat a client with heart failure. Which adverse effect must the nurse watch for **most** carefully?
1. Increase in blood pressure
2. Increase in blood volume
3. Low serum potassium level
4. High serum sodium level

65. A client is admitted to the emergency department after reporting acute chest pain radiating down the left arm. The client is anxious, dyspneic, and diaphoretic. Which laboratory studies would the nurse anticipate preparing the client for? Select all that apply.
1. Hemoglobin and hematocrit (HCT)
2. Serum glucose
3. Creatine kinase (CK)
4. Troponin T and troponin I
5. Myoglobin
6. Blood urea nitrogen (BUN)

66. A client reported chest pain and received sublingual nitroglycerin. Which statement by the client indicates that this drug is producing its therapeutic effect?
1. "I have a bad headache."
2. "My chest pain is decreasing."
3. "I feel a tingling sensation around my mouth."
4. "My blood pressure must be up because my vision is blurred."

67. A client newly diagnosed with heart failure is placed on bed rest and states, "Why do I have to stay in the bed?" What is the nurse's **best** response to this concern?
1. "It will improve the heart's pumping action."
2. "It will enhance arterial oxygenation."
3. "It will decrease fluid volume in the heart."
4. "It will reduce the heart's workload."

63. 2. Violation of confidentiality occurs when client information is discussed with nonmedical persons, such as family or friends, without the client's permission. It is appropriate to discuss a client's diagnosis with other members of the health care team.
CN: Safe, effective care environment; CNS: Coordinated care; CL: Apply; DIFFICULTY: Easy

64. 3. Furosemide is a potassium-wasting diuretic. The nurse must monitor the serum potassium level and assess for signs of low potassium. As water and sodium are lost in the urine, blood pressure decreases, blood volume decreases, and urine output increases.
CN: Physiological integrity; CNS: Pharmacological therapies; CL: Apply; DIFFICULTY: Moderate

65. 3, 4, 5. With myocardial ischemia or infarction, levels of CK, troponin T, and troponin I typically rise because of cellular damage. Myoglobin elevation is an early indicator of myocardial damage. Hemoglobin, HCT, serum glucose, and BUN levels do not provide information related to myocardial ischemia.
CN: Physiological integrity; CNS: Reduction of risk potential; CL: Analyze; DIFFICULTY: Challenge

66. 2. Nitroglycerin, a vasodilator, increases the arterial supply of oxygen-rich blood to the myocardium, thus producing its intended effect: relief of chest pain. Headache is an adverse effect of nitroglycerin. The drug shouldn't cause a tingling sensation around the mouth and should lower, not raise, blood pressure.
CN: Physiological integrity; CNS: Pharmacological therapies; CL: Analyze; DIFFICULTY: Easy

67. 4. Bed rest reduces the heart's workload by decreasing tissue demand for oxygen. Bed rest doesn't improve the heart's pumping action; medications such as digoxin are usually given to achieve this. Oxygen is administered to enhance arterial oxygenation. A diuretic, not bed rest, helps to decrease fluid volume.
CN: Physiological integrity; CNS: Physiological adaptation; CL: Analyze; DIFFICULTY: Easy

68. For a client who has had an acute myocardial infarction (MI), which of the following interventions should be included in the plan of care to assist with bowel elimination and prevent straining?
1. Maintain complete bed rest.
2. Limit fluid intake.
3. Administer a stool softener.
4. Provide a low-fat diet.

69. When collecting data from a client who reports recent chest pain, the nurse obtains a thorough history. Which statement by the client **most** strongly suggests angina pectoris?
1. "The pain lasted about 45 minutes."
2. "The pain resolved after I ate a sandwich."
3. "The pain got worse when I took a deep breath."
4. "The pain occurred while I was mowing the lawn."

70. The nurse is caring for a stable client with digoxin toxicity. Which treatment does the nurse anticipate for this client?
1. Activated charcoal
2. Time and symptomatic treatment
3. Hemodialysis
4. Atropine

71. A nurse is caring for a client who has been administered digoxin 0.125 mg by mouth daily. The client develops sinus bradycardia with a heart rate of 50 beats/minute and other vital signs are stable. Which action should the nurse take **first**?
1. Notify the health care provider.
2. Retake the vital signs in 2 hours.
3. Stop the medication.
4. Have the client turn on the left side.

68. 3. Administering a stool softener helps the client pass stools without straining. Maintaining bed rest and limiting fluids may cause constipation and increase the client's need to strain with each bowel movement. A low-fat diet doesn't assist with elimination.
CN: Physiological integrity; CNS: Basic care and comfort;
CL: Apply; DIFFICULTY: Easy

69. 4. Angina pectoris is chest pain caused by a decreased oxygen supply to the myocardium. Lawn mowing increases the cardiac workload; this, in turn, increases the heart's need for oxygen and may precipitate angina. Anginal pain typically is self-limiting and lasts 5 to 15 minutes. Food consumption doesn't reduce this pain, although it may ease pain caused by a GI ulcer. Deep breathing has no effect on anginal pain.
CN: Physiological integrity; CNS: Physiological adaptation;
CL: Analyze; DIFFICULTY: Moderate

70. 2. Stable clients with digoxin toxicity are best treated with time while their kidneys excrete the metabolites, and with symptomatic treatment for the rhythm disturbances or nausea resulting from the toxicity. Activated charcoal is effective only if the client has taken an overdose of digoxin and if a large amount of unabsorbed drug is in the GI tract, before the serum level is elevated. Hemodialysis is reserved for clients who are extremely unstable despite symptomatic treatment or who have inadequate renal function to excrete the drug. Atropine might be used to treat the bradycardia that results from digoxin toxicity, but it isn't necessarily used to treat the toxicity itself.
CN: Physiological integrity; CNS: Pharmacological therapies;
CL: Apply; DIFFICULTY: Challenge

71. 1. Because bradycardia is an adverse effect of digoxin, the nurse should notify the health care provider and follow prescribed orders. Vital signs should be checked again and the client's heart rate and rhythm should be monitored, but these would not be the first actions. The medication would not be stopped unless the health care provider gave an order to do so. Turning the client on the left side will not increase heart rate.
CN: Safe, effective Care Environment; CNS: Coordinated care;
CL: Apply; DIFFICULTY: Moderate

72. A client has a blockage in the proximal portion of a coronary artery. After learning about treatment options, the client decides to undergo percutaneous transluminal coronary angioplasty (PTCA). During this procedure, the nurse expects which medication to be administered to the client?

1. Antibiotic
2. Anticoagulant
3. Antihypertensive
4. Anticonvulsant

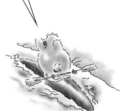

Please keep those arteries open and clear. I will operate so much better.

72. 2. During PTCA, the client receives heparin, an anticoagulant, as well as calcium agonists, nitrates (or both) to reduce coronary artery spasm. An antibiotic isn't given routinely during this procedure; however, because the procedure is invasive, the client may receive prophylactic antibiotics afterward to reduce the risk of infection. An antihypertensive agent may cause hypotension, which should be avoided during the procedure. An anticonvulsant isn't indicated because this procedure doesn't increase the risk of seizures.
CN: Physiological integrity; CNS: Pharmacological therapies; CL: Apply; DIFFICULTY: Easy

73. A client hospitalized for treatment of hypertension is being prepared for discharge. Which statement from the client indicates an understanding of discharge instructions?

1. "I should avoid meat and milk."
2. "I should skip my medication dose if dizziness occurs."
3. "I should only have approximately 2,400 mg of sodium per day."
4. "I should schedule a visit once per week for IV antihypertensive medications."

73. 3. The nurse must teach the hypertensive client how to modify the diet to restrict sodium and saturated fats. In addition, the nurse should explain the actions, dosages, and adverse effects of prescribed antihypertensives. A client receiving antihypertensives also may take a diuretic as part of the drug regimen, should eat a potassium-rich diet including meats and milk, and may require dietary potassium supplements and high-potassium foods to avoid electrolyte disturbances. Instead of skipping medication if dizziness occurs, the client should notify the health care provider of this symptom. The client receiving antihypertensives at home takes them by mouth, not IV
CN: Physiological integrity; CNS: Reduction of risk potential; CL: Apply; DIFFICULTY: Moderate

74. A client is admitted to the cardiac unit with a diagnosis of heart failure. The health care provider prescribes furosemide and digoxin to manage the condition. Which laboratory value should be monitored during hospitalization?

1. Sodium
2. Potassium
3. Chloride
4. Calcium

74. 2. Digoxin may increase the risk of toxicity from furosemide-induced hypokalemia; therefore, potassium levels should be monitored closely. Concurrent administration of digoxin and furosemide doesn't affect sodium, chloride, or calcium levels.
CN: Physiological integrity; CNS: Pharmacological therapies; CL: Analyze; DIFFICULTY: Easy

75. The nurse is obtaining data from a new client in the cardiovascular clinic. When asking about childhood diseases and disorders associated with structural heart disease, the nurse should consider which finding significant?

1. Croup
2. Rheumatic fever
3. Severe staphylococcal infection
4. Medullary sponge kidney

75. 2. Childhood diseases and disorders associated with structural heart disease include rheumatic fever and severe streptococcal (not staphylococcal) infections. Croup—a severe upper airway inflammation and obstruction that typically strikes children ages 3 months to 3 years—may cause latent complications, such as ear infection and pneumonia. However, it doesn't affect heart structures. Likewise, medullary sponge kidney, characterized by dilation of the renal pyramids and formation of cavities, clefts, and cysts in the renal medulla, eventually may lead to hypertension but doesn't damage heart structures.
CN: Health promotion and maintenance; CNS: None; CL: Analyze; DIFFICULTY: Moderate

76. A disaster drill is in progress in the hospital. In preparation for potential admissions, the charge nurse on a cardiac step-down unit asks a nurse which one of the clients could potentially be discharged. Which is the **best** response?
1. A 30-year-old client with recent episodes of ventricular tachycardia scheduled for electrophysiology studies
2. A 75-year-old client who had an inferior myocardial infarction 2 days ago
3. A 52-year-old client who had an endovascular graft placed for an abdominal aortic aneurysm 3 days ago
4. A 62-year-old client who was admitted that morning with heart failure

76. 3. Because endovascular grafting is a minimally invasive procedure for the repair of an abdominal aortic aneurysm, the client is usually discharged from the hospital in 1 to 3 days. It would be unsafe to recommend discharge for any of the other clients.
CN: Safe, effective care environment; CNS: Safety and infection control; CL: Analyze; DIFFICULTY: Difficult

77. A client reports generalized, steady abdominal pain with low back pain. Which finding would indicate that the client might have an abdominal aortic aneurysm?
1. Pulsating mass in the periumbilical area
2. Elevated cardiac enzymes
3. Positive Babinski's sign
4. Pink, frothy sputum

77. 1. Signs of abdominal aortic aneurysm include gnawing, generalized, steady abdominal pain; lower back pain that's unaffected by movement; gastric or abdominal fullness; pulsating mass in the periumbilical area (if the client isn't obese); systolic bruit over the aorta on auscultation of the abdomen; bruit over the femoral arteries; and hypotension (with aneurysm rupture). Elevated cardiac enzymes indicate heart muscle damage. Positive Babinski's sign indicates damage to the pyramidal tract of the central nervous system. Pink, frothy sputum is a sign of pulmonary edema.
CN: Physiological integrity; CNS: Physiological adaptation; CL: Analyze; DIFFICULTY: Moderate

78. Which nursing interventions are appropriate when caring for a client with acute thrombophlebitis?
1. Wrap leg with cool cloth and keep the client's leg lower than the level of the heart.
2. Increase the client's activity level and encourage leg exercises.
3. Administer nitroglycerin and oxygen at 2 LPM.
4. Apply warm soaks and elevate the client's legs higher than the level of the heart.

78. 4. To help treat thrombophlebitis, the nurse should prevent venostasis with measures such as applying warm soaks and elevating the client's legs. The client should remain on bed rest during the acute phase, after which the client may begin to walk while wearing antiembolism stockings. Treatment for thrombophlebitis may also include anticoagulants to prolong clotting time.
CN: Physiological integrity; CNS: Physiological adaptation; CL: Apply; DIFFICULTY: Easy

79. The nurse is obtaining vital signs for a client who is receiving a heparin infusion to treat deep vein thrombosis. The client reports that the gums bleed when brushing the teeth. What should the nurse do **first**?
1. Stop the heparin infusion immediately.
2. Notify the charge nurse
3. Administer a coumarin derivative, as prescribed, to counteract heparin.
4. Reassure the client that bleeding gums are a normal effect of heparin.

79. 2. Because bleeding gums are an adverse effect of heparin that may indicate excessive anticoagulation, the nurse should notify the charge nurse, who will evaluate the client's condition. Laboratory tests, such as partial thromboplastin time, should be performed before concluding that the client's bleeding is significant. The prescribed heparin dose may be therapeutic rather than excessive, so the nurse shouldn't discontinue the heparin infusion, unless the health care provider orders this after evaluating the client. Protamine sulfate, not a coumarin derivative, is given to counteract heparin. Bleeding gums aren't a normal effect of heparin.
CN: Physiological integrity; CNS: Pharmacological therapies; CL: Apply; DIFFICULTY: Moderate

80. On a routine visit to the health care provider, a client with chronic arterial occlusive disease reports stopping smoking after 34 years. To relieve symptoms of intermittent claudication, which suggestions should the nurse recommend?
1. Taking daily walks
2. Engaging in aerobic exercise
3. Reducing daily fat intake to less than 45% of total calories
4. Avoiding foods that increase levels of high-density lipoproteins (HDLs)

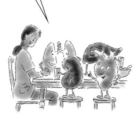

Remember to eat with your whole body in mind, not just your taste buds.

81. A client is receiving captopril for heart failure. Which finding indicates that the medication isn't producing the desired treatment outcome and requires the nurse to notify the health care provider?
1. Skin rash
2. Peripheral edema
3. Dry cough
4. Orthostatic hypotension

82. A client comes to the clinic for a skin assessment from the health care provider. When obtaining data, the nurse knows that which finding increases this client's risk of skin cancer?
1. A deep sunburn
2. A dark mole on the client's back
3. An irregular scar on the client's abdomen
4. White, irregular patches on the client's arm

83. A client with long-standing rheumatoid arthritis has frequent reports of joint pain. The plan of care should be based on the understanding that chronic pain is most effectively relieved when analgesics are administered in which way?
1. Conservatively
2. Intramuscular
3. On an as-needed basis
4. At regularly scheduled intervals

84. Which nursing intervention is appropriate for an adult client with chronic renal failure?
1. Weigh the client daily before breakfast.
2. Offer foods high in calcium and phosphorus.
3. Serve the client large meals and a bedtime snack.
4. Encourage the client to drink large amounts of fluids.

80. 1. Taking daily walks relieves symptoms of intermittent claudication, although the exact mechanism is unclear. Aerobic exercise may make these symptoms worse. Clients with chronic arterial occlusive disease must reduce daily fat intake to 30% or less of total calories. The client should limit dietary cholesterol because hyperlipidemia is associated with atherosclerosis, a known cause of arterial occlusive disease. However, HDLs have the lowest cholesterol concentration, so this client should eat, *not avoid*, foods that raise HDL levels.
CN: Physiological integrity; CNS: Reduction of risk Potential; CL: Apply; DIFFICULTY: Difficult

81. 2. Peripheral edema is a sign of fluid volume overload and worsening heart failure. A skin rash, dry cough, and orthostatic hypotension are adverse reactions to captopril, but they don't indicate that therapy is ineffective.
CN: Physiological integrity; CNS: Pharmacological therapies; CL: Analyze; DIFFICULTY: Moderate

82. 1. A deep sunburn is a risk factor for skin cancer. A dark mole or an irregular scar is benign finding. White, irregular patches are abnormal but aren't a risk factor for skin cancer.
CN: Health promotion and maintenance; CNS: None; CL: Apply; DIFFICULTY: Moderate

83. 4. To control chronic pain and prevent cycled pain, regularly scheduled intervals of analgesia administration are most effective. As-needed and conservative administration aren't effective means to manage chronic pain because the pain isn't relieved regularly. IM administration isn't practical on a long-term basis.
CN: Physiological integrity; CNS: Pharmacological therapies; CL: Apply; DIFFICULTY: Easy

84. 1. Daily weights are obtained to monitor fluid retention. Calcium intake is encouraged, but clients with chronic renal failure have difficulty excreting phosphorus. Therefore, phosphorus must be restricted. To improve food intake, meals and snacks should be given in small portions. Fluids should be restricted for the client with chronic renal failure.
CN: Physiological integrity; CNS: Physiological adaptation; CL: Apply; DIFFICULTY: Easy

85. A client with a recent history of a stroke has been discharged from the rehabilitation facility with a walker. On a return visit to the health care provider, the nurse observes the gait. Which observation indicates the need to reinforce client education about walker use?
1. The client moves the weak leg forward with the walker.
2. When preparing to sit, the client moves hands to the chair armrests before lowering into the chair.
3. The client's arms are fully extended when using the walker.
4. The client backs up to the chair until the legs touch the chair, then sits down.

86. The health care provider prescribes several drugs for a client with hemorrhagic stroke. Which drug order should the nurse question prior to administration?
1. Heparin sodium
2. Dexamethasone
3. Methyldopa
4. Phenytoin

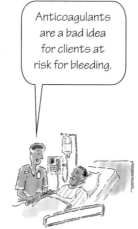

Anticoagulants are a bad idea for clients at risk for bleeding.

87. The nurse is collecting data from a parent regarding the child's behavior. Which behavior is consistent with the diagnosis of conduct disorder in this child?
1. The child is wetting the bed at night.
2. The child has threatened suicide.
3. The child has purposely hurt animals.
4. The child has a fear of attending school.

88. A client has been admitted to the hospital with signs of dehydration. Which intervention would be **most** effective in increasing the client's oral fluid intake?
1. Explain the need for increased fluid intake.
2. Place his choice of beverages at the bedside.
3. Serve small amounts of fluids at frequent intervals.
4. Serve fluids in large amounts at mealtimes.

89. Which outcome developed by the team is appropriate for a client with a diagnosis of depression and attempted suicide?
1. The client will never feel suicidal again.
2. The client will find a group home to live in.
3. The client will remain hospitalized for at least 6 months.
4. The client will verbalize an absence of suicidal ideation, plan, and intent.

85. 3. When using a walker, the client's arms should be slightly bent at the elbow, allowing maximum support from the arms while ambulating. The weak leg is always moved forward first with the walker to provide the maximum support. The client should use the armrests of the chair for support because the armrests are more stable than the walker. When sitting, the client should always back up to the chair and feel the chair with legs before sitting.
CN: Physiological integrity; CNS: Basic care and comfort; CL: Analyze; DIFFICULTY: Moderate

86. 1. Administration of heparin, an anticoagulant, could increase the bleeding associated with hemorrhagic stroke. Therefore, the nurse should question this order to prevent additional hemorrhage in the brain. In a client with hemorrhagic stroke, dexamethasone may be used to decrease cerebral edema and pressure; methyldopa may be used to reduce blood pressure; and phenytoin may be used to prevent seizures.
CN: Physiological integrity; CNS: Pharmacological therapies; CL: Analyze; DIFFICULTY: Easy

87. 3. Cruelty to animals is a symptom of conduct disorder. Enuresis and suicidal ideation aren't usually associated with conduct disorder. Fear of going to school is school phobia.
CN: Psychosocial integrity; CNS: None; CL: Apply; DIFFICULTY: Moderate

88. 3. Fluids should be served in small amounts spread out at frequent intervals. Educating the client about the need for increasing fluids and including the client in the selection of beverages will aid in compliance. It's overwhelming for the client to be expected to drink large amounts of fluids at mealtimes.
CN: Physiological integrity; CNS: Basic care and comfort; CL: Apply; DIFFICULTY: Moderate

89. 4. An appropriate outcome is that the client will verbalize that he no longer feels suicidal. It's unrealistic to expect that he'll never feel suicidal. There's no reason for a group home or 6 months of hospitalization for a client who says he no longer feels suicidal.
CN: Psychosocial integrity; CNS: None; CL: Apply; DIFFICULTY: Easy

90. The nurse is reviewing the proper technique for obtaining a urine specimen from an indwelling urinary catheter. When collecting the urine, which would be the **most** appropriate technique to use?
1. Collect urine from the drainage collection bag.
2. Disconnect the catheter from the drainage tubing to collect urine.
3. Remove the indwelling catheter and insert a sterile straight catheter to collect urine.
4. Clean the tubing's drainage port with alcohol and then insert a sterile needle with syringe to collect the specimen.

90. 4. The nurse should wear clean gloves, clean the drainage port with alcohol, and then obtain the specimen with a sterile needle to ensure that the specimen and the closed urinary drainage system won't be contaminated. A urine specimen must collect new urine, and the urine in the bag could be several hours old and growing bacteria. The urinary drainage system must be kept closed to prevent microorganisms from entering. A straight catheter is used to relieve urine retention, obtain sterile urine specimens, measure the amount of postvoid residual urine, and empty the bladder for certain procedures. It isn't necessary to remove an indwelling catheter to obtain a sterile urine specimen unless the health care provider requests that the whole system be changed.
CN: Safe, effective care environment; CNS: Safety and infection control; CL: Apply; DIFFICULTY: Moderate

91. A registered nurse (RN) is supervising a licensed practical nurse (LPN). The LPN is caring for a client diagnosed with a terminal illness. Which statement by the LPN should the RN correct?
1. "Some clients write a living will indicating their end-of-life preferences."
2. "The law says you have to write a new living will each time you go to the hospital."
3. "You could designate another person to make end-of-life decisions when you can't make them yourself."
4. "Some people choose to tell their health care provider they don't want to have cardiopulmonary resuscitation."

91. 2. One living will is sufficient for all hospitalizations unless the client wishes to make changes. The "No Code" or "Do Not Resuscitate" status is discussed with the health care provider, who then enters this in the client's chart. A living will explains a person's end-of-life preferences. A durable power of attorney for health care can be written to designate who will make health care decisions for the client in the event the client can't make decisions for himself.
CN: Safe, effective care environment; CNS: Coordinated care; CL: Analyze; DIFFICULTY: Easy

92. An older adult client's husband tells the nurse he's concerned because his wife insists on talking about events that happened to her years ago. The nurse finds the client alert, oriented, and answering questions appropriately. Which statement made to the husband is correct?
1. "Your wife is reviewing her life."
2. "A spiritual advisor should be notified."
3. "Your wife should be discouraged from talking about the past."
4. "Your wife is regressing to a more comfortable time in the past."

92. 1. Life review or reminiscing is characteristic of older adults and the dying. A spiritual advisor might comfort the client but isn't necessary for a life review. Discouraging the client from talking would block communication. Regression occurs when a client returns to behaviors typical of another developmental stage.
CN: Health promotion and maintenance; CNS: None; CL: Apply; DIFFICULTY: Challenge

Impressive! You're really rolling through this test.

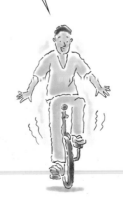

93. A client with a new colostomy asks the nurse how to avoid detachment from the ostomy bag. Which instruction is correct?
1. Limit fluid intake.
2. Eat more fruits and vegetables.
3. Empty the bag when it's about half full.
4. Tape the end of the bag to the surrounding skin.

93. 3. Emptying the bag when partially full prevents the bag from becoming heavy and detaching from the skin or skin barrier. Limiting fluids may cause constipation but won't prevent leakage. Increasing fruits and vegetables in the diet will help prevent constipation, not leakage. Taping the bag to the skin will secure the bag to the skin but won't prevent detachment and could irritate the surrounding skin.
CN: Physiological integrity; CNS: Basic care and comfort; CL: Apply; DIFFICULTY: Easy

CN: Client needs category   CNS: Client needs subcategory   CL: Cognitive level

94. A nurse must obtain the blood pressure of a client in airborne isolation. Which method is **best** to prevent transmission of infection to other clients by the equipment?
1. Dispose of the equipment after each use.
2. Wear gloves while handling the equipment.
3. Use the equipment only with other clients in airborne isolation.
4. Leave the equipment in the room for use only with that client.

94. 4. Leaving equipment in the room for use only with that client is appropriate to avoid organism transmission by inanimate objects. Disposing of equipment after each use prevents the transmission of organisms but isn't cost-effective. Wearing gloves protects the nurse, not other clients. Using equipment for other clients spreads infectious organisms among clients.
CN: Safe, effective care environment; CNS: Safety and infection control; CL: Apply; DIFFICULTY: Easy

95. The nurse is applying an elastic bandage to a client's arm. In order to prevent circulatory impairment, which method is **best**?
1. Wrap the bandage around the arm loosely.
2. Stretch the bandage slightly while wrapping toward the heart.
3. Apply heavy pressure with each turn of the bandage.
4. Start applying the bandage at the upper arm and work toward the lower arm.

95. 2. Stretching the bandage slightly maintains uniform tension on the bandage. Wrapping toward the heart promotes venous return to the heart. Wrapping the bandage loosely wouldn't secure it on the arm and wouldn't be therapeutic. Using heavy pressure would cause circulatory impairment. Wrapping from the upper arm to the lower arm would cause uneven application of the bandage. For example, elastic stockings are applied distal to proximal to promote venous return.
CN: Physiological integrity; CNS: Reduction of risk potential; CL: Application; DIFFICULTY: Moderate

96. The nurse is reinforcing education regarding the use of an incentive spirometer after abdominal surgery in order to prevent complications postoperatively. Which statement made by the client demonstrates an adequate understanding of the use of the spirometer?
1. "If I use this I won't have to get out of the bed so early after surgery."
2. "If I use this, I won't have to take deep breaths to prevent my lungs from collapse."
3. "It won't hurt as bad as deep breathing exercises."
4. "It will help me visualize deep breathing to prevent my lungs from collapse."

96. 4. Incentive spirometry helps the client see inspiratory effort using floating balls, lights, or bellows. Early ambulation is still indicated for this client after abdominal surgery. Incentive spirometry is no more effective than deep breathing without equipment. Deep breathing and incentive spirometry cause equal discomfort during inspiration.
CN: Physiological integrity; CNS: Reduction of risk potential; CL: Apply; DIFFICULTY: Moderate

97. A client reports an inability to sleep while on the medical unit. Which intervention to promote sleep has **priority**?
1. Offer a sedative routinely at bedtime.
2. Give the client a backrub before bedtime.
3. Question the client about sleeping habits.
4. Move the client to a bed farthest from the nurses' station.

97. 3. Interviewing the client about sleeping habits may give more information about the causes of the inability to sleep. Sedatives should be given as a last option. A backrub may promote sleep but may not address this client's problem. Moving the client may not address the client's specific problem.
CN: Physiological integrity; CNS: Basic care and comfort; CL: Apply; DIFFICULTY: Moderate

An allergic reaction to a medication demands immediate attention.

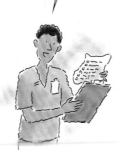

98. The nurse is obtaining vital signs from a client who is receiving an intravenous antibiotic for the first time. Which observations made by the nurse require immediate intervention? Select all that apply.
1. Rash on skin of face, chest, and arms
2. Reports severe itching all over
3. Inspiratory wheezes
4. Heart rate of 86
5. Reports mouth is dry

98. 1, 2, 3. Rash, inspiratory wheezes, and reports of severe itching indicate that the client is having an allergic reaction to the antibiotic. A heart rate of 86 is within normal limits and reports of mouth being dry is not indicative of an allergic reaction.
CN: Physiological integrity; CNS: Pharmacological therapies; CL: Analyze; DIFFICULTY: Easy

99. The nurse is preparing to test function of the optic nerve when obtaining data from a client. Demonstration of the use of which tool used indicates that the nurse is correct in collection of this data?
1. Finger, to test the cardinal fields
2. Flashlight, to test corneal reflexes
3. Snellen chart, to test visual acuity
4. Piece of cotton, to test corneal reflexes

100. The nurse is reinforcing education for a client who will be discharged from the hospital with an indwelling catheter. Which statement made by the client demonstrates an understanding of the education about prevention of infection?
1. "I will limit my fluid intake to 16 oz per day."
2. "I will take a shower instead of a tub bath."
3. "I will open the drainage system if I have to bring a urine specimen to the lab."
4. "I will irrigate the catheter twice daily with sterile saline solution."

101. A nurse wants to use a waist restraint for a client who wanders at night. Which factor or intervention should be considered before applying the restraint?
1. The nurse's convenience
2. The client's reason for getting out of bed
3. A sleeping medication ordered as needed at bedtime
4. The lack of unlicensed assistive personnel (UAP) on the night shift

102. Six months after the death of an infant son, a client is diagnosed with dysfunctional grieving. Which behavior would the nurse expect to find?
1. Going to the infant's grave weekly.
2. Crying when talking about the loss.
3. Overactive without a sense of loss.
4. Stating the infant will always be part of the family.

103. A nurse notices a client has been crying. Which response is the **most** therapeutic?
1. None; this is a private matter.
2. "You seem sad. Would you like to talk?"
3. "Why are you crying and upsetting yourself?"
4. "It's hard being in the hospital, but you must keep your chin up."

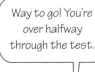

Way to go! You're over halfway through the test.

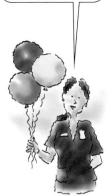

99. 3. The Snellen chart is used to test the function of the optic nerve. Testing the cardinal fields assesses the oculomotor, trochlear, and abducens nerves. Corneal light reflex indicates the function of the oculomotor nerve. Corneal sensitivity is controlled by the trigeminal and facial nerves.
CN: Physiological integrity; CNS: Basic care and comfort; CL: Understand; DIFFICULTY: Challenge

100. 2. A shower would prevent bacteria in the bath water from sustaining contact with the urinary meatus and the catheter, whereas a tub bath may allow easier transit of bacteria into the urinary tract. Increased—not limited—fluid intake is recommended for a client with an indwelling urinary catheter. Opening the drainage system would provide a pathway for the entry of bacteria. Catheter irrigation is performed only with an order from the health care provider to keep the catheter patent.
CN: Physiological integrity; CNS: Reduction of risk potential; CL: Understand; DIFFICULTY: Challenge

101. 2. The nurse should question the client's reason for getting out of bed because the client may be looking for a bathroom. Lack of adequate staffing and convenience aren't reasons for applying restraints. Sleeping medications are chemical restraints that should be used only if the client can't go to sleep and stay asleep.
CN: Safe, effective care environment; CNS: Safety and infection control; CL: Apply; DIFFICULTY: Easy

102. 3. One of the signs of dysfunctional grieving is overactivity without a sense of loss. Going to the grave, tears, and including the infant as a part of the family are all normal responses to the death of an infant son.
CN: Psychosocial integrity; CNS: None; CL: Apply; DIFFICULTY: Moderate

103. 2. Therapeutic communication is a primary tool of nursing. The nurse must recognize that the client's nonverbal behaviors indicate a need to talk. Asking "why" the client is crying might be interpreted as a criticism. Ignoring the client's nonverbal cues or giving opinions and advice are barriers to communication.
CN: Psychosocial integrity; CNS: None; CL: Apply; DIFFICULTY: Easy

104. A nurse gives the wrong medication to a client. What communication should the nurse impart to the risk manager of the facility?
1. A written incident report
2. An oral report
3. A copy of the medication Kardex
4. An order change signed by the health care provider

104. **1.** Incident reports are tools used by risk managers when a client might have been harmed. They're used to determine how future errors can be avoided. An oral report won't serve as legal documentation. A copy of the medication Kardex wouldn't be sent with the incident report to the risk manager. A health care provider won't change an order to cover the nurse's mistake.
CN: Safe, effective care environment; CNS: Coordinated care; CL: Apply; DIFFICULTY: Easy

105. The nurse has been charged by a client with assault and battery. Which action did the nurse perform that caused the client to sue?
1. Taking a necklace that belonged to the client.
2. Entering the client's room several times during the course of treatment.
3. Performing a procedure without obtaining consent.
4. Discussing the client's medical information with another nurse.

105. **3.** Performing a procedure on a client without informed consent can be grounds for charges of assault and battery. Fraud means to cheat, and harassment means to annoy or disturb. Breach of confidentiality refers to conveying information about the client.
CN: Safe, effective care environment; CNS: Coordinated care; CL: Apply; DIFFICULTY: Easy

106. A surgical client newly diagnosed with breast cancer tells a nurse she knows the laboratory made a mistake about her diagnosis. Which term describes this reaction?
1. Denial
2. Intellectualization
3. Regression
4. Repression

106. **1.** Clients with cancer commonly deny this diagnosis when first made. Such a response may benefit the client in that it allows energy for surgical healing. Intellectualization involves speaking of the disease as if reading a textbook. In repression, clients typically don't remember being diagnosed. In regression, clients exhibit childlike behavior.
CN: Psychosocial integrity; CNS: None; CL: Understand; DIFFICULTY: Easy

107. A client who's single and living alone delivers a premature neonate. Which intervention would be included in her treatment plan?
1. An early postpartum health care provider visit
2. Referral to the health department
3. Request for a social service visit in the hospital
4. Request for a home health visit the day after discharge

107. **3.** Because of the client's potential need for support and the premature condition of the neonate, a social service visit is appropriate. The social service visit will determine if there's a need for a referral to the health department. The mother has no physical indications for an early postpartum visit or need for an early home visit.
CN: Safe, effective care environment; CNS: Coordinated care; CL: Analyze; DIFFICULTY: Moderate

108. A client who just gave birth is concerned about her neonate's Apgar scores of 7 and 8. She says she's been told scores lower than 9 are associated with learning difficulties in later life. Which response by the nurse is **most** therapeutic?
1. "You shouldn't worry so much, your infant is perfectly fine."
2. "You should ask about placing the infant in a follow-up diagnostic program."
3. "You're right in being concerned, but there are good special education programs available."
4. "Apgar scores are used to indicate a need for resuscitation at birth. Scores of 7 and above indicate no problem."

Don't think of this as a test ... think of it as an experiment in applying knowledge.

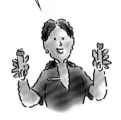

108. **4.** Apgar scores don't indicate future learning difficulties; they provide rapid assessment of the need for resuscitation. Apgar scores of 7 and 8 are normal and don't indicate a need for intervention. It's inappropriate to simply tell a client not to worry.
CN: Health promotion and maintenance; CNS: None; CL: Apply; DIFFICULTY: Easy

109. A pregnant client in her second trimester reveals that she feels very anxious because of a lack of knowledge about giving birth. Which intervention by the nurse is **most** appropriate for this client?
1. Provide her with the information and teach her the skills she'll need to understand and cope during birth.
2. Provide her with written information about the birthing process.
3. Have a more experienced pregnant woman assist her.
4. Do nothing in hopes that she'll begin coping as the pregnancy progresses.

109. **1.** Because the client is in her second trimester, the nurse has ample time to establish a trusting relationship with her and to teach her in a style that fits her needs. Written information would be effective only in conjunction with teaching sessions. Introducing her to another pregnant client may be helpful, but the nurse still needs to teach the client about giving birth. Hoping that the client will begin coping doesn't meet the client's needs.
CN: Health promotion and maintenance; CNS: None; CL: Analyze; DIFFICULTY: Challenge

110. The nurse observes several episodes of late decelerations on the monitor. Which actions are appropriate at this time? Select all that apply.
1. Place the client in the left lateral position.
2. No intervention is required; this is a normal finding.
3. Increase the IV flow rate.
4. Apply oxygen.
5. Have the client sit up on the side of the bed.
6. Notify the charge nurse.

110. **1, 3, 4, 6.** Late decelerations indicate uteroplacental circulatory insufficiency and can lead to fetal hypoxia and acidosis if the underlying cause is not corrected. The client should be turned onto her left side to increase placental perfusion and decrease contraction frequency. In addition, the IV fluid rate may be increased and oxygen administered. The charge nurse should be notified. The client should not sit up on the side of the bed since it will not increase placental perfusion and can cause more pressure on the fetus. Late decelerations are not an expected or normal finding.
CN: Physiological integrity; CNS: Reduction of risk potential; CL: Analyze; DIFFICULTY: Difficult

111. A client in her first trimester of pregnancy reports that she's always tired. Which response by the nurse is **best**?
1. "Needs for rest and sleep typically increase during the first trimester of pregnancy."
2. "I'll inform the health care provider; you'll most likely need some follow-up testing."
3. "Have you tried having a cup of coffee when you awaken in the morning?"
4. "Sometimes a pregnant woman feels fatigued when her baby's sleep pattern is opposite its mother's."

111. **1.** The nurse should allay the client's fears by informing her that needs for sleep and rest normally increase during the first trimester. The nurse should encourage the client to rest whenever possible. No follow-up testing is necessary because feeling tired during the first trimester of pregnancy is a normal occurrence. Caffeine intake should be avoided during pregnancy, so suggesting a cup of coffee in the morning is inappropriate. There isn't evidence to suggest that the baby's rest patterns are opposite the mother's.
CN: Physiological integrity; CNS: Basic care and comfort; CL: Analyze; DIFFICULTY: Easy

112. A postpartum client tells the nurse that she has not had bowel movements in 3 days. Which action taken by the nurse is most effective in relieving constipation?
1. Reduce fluid intake.
2. Maintain bed rest.
3. Add high-fiber foods to her diet.
4. Manual removal of impacted stool.

112. **3.** If a postpartum client has constipation, the nurse should recommend that she eat more high-fiber foods (such as fresh fruits and vegetables, bran, and prunes) and drink plenty of fluids (1 to 2 qt [1 to 2 L] daily to replace fluids lost during labor and birth) to promote peristalsis. Activity and exercise also aid peristalsis. Bed rest decreases peristalsis. There is no indication of impaction and therefore manual removal of impacted stool is not required.
CN: Physiological integrity; CNS: Basic care and comfort; CL: Apply; DIFFICULTY: Easy

113. A parent is planning to enroll a 9-month-old infant in a daycare facility. The parent asks a nurse what to look for as indicators that the facility is adhering to good infection control measures. The nurse identifies which policy as an indication of meeting proper infection control standards? Select all that apply.

1. The facility keeps boxes of gloves in the director's office.
2. Soiled diapers are discarded in covered receptacles.
3. Toys are kept on the floor for the children to share.
4. Disposable papers are used on the diaper-changing surfaces.
5. Facilities for hand hygiene are located in every classroom.
6. Soiled clothing and cloth diapers are sent home in labeled paper bags.

114. A client received a new prescription for oral contraceptives. When reinforcing education, what should the nurse be sure to inform the client to report? Select all that apply.

1. Breast tenderness
2. Breakthrough bleeding within first 3 months of use
3. Decreased menstrual flow
4. Blurred vision and headache
5. Pain in the calf with dorsiflexion of the foot

115. A nurse is monitoring the contractions of a client in the first stage of labor. Order the phases of a uterine contraction from the beginning of contraction to its conclusion. Use all of the options.

1. Relaxation
2. Acme
3. Strong Braxton Hicks contractions
4. Decrement

113. 2, 4, 5. A parent can assess infection control practices at a facility to prevent the spread of disease. Placing soiled diapers in covered receptacles, covering the diaper-changing surfaces with disposable papers, and ensuring that hand sanitizers and sinks are available for personnel to wash their hands after activities are all indicators that infection control measures are being followed. Gloves should be readily available to personnel and, therefore, should be kept in every room—not in an office. Toys typically are shared by numerous children; however, this contributes to the spread of germs and infections. All soiled clothing and cloth diapers should be placed in a sealed plastic bag before being sent home.
CN: Safe, effective care environment; CNS: Safety and infection control; CL: Analyze; DIFFICULTY: Moderate

114. 4, 5. Some adverse effects of birth control pills, such as blurred vision and headaches, and pain in the calf with dorsiflexion of the foot, require a report to the health care provider. Because these two effects in particular may result in cardiovascular compromise and embolus, the client may need to use another form of birth control. Breast tenderness, breakthrough bleeding, and decreased menstrual flow may occur as a normal response to the use of birth control pills.
CN: Physiological integrity; CNS: Pharmacological therapies; CL: Analyze; DIFFICULTY: Moderate

115. Ordered response:

3. Strong Braxton Hicks contractions
2. Acme
4. Decrement
1. Relaxation

Braxton Hicks contractions are contractions which occur before actual labor in preparation for the real labor. A contraction consists of three phases: the increment (when the intensity of the contraction increases), the acme (when the contraction is at its strongest), and the decrement (when the intensity decreases). Between contractions, the uterus relaxes. As labor progresses, the relaxation intervals decrease from 10 minutes early in labor to only 2 to 3 minutes later. The duration of contractions also changes, increasing from 20 to 30 seconds to a range of 60 to 90 seconds.
CN: Health promotion and maintenance; CNS: None; CL: Apply; DIFFICULTY: Easy

116. The mother of a 3-day-old, br[...]t-fed infant expresses concern that her infant has [...]had two recent diapers that contained a lot of lo[...]ose, yellowish stool. Which explanation by the nu[...]rse is best?

1. "It's normal for breast-fed infants to pass three or more loose, yellow stools per day."
2. "Please save the next diaper so the nurses can examine the stools."
3. "New parents tend to worry too much. Infants have frequent stools."
4. "Eliminating dairy products from your diet can help clear this up."

117. A client comes to the office for a routine prenatal visit. After reading the chart entry shown, the nurse should prepare the client for which study?

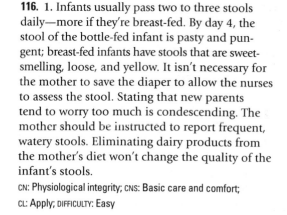

You're really flying through these questions now. Great job!

Progress notes	
4/1/2017	Pt. is 11 weeks pregnant;
1320	urine sample shows
	glycosuria. Pt. has a family
	history of diabetes.
	—Chrissy Franks, LPN

1. Triple screen
2. Indirect Coombs' test
3. 1-Hour glucose tolerance test
4. Amniocentesis

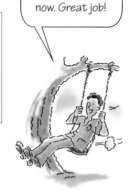

118. The nurse is reinforcing education on how to perform perineal care to reduce the risk of puerperal infection for a postpartum client. Which activity indicates that the client understands proper perineal care?

1. Using a peri bottle to clean the perineum after each voiding or bowel movement
2. Cleaning the perineum from back to front after a bowel movement
3. Spraying water from peri bottle into the vagina
4. Changing perineal pads every 8 hours

119. A neonate begins to gag and turns a dusky color. What should the nurse do first?

1. Calm the neonate.
2. Notify the health care provider.
3. Provide oxygen via a facemask as ordered.
4. Aspirate the neonate's mouth then nose with a bulb syringe.

116. 1. Infants usually pass two to three stools daily—more if they're breast-fed. By day 4, the stool of the bottle-fed infant is pasty and pungent; breast-fed infants have stools that are sweet-smelling, loose, and yellow. It isn't necessary for the mother to save the diaper to allow the nurses to assess the stool. Stating that new parents tend to worry too much is condescending. The mother should be instructed to report frequent, watery stools. Eliminating dairy products from the mother's diet won't change the quality of the infant's stools.
CN: Physiological integrity; CNS: Basic care and comfort; CL: Apply; DIFFICULTY: Easy

117. 3. A 1-hour glucose tolerance test is recommended to screen for gestational diabetes if the client is obese, has glycosuria or a family history of diabetes, lost a fetus for unexplained reasons, or gave birth to a large-for-gestational-age neonate. A triple screen tests for chromosomal abnormalities. The indirect Coombs' test screens maternal blood for red blood cell antibodies. Amniocentesis is used to detect fetal abnormalities.
CN: Physiological integrity; CNS: Reduction of risk potential; CL: Apply; DIFFICULTY: Easy

118. 1. Cleaning with a peri bottle (squirt or spray bottle) should be performed after each voiding or bowel movement. The perineum should be cleaned from *front to back*, to avoid contamination from the rectal area. To keep the perineum clean, perineal pads must be changed when they are soiled. Water from the peri bottle isn't sterile and should never be directed into the vagina.
CN: Physiological integrity; CNS: Basic care and comfort; CL: Apply; DIFFICULTY: Easy

119. 4. The nurse's first action should be to clear the neonate's airway with a bulb syringe. After the airway is clear and the neonate's color improves, the nurse should comfort and calm the neonate. If the problem recurs or the neonate's color doesn't improve readily, the nurse should notify the health care provider. Administering oxygen when the airway isn't clear would be ineffective.
CN: Physiological integrity; CNS: Reduction of risk potential; CL: Apply; DIFFICULTY: Easy

CN: Client needs category   CNS: Client needs subcategory   CL: Cognitive level

120. A client tells th[...]
to sign the hepatiti[...]
because she heard[...]
autism." What's th[...]
interactio[...]

1. Tel[...]
   been[...]
2. Supp[...]
   vacci[...]
3. Encou[...]
   with t[...]
   check-[...]
4. Discussing the purpose of the vaccine and providing the client with written information

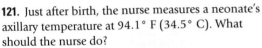

124. 3, 4, 6. Pe[...]
fetus or new[...]
neonate's[...]
soles of[...]
not r[...]
fro[...]

120. 4. There are[...]
cine safety an[...]
provide inf[...]
given, th[...]
reactio[...]
use[...]

[...]many misconceptions about vac-
[...]d complications. The nurse should
[...]ormation about why the vaccine is
[...]e benefits and risks, and common adverse
[...]ons. Health care providers are required to
[...]e a handout that provides all federally required
information about the vaccine because informed consent requires that there has been a full dis-closure of available information. If the client still refuses after full disclosure, the nurse needs to support and document the decision. It's a nursing responsibility to complete client education first, then refer the client with additional questions and concerns to the health care provider.

CN: Safe, effective care environment; CNS: Coordinated care;
CL: Analyze; DIFFICULTY: Easy

---

121. Just after birth, the nurse measures a neonate's axillary temperature at 94.1° F (34.5° C). What should the nurse do?

1. Rewarm the neonate gradually.
2. Rewarm the neonate rapidly.
3. Observe the neonate at least hourly.
4. Notify the health care provider when the neonate's temperature is normal.

121. 1. A neonate with a temperature of 94.1° F (34.5° C) is experiencing cold stress. The nurse must correct cold stress while avoiding hyper-thermia and complications caused by rapid rewarming. The nurse should rewarm the neonate gradually, observing him closely and checking his vital signs every 15 to 30 minutes. Hourly obser-vation isn't frequent enough because cold stress increases oxygen, calorie, and fat expenditure, put-ting the neonate at risk for anabolic metabolism and possibly metabolic acidosis. A neonate with cold stress requires intervention; the nurse should notify the health care provider of the problem as soon as it's identified.

CN: Safe, effective care environment; CNS: safety and infection control; CL: Analyze; DIFFICULTY: Easy

---

122. Which intervention takes **priority** when car-ing for a neonate immediately after birth?

1. Obtaining a Dextrostix result
2. Giving the initial bath
3. Administering a vitamin K injection
4. Covering the neonate's head with a cap

> Keeping the whole body in balance can be challenging. Each system affects all the others.

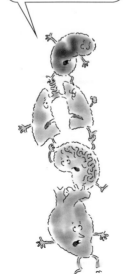

122. 4. Covering the neonate's head with a cap helps prevent cold stress caused by excessive evaporative heat loss from the neonate's wet head. Initial baths aren't given until the neonate's temperature stabilizes. Dextrostix tests, which are performed on neonates at risk for hypoglycemia, are performed 30 minutes to 1 hour after birth. Vitamin K can be administered within 4 hours after birth.

CN: Health promotion and maintenance; CNS: None; CL: Apply;
DIFFICULTY: Challenge

---

123. A nurse is reviewing principles of good body mechanics with a student practical nurse. Which technique should be emphasized?

1. Bending from the waist
2. Pulling rather than pushing
3. Stretching to reach an object
4. Using large muscles in the legs for leverage

123. 4. Keeping one's back straight and using the large muscles in the legs will help avoid back injury, as the muscles in one's back are relatively small compared with the larger muscles of the thighs. Bending from the waist can stress the back muscles, causing a potential injury. Pulling isn't the best option and may cause straining. When feasible, one should push an object rather than pull it. Stretching to reach an object increases the risk of injury.

CN: Safe, effective care environment; CNS: Safety and infection
control; CL: Apply; DIFFICULTY: Easy

CN: Client needs category   CNS: Client needs subcategory   CL: Cognitive level

124. A nurse is obtaining data on a [...] nate in the nursery. Which findings w[...] possible asphyxia in utero? Select all tha[...]
1. The neonate grasps the nurse's finger [...] put in the palm of the neonate's hand.
2. The neonate does stepping movements wh[...] held upright with the sole of the foot touch-ing a surface.
3. The neonate's toes do not curl downward when the soles of the feet are touched.
4. The neonate does not respond when the nurse claps hands.
5. The neonate turns toward the nurse's finger when touching the cheek.
6. The neonate displays weak, ineffective sucking.

[...]natal asphyxia is an insult to the [...]orn due to the lack of oxygen. If the [...]oes do not curl downward when the [...]he feet are touched and the neonate does [...]spond to a loud sound, neurologic damage [...]n asphyxia may have occurred. A normal neuro-logic response would be the downward curling of the toes when touched and extension of the arms and legs in response to a loud noise. Weak, ineffective sucking is another sign of neurologic damage. A neonate should grasp a person's finger when it is placed in the palm of the neonate's hand, do stepping movements when held upright with the sole of the foot touching a surface, and turn toward the nurse's finger when touching the cheek.

CN: Health promotion and maintenance; CNS: None; CL: Apply; DIFFICULTY: Easy

125. A nurse is providing care to a neonate. Place the following steps in the order that the nurse should implement them to properly perform ophthalmia neonatorum prophylaxis. Use all of the options.

1. Gently raise the neonate's upper eyelid with the index finger and pull the lower eyelid down with the thumb.

2. Wash hands and put on gloves.

3. Close and manipulate the eyelids to spread the medication over the eye.

4. Shield the neonate's eyes from direct light, and tilt the head slightly to the side that will receive the treatment.

5. Instill the ointment in the lower conjunctival sac.

6. Repeat the procedure for the other eye.

125. Ordered Response:

2. Wash hands and put on gloves.

4. Shield the neonate's eyes from direct light, and tilt the head slightly to the side that will receive the treatment.

1. Gently raise the neonate's upper eyelid with the index finger and pull the lower eyelid down with the thumb.

5. Instill the ointment in the lower conjunctival sac.

3. Close and manipulate the eyelids to spread the medication over the eye.

6. Repeat the procedure for the other eye.

Ophthalmia neonatorum prophylaxis involves the instillation of 0.5% erythromycin or 1% tetracycline ointment into a neonate's eyes. This procedure is performed to prevent gonorrheal and chlamydial conjunctivitis. All 50 states mandate that this treatment be given within 1 hour after birth to decrease the risk of permanent eye damage and blindness.

CN: Physiological integrity; CNS: Physiological adaptation; CL: Apply; DIFFICULTY: Easy

126. A client reports pain during intercourse. Which statement by the client would be most important for the nurse to report to the health care provider?
1. "I had sex a couple of times when I was 17."
2. "When I was 19 I had a spontaneous abortion."
3. "My second pregnancy was complicated with eclampsia."
4. "I had a human papillomavirus infection at age 32."

126. 4. Like other viral and bacterial venereal infections, human papillomavirus is a risk factor for cervical cancer. Other risk factors for this disease include frequent sexual intercourse before age 16, multiple sex partners, and multiple pregnancies. A spontaneous abortion and pregnancy complicated by eclampsia aren't risk factors for cervical cancer.

CN: Health promotion and maintenance; CNS: None; CL: Apply; DIFFICULTY: Easy

120. A client tells the nurse that she doesn't want to sign the hepatitis B vaccination consent form because she heard that, "vaccinations can cause autism." What's the most appropriate nursing interaction?
1. Telling the client that such information hasn't been substantiated
2. Supporting the client's decision because all vaccines have associated risks
3. Encouraging the client to discuss the issue with the pediatrician at the infant's 2-week check-up
4. Discussing the purpose of the vaccine and providing the client with written information

120. 4. There are many misconceptions about vaccine safety and complications. The nurse should provide information about why the vaccine is given, the benefits and risks, and common adverse reactions. Health care providers are required to use a handout that provides all federally required information about the vaccine because informed consent requires that there has been a full disclosure of available information. If the client still refuses after full disclosure, the nurse needs to support and document the decision. It's a nursing responsibility to complete client education first, then refer the client with additional questions and concerns to the health care provider.
CN: Safe, effective care environment; CNS: Coordinated care; CL: Analyze; DIFFICULTY: Easy

121. Just after birth, the nurse measures a neonate's axillary temperature at 94.1° F (34.5° C). What should the nurse do?
1. Rewarm the neonate gradually.
2. Rewarm the neonate rapidly.
3. Observe the neonate at least hourly.
4. Notify the health care provider when the neonate's temperature is normal.

121. 1. A neonate with a temperature of 94.1° F (34.5° C) is experiencing cold stress. The nurse must correct cold stress while avoiding hyperthermia and complications caused by rapid rewarming. The nurse should rewarm the neonate gradually, observing him closely and checking his vital signs every 15 to 30 minutes. Hourly observation isn't frequent enough because cold stress increases oxygen, calorie, and fat expenditure, putting the neonate at risk for anabolic metabolism and possibly metabolic acidosis. A neonate with cold stress requires intervention; the nurse should notify the health care provider of the problem as soon as it's identified.
CN: Safe, effective care environment; CNS: safety and infection control; CL: Analyze; DIFFICULTY: Easy

122. Which intervention takes **priority** when caring for a neonate immediately after birth?
1. Obtaining a Dextrostix result
2. Giving the initial bath
3. Administering a vitamin K injection
4. Covering the neonate's head with a cap

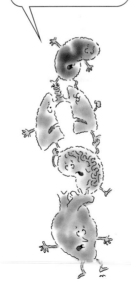

Keeping the whole body in balance can be challenging. Each system affects all the others.

122. 4. Covering the neonate's head with a cap helps prevent cold stress caused by excessive evaporative heat loss from the neonate's wet head. Initial baths aren't given until the neonate's temperature stabilizes. Dextrostix tests, which are performed on neonates at risk for hypoglycemia, are performed 30 minutes to 1 hour after birth. Vitamin K can be administered within 4 hours after birth.
CN: Health promotion and maintenance; CNS: None; CL: Apply; DIFFICULTY: Challenge

123. A nurse is reviewing principles of good body mechanics with a student practical nurse. Which technique should be emphasized?
1. Bending from the waist
2. Pulling rather than pushing
3. Stretching to reach an object
4. Using large muscles in the legs for leverage

123. 4. Keeping one's back straight and using the large muscles in the legs will help avoid back injury, as the muscles in one's back are relatively small compared with the larger muscles of the thighs. Bending from the waist can stress the back muscles, causing a potential injury. Pulling isn't the best option and may cause straining. When feasible, one should push an object rather than pull it. Stretching to reach an object increases the risk of injury.
CN: Safe, effective care environment; CNS: Safety and infection control; CL: Apply; DIFFICULTY: Easy

CN: Client needs category   CNS: Client needs subcategory   CL: Cognitive level

124. A nurse is obtaining data on a 1-day-old neonate in the nursery. Which findings would indicate possible asphyxia in utero? Select all that apply.
1. The neonate grasps the nurse's finger when put in the palm of the neonate's hand.
2. The neonate does stepping movements when held upright with the sole of the foot touching a surface.
3. The neonate's toes do not curl downward when the soles of the feet are touched.
4. The neonate does not respond when the nurse claps hands.
5. The neonate turns toward the nurse's finger when touching the cheek.
6. The neonate displays weak, ineffective sucking.

124. **3, 4, 6.** Perinatal asphyxia is an insult to the fetus or newborn due to the lack of oxygen. If the neonate's toes do not curl downward when the soles of the feet are touched and the neonate does not respond to a loud sound, neurologic damage from asphyxia may have occurred. A normal neurologic response would be the downward curling of the toes when touched and extension of the arms and legs in response to a loud noise. Weak, ineffective sucking is another sign of neurologic damage. A neonate should grasp a person's finger when it is placed in the palm of the neonate's hand, do stepping movements when held upright with the sole of the foot touching a surface, and turn toward the nurse's finger when touching the cheek.

CN: Health promotion and maintenance; CNS: None; CL: Apply; DIFFICULTY: Easy

125. A nurse is providing care to a neonate. Place the following steps in the order that the nurse should implement them to properly perform ophthalmia neonatorum prophylaxis. Use all of the options.

1. Gently raise the neonate's upper eyelid with the index finger and pull the lower eyelid down with the thumb.

2. Wash hands and put on gloves.

3. Close and manipulate the eyelids to spread the medication over the eye.

4. Shield the neonate's eyes from direct light, and tilt the head slightly to the side that will receive the treatment.

5. Instill the ointment in the lower conjunctival sac.

6. Repeat the procedure for the other eye.

125. Ordered Response:

2. Wash hands and put on gloves.

4. Shield the neonate's eyes from direct light, and tilt the head slightly to the side that will receive the treatment.

1. Gently raise the neonate's upper eyelid with the index finger and pull the lower eyelid down with the thumb.

5. Instill the ointment in the lower conjunctival sac.

3. Close and manipulate the eyelids to spread the medication over the eye.

6. Repeat the procedure for the other eye.

Ophthalmia neonatorum prophylaxis involves the instillation of 0.5% erythromycin or 1% tetracycline ointment into a neonate's eyes. This procedure is performed to prevent gonorrheal and chlamydial conjunctivitis. All 50 states mandate that this treatment be given within 1 hour after birth to decrease the risk of permanent eye damage and blindness.

CN: Physiological integrity; CNS: Physiological adaptation; CL: Apply; DIFFICULTY: Easy

126. A client reports pain during intercourse. Which statement by the client would be most important for the nurse to report to the health care provider?
1. "I had sex a couple of times when I was 17."
2. "When I was 19 I had a spontaneous abortion."
3. "My second pregnancy was complicated with eclampsia."
4. "I had a human papillomavirus infection at age 32."

126. **4.** Like other viral and bacterial venereal infections, human papillomavirus is a risk factor for cervical cancer. Other risk factors for this disease include frequent sexual intercourse before age 16, multiple sex partners, and multiple pregnancies. A spontaneous abortion and pregnancy complicated by eclampsia aren't risk factors for cervical cancer.

CN: Health promotion and maintenance; CNS: None; CL: Apply; DIFFICULTY: Easy

127. A client's gestational diabetes is poorly controlled throughout her pregnancy. She goes into labor at 38 weeks and delivers a baby boy. Which priority intervention should be included in the plan of care for the baby during his first 24 hours?

1. Administer insulin subcutaneously.
2. Administer a bolus of dextrose IV.
3. Provide frequent early feedings with formula.
4. Avoid oral feedings.

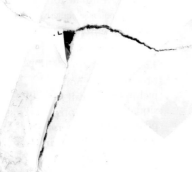

128. A 6-year-old child is diagnosed with diabetes and requires education along with the family. Which factor is considered when the nurse assists in the planning of the education?

1. Another child with diabetes can educate the client
2. The child can educate the parents after the nurse educates the child.
3. The child and parents should be educated together.
4. Education should be directed to the parents, who then can educate the child.

129. After delivering a neonate with a cleft palate and cleft lip, a client has minimal contact with her neonate and asks the nurse to do most of the neonate's care. What is the **best** response by the nurse?

1. "You can't stop caring for the child because of a deformity."
2. "I will take care of your baby while in the hospital but then you will have to take over."
3. "I understand that you may be nervous about taking care of your baby. Let's go over some of the care."
4. "Do you have anyone else that can take care of the baby for you while you are at home?"

130. A client reports excessive flatulence. Which foods, reported by the client as consumed regularly, may be responsible for this? Select all that apply.

1. Cauliflower
2. Ice cream
3. Meat
4. Potatoes
5. Cabbage

127. 3. The neonate of a mother with gestational diabetes may be slightly hyperglycemic immediately after birth because of the high glucose levels that cross the placenta from mother to fetus. During pregnancy, the fetal pancreas secretes increased levels of insulin in response to this increased glucose amount that crosses the placenta from the mother. However, during the first 24 hours of life, this combination of high insulin production in the neonate coupled with the loss of maternal glucose can cause severe hypoglycemia. Frequent, early feedings of formula given orally can prevent hypoglycemia. Insulin shouldn't be administered because the neonate of a mother with gestational diabetes is at risk for hypoglycemia. A bolus of dextrose given IV may cause rebound hypoglycemia. If dextrose is given IV, it should be administered as a continuous infusion.

CN: Physiological integrity; CNS: Reduction of risk potential; CL: Apply; DIFFICULTY: Easy

128. 3. The parents and child should participate in the nurse's education together to ensure an understanding and that the child has adult caregivers who are knowledgeable. Another child with diabetes shouldn't be entrusted to educate this child, although input would be valuable. The school-age child shouldn't be the sole teacher for the parents. Parents should be included in the education plan but shouldn't be responsible for educating their child.

CN: Health promotion and maintenance; CNS: None; CL: Apply; DIFFICULTY: Easy

129. 3. Talking to the mother in a nonjudgmental manner and making sure she understands that the nurse will help her with care during the hospital stay are therapeutic responses. Telling the mother that she can't stop caring for the child is nontherapeutic and is giving advice. Taking over the care of the child while hospitalized and not allowing the mother to perform any care will not allow the nursing staff to determine if the child is being released into a safe home environment. Asking the client if someone else can perform the care is nontherapeutic and infers that the mother should not care for the child.

CN: Health promotion and maintenance; CNS: None; CL: Apply; DIFFICULTY: Easy

130. 1, 5. Cauliflower and cabbage are the only foods listed that commonly result in flatulence.

CN: Physiological integrity; CNS: Basic care and comfort; CL: Understand; DIFFICULTY: Difficult

131. The care plan for an older adult client who has had a stroke and is paraplegic indicates that the client should be turned at least every 2 hours. What outcome does the nurse hope to achieve with this intervention?
1. The client will receive needed physical and emotional stimulation.
2. The client will not develop venous stasis
3. The client will not develop skin breakdown, pneumonia, and urinary tract infections (UTIs).
4. The client will be comfortable and safe.

132. A prenatal client says she can't believe she has such mixed feelings about being pregnant. She tried for 10 years to become pregnant and now feels guilty for her conflicting reactions. Which response by the nurse is **best**?
1. "You need to talk to your midwife about these feelings."
2. "You're experiencing the normal ambivalence pregnant mothers feel."
3. "These feelings are expected only in women who have had difficulty becoming pregnant."
4. "Let's make an appointment with a counselor."

133. A client with terminal cancer tells a nurse, "I've given up. I have no hope left. I'm ready to die." Which response is **most** therapeutic?
1. "You've given up hope?"
2. "We should talk to a social worker about the subject of dying."
3. "You should talk to your health care provider about your fears of dying so soon."
4. "Now, you shouldn't give up hope. There are cures for cancer found every day."

134. Three days after discharge, a client bottle-feeding her neonate calls the postpartum floor to ask what she can do for breast engorgement. Which instruction by the nurse is correct?
1. "Wear a supportive bra."
2. "Get under a warm shower and let the water flow on your breasts."
3. "Stop drinking milk because it contributes to breast engorgement."
4. "Contact your health care provider; you shouldn't be engorged at this late date."

135. The infection control nurse is making rounds to ensure that airborne precautions are being observed while caring for clients with tuberculosis. Which action by the staff nurse requires further education?
1. The nurse double-bags respiratory secretions.
2. The nurse dons a surgical isolation mask when entering the client's room.
3. The nurse gathers disposable client care items.
4. The client's meals are served on disposable trays.

131. 3. Immobility can lead to severe physiologic problems such as skin breakdown, pressure ulcers, pneumonia, and UTIs. Therefore, frequent turning helps to minimize the effects of immobility. Immobility doesn't necessarily mean there's lack of stimuli. Although venous stasis can occur with immobility, heart failure doesn't develop as a result of venous stasis. Turning the client may improve how the client feels, but this isn't the primary rationale for this intervention.
CN: Physiological integrity; CNS: Basic care and comfort; CL: Analyze; DIFFICULTY: Easy

132. 2. Conflicting ambivalent feelings regarding pregnancy are normal for pregnant women. These feelings don't call for counseling or other professional interventions. Ambivalence is felt by most pregnant women, not exclusively mothers who had difficulty becoming pregnant.
CN: Psychosocial integrity; CNS: None; CL: Apply; DIFFICULTY: Moderate

133. 1. The use of reflection invites the client to talk more about his concerns. Deferring the conversation to a social worker or health care provider closes the conversation. Telling the client that cures for cancer are found every day gives false hope.
CN: Psychosocial integrity; CNS: None; CL: Apply; DIFFICULTY: Moderate

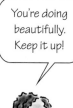

You're doing beautifully. Keep it up!

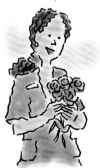

134. 1. A supportive bra or breast binder is recommended for the client who is bottle-feeding her neonate to reduce engorgement. A warm shower will stimulate milk production; cold compresses may provide relief. It's normal to become engorged during the first few days after birth; drinking milk isn't the cause. It isn't necessary to contact the health care provider.
CN: Physiological integrity; CNS: Basic care and comfort; CL: Apply; DIFFICULTY: Challenge

135. 2. When entering the room of a client with tuberculosis, the nurse should wear an N95 particulate respirator mask because surgical isolation masks allow tubercle bacilli to pass through. All trash and waste should be disposed of as infectious waste. All client care items and meal trays should be disposable.
CN: Safe, effective care environment; CNS: Safety and infection control; CL: Apply; DIFFICULTY: Moderate

136. When obtaining data from a client who just gave birth, a nurse finds the following: blood pressure, 110/70 mm Hg; pulse, 60 beats/minute; respirations, 16 breaths/minute; lochia, moderate rubra; fundus, above the umbilicus to the right; and negative Homans sign. Which intervention is correct?
1. No action is required since findings are normal
2. Ask the client to void and recheck the fundus.
3. Turn the client on her left side to decrease the blood pressure.
4. Massage the fundus to decrease lochia flow and prevent hemorrhage.

137. A client with diabetes delivers a 9-lb, 6-oz (4,250 g) neonate. The nurse should be alert for which condition in the neonate?
1. Hyperglycemia
2. Hypoglycemia
3. Hyperthermia
4. Hypothermia

138. An adolescent prenatal client asks about getting fat while pregnant. A nurse tells her she needs to gain enough weight to be in the upper portions of her recommended weight due to her age to prevent which condition?
1. Birth of a premature neonate
2. A difficult birth
3. Birth of a low-birth-weight neonate
4. Gestational hypertension

139. A nurse is preparing to bathe a client hospitalized for emphysema. Which nursing intervention is correct?
1. Remove the oxygen and proceed with the bath.
2. Increase the flow of oxygen to 6 L/minute by nasal cannula.
3. Keep the head of the bed slightly elevated during the procedure.
4. Lower the head of the bed and roll the client to his left side to increase oxygenation.

140. A client who is 36 weeks' pregnant chokes on her food while eating at a restaurant. Which actions would be appropriate for this pregnant client?
1. Chest thrusts are used when the client is pregnant.
2. Only back thrusts are used when the client is pregnant.
3. Abdominal thrusts are performed the same as for a nonpregnant client.
4. Abdominal thrusts can't be performed on a pregnant client.

136. 2. Placement of ... and to the right of the uterus at the umbilicus a full bladder ... isn't a normal finding. It indicates ... and be ... er. The client should empty her bladder are no ... checked. Lochia flow and blood pressure ... CN: P... rmal.
CN: Physiological integrity; CNS: Reduction of risk potential; CL: Analyze; DIFFICULTY: Moderate

137. 2. Neonates of mothers with diabetes and large neonates are at risk for hypoglycemia related to increased production of insulin by the neonate in utero. Hyperglycemia, hyperthermia, and hypothermia aren't primary concerns.
CN: Physiological integrity; CNS: Reduction of risk potential; CL: Apply; DIFFICULTY: Challenge

138. 3. Adolescent girls, especially those younger than age 15, are at higher risk for delivering low-birth-weight neonates unless they gain adequate weight during pregnancy. Gaining weight isn't associated with preventing a difficult birth, risk of gestational hypertension, or a premature neonate.
CN: Physiological integrity; CNS: Reduction of risk potential; CL: Apply; DIFFICULTY: Easy

139. 3. The elasticity of the lungs is lost for clients with emphysema. Therefore, these clients can't tolerate lying flat because the abdominal organs compress the lungs. The best position is one with the head slightly elevated. Discontinuing oxygen or altering the oxygen delivery rate should never be done without an order from the health care provider. Increasing oxygen flow on a client with emphysema may suppress the hypoxic drive to breathe. Positioning the client on the left side with the head of the bed flat would decrease oxygenation.
CN: Physiological integrity; CNS: Physiological adaptation; CL: Apply; DIFFICULTY: Easy

140. 1. During pregnancy, chest thrusts are used instead of abdominal thrusts because abdominal thrusts compress the abdomen and would harm the fetus. To perform a chest thrust, a fist is made with one hand, placing thumb side against the center of the breastbone. The fist is grabbed with the other hand and thrust inward. Avoid the lower tip of the breastbone. Back thrusts aren't done as they may dislodge the obstruction, further blocking the airway.
CN: Physiological integrity; CNS: Reduction of risk potential; CL: Apply; DIFFICULTY: Moderate

CN: Client needs category   CNS: Client needs subcategory   CL: Cognitive level

141. A client with an alcohol use p... ...lity. When discharged from a mental health fac... interven-assisting with discharge planning which ...tion should be included?
1. Referral to Al-Anon
2. Weekly urine testing for drug use
3. Day hospital treatment for 6 months
4. Participation in a support group like Alcoholics Anonymous (AA)

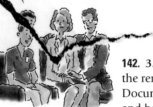

Support is a critical part of preventing relapse of substance use.

141. 4. AA is a major support group for alcoholics after treatment. Membership in AA is associated with relapse prevention. Al-Anon is a support group for the family of the user of alcohol. Weekly urine testing or day hospital treatment isn't usual.
CN: Safe, effective care environment; CNS: Coordinated care; CL: Apply; DIFFICULTY: Easy

142. A nurse is removing an indwelling urinary catheter. Which nursing action reflects the **best** technique?
1. Wear sterile gloves.
2. Cut the lumen of the balloon.
3. Document the time of removal.
4. Position the client on his left side.

142. 3. The client should void within 8 hours of the removal of an indwelling urinary catheter. Documenting the time of removal allows the nurse and health care provider to verify the duration of elapsed time since removal, thus contributing to continuity of care. Clean, disposable gloves are required because it isn't a sterile procedure. If the balloon is cut from the lumen and the catheter isn't secured, the catheter may retrograde into the bladder, requiring surgical removal. The client should be positioned comfortably on his back, and privacy should be provided.
CN: Safe, effective care environment; CNS: Safety and infection control; CL: Apply; DIFFICULTY: Moderate

143. A client is scheduled to retire in the next month and phones the nurse therapist stating, "I can't cope." Which reaction is this client exhibiting?
1. Panic reaction
2. Situational crisis
3. Normal separation anxiety
4. Maturational crisis

143. 4. A maturational (developmental) crisis is one that occurs at a predictable milestone during a life span; birth, marriage, and retirement are examples. A panic reaction would also involve physical symptoms. A situational crisis is caused by events such as an earthquake. Separation anxiety is a childhood disorder.
CN: Health promotion and maintenance; CNS: None; CL: Analyze; DIFFICULTY: Challenge

144. A client with a phobia is being treated with behavior modification therapy. The client asks the nurse which treatment he should expect with this therapy. The nurse should tell the client to expect which treatment?
1. Dream analysis
2. Free association
3. Systematic desensitization
4. Electroconvulsive therapy (ECT)

144. 3. Systematic desensitization is a behavior therapy used in the treatment of phobias. Dream analysis and free association are techniques used in psychoanalytic therapy. ECT is used with depression.
CN: Psychosocial integrity; CNS: None; CL: Apply; DIFFICULTY: Moderate

145. A severely depressed client rarely leaves the chair. To prevent physiologic complications associated with psychomotor retardation, which action is appropriate?
1. Restrict coffee intake.
2. Increase calcium intake.
3. Encourage resting in bed three times per day.
4. Encourage emptying the bladder on a schedule.

145. 4. To prevent bladder infections associated with stasis of urine, the client should be encouraged to routinely empty the bladder. Neither calcium nor coffee intake are directly related to the psychological effects associated with this condition. Resting in bed is another form of psychomotor retardation.
CN: Health promotion and maintenance; CNS: None; CL: Apply; DIFFICULTY: Moderate

CN: Client needs category   CNS: Client needs subcategory   CL: Cognitive level

146. A hospitalized client becomes angry and belligerent toward a nurse after speaking on the phone with a parent. The nurse learns that the parent cannot visit as expected. Which interventions might the nurse use to help the client deal with the displaced anger? Select all that apply.
1. Explore the client's unmet needs.
2. Avoid the client until he apologizes.
3. Suggest that the client direct the anger at a parent.
4. Invite the client to a quiet place to talk.
5. Assist the client in identifying alternate ways of approaching the problem.

147. An 8-year-old child, diagnosed with obsessive-compulsive disorder, is admitted by the nurse to a psychiatric facility. When obtaining data, which behaviors would be characterized as compulsions? Select all that apply.
1. Checking and rechecking that the television is turned off before going to school.
2. Repeatedly washing the hands.
3. Brushing teeth three times per day.
4. Routinely climbing up and down a flight of stairs three times before leaving the house.
5. Feeding the dog the same meal every day.
6. Wanting to play the same video game each night.

148. During the termination phase of a therapeutic nurse–client relationship, which intervention is **most** appropriate?
1. Tell the client there is no need for support groups now.
2. Address new issues with the client.
3. Review what has been accomplished during this relationship.
4. Avoid discussing the client's emotions.

149. The behavior of a client with borderline personality disorder causes a nurse to feel angry toward the client. Which response by the nurse is the **most** therapeutic?
1. Ignore the client's irritating behavior.
2. Restrict the client to her room until supper.
3. Report feelings to the client's health care provider.
4. Tell the client how this behavior makes the nurse feel.

150. A client with a panic disorder is having difficulty falling asleep. Which nursing intervention should be performed **first**?
1. Call the client's psychotherapist.
2. Educate the client about progressive relaxation.
3. Allow the client to stay up and watch television.
4. Obtain an order for a sleeping medication as needed.

146. 1, 4, 5. Feelings of displacement or directing anger toward the nurse need to be identified and understood by the client before the nurse can help guide the client to choose appropriate actions. Avoiding the client or having them direct anger at another person is inappropriate. Approaching the client in a calm manner and offering to assist in the problem-solving process allows the client to identify needs that are not being met and explore constructive ways of dealing with anger.
CN: Psychosocial integrity; CNS: None; CL: Apply; DIFFICULTY: Moderate

147. 1, 2, 4. Compulsions involve symbolic rituals that relieve anxiety when they are performed. The disorder is caused by anxiety from obsessive thoughts, and acts are seen as irrational. Examples include repeatedly checking the television set, washing hands, or climbing stairs. An activity such as playing the same video game each night may be indicative of normal development for a school-age child. Frequent brushing of the teeth and feeding the dog a consistent meal are not abnormal.
CN: Psychosocial integrity; CNS: None; CL: Analyze; DIFFICULTY: Easy

148. 3. Reviewing what has been accomplished is a goal of the termination phase of a therapeutic nurse–client relationship. It's appropriate to refer the client to support groups. During the termination phase, new issues shouldn't be explored. Discussing the client's emotions during this phase is appropriate.
CN: Psychosocial integrity; CNS: None; CL: Apply; DIFFICULTY: Easy

149. 4. A nursing intervention used with personality disorders is to help the client recognize how her behavior affects others. The nurse should tell the client that this behavior is making the nurse angry. Ignoring the client, restricting the client, and reporting feelings to the health care provider aren't therapeutic interventions at this time.
CN: Psychosocial integrity; CNS: None; CL: Apply; DIFFICULTY: Moderate

150. 2. Relaxation techniques work very well with a client showing anxiety. If this doesn't help the client fall asleep, then pharmacologic interventions, diversion activities, and contacting the psychotherapist would be in order.
CN: Psychosocial integrity; CNS: None; CL: Apply; DIFFICULTY: Easy

CN: Client needs category   CNS: Client needs subcategory   CL: Cognitive level

151. A client with major depression hasn't responded to antidepressants. Which intervention should the nurse prepare the client for?
 1. Electroconvulsive therapy (ECT)
 2. Electroencephalography (EEG)
 3. Electromyography (EMG)
 4. Tranquilizers

152. A client diagnosed with bipolar disorder is receiving a maintenance dosage of lithium carbonate. The client is reported by a family member to be hyperactive and hyperverbal. Which intervention is appropriate?
 1. Obtain data regarding mental status.
 2. Prepare the client for lithium blood levels.
 3. Have the client brought to the local emergency department.
 4. Prepare the client for admission to the hospital.

153. A client is receiving electroconvulsive therapy (ECT) for the treatment of severe depression. After ECT, what is the **priority** nursing intervention?
 1. Assess the client's vital signs.
 2. Let the client sleep undisturbed.
 3. Allow the family to visit immediately.
 4. Restrain the client until completely awake.

154. A client recently placed on a cardiac monitor has a heart rate of 170 beats/minute, with frequent premature contractions. Which nursing action is **best**?
 1. Call the client's health care provider immediately.
 2. Check the client and make a full assessment.
 3. Delegate one of the unlicensed assistive personnel (UAP) to take the client's vital signs.
 4. Notify the supervisor about the change in the client's condition.

155. A client who has been deemed competent and requires long-term mechanical ventilation privately tells a nurse that she wants the ventilator withdrawn. Which response by the nurse is **best**?
 1. "Tell me how you are feeling."
 2. "What about your family?"
 3. "You are asking us to do something we can't do."
 4. "You have been doing so well."

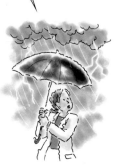

Some treatments sound a lot worse than they actually are.

151. **1.** ECT is commonly used for treatment of major depression for clients who haven't responded to antidepressants or who have medical problems that contraindicate the use of antidepressants. EEG is a tool used in the diagnosis and management of clients with anxiety, seizure disorder, sleep disorders, degenerative disorders, and others. EMG is used to assess muscles and the nerves that control them. Tranquilizers are used to treat schizophrenia or anxiety disorders.
CN: Physiological integrity; CNS: Physiological adaptation;
CL: Understand; DIFFICULTY: Easy

152. **2.** Hyperactive activity might indicate that the client's lithium levels are subtherapeutic; blood lithium levels will determine this. This client doesn't need to have a mental status examination, go to the emergency department, or be admitted to the hospital at this time.
CN: Physiological integrity; CNS: Pharmacological therapies;
CL: Analyze; DIFFICULTY: Moderate

153. **1.** Vital signs are monitored carefully for approximately 1 hour after ECT or until the client is stable. The client shouldn't be restrained or left alone. Visitors should be allowed when the client is awake and alert.
CN: Physiological integrity; CNS: Reduction of risk potential;
CL: Apply; DIFFICULTY: Easy

154. **2.** Because a change has occurred in the client's status, the nurse must assess the client first. This shouldn't be delegated to unlicensed assistive personnel. Before the health care provider or supervisor is notified, a full assessment by the nurse must be made.
CN: Health promotion and maintenance; CNS: None; CL: Apply;
DIFFICULTY: Challenge

155. **1.** Asking about the client's state of well-being is an open-ended response that encourages the client to express her feelings. Asking if the client's family will agree with the decision is judgmental and inappropriate. Telling the client that the ventilator can't be withdrawn is not true; ventilation can be withdrawn according to the client's wishes. Telling the client, "You have been doing so well" in order to have her continue the ventilator treatment is judgmental and dismisses the client's concerns.
CN: Safe, effective care environment; CNS: Coordinated care;
CL: Analyze; DIFFICULTY: Easy

156. A client reports feelings of hopelessness, depression, poor appetite, insomnia, low self-esteem, and difficulty making decisions. The client tells the nurse that these symptoms began at least two years ago and have been ongoing. The nurse recognizes that the client's signs and symptoms are consistent with which disorder?
1. Major depression
2. Dysthymic disorder
3. Cyclothymic disorder
4. Atypical affective disorder

156. **2.** Dysthymic disorder is marked by feelings of depression lasting at least two years, accompanied by at least two of the following symptoms: sleep disturbance, appetite disturbance, low energy or fatigue, low self-esteem, poor concentration, difficulty making decisions, and hopelessness. Major depression is a recurring, persistent sadness or loss of interest or pleasure in almost all activities, with signs and symptoms recurring for at least two weeks. Cyclothymic disorder is a chronic mood disturbance of at least two years, marked by numerous periods of depression and hypomania. Manic signs and symptoms characterize atypical affective disorder.
CN: Psychosocial integrity; CNS: None; CL: Analyze; DIFFICULTY: Challenge

157. A client is postoperative after abdominal surgery. When reinforcing education for coughing and deep breathing, which technique should be used?
1. Splint the incision and cough.
2. Splint the incision, take a deep breath, and then cough.
3. Lie prone, splint the incision, take a deep breath, and then cough.
4. Lie supine, splint the incision, take a deep breath, and then cough.

157. **2.** Splinting the incision with a pillow will protect the incision while the client coughs. Taking a deep breath will help open the alveoli, which promotes oxygen exchange and prevents atelectasis. Coughing and deep-breathing exercises are best accomplished in a sitting or semi-sitting position. Expectoration of secretions will be facilitated in a sitting position, as will splinting and taking deep breaths.
CN: Physiological integrity; CNS: Reduction of risk potential; CL: Apply; DIFFICULTY: Easy

158. The health care provider's order reads 2 g of cephalexin PO daily in equally divided doses of 500 mg each. How many times per day should the nurse administer this medication? Record your answer using a whole number.

_____ times per day

158. **4.**
The nurse would administer the medication four times per day. Two grams is equivalent to 2,000 mg. To give equally divided doses of 500 mg, divide the desired dose of 500 mg into the total daily dose of 2,000 mg. This gives an answer of four times per day. The nurse would give 500 mg every 6 hours for a total of four times per day.
CN: Physiological integrity; CNS: Pharmacological therapies; CL: Analyze; DIFFICULTY: Easy

159. The nurse suspects that a client is in cardiac arrest. According to the 2013 American Heart Association (AHA) guidelines, the nurse would perform the following actions. Place the actions listed below in ascending chronologic order. Use all of the options.

1. Activate the emergency response system.
2. Assess responsiveness.
3. Call for a defibrillator.
4. Provide two breaths.
5. Assess pulse.
6. Begin cycles of 30 compressions.

159. Ordered response:

2. Assess responsiveness.
1. Activate the emergency response system.
3. Call for a defibrillator.
5. Assess pulse.
4. Provide two breaths.
6. Begin cycles of 30 compressions.

According to the 2013 AHA guidelines, the nurse should first assess responsiveness. If the client is unresponsive, the nurse should activate the emergency response team and call for a defibrillator. Next, the nurse should assess the carotid pulse for no more than 10 seconds. If no pulse is present, the nurse should start cycles of 30 chest compressions and two breaths.
CN: Physiological integrity; CNS: Physiological adaptation; CL: Apply; DIFFICULTY: Difficult

160. Which symptoms reported by an adolescent's parents would suggest to the nurse that the adolescent is using amphetamines? Select all that apply.
1. Restlessness
2. Fatigue
3. Excessive perspiration
4. Talkativeness
5. Watery eyes
6. Excessive nasal drainage

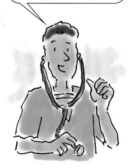

Remember that amphetamines are stimulants, and symptoms of use would reflect this.

160. 1, 3, 4. Amphetamines are central nervous system stimulants. Symptoms of amphetamine use include marked nervousness, restlessness, excitability, talkativeness, and excessive perspiration. CN: Health promotion and maintenance; CNS: None; CL: Analyze; DIFFICULTY: Difficult

161. A client in the terminal stage of cancer is receiving a continuous infusion of morphine for pain management. Which data collection finding suggests that the client is experiencing an adverse effect of this drug?
1. Voiding of 350 mL of concentrated urine in 8 hours
2. Respiratory rate of 8 breaths/minute
3. Irregular heart rate of 82 beats/minute
4. Pupils constricted and equal

161. 2. A respiratory rate of 8 breaths/minute is below normal and suggests respiratory depression, a common adverse effect of morphine. Voiding 350 mL of concentrated urine in 8 hours signals dehydration, and an irregular heart rate of 82 beats/minute signals a cardiac problem—neither of which typically results from morphine. Constricted and equal pupils are an expected, but not necessarily adverse, effect of opioids. CN: Physiological integrity; CNS: Pharmacological therapies; CL: Apply; DIFFICULTY: Easy

162. A client receiving chemotherapy has a deficiency of diversional activities related to decreased energy. Which statement by the client indicates an understanding of appropriate ways to deal with this deficit?
1. "I'll play card games with my friends."
2. "I'll take a long trip to visit my aunt."
3. "I'll bowl with my team after discharge."
4. "I'll eat lunch in a restaurant every day."

162. 1. During chemotherapy, playing cards is an appropriate diversional activity because it doesn't require a great deal of energy. To conserve energy, the client should avoid such activities as taking long trips, bowling, and eating in restaurants every day. However, the client may take occasional short trips and can dine out on special occasions. CN: Physiological integrity; CNS: None; CL: Apply; DIFFICULTY: Moderate

163. A client received chemotherapy 24 hours ago. Which precautions are necessary when caring for this client?
1. Wearing sterile gloves
2. Placing incontinence pads in the regular trash can
3. Wearing personal protective equipment (PPE) when handling blood, body fluids, or feces
4. Using a urinal or bedpan to decrease the likelihood of soiling linens

163. 3. Chemotherapy drugs are present in the client's waste and body fluids for 48 hours after administration. The nurse should wear personal protective equipment, including a face shield, gown, and gloves when exposure to blood, body fluid, or feces is likely. Gloves alone offer minimal protection against exposure. Placing incontinence pads in the regular trash can and using a urinal or bed pan don't protect the nurse from exposure to chemotherapy drugs. CN: Safe, effective care environment; CNS: Safety and Infection Control; CL: Apply; DIFFICULTY: Easy

164. The nurse is speaking to a group of women about early detection of breast cancer. The average age of the women in the group is 47. Following the American Cancer Society guidelines, what information would be the **most** important for the nurse to give the women?
1. "All women should perform breast self-examination two to three times yearly."
2. "Every woman should have a mammogram every 2 years beginning at age 40."
3. "After the age of 50 you should have a hormonal receptor assay once yearly."
4. "Women older than age 40 should have a mammogram and clinical examination every year."

164. 4. The American Cancer Society guidelines state, "Women older than age 40 should have a mammogram annually and a clinical examination at least annually [not every 2 years]; all women should perform breast self-examination monthly [not annually]." The hormonal receptor assay is done on a known breast tumor to determine whether the tumor is estrogen- or progesterone-dependent. CN: Health promotion and maintenance; CNS: None; CL: Apply; DIFFICULTY: Easy

CN: Client needs category   CNS: Client needs subcategory   CL: Cognitive level

165. A client is undergoing a left modified radical mastectomy for breast cancer. Postoperatively, blood pressure should be obtained from the client's right arm, and the left arm and hand should be elevated as much as possible to prevent which condition?
1. Lymphedema
2. Trousseau sign
3. IV infusion infiltration
4. Muscle atrophy related to immobility

166. The nurse is caring for a client who was admitted with rectal bleeding. The client is at high risk for having colorectal cancer. The nurse anticipates preparing the client for which diagnostic test to confirm this suspicion?
1. Stool Hematest
2. Carcinoembryonic antigen (CEA)
3. Colonoscopy
4. Abdominal computed tomography (CT) scan

167. A client in the final stages of terminal cancer tells his nurse: "I wish I could just be allowed to die. I'm tired of fighting this illness. I have lived a good life. I only continue my chemotherapy and radiation treatments because my family wants me to." What is the nurse's **best** response?
1. "Would you like to talk to a psychologist about your thoughts and feelings?"
2. "Would you like to talk to your minister about the significance of death?"
3. "Would you like to meet with your family and your health care provider about this matter?"
4. "I know you are tired of fighting this illness, but death will come in due time."

168. A client with newly diagnosed breast cancer asks the nurse, "Why me? I've always been a good person. What have I done to deserve this?" Which response by the nurse would be **most** therapeutic?
1. "Don't worry. You'll probably live longer than I will."
2. "I'm sure a cure will be found soon."
3. "You seem upset. Let's talk about something happy."
4. "Would you like to talk about this?"

165. 1. Lymphedema is a common postoperative adverse effect of modified radical mastectomy and lymph node dissection. Elevation of the arm on the affected side will allow gravity to assist lymph drainage. Other preventive measures include exercises in which the arms are elevated. Trousseau sign is a sign of hypocalcemia and wouldn't be expected in this situation. Neither IV infusions nor venipunctures should be given in the left arm. Although muscle atrophy is a potential adverse effect if the client doesn't exercise her left arm, it wouldn't be prevented by elevating the arm.
CN: Physiological integrity; CNS: Reduction of risk potential; CL: Apply; DIFFICULTY: Easy

166. 3. Used to visualize the lower GI tract, colonoscopy aids in detecting two-thirds of all colorectal cancers. Stool Hematest detects blood, which is a sign of colorectal cancer; however, the test doesn't confirm the diagnosis. CEA may be elevated in colorectal cancer but isn't considered a confirming test. An abdominal CT scan is used to stage the presence of colorectal cancer.
CN: Health promotion and maintenance; CNS: None; CL: Apply; DIFFICULTY: Easy

167. 3. The nurse has a moral and professional responsibility to advocate for clients who experience decreased independence, loss of freedom of action, and interference with their ability to make autonomous choices. Coordinating a meeting between the health care provider and family members may give the client an opportunity to express his wishes and promote awareness of feelings as well as influence future care decisions. All the other options are inappropriate.
CN: Psychosocial Integrity; CNS: None; CL: Apply; DIFFICULTY: Moderate

168. 4. Listening, responding quickly, and providing support promote therapeutic communication. Offering to talk about the client's feelings validates those feelings and allows the client to express them. Saying not to worry or that a cure will be found soon ignores the client's feelings. Saying "you seem upset" then changing the subject identifies the client's feelings but doesn't follow through by exploring them.
CN: Psychosocial Integrity; CNS: None; CL: Apply; DIFFICULTY: Easy

169. A multidisciplinary oncology team of health care providers, nurses, and the social worker notes that a client who has been undergoing chemotherapy is now experiencing pancytopenia. When reviewing the laboratory data, which values support this diagnosis? Select all that apply.

1. Decreased white blood cells
2. Increased white blood cells
3. Decreased platelets
4. Increased platelets
5. Decreased RBCs
6. Increased RBCs

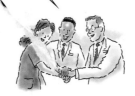

Health care is a team sport. Remember to communicate well with your teammates.

170. A client states to the nurse "I know that I'm going to die." Which response by the nurse would be **best**?

1. "We have special equipment to monitor you and your problem."
2. "Don't worry. We know what we're doing and you aren't going to die."
3. "Why do you think you're going to die?"
4. "Oh no, you're doing quite well considering your condition."

171. A client with metastatic brain cancer is admitted to the oncology floor. According to the Patient Self-Determination Act of 1991 (PSDA), what is the hospital required to do concerning the execution of advance directives?

1. Decide on a treatment plan if the client can't.
2. Inform the client or legal guardian of his right to execute an advance directive.
3. Respect individuals' moral rights.
4. Advise clients not to execute an advance directive because it limits treatment options.

172. A client with acne vulgaris is seeking treatment. The nurse will reinforce education on nightly apply of which medication?

1. Minoxidil
2. Tretinoin
3. Zinc oxide gelatin
4. Fluorouracil

173. A nurse is instructing a group of unlicensed assistive personnel (UAP) about client care. The nurse tells them to turn clients how often to prevent skin breakdown?

1. Every 2 hours
2. Hourly
3. Once per shift
4. Each time the nurse enters a client's room

169. 1, 3, 5. Pancytopenia is a deficiency of all blood cells, which includes a state of simultaneous leukopenia (decreased white blood cells), thrombocytopenia (decreased platelets), and anemia (decreased RBCs). Pancytopenia has widespread effects on the body by leading to oxygen shortage and immune function.

CN: Physiological integrity; CNS: Physiological adaptation; CL: Analyze; DIFFICULTY: Easy

170. 3. A therapeutic approach would be to reflect on the client's comments, focusing on his specific words. Telling the client that special equipment is available, not to worry because nurses have training and knowledge to handle care, and that he's doing quite well are nontherapeutic responses. Such statements offer false reassurance and ignore the client's needs.

CN: Psychosocial integrity; CNS: None; CL: Apply; DIFFICULTY: Easy

171. 2. The PSDA of 1991 requires all health care facilities to notify clients upon admission of their right to execute an advance directive. The facility's ethics committee can decide on a treatment plan if the client is unable to do so, and if a durable power of attorney hasn't been appointed. Hospitals aren't required by law to respect individuals' moral rights; however, health care professionals should do so as part of their professional responsibility. Health care professionals are sometimes concerned that advance directives prevent treatment that might help the client. However, the hospital shouldn't advise clients not to execute an advance directive.

CN: Safe, effective care environment; CNS: Coordinated care; CL: Apply; DIFFICULTY: Easy

172. 2. Tretinoin is a topical agent applied nightly to treat acne vulgaris. Minoxidil is used to promote hair growth. Zinc oxide gelatin is used for abrasions on the lower arms or legs; the affected area must be covered with a bandage for about 1 week. Fluorouracil is an antineoplastic topical agent used to treat superficial basal cell carcinoma.

CN: Physiological integrity; CNS: Pharmacological therapies; CL: Remember; DIFFICULTY: Moderate

173. 1. The nurse should instruct UAP to turn a client every 2 hours to prevent skin breakdown. Turning a client more frequently disturbs his rest and isn't necessary. Waiting longer than 2 hours increases the risk of skin breakdown. The schedule for turning clients shouldn't be based on when the nurse enters the client's room.

CN: Safe, effective care environment; CNS: Coordinated care; CL: Apply; DIFFICULTY: Easy

174. A client has just been diagnosed with terminal cancer and is being transferred to home hospice care. The client's daughter tells the nurse, "I don't know what to say to my mother if she asks me if she's going to die." Which responses by the nurse would be appropriate? Select all that apply.
1. "Tell your mother not to worry. She still has some time left."
2. "Let's talk about your mother's illness and how it will progress."
3. "You sound like you have some questions about your mother dying. Let's talk about that."
4. "Don't worry, hospice will take care of your mother."
5. "Tell me how you're feeling about your mother dying."

175. A nurse is obtaining data from a client who has a rash on the chest and upper arms. Which questions should the nurse ask in order to gain further information about the client's rash? Select all that apply.
1. "When did the rash start?"
2. "Are you allergic to any medications, foods, or pollen?"
3. "How old are you?"
4. "What have you been using to treat the rash?"
5. "Have you recently traveled outside the country?"
6. "Do you smoke cigarettes or drink alcohol?"

176. The health care provider orders contact precautions for a client with a draining wound. Which action should the nurse take to initiate these precautions?
1. Pull the curtain to separate the client from the roommate.
2. Place a box of masks outside the client's room.
3. Place an isolation cart containing gloves and gowns outside the client's room.
4. Store the client's belongings at the nurses' station.

177. A family member is observed looking at the blood glucose flow sheet for a client in the next bed. Which action would be an appropriate measure for the nurse to take?
1. Call security.
2. Notify the charge nurse about this breach in the client's personal health information.
3. Do nothing.
4. Ask the family member not to tell the client what his blood glucose levels have been.

174. 2, 3, 5. Talking about death is an uncomfortable situation. Conveying information clearly and openly can alleviate fears and strengthen the individual's sense of control. Encouraging verbalization of feelings helps build a therapeutic relationship based on trust and reduces anxiety. Advising the daughter not to worry, or having the daughter tell her mother that, ignores her feelings and discourages further communication.
CN: Psychosocial integrity; CNS: None; CL: Analyze; DIFFICULTY: Moderate

175. 1, 2, 4, 5. The nurse should first find out when the rash began; this can assist with the correct diagnosis. The nurse should also ask about allergies; rashes can occur when a person changes medications, eats new foods, or contacts pollen. It is also important to find out how the client has been treating the rash; some topical ointments or oral medications may worsen it. The nurse should ask about recent travel; exposure to foreign foods and environments can cause a rash. The client's age and smoking and drinking habits would not provide further insight into the rash or its cause.
CN: Physiological integrity; CNS: Physiological adaptation; CL: Analyze; DIFFICULTY: Moderate

176. 3. Any type of transmission-based precaution requires that gloves be worn for client care, and a gown as well if soiling is possible. Placing an isolation cart outside the client's room makes isolation equipment readily available to those health care workers who must enter the client's room. Clients who require isolation precautions should be placed in a private room when possible. Masks aren't required for clients on contact precautions. The client's personal belongings should remain in the client's room.
CN: Safe, effective care Environment; CNS: Safety and infection control; CL: Apply; DIFFICULTY: Easy

177. 2. The family member was in violation of the other client's personal health information rights. Therefore, the nurse should notify the charge nurse of the breach in client confidentiality. The nurse shouldn't call security. Doing nothing is inappropriate. Asking the family member not to tell the client about glucose readings isn't appropriate.
CN: Safe, effective care environment; CNS: Coordinated care; CL: Analyze; DIFFICULTY: Easy

178. To evaluate a client's chief concern, the nurse practitioner (NP) performs deep palpation. The nurse recognizes the purpose of deep palpation is to assess which of the following?
1. Skin turgor
2. Hydration
3. Organs
4. Temperature

178. 3. The purpose of deep palpation, in which the nurse indents the client's skin approximately 1.5 in (3.8 cm), is to assess underlying organs and structures, such as the kidneys and spleen. Skin turgor, hydration, and temperature can be assessed by using light touch or light palpation.
CN: Health promotion and maintenance; CNS: None; CL: Apply; DIFFICULTY: Easy

179. The nurse is caring for a client on the orthopedic unit. When preparing the client for discharge, which instructions should the nurse reinforce after surgical repair of a hip fracture?
1. "Do not flex the hip more than 30°, do not cross your legs, and get help putting on your shoes."
2. "Do not flex the hip more than 60°, do not cross your legs, and get help putting on your shoes."
3. "Do not flex the hip more than 90°, do not cross your legs, and get help putting on your shoes."
4. "Do not flex the hip more than 120°, do not cross your legs, and get help putting on your shoes."

179. 3. Discharge instructions should include not flexing the hip more than 90°, not crossing the legs, and getting help to put on shoes. These restrictions prevent dislocation of the new prosthesis.
CN: Safe, effective care environment; CNS: coordinated care; CL: Apply; DIFFICULTY: Moderate

180. The nurse is caring for a client who is experiencing an exacerbation of gout. When providing instruction, which dietary modifications are stressed? Select all that apply.
1. Eat a low-purine diet.
2. Limit fluid intake to no more than 1 L/day.
3. Eat a high-protein diet, with at least two servings of lean meat per day.
4. Eat a high-purine diet.
5. Limit alcohol intake.

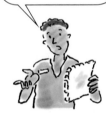

Remember to "select all that apply" in question #180.

180. 1, 5. Gout is characterized by an abnormal metabolism of uric acid. Individuals either produce too much uric acid or their body is unable to metabolize and excrete it. Purines are metabolized into uric acid. The client who suffers from gout should be placed on a low-purine diet with foods such as peanut butter, cherries, rice, pasta, fruits, and vegetables. Fluids do not have to be limited. Alcohol intake should be limited as it is thought to trigger an exacerbation.
CN: Physiological integrity; CNS: Basic care and comfort; CL: Apply; DIFFICULTY: Difficult

181. The nurse is caring for an older adult resident with a cough. The resident has standing orders for guaifenesin syrup 200 mg, PO, every 4 hours. The nurse has a dosage of 100-mg/5-mL. Mark on the medicine cup the amount of syrup the nurse would pour.

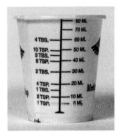

181. The correct formula to calculate a drug dosage is:

$$\text{Dosage} = \frac{\text{Dose desired}}{\text{Dose on hand}} \times \text{Quantity}$$

In this example, the equation is:

$$\text{Dosage} = \frac{200 \text{ mg}}{100 \text{ mg}} \times 5 \text{ mL}$$

$$\text{Dosage} = 10 \text{ mL}.$$

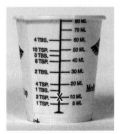

CN: Physiological integrity; CNS: Pharmacological therapies; CL: Apply; DIFFICULTY: Easy

182. A client has been admitted to the emergency department with severe right upper quadrant pain. Based on the signs and symptoms and laboratory data documented in the chart shown, the nurse would expect the client to have which diagnosis?

Progress notes	
4/1/17 0730	Client admitted to the emergency department with severe right upper quadrant pain radiating to the back, nausea and vomiting, and fever. Laboratory results received via telephone as follows: glucose 462 mg/dL, WBC 14,000 cells/mm3, lipase 214 units/L, and calcium 6.5 mg/dL. — Andrea Nichols, LPN

1. Peptic ulcer
2. Crohn disease
3. Pancreatitis
4. Irritable bowel syndrome

183. A client who is 28 weeks pregnant is admitted for testing. After reading the nursing notes below, which rationale best explains why a pregnant client should lie on her left side when resting or sleeping in the later stages of pregnancy?

Progress notes	
4/1/17 1430	Pt. admitted to short-term procedure unit for testing. States "I'm feeling a little faint." Skin slightly diaphoretic to touch. Pt. assisted to left side. VS stable. States "I'm feeling better now." — S. Brown, LPN

1. To facilitate digestion
2. To facilitate bladder emptying
3. To prevent compression of the vena cava
4. To prevent development of fetal anomalies

182. 3. The assessment findings combined with the laboratory results suggest pancreatitis. Signs and symptoms of pancreatitis include severe right upper quadrant pain, fever, nausea, and vomiting. Inflammation of the pancreas results in leukocytosis. Injured beta-cells are unable to produce insulin, leading to hyperglycemia, which may be as high as 500 to 900 mg/dL. Lipase and amylase levels become elevated as the pancreatic enzymes leak from injured pancreatic cells. Calcium becomes trapped as fat necrosis occurs, leading to hypocalcemia. Peptic ulcer, Crohn disease, and irritable bowel syndrome do not cause amylase or lipase levels to increase.
CN: Physiological integrity; CNS: Reduction of risk potential; CL: Analyze; DIFFICULTY: Easy

183. 3. The weight of the pregnant uterus is sufficiently heavy to compress the vena cava, which could impair blood flow to the uterus, possibly decreasing oxygen to the fetus. The client may experience supine hypotension syndrome (faintness, diaphoresis, and hypotension) from the pressure on the inferior vena cava. The side-lying position puts the weight of the fetus on the bed, not on the woman. The side-lying position has not been shown to prevent fetal anomalies, nor does it facilitate bladder emptying or digestion.
CN: Physiological integrity; CNS: Reduction of risk potential; CL: Analyze; DIFFICULTY: Easy

184. A nurse is caring for a client in the fourth stage of labor. Based on the nurse's note, which postpartum complication has the client developed?

Progress notes	
4/1/17	Pt.'s 24-hour blood loss is 600 mL. Uterus
1745	is soft and relaxed on palpation and pt.
	has a full bladder. Assisted pt. in emptying
	bladder and notified Dr. G. McMann of
	findings. Vital signs stable at present. See
	graphic sheet for ongoing assessments and
	perineal pad weights.
	— S. Jones, LPN

1. Postpartum hemorrhage
2. Puerperal infection
3. Deep vein thrombosis (DVT)
4. Mastitis

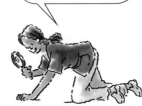

Focus on the blood loss of "600 mL" and the uterus being "soft" in question #184.

185. A licensed practical nurse is assisting a triage nurse in the emergency department. They are admitting a client with second-degree burns on the anterior and posterior portions of both legs. Based on the Rule of Nines, which percentage of the body is burned? Record your answer using a whole number.

_____ %

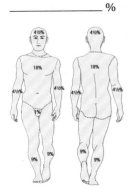

186. A client has an IV line in place for 3 days and begins to report discomfort at the insertion site. Based on the client's progress notes shown, which condition has most likely occurred?

Progress notes	
4/1/17	IV site assessed and found to have blanching
0730	around the site, swelling, and coolness to
	the touch. Laboratory results include a white
	blood cell count within normal limits.
	— Sue Thompson, LPN

1. Infiltration
2. Phlebitis
3. Infection
4. Infection and infiltration

184. 1. Blood loss from the uterus that exceeds 500 mL in a 24-hour period is considered postpartum hemorrhage. If uterine atony is the cause, the uterus feels soft and relaxed. A full bladder can prevent the uterus from contracting completely, increasing the risk of hemorrhage. Puerperal infection is an infection of the uterus and structures above; its characteristic sign is fever. Two major types of DVT occur in the postpartum period: pelvic and femoral. Each has different signs and symptoms, but both occur later in the postpartum period (femoral, after 10 days postpartum; pelvic, after 14 days). Mastitis is an inflammation of the mammary glands that disrupts normal lactation and usually develops 1 to 4 weeks of postpartum. Uterine rupture is a potentially catastrophic event during birth where the wall of the uterus ruptures. A uterine rupture is a life-threatening event for the mother and fetus.

CN: Physiological integrity; CNS: Reduction of risk potential; CL: Analyze; DIFFICULTY: Easy

185. 36.
The anterior and posterior portions of one leg amount to 18%. Because both legs are burned, the total is 36%.

CN: Physiological integrity; CNS: Physiological adaptation; CL: Analyze; DIFFICULTY: Easy

186. 1. The assessment findings of pallor, swelling, skin that is cool to the touch at the IV insertion site, and a normal WBC count all indicate infiltration. The infusion should be discontinued and restarted in a different site. Phlebitis would be evidenced by redness at the cannula tip and along the vein. Infection would be evidenced by an elevated WBC count.

CN: Physiological integrity; CNS: Physiological adaptation; CL: Apply; DIFFICULTY: Easy

CN: Client needs category   CNS: Client needs subcategory   CL: Cognitive level

187. The nurse is caring for a diabetic adolescent who admits to consuming many simple sugars and carbohydrates at a graduation party. The parents brought the client to the emergency room with unusual behavior. The serum glucose level was 375 mg/dL. The health care provider provided a coverage schedule:

150 to 200 mg/dL—2 units of Humulin R.
201 to 250 mg/dL—4 units of Humulin R.
251 to 300 mg/dL—6 units of Humulin R.
301 to 350 mg/dL—8 units of Humulin R.
351 to 399 mg/dL—10 units of Humulin R.
Over 400 mg/dL—call the health care provider.

Mark the amount of insulin the nurse should draw into the low-dose insulin syringe.

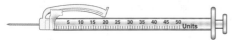

188. The nurse is caring for an infant in the Emergency Department (ED) who has symptoms of irritability and a high fever. Identify the area where a nurse should palpate when assessing for increased intracranial pressure using the anterior fontanel.

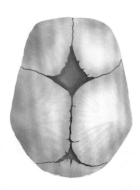

189. A nurse places electrodes on a collapsed individual who was visiting a hospitalized family member. The monitor displays the following.

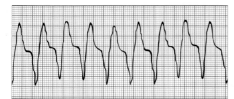

Which intervention should the nurse do **first**?
1. Place the client on oxygen.
2. Confirm the rhythm with a 12-lead ECG.
3. Begin chest compressions.
4. Assess the client's airway, breathing, and circulation.

187. The adolescent's blood sugar is 375 mg/dL, thus falling within the 10 unit range (351 to 399 mg/dL). The nurse would drawn up 10 units of Humulin R to administer as per health care provider's orders.

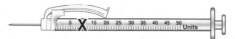

CN: Physiological integrity; CNS: Pharmacological therapies; CL: Apply; DIFFICULTY: Easy

188. The anterior fontanel is formed by the junction of the sagittal, frontal, and coronal sutures. It is shaped like a diamond and normally measures 4 to 5 cm at its widest point. The posterior fontanel closes during the first several months of life and the anterior fontanel closes around 2 years of age. A widened, bulging fontanel is a sign of increased intracranial pressure.

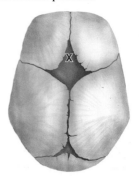

CN: Health promotion and maintenance; CNS: None; CL: Apply; DIFFICULTY: Easy

189. 4. The rhythm the client is experiencing is ventricular tachycardia (VT). The nurse must first assess the airway, breathing, and circulation, and level of consciousness to establish the client's stability and obtain further help from nursing staff. Different actions are required if the client's VT is unstable or pulseless.

CN: Physiological integrity; CNS: Reduction of risk potential; CL: Analyze; DIFFICULTY: Moderate

Hang in there— you're almost done.

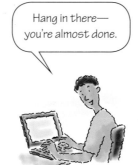

190. A nurse is caring for a client who is recovering from an illness requiring prolonged bed rest. Based on the nursing documentation below, which procedure would the nurse implement next?

Progress notes	
4/1/17	Pt. instructed in contraction of back
1015	extensors, hip extensors, knee extensors,
	and ankle flexors and extensors. Pt. able
	to demonstrate correct technique without
	joint motion or muscle lengthening. C/O
	being "a little tired" after holding each
	contraction 5 seconds and repeating three
	times. Instructed to repeat exercises three
	times daily; pt. verbalized understanding of
	all information given.
	— F. Brown, LPN

1. Performing active range-of-motion exercises of the legs
2. Performing isometric exercises of the legs
3. Providing assistance walking the client to the bathroom
4. Performing passive range-of-motion exercises of the legs

190. 1. Active range-of-motion exercises involve moving the client's joints through their full range of motion; they require some muscle strength and endurance. The client should have received passive range-of-motion exercises since admission to maintain joint flexibility and should have been taught isometric exercises to build strength and endurance for transfers and ambulation. Walking to the bathroom would be unsafe without the ability to first dangle the legs over the bedside and transfer from bed to chair.
CN: Physiological Integrity; CNS: Reduction of Risk Potential; CL: Analyze; DIFFICULTY: Moderate

191. At the beginning of the shift, the nurse is assigned a client with an ascending colostomy. Which picture identifies the correct placement where the nurse will assess the stoma?

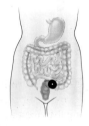
1.   2.

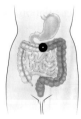 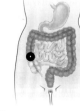
3.   4.

191. 4. A colostomy can be performed along any site of the colon. The location of an ascending colostomy is on the right side of the abdomen. An ostomy located in the ascending colon would likely produce continuous liquid output because feces in this section contain the most water and, therefore, have a liquid consistency. A sigmoid colostomy is located on the sigmoid colon and located close to the location of a descending colostomy in the left side of the abdomen. The transverse colostomy is horizontal across middle abdomen or toward the right side of the body across the abdomen.
CN: Physiological integrity; CNS: Physiological adaptation; CL: Apply; DIFFICULTY: Easy

CN: Client needs category   CNS: Client needs subcategory   CL: Cognitive level

192. A nurse is obtaining data from a client with right flank pain, fever, and chills. A urine culture is obtained, and a diagnosis of suspected right pyelo-nephritis is documented. When instructing the client on the diagnosis, the nurse uses a diagram of the urinary structures. Mark the area associated with the diagnosis.

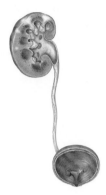

192. Pyelonephritis is a type of urinary tract infection that affects one or both kidneys. Right pyelonephritis is on the right side of the client's body but would be documented on the left in the anatomical position. Bacteria and viruses can move to the kidneys from the bladder or can be carried from other body systems through the bloodstream causing the disease process.

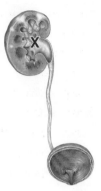

CN: Physiological integrity; CNS: Physiological adaptation; CL: Apply; DIFFICULTY: Easy

193. A nurse assesses a client's vaginal discharge on the first postpartum day and describes it in the progress note (shown). Which term **best** identifies the discharge?

Progress notes	
4/1/17	Perineal pad changed two times this shift for
1645	moderate amount of red discharge.
	— J. Jones, LPN

1. Lochia alba
2. Lochia
3. Lochia serosa
4. Lochia rubra

193. 4. For the first 3 days after birth, the discharge is called lochia rubra. It consists almost entirely of blood, with only small particles of decidua and mucus. Lochia alba is a creamy white or colorless discharge that occurs 10 to 14 days postpartum. Lochia serosa is a pink or brownish discharge that occurs 4 to 14 days postpartum. The term lochia alone is not a correct description of the discharge.
CN: Physiological integrity; CNS: Physiological adaptation; CL: Apply; DIFFICULTY: Easy

194. Which action should a nurse take when administering a new blood pressure medication to a client?
1. Administer the medication to the client without explanation.
2. Inform the client of the new drug only if he asks about it.
3. Inform the client of the new medication, its name, use, and the reason for the change.
4. Administer the medication and inform the client that the health care provider will explain the medication later.

194. 3. Informing the client about the medication, its use, and the reason for the change is important to the care of the client. Educating the client about the treatment regimen promotes compliance. The other responses are inappropriate.
CN: Safe, effective care environment; CNS: Safety and infection control; CL: Apply; DIFFICULTY: Easy

195. An 11-year-old girl comes into the health care provider's office reporting dysuria. Which findings on the laboratory report are consistent with a urinary tract infection?

Laboratory Results	
Test: Urinalysis	
Date: 04/01/2017	
Time collected: 0700	
Parameter	Results
Color	Pale yellow
Turbidity	Clear
pH	7.8
Specific gravity	1.015
Protein	Negative
Glucose	Positive
Ketones	Positive
Red blood cells	<1 per high-power field
White blood cells	20 per high-power field
Casts	None

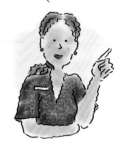

Look for the result that is abnormal.

1. WBCs: 20 per high-power field
2. pH 7.8
3. Ketones: positive
4. Glucose: positive

195. **1.** Urinary tract infections are more common in school-aged girls than in school-aged boys. A normal urinalysis would show less than 5 WBCs per high-power field. An elevated WBC count of 20 is an indication of bacteria and urinary tract infection. The normal range of urinary pH is 4.6 to 8.0. The presence of glucose or ketones in the urine does not indicate a urinary tract infection, but may indicate diabetes mellitus.

CN: Physiological integrity; CNS: Reduction of risk potential; CL: Analyze; DIFFICULTY: Moderate

196. A client exhibits signs of heightened anxiety. Which response by the nurse is **most** likely to reduce the client's anxiety?
1. "Everything will be fine. Don't worry."
2. "Read this manual and then ask me any questions you may have."
3. "Why don't you listen to the radio?"
4. "Let's talk about what is bothering you."

We hope the nurse's response gets us out of here and helping the client.

196. **4.** Anxiety may result from feelings of helplessness, isolation, or insecurity. This response helps reduce anxiety by encouraging the client to express feelings. The nurse should be supportive and develop goals together with the client to give the client some control over an anxiety-inducing situation. Because the other options ignore the client's feelings and block communication, they wouldn't reduce anxiety.

CN: Psychosocial integrity; CNS: None; CL: Apply; DIFFICULTY: Easy

197. Which statement made by a client with a chlamydial infection indicates understanding of the potential complications?
1. "I'm glad I'm not pregnant; I'd hate to have a malformed baby from this disease."
2. "I hope this medicine works before this disease gets into my urine and destroys my kidneys."
3. "If I had known a diaphragm would put me at risk for this, I would have taken birth control pills."
4. "I need to treat this infection so it doesn't spread into my pelvis because I want to have children someday."

197. **4.** Chlamydia is a common cause of pelvic inflammatory disease and infertility. It doesn't affect the kidneys or cause birth defects. It can cause conjunctivitis and respiratory infection in neonates exposed to infected cervicovaginal secretions during birth. Use of a diaphragm isn't a risk factor.

CN: Physiological integrity; CNS: Reduction of risk potential; CL: Apply; DIFFICULTY: easy

CN: Client needs category   CNS: Client needs subcategory   CL: Cognitive level

198. A client is injected with radiographic contrast medium and immediately shows signs of dyspnea, flushing, and pruritus. Which intervention should take **priority**?
1. Check vital signs
2. Make sure the airway is patent
3. Apply a cold pack to the IV site
4. Call the health care provider

199. A client is admitted to the medical-surgical floor with a suspected diagnosis of acute myeloid leukemia. A nurse discusses the client's condition in the hallway. This action by the nurse jeopardizes which principle?
1. Plan of care
2. Client safety
3. Client's right to know
4. Confidentiality

200. A client reports urinary frequency and burning. The health care provider diagnoses cystitis and prescribes sulfamethoxazole-trimoxazole. Which instruction should the nurse give the client?
1. "Expect your urine to be dark green."
2. "Discontinue the medication when your symptoms are gone."
3. "Take the medication with 6 to 8 oz (180 to 240 mL) of water."
4. "Get some sun to help with vitamin D absorption."

201. The nurse is caring for a client with a postoperative wound evisceration. Which action should the nurse perform **first**?
1. Explain to the client what is happening and provide support.
2. Cover the protruding internal organs with sterile gauze moistened with sterile saline solution.
3. Push the protruding organs back into the abdominal cavity.
4. Ask the client to drink as much fluid as possible.

202. A nurse is caring for a 12-year-old child with a diagnosis of eczema. Which nursing interventions are appropriate for a child with eczema?
1. Administer antibiotics as prescribed.
2. Administer antifungals as ordered.
3. Administer tepid baths, and use moisturizers immediately after the bath.
4. Administer hot baths, and pat dry or air-dry the affected areas.

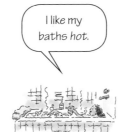
I like my baths hot.

198. 2. The client is showing symptoms of an allergy to the iodine in the contrast medium. The first action is to make sure the client's airway is patent. If compromised, call a cardiac arrest code. Checking vital signs and calling for the health care provider are important nursing actions but checking for a patent airway should come first. A cold pack isn't indicated.
CN: Physiological integrity; CNS: Physiological adaptation; CL: Apply; DIFFICULTY: Easy

199. 4. Discussing the client's condition in the hallway jeopardizes the client's right to confidentiality. This action shouldn't jeopardize the plan of care. Statutory law and common law support the client's right to have information about his condition and treatment. Discussing the client's condition in the hallway doesn't jeopardize this right or client safety.
CN: Safe, effective care environment; CNS: Coordinated care; CL: Apply; DIFFICULTY: Easy

200. 3. Adequate fluid intake is required with sulfa drugs to prevent crystalluria. The client's urine shouldn't turn green from use of sulfamethoxazole-trimoxazole. The nurse should stress the importance of taking the entire prescription, warning that symptoms typically disappear before bacteria are eliminated from the system. The client should avoid prolonged sun exposure because sulfamethoxazole-trimoxazole may cause a photosensitivity reaction.
CN: Physiological integrity; CNS: Basic care and comfort; CL: Apply; DIFFICULTY: Easy

201. 2. The nurse should first cover the wound with moistened gauze to prevent the organs from drying. Both the gauze and the saline solution must be sterile to reduce the risk of infection. The nurse should provide support that will reduce the client's anxiety, but covering the wound is the top priority. The organs shouldn't be pushed back into the abdomen because doing so may tear or damage them. Evisceration requires emergency surgery; therefore, the nurse should place the client on nothing-by-mouth status immediately.
CN: Physiological integrity; CNS: Physiological adaptation; CL: Apply; DIFFICULTY: Easy

202. 3. Tepid baths and moisturizers are indicated for eczema to keep the infected areas clean and to minimize itching. Antibiotics are given only when superimposed infection occurs. Antifungals aren't usually administered in the treatment of eczema. Hot baths can exacerbate the condition and increase itching.
CN: Physiological integrity; CNS: Physiological adaptation; CL: Apply; DIFFICULTY: Easy

CN: Client needs category   CNS: Client needs subcategory   CL: Cognitive level

203. The nurse is caring for a wheelchair-bound client. Which piece of equipment impedes circulation to the area it's meant to protect?
1. Air-fluidized bed
2. Ring or donut
3. Gel flotation pad
4. Water bed

204. A client is prescribed clozapine 250 mg by mouth daily. How many tablets should the nurse administer if each tablet contains 100 mg? Record your answer using one decimal place.

_____ tablets

205. The nurse is caring for a client that is postoperative after abdominal surgery and reporting "gas pains." What action by the nurse can assist the client with alleviating the discomfort associated with gas?
1. Encourage the client to ambulate.
2. Administer opioid analgesics.
3. Encourage the client to drink iced liquids
4. Have the client turn to the right side.

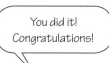
You did it! Congratulations!

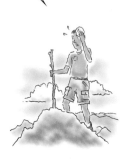

203. 2. Rings or donuts aren't to be used because they restrict circulation. An air-fluidized bed contains beads that move under an airflow to support the client, thus reducing shearing force and friction. Gel pads redistribute with the client's weight. The water bed also distributes pressure over the entire surface.
CN: Physiological integrity; CNS: Reduction of risk potential; CL: Apply; DIFFICULTY: Moderate

204. 2.5.
The correct formula to calculate a drug dosage is:

$$\text{Dose on hand} = \frac{\text{Dose desired}}{X}$$

In this example, the equation is:

$$100\frac{\text{mg}}{1}\text{tablet} = \frac{250\text{ mg}}{X}$$

$$X = 2.5 \text{ tablets}$$

CN: Physiological integrity; CNS: Pharmacological therapies; CL: Apply; DIFFICULTY: Easy

205. 1. The nurse should encourage the client to ambulate to increase peristaltic movement of the bowel to alleviate gas and promote bowel function. Opioid analgesics often make the problem of gas worse by slowing motility. Hot liquids and not cold promote the elimination of gas. The client should lay on the left side to promote evacuation of gas.
CN: Physiological integrity; CNS: Reduction of risk potential; CL: Apply; DIFFICULTY: Challenge

---